NEZHAT'S OPERATIVE GYNECOLOGIC LAPAROSCOPY AND HYSTEROSCOPY

During the past 25 years, gynecologic endoscopy has evolved into a major surgical tool used to treat a multitude of gynecologic indications. Laparoscopy and hysteroscopy are the most common surgical procedures performed by gynecologists today.

This book catalogs the full spectrum of laparoscopic and hysteroscopic procedures in gynecology, oncology, and infertility treatment. The authors describe different techniques in minimally invasive surgery and review the evidence-based medical literature supporting these techniques. The book includes sections on the management of complications during laparoscopy, ranging from vascular injury to bladder or bowel injury. It contains expanded chapters on laparoscopic anatomy, infertility procedures, operative hysteroscopy, pelvic floor repair, and laparoscopic management of gynecologic malignancy. High-quality color pictures supplement many of the presentations.

The three editors have pioneered some of the most important laparoscopic procedures used today. Their work has opened up the field of operative endoscopy for surgeons worldwide. The contributors have extensive experience in laparoscopy and hysteroscopy, and many of them have established some of the surgical techniques discussed.

Dr. Camran Nezhat is Clinical Professor of Obstetrics and Gynecology at the University of California, San Francisco, and Stanford University Medical Schools and Fellowship Director of the Center for Special Minimally Invasive and Robotic Surgery. He has served as president of the Society of Laparoendoscopic Surgeons. He is coauthor of *Endometriosis: Advanced Management and Surgical Techniques* (1995) and has published articles in numerous journals.

Dr. Farr Nezhat is Professor and Director of the Gynecologic Minimally Invasive Surgery, Robotic, and Gynecologic Oncology Fellowship Program in the Department of Obstetrics and Gynecology at Mount Sinai School of Medicine. He is coauthor of *Endometriosis: Advanced Management and Surgical Techniques* (1995) and has published extensively.

Dr. Ceana Nezhat is Director of the Nezhat Medical Center in Atlanta and Associate Clinical Professor of Obstetrics and Gynecology at the Stanford University School of Medicine. He is coauthor of *Endometriosis: Advanced Management and Surgical Techniques* (1995) and has published articles in multiple journals.

NEZHAT'S OPERATIVE GYNECOLOGIC LAPAROSCOPY AND HYSTEROSCOPY

Third Edition

EDITED BY

Camran Nezhat
Stanford University Medical School, Palo Alto

Farr Nezhat
Mount Sinai Hospital, New York

Ceana Nezhat
Nezhat Medical Center, Atlanta

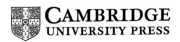

CAMBRIDGE
UNIVERSITY PRESS

CAMBRIDGE UNIVERSITY PRESS
Cambridge, New York, Melbourne, Madrid, Cape Town, Singapore, São Paulo, Delhi

Cambridge University Press
32 Avenue of the Americas, New York, NY 10013-2473, USA

www.cambridge.org
Information on this title: www.cambridge.org/9780521862493

First published 2008

Printed in Hong Kong by Golden Cup

A catalog record for this publication is available from the British Library.

Library of Congress Cataloging in Publication Data

Nezhat's operative gynecologic laparoscopy and hysteroscopy / edited by
Camran Nezhat, Farr Nezhat, Ceana Nezhat–3rd ed.
        p. ; cm.
Rev. ed. of: Operative gynecologic laparoscopy. 2nd ed. c2000.
Includes bibliographical references and index.
ISBN: 978-0-521-86249-3 (hardback)
1. Generative organs, Female—Endoscopic surgery.   2. Laparoscopic surgery.   3. Hysteroscopy.
I. Nezhat, Camran.   II. Nezhat, Farr R.   III. Nezhat, Ceana.   IV. Operative gynecologic laparoscopy.
V. Title: Operative gynecologic laparoscopy and hysteroscopy.
[DNLM: 1. Genital Diseases, Female—surgery.   2. Hysteroscopy—methods.   3. Laparoscopy—methods.
WP 660 N575 2008]
RG104.7.O64   2008
618.1′059—dc22

2007038682

ISBN 978-0-521-86249-3 hardback

Contents

Contributing Authors

OSCAR J. ABILEZ, MD
Postdoctoral Fellow
Department of Vascular Surgery
Division of Vascular Surgery
Stanford University Medical Center
Palo Alto, CA

NADEEM R. ABU-RUSTUM, MD, FACOG
Associate Professor
Department of Obstetrics and Gynecology
Weill Medical College of Cornell University
Director, Minimally Invasive Surgery
Gynecology Service, Department of Surgery
Memorial Sloan-Kettering Cancer Center
New York, NY

ARNOLD P. ADVINCULA, MD
Associate Professor
Director, Minimally Invasive Surgery Program & Fellowship
Department of Obstetrics and Gynecology
University of Michigan Medical Center
Ann Arbor, MI

CRAIG T. ALBANESE, MD, MBA
Professor and Chief
Department of Surgery, Division of Pediatric Surgery
Stanford University Medical Center
John A. and Cynthia Fry Gunn Director of
    Surgical Services
Lucile Packard Children's Hospital
Stanford, CA

CHANDRAKANTH ARE, MD, FRCS, FACS
Assistant Professor
Department of General Surgery
University of Nebraska Medical Center
Omaha, NE

CHARLES J. ASCHER-WALSH, MD
Assistant Professor
Department of Obstetrics, Gynecology, and Reproductive Science
Mount Sinai School of Medicine
New York, NY

AMR M. A. AZIM, MD, MSc, FACOG
Fellow
Center for Reproductive Medicine and Infertility
Weill Medical College of Cornell University
New York, NY

BULENT BERKER, MD
Associate Professor
Department of Obstetrics & Gynecology
Ankara University School of Medicine
Ankara, Turkey

NICOLA BERLANDA, MD
Department of Obstetrics and Gynecology
San Paolo Hospital
University of Milan
Milan, Italy

STEFANO BIANCHI, MD
Department of Obstetrics and Gynecology
San Paolo Hospital
University of Milan
Milan, Italy

ERIC J. BIEBER, MD, MSHCM
Chairman
Department of Obstetrics and Gynecology
Geisinger Health Systems
Danville, PA

WILLIAM H. BRADLEY, MD
Division of Gynecologic Oncology
Department of Obstetrics and Gynecology
Mount Sinai School of Medicine
New York, NY

MICHAEL BRODMAN, MD
Professor and Chairman
Department of Obstetrics, Gynecology, and
    Reproductive Science
Mount Sinai School of Medicine
New York, NY

PHILIP G. BROOKS, MD
Clinical Professor
Department of Obstetrics and Gynecology
David Geffen School of Medicine at UCLA
Attending Physician
Department of Obstetrics and Gynecology
Cedars-Sinai Medical Center
Los Angeles, CA

ALESSANDRO BULFONI, MD
Department of Obstetrics and Gynecology
San Paolo Hospital
University of Milan
Milan, Italy

RICHARD O. BURNEY, MD, MSc
Clinical/Research Fellow
Division of Reproductive Endocrinology and Infertility
Department of Obstetrics and Gynecology
Stanford University School of Medicine
Stanford, CA

JAMES E. CARTER, MD†
Clinical Professor
Department of Obstetrics and Gynecology
University of California at Irvine School of Medicine
Irvine, CA

JÉRÔME CAU
Department of Vascular Surgery
University Hospital
Poitiers, France

VENITA CHANDRA, MD
Resident
Department of Surgery
Stanford University Medical Center
Palo Alto, CA

ROBERT L. COLEMAN, MD
Associate Professor
Department of Gynecologic Oncology
The University of Texas M. D. Anderson Cancer Center
Houston, TX

ALAN B. COPPERMAN, MD
Associate Clinical Professor
Director, Reproductive Endocrinology
Department of Obstetrics, Gynecology, and
    Reproductive Science
Mount Sinai School of Medicine
New York, NY

MYRIAM J. CURET, MD
Professor
Director, Minimally Invasive Surgery Program
Department of Surgery
Stanford University Medical Center
Palo Alto, CA

M. SHOMA DATTA, MD
Department of Obstetrics and Gynecology
St. Luke's–Roosevelt Hospital
New York, NY

ANDREW DEFAZIO, MD
Clinical Fellow
Atlanta Center for Specialty Pelvic Surgery
Atlanta, GA

EDIE L. DERIAN, MD
Department of Obstetrics and Gynecology
Geisinger Medical Center
Danville, PA

SANJEEV DUTTA, MD, MA
Assistant Professor
Division of Pediatric Surgery
Department of Surgery
Stanford University Medical Center
Lucile Packard Children's Hospital
Palo Alto, CA

TOMMASO FALCONE, MD
Professor and Chairman
Department of Obstetrics and Gynecology
Cleveland Clinic Foundation
Cleveland, OH

LUIGI FEDELE, MD
Professor
Department of Obstetrics and Gynecology
San Paolo Hospital
University of Milan
Milan, Italy

ROGER FERLAND, MD
Associate Clinical Professor
Department of Obstetrics and Gynecology
Brown University School of Medicine
Providence, RI

DEIDRE T. FISHER, MD, MHA, FACOG
Clinical Fellow
Atlanta Center for Special Pelvic Surgery
Nezhat Medical Center
Associate
The Center for Endometriosis Care
Atlanta, GA

ERIC FLISSER, MD
Medical Director, Long Island Office
Reproductive Medicine Associates of New York
New York, NY

ELEONORA FONTANA, MD
Department of Obstetrics and Gynecology
San Paolo Hospital
University of Milan
Milan, Italy

ALAN D. GARELY, MD
Vice-Chairman and Chief of Gynecology
Director, Urogynecology and Pelvic Reconstructive Surgery
Department of Obstetrics and Gynecology
Winthrop-University Hospital
Mineola, NY
Clinical Associate Professor
Department of Obstetrics and Gynecology
School of Medicine in the State University
    of New York at Stony Brook

†Deceased

LINDA C. GIUDICE, MD, PhD, MSc
The Robert B. Jaffe MD Professor and Chair
Department of Obstetrics, Gynecology,
   and Reproductive Sciences
University of California, San Francisco
School of Medicine
San Francisco, CA

MARK H. GLASSER, MD
Chief
Department of Obstetrics and Gynecology
Kaiser Permanente Medical Center
San Rafael, CA

OLIVIER GOËAU-BRISSONNIÈRE, MD, PhD
Department of Vascular Surgery
Ambróise Pare University Hospital
Boulogne-Billancourt, France

JEFFREY M. GOLDBERG, MD
Head, Division of Reproductive Endocrinology and Infertility
Department of Obstetrics and Gynecology
Cleveland Clinic
Cleveland, OH

JAMIE A. GRIFO, MD, PhD
Professor
Director, Division of Reproductive Endocrinology
Department of Obstetrics and Gynecology
New York University School of Medicine
Attending Physician
Department of Obstetrics and Gynecology
Tisch Hospital
New York, NY

WM. LeROY HEINRICHS, MD, PhD
Past Chair
Department of Obstetrics and Gynecology
Stanford University Medical Media and Information
   Technologies (SUMMIT)
Stanford University School of Medicine
Stanford, CA

THOMAS HERZOG, MD
P & S Alumni Professor of Clinical Obstetrics and Gynecology
Director, Division of Gynecologic Oncology
Department of Obstetrics and Gynecology
Columbia University Medical Center
New York, NY

GEORGIOS E. HILARIS, MD
Clinical Instructor
Department of Obstetrics and Gynecology
Center for Special Minimally Invasive Surgery
   (Laparoscopic and Robotic)
Stanford University Medical Center
Palo Alto, CA
Gynecologic and Oncologic Surgery
Paradeisos Amarousion
Athens, Greece

SENZAN HSU, MD
Clinical Fellow
Center for Special Minimally Invasive Surgery
Stanford University Medical Center
Palo Alto, CA

THOMAS H. S. HSU, MD
Assistant Professor
Director, Laparoscopic and Minimally Invasive Surgery
Department of Urology
Stanford University School of Medicine
Palo Alto, CA

KEITH ISAACSON, MD
Director, Minimally Invasive Gynecological Surgery Unit
   and Infertility
Newton-Wellesley Hospital
Associate Professor of Obstetrics and Gynecology
Harvard Medical School
Boston, MA

MARY JACOBSON, MD
Clinical Assistant Professor
Department of Obstetrics and Gynecology
Stanford University School of Medicine
Palo Alto, CA

THOMAS M. KRUMMEL, MD, FACS
Professor and Chair
Department of Surgery
Stanford University School of Medicine
Susan B. Ford Surgeon in Chief
Lucile Packard Children's Hospital
Palo Alto, CA

KEITH L. LEE, MD
Resident
Department of Urology
Stanford University Medical Center
Palo Alto, CA

CHARLES LEVENBACK, MD
Professor
Department of Gynecologic Oncology
The University of Texas M. D. Anderson Cancer Center
Houston, TX

SHARYN N. LEWIN, MD
Fellow
Gynecologic Oncology
Memorial Sloan-Kettering Cancer Center
New York, NY

ANTHONY A. LUCIANO, MD
Director of Center for Fertility and Women's Health, P.C.
Director of Endoscopic Surgery
The Center for Advanced Reproductive Services
Professor, Obstetrics and Gynecology
University of Connecticut School of Medicine
Farmington, CT

JAVIER F. MAGRINA, MD
Professor
Department of Gynecology
Director, Gynecologic Oncology
Barbara Woodward Lips Professor
Mayo Clinic Arizona
Scottsdale, AZ

PAUL M. MAGTIBAY, MD
Assistant Professor and Chairman
Department of Gynecology and Gynecologic Surgery
Mayo Clinic Arizona
Scottsdale, AZ

ALI MAHDAVI, MD
Clinical Fellow and Instructor
Division of Gynecologic Oncology
Department of Obstetrics and Gynecology
University of California at Irvine Medical Center
Orange, CA

ANDREA MARIANI, MD
Assistant Professor
Department of Gynecology
Mayo Clinic Rochester
Rochester, MN

AMIN A. MILKI, MD
Professor
Director, Reproductive Endocrinology and Infertility
Department of Obstetrics and Gynecology
Stanford University School of Medicine
Palo Alto, CA

ROSA MOGHADAM, MD
Clinical Research Fellow
Reproductive Medicine and Advanced Laparoscopic
    Surgery
Center for Special Minimally Invasive Surgery
Palo Alto, CA

STEPHANIE N. MORRIS, MD
Clinical Instructor
Harvard Medical School
Associate Medical Director, Minimally Invasive Gynecologic
    Surgery Center
Newton-Wellesley Hospital
Boston, MA

CAMRAN NEZHAT, MD, FACOG, FACS
Fellowship Director, Center for Special Minimally Invasive
    and Robotic Surgery
Stanford University Medical Center
Clinical Professor
Department of Obstetrics and Gynecology
University of California at San Francisco
    School of Medicine
Departments of Obstetrics and Gynecology
    and Surgery
Stanford University School of Medicine
San Francisco/Palo Alto, CA

CEANA NEZHAT, MD, FACOG, FACS
Fellowship Director
Atlanta Center for Special Minimally Invasive Surgery
    and Reproductive Medicine
Atlanta, GA
Director, Nezhat Medical Center
Adjunct Clinical Associate Professor of Obstetrics
    and Gynecology
Stanford University School of Medicine
Palo Alto, CA

FARR NEZHAT, MD, FACOG, FACS
Professor of Obstetrics and Gynecology
Chief, Minimally Invasive Surgery and Robotics
Fellowship Programs
Division of Gynecologic Oncology
Department of Obstetrics, Gynecology, and Reproductive Science
Mount Sinai School of Medicine
New York, NY

MARIO NUTIS, MD
Clinical Fellow
Center for Special Minimally Invasive Surgery
Stanford University Medical Center
Palo Alto, CA

JAIME OCAMPO, MD
Clinical Fellow
Center for Special Minimally Invasive Surgery
Stanford University Medical Center
Palo Alto, CA

CEDRIC K. OLIVERA, MD
Fellow
Division of Female Pelvic Medicine and Reconstructive Surgery
Department of Obstetrics and Gynecology
Mount Sinai Medical Center
New York, NY

KUTLUK OKTAY, MD, FACOG
Professor of Obstetrics and Gynecology
Medical Director, Institute for Fertility Preservation
Center for Human Reproduction
New York, NY
Director, Division of Reproductive Medicine and Infertility
Department of Obstetrics and Gynecology
New York Medical College
Valhalla, NY

BARBARA J. PAGE
University of California at Berkeley
Berkeley, CA

TANJA PEJOVIC, MD, PhD
Assistant Professor
Department of Obstetrics and Gynecology
Oregon Health & Science University
Portland, OR

JEAN PICQUET, MD
Division of Vascular and Thoracic Surgery
University Hospital of Angers
Angers, France

MARK R. PRESTON, MD
Director, Center for Female Continence and Minimally Invasive
    Pelvic Surgery
The GYN Center for Women's Health
Waterbury, CT
Clinical Instructor
Department of Obstetrics and Gynecology
University of Connecticut School of Medicine
Farmington, CT

PEDRO T. RAMIREZ, MD
Associate Professor
Director of Surgical Research and Education
Department of Gynecologic Oncology
The University of Texas M. D. Anderson Cancer Center
Houston, TX

MAHMOOD K. RAZAVI, MD
Director, Center for Clinical Trials and Research
St. Joseph Vascular Institute
Orange, CA

JIM W. ROSS, MD, PhD
Director, Center for Female Continence
Salinas, CA
Clinical Professor
Department of Obstetrics and Gynecology
David Geffen School of Medicine
University of California, Los Angeles
Los Angeles, CA

SOPHIA ROTHBERGER, MD
Resident
Department of Obstetrics and Gynecology
Oregon Health and Science University
Portland, OR

NAGHMEH SABERI, MD
Assistant Clinical Professor
Department of Obstetrics and Gynecology
University of California at Irvine School of Medicine
Irvine, CA

DANIEL S. SEIDMAN, MD
Professor
Department of Obstetrics and Gynecology
Sackler School of Medicine, Tel-Aviv University
Tel-Aviv, Israel

BABAC SHAHMOHAMADY, MD
Clinical Assistant Professor
Department of Obstetrics and Gynecology
University of Miami School of Medicine
Miami, FL

ANDREW A. SHELTON, MD
Assistant Professor
Department of Surgery
Stanford University School of Medicine
Palo Alto, CA

YUKIO SONODA, MD
Assistant Attending Surgeon
Gynecology Service, Department of Surgery
Memorial Sloan-Kettering Cancer Center
New York, NY

TATUM TARIN, MD
Resident
Department of Urology
Stanford University Medical Center
Palo Alto, CA

SALLI TAZUKE, MD
Department of Obstetrics and Gynecology
Palo Alto Medical Foundation
Portola Valley, CA

MAUREEN M. TEDESCO, MD
Resident
Department of Surgery
Stanford University School of Medicine
Stanford, CA

MICHELLE THAM, MD
Obstetrics and Gynecology Attending Physician
New York University Medical Center
New York, NY

TOGAS TULANDI, MD, MHCM
Professor and Milton Leong Chair in
    Reproductive Medicine
Department of Obstetrics and Gynecology
McGill University
Montreal, Canada

RAFAEL F. VALLE, MD
Professor Emeritus
Department of Obstetrics and Gynecology
Northwestern University Feinberg School of Medicine
Chicago, IL

LINDSEY VOKACH-BRODSKY, MB, CHB
Clinical Associate Professor
Department of Anesthesia
Stanford University School of Medicine
Palo Alto, CA

JYOTI YADAV, MD
Department of Obstetrics and Gynecology
Our Lady of Mercy Medical Center
Bronx, NY

PATRICK YEUNG, MD
Clinical Fellow
Department of Obstetrics and Gynecology
University of Louisville School of Medicine
Louisville, KY

CHRISTOPHER K. ZARINS, MD
Professor
Director, Division of Vascular Surgery
Department of Surgery
Stanford University School of Medicine
Palo Alto, CA

Forewords

Progress in surgical science has been characterized by a continuous cycle of innovation from bedside to bench and back to bedside. Beginning 30,000 years ago with the first bone needles to the current armamentarium today, each quantum leap has resulted from the convergence of technical advances and creative surgeons.

Some surgical capability has been enhanced by relatively simple or more complex tool manufacture or modification, usually for a single purpose. Kocher's addition of a tooth to a straight clamp facilitated the grasping of a thyroid goiter; the more modern fixed-ring retractors have added considerable utility in abdominal retraction.

A few very special tools or techniques revolutionize our work. The development of the simple balloon catheter by Fogarty was the seminal event in initiating the concept of all endovascular procedures, beginning with the procedure of intra-luminal thrombectomy. It has expanded to balloon dilatation, angioplasty, stent placement, and now drug delivery systems in the form of drug-eluting stents.

Dr. Camran Nezhat's creative and ingenious contribution to the field of laparoscopic surgery has been similarly revolutionary. Operating off the video monitor during endoscopic surgery by the addition of a video camera to the laparoscope as developed by Camran Nezhat was a critical step in facilitating the entire field of minimal access surgery, moving it out of its initial realm in gynecologic and pelvic surgery to the entire abdomen, the chest, and beyond. He further demonstrated for the first time that even the most advanced pathology, including bowel, bladder, and ureter diseases, can successfully be managed laparoscopically. (Surgical treatment of endometriosis via laser laparoscopy, *Fertility & Sterility* 1986; Safe laser and endoscopic excision or vaporization of peritoneal endometriosis, *Fertility & Sterility* 1989; Operative laparoscopy (minimally invasive surgery): state of the art, *Journal of Gynecological Surgery*, 1992.)

The laparoscopic revolution has been startlingly rapid. In the early days of my surgical career, I heard three quotations that described surgeons' views of themselves.

"If it's easy for me, it's easy for the patient."

"Incisions heal side-to-side, not end-to-end."

"Big hole, big surgeon."

In other words, the collateral damage of incisions for access was either not relevant to the surgeon or even defined the surgeon. Dr. Nezhat's contributions began a revolution, where bigger is no longer better, and what is easy for the patient dominates our thinking. The entire field of minimal access surgery and its application is not just a set of tools and technologies but a new way of thinking. No longer is the default procedure an open one; it is fair to say that the current state of the art in most surgical arenas makes the default procedure one done with scopes.

Accordingly, this textbook, written and edited by the genius pioneers in the field, reflects that way of thinking. As such, it is both a masterpiece and a treasure.

Thomas M. Krummel, MD, FACS
Professor and Chair
Department of Surgery
Stanford University School of Medicine
Susan B. Ford Surgeon in Chief
Lucile Packard Children's Hospital
Palo Alto, CA

Laparoscopic surgery has revolutionized medicine – in gynecology and in multiple other disciplines – and offers additional opportunities to address surgical conditions through a minimally invasive approach. Camran Nezhat and his brothers, Farr and Ceana, have been and continue to be the pioneers in this effort, and this edition of *Nezhat's Operative Gynecologic Laparoscopy and Hysteroscopy* has advanced applications of the laparoscope and the hysteroscope in surgical therapies to new heights. In particular, the title and text have added *hysteroscopy* – a valuable approach to evaluate the uterine cavity and for surgical cor-

rection of abnormalities contained therein. In addition to the detailed and beautiful illustrations and clear and precise text, new sections have been added, such as the role of the laparoscope and hysteroscope in fertility evaluation and treatment, management of adnexal masses, pathogenesis and treatment of endometriosis, uterine fibroid embolization, and multiple procedures to address pelvic floor disorders. Furthermore, as experience has been derived in the minimally invasive approach to treat gynecologic malignancies, the section on gynecologic cancer has been expanded to include a comprehensive presentation of the laparoscopic approach to lymph node dissection, radical hysterectomy, and endometrial and ovarian cancer. Furthermore, the issue of trocar metastases has a dedicated section for this relatively uncommon complication of surgery. Other pioneering applications of laparoscopic surgery are discussed in detail and with accompanying informative illustrations, including laparoscopic surgery during pregnancy and in the pediatric patient and the use of the laparoscope in vascular surgery. Experience derived from performing laparoscopic procedures can, in well-trained and well-experienced surgeons, be expanded to a minimally invasive approach to gastrointestinal and genitourinary disorders. The sections on these procedures are also detailed and well illustrated. The book also includes a unique chapter on the use of simulators in laparoscopy and a visionary, multidisciplinary approach to the use of robotics and computer-assisted surgery in the treatment of surgically amenable disorders.

Laparopscopy has come a long way from the operator looking through the laparoscope. It now uses adjunctive surgical approaches and new technologies and instruments. This book says it all and says it well!

Linda C. Giudice, MD, PhD, MSc
The Robert B. Jaffe Professor and Chair
Department of Obstetrics, Gynecology
 and Reproductive Sciences
University of California, San Francisco
School of Medicine
San Francisco, CA

In his foreword to the first edition of *Operative Gynecologic Laparoscopy: Principles and Techniques*, Alan DeCherney predicted that because of its then encyclopedic scope and the skill and experience of the authors, the volume would "become a classic." The first edition was essentially a family affair, arranged as a tabulation of the vast experience of three Nezhats, led by Camran, the senior pioneer in the group. At the time of publication of the original edition, the Nezhats had been either primary innovators or major contributors to most aspects of the progressively evolving field of minimally invasive abdominal surgery. This ranged from the introduction of video-laparoscopy through instrument design, and extension of the minimally invasive technique to include applications conventionally considered contraindicated or at best reserved for open laparotomy. They wisely archived their video recordings of each procedure for their own analysis and personal education, and ultimately, for teaching others. They also documented their observations, outcomes, and modification of techniques to recommend best practices. Alan DeCherney was prescient!

The second edition, with somewhat expanded but only jointly attributed authorship, broadened the scope and offered the reader an expert review of new developments. This remained a reliable standard for the ensuing seven years.

The new title retains the Nezhat imprimatur but is dramatically enlarged in scope, so that the encyclopedic character embraces not only history, details of equipment, power sources, and clearly illustrated surgical technique with profit for both the novice and the senior surgeon, but there are now chapters and sections that include the patho-physiology and surgical remedy for anatomic, endocrine, and neoplastic disorders that can reasonably stand alone as reliable and eloquent treatises. By further expanding authorship and including experts who are authoritative and scholarly, this edition has become an even more essential resource.

Ever mindful of the responsibility of the complete educator, the Nezhats have included excellent chapters on the skills and disciplines ancillary but essential to successful surgical adventures, even including specialized anesthesia. They have also addressed the issues of training and have expanded the section dealing with complications, their prevalence, causes, prevention, and remedies. While all of the chapters dealing with surgical procedures are careful to describe and beautifully illustrate approaches and engagements designed to reduce risk, special emphasis in a section on complications is wise.

Discrete sections dealing with special populations, namely the pediatric or pregnant patient, or the patient with chronic and often unexplained pelvic pain, extend the scope of this edition, further informing the consultant who will certainly be called upon for opinion or intervention in these circumstances.

Finally, the new edition, typical of the authors, addresses the most recent driving trend: computer-assisted surgery, thus bridging the gap between the frontiers of accomplishment and the promise of larger unrealized achievement.

It is a pleasure to read this remarkable resource. Its design, style, and content will certainly evoke the same satisfaction for anyone considering surgical intervention as part of the remedy for any gynecologic disorder.

Carmel J. Cohen, MD
Professor of Clinical Obstetrics and Gynecology
Division of Gynecologic Oncology
Department of Obstetrics and Gynecology
Columbia University Medical Center
New York, NY

The surgical discipline of gynecologic endoscopy has progressed substantially in the seventy years since the development of the first laparoscope for gynecology. The technology has evolved to include sophisticated innovations that dramatically improve its utility. As the knowledge of the advantages and limitations of these operations has grown, the application of these surgical tools has been progressively improved. Therefore, it is appropriate to dedicate a textbook to the thorough description of the standard practice, indications, and techniques of these operations.

As with any surgical instrument, a thorough understanding of the requisite operative principals governing the use of the laparoscope is essential. The surgeon's goal is to apply those tenets in the most careful manner to ensure that the operations are truly "minimally invasive." Laparoscopy is still major surgery and must be offered judiciously in those circumstances where it is clearly necessary and appropriate.

The editors have made important contributions to our understanding of the principles and techniques for endoscopic operations in gynecology. *Nezhat's Operative Gynecologic Laparoscopy and Hysteroscopy* provides gynecologic surgeons with a current and extraordinarily clear summary of the topic.

The purpose of any contributed medical text is to bring together highly qualified experts in the field and deliver a consensus report that permits a greater understanding of the topical issues. This book accomplishes that goal. It helps us to refine our technique, to make wise use of our skills, and to provide the best possible care to our patients.

Jonathan S. Berek, MD, MMS
Professor and Chair
Department of Obstetrics and Gynecology
Stanford University School of Medicine
Palo Alto, CA

Forewords to the Second Edition

Once again the Nezhats have provided, in their second edition, an excellent text in operative gynecologic laparoscopy. Not only has this group been clinically active and leaders in the field for many years, but the fact that they document their experiences and techniques is extremely laudatory. They have been not only innovators, demonstrating great creativity and imagination, but also have studied their patients prospectively and retrospectively to draw conclusions based on experience and numbers of cases. Their knowledge of the technology that they employ, that is, lasers, electrosurgery, and Harmonic scalpel instrumentation, is profound and they freely share it in this text.

The scope of the book covers all aspects of the leading surgical procedure in gynecology that can be carried out by endoscopy. Areas covered include adhesiolysis, ovarian cystectomy, ectopic pregnancy, and operations on the uterus, but there are also portions on anesthesia and office microlaparoscopy, to cite a few. The authors have made a tremendous number of revisions, demonstrating their care to detail, their awareness of this rapidly changing and developing field.

It is great that this group has produced a second edition because there are many changes that have occurred since the first edition, including work on stress incontinence and the revisiting of presacral neurectomy. Each chapter is well referenced. Any surgical text must have excellent illustrations, as this one does. This text is an excellent atlas as well.

I found this a comprehensive text for its knowledge, informative because of its insight and imagination, and practical because of its illustrations and explanations. This is a proud testimony to a work well done.

Alan H. DeCherney, MD
Professor and Chairman
Department of Obstetrics and Gynecology
UCLA School of Medicine
Los Angeles, CA

Drs. Nezhat embody the entire spectrum of current knowledge regarding laparoscopy. This book is a reference book in laparoscopy for advanced surgeons and beginners alike. The Nezhats' genius in the operating room is reflected in the writing of this book, especially in descriptions of new techniques and the lucid explanations of the advantages of laparoscopy over laparotomy in a growing list of gynecologic procedures.

As a gynecologist from Germany, I began promoting laparoscopy in 1963. At that time the thinking was that laparoscopy was only performed by gastroenterologists and hepatologists under local anesthesia, and was a procedure to be avoided by all gynecologists. It was believed that turning the laparoscope toward the lower pelvis instead of the upper abdomen would be too dangerous. Structures such as the aorta, common iliac veins, intestines, and ureters were of great concern. There were fatal complications in early gynecologic laparoscopy cases, rendering the procedure obsolete in gynecology at the beginning of the 1960s. Because of these negative connotations and in order to market this innovative technology, I changed the name to "Pelviscopy." My scientific publications and my books were printed under this name.

Dr. Camran Nezhat never criticized any of my elaborate endoscopic procedures. Instead, with his genius, he widened the operative field, creating new techniques, employing new instruments and apparatuses. In my opinion, with the cooperation of his two brothers, Camran Nezhat has enlivened and enriched the entire field of surgical laparoscopy.

Since its inception, endoscopy has changed and the authors have written about a new endoscopic world. The general surgeons have now accepted surgical laparoscopy completely. Years ago, if a gynecologist was unlucky in a pelviscopic procedure, the surgeons condemned this person as an unethical surgeon who used techniques which were as yet unproven and against the current surgical rules.

This book is indeed a bible in surgical laparoscopy. At the end of each chapter an extended bibliography is included. A lengthy chapter is dedicated to complications and how they can be avoided. This is invaluable to all: Everybody can use it: the clinician, student, scientist, and lawyer. This manual should not be missed in any library.

On June 30, 1980, I performed a laparoscopic appendectomy, which ultimately opened the door for general surgeons to perform endoscopic surgery, especially since the appendix was a holy grail of surgery. Today this book opens a new door to a whole new era of endoscopic surgery.

Prof. Dr. H. C. Mult Kurt Semm

Forewords to the First Edition

This textbook on endoscopic surgery is a timely contribution and has all the trappings of being extremely successful. The competition is keen at this point in time with regards to textbooks and atlases on endoscopic surgery but none will rival this one.

In the past decade, gynecologic surgery, because of endoscopic surgery, has undergone a tremendous revolution. There are few cases now remaining in the gynecologist's surgical armamentarium that cannot be carried out through an endoscopic approach. Many of these changes are due to the courage, innovativeness, and technical skill of Dr. Camran Nezhat. Just as in *Star Trek*, he dared to go where no man went before and, by doing this, he opened up unimagined vistas to endoscopic surgeons all over the world. For his courage, Camran has over the years suffered, but he has persevered.

This book brings to a culmination many of Dr. Nezhat's techniques, innovations, and, most importantly, thought processes. All of the characteristics necessary for an excellent textbook of surgery are included. The text is well written, provocative, and clear, and it demonstrates editorial consistency. The illustrations are superb and would provide the novice in endoscopic surgery enough information to carry out many of the procedures proposed.

I have chosen as an illustrative chapter the chapter on endometriosis. It demonstrates many of the things that have been conjured up by Dr. Nezhat and have become part of what we do as endoscopic surgeons. These include hydrodissection, ureteric resection, and reanastomosis with a stapler. If one could learn all of the techniques suggested in the chapter on endometriosis, one could become, as Dr. Nezhat has, a master endoscopic surgeon.

The book is encyclopedic in that it covers not only all surgical techniques, but also various kinds of equipment, laser and electrosurgical physics, adhesion formation, and, most importantly, complications.

Dr. Nezhat has synthesized his years of experience in this text. It will become a classic in the field and is a testimony to his skill, intelligence, and perseverance.

Alan H. DeCherney, MD
Louis E. Phaneuf Professor and Chairman
Department of Obstetrics and Gynecology
Tufts University
Boston, MA

Excellence in any human activity always commands admiration and respect. In the case of surgical techniques, excellence commands not only the admiration and respect of professional colleagues, but the gratitude of patients as well. Those who have had the opportunity to see the "Nezhat Orchestra" operate and simultaneously conduct the endoscopic operating team, recognize that they have seen a performance of excellence. It is a unique combination of manual dexterity, innovation, creativity, and teamwork.

The rapid proliferation of laparoscopic procedures in the last two decades originated in gynecology, but crossed the borders of this discipline to several other applications below and above the diaphragm. Many new devices have been introduced into the armamentarium of the endoscopic operating room. However, if there was a single factor that contributed to the increased interest, quality of patient care, and education of new generations of surgeons, it was the incorporation of video equipment as an integral part of the standard endoscopic set. This was promulgated and pioneered by Dr. Camran Nezhat. In so doing, the

secrets behind the curtain of the "single eye–single hand" procedures were revealed and broadened the horizons of operative laparoscopy.

In this book, "the Nezhats" review the instrumentation and general principles of laparoscopy and elucidate the management of various procedures in gynecology and gastrointestinal and genitourinary surgery. The uniformity of text and illustration format of this book contribute to the clear message that comes from the "Nezhat School of Laparoscopic Surgery," and is complementary to the high-quality educational video library that originated in the same school.

I regard it as an honor to have this opportunity to be associated with this special project that will find an important place in the literature of our specialty.

Yona Tadir, MD
Department of Surgery
Beckman Laser Institute & Medical Clinic
Irvine, CA

Preface

This is an exciting time to be a surgeon. The field of reproductive medicine has undergone many changes over the past three decades. Gynecologic endoscopic surgery, in particular, has seen tremendous advances during this period. Breakthroughs in video technology, instrumentation, adhesion prevention, and computer-enhanced technology have certainly allowed surgeons to routinely perform a number of procedures endoscopically rather than by laparotomies. These innovations have contributed to faster recovery time, smaller scars, less adhesion formation, fewer complications, lower cost, and, most importantly, better results.

The editors deemed it necessary to update their previous edition due to popular demand and to reflect the rapid advancement in this field. With the contributions of authoritative figures in their respective areas of expertise, many new additions can be found in this book. The inclusion of hysteroscopy in the title and the dedication of a new section on hysteroscopy are meant to emphasize the importance of such surgery in the gynecologic practice today. A new section on fertility treatment and procedures reflects the rapid development in this area. As minimally invasive surgery and natural orifice surgery are becoming more and more accepted and applied in the management of gynecologic malignancy, a significant portion of the book is devoted to this topic to bring the latest information and controversies to our readers. New chapters have also been added on the emerging technologies in simulation and robotic surgery that have brought thought-provoking changes to the practice of surgery in general.

As predicted by the editors more than two decades ago, advanced laparoscopic procedures, which originated in gynecology, have now proliferated into other disciplines such as general surgery, urology, and cardiothoracic surgery. The expansion of such boundaries into the use of laparoscopy in pediatric and vascular surgery arenas is featured in this edition.

The compilation of *Nezhat's Operative Gynecologic Laparoscopy and Hysteroscopy* would certainly not have been possible without the tremendous enthusiasm and support of the contributors. The editors are deeply indebted to them for making this project successful. It is the editors' hope that this book would be able to impart to our readers both the depth and breadth of the experts' knowledge in the exciting field of minimally invasive gynecologic procedures.

Progress in medicine is made when different disciplines collaborate. The work of the editors would not have been possible without the selfless, dedicated support of the following friends and colleagues at Stanford University Medical Center:

Drs. Christopher Payne, Harcharan Gill, and Thomas Hsu of the Department of Urology; Drs. Mark Welton and Andy Shelton of the Division of Colorectal Surgery; Drs. Myriam Curet and John Morton from the Department of General Surgery; Drs. Amin Milki and Ruth Lathi of the Department of Obstetrics and Gynecology; and Drs. Mary Lake Polan and Jonathan Berek, past and present Chairmen of the Department of Obstetrics and Gynecology, respectively.

The editors would like to thank their colleagues in New York for their assistance and encouragement: Dr. Carmel Cohen from Columbia University; Dr. Michael Brodman, Chairman of the Department of Obstetrics and Gynecology; and Dr. Joel Bauer of the Department of Colorectal Surgery at Mount Sinai Medical Center, as well as Dr. Perkash Saharia from Mercy Medical Center.

The editors would also like to express their gratitude to their collaborators in Atlanta for their tremendous support for this work: Dr. Earl Pennington, colorectal surgeon, and Dr. Howard Rottenberg, urologist.

We would like to thank our current Fellows: Drs. Radamila Kazanegra, Madeleine Lemyre, Senzan Hsu, Connie Liu, and Vadim Morozov.

The editors thank all the clinical Fellows in Advanced Laparoscopy, especially Drs. Eve Zaritsky and Jaime Ocampo, for their diligence and patience in completing this project. Eve and Jaime each spent one year reviewing, updating, and critiquing the chapter manuscripts. Without their help, this project would certainly be unfinished still. We are immensely grateful to Dr. Senzan Hsu for his enormous contribution and dedication in making this project a reality. We would also like to recognize Mr. Nat Russo, for his enthusiastic support of this project since it started more than 15 years and 2 editions ago. Without his foresight, these volumes would not have been published. The editors greatly appreciate the exceptional efforts of Ms. Barbara Walthall at Aptara Inc. and Mr. Marc Strauss at Cambridge University Press in making the publishing process as smooth as it could be. The editors would like to thank Dr. David Stevenson, Senior Dean at Stanford University Medical School, and Dr. Linda Giudice, Chairman of the Department of Obstetrics and Gynecology at the University of California at San Francisco, with whom they have enjoyed a long and fruitful collaboration. Finally, the editors are very grateful to Dr. Thomas Krummel, Professor and Chairman of the Department of Surgery at Stanford University Medical Center, and Susan B. Ford Surgeon in Chief, Lucile Packard Children's Hospital, for his continuous and unwavering support and friendship.

1 | HISTORY OF MODERN OPERATIVE LAPAROSCOPY

Barbara J. Page, Jaime Ocampo, Mario Nutis, and Anthony A. Luciano

UNREASONABLENESS REDEFINED

The reasonable man adapts himself to the world; the unreasonable one persists in trying to adapt the world to himself. Therefore all progress depends on the unreasonable man. –George Bernard Shaw

One of the greatest transformations within the history of surgery has been the paradigmatic shift away from open surgery and into the realm of operative video-laparoscopy, an approach that truly captured all that minimally invasive surgery was meant to mean. Many have described the advent of operative video-laparoscopy as a change to surgery as "revolutionary to this century as the development of anesthesia was to the last century."[1]

Indeed, video-endoscopy is today the most common surgical procedure performed by gynecologists, colonoscopists, and gastroendoscopists.[2] As for our own discipline, gynecologic laparoscopists were some of the earliest believers in the new way. Indeed, by 1986, it was estimated that more than 1 million laparoscopic sterilizations were being performed in the United States alone.[3] Today, gynecologic operative video-laparoscopy has freed millions of women from the era when debilitating, multiple laparotomies were the norm for even mild pelvic pathologies.

NEZHAT AND THE ADVENT OF ADVANCED OPERATIVE VIDEO-LAPAROSCOPY

However, getting to this point of general acceptance – a process that is not even complete yet – actually took years of persistent insistence and ingenuity. To actually breathe life into video-laparoscopy, an entirely new way of operating had to be envisioned and accepted into the fold of convention. Yet, to convince an entire surgical discipline to relearn how to perform surgery was no walk in the park. We all know, of course, that attempting to convince surgeons to do anything against their will is a headache in the making. But especially to force upon their heads a change so radical – that of shifting their sacred line of vision – was like courting a collision with catastrophe.

An outsized catalyst was needed to rend surgeons loose from the mighty clasp of custom. It was Camran Nezhat, considered the "founding father" of operative video-laparoscopy, who would use his visionary foresight and virtuoso surgical skill to bring this concept clamoring out of its dream-state and headlong into the realm of reality.

To achieve this, Nezhat rigged together video cameras intended for other uses and began operating off the monitor in the late 1970s, which then allowed him to perform advanced procedures never before done by the laparoscope. For the first time, laparoscopic treatment of extensive endometriosis involving extragenital organs was shown to be possible when Nezhat presented his work at the Annual Meeting of the American Fertility Society in 1985. A year later, his early clinical results on the subject were published in the *Journal of Fertility & Sterility* under the title of "Surgical treatment of endometriosis via laser laparoscopy." After demonstrating the safety and feasibility of performing these complicated surgeries laparoscopically, Nezhat predicted that if such a complicated and extensive disease as endometriosis could be treated laparoscopically, then almost all other pathologies could be managed in that way, too, as long as a cavity existed or could be created in the body.

When all was said and done, Nezhat's conceptual breakthrough would revolutionize modern abdominal and pelvic surgery, overturning in its wake almost 200 years of endoscopic tradition. Talk about rocking the boat; boy would there be dues to pay before this uber-idea could claim its place at the helm of the minimally invasive movement.

THE NATURAL ORDER OF THINGS?

Of course, today all of this may seem so natural, so evolutionarily inevitable, like the story of man walking upright. Yet, operative video-laparoscopy, a concept that now seems almost prosaic in its self-evident appeal, was not so obvious a solution during the late 1970s, nor was it an idea that came gently into being.

Looking back, one actually finds that the opposite was true. Rather, the birth of operative video-laparoscopy was more like a case of gravity defied. It was like suggesting a baseball player look the other way right when the ball is pitched, totally counter-intuitive.

To get a feel for just what Nezhat was up against in trying to convince the surgical world to believe in his ideas, let us take a quick trip back in time to review the status of operative laparoscopy as it stood in the 1970s, in terms of the types of procedures being performed, available technologies, and cultural mindsets that hindered its development.

MAROONED IN MEDIOCRITY: THE EARLY 1970S JUST BEFORE VIDEO-LAPAROSCOPY

Powerful indeed is the empire of habit. –Publilius Syrus

Operative Procedures Achieved by the 1970s

The late 1970s skepticism concerning gynecologic operative laparoscopy is not so clearly spelled out in other historical accounts. Many have made the inaccurate claim that gynecologists had "fully embraced" laparoscopy as a standard modality by the 1970s.[4,5] While there is a grain of truth in this with respect to diagnostic laparoscopy, for advanced operative procedures, the story was quite different. This can be established by reviewing the literature and textbooks of this era, where one can plainly see that operative laparoscopic procedures being performed were essentially no more advanced than those which had been introduced nearly 50 years earlier by endoscopy's early-20th-century pioneers: draining cysts, lysis of adhesions, taking biopsies, electrocautery, and tubal ligations.

Aspiration of Ovarian Cysts – But Not Their Removal

The history of draining cysts laparoscopically serves as a perfect example to track these operative plateaus. As early as the 1920s, the American laparoscopic pioneers Ordnoff and Bernheim were some of the first to demonstrate how successful the "peritoneoscope" (aka, laparoscope) was for this procedure. Jacobaeus was also able to drain ascites in the abdomen in the 1910s, a laparoscopic procedure similar in nature. Yet, more than 50 years later, some of the most popular manuals and textbooks of the 1970s and 1980s – Frangeheim's *Endoscopy and Gynecology*, TeLinde's *Operative Gynecology*, AAGL *Manual of Endoscopy*, Hulka's *Textbook of Laparoscopy*, Baggish's *Atlas of Contract Hysteroscopy and Endoscopy*, Wheeless' *Atlas of Pelvic Surgery* – all specifically direct laparoscopists to focus only on aspiration as the standard practice.[6–11] Surgical removal was made possible as a routine practice as a result of video-laparoscopy. Today, of course, clinical data demonstrate that up to 40% of these cysts do refill, indicating, therefore, that surgical removal is the preferred standard.[12]

Tubal Sterilizations

As for the endoscopic superstar of the 1970s – tubal sterilizations – it actually got its start back in 1936, when Boesch performed the world's first documented laparoscopic tubal sterilization using electro-cauterization.[13] Naturally, the technique has been per-

fected over the years. Yet, by the 1970s, conceptually the procedure had not changed much from its 1930s debut.

Indeed, with the exception of contributions from the era's few virtuosos, such as Palmer, Semm and Mettler, Steptoe, Cohen, and Gomel, our entire discipline seemed stalled for what felt like was going to be forever at tubal sterilizations, as if it were the final frontier.

Близок локоток, да не укусишь – *Blizok lokotok, da ne ukusish*

Impossible, you might say! Fifty years without a new operative procedure? How could this be? After all, eye-popping technological advances were proliferating at an astonishing clip during this era; fiber optics, automatic insufflators, electronically controlled thermo-coagulators. Yet, here we were, in the late 20th century, with men and monkeys flying to the Moon and back, while we laparoscopists were still stuck back at the farm, doing mainly routine diagnostics. It seemed to be a clear case of *Blizok lokotok, da ne ukusish*. This old Russian proverb, translated as "your elbow is close, yet you can't bite it," was an apt description for the times because, with the new technologies enabling video-laparoscopy even more, we were so elbow-close to breaking through and past the old ways. Yet, paradoxically, we were so far away from the "bite" because, as Nezhat and other pioneering laparoscopists of this era soon discovered, confronting psychological resistance to change was the far more difficult task to overcome.[14]

ANOTHER CONUNDRUM

There was another conundrum to overcome: New surgical techniques had to be invented that could accommodate being done in the new closed, video-laparoscopic manner. Doing a procedure endoscopically that was actually designed to be done via laparotomy presented one of the most formidable problems. In short, there were essentially no textbooks or protocols established that would have demonstrated how to make these procedures feasible laparoscopically. Some innovations were beginning to pour through the pipeline; Semm and Mettler's extracorporeal Roeder's loop was one such example.[15,16] Yet these contributions still did not resolve the majority of the problems having to do with achieving more advanced procedures.

In short, each procedure normally done via laparotomy would have to be re-invented. This process was naturally one of trial and error, a factor that especially exposed Nezhat and other laparoscopic pioneers to some harsh criticism in the early days.

An Overview of the Times – TV, Video, and Light Source Technologies

As for the nature of endoscopic technologies, many precursors to video had been established for many years prior to the 1970s. Cinematography and television had actually been used modestly in a handful of surgical centers since the late 1930s. By the 1950s, Japanese pioneers from Hayashida Hospital, Uji, Fukami, and Suginara, developed one of the earliest endoscopic cameras, the gastrocamera,[17] while in 1953 Cohen and Guterman introduced their Cameron cavicamera.[18]

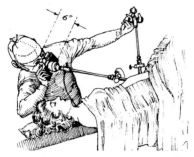

With camera attached, the surgeon's head and body are 4" to 6" farther away from his instruments: surgical reach is awkward.

Figure 1.1. Surgeon with old laparoscopic setup still being published in laparoscopic books in the 1980s. Picture adopted from *Textbook of Laparosopy* by Jaroslav Hulka, 1985.

Some of the most sensational moments in endoscopy's history came with the debuts of the world's first television and color film broadcasts by French pioneers; Palmer's 1955 color film debut of the first live laparoscopy; and, in the same year, the world's first television broadcasts of live bronchoscopies, achieved separately by the French bronchoscopists Soulas and Dubois de Montreynaud.[19] Within a few years, Frangenheim of Germany would produce his famous 1958 color film of a gynecologic laparoscopic surgery, a feat that reverberated throughout the world of gynecologic laparoscopists for years to come.[20]

By 1960, Inui, Berci, and others had either invented or collaborated with industry to bring miniaturized video endo-cameras into endoscopy. However, all of these systems were definitely not designed with advanced operative video laparoscopy in mind. For instance, Berci's 1962 article was one of the earliest to mention both "TV" and endoscopy" in the title. While this article did an excellent job of delineating the latest TV technologies, nevertheless its singular focus was on the ways in which the new imaging technologies would enhance documentation and teaching capabilities; there is no mention of changing the method of performing endoscopic procedures, with the goal of advancing laparoscopy's operative potential.[21]

Even as late as 1977, Berci revisited the role of TV and video devices – referred to as "teaching attachments" – as technologies to enhance teaching only.[22,23] Figures 1.1 through 1.5 from this same 1977 article also clearly show that the most recent camera-equipped endoscopes were still designed to be used in the old way, with endoscopists peering awkwardly through the scope. A similar attachment, called a "multiple tube medical television camera," highlighted in a 1977 American Association of Gynecologic Laparoscopists (AAGL) conference also demonstrates this well-entrenched trend.[24–25]

In other words, while some of the technological rudiments to support video-laparoscopy had been in existence for at least 40 years, the most crucial missing link was not technological in nature, but rather was an issue of missing imagination. The conceptual idea of combining these technologies and using them in an entirely different way had been entirely overlooked until Nezhat's unique contribution.

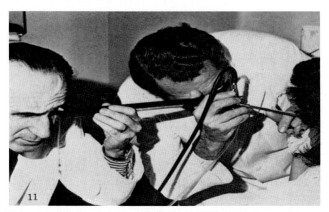

Figure 1.2. Dr. Berci peering through a teaching attachment in 1977. Although Dr. Berci had very innovative ideas, Dr. Nezhat was the first person to operate off a videomonitor. Photo adopted from Berci, G. (1977). Present and future developments in endoscopy. Proceedings of the Royal Society of London.

A PARADOX – POOR RESOLUTION ALMOST FOILS THE THOUGHT

This background review has missed one vital but paradoxical point: Even with these newly emerging optic and video technologies, Nezhat's idea was still too advanced for the era's technologies to support. At the time of Nezhat's awakening to the magic of operating upright, operating off the monitor was barely feasible. The early generation optics and video systems (before digital was perfected) did not yet produce the level of high pixel resolution that we have become accustomed to today. And, despite the superior illumination afforded by the most recent fiber optics and Hopkins lens systems, the quality of light had not advanced to a level where images could be efficiently split toward the monitor. As recently as 1977, Berci made a point to mention the inadequate nature of light sources, stating that "Illumination sources are in a chaotic state."[26] These combined technical deficiencies meant that the images shown on the monitor were so grainy that for most they proved to be indiscernible; definitely not clear enough to support the notion of operating off images. This is why so many surgeons were initially against the idea, because it was quite disorienting to view barely discernible images emanating from a low-resolution, two-dimensional screen positioned several feet away from both surgeon and patient!

BACKLASH TO LAPAROSCOPY FOR SECOND TIME IN THE 20TH CENTURY

As if these obstacles were not enough, gynecologic laparoscopy in the United States was experiencing another season of discontent, just beginning to surface in the late 1970s. Of course, as usual with the story of laparoscopy, this is completely paradoxical, for the discipline did experience some very dramatic leaps forward during this era, at least symbolically. For example, by the mid-1970s training in laparoscopy had been added to "all major gynecologic residency programs" in Europe.[27] By 1981, the American Board of Obstetricians and Gynecologists followed suit and made laparoscopic training a required component of U.S. residency programs. The number of procedures being performed annually also skyrocketed. By about 1973, some sources state that between 6 million and 7 million endoscopic procedures were being performed annually in the United States alone.[28] Other reports show that from 1971 to 1976, laparoscopic sterilizations increased from a mere 1% to an astonishing 60%. [29] Although such statistics on the quantity of surgical procedures are notoriously difficult to verify, based on our research these appear to be reasonable estimates.

Yet at the end of the day, the majority of operative procedures were still limited to simple tasks, which translated to millions of female patients continuing to be subjected to multiple laparotomies for even mild cases of endometriosis. This stall in the progression toward more advanced procedures was, in part, caused by growing concerns about complication rates associated with out-patient laparoscopic sterilizations, which had rapidly grown in popularity in just a few short years.

A growing backlash toward all things laparoscopic developed in earnest, and articles forewarning of high complication rates began to seep into the literature. One of the first such articles to gain national attention was published by the well-respected

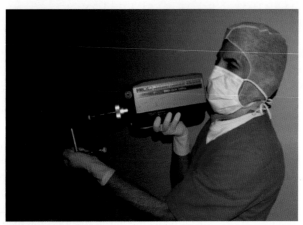

Figure 1.3. One of the first cameras used for video-laparoscopic surgery by Cameron Nezhat, MD.

founder of the AAGL, Jordan Phillips, whose 1977 report outlining in stark detail the estimated complication rates associated with laparoscopic tubal sterilizations struck a raw nerve within surgical communities and served for a time to temper enthusiasm.[30] Indeed, failed sterilizations became the second leading cause of lawsuits for ob-gyns in the United States, only after those associated with pregnancy complications.[31]

Another example of the ambivalence over the scope's role in more advanced operative procedures can be found in one of AAGL's most memorable meetings, at which Semm had been invited to demonstrate the types of operative procedures he envisaged for his "pelviscopy." "Kurt Semm's pelviscopy presentation struck people in that meeting as going too far," recalls Soderstrom, one of the founding members of AAGL. The title of this debate, called "Laparoscopy is replacing the clinical judgment of the gynecologist," also perfectly captured the unease about allowing the scope to advance beyond diagnostics.[32]

Soon thereafter, urgent congressional hearings and other governmental advisory panels were called into session to address concerns about the rapid technological changes affecting endoscopic medical devices, in particular, and medical technologies, in general. Symbolic actions were taken against laparoscopy, beginning most conspicuously with the Congressional Health Device Act passed in 1976. Later, in 1981, the Centers for Disease Control (CDC) in Atlanta issued a very strong public rebuke over patient deaths apparently linked to unipolar laparoscopic sterilization procedures.[29] Because the medical community tends to err on the side of caution, such adverse reports – whether exaggerated or not – were nearly the death-knell for laparoscopic innovation in those days.

THE FROZEN TUNDRA OF BUFFALO – THIS IS YOUR BRAIN ON IMAGINATION

Necessity knows no law except to conquer. – Publilius Syrus

And thus it unfolded that, for the second time in the 20th century, interest in laparoscopy had soared to the heights of unfathomable popularity, only to plunge back down to Earth once its inherent limitations were revealed after the veil had been lifted. An epic tale

indeed was in the making, as it seemed our laparoscope's once rising star of shiny, happy brilliance was on the verge of being reduced to a garish glare. The revivalist hey-day that American laparoscopists had so enjoyed from 1965 to 1975 had been nearly neutralized by the end of the 1970s. [32]

In other words, the timing could not have been worse to introduce such a radically new concept as that of advanced operative video-laparoscopy!

All the same, Nezhat remained imperturbable. These heavy realities were no match for his hidden reserves of moxie; he boldly pushed past the raucous ramble of naysayers, forcing a reckoning with minimally invasive surgery as the new reality. So, how did it all begin?

Amidst the frozen tundra that is Buffalo, New York, in midwinter, there was a kindling mind, ablaze with great visions that soon would take the surgical world by storm. But how did video-laparoscopy develop from the imagination of this young physician just starting his residency? And, by the way, what audacity! How did he find the courage to disagree with senior surgeons – at risk to his own just-blooming career – and take on the entire surgical world? Very gracefully, of course.

More than anything, the "how" came from the "why": Nezhat was driven to help ease the pain of his patients, who had been forced to endure 6- to 12-inch incisions into their abdomens for even the mildest of pathologies. In witnessing the extreme pain and suffering of his patients, their long convalescence, and the serious and numerous complications arising out of laparotomies, Nezhat believed that with just minor alterations almost all of this unnecessary suffering could be averted. It seemed clear to Nezhat that one of the most significant hindrances was the positioning of the surgeon in relation to the scope. The whole contraption left him contorted in the most unnatural of positions: bent-over sideways, with an assistant blindly holding the scope in place while the surgeon tried in vain to verbally direct its positioning.

He knew that if only he could find a way to circumvent the physical limitations posed by peering through the scope's singular eyepiece that the scope's surgical capabilities could then be extended into more advanced operative procedures. Practicing in the lab late at night, he realized that one might be able to perform surgery standing upright by watching the monitor.

With the concept now firmly in his head, Nezhat began the art of rigging together whatever equipment he could find to make this vision come true.

Nezhat recounts those early days:

> Early on, vascular and neurosurgeons had had success using cameras for microsurgery. So, hoping to learn from their successes, I approached my colleagues in these disciplines. Their willingness to spend time demonstrating this technology was very fruitful. Of course, we ran into unusual logistical dilemmas trying to adapt this technology. Many strange configurations were attempted before achieving any degree of success. [Eventually though], we were able to convert an old camera used in their disciplines into an awkward but nevertheless functioning addition to the scope. – Nezhat, C, Presidential Speech, September 2005, JSLS (Figure 1.3)

Despite this precarious start, Nezhat was able to collaborate with other disciplines, a factor which became crucial in further developing these ideas.[34] Nezhat attributes this multidisciplinary facet as having been a vital source of endless inspiration. Endometriosis especially led him to work with other specialties because it commonly affects many different organs, especially the gastrointestinal (GI) and genitourinary (GU) tracts. The contributions of Dr. Earl Pennington, a pioneering colorectal surgeon, and Drs. Rottenberg and Green, both urologists, were especially noteworthy, as they guided Nezhat through very challenging procedures that had never been achieved laparoscopically before.[34] Nezhat recalls, "Colorectal surgeon, Earl Pennington, and urologist, Howard Rottenberg, were always at our side." Also, patients with endometriosis have high rates of endometriomas that sometimes can have the appearance of malignancy. Therefore, from the very beginning, contributions from colleagues in gynecologic oncology were of critical importance. In this area, the guidance of Drs. Benedict Benigno and Matthew Burrell was absolutely invaluable. Through their vision and willingness to share their expertise, a better understanding of how to recognize and manage malignancies laparoscopically was achieved.[35]

As for new suturing methods, only a few modifications were needed. For the most part, Nezhat was able to convert the same microsurgical techniques for open surgeries as were taught by pioneers in treating endometriosis such as Drs. Robert Frankling of Houston, Texas, and Ron Batt of Buffalo.[37] Before switching to video-laparoscopy, suturing laparoscopically was a feat extraordinarily difficult to achieve while hunched over the scope. In fact, this factor was one of the main hindrances that had made earlier attempts at operative laparoscopy so awkward, unsuccessful, and, ultimately, unpopular.

"FOREVER-SCOPY"

Operative video-laparoscopy was certainly not without its flaws. And we would not want to delude the reader by providing only the pretty pictures of its past. Indeed, one of its least attractive features initially was the extra time it took to perform some of the advanced procedures. As Nezhat recalled, "They used to call laparoscopy 'forever-scopy.'" For instance, laparoscopic ectopic pregnancy surgeries were taking 4–5 hours initially, while Nezhat recalls that his first – and also the world's first – radical hysterectomy and paraeortic and pelvic lymphadenectomy by video-laparoscopy actually took 7 hours. This added time factor was not helping convince anyone that the video-laparoscopic method was better or safer than open surgery.[36] Of course, even some laparotomies took up to 7 hours. But, the new method naturally was judged more harshly than classical standards.

Because of this time factor stemming from the very steep learning curve, the effectiveness of video-laparoscopy was difficult to assess at first. Early reports showed laparoscopy to have higher complication rates than laparotomies, although these results were attributable mainly to inexperience.

COLLABORATION WITH INSTRUMENT MAKERS

To overcome these inherent deficiencies standing in the way of the new technique, Nezhat began a fruitful relationship of collaboration with Karl Storz and other surgical instrument companies.

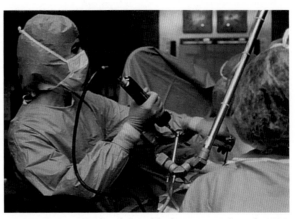

Figure 1.4. Camran Nezhat doing videolaparoscopy in early 1980.

Using those same old clunky cameras borrowed from the neuro and vascular surgeons, Nezhat was able to show the company representatives that operating off the monitor could work. After hours in the operating room, eventually Storz and other company representatives were also convinced of the scope's greater potential and they began producing new cameras and light sources customized for operative video-laparoscopy.

Today, working together with companies in this fashion might be discouraged. Yet, without this early support and free-spirited exchange of ideas between engineers and surgeons, poor visualization and other technological hindrances certainly would have persisted as formidable conceptual and technological divides.[37]

DELAYS IN PUBLICATIONS

Despite collecting verifiable clinical proof to the safety and efficacy of video operative laparoscopy, at first no journal would accept Nezhat's early manuscripts on the subject.[12]

It took several years, but finally his debut articles on these never-before-seen laparoscopic surgeries were published in 1986. [13,38] From this point, Nezhat was able to continue to demonstrate –this time to a larger audience – that other complex surgeries were finally possible (Figure 1.4). Indeed, between the years of 1984 and 1989, Nezhat forced a reconsideration of all that was thought possible when he and his colleagues became the first to successfully perform such complex surgeries as:

- the first laparoscopic treatment of multi-organ, extensive, stage iv endometriosis, affecting the GI and GU;[39–49]
- the first laparoscopic bowel surgery and resection with Pennington;[39,42, 44, 45, 49, 50]
- the first laparoscopic ureter resection and ureterouretrostomy with H. Rottenberg and B. Green;[43, 45, 48]
- the first laparoscopic radical hysterectomy with paraortic and pelvic node dissection with M. Burrell and B. Benigno;[51, 52]
- the first laparoscopic bladder resection with H. Rottenberg; [43, 45, 48]
- the first laparoscopic vesicovaginal fistula repair with H. Rottenberg;[53]
- the first laparoscopic rectovaginal fistula repair with J.A. Bastidas;

- the first laparoscopic ovarian cystectomy in second and third trimesters of pregnancy;[54]
- the first laparoscopic-assisted surgery (laparoscopically assisted myomectomy);
- the first laparoscopic Burch procedure;[55]
- the first laparoscopic treatment of ovarian remnant with E. Pennington and H. Rottenberg;[56]
- the first laparoscopic sacral colpopexy;[57]
- the first laparoscopic treatment of diaphragmatic endometriosis lesions with H. Brown;[58]
- the first laparoscopic management of a leaking inferior mesenteric artery with C. Zarins;[59]
- the first laparoscopic coronary reanastomosis in a porcine model;[49]
- and the first laparoscopic management of dermoid cyst.[60]

Acceptance and publications on these firsts by Nezhat and his colleagues often faced numerous rejections and/or lagged 3 to 5 years after the initial procedures were performed, due to either resistance from journal editors to such new-fangled ideas, or for preference to publish the work of those in academia rather than those in private practice. In any case, before 1990, Nezhat and his colleagues had already performed laparoscopically nearly all the major procedures involving the bowel, bladder, and ureter, which in the past had only been accomplished via laparotomy.

"AGONY IN THE GARDEN" – THE ERA OF HOSTILITY

Scandal has ever been the doom of beauty. – book ii, properties

Like a rite of passage, the quintessential pioneer story would not be complete without an element of abject suffering to startle us out of our imaginative reverie. Like Semm, Muhe, and others, Nezhat endured many years of doubt before his ideas became accepted. In terms of endoscopy's long history, this was not surprising. There had always existed an element of resistance since the time of Bozzini, if not earlier. Resistance to operative video-laparoscopy was especially fierce for it forced surgeons – for the second time in the 20th century – to lose two vital sensory mechanisms: tactile and direct visualization.[61] These changes seemed to be the tipping point that drove the final stake into ancient surgical practices, bringing to the fore a 21st-century approach that few were actually ready to embrace. Indeed, so suspect was the new surgical revolution that Nezhat and his brothers had their academic integrity called into question.

Just a few years ago, in 2002, a lay media frenzy went so far as to label Nezhat's work "bizarre," "barbaric," and akin to "medical-terrorism." Forced now to answer to this misinformed media frenzy, Stanford University was essentially left with no choice but to act in the most politically expedient manner by launching a highly publicized, formal investigation of Nezhat's work, issuing in the process a temporary suspension to appease the public outcry. After lengthy investigations – and to the surprise of no one in the know – Nezhat's work was found to be free of any misconduct whatsoever, cleared by the highest authorities from Stanford University, the U.S. State Supreme Court, and the California and Georgia State Medical Boards. How ironic it is today that, quietly, all the studies are pouring forth which confirm

Nezhat's initial impressions of the advantages of operative video-laparoscopy. Those same procedures, pioneered by Nezhat and his team considered so controversial just a few years ago, are now encouraged to be performed by the most prestigious journals. A 2004 editorial from the *New England Journal of Medicine* states, "Surgeons must progress beyond the traditional techniques of cutting and sewing . . . to a future in which . . . minimal access to the abdominal cavity [is] only the beginning."[62]

CONCLUSION

History may be servitude, history may be freedom – from "Little Gidding," TS Eliot

Sometimes history can become an unbearable weight. Operating off the monitor and inventing the accompanying advanced procedures were the crucial links which allowed our discipline to be set free from hundreds of years of history, peering directly through a tube, specula, or scope. By demonstrating the scope's boundless potential, Nezhat hit the groundbreaking grand slam that drove laparoscopy home toward its true operative potential.

Perhaps of even more lasting significance, switching to the monitor set off an intense scientific and philosophical debate about just where the upper bounds – if any – of operative laparoscopy should end. It forced a reconsideration of the entire field of surgery, a change that called for every aspect of surgical methodologies to be thoroughly scrutinized. And it was not strictly the category of surgery that was reevaluated. Rather, questions arose having to do with a wide range of aspects concerning medicine, patient rights, and disease-states. New concepts relating to pain management for patients emerged as one of the most important changes to have come about due to the minimally invasive movement. As well, an eventual rethinking in expectations about surgical outcomes arose. Complications once considered unavoidable in the days of open surgery were suddenly reevaluated and revised in the minimally invasive era.

Still, as gynecologic laparoscopists, our advocacy work to perfect and promote minimally invasive surgery is not done. There are still too many patients who are enduring needless open procedures. For example, in 1997 66.8% of hysterectomies performed in the United States were done via laparotomy. Nevertheless, humankind is closer than ever to truly being able to perform the most advanced operative surgeries through the least traumatic incisions. For this reason, the nearly complete triumph of minimally invasive surgery – with video-laparoscopy leading the way – has turned out to be one of the greatest achievements of 20th-century medicine. More than that, it transformed into one of the world's most important human rights movements by insisting on greater and more democratized standards in healthcare, a change that touched the lives of millions of patients who had suffered too long in the shadows of silence.

REFERENCES

1. www.sls.org, Marelyn Medina, MD, Rio Grande Regional Hospital (McAllen, TX).
2. www.sls.org, Marelyn Medina, MD, Rio Grande Regional Hospital (McAllen, TX). The trouble with trocars, quote from M. Kavic in Nov 2001.

3. Gomel, V. Surgical textbook introduction.

4. Sgambati, SA & Ballantyne, GH. Minimallyinvasive surgery in the diseases of the colon and rectum: the legacy of an ancient tradition. In: Jager RM Wexner S, *Laparoscopic Colectomy*, Churchill & Livingstone. New York. 1995. pp 13–23.

5. Gunning, JE. The history of laparoscopy. *Jour of Repr Med*, 1974, 12:6.

6. Frangeheim H. Endoscopy and gynecology. In *The Range and Limits of Operating Laparoscopy in the Diagnosis of Sterility*, Phillips, JM, ed. Downey, CA: AAGL, 1978.

7. TeLinde's Operative Gynecology, Lippincott Williams & Wilkins,

8. Martin DC, ed. *AAGL Manual of Endoscopy*. , 1988.

9. Hulka, JF *Textbook of Laparoscopy*, Orlando, FL:Grune and Stratton, Inc., 1985.

10. Baggish, MS. *Atlas of Contact Hysteroscopy and Endoscopy*. Urban & Schwarzenberg, 1982.

11. Wheeless, CR. *Atlas of Pelvic Surgery*, Lippincott Williams & Wilkins, 1988.

12. Nezhat C, Crowgey S, Garrison C. Surgical treatment of endometriosis via laser laparoscopy. *Fertility and Sterility*, 1986; Vol 25, No 6, pp 778–783.

13. Boesch PF. Laproskopie. *Schweiz Z Krankenh Anstaltw* 1936; 6:62.

14. Bruhat MA, Mage G, Manhes H.: Use of CO_2 laser by laparoscopy. In Laser Surgery III. *Proceedings of the Third International Congress on Laser Surgery*, I. Kaplan, editor. Tel Aviv, Jerusalem Press, 1979, p 225.

15. Semm K, Mettler L. Technical progress in pelvic surgery via operative laparoscopy. *Am J Obstet Gynecol*. 1980;138(2):121–7.

16. Semm K: The endoscopic intra-abdominal suture. *Geburtshilfe Frauenheilkd*. 42:56, 1982.

17. Uji T, Shirotokoro T and Hayashida T: Gastrocamera. *Tokyo Med. J.*, 61:135, 1953 *J. Japan Med. Ass.*, 1954; 31:681.

18. Cohen M. *Laparoscopy, Culdoscopy, and Gynecolography*. Philadelphia:WB Saunders, 1970.

19. Soulas A.: *Televised bronchoscopy*. Presse Med. 1956; 64:97.

20. Frangenheim H. *Laparoscopy and Culdoscopy in Gynaecology*. 1972; London: Butterworth, 1972.

21. Berci G., Davids J.: Endoscopy and television. *B.M.J.* 1962; 1: 1610.

22. Berci G. Present and future developments in endoscopy. Proc. R. Soc. *Lond*. 1977. B. 195, 235–242

23. Olsen V, Berci G. *Teaching attachments. Endoscopy*. 1976. New York: Appleton-Century-Crofts.

24. Phillips, JM. Endoscopy in Gynecology. *AAGL* Proceedings of the Third International Congress on Gynecologic Endoscopy, 1977; 488–489.

25. Berci G. Flexible fiber endoscopes, Figure 2, *Endoscopy Today*. Mar 1972; 111–113.

26. Berci G. Present and future developments in endoscopy. Proc. R. Soc. *Lond*. 1977. B. 195, 235–242.

27. Litynski GS. *Highlights in the history of laparoscopy*.1996; Barbara Bernert Verlag.

28. Berci G. *Endoscopy Today*, 1972; vol 51, Nos 2 and 3: 64–70.

29. Soderstrom RM. A history of the American Association of Gynecologic Laparoscopists. *The Journal of the American Association of Gynecologic Laparoscopists*; 2001;Vol 8(4).

30. Phillips JM. Complications in laparoscopy. *Int J Gynaecol Obstet*. 1977;15:157–162.

31. Hulka JF. Foreword to Textbook of Laparoscopy. 1985; Grune & Stratton.

32. Nezhat C. Personal correspondence files; rejection letters for the technique of video-laparoscopy and operating off the monitor.

33. Mahnes H. A History of Laparoscopy, Acceptance Speech, *Recipient of SLS Excel Award*, 2003.

34. Nezhat F, Nezhat C, Pennington E, Ambroze W, Jr.: Laparoscopic segmental resection for infiltrating endometriosis of the rectosigmoid colon: a preliminary report. *Surg Laparosc Endosc*, 1992, 2(3):212–216.

35. Journal of Society of Laparoendoscopic Surgeons, Presidential Speech, C. Nezhat, Sept 2005.

36. Shushan A, Mohamed H, Magos AL. How long does laparoscopy surgery really take? Lessons learned from 1000 operative laparoscopies. *Hum Reprod*. 1999; 14(1):39–43.

37. Nezhat C. Videolaseroscopy: A new modality for the treatment of endometriosis and other diseases of reproductive organs. *Colposcopy & Gynecologic Laser Surgery*, 1986, 2(4): 221–224.

38. Nezhat C, Crowgey S, and Nezhat F. Videolaseroscopy for the treatment of endometriosis associated with infertility. *Fertility and sterility*. 1989; 51(2): 237–40.

39. Nezhat C, and Nezhat FR. Safe laser endoscopic excision or vaporization of peritoneal endometriosis. *Fertility and sterility*, 1989; 52(1), 149–51.

40. Nezhat CR, Nezhat FR, and Silfen, SL. Videolaseroscopy. *The CO_2 laser for advanced operative laparoscopy. Obstetrics and gynecology clinics of North America*. 1991; 18(3), 585–604.

41. Nezhat F, Nezhat C, & Pennington E. Laparoscopic proctectomy for infiltrating endometriosis of the rectum. *Fertility and sterility*, 1992;57(5), 1129–32.

42. Nezhat CR, and Nezhat FR.. Laparoscopic segmental bladder resection for endometriosis: a report of two cases. *Obstetrics and gynecology*, 1992; 81(5 (Pt 2)), 882–4.

43. Nezhat C, Nezhat F, Pennington E, et al. Laparoscopic disk excision and primary repair of the anterior rectal wall for the treatment of full-thickness bowel endometriosis. *Surgical endoscopy*. 1994;8(6), 682–5.

44. Nezhat, Camran. A safe approach to Laparoscopic Excision of Serosal and Subserosal Endometriosis, Endometriosis of the Bladder, Ureter, Rectovaginal Septum and Rectum. Annual Meeting of AAGL September 1989.

45. Nezhat C. Advanced Laparoscopic Treatment of Endometriosis. *Annual Meeting of AAGL*, Sept 1989.

46. Nezhat F, Nezhat C, Videolaseroscopy for the treatment of infiltrative rectovaginal septum, *endometriosis and posterior cul-de-sac nodularity. Annual Meeting of AAGL*, Nov 1990.

47. Nezhat CR, Nezhat F, Nezhat CH. Operative Laparoscopy (minimally invasive surgery): State of the art. J. *Gynecol Surg* 1992;8:111–141.

48. Seidman DS, Nezhat C. Letter-to-the-Editor: Is the laparoscopic bubble bursting? *The Lancet*, Feb 24 1996.

49. Nezhat, C, Nezhat, F, Ambroze, W, et al. (1993). Laparoscopic repair of small bowel and colon. *A report of 26 cases. Surgical endoscopy*, 7(2), 88–9.

50. Nezhat, CR, Nezhat, FR, Burrell, MO, et al. (1993). Laparoscopic radical hysterectomy and laparoscopically assisted vaginal radical hysterectomy with pelvic and paraaortic node dissection. *Journal of gynecologic surgery*, 9(2), 105–20.

51. Nezhat, CR, Burrell, MO, Nezhat, FR, et al. (1992). Laparoscopic radical hysterectomy with paraaortic and pelvic node dissection. *American journal of obstetrics and gynecology*, 166(3), 864–5.

52. Nezhat, CH, Nezhat, F, Nezhat, C, et al. (1994). Laparoscopic repair of a vesicovaginal fistula: a case report. *Obstetrics and gynecology*, 83(5 Pt 2), 899–901.

53. Nezhat, F, Nezhat, C, Silfen, SL, et al. (1991). Laparoscopic ovarian cystectomy during pregnancy. *Journal of laparoendoscopic surgery*, 1(3), 161–4.

54. Nezhat C, Nezhat F, Nezhat CH. Laparoscopic Burch procedure. *Operative laparoscopy (minimally invasive surgery): state of the art. J Gynecol Surg*. 1992; 8:111–141.

55. C Nezhat, F Nezhat. Videolaseroscopy for the treatment of ovarian remnant attached to bowel and ureter Annual Meeting of AAGL November 1990.

56. Nezhat F, Nezhat C, Nezhat CH. Laparoscopic sacral colpopexy for vaginal wall prolapse. *Obstet Gynecol.* 1994; 84:885–888.

57. Nezhat F, Nezhat C, Levy JS. Laparoscopic treatment of symptomatic diaphragmatic endometriosis: A case report. *Fertil Steril.* 1992;58:614–616.

58. Nezhat C, Childers J, Nezhat F, et al. Major retroperitoneal vascular injury during laparoscopic surgery. *Hum Reprod.* 1997; 12:480–483.

59. Nezhat C, Winder WK, Nezhat F. Laparoscopic removal of dermoid cysts, *Obst Gynecol.* 1989;73(2):278–281.

60. Seidman DS, Nezhat C. Letter-to-the-Editor: Is the laparoscopic bubble bursting? *The Lancet*, Feb 24 1996.

61. Pappas, Joacobs, NEJM, May 2004.

2 | EQUIPMENT

Jaime Ocampo, Mario Nutis, Camran Nezhat, Ceana Nezhat, and Farr Nezhat

Successful operative laparoscopy requires the proper basic and specialized equipment to make difficult procedures technically possible and safe. Most operations can be done with two or three forceps, a suction–irrigator probe, a bipolar electrocoagulator, and a CO_2 laser. With the rapid growth of operative laparoscopy, disposable, semireusable, and reusable instruments have become available. In selecting the appropriate instruments, their cost and effectiveness should be considered because too many instruments clutter the field and increase operative time.

With videolaseroscopy, the operation is observed by the surgeon and operating room staff on video monitors. The CO_2 laser is used through the operative channel of the laparoscope for cutting and establishing hemostasis of small blood vessels.[1] Electrocoagulation with a bipolar forceps is used to control bleeding from larger vessels. These instruments enable surgeons to increase the diversity of laparoscopic procedures. Some of them have multiple functions, whereas others are specialized. Most are designed to fit through trocar sleeves between 2 mm and 33 mm in diameter.

THE BASIC INSTRUMENTS

The Laparoscope

The endoscope allows one to view the abdominal and pelvic cavities and is the most important piece of equipment. It must be in optimal condition. Although the diameter of laparoscopes varies from 2 to 12 mm and the angle of view varies from 0° to 90°, the most commonly used laparoscopes are straight diagnostic (Figure 2.1A) and angled operative laparoscopes (Figure 2.1B,C). A direct 10-mm, 0° diagnostic laparoscope and an 11-mm, 0° operative laparoscope with a channel for the CO_2 laser are preferable (Figure 2.2A,B). The image transmitted by the diagnostic scope is better. The operative channel requires a reduction in the size of the lens system and the number of fiberoptic bundles. With a Hopkins rod lens system, the shaft of the laparoscope contains quartz rods with concave ends that provide excellent clarity. This type of lens rarely is dislodged during handling. Endoscopes are either rigid or flexible. Most rigid scopes are focused with the camera coupler. With a videoscope (camera and scope together), either there will be a focus control on the scope or the focus will occur automatically inside the camera. The image is magnified and appears larger on the monitor.

Flexible scopes rely on many fiberoptic bundles. As the image is magnified, so are the bundles, making the ends of the bundles visible along with the image. The scopes are relatively fragile, and small cracks allow water to seep through the lens and distort the image.

Another breakthrough in medical cameras is "chip-on-a-stick," a technology that combines the camera and the scope in one piece of equipment. The camera chip is taken out of the camera head and placed at the distal end of the scope. This technology does away with the optical lenses an image passes through when the chip is in the camera head. Chip-on-a-stick cameras require less light than do standard cameras because light is not lost in the light cord and rod lens.

There are multiple manufacturers of laparoscopes, all of which have slightly different variations. We recommend that you try laparoscopes from different manufacturers so that you can find the most comfortable one for you.

Primary Trocars

Reusable and disposable trocars are constructed of a combination of metal and plastic (Figure 2.3A,B). A feature common to all of them is a flapper or trumpet valve that is designed to prevent gas leakage as the laparoscope or other instruments are removed from the abdomen. With reusable trocars, this mechanism creates friction on the laparoscope. After a prolonged procedure, the trocar moves with the laparoscope. This phenomenon causes inadvertent removal of the trocar from the abdominal cavity and a loss of pneumoperitoneum. When the spring is removed from the valve, there is less friction and that problem can be avoided. A feature of disposable cannulas is a new stability thread design that provides greater fixation of the abdominal wall. A radially expanding outer sheath has been developed to allow safer trocar insertion (Step, InnerDyne, Sunnyvale, CA). The radially expanding dilation is supposed to leave a 50% smaller scar while securely anchoring the cannula and virtually eliminating abdominal wall bleeding (Figure 2.4).

Another approach to improving the safety of primary trocar insertion is the observing or optical trocar (Ethicon; Figure 2.3B). The obturator of this trocar is hollow except for a clear plastic conical tip with two external ridges. The trocar–cannula assembly is passed through tissue layers to enter the operative space under direct vision from a 10-mm or a 5-mm 0° laparoscope placed into the trocar. Initial experience suggests that this technique represents a safe alternative to Veress needle placement when laparoscopic access could be hazardous or difficult.[2,3] The optical device requires some additional training so that the operator can identify the various anatomic layers upon entry into the abdomen through the contact view. This device is no substitute for proper training, and its cost-effectiveness for an experienced laparoscopist is doubtful.

A fiberglass optic–equipped safety needle has been developed for visually controlled access in laparoscopic procedures. This device can allow immediate diagnosis of small bowel perforation by endoscopy.[4]

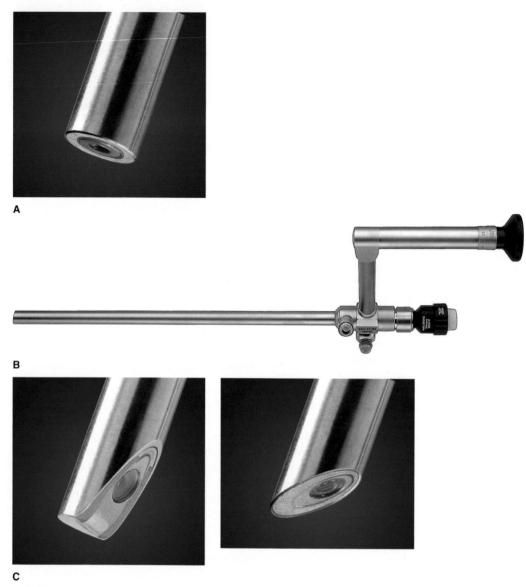

Figure 2.1. (**A**) A 5-mm straight diagnostic laparoscope. (**B**) A 10-mm diagnostic laparoscope. (**C**) Angled laparoscopes.

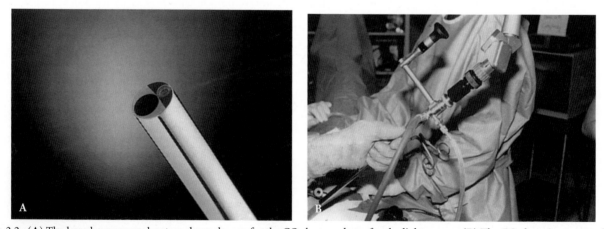

Figure 2.2. (**A**) The laser laparoscope has two channels: one for the CO_2 laser and one for the light source. (**B**) The CO_2 laser is connected to the operative channel of the laparoscope.

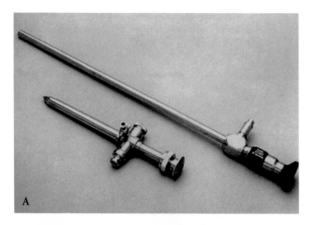

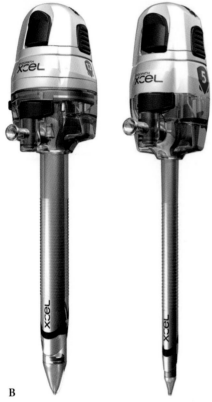

Figure 2.3. (**A**) A reusable 11-mm trocar with a 10-mm laparoscope. (**B**) A 5-mm and 10-mm trocar with a bladeless obturator (Ethicon). Both of these trocars also allow for the insertion of the camera in order to have visualization on insertion of the trocar.

Various disposable trocar tips are available. Spring-loaded safety shields (Ethicon) retract into the cannula as the trocar is inserted into the abdomen. This exposes the sharp trocar for entry and automatically releases the plastic shield inside the peritoneal cavity to cover the sharp tip and protect intra-abdominal organs. Another trocar uses the same principle as the Veress needle. The trocar tip has a hollow core with a spring-loaded blunt stylet (Dexide). After the peritoneal cavity is penetrated, the blunt stylet moves beyond the tip to prevent injury. Bullet blunt-tip disposable trocars (Ethicon) lessen the possibility of tissue being caught between the trocar and the sleeve. In the presence of adhesions to the anterior abdominal wall, under the umbilicus, the reusable devices have no proven advantage.

There has been great debate over the decreased risk of trocar injury with radially expanding (blunt) trocars versus sharp trocars. Both these types of trocars are available on the market today. Bhoyrul et al. [5] compared the complication rates in two groups of patients who had procedures using sharp trocars versus blunt trocars. There was a decrease in the rate of intraoperative cannula site bleeding and operative wound complications in the blunt trocar group. Pain scores were lower in the blunt trocar group, but these did not reach statistical significance. In these studies, the investigators opted for no closure of the 12-mm trocar sites when using blunt trocars. No incisional hernias were reported during a follow-up period of 18 months. Decreased risk of incisional hernias, even in nonapproximated port sites of 12 mm, was also shown by a study done by Johnson et al.[6] In this retrospective review, 747 patients with 3735 trocar sites were studied. There were no incisional hernias reported with the use of the VersaStep blunt trocars. These results were compared to the 1.2% rate of incisional hernias when the Hassan trocar was used.

Whether or not blunt trocars decrease the risk of vascular injury remains unknown. The Office of Surveillance and Biometrics, U.S. Food and Drug Administration keeps records through the Manufacturer and User Facility Device Experience (MAUDE) database.[6] In most cases of vascular injury, the trocar involved was either a shielded trocar (which has a retractable shield that covers the trocar blade before and after insertion to help protect abdominal and pelvic organs from inadvertent puncture) or an optical trocar (which allows the laparoscopist to view the cutting tip as it penetrates the tissues). However, no studies looking at this issue have been done.

Secondary Trocars

Reusable and disposable accessory trocars and sleeves come in a variety of lengths and range in diameter from 2 to 30 mm; the most common size is 5 mm. Some are threaded and are screwed into the abdominal wall, making them relatively immobile during manipulation. The use of "fascial screws" is associated with an increased incidence of omental and bowel herniation after laparoscopy.[7]

Veress Needle

Disposable and reusable Veress needles consist of a blunt-tipped, spring-loaded inner stylet and a sharp outer needle (Figure 2.5). A lateral hole on this stylet enables CO_2 gas to be delivered. As the needle passes through the abdominal layers, the stylet retracts to allow penetration into the peritoneal cavity. The absence of tissue resistance allows the blunt stylet to protrude intra-abdominally. The disposable Veress needle has several added safety points, related mainly to the sharp tip of the outer needle and the smooth operation of the spring mechanism.

Many laparoscopists continue to use the Veress needle to create pneumoperitoneum, mainly because of preference for and comfort with this technique. They also claim that a vascular or organ injury would be less severe with a smaller-caliber instrument. However, multiple studies have shown that direct trocar insertion is a safe alternative to Veress needle insertion technique for the creation of pneumoperitoneum; it has lower complication rates, has less cost/instrumentation, and allows rapid creation of pneumoperitoneum.[8,9]

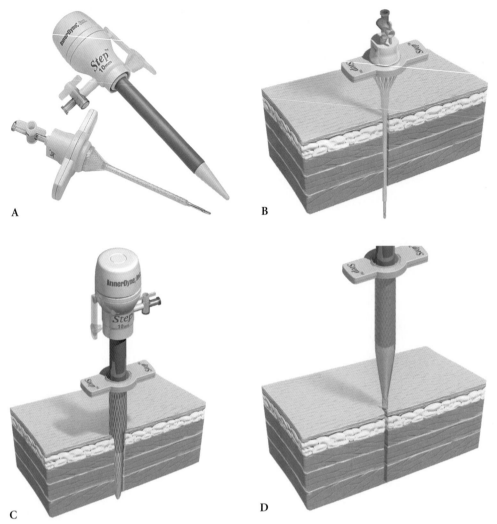

Figure 2.4. (**A**) A radially expanding 10-mm cannula/dilator. (**B**) After insufflation, intra-abdominal entry is made by using an insufflation and access needle with a radially expandable sleeve. The needle is withdrawn, leaving the expandable sleeve in place. (**C**) A tapered blunt dilator is inserted, expanding the sleeve and tissue tract. Radial dilation of the tract splits each layer of tissue along a path of least resistance. (**D**) After the cannula is removed, a small slit-like defect remains when the layers of muscle in the abdominal wall collapse.

Insufflator

To adequately observe the contents of the abdominal and pelvic cavity, the abdomen is distended with insufflated CO_2. Some operations require an automatic electric insufflator that can

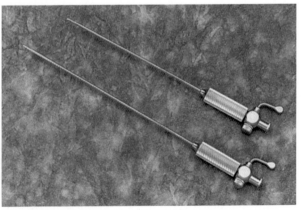

Figure 2.5. Reusable Veress needles.

deliver up to 40 L of gas per minute. The insufflator compensates for changes in intra-abdominal pressure. To avoid complications such as subcutaneous emphysema, intra-abdominal pressures should not exceed 15 mm Hg. The Stryker Endoscopy Insufflator (Stryker Corporation, Kalamazoo, MI) (Figure 2.6) uses heated carbon dioxide (37°C/99°F) immediately before it enters the patient's abdominal cavity, and this may help maintain body temperature, decrease the risk of hypothermia, and reduce endoscope fogging.

The Light Cord

The light cord is as important as a high-resolution camera and a precision scope. If light does not move properly from the light source to the scope through the cord, the value of the camera is limited and images are poor. Light dispersed evenly across the cord's diameter is preferred. Light cords are either fiberoptic or liquid filled. Fiberoptic cables are available in varying lengths (6, 8, and 10 ft) with little light loss. Light cords are fragile and should not be wound into small bundles. Liquid-filled light guide cables transmit more light and are more durable than fiberoptic cables.

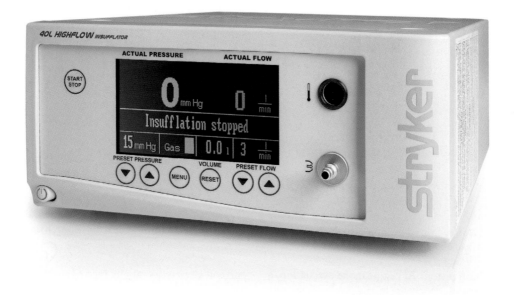

Figure 2.6. High flow insuflattors (like this Stryker unit) warm CO_2 gas(37°C/99°F) immediately before it enters the patient's abdominal cavity. These insufflators can provide flow up to 40 L /min.

They are more expensive, produce more heat at their connection to the endoscope, and are limited to a standard 6-ft length.

Light Sources

All light sources use xenon, halogen, or mercury bulbs. Each type generates light of a different color and intensity. The most common bulbs are halogen and xenon, with xenon available in 150, 175, and 300 W (Figure 2.7). Xenon bulbs generate a higher intensity of light, last longer, and are more expensive to replace. They provide consistent levels of light intensity and can generate even higher levels of light as needed.

Suction–Irrigator Probe and Hydrodissection Pump

A suction–irrigator probe is a versatile instrument. Controlled suction and irrigation enhance observation and improve operative technique. This device serves as an extension of the surgeon's fingers, serves as a backstop for the CO_2 laser, and helps with hydrodissection, division of tissue planes and spaces, lavage, blunt dissection, and smoke and fluid evacuation. A properly designed suction–irrigation system has the following characteristics:

1. The trumpet valve is designed ergonomically and is versatile, so electrosurgical accessories, lasers, and hand instruments can be inserted through the probe (Figure 2.8A,B)
2. The trumpet valve is easy to use and provides constant control of fluid or suction, including valve regulation, rather than an on/off mechanism.
3. The internal valve diameters are large enough to allow blood and tissue to pass easily through the canister and provide sufficient irrigation flow.
4. Probe tips are smooth, strong, and nonreflective so that they can be used for blunt dissection and serve as a backstop for the CO_2 laser (Figure 2.9).
5. The irrigation pump provides precise and variable irrigation pressures.

A trumpet valve can incorporate a metered adjustment feature, allowing smoke evacuation without manual intermittent

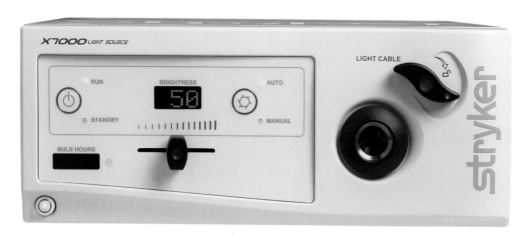

Figure 2.7. Xenon light source by Stryker.

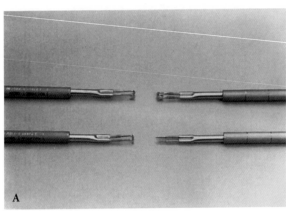

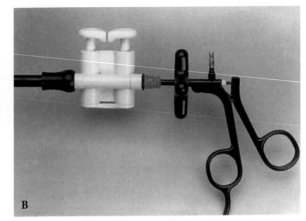

Figure 2.8. (**A**) Nezhat-Dorsey hydrodissection suction–irrigator probes with different electrosurgical accessories. (**B**) A hydrodissection probe can accommodate hand instruments.

depression of the suction piston. To begin smoke evacuation, a control pad is rotated counterclockwise by the surgeon, allowing variable evacuation up to 10 L per minute (Figure 2.10). Additional suction capability can be accessed by depressing the suction piston button. Laser or electrosurgical accessories inserted through the rear access port simultaneously can be combined with smoke evacuation, maintaining a clear field of vision. Several probe tips are available in various lengths and shapes (Figure 2.11). A quick mechanism-disconnect probe tip speeds the changing of the tips. An aspiration–injection needle accessory with nonfenestrated 5-mm/28-cm probe tips allows precise closed-chambered aspiration of ovarian cysts or injection of fluid (Figure 2.12). This system has reusable probe tips. Although the pump can deliver fluid with a pressure up to 775 mm Hg, 300 mm Hg is used for routine irrigation. Higher pump pressures are used to dissect areas near the bowel, bladder, major blood vessels, and ureters. The irrigation fluid consists of warmed 1-L bottles of lactated Ringer's solution (Travenol Laboratories, Deerfield, IL), and wall suction is used as the aspirated material initially enters a Vac-Rite canister. A laser plume filter removes particles that might clog the wall suction. A higher pneumatically powered pump pressure with adjustable pulsations has been developed (Davol X-Stream Irrigation System [previously American Hydro-Surgical Instruments]). It incorporates the effectiveness and convenience of bag irrigation with the precision and effective delivery of pressurized pump irrigation (Figure 2.13). It does not use electric

current, electronics, or any type of computer software but offers irrigation control. It has a "pump cartridge chamber" into which a disposable cartridge is inserted. As compressed gas does not contact the irrigation fluid at any time, this design eliminates the potential for procedural contamination during setup and the possibility of inadvertently entering the abdominal cavity. Irrigation bags replace bottled solutions. As the bag is depleted, it collapses on itself, stopping the pump and alerting the staff to switch to the second fluid supply. The fluid is delivered in a continuous flow or in a pulsed irrigation mode. The rates of pulsation and irrigation pressure are adjustable. The latter setting ranges from 0 to 2500 mm Hg. Pulsatile irrigation cleanses the surgical site more effectively than does normal continuous flow, enabling a more thorough removal of blood clots and char. The use of irrigation fluid warmed to 39°C has been advocated to decrease the drop in core temperature commonly observed in laparoscopy.[10]

Forceps

Atraumatic and grasping forceps with jaws are available in sizes from 3 to 10 mm (Figure 2.14). Atraumatic stabilization of structures is important in many procedures, and several types of forceps are available for this purpose. The preferred type is medium sized, with a rounded tip and serrated jaws. It can grasp tissue for exposure, act as a blunt probe with the jaws closed, affect traction

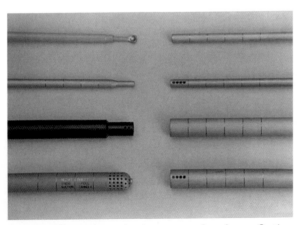

Figure 2.9. Different size probe tips are smooth and nonreflective and can be used for blunt dissection and as laser backstops.

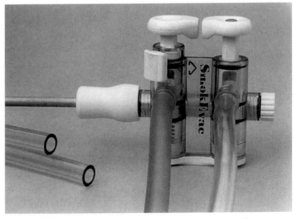

Figure 2.10. A trumpet valve has a control-metered adjustment pad that permits smoke evacuation.

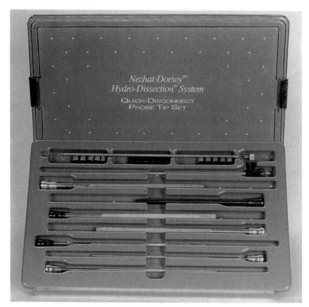

Figure 2.11. Designed specifically for use with the Nezhat-Dorsey hydrodissection system, the "Quick-Disconnect" probe tip set contains one 5-mm probe tip without irrigation holes, one Micro-Probe tip, one 10-mm probe tip with irrigation holes, one suction cannula, one instrument insert probe, 12 instrument insert adapters, and six "Quick-Disconnect" adapters. All probe tip sets are available in 23-cm, 28-cm, and 33-cm lengths.

with the jaws open for more tissue surface area, serve as a needle holder, and tie sutures (Figure 2.15A).

Forceps can grasp tissue and remove tissue from the peritoneal cavity. Those made of titanium with a polished finish can serve as a backstop for the CO_2 laser, whereas others have monopolar electrocoagulating ability. The Remorgida 3-in-1 bipolar forceps (Karl Storz, Culver City, CA) features two jaws of atraumatic grasping teeth and a scalpel-like blade between the forceps, enabling surgeons to grasp, cut, and coagulate tissue with one instrument (Figure 2.15B). Creating a neosalpingostomy in a hydrosalpinx requires two grasping forceps for traction and countertraction. Fine forceps are used for delicate work such as ovariolysis, fimbrioplasty, and tubal exploration during salpingostomy for ectopic pregnancy (Figure 2.16).

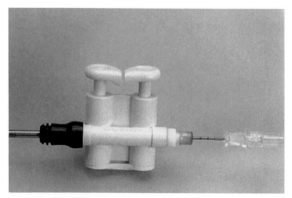

Figure 2.12. The aspiration–injection needle is inserted through the back of the trumpet valve. At the distal end of the needle, there is a Luer-Lock that allows connection to a syringe so that suction and irrigation are not interrupted.

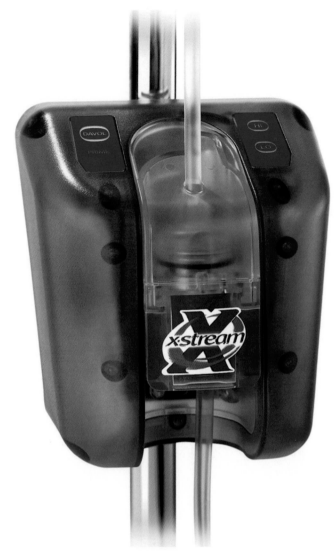

Figure 2.13. The X-Stream Irrigation System (Davol Inc., New Jersey) uses bag irrigation. It uses a "pump cartridge chamber" into which a disposable cartridge is inserted.

Scissors

Scissors are curved, straight, or hooked (Figure 2.17). Some have an electrical adaptor so that they can be combined with unipolar or bipolar electrocoagulation (Figure 2.18). Scissors are inserted into the secondary trocar under direct observation to avoid injury to pelvic structures. Hooked scissors have overlapping tips and can cause damage even when closed. Scissors can lyse adhesions, divide coagulated tissue, cut sutures, and open a fallopian tube for salpingostomy. If they become dull, they are discarded because sharpening is ineffective. Disposable scissors are particularly useful for patients who have extensive adhesions.

Biopsy Forceps

Biopsy forceps can sample suspected endometrial implants, ovarian lesions, and peritoneum (Figure 2.19). The jaws should be sharp and overlap when closed to avoid tearing tissue and causing unnecessary bleeding. Some have a small tooth on the upper or lower jaw and are ideal for taking a tissue sample from hard or slippery surfaces (Figure 2.20). Bleeding from the biopsy site is controlled by a defocused laser or bipolar electrocoagulation.

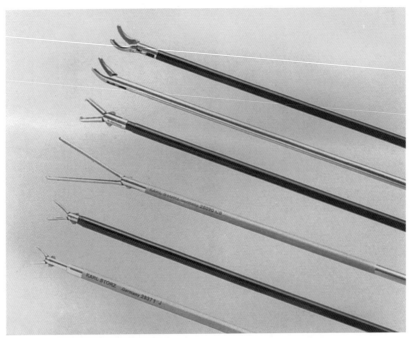

Figure 2.14. Straight and curved laparoscopic grasping forceps.

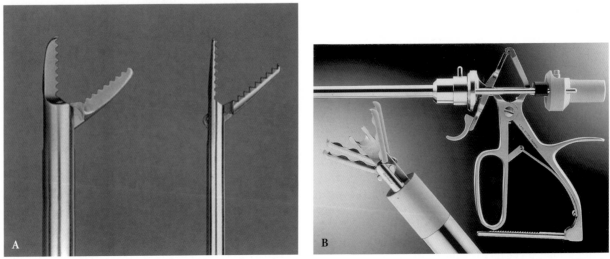

Figure 2.15. (**A**) Serrated jaws of 5-mm (left) and 3-mm (right) needle holders. (**B**) The Remorgida 3-in-1 bipolar forceps (Storz).

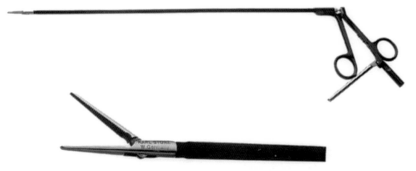

Figure 2.16. Fine forceps can be used for delicate procedures such as ovariolysis, fimbrioplasty, and tubal exploration for ectopic pregnancy.

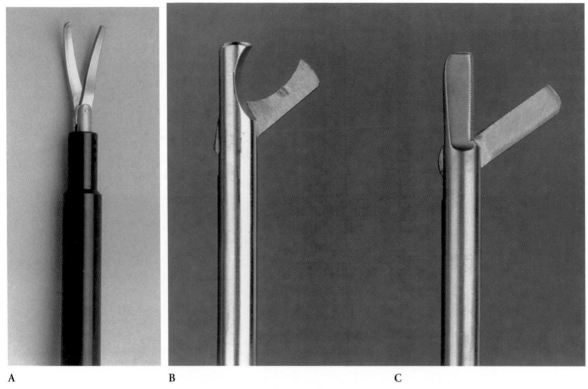

Figure 2.17. Laparoscopic scissors. (**A**) Curved. (**B**) Hooked. (**C**) Straight.

Electrosurgical Generator and Bipolar Forceps

The primary instrument used for hemostasis during operative laparoscopy is the bipolar electrocoagulator (Figure 2.21). One should prepare and test this instrument before the operation begins because it is essential for hemostasis during oophorectomy, hysterectomy, or even bowel resection to desiccate the mesenteric artery. Several types of bipolar forceps are available (Figures 2.21, 2.22). Fine tips are used for coagulating small blood vessels during delicate operations involving the tubes, bowel, or ureter. Flatter jaws are appropriate for use on large blood vessels or pedicles, including the uterine artery and the infundibulopelvic ligaments. A 3-mm bipolar forceps is available and is useful for tubal coagulation under local anesthesia. The main advantage of bipolar energy to monopolar energy is more controlled spread of energy

because energy travels only between the small space of the two jaws. The thermal spread of bipolar forceps has been reported to be between 2.0 mm and 3.5 mm when sealing arteries and 4.0 mm to 6.0 mm when sealing veins.[11] This thermal spread is the highest among devices using bipolar energy.

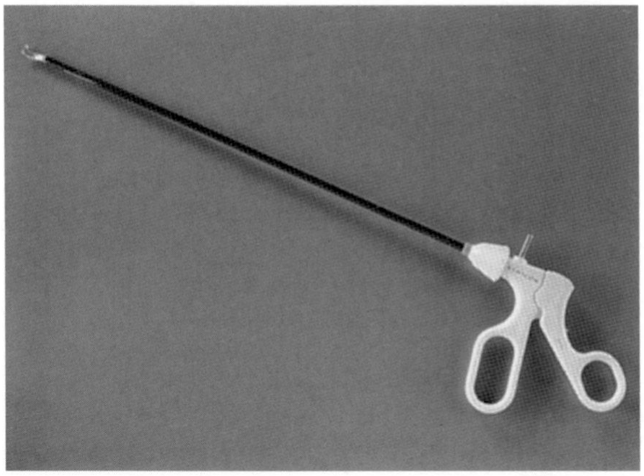

Vessel-Sealing Systems

The ever-present need to facilitate advanced laparoscopic procedures has brought about the invention of new modalities for achieving hemostasis. Besides titanium clips and laparoscopic stapling devices, there are two other modalities available on the market: bipolar vessel-sealing devices and ultrasonic energy.

Bipolar Vessel-Sealing Devices

Modern feedback-controlled bipolar devices include the LigaSure (LS) sealing device (Valleylab, Boulder, CO; Figure 2.23A,B)and the PlamaKinetics (PK) sealer (Gyrus Medical, Maple Grove, MN; Fig. 2.23C). Both of these devices use radiofrequency bipolar energy and both have an impedance-based feedback loop that modifies the bipolar energy delivered. Delivery of bipolar energy differs in that the LS device provides a continuous bipolar waveform whereas the PK sealer delivers a pulsed bipolar waveform, allowing for a cooling-off period for cooling of the blades.[12] These devices are recommended for sealing vessels up to 7 mm in diameter.

Both devices have been thoroughly tested and provide supra-physiologic burst pressures (burst pressure is the capacity to seal vessels) equivalent to the gold standard burst pressures of sutures and clips or staples.[11]

Figure 2.18. Laparoscopic scissors have unipolar electrocoagulation capability.

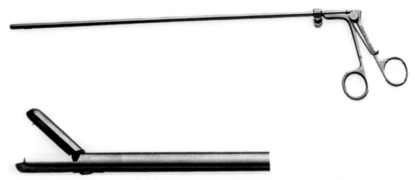

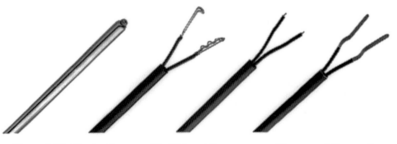

Figure 2.19. A 5-mm biopsy forceps is used to obtain tissue from endometrial ovarian implants.

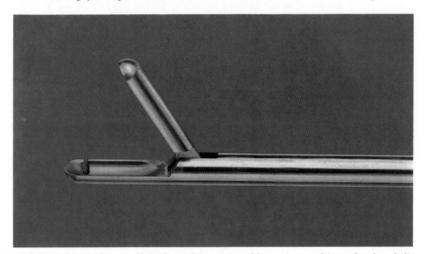

Figure 2.20. A biopsy forceps has small teeth on the upper and lower jaws to biopsy hard and slippery tissue surfaces.

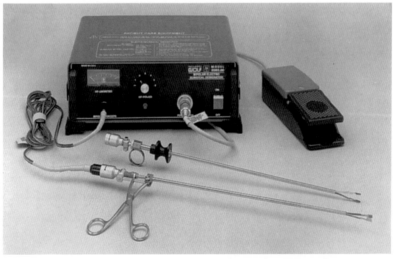

Figure 2.21. An electrogenerator with different types of bipolar forceps.

Figure 2.22. Bipolar forceps with different tips are seen with a coagulating probe.

heat causes the proteins to denature. The harmonic scalpel may limit the number of steps required for desiccation and transection of vascular pedicles such as the infundibulopelvic ligaments, reducing overall operating time. It is available in both 5-mm and 10-mm sizes. Several additional interchangeable tips, such as those useful during linear salpingotomy for the treatment of ectopic pregnancies, are available, allowing the surgeon to tailor the use of the harmonic scalpel to the specific task (Figure 2.24A,B,C).

A few studies have also compared the efficacy of the harmonic scalpel with bipolar vessel-sealing devices. Although the harmonic scalpel also provides supraphysiologic burst pressures, it has been found to be less effective in sealing vessels greater than 4 mm in diameter.[11] However, thermal spread of this device was found to be the least of the group, with a range of thermal damage of 0 to 2.4 mm.[11,13] Another advantage of the harmonic scalpel is that its active blade can be used as a surgical knife, which allows for transection of tissues that do not need to be desiccated.

SPECIALIZED INSTRUMENTS

Claw-Tooth and Spoon Forceps

Claw-tooth and spoon forceps are 10-mm graspers that require a 10- to 11-mm sleeve and are used during myomectomy to remove large pieces of tissue, such as a section of tube and ovary, or an ectopic pregnancy (Figure 2.25).

Clips

Laparoscopic clip applicators are used through 5- to 11-mm sleeves for reapproximation of peritoneal surfaces or hemostasis of medium-sized vessels. A disposable loaded applicator and reusable single-clip applicators are available (Figures 2.26, 2.27).

Linear Stapler

The stapler designed for gynecologic use is similar to the one used for bowel operations and fits through a 12-mm trocar sleeve (Figure 2.28). [14] Ethicon and U.S. Surgical produce endoscopic surgical staplers with different designs, but their function is essentially the same. The available staplers are disposable and can be reloaded with cartridges for use in gynecologic, general, and thoracic surgery (Figure 2.29). Each cartridge contains 54 (Ethicon) or 48 (U.S. Surgical) titanium staples that are arranged in two sets of triple-staggered rows. The instrument also contains a push-bar knife assembly, which cuts between the two sets of triple rows, ligating both ends of the incised tissue. The cut line usually is shorter than the staple line. For example, the laparoscopic linear cutter 35 (Ethicon) cut line is approximately 33 mm, with a staple line of 37 mm.

Tissue to be clipped is placed on stretch with grasping forceps, and the applicator's jaws are placed at the desired incisional site. When fired, it simultaneously places six rows of small titanium clips and cuts along the center, leaving three rows of clips on the edge of each pedicle (Figure 2.30). This instrument is used to seal blood vessels and cut pedicles, but it should be used with caution. Several complications have resulted from the use of this device.[15]

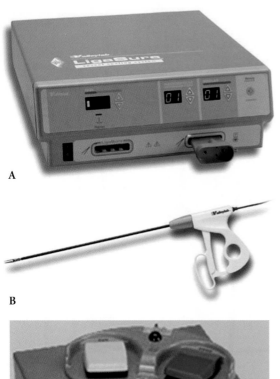

Figure 2.23. (**A**) LigaSure generator is shown along with (**B**) ligasure laparoscopic device (Valley Lab). (**C**) Gyrus generator.

In a study conducted by Carbonell et al. [12], the LS device was shown to provide significantly higher burst pressures. As vessel size increased, burst pressures became progressively weaker with the PK versus the LS (397 vs. 326 mm Hg in vessels 2 to 3 mm, 389 vs. 573 mm Hg in vessels 4 to 5 mm, and 317 vs. 585 mm Hg in vessels 6 to 7 mm). Although this difference was statistically significant, it is unclear whether this difference is clinically important because these burst pressures remain supraphysiologic and on par with the gold standard. Thermal spread with the LS system was not significantly different from that of PK (2.5 vs. 3.2 mm when sealing vessels 6 to 7 mm).

Ultimately, both instruments seem to be equally effective for achieving hemostasis, and choice of instrument will depend on the surgeon's preference.

Harmonic Scalpel

The ultrasonically activated vibrating blade of the harmonic scalpel (Ethicon) moves longitudinally at 55,000 vibrations per second, cutting tissue while simultaneously providing hemostasis. The vibration of the ultrasonic scalpel is thought to generate low heat at the incision site. This combination of vibration and

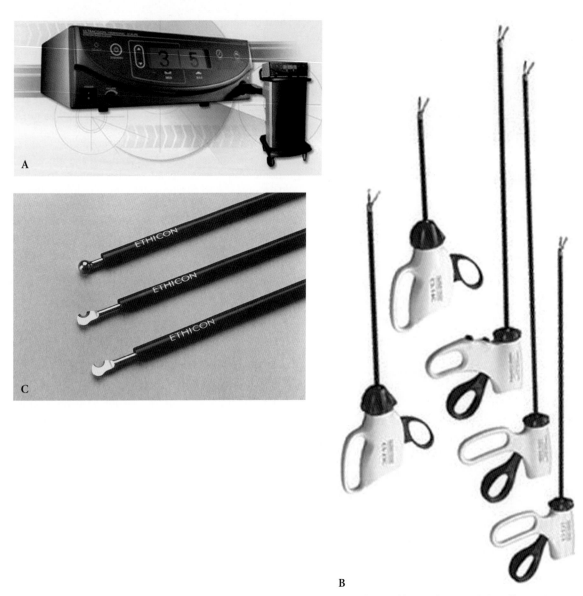

B

Figure 2.24. The harmonic scalpels (Ethicon). (**A**) Generator. (**B**) Interchangeable attachments. (**C**) Different tips.

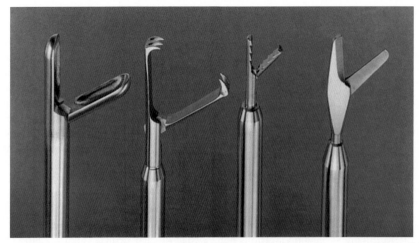

Figure 2.25. Different 10-mm instruments are used during operative laparoscopy. From left to right: spoon forceps, claw graspers, serrated grasper, and scissors.

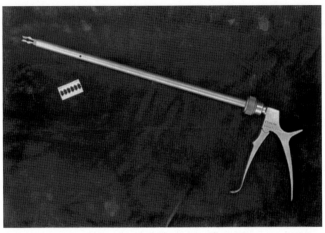

Figure 2.26. A reusable 10-mm laparoscopic clip applicator with clips.

Myoma Screw

When one is doing a laparoscopic myomectomy, it is difficult to stabilize a smooth, hard fibroid. Five- and 10-mm myoma screws allow the surgeon to maneuver the myoma and apply traction with improved visibility and access (Figure 2.31).

Morcellator

Morcellators grasp, core, and cut the tissue to be removed into small bits. These fragments are forced into the hollow part of the instrument. The morcellator is designed for the removal of fragments of myomas and ovaries through 5- or 10-mm trocar sleeves or through a colpotomy incision. If the removal of a large myoma is attempted, the effort to morcellate it mechanically may outweigh the amount of time saved, particularly if the myoma is calcified.

Electromechanical morcellators, such as the Steiner electromechanical morcellator (Karl Storz, Tuttlingen, Germany), consist of a motor-driven cutting cannula that can be inserted directly into the peritoneal cavity or introduced through a standard trocar (Figure 2.32). Tissue is morcellated and removed by applying uniform traction and varying the speed and direction of the cannula's rotation. This technique facilitates the rapid removal of even large sections of tissue through the minimal access ports.

Carter and McCarus [16] compared electromechanical to manual morcellation in doing laparoscopic myomectomies. The use of the electromechanical morcellator reduced the average

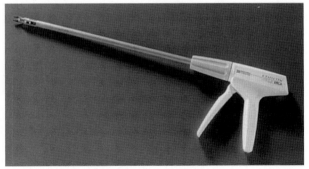

Figure 2.27. A disposable loaded 10-mm laparoscopic clip applicator.

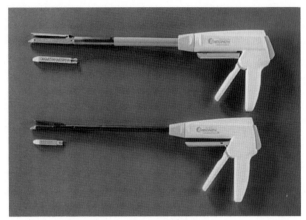

Figure 2.28. Endo-path linear cutters (Ethicon) are used in intestinal operations and gynecologic laparoscopy.

time for extraction of myomas less than 100 g by 15 minutes and 401 to 500 g by 150 minutes. The average time saved for all myomectomies was 53 minutes. It was estimated that with operating room charges of $10 per minute, the $14,000 cost of the morcellator was recovered by the 21st case. The authors concluded that electromechanical morcellation results in significant time savings compared with the manual technique, with financial savings accruing rapidly after the 21st case.

The serrated edged macro morcellator (SEMM) has been used during laparoscopic myomectomy.[17] It allows rapid morcellation of even large myomas, up to 418 g, and their removal by means of a 15-mm trocar. This morcellator has been used extensively in Germany to do endoscopic intrafascial supracervical hysterectomy.[18] It is available with a battery-operated motor (WISAP Moto-Drive) in diameters of 10, 15, 20, and 24 mm.

A powered disposable morcellator (Gynecare, Sunnyvale, CA) has been used successfully during laparoscopic supracervical hysterectomy to morcellate the entire uterus for easy removal through a 15-mm cannula (Figure 2.33).[19]

The use of the automatic tissue morcellator does not interfere with proper histologic evaluation of solid pediatric malignant tumors, in which accurate histologic assessment is important for prognosis and staging.[20]

Specialized Graspers

Three-pronged forceps specifically designed to atraumatically immobilize adnexal structures [21] hold the ovary, whereas four-pronged forceps are designed to hold fallopian tubes. The force applied by the prongs is adjustable and is maintained by tightening a screw in the handle. Three-pronged graspers with teeth also are available. Large spoon forceps are used to extract tissue excised during the procedure.

Laparoscopic Specimen Retrieval Bag

To simplify the retrieval of specimens from the abdominal cavity and avoid contamination of the abdominal and pelvic cavities with cyst contents, a disposable retrieval bag (Endopouch, Ethicon) has been developed (Figure 2.34). It is composed of a flexible plastic bag with a cannula, introduction sleeve, and introduction cap (Figures 2.35–2.41). The bag is pushed by hand

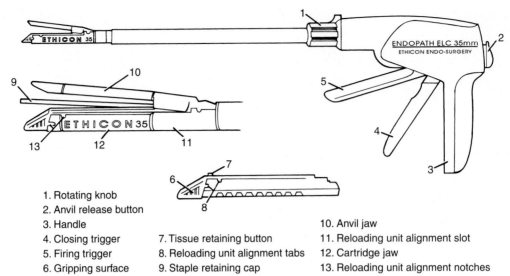

1. Rotating knob
2. Anvil release button
3. Handle
4. Closing trigger
5. Firing trigger
6. Gripping surface

7. Tissue retaining button
8. Reloading unit alignment tabs
9. Staple retaining cap

10. Anvil jaw
11. Reloading unit alignment slot
12. Cartridge jaw
13. Reloading unit alignment notches

Figure 2.29. Schematic representation of the Endo-path linear cutter 35 (ELC 35, Ethicon).

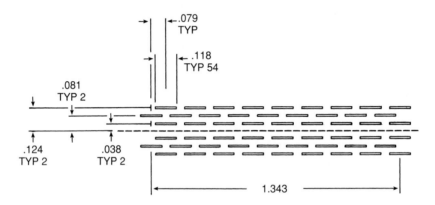

Figure 2.30. The stapler can place six rows of small titanium staples (54 staples).

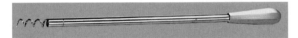

Figure 2.31. A myoma screw (Circon).

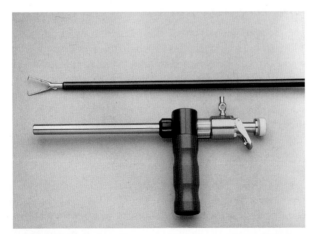

Figure 2.32. Steiner electromechanical morcellator (Storz).

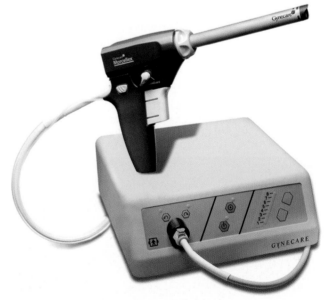

Figure 2.33. The Gynecare disposable morcellator (Gynecare).

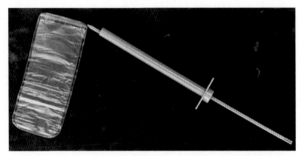

Figure 2.34. Specimen retrieval bag (Endopouch, Ethicon).

into the introducer before being loaded into a 10-/11-mm trocar (Figures 2.35 and 2.36A). During loading, the cannula should not be pulled to retract the Endopouch bag. The introducer cap and introducer sleeve are inserted into the abdomen through the trocar (Figure 2.36B). The introducer cap should remain flush against the top of the trocar. The cannula is pushed until the bag is exposed fully. A closed grasper is used to expand the bag opening (Figure 2.37). A specimen is placed in the bag (Figure 2.38A) and the cannula is broken at the scored point (Figure 2.38B), allowing the suture to be pulled through the cannula and closing the top of the bag (Figure 2.39). The bag is retracted to the base of the trocar sleeve by carefully pulling the suture strand. Small masses are retracted into the introducer and extracted through the trocar sleeve. If the bag and contents cannot be extracted, the bag is pulled into the trocar until resistance is felt (Figure 2.40). The trocar is removed, and the bag is brought to the incision. The contents are aspirated or removed with forceps (Figure 2.41). A larger incision may be required to remove the bag with its contents from the body.

Instruments for Trocar Port Dilation

Occasionally a 10- or 12-mm instrument must be inserted through incisions made for 5-mm instruments. Dilator rods for this purpose allow the placement of a 10- or 12-mm trocar. The operator withdraws the smaller trocar and replaces it with a larger one.

Aspiration–Injection Needle

A 16- or 22-gauge calibrated aspiration–injection needle can be used to precisely aspirate and inject fluids (Figure 2.42). When it is used with a 28-cm probe tip without fenestrations, close-chambered ovarian cyst aspiration can be done. When the suction

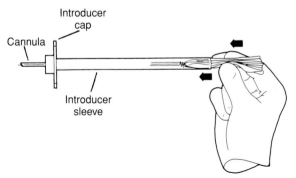

Figure 2.35. The bag is put into the introducer.

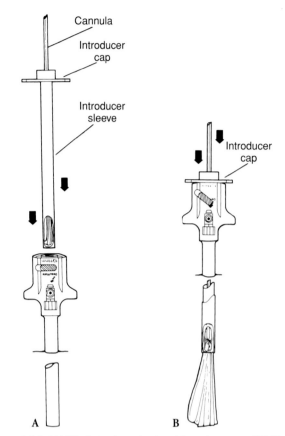

Figure 2.36. (**A**) The introducer is placed into the trocar. (**B**) The bag can be pushed into the abdominal cavity.

is started and the probe tip is placed on tissue, suction–retraction of that tissue results. The needle is inserted into the cyst, and leakage of contents is avoided. The 2.0-cm exposed portion of the needle is etched with 0.5-cm markings to accurately gauge tissue penetration. When a 60-mL syringe is attached to the needle, the fluid from the aspirated cyst is sent for cytologic examination.

This needle also is used to inject dilute vasopressin into the base of fibroids before myomectomy or into the mesosalpinx or tube before salpingostomy for tubal pregnancy. A syringe is attached to the needle by a connecting tube before injection to verify that intravascular injection does not occur.

Uterine Manipulators

Safe, effective endoscopy requires adequate mobilization and stabilization of the uterus and associated organs. Various combinations of uterine sounds, cannulas, and dilators are available. The most useful types of manipulators are the HUMI (Unimar, Wilton, CT) and the Cohen cannula in combination with a single-toothed tenaculum applied to the anterior cervical lip (Figure 2.43). The HUMI has a balloon at its tip to minimize the chance of uterine perforation, but when uterine manipulation is vigorous, the HUMI can twist within the uterine cavity, making it difficult to stabilize the uterus. The Cohen cannula is inserted as far as the internal os and is rigid, allowing excellent control of the uterine position. Although a large acorn tip limits its uterine entry, the cervix may dilate, resulting in uterine perforation by the acorn tip. It is crucial to monitor the position of uterine manipulators continually.

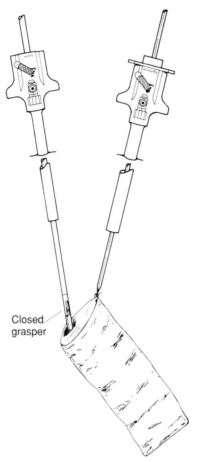

Closed grasper

Figure 2.37. A closed grasper is used to open the bag.

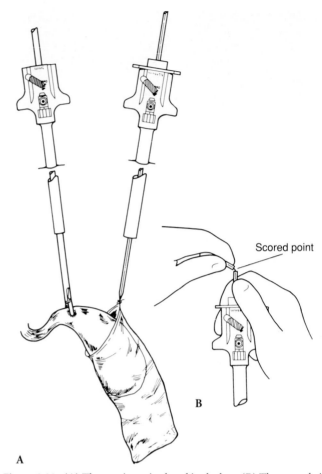

Scored point

B

A

Figure 2.38. (**A**) The specimen is placed in the bag. (**B**) The cannula is broken at the scored point.

Valtchev and Papsin (Conkin Surgical Instruments, Ltd., Toronto, Canada) [22] devised an instrument consisting of an acorn-shaped head with a cannula connected to a rod by an articulation point. This arrangement allows the angle between the rod and the cannula to be changed, providing various degrees of uterine anteversion, which is adjusted with a screw. The Hulka tenaculum and sound combination is a good uterine manipulator but lacks a channel for chromopertubation.

More elaborate systems specifically designed to simplify total laparoscopic hysterectomy are available. For instance, the Koh Colpotomizer system (Cooper Surgical) is designed to be used with the RUMI uterine manipulator and consists of a vaginal extender to delineate the vaginal fornices and a pneumo-occluder (Figure 2.44).[23]

Another uterine manipulator that includes a vaginal cup to define the dissecting plane of colpotomy, as well as to prevent the loss of pneumoperitoneum, is the Vcare uterine manipulator (ConMed, Utica, NY; Figure 2.45).

Ceana Glove

Laparoscopic procedures that involve incision of the vaginal apex result in the loss of the pneumoperitoneum. A simple cost-effective technique has been developed by Ceana Nezhat that effectively preserves pneumoperitoneum. Two 4-inch by 4-inch sponges are folded (Figure 2.46) and submerged in sterile water or saline for several seconds. The sponges are placed in a latex

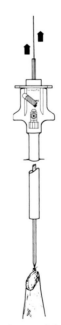

Figure 2.39. The bag is closed around the specimen.

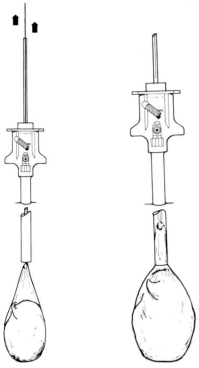

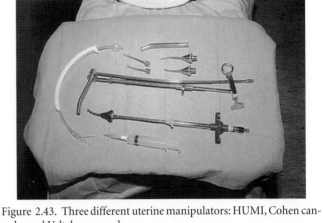

Figure 2.43. Three different uterine manipulators: HUMI, Cohen cannula, and Valtchev cannula.

Figure 2.40. The bag is pulled to the base of the trocar sleeve until resistance is felt.

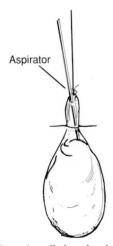

Aspirator

Figure 2.41. The specimen is pulled to the abdominal wall and aspirated.

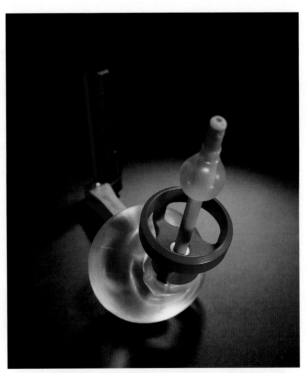

Figure 2.44. The Koh Colpotopmizer system.

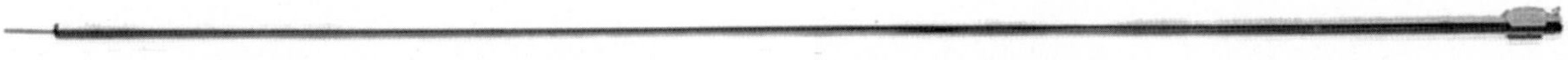

Figure 2.42. A laparoscopic aspiration–injection needle is used for aspiration of ovarian cysts (16- or 18-gauge), injection of diluted vasopressin in the base of a myoma, or hydrodissection (22-gauge).

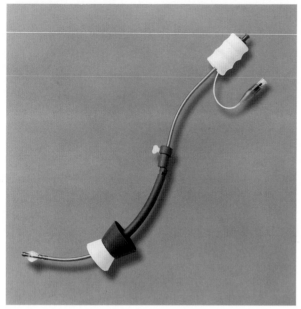

Figure 2.45. The Vcare uterine manipulator.

surgical glove, usually trapping some air in the glove fingers (Figure 2.46B,C).[24–28] The top of the glove is tied shut and placed in the vagina or minilaparotomy incision, acting as a flexible air block for preservation of pneumoperitoneum (Figure 2.46D). This device, which is called the Ceana glove, can be prepared in any operating room and has been found to be both safe and effective in numerous laparoscopic procedures.

Instruments for Port Closure

The use of a new device for the closure of subcutaneous tissue in laparoscopic sites was reported by Airan and Sandor.[29] The use of such instruments is gaining in popularity with the widening recognition of the risk of incisional hernia at trocar sites. These instruments are similar to the device described as the Carter–Thomason device.[30] Both instruments operate as a needle and a grasper that serve as a suture passer. The conical suture passer guide frequently aids in introducing the suture at the proper angle for the closure of fascia, muscle, and peritoneum. The conical guide has the additional benefit of maintaining pneumoperitoneum once the laparoscopic trocar has been removed. The Carter–Thomason suture passer (Figure 2.47) has been recommended for use without the guide if that is deemed more appropriate, for instance, in ligating epigastric arteries. Because the proper closing of the abdominal layers occasionally presents a challenge, the growing interest in instruments designed to assist

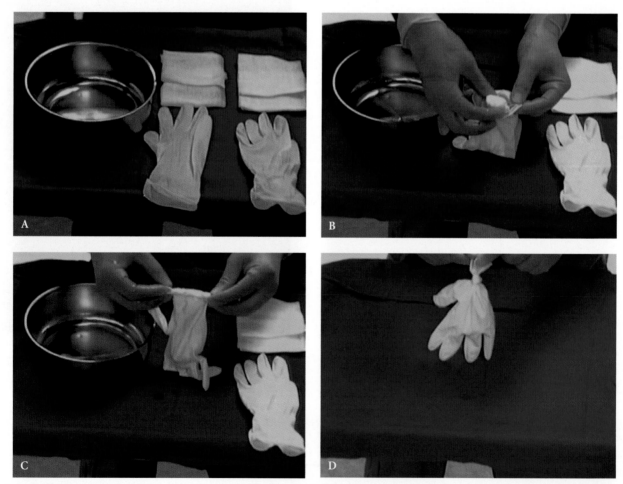

Figure 2.46. The Ceana glove. (**A**) The materials for a Ceana glove are available in the operating room and can be prepared easily. (**B**) Two 4 × 4 sponges are folded and emerged in sterile water. (**C**) They are inserted inside a sterile glove. (**D**) The glove is closed at the top, and is placed in the vagina to block the loss of pneumopertioneum.

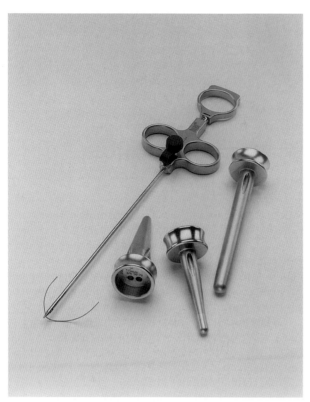

Figure 2.47. The Carter–Thomason device.

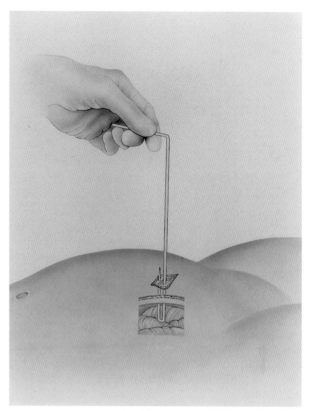

Figure 2.48. J-needle.

the surgeon is encouraged. The J-needle allows for port closure that incorporates all layers of the abdominal wall under direct observation (Figure 2.48).

ENDOSCOPIC ULTRASOUND

Intraoperative ultrasound has gained an established role in many surgical procedures. Laparoscopic ultrasound and thoracoscopic ultrasound are the latest modes of intraoperative sonography. They have been introduced mainly to overcome the two major drawbacks of laparoscopy: the ability to show only the surface of the organs and the lack of manual palpation of the anatomic structures. The technology, new indications, and results of intraoperative and laparoscopic ultrasound were reviewed by Bezzi and associates [31] during more than 500 operative procedures. Intraoperative ultrasound and laparoscopic ultrasound are helpful in confirming preoperative studies and acquiring new data not available otherwise. An important role of these techniques is to ascertain the anatomy of the involved organs, thus providing guidance for surgery. Both techniques play an important role in surgical decision making, particularly with respect to hepatic, biliary, and pancreatic malignancies. In some series, the rate of major changes in the surgical strategy can be as high as 38%. A relatively new application of intraoperative ultrasound is the ability to do interstitial therapy for tumors at the time of the initial surgery. This may be useful, for example, in patients undergoing liver resection when other unresectable lesions are found in a different segment or in the contralateral lobe. Finally, laparoscopic sonography plays an important role in staging abdominal neoplasms, providing more information than do preoperative imaging and laparoscopic exploration. This feature may be used to effectively stage gastrointestinal malignancies, pancreatic carcinomas, and abdominal lymphomas. It may be expected that a

variety of open procedures will be done with videolaparoscopic monitoring and will need guidance from laparoscopic sonography. In the future, the staging of abdominal neoplasms may be improved by laparoscopy combined with laparoscopic ultrasound. A cost–benefit analysis of these techniques and a comparison with preoperative tests should be carried out. High-resolution images may be obtained to delineate abnormalities such as suspected ovarian cysts and uterine myomas. Endoscopic ultrasound is a new instrument that allows the surgeon to evaluate and define pelvic abnormalities suspected at laparoscopy. Endoscopic ultrasound may augment the diagnosis of subtle pathologic findings during laparoscopy.[32,33]

Laparotomy-Type Instruments

Babcocks, atraumatic bowel grasping forceps, Allis clamps, and Metzenbaum scissors have been adapted for laparoscopic use. The acquisition of these instruments depends on whether they will improve a procedure's efficiency.

Standard grasping forceps hold needles for most procedures, but stronger needle holders are necessary if precise placement is required and for suturing thick tissue (i.e., myometrium or periosteum). Some needle holders have handles similar to those used in laparotomy (Figure 2.49). Straight and curved narrow-tip needle holders are available for fine intra-abdominal suturing (Figure 2.50).

THE CAMERA

The camera includes the camera head with its cable and the camera control unit (CCU) or camera controller. The cable is plugged into the camera controller. The lens on the medical camera is

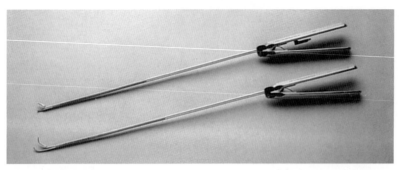

Figure 2.49. This needle holder is similar to that used at laparotomy with locking capability.

called a coupler. The coupler screws onto the camera head and is available in several sizes that magnify the image. A 24-mm coupler will produce a larger image on the monitor than will a 20-mm coupler. With a direct coupler, the image travels directly to the camera and is the most widely used style of coupler. A beam splitter coupler has a 90° angle; part of the image travels to the camera and part travels to a porthole or eye cup. The porthole allows the surgeon to view the image directly and is typically used in urology cases. In addition, urologists usually prefer the 20-mm coupler to prevent part of the anatomy from being cut off by the bottom of the monitor. One example is Stryker's new urology camera head, which has a built-in 20-mm rotating coupler with a beam splitter.

Couplers are mounted and fixed on the camera head. Removable couplers, also known as c-mount couplers, allow the purchase of a camera with interchangeable direct couplers and beam splitters. The removable coupler provides flexibility and economy. Being removable is a potential problem because the coupler is screwed to the camera head, and if it is not attached securely or if its O-ring is worn, liquids may seep between the coupler and the camera head, causing internal fog. A coupler with internal fog is not usable and must be repaired. A fixed coupler eliminates this problem.

Cameras are either single chip (red, green, and blue on the same chip) or three chip (each chip is dedicated to red, green, or blue). Three-chip cameras have better color separation and take in more information, which is beneficial in procedures in which color is important. The production of a unique video camera (Circon) has proprietary red–green–blue (RGB) 24-bit digital

enhancement circuits. The signals coming from the charged coupled device (CCD) sensor are sampled at equal time intervals, and the amplitude of each sample is classified into a discrete level system and converted to a binary code. All the video information is encoded into a stream of noise-free digital numbers. These numbers are used as variables in mathematical equations (algorithms) to manipulate and shift in time and value through digital signal processing. Digital electronics are the leading edge in video technology and will be the new standard of performance just as digital compact discs have replaced LP records and audiocassettes. Digital signals take up less bandwidth than do the analog signals currently in use. Moreover, digitally processed signals can be applied to three-chip and high-definition television (HDTV).

One camera on the market with high definition technology is made by Stryker (Figure 2.51A,B). It is a three-chip camera with a format of 1280 × 1024. This high-definition camera also uses progressive scan technology versus interlace technology. Progressive scan is a process in which a camera sends a complete picture back to the monitor 60 times per second. Interlace cameras take half a picture (every other line) and send the partial image back for a total of 30 complete pictures a second. Progressive scan is useful for sending a lot of information to the monitor at once and keeping pace with a live image; a high-definition camera is necessary when there is much more information being scanned.

One feature of the camera head is its ability to manipulate peripheral equipment by using buttons to accomplish a variety of tasks, including activation of the video printer and videocassette recorder (VCR). Some cameras have a single button to start both the video printer and the VCR. With a main control switch, several desired functions can be manipulated. Another variation includes separate buttons on the camera head to increase or decrease the camera gain level. With this arrangement, the first button can operate the video printer, the VCR, and additional components. An infrared remote control is required for all components to make the buttons operable. Another camera with two buttons on the camera head can control any two components. This system has cables running from the CCU (camera box) to two selected components, the video printer and VCR, or to the video printer and the still video recorder. With this system, infrared remote control is not required. The most prevalent camera sold on the market (Stryker) has a four-button design in which surgeons are able to control the gain, record video, take pictures, digitally zoom, and white balance. Another camera feature is field-replaceable camera cables. Because most camera problems occur in the camera cable, replacing cables at the hospital rather than sending a camera out for repair saves time and expense.

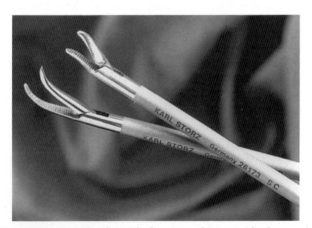

Figure 2.50. Curved and straight fine serrated tips provide a better grip of straight or curved needles.

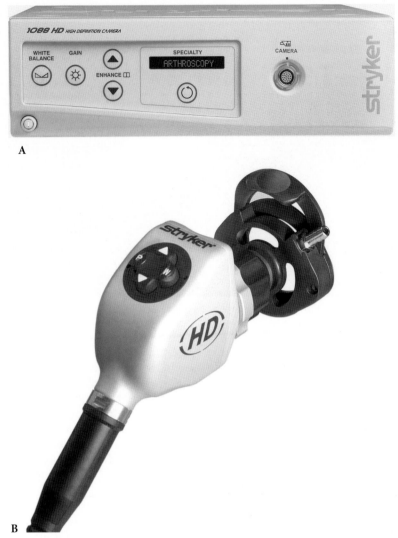

Figure 2.51. The Stryker camera provides a picture with a definition of 1280 × 1024 pixels. (**A**) Camera CCU. (**B**) Camera lens.

Camera Equipment

The first medical camera (Circon Corporation), which was developed in 1972, had three tubes and weighed 18 lb. It used a fiberoptic image guide to transfer a microscopic image to the camera that transferred the image to a video monitor. In 1973, a single-tube camera was designed weighing 3.8 lb (Figure 2.53). Although the weight was reduced, the camera remained heavy and counterweights were needed. This camera was attached directly to the endoscope without using a fiberoptic image guide. The single 1-inch tube had a specially striped filter to produce a full-color picture. Video camera manufacturers continued to make improvements in size, weight, and image quality. In 1975, a camera weighing 1.25 lb was developed, and in the following year, a low-light feature enabled it to be 10 times more light sensitive. In 1980, a new 6-oz camera was small enough to be held in the palm of the surgeon's hand. It produced excellent color separation and image resolution (Figure 2.53). Another milestone was achieved 2 years later with the first solid-state CCD camera. This camera weighed 3 oz, and with the change from tubes to solid-state CCD sensors, two major achievements were accomplished.

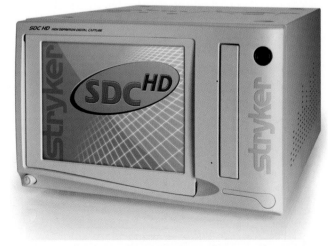

Figure 2.52. The Stryker capturing device digitizes video or picture images. These can then be transferred to a DVD/CD or downloaded directly into a portable hard drive.

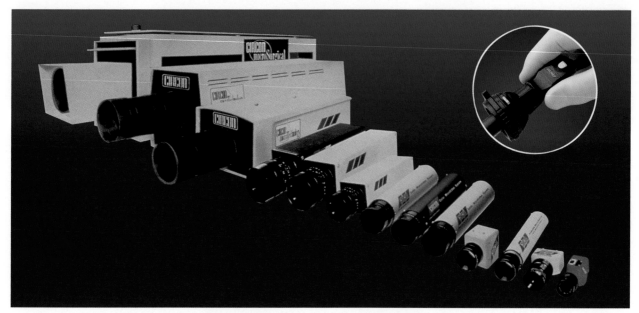

Figure 2.53. The decrease in size of video cameras over the years is illustrated. The inset shows a contemporary camera head.

First, the camera could be disinfected in solutions so that there was no need to "bag the camera." Second, the colors produced by solid-state construction were more reliable than were colors produced by tube cameras (Figure 2.54).

Since 1982, all surgical camera manufacturers have switched to solid-state construction. Developments include low lux levels (enhancing the quality of the image in low-light situations), buttons on the cameras to start and stop VCRs, field-replaceable camera cables, and increased lines of resolution (S-Video and RGB signal output as opposed to National Television Systems Committee [NTSC]). Cameras also became more durable. The technologies of the 1990s added digitally processed signals, three-chip cameras, and chip-on-a-stick to surgical video. Currently digital technology has replaced VCRs in many operating rooms.

Basic Video Information

Within the camera is a CCD that "sees" an optical image through the lens and converts it into an electrical image. A CCD is composed of rows of tiny picture elements called pixels. Each pixel can sense red, green, or blue light to produce color. The more

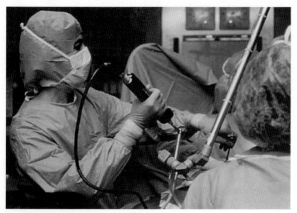

Figure 2.54. Initial camera that Camran Nezhat used for video-laparoscopy in early 1980.

pixels, the better the picture. The most pixels on a camera to date are in the Stryker 1088 HD camera in which each CCD in the camera is in a format of 1280×1024 (pixels) (Figure 2.51A, B).

An image is sent through camera cables to the CCU to the monitor input. The monitor converts the electrical image to the original optical image seen by the human eye. The electrical image also is directed to components other than the monitor after leaving the CCU. It is relayed by a cable to a VCR or a digital capturing device (Figure 2.52), to a printer and onto a monitor.

Scanning Formats

Video information is scanned to generate a signal frequency. The scanning is done at a rate of 525 lines per frame; there are 30 frames per second of video information, with the exception of the Stryker camera, which scans at 60 frames per second via the progressive scan technology. This scanning rate is like a television broadcast standardized by the National Television Systems Committee (NTSC). NTSC scanning rates are used in the United States, Canada, Japan, South America, and Asia. Russia and France use a different scanning rate called SECAM (*séquentiel couleur à mémoire*). PAL (phase alternation lines), a third type of scanning rate, is used in other European nations. These scanning rates are not compatible with NTSC standards. Videotapes made in the United States must be converted before they can be viewed in countries with non-NTSC scanning rates. The process of converting one scanning rate to another is expensive. When the NTSC scanning rates were created, technicians used a limited bandwidth to send the video signal to color and light information simultaneously. The first format of the NTSC signal is called a composite signal. There are inherent problems with this method of transference because a camera first processes color and light separately and then combines the two to create a signal. Cross-talk is a signal noise that generates grainy images with soft edges and causes colors to be less consistent. The signal-to-noise ratio is a measurement that differentiates between video noise (cross-talk) and useful video information. The higher the signal-to-noise ratio, the better the detail at the edge and the better the total image. Signal noise is measured in decibels. A quick way to evaluate noise is not to allow any light to reach the camera chip. With the absence of picture information, the image contains only noise. Another way to see picture noise is to adjust the camera to place color bars on the monitor screen. One selects first an NTSC signal, then a Y/C signal, and finally an RGB signal. One looks at the edge of each bar color and notes that movement from NTSC to Y/C to RGB makes the edges progressively sharper because NTSC has the most noise and RGB has the least. Specifications (lines of resolution, pixels, signal-to-noise ratios) set the parameters of the video components, but one should always test the monitor.

The second format, called a component signal, carries the color and light separately. There is less cross-talk, so pictures generated by component signals have sharper edges and truer colors than do pictures generated by composite signals. The Y/C format and NTSC format carry the video signal in a single cable. Y/C (Y stands for light brightness, and C refers to color) is the name for the format. SVHS and Super VHS are tape formats that accept this type of signal.

The third format, RGB, is also a component signal. Video information is separated into four signals: red, green, blue, and a timing signal. Each signal carries its own light. Separation occurs in the camera head and is done electrically. Because the colors and light are separate, this format requires less electronic processing. There are four separate cables from the camera box. A monitor that accepts RGB input is needed. Although these monitors are more expensive, they have higher resolution capabilities. Thus, of the three signal-carrying formats, the first format, NTSC, is the least desirable. The second and third formats carry much clearer signals with less noise.

Resolution

The clarity and detail of the video image depend on the number of horizontal lines of resolution, which are detected by the number of distinct vertical lines seen in a picture. Resolution is set forth by the camera's pixel count and by a formula used to achieve the resolution number. The HD camera made by Stryker has more than 1000 lines of resolution with a pixel. No resolution number can be higher than the pixel count. Each line of resolution is composed of pixels, and the more pixels per line, the better the image. Another way to understand the pixel effect is to compare a large-screen television with a small (13-inch) monitor. Smaller monitors have a sharper, crisper image, especially at the edges of an image, because pixels are placed closer together on a small screen. The ability of the video system to carry and process signals, the components that transmit signals, and the resolution numbers of the monitor together determine the ultimate picture quality. The industry standard is to measure horizontal resolution using 75% of the chip. However, some manufacturers have been known to use 100% of the chip, resulting in a higher resolution number.

The Camera Box (CCU)

The most common features include a color bar button and a white balance button. Some CCUs have manual and automatic white balance features. The most important feature for the CCU is to provide an automatic shutter because it adjusts each pixel's exposure time up to 1/15,000 of a second. The circuit can react to varying light conditions as fast as the human eye can. An electronic shutter is essential for a surgical video camera.

The Monitor and Accessories

The sizes of the screens vary from 19 to 20 inches. Over the past 5 years, the medical industry has adopted flat panel technology to accommodate the high-definition video cameras. The native resolution of the flat panel monitors should be no less than 1280 × 1024 and should accept a DVI (digital visual interface) video signal along with standard definition analog signals.

The preferred method of capturing both still and live images has been through digital capture devices. Stryker Endoscopy's SDC HD captures still images in native resolution 1280 × 1024 and can record videos in multiple mpeg formats. Digital capture devices allow surgeons to archive information to DVDs, USB hard drives, and hospital networks while printing pictures for medical records.

Equipment Problems and Troubleshooting

After the video system is moved to the operating room, it is plugged in and the components are tested. The following steps will reduce the chance of unexpected events:

1. Note the image, put color bars on the monitor screen, and evaluate the accuracy of the colors.
2. Look at the monitor, check the buttons, turn on the light source, and check the light cord for damaged light bundles.
3. Look through the scope before it is hooked up and illuminated because light hides defects.
4. Hold the scope with the distal end pointed at a normal ceiling light and then look through the eyepiece. Is the scope clear?
5. Check both the distal end and the eyepiece for cracks or other visible damage.

If a problem with the image occurs during an operation, the scope should be checked initially, then the light cord, and then the camera. If the picture is poor, the color and light level should be examined to search for the cause. If there is no picture, the operator should be certain that the light source is turned on. If none of the preceding steps solves the problem, the camera should be detached from the scope and focused on an object in the room. If the picture is good, the camera is functioning properly and the scope or the light cord is at fault. If the picture is poor, the camera may be defective or the lens may be fogged; a button on the CCU may have to be changed, or a new camera may be required. A methodical piece-by-piece examination of the components makes it easier to locate the fault so that it can be fixed or replaced.

ROBOTICS

Efforts to improve surgical efficiency have led to the development of robotically assisted laparoscopic procedures. The Animated Endoscopic System for Optimal Positioning (AESOP) was designed to hold and maneuver the laparoscope under the direct control of the surgeon. The elimination of the camera holder allows two doctors to do complex laparoscopic operations faster than they could without the robotic arm. This technology also may allow the surgeon to carry out some procedures without the aid of an assistant. The AESOP system can be activated by voice or by foot or hand control. For 50 patients undergoing routine gynecologic endoscopic procedures, the operating time

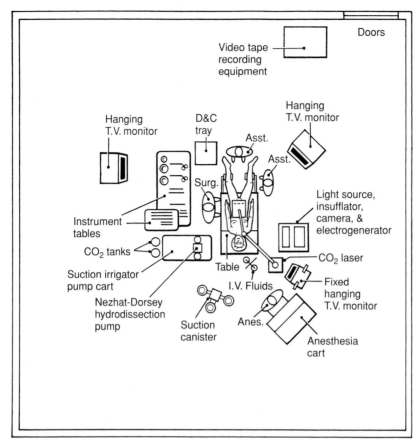

Figure 2.55. Positions of patient, assistants, surgeon, and equipment.

using voice control was compared with that using foot or hand control. The voice control worked more efficiently and faster than did hand or foot control.[34] In a comparison of the findings of five studies evaluating the need for a human camera holder assistant, the robotic man outperformed the human camera holder, and reduced laparoscopic operating time, resulting in efficiency and cost savings.[35] AESOP company is now part of intuitive surgical, which owns the da Vinci "Robotic Arm."

OPERATING ROOM SETUP

An organized and well-equipped operating room is essential for successful laparoscopy.[36, 37] The surgical team and the operating room staff should be familiar with the instruments and their functions. Each instrument is inspected periodically. Scissors, graspers, trocars, trocar sleeves, and the like are checked for loose or broken tips, even if the same instruments were used during a previous procedure. Before a new instrument is used, it is tested by the surgeon. Although the total cost of operative laparoscopy is decreased by the shortened hospital stay and recovery, the cost of the operating room is higher for operative laparoscopy because of the higher cost of instruments and the longer operating time.[38, 39]

Position of Equipment

Equipment positioning (Figure 2.55) varies according to the surgeon's preference. The following arrangements are suggested.

Operating Tables

Before the patient is brought to the operating room, the operating tables are set.

1. Mayo stand 1 contains a dilation and curettage setup with instruments for video-augmented hysteroscopy (videohysteroscopy). Included are a long-bladed weighted speculum, a double-or single-toothed tenaculum, dilators, a uterine sound, a small Kevorkian curette, a uterine manipulator, Raytec sponges (Baxter Healthcare, Deerfield, IL), Telfa pads, and a Foley catheter. The videohysteroscopy equipment includes a Circon (Circon-ACMI, Santa Barbara, CA) or a Storz (Karl Storz, Culver City, CA) diagnostic and operative hysteroscope along with its appropriate scissors and grasper. An adaptive sleeve is available for passing a scissors, grasper, or the fiber laser when it is used in the uterus. For more complicated procedures, such as resection of an intrauterine leiomyoma and endometrial ablation, electrosurgical wire loops and roller balls (Circon, Karl Storz) are added.

2. The back table is positioned behind the surgeon and next to the first assistant. The table contains a Veress needle, a scalpel, an Allis clamp, an 11-mm trocar and sleeve, a 10-mm laparoscope, a fiberoptic light cord, 5.5-mm secondary trocars and sleeves, a suction–irrigator probe (American Hydro-Surgical Instruments) with irrigation and suction tubing, tubing for the CO_2 insufflator with a CO_2 connector, atraumatic grasping forceps with teeth, bipolar forceps with cord, aspirating needles each with a 60-mL syringe, and Telfa pads and Raytec sponges. A small amount of dilute vasopressin (Pitressin, Monarch Pharmaceuticals) is made available (one ampule

in 100 mL of bacteriostatic sterile water). This solution (1 to 2 mL) is injected through the laparoscopic needle before the removal of a large fibroid or endometrioma to reduce bleeding. Vicryl suture (3–0) on a cutting needle for closing the primary trocar site, 1.5-inch Steri-Strips (3M) to be used with Mastisol (Ferndale Laboratories, Inc., Ferndale, MI), eye pads, and 3M tape for dressing care are placed on the back table.

3. Mayo stand 2 is positioned so that the surgeon and first assistant can reach the endoscopic scissors and grasping forceps with and without teeth.

Hydrodissection Pump

The Nezhat–Dorsey hydrodissection pump or any of the recent powerful suction irrigation pumps provide pressure during hydrodissection and is located behind the surgeon on a cart or specially designed stand. The plastic tubing is connected to the pump, brought to the operative field, and attached to the suction–irrigator probe.

Light Sources, Insufflator, and Electrogenerator

Other items kept on the side of the room opposite the surgeon include a storage table that holds the insufflator, electrosurgical equipment, camera boxes, and light sources. This equipment is stored in a specially designed stand opposite the surgeon and close to the patient, toward her head. This cart is placed so that it does not interfere with the assistants' position and does not obstruct the surgeon's view of the insufflator and light source. The camera is covered with a sterile cover, connected to the camera box, brought to the operative field, and attached to the laparoscope. Video cabinets are manufactured with removable backs, making adjustment of the machines easy.

Video Monitors

Video monitors should be positioned within view of the surgeon and the two assistants; one assistant stands between the patient's legs, and the other one opposite the surgeon. Three video monitors provide adequate views for the surgeon, the assistants, and other observers. The monitor provides the surgeon's view of the operative site and should be set for maximal clarity and true color transmission. The video monitors can be fixed to the ceiling, placed on a portable stand, or attached to a mobile stand with an articulating arm. The monitors are positioned for optimal viewing from any area in the operating room and are pushed from the operative area at the end of the day.

Video Recording

Depending on the surgeon's preference, the digital capture devices should be turned on at the start of the case. One capture device is sufficient as it will provide multiple ways to archive the information. The digital capture device is also ideal for surgeons who videotape procedures for educational purposes.

Lasers and Laser Equipment

Three different lasers are available in the operating room: a CO_2 laser (with a coupler), an argon or potassium titanyl phosphate (KTP) laser, and a neodymium:yttrium–aluminum–garnet (Nd:YAG) laser. They are used through the operative channel of the laparoscope or a suprapubic trocar. The CO_2 laser is on the patient's side, opposite the surgeon. The articulating arm is extended appropriately so that it does not weigh too heavily on the surgeon's hand. YAG and argon lasers are used less frequently than is the CO_2 laser and are located behind the first assistant, who stands between the patient's legs. This allows laser fibers to be passed from the back table through the second puncture site. Appropriate electrical outlets and special water connections are necessary when one uses fiber lasers. Typically, an outlet supplying a 220-V 30-A circuit is required. The YAG laser may be either three phase or single phase and air or water cooled, depending on the peak wattage required for a particular procedure. The CO_2 laser can be operated from a 100-V circuit supplied by any standard electrical outlet. Individually wrapped sterile fibers are kept with the fiber lasers, each with its own cleaver for sharpening fiber tips. Because the fibers break easily, they are handled carefully and checked repeatedly. Safety precautions are followed strictly when one is using lasers. One risk of fiber-equipped lasers that does not exist with a CO_2 laser is the possibility of fiber breakage in or outside the patient's abdomen. In the CO_2 laser, the beam is transmitted through and reflected by mirrors contained in the articulating arm. When fiber lasers are used, the appropriate tinted eye protection is worn by both the patient and the staff. Regular glasses may be worn when one is using the CO_2 laser but are not necessary during videolaseroscopy. The patient's eyes are covered with moistened eye pads when the CO_2 is used and with the appropriate tinted goggles when other lasers are used.

Preparation and Termination of the Procedure

All the setup tables are brought close to the operating table, and both the hysteroscope and the laparoscope are connected to the light sources and cameras. After they are checked and functioning, they are placed over the patient. After the videohysteroscopy is completed and as the laparoscopic portion begins, the first Mayo stand is moved out of the way and the surgeon moves to the side of the patient for the laparoscopy.

The anesthesiologist covers the patient's eyes with moistened 4×4 pads when the laser is used and places a foam pad over her neck to protect her if lightweight camera equipment is placed on the sterile field during the procedure.

When the procedure is completed, instruments are handled carefully so that laparoscopes and other delicate equipment are not damaged. The disposable equipment is discarded, and the reusable instruments are given to the circulating nurses for cleaning. Care is taken to ensure that reusable instruments are not mixed with disposables and inadvertently thrown out.

The patient's abdomen is washed thoroughly, and her legs are lowered. Although the patient is not fully alert, she often can hear conversation as she is being extubated and while awakening. A professional demeanor is maintained, and conversation is limited.

MANAGED HEALTH CARE

New endoscopic procedures are done with increasing frequency, so hospitals need more video equipment to keep up with demand, and purchases must justify their cost. As medical services move from a large hospital-based facility to smaller community-based surgical centers, patients residing 2 hours from the main hospital could have a knee arthroscopy or laparoscopy done closer to home. The leading edge of technology includes three-dimensional (3-D) equipment, virtual reality, and HDTV. HDTV can expand the scanning rate from 525 lines of resolution to 1100 or 1200 lines per frame, and the quality of current pictures will more than double. One challenge is to reduce the cost to make it affordable for hospitals.

With virtual reality, a 3-D computer image is presented to the user through liquid crystal glasses. This technique is used in the United States by public institutions such as the Central Intelligence Agency and by architects so that clients can "see" a building inside and out before its construction. In a way, this is similar to a surgeon's use of virtual reality, but cost continues to be a major obstacle. The 3-D technology attempts to provide depth to the image that is not available with monocular endoscopic systems. The increased perception of depth of field enables the surgeon to locate instruments in relation to tissues and organs. These systems rely on special optical devices.

REFERENCES

1. Nezhat F, Nezhat C, Silfen SO. Videolaseroscopy for oophorectomy. *Am J Obstet Gynecol.* 1991;165:1323.

2. Wolf JS Jr. Laparoscopic access with a visualizing trocar. *Tech Urol.* 1997;3:34.

3. Kaali SG. Establishment of primary port without insertion of a sharp trocar. *J Am Assoc Gynecol Laparosc.* 1998;5:193.

4. Schaller G, Kuenkel M, Manegold BC. The optical "Veress-needle" – initial puncture with a minioptic. *Endosc Surg Allied Technol.* 1995;3:55.

5. Bhoyrul S, Payne J, Steffes B, et al. A randomized prospective study of radially expanding trocars in laparoscopic surgery. *J Gastrointest Surg.* 2000;4(4):392–397.

6. Fuller J, Ashar BS, Carey-Corrado J. Trocar-associated injuries and fatalities: an analysis of 1399 reports to the FDA. *J Minim Invasive Gynecol.* 2005;12(4):302–307.

7. Boike GM, Miller CE, Spiritos NM, et al. Incisional bowel herniations after operative laparoscopy: a series of nineteen cases and review of the literature. *Am J Obstet Gynecol.* 1995;172:1726.

8. Yerdel MA, Karayalcin K, Koyuncu A, et al. Direct trocar insertion versus Veress needle insertion in laparoscopic cholecystectomy. *Am J Surg.* 1999;177(3):247–249.

9. Nezhat FR, Silfen SL, Evans D, Nezhat C. Comparison of direct insertion of disposable and standard reusable trocars and previous pneumoperitoneum with Veress needle. *Obstet Gynecol.* 1991;78:148–150.

10. Moore SS, Green CR, Wang FL, et al. The role of irrigation in the development of hypothermia during laparoscopic surgery. *Am J Obstet Gynecol.* 1997;176:598.

11. Landman J, Kerbl K, Rehman J, et al. Evaluation of a vessel sealing system, bipolar electrosurgery, harmonic scalpel, titanium clips, endoscopic gastrointestinal anastomosis vascular staples and sutures for arterial and venous ligation in a porcine model. *J Urol.* 2003;169:697–700.

12. Carbonell AM, Joels CS, Kercher KW, et al. A comparison of laparoscopic bipolar vessel sealing devices in the hemostasis of small-, medium-, and large-sized arteries. *J Laparoendosc Adv Surg Tech A.* 2003;13(6):377–380.

13. Harold KL, Pollinger H, Matthews BD, et al. Comparison of ultrasonic energy, bipolar thermal energy, and vascular clips for the hemostasis of small-, medium-, and large-sized arteries. *Surg Endosc.* 2003;17(8):1228–1230.

14. Nezhat C, Nezhat F, Silfen SO. Laparoscopic hysterectomy and bilateral salpingo-oophorectomy using multifire GIA surgical stapler. *J Gynecol Surg.* 1990;6:287.

15. Nezhat C, Nezhat F, Bess O, et al. Injuries associated with the use of a linear stapler during operative laparoscopy: review of diagnosis, management, and prevention. *J Gynecol Surg.* 1993;9:145.

16. Carter JE, McCarus SD. Laparoscopic myomectomy: time and cost analysis of power vs. manual morcellation. *J Reprod Med.* 1997;42:383.

17. Mecke H, Wallas F, Brocker A, Gertz HP. Pelviscopic myoma enucleation: technique, limits, complications. *Geburtshilfe Frauenheilkd.* 1995;55:374.

18. Mettler L, Semm K, Lehmann-Willenbrock L, et al. Comparative evaluation of classical intrafascial-supracervical hysterectomy (CISH) with transuterine mucosal resection as performed by pelviscopy and laparotomy – our first 200 cases. *Surg Endosc.* 1995;9:418.

19. Kresch AJ, Lyons TL, Westland AB, et al. Laparoscopic supracervical hysterectomy with a new disposable morcellator. *J Am Assoc Gynecol Laparosc.* 1998;5:203.

20. Lobe TE, Schropp KP, Joyner R, et al. The suitability of automatic tissue morcellation for the endoscopic removal of large specimens in pediatric surgery. *J Pediatr Surg.* 1994;29:232.

21. Hasson HM. Ovarian surgery. In: Sanfilippo JS, Levine RL, eds. *Operative Gynecologic Endoscopy.* New York: Springer-Verlag;1989.

22. Valtchev KL, Papsin FR. A new uterine mobilizer for laparoscopy: its use in 518 patients. *Am J Obstet Gynecol.* 1977;127:738.

23. Koh CH. A new technique and system for simplifying total laparoscopic hysterectomy. *J Am Assoc Gynecol Laparosc.* 1998;5:187.

24. DesCoteaux JG, Tye L, Poulin EC. Reuse of disposable laparoscopic instruments: cost analysis. *Can J Surg.* 1996;39:133.

25. DesCoteaux JG, Blackmore K, Parsons L. A prospective comparison of the costs of reusable and limited-reuse laparoscopic instruments. *Can J Surg.* 1998;41:136.

26. DesCoteaux JG, Poulin EC, Lortie M, et al. Reuse of disposable laparoscopic instruments: a study of related surgical complications. *Can J Surg.* 1995;38:497.

27. Schaer GN, Koechli OR, Haller U. Single-use versus reusable laparoscopic surgical instruments: a comparative cost analysis. *Am J Obstet Gynecol.* 1995;173:1812.

28. Nezhat C, Bess O, Admon D, et al. Hospital cost comparison between abdominal, vaginal, and laparoscopy-assisted vaginal hysterectomy. *Obstet Gynecol.* 1994;83:713.

29. Airan MC, Sandor J. A simple subcutaneous tissue closure device for laparoscopic procedure. *Minim Invasive Ther Allied Technol.* 1996;5:35.

30. Carter JE. A new technique of fascial closure for laparoscopic incisions. *J Laparosc Surg.* 1994;4:143.

31. Bezzi M, Silecchia G, De Leo A, et al. Laparoscopic and intraoperative ultrasound. *Eur J Radiol.* 1998;27(suppl 2):14.

32. Nezhat F, Nezhat C, Nezhat CH, et al. Use of laparoscopic ultrasonography to detect ovarian remnants. *J Ultrasound Med.* 1996;15:487.

33. Hurst BS, Tucker KE, Awoniyi CA, Schlaff WD. Endoscopic ultrasound. A new instrument for laparoscopic surgery. *J Reprod Med.* 1996;41:67.

34. Dunlap KD, Wanzwe L. Is the robotic arm a cost effective surgical tool? *Am Oper Room Nurs J.* 1998;68:265.

35. Mettler L, Ibrahim M, Jonar W. One year experience working with the aid of a robotic assistant (the voice controlled optic holder, AESOP) in gynecological endoscopic surgery. *Hum Reprod.* 1998;13:2748.

36. Berguer R, Rab GT, Abu-Ghaida H, et al. A comparison of surgeon's posture during laparoscopic and open surgical procedures. *Surg Endosc.* 1997;11:139.

37. Nezhat C, et al. Reduce fatigue and discomfort: tips to improve operating room set-up. *Laparosc Surg Update.* 1997;5:97.

38. Hurd WW, Diamond MP. There's a hole in my bucket: the cost of disposable instruments. *Fertil Steril.* 1997;67:13.

39. Dorsey JH, Holtz PM, Griffiths RI, et al. Costs and charges associated with three alternative techniques of hysterectomy. *N Engl J Med.* 1996;335:476.

3 | ANESTHESIA

Lindsey Vokach-Brodsky

Pneumoperitoneum and patient positioning during laparoscopy induce certain pathophysiologic changes. These must be understood for the anesthesiologist to provide the best perioperative care, particularly for patients with coexisting medical problems.

In this chapter, the changes induced by raised CO_2 pneumoperitoneum and head-down tilt are reviewed. The complications of laparoscopy that are of immediate concern to the anesthesiologist are discussed, followed by a brief description of anesthetic techniques and postoperative management. Recent research involving anesthesia for nongynecologic laparoscopy is included when relevant.

HEMODYNAMIC CHANGES DURING LAPAROSCOPY

The hemodynamic effects of gynecologic laparoscopy are the result of raised intra-abdominal pressure, insufflation of CO_2, and head-down positioning.

After CO_2 insufflation to an intra-abdominal pressure greater than 10 mm Hg, cardiac output falls 10% to 30%, arterial pressure increases, and both systemic and pulmonary vascular resistance increase.[1,2] Heart rate is unchanged. The fall in cardiac output is related to reduced flow in the inferior vena cava, pooling of blood in the legs, and an increase in venous resistance. Although venous return falls, cardiac filling pressures increase, which is consistent with the observed rise in intrathoracic pressure.[2,3] There is an increase in intrathoracic blood volume.[4] Systemic vascular resistance (SVR) increases because of an increase in the vascular resistance of intra-abdominal organs and increased venous resistance. This increase in SVR is reduced by a head-down tilt.[3] After pneumoperitoneum has been established, placing the patient in a 10° to 30° head-down position increases preload, pulmonary capillary wedge pressure (PCWP), and pulmonary artery pressure (PAP) while returning afterload toward normal.[2,3]

These hemodynamic changes appear to be more marked in patients with severe heart disease, particularly congestive heart failure. These patients require careful preoperative evaluation, more extensive intraoperative monitoring, and close hemodynamic control extending into the postoperative period.[5]

Vagal stimulation resulting in bradycardia and bradyarrhythmias may be provoked by mechanical distention of the peritoneum or manipulation of pelvic organs.[6] Surgery should be interrupted while atropine is administered and the level of anesthesia is deepened.

VENTILATORY CHANGES DURING LAPAROSCOPY

Pneumoperitoneum causes a cephalad shift in the diaphragm, stiffens the lower chest wall, and restricts lung expansion. There is a resultant 30% to 50% decrease in thoracopulmonary compliance, which occurs in all patients: healthy, obese, and American Society of Anesthesiology (ASA) class III and IV. A subsequent change in position does not affect compliance.[2,7–12] Functional residual capacity is also decreased. Physiologic dead space and shunt are unchanged in the absence of significant cardiac disease.

Peak inspiratory pressure (PIP) and mean airway pressure increase during pneumoperitoneum.[9] Mechanical ventilation may become difficult in the obese or in patients with lung disease.[10]

Pneumoperitoneum has been shown to shift the carina cephalad sufficiently to result in endobronchial intubation in some patients.[13,14] Increased PIP and decreased oxygen saturation (SaO_2) result. After positioning the patient, endotracheal tube placement should be rechecked by auscultation.

CO_2 is used commonly to provide a pneumoperitoneum. As CO_2 is absorbed from the peritoneal cavity, the CO_2 load increases over the first 20 minutes of pneumoperitoneum before reaching a plateau about 25% above preinsufflation values.[15,16] CO_2 absorption is probably limited by reduced peritoneal perfusion as the result of increased intra-abdominal pressure. An increase in minute ventilation of about 30% has been shown to maintain a normal end-tidal CO_2 partial pressure ($PetCO_2$).[7,16] Increasing respiratory rate rather than tidal volume tends to minimize the rise in PIP. Investigations of arterioalveolar CO_2 partial pressure differences have not shown a consistent change, but the differences may increase over time in prolonged operations. $PetCO_2$ therefore may not be a reliable measure of arterial CO_2 partial pressure ($PaCO_2$), particularly in prolonged procedures or in patients with underlying lung disease.[8,9,15]

METABOLIC AND RENAL RESPONSE TO LAPAROSCOPY

Endocrine responses to laparoscopy do not appear to differ from those seen with open surgery.[17,18] Increases in circulating catecholamines, cortisol, renin, and aldosterone are similar whether cholecystectomy is open or laparoscopic. However, the metabolic response to surgery is reduced. Acute phase proteins, hyperglycemia, and leukocytosis are lower following laparoscopic cholecystectomy, compared with an open procedure.[18,19]

Pneumoperitoneum is associated with a 50% reduction in the glomerular filtration rate and urine output. Urine output recovers promptly after release of the pneumoperitoneum.[20]

INTRAOPERATIVE COMPLICATIONS

CO_2 Embolism

CO_2 embolism is a rare but potentially fatal event.[21] It occurs most commonly during initial insufflation of gas as a result of inadvertent insertion of the trocar or Veress needle into a vessel or abdominal organ. The severity of the response depends on the volume of gas entering the circulation and the speed of entrainment. Small CO_2 emboli appear to follow a more benign and transient course than do air emboli because of the high solubility of CO_2 in blood and tissues and the large buffering capacity of blood, which leads to rapid elimination.[21] The lethal dose of CO_2 is about five times that of air (25 mL/kg for CO_2 and 5 mL/kg for air) in dogs.[22] The expansion of an air embolus caused by diffusion of nitrous oxide into the bubble of air does not occur with CO_2 emboli because CO_2 has a solubility similar to that of N_2O. Unlike air embolus, CO_2 embolus does not cause bronchospasm. Large volumes of gas injected under pressure, however, can cause an "air lock" in the vena cava or right atrium, causing sudden cardiovascular collapse.[21]

Paradoxic embolus occurs when gas passes through a patent foramen ovale into the systemic circulation, driven by high right atrial pressures.[2] About 25% of normal individuals have a probe patent foramen ovale.

Transesophageal echo and esophageal or precordial Doppler probes are the most sensitive detectors of CO_2 emboli. However, the low incidence of this complication during laparoscopy does not justify their routine use. Capnography is the most sensitive detector of CO_2 embolism normally in use during laparoscopy. In case reports, capnography showed an initial small sharp rise in end-tidal CO_2 concentration in expiratory air ($ETCO_2$) with a subsequent fall caused by an increase in dead space in the lung. [23,24] Saturation of peripheral oxygen (SpO_2) and mean arterial pressure (MAP) fall, with the magnitude of the fall depending on the size of the embolus. Bradycardia or other arrhythmia may occur, and a characteristic "mill wheel" murmur may be heard over the precordium. The alveolar–arterial CO_2 difference will increase. Treatment involves stopping insufflation, releasing the pneumoperitoneum immediately, and giving 100% oxygen. Turning the patient head down on the left side is recommended to displace the gas bubbles from the outflow tract of the right heart. Cardiopulmonary resuscitation should be instituted as necessary. Aspiration of gas through a central venous pressure (CVP) line may be attempted. Cardiopulmonary bypass has been used successfully after massive CO_2 embolus.[23] Hyperbaric oxygen has been recommended to treat suspected cerebral embolism.[25]

Pneumothorax, Pneumomediastinum, and Subcutaneous Emphysema

Although pneumothorax is a complication that is more commonly associated with upper abdominal laparoscopy, it has been reported during gynecologic procedures.[26] A congenital diaphragmatic defect may allow peritoneal gas to pass into the pleural cavity. An increase in PIP, a fall in SpO_2, and decreased breath sounds on one side point to the diagnosis, which should be confirmed by chest radiograph. The laparoscopist may be able to show abnormal motion of one hemidiaphragm. Reduced QRS amplitude in precordial ECG leads supports the diagnosis.[27] Falling MAP and SpO_2 suggests the presence of a tension pneumothorax that requires immediate decompression. In the absence of tension, unless there is a pulmonary cause (such as a ruptured bulla), pneumothorax resolves spontaneously after 30 to 60 minutes in the recovery period. If the patient is stable, Joris [27] suggests conservative intraoperative management. Chest tube drainage should be avoided during surgery because it will make it difficult to maintain the pneumoperitoneum. Increasing fraction of inspiratory oxygen (FiO_2), the addition of 5 cm of positive end-expiratory pressure (PEEP), and reduction of intra-abdominal pressure will maintain oxygenation and allow surgery to be completed.[29]

Subcutaneous CO_2 emphysema may accompany pneumothorax or occur in isolation. An abrupt and severe rise in $ETCO_2$ is characteristic. This occurs when CO_2 tracks into tissue planes, increasing the surface area for uptake into the circulation. A higher than normal increase in minute ventilation is required for control. $ETCO_2$ may increase to very high levels. Rarely, it may become necessary to discontinue surgery and release the pneumoperitoneum until control of $ETCO_2$ is achieved. The possibility of pneumothorax and pneumomediastinum always should be considered when subcutaneous emphysema is present. Subcutaneous emphysema resolves over several hours. Explanation and reassurance may be necessary for the patient in the postoperative care unit.

Nerve Injury

The common peroneal and sciatic nerves are at risk for injury during laparoscopy in the lithotomy position. Femoral neuropathy has also been reported.[30] The brachial plexus may be injured by pressure or stretching from shoulder restraints, especially in the steep head-down position. Meticulous care is necessary when positioning the patient to minimize the risk of injuring these vulnerable nerves. Lower limb compartment syndrome has complicated prolonged laparoscopy performed in the lithotomy position.[31,32]

Fluid Balance

A patient who has undergone a preoperative bowel preparation and a prolonged fast may be dehydrated on arrival in the operating room. Intraoperative blood loss may be difficult to assess during laparoscopy because of dilution in large volumes of irrigation fluid. Pulmonary edema has been described after the absorption of intra-abdominal irrigating fluid, resulting in dyspnea and hypoxemia in the recovery room.[33] Maintaining a careful record of irrigating fluid balance intraoperatively will alert the anesthesiologist when large deficits are accumulating.

Heat Loss

Postoperative hypothermia has been associated with an increased incidence of wound infection and prolonged hospital stay after laparotomy.[34] In patients with cardiac risk factors, perioperative myocardial events are increased in the presence of mild hypothermia.[35] Peritoneal gas insufflation and the use of large volumes of peritoneal irrigation predispose a patient to hypothermia during laparoscopy.[36] Warming of insufflation gas has not proved useful.[37] Warming of irrigation fluids and the use of a forced-air warming blanket reduce the incidence of the undesirable postoperative effects of hypothermia.

ANESTHESIA CONSIDERATIONS

Preoperative Evaluation and Premedication

Most patients for gynecologic laparoscopy are young, healthy women, requiring routine preoperative evaluation and few laboratory investigations.[38] A complete blood count and pregnancy test may be performed when indicated.

Patients with coexisting medical problems should be evaluated appropriately. In particular, patients with severe cardiac disease, particularly congestive heart failure, require careful workup. These patients may be unable to tolerate the cardiovascular changes of laparoscopy, and open procedure may be a better choice.

Laparoscopy has few contraindications, but pneumoperitoneum should be avoided in patients with raised intracranial pressure and in those with ventriculoperitoneal or peritoneojugular shunts.

Premedication with a small dose (1 to 2 mg) of the short-acting benzodiazepine midazolam allays anxiety without contributing to postoperative sedation. For patients with a history of severe postoperative nausea and vomiting, transdermal scopolamine is an effective adjunct to antiemetic medication given intraoperatively. It must be given at least 4 hours before the end of surgery to be effective.[39] In patients at risk for regurgitation of gastric contents, preoperative administration of a nonparticulate antacid increases gastric pH. Metoclopramide and H_2 receptor blockers may be given to reduce gastric volume and acidity.

Choice of Anesthesia

Although regional and local anesthesia have been used successfully for laparoscopy, they are suitable only for brief procedures with minimal intra-abdominal gas and few incisions. Operative gynecologic laparoscopy necessitates optimal surgical conditions, steep head-down positioning, muscle relaxation, a large pneumoperitoneum, and multiple incisions. These considerations make general anesthesia the safest and most comfortable choice. Similarly, although the laryngeal mask airway has been used successfully for laparoscopy [40], endotracheal intubation protects the airway from aspiration of gastric contents and facilitates the delivery of increased minute ventilation in the presence of increased airway pressures.[41]

Propofol anesthesia in outpatient surgery is associated with better postoperative recovery.[42] After the administration of the muscle relaxant, care must be taken during mask ventilation not to inflate the stomach with gas. Once the endotracheal tube is secured, an orogastric tube is passed to decompress the stomach. Balanced anesthesia with oxygen-enriched air, an inhalational agent, a muscle relaxant, and a narcotic such as fentanyl is suitable. Total intravenous anesthesia has also been used successfully. Intra-abdominal pressure can be kept as low as possible by controlled ventilation, maintaining muscle relaxation, and a relatively deep plane of anesthesia.

The role of nitrous oxide in anesthesia for laparoscopy remains controversial. Several studies have failed to show a difference in operating conditions or bowel distention during laparoscopy with and without nitrous oxide.[43,44] These procedures were less than 3 hours in duration. Studies of nonlaparoscopic colonic surgery lasting 3 hours or longer have demonstrated a deleterious effect on bowel function when nitrous oxide is used.[45] Avoidance of nitrous oxide may be most useful in procedures of long duration.

Continuous intraoperative monitoring should include pulse oximetry, ECG, $ETCO_2$, blood pressure, temperature, muscle relaxation, minute ventilation, and airway pressure. Patients with cardiac disease may benefit from transesophageal echo or invasive hemodynamic monitoring.[5]

RECOVERY FROM ANESTHESIA

Postoperative Nausea and Vomiting

Nausea with or without vomiting is a common postoperative occurrence and is distressing to patients. The incidence of postoperative nausea and vomiting (PONV) overall is about 30%; after laparoscopy, it is about 50%.[46] Younger, nonsmoking women with a history of motion sickness or previous PONV have the highest risk. The use of prophylactic antiemetic medication may be justified in laparoscopy because of this high probability of PONV. The optimal prophylactic regimen remains a matter of debate. Given the complex causes of vomiting, it seems likely that the use of a combination of medications will produce better results than will one alone. Several prophylactic and rescue algorithms have been proposed.[47,48]

Pain Management

Postoperative pain occurs in the abdomen, shoulders, and back. Shoulder pain, presumably from diaphragmatic irritation and phrenic nerve stimulation, tends to become more significant on the second postoperative day.[49] Many studies have examined the effect of nonsteroidal anti-inflammatory drugs (NSAIDs) on pain after laparoscopy. The intensity and duration of pain relief are improved by adding ketorolac to a short-acting opioid, but NSAIDs alone provide inadequate pain relief. There is evidence of increased postoperative bleeding associated with NSAIDs.[50] Various local anesthetic techniques have been used, including infiltration of the abdominal wounds and rectus sheath block. A combination of narcotics, local anesthesia, and an NSAID may offer the best relief.[51]

REFERENCES

1. Johansen G, Anderson M, Juhl B. The effect of general anesthesia on the hemodynamic events during laparoscopy with CO_2 insufflation. *Acta Anaesthesiol Scand.* 1989;33:132.
2. Hirvonen EA, Nuutinen LS, Kauko M. Hemodynamic changes due to Trendelenburg positioning and pneumoperitoneum during laparoscopic hysterectomy. *Acta Anaesthesiol Scand.* 1995;39:949.

3. Odeburg S, Ljungqvist O, Svenberg T, et al. Haemodynamic effects of pneumoperitoneum and the influence of posture during anaesthesia for laparoscopic surgery. *Acta Anaesthesiol Scand.* 1994;38:276.

4. Hofer CK, Zalunardo MP, Klaghofer R, Spahr T, Pasch T, Zollinger A. Changes in intrathoracic blood volume associated with pneumoperitoneum and positioning. *Acta Anaesthesiol Scand.* 2002;46:303.

5. Safran D, Sgambati S, Orlando R. Laparoscopy in high risk cardiac patients. *Surg Gynecol Obstet.* 1993;176:584.

6. Sprung J. Recurrent complete heart block in a healthy patient during laparoscopic electrocauterization of the fallopian tube. *Anesthesiology.* 1998;88:1401.

7. Hirvonen EA, Nuutinen LS, Kauko M. Ventilatory effects, blood gas changes, and oxygen consumption during laparoscopic hysterectomy. *Anesth Analg.* 1995;80:961.

8. Monk TG, Weldon BC, Lemon D. Alterations in pulmonary function during laparoscopic surgery [abstract]. *Anesth Analg.* 1994;76:S274.

9. Wahba RW, Mamazza J. Ventilatory requirements during laparoscopic cholecystectomy. *Can J Anaesth.* 1993;40:206.

10. Sprung J, Whalley D, Falcone T, Warner D, Hubmayr RD, Hammel J. The impact of morbid obesity, pneumoperitoneum, and posture on respiratory system mechanics and oxygenation during laparoscopy. *Anesth Analg.* 2002;94:1345.

11. Rauhr R, Hemmerling TM, Rist M, et al. Influence of pneumoperitoneum and patient positioning on respiratory system compliance. *J Clin Anesth.* 2001;13:361.

12. Oikkonen M, Tallgren M. Changes in respiratory compliance at laparoscopy: measurements using sidestream spirometry. *Can J Anaesth.* 1995;42:495.

13. Lobato EB, Paige GB, Brown MM, et al. Pneumoperitoneum as a risk factor for endobronchial intubation during laparoscopic gynecologic surgery. *Anesth Analg.* 1998;86:301.

14. Ezri T, Hazin V, Warters D, Szmuk P, Weinbroum AA. The endotracheal tube moves more often in obese patients undergoing laparoscopy compared with open abdominal surgery. *Anesth Analg.* 2003;96:278.

15. Puri GD, Singh H. Ventilatory effects of laparoscopy under general anaesthesia. *Br J Anaesth.* 1992;68:211.

16. Tan PL, Lee TL, Tweed WA. Carbon dioxide absorption and gas exchange during pelvic laparoscopy. *Can J Anaesth.* 1992;39:677.

17. Hirvonen EA, Nuutinen LS, Vuolteenaho O. Hormonal responses and cardiac filling pressures in head up or head down position and pneumoperitoneum in patients undergoing operative laparoscopy. *Br J Anaesth.* 1997;78:128.

18. Joris J, Cigarini I, Legrand M, et al. Metabolic and respiratory changes after cholecystectomy performed via laparotomy or laparoscopy. *Br J Anaesth.* 1992;69:341.

19. Karayiannakis AJ, Makri GG, Mantzioka A. Systemic stress response after laparoscopic or open cholecystectomy: a randomized trial. *Br J Surg.* 1997;84:467.

20. Hashikura Y, Kawasaki S, Munakata Y, et al. Effects of peritoneal insufflation on hepatic and renal blood flow. *Surg Endosc.* 1994;8:759.

21. Wahba RW, Tessler MJ, Kleiman SJ. Acute ventilatory complications during laparoscopic upper abdominal surgery. *Can J Anaesth.* 1995;43:77.

22. Graff TD, Arbegast NR, Philips OC, et al. Gas embolism: a comparative study of air and carbon dioxide as embolic agents in the systemic venous system. *Am J Obstet Gynecol.* 1959;78:259.

23. Shulman D, Aronson HB. Capnography in the early diagnosis of carbon dioxide embolism during laparoscopy. *Can J Anaesth.* 1984;31:31.

24. Diakun TA. Carbon dioxide embolism: successful resuscitation with cardiopulmonary bypass. *Anesthesiology.* 1991;74:1151.

25. McGrath BJ, Zimmerman JE, Williams JF, Parmet J. Carbon dioxide embolism treated with hyperbaric oxygen. *Can J Anaesth.* 1989;36:586.

26. Perko G, Fernandes A. Subcutaneous emphysema and pneumothorax during laparoscopy for ectopic pregnancy removal. *Acta Anaesthesiol Scand.* 1997;41:792.

27. Ludemann R, Krysztopik R, Jamieson G, Watson DI. Pneumothorax during laparoscopy. *Surg Endosc.* 2003;17:12.

28. Joris JL. Anesthetic management of laparoscopy. In: Miller RD, ed. *Anesthesia.* 4th ed. New York: Churchill Livingstone; 1994.

29. Chiche JD, Joris J, Lamy M. PEEP for treatment of intra-operative pneumothorax during laparoscopic fundoplication. *Br J Anaesth.* 1994;72:A38.

30. Gombar KK, Gombar S, Singh B, et al. Femoral neuropathy: a complication of the lithotomy position. *Reg Anaesth.* 1992;17:306.

31. Lydon JC, Spielman FJ. Bilateral compartment syndrome following prolonged surgery in the lithotomy position. *Anesthesiology.* 1984;60:236.

32. Montgomery CJ, Ready LB. Epidural opioid analgesia does not obscure diagnosis of compartment syndrome resulting from prolonged lithotomy position. *Anesthesiology.* 1991;75:541.

33. Healzer JM, Nezhat C, Brodsky JB, et al. Pulmonary edema after absorbing crystalloid irrigating fluid during laparoscopy. *Anesth Analg.* 1994;78:1207.

34. Kurz A, Sessler DI, Lenhardt R. Peri-operative normothermia to reduce the incidence of surgical wound infection and shorter hospitalization. *N Engl J Med.* 1996;334:1209.

35. Frank SM, Fleisher LA, Breslow MJ, et al. Perioperative maintenance of normothermia reduces the incidence of morbid cardiac events. *JAMA.* 1997;277:1127.

36. Moore SS, Green CR, Wang FL, et al. The role of irrigation in the development of hypothermia during laparoscopic surgery. *Am J Obstet Gynecol.* 1997;176:598.

37. Nelskaya K, Yli-Hankala A, Sjoberg J, Korhonen I, Kortila K. Warming of insufflation gas during laparoscopic hysterectomy: effect on body temperature and the autonomic nervous system. *Acta Anaesthesiol Scand.* 1999;43:10.

38. Roizen MF, Cohn S. Preoperative evaluation for elective surgery – what laboratory tests are needed? *Adv Anesth.* 1993;10:25.

39. Kranke P, Morin AM, Roewer N, Wulf H, Eberhart LH. The efficacy and safety of transdermal scopolamine for the prevention of postoperative nausea and vomiting: a quantitative systematic review. *Anesth Analg.* 2002;95:133.

40. Maltby JR, Beriault MT, Watson NC, Liepert DJ, Fick GH. LMA-Classic and LMA Pro-Seal are effective alternatives to endotracheal intubation for gynecologic laparoscopy. *Can J Anaesth.* 2003; 50:1.

41. Ho BY, Skinner HJ, Mahajan RP. Gastro-oesophageal reflux during day case gynaecological laparoscopy under positive pressure ventilation: laryngeal mask vs. tracheal intubation. *Anaesthesia.* 1998;53:910.

42. De Grood RM, Habers JB, van Egmond J, Crul JF. Anesthesia for laparoscopy: a comparison of 5 techniques including propofol, etomidate, thiopentone and isoflurane. *Anaesthesia.* 1987;42:815.

43. Brodsky JB, Lemmens HJ, Collins JS, et al. Nitrous oxide and laparoscopic bariatric surgery. *Obes Surg.* 2005;15:4.

44. Taylor E, Feinstein R, White PF, Soper N. Anesthesia for laparoscopic cholecystectomy. Is nitrous oxide contraindicated? *Anesthesiology.* 1992;76:541.

45. Akca O, Lenhardt R, Fleischman E, et al. Nitrous oxide increases the incidence of bowel distension in patients undergoing elective colon resection. *Acta Anaesthesiol Scand.* 2004;48:894.

46. Beattie WS, Linblad T, Buckley DN, Forest JB. Menstruation increases the risk of nausea and vomiting after laparoscopy. *Anesthesiology*. 1993;78:272.

47. Habib AS, Gan TJ. Evidence-based management of postoperative nausea and vomiting: a review. *Can J Anaesth*. 2004;51:326.

48. Gan TJ, Meyer T, Apfel CC, et al. Consensus guidelines for managing postoperative nausea and vomiting. *Anesth Analg*. 2003;97:62.

49. Alexander JI. Pain after laparoscopy. *Br J Anaesth*. 1997;79:369.

50. Forrest JB, Camu F, Greer IA, et al. Ketorolac, diclofenac, and ketoprofen are equally safe for pain relief after major surgery. *Br J Anaesth*. 2002;88:227.

51. Michalolaikou C, Chung F, Sharma S. Preoperative multimodal analgesia facilitates recovery after ambulatory laparoscopic cholecystectomy. *Anesth Analg*. 1996;82:44.

4 | LAPAROSCOPIC ACCESS
Section 4.1. Principles of Laparoscopy

Camran Nezhat, Ceana Nezhat, Farr Nezhat, and Roger Ferland

The modern era of laparoscopy began in 1954, when Palmer [1] reported the results of endoscopic procedures in 250 patients without sequelae. He produced a pneumoperitoneum with CO_2 at a rate of 300 to 500 mL/min and cautioned that the intra-abdominal pressure should not exceed 25 mm Hg. The claimed advantages of laparoscopy over culdoscopy were a decreased chance of infection, a better view of the pelvis, improved access to the pelvic organs and cul-de-sac, and easier application of surgical techniques.

Although the basic principles of laparoscopy are the same, the instruments and the complexity of operative procedures have changed significantly since 1954. This chapter presents information for residents learning laparoscopic operations and clinicians who are updating their knowledge of operative laparoscopy.

PREOPERATIVE EVALUATION

Advanced operative laparoscopy is a major intra-abdominal procedure. Careful preoperative evaluation optimizes the operative outcome and decreases the incidence of injuries and complications. Preoperative consultations with surgeons in other disciplines (colorectal, urologic, oncologic) sometimes are necessary. The patient is informed about the possible outcome and results of the planned operation, possible complications, and the surgeon's experience in doing the particular procedure. The following preoperative work-up is suggested:

1. History and physical
2. Complete blood count (CBC) with differential
3. Serum electrolytes
4. Urinalysis
5. Papanicolaou smear
6. Thrombin time, partial thrombin time, bleeding time
7. Transvaginal sonography (TVS)

In special situations, an endometrial biopsy, cervical culture, hysterosalpingogram, barium enema, intravenous pyelogram, blood type and screen or type and crossmatch, and bowel preparation are indicated.[2] Two bowel preparations are suggested (Tables 4.1.1 and 4.1.2).

Women who have had a previous laparotomy or have an adnexal mass, pelvic endometriosis, or adhesions are given instructions for the 1-day preparation. The 3-day regimen is used for a patient who may need an extensive laparoscopic procedure, such as a bowel resection.

PATIENT PREPARATION AND POSITION

The anesthesiology team and circulating nurses coordinate the patient's transfer onto the operating table. The operative site is cleansed and shaved preoperatively by an operating room (OR) nurse. Operating tables must be designed to provide a 25° Trendelenburg position. After the induction of endotracheal anesthesia, the patient's legs are placed in padded Allen stirrups to provide good support and proper position. Padding near the peroneal nerve is essential. To avoid nerve compression, no leg joint is extended more than 60°. The buttocks must protrude a few centimeters from the edge of the table to allow uterine manipulation. The patient's arms are placed at the side, padded with foam troughs, and secured by a sheet. This allows the surgeon and assistants to stand unencumbered next to the patient. The anesthesiologist should have easy access to the patient's arm (Figure 4.1.1).

Once the patient is positioned, her abdomen, perineum, and vagina are prepared with a suitable bactericidal solution and a Foley catheter is inserted. She is draped to expose the abdomen and perineum, and a pelvic examination is done. Diagnostic hysteroscopy may be indicated for patients undergoing diagnostic and operative laparoscopy. After withdrawal of the hysteroscope, a uterine manipulator is inserted into the cervical os to manipulate the uterus and for chromopertubation. Rectal and vaginal probes can help separate the tissue planes of the cul-de-sac. The assistant can do a simultaneous rectal and vaginal examination for the same purpose. A sponge on a ring forceps is placed in the posterior fornix to outline the posterior cul-de-sac or anteriorly to identify the vesicouterine space. In patients who are suspected of having rectosigmoid endometriosis, a sigmoidoscopic examination is suggested. The rectum is insufflated to look for bubbles as they pass into the posterior cul-de-sac filled with irrigation fluid.[3]

PLACEMENT OF THE VERESS NEEDLE

Insertion of the Veress needle, the primary trocar, and the secondary trocar is an important aspect of diagnostic and operative laparoscopy. Serious complications and injuries may occur during these procedures. The following factors increase the risk of injury:

1. Previous abdominal and pelvic operations
2. Body weight (whether patient is obese or very thin)
3. A large uterus and the presence of a large pelvic mass

Table 4.1.1: One-Day Bowel Preparation

1. Clear liquid the day before the operation
2. One gallon of GoLYTELY (Braintree Laboratories) consumed over 3 hours the evening before the laparoscopy or 45 mL of Fleet Phospho-Soda (C. B. Fleet Co.) orally at bedtime
3. One Fleet enema at bedtime and in the morning
4. 1 g metronidazole (Flagyl; Pfizer) by mouth at 11 PM
5. 1 g cefoxitin one-half hour before the procedure (intravenously)

Table 4.1.2: Three-Day Bowel Preparation

Day 1
100 mL Fleet Phospho-Soda by mouth at bedtime

Day 2
Clear liquid diet

Day 3
Clear liquid diet
10 mg prochlorperazine by mouth at noon
Begin drinking 1 gallon of GoLYTELY at 2 PM
1 g neomycin by mouth at 6 PM and 11 PM
1 g erythromycin base by mouth at 6 PM and 11 PM
One Fleet enema at bedtime

Day of surgery
Two tap water enemas before reporting to the hospital

The optimal location for the Veress needle and primary trocar is the umbilicus because the skin is attached to the fascial layer and anterior parietal peritoneum with no intervening subcutaneous fat or muscle (Figure 4.1.2). The transumbilical approach accounts for the shortest distance between the skin and the peritoneal cavity even in obese patients. These sites sometimes are modified. The primary trocar is inserted approximately 4 to 6 cm above the umbilicus in patients who have an enlarged uterus caused by a uterine leiomyoma or pregnancy or for para-aortic lymph node dissection.

Before the needle is inserted, a transverse or vertical cutaneous incision is made large enough to accommodate the primary trocar. A vertical umbilical incision provides better cosmetic results.[4] When one is incising the umbilicus, an Allis clamp or skin hook is used to grasp and evert the base of the umbilicus, raising it from the abdominal structures.

One should check the patency of the needle before it is inserted. Traditionally, the angle of insertion is approximately 45° for an infraumbilical placement while the patient is horizontal; a premature Trendelenburg position alters the usual landmarks (Figure 4.1.3). Transumbilical placement with a 90° angle of insertion is recommended after adequate training with this technique. Palpating the abdominal aorta and the sacral promontory is performed first. The patient is completely flat and the operating table is all the way down to maximize the surgeon's upper body control during insertion of the Veress needle (Figure 4.1.4). The Veress needle, held at the shaft, is directed toward the sacral promontory (Figure 4.1.5). The surgeon and assistants apply countertraction by grasping the skin and fat on each side of the umbilicus with a towel clip (Figure 4.1.6).[5] In obese patients, a 90° angle is necessary initially to enter the peritoneal cavity. In thin individuals, vital structures are closer to the abdominal wall, so the surgeon makes certain that the abdominal wall is elevated and only a small portion of the needle is inserted into the abdominal cavity. That is rarely more than 2 to 3 cm of the Veress needle or trocar. A prospective study involving 97 women undergoing operative laparoscopy showed that the position of the aortic bifurcation is more likely to be caudal to the umbilicus in the Trendelenburg position, compared with the supine position, regardless of body mass index.[6] Its presumed location may be misleading during Veress needle or primary cannula insertion. The physician must be careful to avoid major retroperitoneal vascular injury during this procedure.

Verification of Intraperitoneal Location

Failure to achieve and maintain a suitable pneumoperitoneum predisposes the patient to complications.

Hanging Drop Method

Correct needle placement is verified by the "hanging drop" technique. A drop of saline is placed on the hub of the Veress needle after insertion through the abdominal wall; lifting the abdominal wall establishes negative pressure within the abdomen, drawing the drop of fluid into the needle. Absence of this sign indicates improper placement of the Veress needle.

The Syringe Test

Alternatively, a 10-mL syringe with normal saline is attached to the Veress needle and aspiration verifies the absence of bowel contents or blood (Figure 4.1.7). The saline is injected into the peritoneal cavity, and if the needle placement is correct, the fluid cannot be withdrawn because it is dispersed intraperitoneally. If the needle is placed within adhesions or the preperitoneal space, the fluid usually is recovered by aspiration. If the needle has been placed intravascularly or in the intestine or bladder, characteristic contents are obtained. Additional methods of verifying proper placement of the Veress needle are summarized in Table 4.1.3. Once correct intraperitoneal placement of the Veress needle is assured, trocar-related injuries can be avoided by employing the technique of abdominal mapping before the insertion of the initial trocar. Mapping of the abdomen at the site of the trocar placement requires an 18-gauge spinal needle attached to a

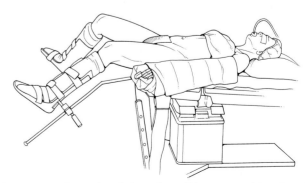

Figure 4.1.1. The patient is in a dorso-lithotomy position, but the thighs are not flexed so that the suprapubic trocars may be maneuvered.

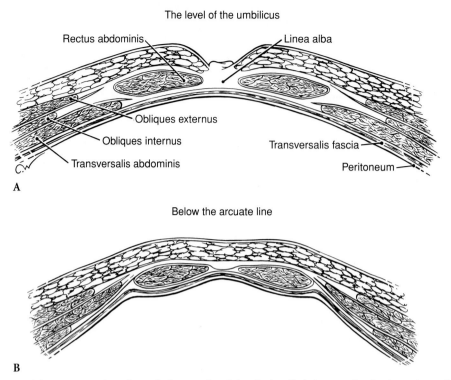

The level of the umbilicus

Rectus abdominis

Linea alba

Obliques externus

Obliques internus

Transversalis abdominis

Transversalis fascia

Peritoneum

A

Below the arcuate line

B

Figure 4.1.2. Transverse sections through the anterior abdominal wall. (**A**) Immediately above the umbilicus. (**B**) Below the arcuate line.

syringe partially filled with saline. Pneumoperitoneum is maintained through the Veress needle by using low-flow insufflation with CO_2 gas. The needle is placed transabdominally into the peritoneal cavity at several points surrounding the proposed trocar insertion site. Usually this is periumbilical. If the needle is placed in an area free of viscera or adhesions, bubbles of CO_2 gas should be seen rising through the fluid into the syringe. Mapping the abdomen will demonstrate the safest direction in which to place the primary trocar.

Alternative Sites for Insertion

Different sites may be used for insertion of the Veress needle (Figure 4.1.8), such as the left subcostal margin in the midclavicular line. This site is palpated and percussed to rule out splenomegaly or an insufflated stomach from a misplaced endotracheal tube. This site is useful, especially in patients who have had multiple previous laparotomies. The transvaginal approach is used through the posterior cul-de-sac as long as there is no evidence of pelvic thickening or masses in the cul-de-sac and the uterus is mobile.[7] This technique is effective in patients who have developed preperitoneal emphysema from unsuccessful attempts to insert the needle through the umbilicus or other abdominal sites.

Another technique is the transabdominal route through the uterine fundus.[8,9] The fundus is pushed up against the abdominal wall by using the uterine manipulator. A needle is passed through all layers of the abdomen and into the uterine fundus. As the uterus is pulled away from the tip of the needle, intra-abdominal placement is achieved. Alternatively, the Veress needle is inserted transcervically through the fundus into the abdominal cavity. These alternative methods have uncertain margins of

safety. Puncture of the uterus with this technique may result in persistent low-grade bleeding throughout the laparoscopy. Inadvertent perforation of the bladder, broad ligament perforation, and hemorrhage are possible. An intrauterine or intramyometrial position during insufflation may cause gas embolism. The technique is contraindicated if fundal adhesions are anticipated or chromopertubation is necessary.[10]

In an obese patient, proper placement of the Veress needle is difficult to achieve. If it is placed below instead of within the umbilicus at 45° to the abdominal wall, it can dissect into the preperitoneal space. It is preferable to insert the needle and trocar transumbilically and at 90°, using towel clips for traction and abdominal wall elevation (Figure 4.1.9).[11]

A survey of the existing data on the rates of failure and complications for each of the available methods of creating pneumoperitoneum showed that no technique was superior. Laparoscopists should be familiar with at least two of these techniques.[12]

PNEUMOPERITONEUM

A pneumoperitoneum is a prerequisite for laparoscopic observation and exposure to do intraperitoneal manipulations for endoscopic operations. Unless the surgeon is confident about the proper position of the Veress needle, the high flow is not used. The pressure recorded within the abdomen initially should be no greater than 9 or 10 mm Hg. If higher pressures are recorded, the needle has been placed improperly. The tip could be lodged in the omentum and can be dislodged by gently elevating and shaking the lower abdominal wall. If this maneuver fails, the needle hub is manipulated in a different direction because its distal

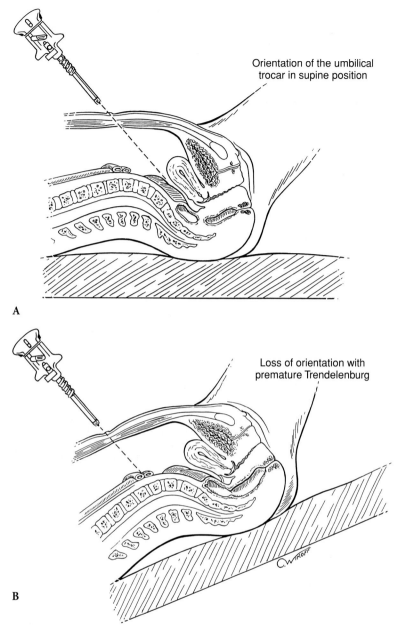

Orientation of the umbilical trocar in supine position

A

Loss of orientation with premature Trendelenburg

B

Figure 4.1.3. Angle of trocar insertion with operating table in flat (**A**) and Trendelenburg (**B**) positions.

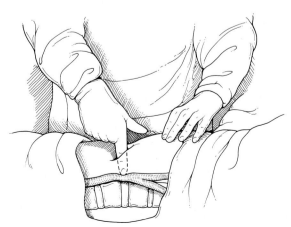

Figure 4.1.4. The aorta and sacral promontory are palpated.

hole could impinge on the anterior abdominal wall. If neither of these techniques relieves the increased recorded pressure, the Veress needle is removed and reinserted. Occasionally, while it is passing through the different layers of the abdomen, tissue lodges in the tip, obstructing the opening. Whenever the Veress needle is withdrawn because of high recorded pressures, the surgeon should check its patency.

After 1 L of CO_2 is insufflated, the surgeon percusses the right costal margin to check for loss of liver dullness. If liver dullness is detected, the Veress needle may be positioned improperly and is withdrawn and reinserted. The surgeon should use palpable abdominal distention and the pressure reading rather than the volume of gas insufflated because they more accurately reflect the adequacy of the pneumoperitoneum. After insertion of the trocars, the intra-abdominal pressure should be preset between 12 and 16 mm Hg during the operative procedure. Higher

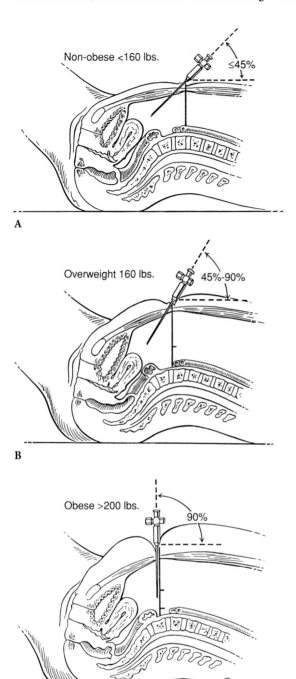

Figure 4.1.5. Note the anatomic location of the umbilicus and abdominal aorta in nonobese (**A**), overweight (**B**), and obese (**C**) patients.

pressures for long periods may cause subcutaneous emphysema.

PLACEMENT OF THE PRIMARY TROCAR

The sharp primary trocar is aimed toward the sacral promontory. Dull trocars require increased force during insertion, multiple insertions, and excessive instrument manipulation. The insertion of a disposable shielded trocar in the presence of a pneu-

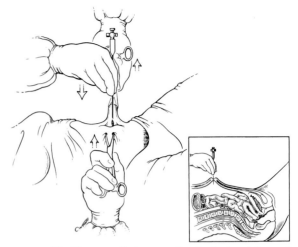

Figure 4.1.6. The Veress needle is grasped by the shaft and directed posteriorly at a 90° angle. Inset shows elevation of skin and subcutaneous tissue.

moperitoneum requires half the force needed for the insertion of a reusable sharp trocar. The disposable trocar shield does not prevent injury completely.[13] Using these new devices may inflict injury because of the unexpected ease of their insertion. Numerous mesenteric, bowel, and vascular injuries have been reported with the use of disposable trocars.

A pneumoperitoneum reduces the proximity of the abdominal wall to the spine and the potential for damage to bowel and vessels.[14] Whether a pneumoperitoneum is associated with a lower incidence of trocar-related injuries is unproved.

Conventional Technique

The direction of trocar insertion is 90° to the abdominal wall plane toward the sacral promontory. Control of the laparoscopic trocar is essential as it penetrates each layer of the anterior abdominal wall. The trocar is inserted with the patient in a horizontal position because viscera tend to slide away from the advancing trocar. A premature Trendelenburg position does not prevent visceral injury, even if significant adhesions are present. Altering the patient's position affects the surgeon's view of important landmarks such as the sacral promontory and sacral hollow. The major anatomic landmarks include the umbilicus, located at the level of L3 and L4. The abdominal aorta bifurcates between L4 and L5 (Figure 4.1.4).

Recent studies measuring the thickness of the abdominal wall at the umbilicus favor a vertical orientation and insertion through the base of the umbilicus while elevating the periumbilical skin with towel clips. Roy [15] measured the thickness of the abdominal wall at the base of the umbilicus and at the lower margin of the umbilicus. His group determined the trocar traverses a shorter distance when oriented perpendicular to the abdominal wall in the base of the umbilicus. Additionally, omental and bowel adhesions to the anterior abdominal wall are often seen extending inferiorly from the umbilicus following pelvic surgery. Orientation of the trocar at 45° will direct the instrument into this area, whereas a perpendicular orientation may enter cephalad to the adhesions. Performed with care, a controlled entry in this

Table 4.1.3: Tests to Confirm the Proper Position of the Veress Needle

1. Injection and aspiration of fluid through the Veress needle
2. Loss of liver dullness early in insufflation
3. Hanging drop test
4. An unimpeded arc of rotation of the needle to detect anterior abdominal wall adhesions
5. Sound of air entering Veress needle with elevation of the abdominal wall
6. Free flow of gas through the Veress needle
7. Observation of the fluctuation of pressure gauge needle with inspiratory and expiratory diaphragmatic motions

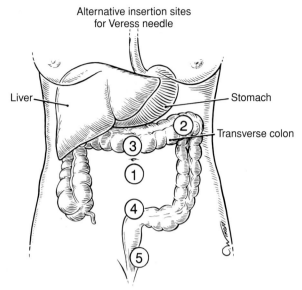

Figure 4.1.8. Alternative sites for Veress needle insertion. (1) Infra- or intraumbilical. (2) Left upper quadrant, midclavicular. (3) Supraumbilical. (4) Midline suprapubic. (5) Transcervical through the uterine fundus or transvaginal through the posterior fornix into the abdominal cavity.

fashion will prevent injury to the great vessels at the level of the sacral promontory.

In a program for laparoscopic sterilization, Soderstrom and Butler [16] revealed that the complication rate was reduced 10-fold when a consistent operating format was used. Successful insertion depends on an adequate skin incision; trocars in good working condition (disposable trocars should be checked to be sure they are not locked); proper orientation of the trocar, sheath, and surgeon's hand; and control over the instrument's force and depth of insertion.

With all trocar insertions, the surgeon must hold the instrument properly, with the patient in a supine position at the height of the surgeon's waist or slightly below it. The trocar and its sleeve are held with the index finger extended to the level of the maximal planned penetration to prevent the sharp trocar tip from

thrusting too deeply. The trocar is palmed, and the dominant hand is used for this procedure. It is rotated in a semicircular fashion with its long axis as controlled, firm downward pressure is applied (Figure 4.1.9). As the trocar is advanced, the operator senses when the fascia is traversed; the force is reduced as the

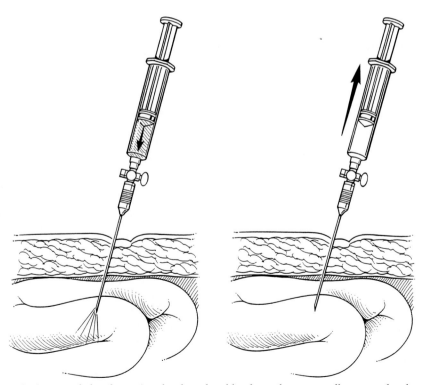

Figure 4.1.7. Syringe test helps determine that bowel or blood vessels are not adherent under the umbilicus before trocar insertion. A 10-mL syringe with 5 mL of normal saline is attached to the Veress needle, and aspiration verifies the absence of bowel contents or blood.

Table 4.1.4: Comparison of Veress Needle and Direct Trocar Insertion

	Veress Needle (n = 100)	Direct Trocar Insertion (n = 100)
Complications	22	3
Two insertions required	20	20
Failed insertions	3	6

Table 4.1.5: Comparison of Reusable and Disposable Trocars

	Reusable (n = 50)	Disposable (n = 50)
Complications	3	0
Two insertions required	10	10
Failed insertions	4	s2

trocar is advanced slowly to enter the peritoneum. Disposable bullet-tip trocars are preferable. A disposable shielded trocar has two advantages: a safety shield that snaps into position after the peritoneum is entered and a sharp instrument for each operation.

Direct Insertion

Trocar insertion without creating a pneumoperitoneum initially reduces the number of preliminary procedures, saving operative time and preventing potential complications. Direct insertion is a safe alternative to initially creating a pneumoperitoneum.[17–24] Nezhat and associates [17] compared the ease and safety of creating a pneumoperitoneum with those of direct insertion of either a reusable trocar or a disposable shielded trocar in 200 patients in a randomized, prospectively controlled study. Complications of 22%, 6%, and 0%, respectively, were observed. Although there were fewer complications from direct insertion, no differences were noted in the ease of insertion or the frequency of multiple attempts (Tables 4.1.4 and 4.1.5).

The technique is done by elevating the abdominal wall with towel clips applied close to the umbilicus. After the trocar is inserted into the peritoneal cavity, the laparoscope is introduced to verify its correct intraperitoneal placement. A pneumoperi-

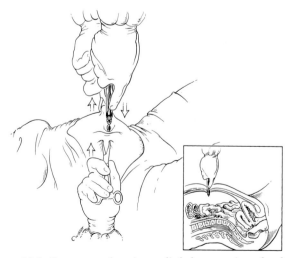

Figure 4.1.9. Countertraction is applied by grasping the lower abdomen; the surgeon inserts the trocar into the abdomen by palming it and using the index finger as a guard against sudden entry into the abdomen. Inset shows the portion of the trocar and intestines.

toneum is created with high-flow insufflation. At our centers in Atlanta, Georgia, and Palo Alto, California, direct trocar insertion is used, except in patients who have had multiple laparotomies. Since 1989, more than 4500 direct trocar insertions have been done without major complications.

In a randomized comparison of Veress needle and direct trocar insertion, Byron and Markenson [24] reported no major complications with either technique. Complications such as preperitoneal insufflation, failed entry, and needing more than three attempts to enter the peritoneal cavity were more common ($P < 0.05$) in the Veress needle group. Additionally, the mean times for doing the laparoscopic procedure using the direct insertion and Veress needle techniques were 15.3 and 19.6 minutes ($P < 0.01$), respectively, in 113 patients who underwent sterilization procedures.

Open Laparoscopy

In 1971, Hasson [25] introduced the concept of open laparoscopy to eliminate the risks associated with insertion of the Veress needle and trocar. This technique involves direct trocar insertion through a small skin incision without prior pneumoperitoneum. Specially designed equipment consists of a cannula and trumpet valve fitted with a cone-shaped stainless steel sleeve. A blunt obturator protrudes 1 cm from the tip of the cannula. The cone sleeve seals the peritoneal and fascial gap.

A small transverse, curved, or vertical incision is made at the umbilicus. Two Allis clamps, a knife handle with a small blade, a straight scissors, a tissue forceps with teeth, a right-angle skin hook, four S-shaped retractors, a needle holder, two curved Kocher clamps, and four small curved hemostats are needed. As the incision is made, Allis clamps or a self-retaining retractor are used to provide adequate exposure. Once the fascia is cut, a 1-cm incision is made in the peritoneum. One suture of 0 polydioxanone (Ethicon) is passed through each peritoneal edge and fascia and tagged. The corklike cannula carrying the blunt obturator is inserted through the opening into the peritoneal cavity. The obturator is withdrawn, and CO_2 is insufflated through the cannula, which is inserted as deep as required to prevent leakage. The previously placed sutures are used to fix the trocar sleeve so that the laparoscope can move freely within the abdominal cavity. At the end of the procedure, the abdominal wall is closed, using the previously placed sutures.

Open laparoscopy usually takes about 5 to 10 minutes longer than closed laparoscopy done by operators with comparable expertise. In more than 1000 consecutive operations done by Hasson [25], the frequency of minor wound infection was 0.6% and that of small bowel injury was 0.1%. In a review of the laparoscopic complications, the open techniques reduced the incidence of failed procedures, inappropriate gas insufflation, gas embolism, bladder and pelvic kidney punctures, major vessel injuries, and postoperative herniations.[26]

In a survey conducted by Penfield [27], intestinal laceration was the most serious complication of open laparoscopy, and most of those lacerations occurred during the early use of this technique. In 10,840 open laparoscopies attempted by 18 board-certified obstetrician/gynecologists, six bowel lacerations were reported, four were recognized and repaired, and two were not suspected until several days postoperatively.

To reduce the risk of bowel laceration, the surgeon should use a focus spotlight, work with an experienced assistant, make a vertical incision to facilitate exposure, grasp and elevate the fascia with small Kocher clamps, and cut between the clamps. A gynecologist who attempts open laparoscopy only in special situations will find that the procedure is slow and cumbersome because of difficulty in exposing and identifying each layer of the abdominal wall.

ACCESSORY TROCARS

Additional cannulas are needed through which various instruments are inserted into the abdomen for manipulation and operative procedures. Placement sites depend on the patient's anatomy, the contemplated procedure, and the surgeon's preference. For diagnostic purposes, an incision generally is made 4 to 5 cm above the symphysis pubis in the midline. This area, delineated by the two umbilical ligaments and the bladder dome, is safe and usually avascular.

For operative laparoscopy, two accessory trocars (5 mm) are placed 4 to 5 cm above the symphysis pubis at the outer border of the rectus muscle, 3 to 4 cm below the iliac crest, 2 to 3 cm lateral to the deep inferior epigastric vessels. These trocars are inserted under direct vision to lessen the risk of intra-abdominal visceral, uterine, and vascular injury and to provide free access to the posterior cul-de-sac. Vascularization of the lower abdomen is provided by two vessels: the deep inferior epigastric originating from the external iliac artery and the superficial epigastric, a branch of the femoral artery. Transillumination helps identify the superficial vessels, but they are difficult to see in obese patients. The deep inferior epigastric vessels run lateral to the umbilical ligaments (Figure 4.1.10) and are seen intraperitoneally and identified easily. These vessels pass the round ligament, proceed to the anterior abdominal wall, and are seen above the peritoneum. To avoid injuring these vessels, the trocar is inserted medial or lateral to the umbilical ligaments by viewing the underside of the abdomen wall laparoscopically (Figure 4.1.11). Despite these precautions, aberrant vascular branches occasionally are traumatized, and the operator must be able to manage this type of injury.

To reduce the chance of trauma to the abdominal structures, the proposed site for the secondary puncture is indented by applying abdominal pressure with the index finger and observing the peritoneal surface with the laparoscope. Next, mapping of the potential sites for accessory trocar placement is done by advancing the tip of an 18-gauge needle attached to a syringe transabdominally through the peritoneum, revealing the exact course and placement of the accessory trocar. This allows optimal placement. These maneuvers are important, particularly in a patient

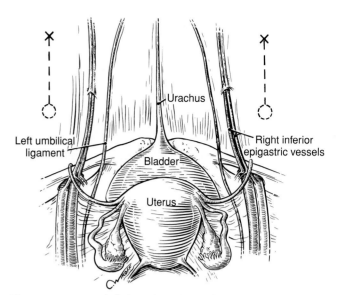

Figure 4.1.10. Deep inferior epigastric vessels run lateral to the umbilical ligaments.

with evidence of abdominal wall adhesions, and help ensure safe access.

The trocar, held with the index finger extended on the sheath to control the depth of penetration, is inserted through the skin, fat, and fascia. Further advancement is controlled under a laparoscopic view (Figure 4.1.11). The trocar is aimed toward the center of the abdomen and hollow of the sacrum. If it is aimed laterally, it can slide down the pelvic side wall without being seen through the laparoscope, resulting in injury to the iliac vessels. The accessory trocars are never inserted without laparoscopic observation of their indentation on the abdominal wall or before mapping the abdomen. When insertion of the trocars is viewed directly from the monitor, the surgeon should be sure the camera has not been rotated so that it shows the wrong view of the pelvis. Most laparoscopic procedures do not require more than two or three accessory trocars. Other sites of entry include the midpoint between the symphysis pubis and the umbilicus and McBurney's point.

Some accessory trocar sleeves are too long to allow free access to the pelvic structures and tend to slip out of the peritoneal cavity. The presence of trap valves may interfere with efficient instrument exchange, prevent the introduction and removal of suture material, and prevent the removal of tissue. Several accessory trocar sleeves either screw in or have an umbrella to secure them to the abdominal wall. Radially expanding trocars may reduce laparoscopic complications, lessen a surgeon's exposure to liability, and improve patient outcomes.[28] Two hundred twelve women underwent various laparoscopic procedures involving the placement of 541 radially expanding access cannulas, and no major complications occurred. One patient developed a postoperative mesenteric hematoma that was assumed to be secondary to a venous injury from the Veress needle. Despite the absence of fascial anchoring devices, only six cannulas (1%) slipped.

Accessory Sites

Examples of single accessory site procedures include tubal sterilization, aspiration of an ovarian cyst, and mild peritubal and

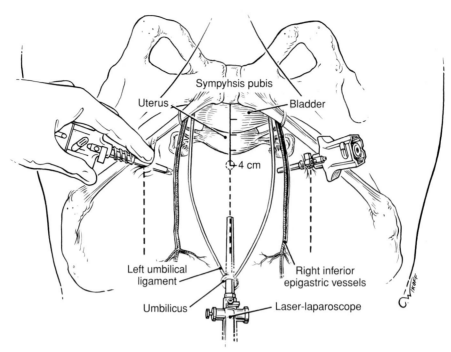

Figure 4.1.11. Accessory trocars are placed under direct vision to avoid injury to the inferior epigastric vessels and any organs that may be adherent to the pelvic side wall or the anterior abdominal wall. The trocar is inserted lateral to the left umbilical ligament, avoiding inferior epigastric vessels that are invariably lateral to umbilical ligaments.

peri-ovarian adhesiolysis. The suction–irrigator probe is placed through a suprapubic trocar site. Two accessory sites are suggested for lysing peritubal and peri-ovarian adhesions, doing a salpingectomy, removing an ectopic pregnancy, or excising moderate pelvic endometriosis. The suction–irrigator and one additional instrument are needed. Traction is required for these procedures. The suction–irrigator is used for manipulation and smoke evacuation. Bipolar forceps replace the grasping instruments if necessary to achieve hemostasis. For procedures requiring traction, hemostasis, and suturing almost simultaneously, three sites are necessary. Examples are salpingo-oophorectomy, hysterectomy, repair of an ovarian or uterine incisional defect, lysis of extensive abdominal or pelvic adhesions, myomectomy, and cystectomy. During oophorectomy, the infundibulopelvic ligament is grasped with forceps for traction. The assistant holds the grasping forceps, and the surgeon uses the bipolar electrocoagulator to desiccate the infundibulopelvic ligament. The forceps are removed and held by an assistant. The surgeon uses the suction–irrigator probe, and while the plume is suctioned, the CO_2 laser is used for excision. During reconstructive procedures, the operator can give the videolaparoscope to the assistant, freeing the operator's hands for applying traction and suturing. An assistant maintains traction with the grasping forceps as the surgeon uses the needle driver. As with other techniques, surgeons modify procedures as they gain experience.

Operative laparoscopy enables a physician to do complex, delicate procedures through small incisions, thus decreasing the patient's discomfort, morbidity, expense, and duration of convalescence.[29] Laparoscopy is a technique for accessing the patient's diseased organs and gives the surgeon an opportunity to remove abnormal tissue and reconstruct damaged organs.

HIGH-RISK PATIENTS

Body Habitus

Special considerations are required for obese patients because the trocar is inserted almost vertically. The distance between the sacral promontory and the trocar tip is relatively small, and there is a risk to the major vessels. In thin patients, it is safer to overdistend the abdomen with CO_2 before trocar insertion. The force required to introduce the trocar is less than anticipated because the fascia is thin and offers little resistance.

Bowel Distention

Bowel distention secondary to obstruction is a relative contraindication to laparoscopy. This condition may be iatrogenic, resulting from the placement of the Veress needle within the bowel lumen. The filling pressure of the small bowel is the same as that of the abdominal cavity because of the intestine's large capacity. The operator, unaware of the possibility of an "apparent" pneumoperitoneum, might lacerate the distended bowel during the insertion of the trocar.

Previous Laparotomy

In women who have had previous laparotomies, the underlying intra-abdominal anatomy may be altered. Inflexible adhesive bridging between the intestine and the abdominal wall can nullify any protection from trocar injury afforded by elevating the abdominal wall, creating a pneumoperitoneum, using the Trendelenburg position, and maintaining intestinal mobility. In some patients, injury will occur to adherent omental vessels or directly

Table 4.1.6: Patients by Type and Number of Incisions

Incision Type	1	2	3	4	5	6	Total Patients
Pfannenstiel	180	51	19	4	4	0	258
Midline below umbilicus	55	18	9	4	0	1	87
Midline above umbilicus	10	2	1	2	0	0	15

No. Incisions spans columns 1–6.

Table 4.1.7: Incidence of Adhesions after Previous Laparotomy

Type of Incision	No.	Percent	Omental,%	Bowel,%
Pfannenstiel	258	72	23	4
Midline below umbilicus	87	24	46	9
Midline above umbilicus	15	4	40	27
Total	360	100		

Table 4.1.8: Patients by Clinical Indication and Incision Type

Incision Type	Gynecologic	Obstetric
Pfannenstiel	186	43
Midline above or below umbilicus	73	12
Total	259	55

to the bowel wall. The patients at the highest risk are those who have undergone major abdominal surgery, such as bowel resection, or an exploratory laparotomy for abdominal trauma or ovarian carcinoma.[5] Women who have had an uncomplicated abdominal operation are not at increased risk.

The association between intestinal and omental adhesions and injury to those structures during operative laparoscopy was evaluated in 360 patients who previously had undergone a variety of abdominal operations (Tables 4.1.6 through 4.1.8).[30]

The following approach is recommended:

1. Patients with prior midline incisions have more adhesions than do those with prior Pfannenstiel incisions.
2. Patients with multiple prior incisions do not have more adhesions than do those with a single prior incision.
3. The presence of adhesions does not have a linear correlation with increasing numbers of prior incisions.
4. Women with prior midline or Pfannenstiel incisions for gynecologic operations have more adhesions than do those who have undergone obstetric operations.
5. Patients with prior midline incisions for obstetric operations do not have more adhesions than do those with a prior Pfannenstiel incision for obstetric operations.

The following conditions were associated with severe adhesions:

1. Generalized peritonitis
2. Bowel resection after intestinal obstruction
3. Oncologic procedure with omentectomy
4. Previous radiation and intraperitoneal chemotherapy
5. Previous adhesions

During insertion of the primary trocar and entry into the abdominal cavity, intestinal injuries occurred in 21 instances (6%; Table 4.1.9). Of these injuries, six were to the small bowel. Only one patient had a single incision; the remaining five had multiple incisions and complicated surgical histories. Two small bowel injuries occurred during open laparoscopy. In these two patients, the small bowel was attached to the anterior abdominal wall, directly under the umbilicus. It was entered during incision of the fascia that was attached to the intestine. With the exception of 32 patients in whom open laparoscopy was done, the closed technique with prior establishment of pneumoperitoneum was used. The use of open laparoscopy was based on the patients' surgical history (bowel resection, bowel obstruction, ovarian cancer surgery) and the surgeons' preoperative judgment.

The attachment of the bowel and omentum to the abdominal wall is primarily distal to the umbilicus (Figure 4.1.12A). If the insertion of the trocar is more vertical than oblique, the possibility of bowel injury is low if a disposable trocar with a shield is used. In patients who have had complicated abdominal operations (bowel resection, bowel obstruction, etc.), the bowel may be attached under, very close to, or occasionally above the umbilicus (Figure 4.1.12B).

In a subsequent study, the safety of direct trocar insertion was evaluated in 246 consecutive women with previous uncomplicated Pfannenstiel or midline incisions. All of them underwent bowel preparation and understood that laparotomy was possible. Trocar insertion was almost at a 90° angle while the operator and the assistant elevated the abdominal wall, lateral to the umbilicus. Fifty patients had omental adhesions, and 34 had bowel adhesions to the anterior abdominal wall. There were no small bowel injuries. There were five omental injuries; in one, the injury was associated with bleeding and was managed laparoscopically.

On the basis of these findings, it can be concluded that the incidence of subumbilical bowel adhesions and subsequent bowel injury is related to the indication for previous laparotomy rather than to the type or number of previous laparotomies. The incidence of bowel injuries during insertion of the primary trocar is low. The closed technique with or without prior establishment of a pneumoperitoneum is used in most instances without increasing the chance of bowel injury.

Special Techniques

Several procedures have been described to assess the anterior abdominal wall for intestinal adhesions. DeCherney [31] advocates using a small-gauge needle laparoscope 2 to 3 mm in diameter. The needle scope is inserted instead of the Veress needle under direct vision through the umbilical, preperitoneal, and subperitoneal structures. The Veress needle is inserted intra-abdominally, and insufflation proceeds under direct observation.

Table 4.1.9: Incidence of Injury – 21/360 (6%)

Type of Injury	Omental Hematoma (Closed Technique)		Omental Bleeding (Closed Technique)		Small Bowel Injury (Closed, 6; Open, 2)	
	Single	Multiple	Single	Multiple	Single	Multiple
Number	1	5	7	2	1	5
Percent	0.3	1.4	1.9	0.6	0.3	1.4

Exploring the periumbilical area with an 18-gauge needle attached to a syringe after establishing the pneumoperitoneum (Figure 4.1.13) also is possible. If adhesions are detected by these techniques, the options include open laparoscopy and alternative sites of abdominal entry. The primary trocar is inserted in the midline between the xiphoid and the pubic symphysis provided that care is taken to remain at least 5 cm below the xiphoid and 5 cm above the pubic symphysis (Figure 4.1.8).[16] Although these techniques help detect periumbilical adhesions, they are not definitive and are time consuming. Based on these observations, the following approach is recommended:

1. Patients who have had a previous laparotomy are allocated to noncomplicated and complicated groups.
2. One-day or 3-day bowel preparation is administered, based on the patient's history. All patients must understand that bowel injury is possible and must consent to a possible conversion of the procedure to laparotomy.
3. In the noncomplicated group, open or closed techniques are used. If the closed technique is used, a disposable trocar with a bullet shield is preferable. Trocar entry is controlled, and the placement angle is vertical rather than oblique (Figure 4.1.14). Either previous establishment of a pneumoperitoneum by a Veress needle or direct trocar insertion is used. If the Veress needle is used, the subumbilical area is searched for bowel adhesions before trocar insertion. If adhesions are suspected, other locations are explored until a safe area is detected and the trocar is inserted. In patients at risk for significant adhesions, a pneumoperitoneum is created by inserting the Veress needle transumbilically or in the left subcostal area in the midclavicular line after aspirating with a syringe to rule out bowel entry. The abdomen is insufflated with CO_2. The area is explored with a 20-gauge needle to inject saline (Figure 4.1.13). If no fluid is aspirated (the conditions are favorable), a 5-mm trocar is inserted and a 4-mm laparoscope is placed to observe the peritoneal cavity (Figure 4.1.14). If there is no intestinal injury, the 5-mm trocar is replaced with the 10-mm trocar. If intestinal entry occurs, the 5-mm trocar is left in place and a safe area is found to insert the 10-mm trocar and laparoscope. The loops of injured bowel are mobilized and repaired laparoscopically or through a minilaparotomy.[2] Since this approach was adopted, no bowel injuries have

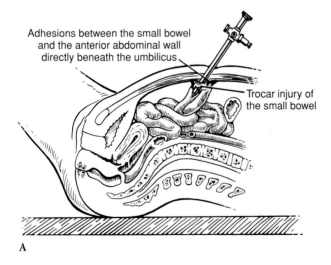

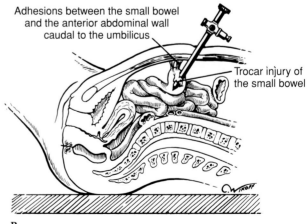

Figure 4.1.12. The bowel is attached to the anterior abdominal wall. (**A**) The bowel is attached directly under the umbilicus. (**B**) The attachment is below and distal to the umbilicus.

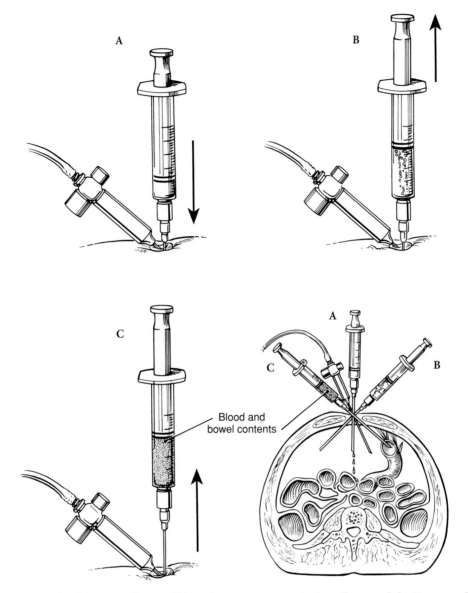

Figure 4.1.13. The abdomen is "mapped" by using an 18-gauge spinal needle around the Veress needle. A 20-gauge needle is inserted under negative pressure at several cardinal points of a 20-mm circle around the umbilicus. If blood or bowel content is aspirated instead of CO_2 gas at any of these points, alternative sites for trocar insertion should be chosen.

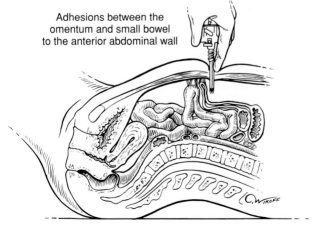

Figure 4.1.14. This patient had bowel adhesions from a previous laparotomy.

been observed resulting from trocar insertion in more than 700 patients with different types of laparotomies for different indications. Another instrument that may be helpful is the 2-mm microlaparoscope for initial intra-abdominal evaluation. If the patient has undergone an adequate bowel preparation, an incidental bowel perforation can be managed conservatively after thorough and extensive irrigation of the abdominal cavity, unlike similar injuries caused by the 4-mm laparoscope.

4. For patients in the complicated group, a mapping technique is used to lessen the chance of sequelae. After insertion of the laparoscope, the abdominal wall with adherent bowel or omentum is explored. If the adhesions are severe and no clear space for accessory trocar insertion is seen, the abdominal wall is observed through the laparoscope and gentle external compression is done, marking areas that seem free of adhesions.

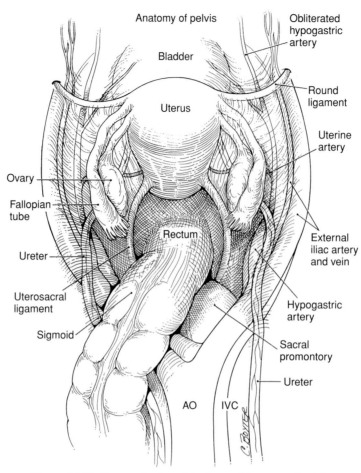

Figure 4.1.15. Panoramic view of the lower abdomen and pelvis.

Before inserting the trocar, the surgeon should simulate its track with a 21-gauge spinal needle. If this identifies a clear path, the trocar is introduced next to the needle, or the needle is removed and the trocar is introduced. An advantage of first inserting the 21-gauge needle is its small diameter, because the injury incurred does not require repair. As the needle's placement is seen, there is little risk of missing a visceral injury. The insertion of the needle through the skin of the abdominal wall is easy, so the surgeon can control the needle precisely and prevent any deviation from the present course.

PELVIC EXPLORATION

The initial phase of laparoscopy is done to assess the extent of disease, document it with photographs or video recordings, and identify anatomic landmarks. The characteristics of the bladder, ureters, colon, rectum, uterosacral ligaments, and major blood vessels are noted (Figure 4.1.15). The appendix is inspected for endometriosis. The upper abdomen, including the abdominal walls, liver, gallbladder, and diaphragm, is examined for any abnormality that could contribute to the patient's symptoms. As the laparoscope is turned toward the left, the intestine is evaluated, and then the laparoscope is returned to view the pelvic cavity. The omentum and intestines are examined to confirm

that they were not injured during insertion of the Veress needle and trocar.

After the posterior cul-de-sac is filled with irrigation fluid, the right adnexa are assessed. The fimbriae are lifted, and the posterior aspect of the ovary and the ovarian fossa are evaluated. The ureter is seen, and its direction is traced from the pelvic brim to the bladder. The uterus is anteverted, and the uterosacral ligaments, posterior cul-de-sac, and rectum are examined. The patient is placed in a 30° Trendelenburg position to allow the surgeon to push the small bowel into the upper abdomen to aid in viewing the posterior cul-de-sac (Figure 4.1.16). The rectosigmoid colon and its folds are evaluated, and after the rectosigmoid colon is pushed laterally, the left and right pararectal areas are examined. The left ovary and tube are evaluated. In the presence of extensive adhesions, this technique is modified. The gynecologist ascertains the approximate location of the normal structures, assesses the type of adhesion, plans the procedure, and decides whether the procedure is to be done by laparoscopy or laparotomy. This decision depends on the abnormalities, the time needed to correct them, and the surgeon's experience.

END OF THE OPERATION

Chromopertubation is done in all infertility patients intraoperatively. The patient's position is changed from Trendelenburg

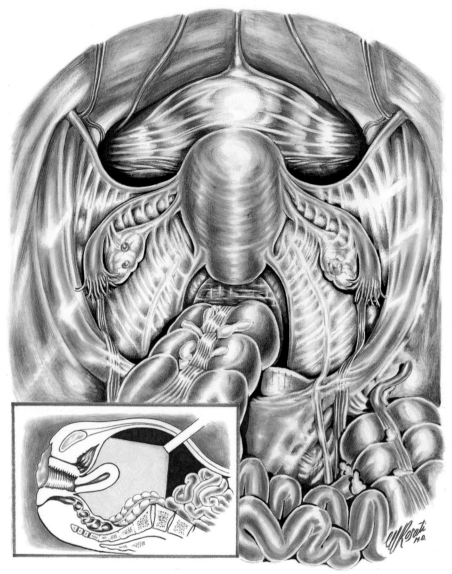

Figure 4.1.16. The patient is placed in a Trendelenburg position. Inset shows the elevation of the pelvis.

to horizontal to allow fluid from the upper abdomen to collect in the pelvic cavity. The entire peritoneal cavity is irrigated copiously with isotonic fluid, usually lactated Ringer's solution, and inspected for blood clots, pieces of adhesions, cyst wall, endometriosis implants, and bleeding. Bleeding points are identified and coagulated with bipolar forceps. Because the intra-abdominal pressure created by the pneumoperitoneum can tamponade bleeding from small vessels, the gas is evacuated temporarily and the operative sites are inspected for bleeding before the abdominal cavity is reinsufflated. The presence of clear irrigating fluid confirms adequate hemostasis. The procedure is concluded by evacuating the CO_2 from the abdomen.

Release of Pneumoperitoneum

The CO_2 used to distend the abdomen is evacuated to reduce postoperative shoulder pain caused by gas trapped under the diaphragm. The patient is put in a straight, supine position as the gas escapes from the umbilical and suprapubic trocars. Suprapu-

bic trocars are removed under low pneumoperitoneal pressure to search for possible inferior epigastric vessel injury. The umbilical trocar is removed, and the skin incisions are inspected for bleeding. Except for patients in whom Interceed (Ethicon) is applied, 300 to 400 mL of lactated Ringer's solution is left in the abdominal cavity to aid in displacing the gas and possibly to decrease postoperative adhesions.[32] Since this procedure was instituted, the prevalence of postoperative shoulder pain has decreased.

Closure of Incisions

The trocar incisions are closed using Steri-Strips or inverted subcutaneous 4–0 polyglactin (Ethicon) sutures. Incisions made for trocars larger than 5 mm are closed in layers, especially in older or thin women, because failure to close the fascia has been associated with small bowel strangulation and hernia. Several instruments, including the J-needle and the Carter–Thomason needle (Figure 4.1.17), have been developed to allow for fascial and peritoneal closure of the trocar site incisions under direct observation.

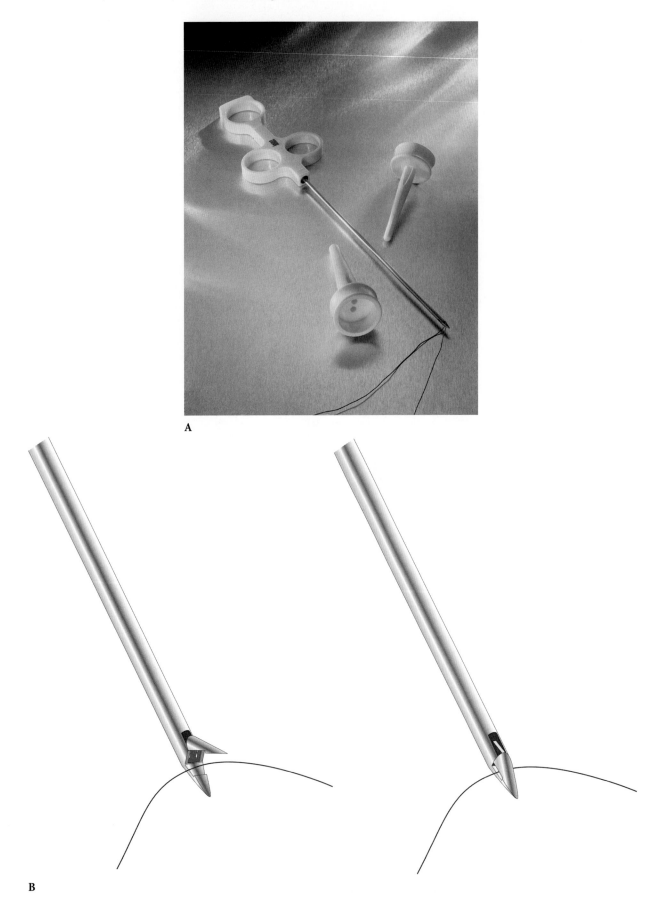

A

B

Figure 4.1.17. The Carter–Thomason needle. The system allows the passage of suture through soft tissue and then retrieval from a separate entry with the same device. (**A**) The CloseSure Procedure Kit (Inlet Medical Inc.) contains the Carter–Thomason suture passer and the Pilot suturing guides. (**B**) A stepdown from the distal to proximal segment of the jaws allows the distal tip to close completely with the suture in the proximal stepdown segment. (*Continued*)

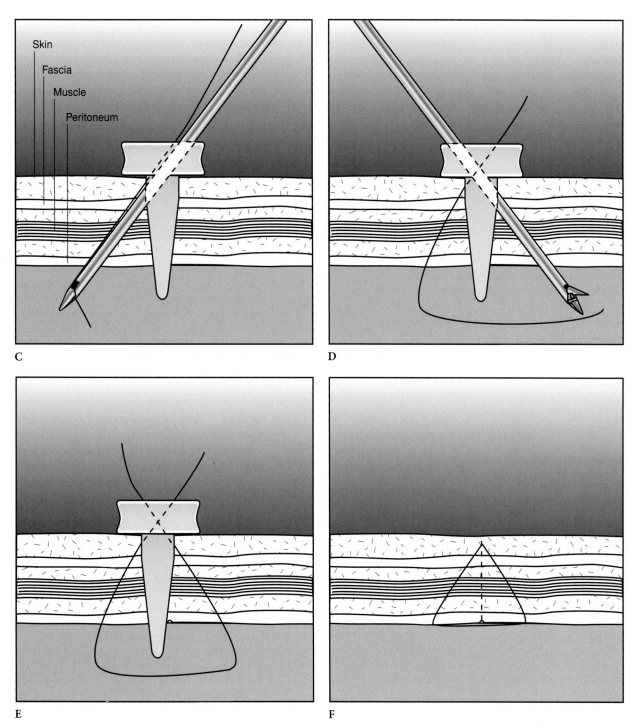

C

D

E

F

Figure 4.1.17. (continued) (**C**) A suture passer is used to push suture material through the Pilot guide, fascia, muscle, and peritoneum and into the abdomen. The suture is dropped, and the suture passer is removed. (**D**) The suture passer is pushed through opposite side of the Pilot guide and used to pick up the suture. (**E**) The suture passer is removed, pulling the suture through the peritoneum, muscle, fascia, and guide. (**F**) The guide is removed, and the suture is tied to complete the closure.

POSTOPERATIVE CARE

Patients are provided with postoperative instructions before the operation to prepare them for the postoperative experience. The gynecologist sees the patient in the outpatient extended recovery room to explain the operative findings and the expected postoperative course. Before discharge, patients are given prescriptions for pain medications (usually Tylenol with codeine) as needed and routine postoperative instructions. Outpatient nurses or office nurses contact the patient 1 or 2 days postoperatively to answer additional questions and monitor her recovery. If a patient complains of pain, fever, or bowel or bladder symptoms, she is examined promptly. Patients routinely are seen 1 to 6 weeks postoperatively. Most women return to normal activity within 1 week. The time required for full recovery is between 1 and 3 weeks, depending on the extent of the operation.

Common Postoperative Complaints

Nausea and vomiting most likely are related to intra-abdominal CO_2 and the narcotics frequently used perioperatively. Usually these symptoms respond to parenteral antiemetic medication, but patients occasionally are admitted overnight for continued care. Shoulder pain referred from the collection of CO_2 under the diaphragm is the most common complaint and generally resolves within 48 hours. Resting on the abdomen with pillows under it is helpful. Elevating the lower pelvis also will alleviate this pain.

Occasionally a patient develops hypotension unrelated to blood loss. These patients are cured promptly after a bolus of intravenous fluid is given.

Postoperative incisional pain is usually mild and is managed by using a heating pad and analgesics. A randomized, double-blinded trial of preemptive analgesia in laparoscopy patients concluded that the administration of bupivacaine before laparoscopy results in decreased postoperative pain compared with the popular practice of infiltrating bupivacaine at the time of incision closure.[33] Patients who undergo extensive intra-abdominal procedures may have severe visceral pain. Narcotic or nonsteroidal anti-inflammatory agents are needed in addition to a heating pad. Persistent pain for more than a few hours after release from the hospital requires that the patient be examined.

When large amounts of isotonic fluid are left in the abdomen, the patient tends to drain pinkish fluid through the abdominal puncture wounds. This ceases within 24 to 48 hours. Reassurance allays the patient's concern.

To become proficient with operative laparoscopy, a gynecologist must understand the learning curve and begin with simple procedures before gradually advancing to more complicated ones. Complications may occur during the simplest procedures. The primary steps are exposure (by identifying the anatomy and pathology), traction, and action (cutting, vaporization, hemostasis, or suturing). The gynecologist holds the video-laproscope with the dominant hand. Most procedures require only one or two accessory instruments.

REFERENCES

1. Palmer R. La coelioscopie gynecologique, ses possibilities et ses indications actuelles. *Semin Hop Paris*. 1954;30:4441.
2. Nezhat CR, Nezhat FR, Silfen SL. Videolaseroscopy: the CO_2 laser for advanced operative laparoscopy. *Obstet Gynecol Clin North Am*. 1991;18:585.
3. Nezhat C, Nezhat F, Pennington E. Laparoscopic treatment of infiltrative rectosigmoid colon and rectovaginal septum endometriosis by the technique of videolaseroscopy and the CO_2 laser. *Br J Obstet Gynaecol*. 1992;99:664.
4. East MC, Steele PRM. Laparoscopic incisions at the lower umbilical verge. *Br Med J*. 1988;296:753.
5. Loffer FD. Endoscopy in high risk patients. In: Martin DC, ed. *Manual of Endoscopy*. Santa Fe Springs, CA: American Association of Gynecologic Laparoscopists; 1990.
6. Nezhat F, Brill AI, Nezhat CH, et al. Laparoscopic appraisal of the anatomic relationship of the umbilicus to the aortic bifurcation. *J Am Assoc Gynecol Laparosc*. 1998;5:135.
7. Neely MR, McWilliams R, Makhlouf HA. Laparoscopy: routine pneumoperitoneum via the posterior fornix. *Obstet Gynecol*. 1975;45:459.
8. Wolfe WM, Pasic R. Transuterine insertion of Veress needle in laparoscopy. *Obstet Gynecol*. 1990;75:456.
9. Morgan HR. Laparoscopy: induction of pneumoperitoneum via transfundal puncture. *Obstet Gynecol*. 1979;54:260.
10. Awadalla SG. Letter to the editor. *Obstet Gynecol*. 1990;76:314.
11. Loffer FD, Pent D. Laparoscopy in the obese patient. *Am J Obstet Gynecol*. 1976;125:104.
12. Rosen DM, Lam AM, Chapman M, et al. Methods of creating pneumoperitoneum: a review of techniques and complications. *Obstet Gynecol Surv*. 1998;53:167.
13. Corson SL, Batzer FR, Gocial B, Maislin C. Measurement of the force necessary for laparoscopic entry. *J Reprod Med*. 1989;34:282.
14. Phillips JM. *Laparoscopy*. Baltimore: Williams & Wilkins; 1977.
15. Roy G, Bazzurini L, Solima E, Luciano A. Safe technique for laparoscopic entry into the abdominal cavity. *J Am Assoc Gynecol Laparosc*. 2001;8:519–528.
16. Soderstrom RM, Butler JC. A critical evaluation of complications in laparoscopy. *J Reprod Med*. 1973;10:245.
17. Nezhat FR, Silfen SL, Evans D, Nezhat C. Comparison of direct insertion of disposable and standard reusable laparoscopic trocars and previous pneumoperitoneum with Veress needle. *Obstet Gynecol*. 1991;78:148.
18. Borgatta L, Gruss L, Barad D, Kaali SG. Direct trocar insertion versus Veress needle use for laparoscopic sterilization. *J Reprod Med*. 1990;35:891.
19. Jarrett JC. Laparoscopy: direct trocar insertion without pneumoperitoneum. *Obstet Gynecol*. 1990;75:725.
20. Kaali SG, Bartfai G. Direct insertion of the laparoscopic trocar after an earlier laparotomy. *J Reprod Med*. 1988;33:739.
21. Saidi MH. Direct laparoscopy without prior pneumoperitoneum. *J Reprod Med*. 1986;31:684.
22. Copeland C, Wing R, Hulka JF. Direct trocar insertion at laparoscopy: an evaluation. *Obstet Gynecol*. 1983;62:655.
23. Dingfelder JR. Direct laparoscopic trocar insertion without prior pneumoperitoneum. *J Reprod Med*. 1978;21:45.
24. Byron JW, Markenson GA. Randomized comparison of Veress needle and direct trocar insertion for laparoscopy. *Surg Gynecol Obstet*. 1993;177:259.
25. Hasson HM. Open laparoscopy versus closed laparoscopy: a comparison of complication rates. *Adv Plan Parent*. 1978;13:41.
26. Gomel V, Taylor PJ, Yuzpe AA, Rioux JE. The technique of endoscopy. In: *Laparoscopy and Hysteroscopy in Gynecologic Practice*. Chicago: Year Book; 1986.
27. Penfield AJ. How to prevent complications of open laparoscopy. *J Reprod Med*. 1985;30:660.
28. Galen DI, Jacobson A, Weckstein LN, et al. Reduction of cannula-related laparoscopic complications using a radially expanding access device. *J Am Assoc Gynecol Laparosc*. 1999;6:79.
29. Luciano AA, Lowney J, Jacobs SL. Endoscopic treatment of endometriosis-associated infertility: therapeutic, economic and social benefits. *J Reprod Med*. 1992;37:573.
30. Brill AI, Nezhat F, Nezhat CH, Nezhat CR. The incidence of adhesions after prior laparotomy: a laparoscopic appraisal. *Obstet Gynecol*. 1995;85:269.
31. DeCherney AH. Laparoscopy with unexpected viscous penetration. In: Nichols DH, ed. *Clinical Problems, Injuries and Complications of Gynecologic Surgery*. Baltimore: Williams & Wilkins; 1988.
32. Pagidas K, Tulandi T. Effects of Ringer's lactate, Interceed (TC7) and Gore-Tex Surgical Membrane on postsurgical adhesion formation. *Fertil Steril*. 1992;57:199.
33. Ke RW, Portera SG, Bagous W, Lincoln SR. A randomized, double-blinded trial of preemptive analgesia in laparoscopy. *Obstet Gynecol*. 1998;92:972.

Section 4.2. Laparoscopic Trocars and Complications

Roger Ferland

The key to successful laparoscopic surgery depends on safe access to the peritoneal cavity. Proper trocar placement and position will set the tone for the remainder of the procedure. Poor placement or injury to the abdominal wall or intraperitoneal structures will limit visualization, impair instrument handling, and seriously complicate laparoscopic surgery.

Advances in trocar design have reduced the potential for such trauma, allow for easier placement, and facilitate performance of laparoscopic surgery. In spite of these advances, the U.S. Food and Drug Administration (FDA) received more than 1300 trocar injury reports resulting in 30 deaths over a 5-year period from 1997 to 2002.[1] This section reviews different trocar designs, discusses proper placement, and reviews management of complications resulting from trocar placement.

DESIGNS

Trocars available in the late 1970s through the mid-1980s were typically constructed from reusable stainless steel or composite materials with a cutting tip. Their design was patterned after trocars used for thoracentesis. Trumpet valves reduced pneumoperitoneum leakage as scopes were passed, but complete seals depended on rubber gaskets at the top of the trocar. Insufflation valves were of a stopcock design and could be dismantled for cleaning (Figure 4.2.1).

Multiple parts, all with a potential for failure, made maintenance difficult and at times limited the surgeon's laparoscopic capabilities. Cutting tips would dull over time, causing the surgeon to use excessive force for placement. Gaskets and trumpet or insufflation valves would fail intraoperatively, leading to leakage of pneumoperitoneum.

The use of conductive stainless steel sleeves created the potential for direct and indirect coupling of electrosurgical energy. These trocars were typically inserted in a blind fashion after establishment of pneumoperitoneum by Veress needle. The historical record indicates an injury is most likely with the primary trocar placement.

The first major change in trocar placement technique occurred in 1971. Hasson [2] reported 14 cases of successful laparoscopy by opening a small subumbilical incision under direct vision and later suturing a cannula sheathed in a cone-shaped sleeve (Figure 4.2.2) to the fascia to maintain pneumoperitoneum. He theorized this would reduce the risks of bowel injury and failed pneumoperitoneum. However, in Molloy's [3] 2002 meta-analysis of entry techniques, open laparoscopic access resulted in a 1.1/1000 incidence of bowel injury but no vascular injuries. Hanney [4] reported two cases of aortic laceration when placing a Hassan cannula for laparoscopic cholecystectomy, one thought to result from the initial skin incision and the other from the end of the trocar resting against the aorta. Although bowel injuries have been reported with this technique, it remains a viable option for peritoneal access. It is clear that if bowel is firmly adherent to the abdominal wall at the incision, the site is at risk, even with the open approach.

Another change in technique was described by Dingfelder [5] in 1978. He demonstrated safe peritoneal access with sharp primary trocars without the prior establishment of a pneumoperitoneum. Subsequently, multiple authors [6–8] show similar rates of bowel or vascular injuries with direct placement versus placement following pneumoperitoneum.

These limitations became more problematic with the advent of video-laparoscopy in the late 1980s. As leaders in the field expanded the horizons of cases managed laparoscopically, the need for better trocars became greater. The increased number and complexity of cases caused the reusable trocars to have a shorter utility cycle and increased maintenance costs. Additionally, Corson [9] demonstrated reusable trocars that required great force for placement because of the inability to maintain a sharp cutting surface at the tip.

It was in this environment that disposable trocars were introduced. They had several advantages: (1) consistently sharp tips; (2) simpler valve designs, reducing the failure of gas seals; (3) faster turnover of cases as reprocessing was eliminated; (4) nonconductive materials that eliminated risks of electrosurgical coupling; and (5) safety shields that may reduce but not eliminate injuries.

Initially, the cost of disposable trocars was concerning. However, decreased costs, increasing case volume, and the elimination of reprocessing costs have created a favorable cost/benefit ratio in most hospitals.

When disposable trocars were first introduced in the mid- to late 1980s, a retractable shield would expose the sharp cutting surfaces of the tip, then drop down to cover the tip when the shield cleared the peritoneum. This feature was held out as an improvement in patient safety in marketing efforts by the manufacturers. However, the literature is replete with case reports of bowel or vascular injuries from using such trocars.[10,11] The limitation stems from the exposure of the sharp tip until the shield passes through the peritoneum, leaving the tip exposed during placement. Other case reports describe a "cookie cutter" injury to bowel or vessels resulting from the shield dropping down coincident with the force advancing the trocar.

Additional modifications allowed for secure placement without incidental removal during instrument changes, as well as better gas seals during laparoscopic suturing. Integral designs

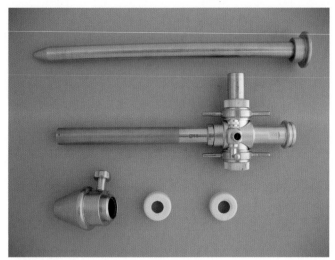

Figure 4.2.1. Hassan cannula disassembled. Note the multiple parts and gaskets.

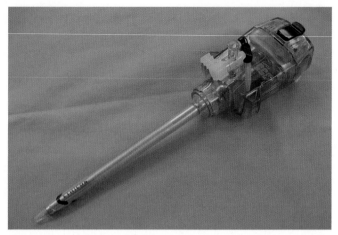

Figure 4.2.3. Endopath bladeless optical trocar (Ethicon Endo-Surgery).

such as the reverse "Christmas tree" pattern on the trocar sleeve (Ethicon Endo-Surgery [EES]) or the inflatable balloons at the trocar mouth largely prevent the accidental dislodgement of trocars (SAC, Marlow Medical).

Optical trocars that allow visualization during placement have had mixed success. Early versions included a sharp blade that passed over the leading surface by squeezing a trigger mechanism, thereby cutting through the abdominal wall (Visiport, United States Surgical). These devices were associated with complications related to failure to recognize peritoneal entry and continued cutting into organs or vessels.[12–15]

The more recent designs, such as that of Endopath (EES; Figures 4.2.3 and 4.2.4), allow for good visualization of the layers of the abdominal wall during entry and minimize trauma and caliber of defect in the fascia. However, peritoneal entry may still be unrecognized in the event of omental or bowel adhesions to the abdominal wall at the entry site.

Several trocar tip designs (Figure 4.2.5) have been manufactured to minimize the risk of placement and reduce the size of the

defect in the fascia. This would eliminate the need for fascial closure or associated risk of hernia formation. Conical or bladeless trocar tips may require more force for placement but produce a smaller defect at the fascial level. This appears to be the case based on the study of Xcel bladeless optical trocars (EES) by McCarus [16], who demonstrated an incidence of hernias of 0.2% or less (1/500) with these trocars, even with diameters greater than 10 mm, in the absence of closing the fascia. The defect in the fascia is smaller than the peritoneal defect because of the dilating action of the bladeless trocar (Figure 4.2.5).[16]

Radially expanding trocars (Step, InnerDyne) have the advantage reported of secure placement, smaller defects in the fascia, and ease of placement.[17,18] This device is introduced as a sheath over the Veress needle and later expanded to accommodate the scope and operative instruments.

COMPLICATIONS AND THEIR MANAGEMENT

The commonly accepted incidence of major complications from trocar injuries was similar among several authors. Bowel injuries are more common (0.7 to 1.1/1000) than vascular injuries (0.4/1000).[3,10,19–21]

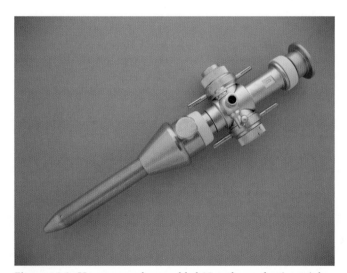

Figure 4.2.2. Hassan cannula assembled. Note the conductive stainless steel sleeve.

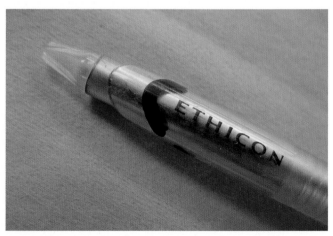

Figure 4.2.4. Endopath bladeless optical trocar; detail of bladeless tip design (Ethicon Endo-Surgery).

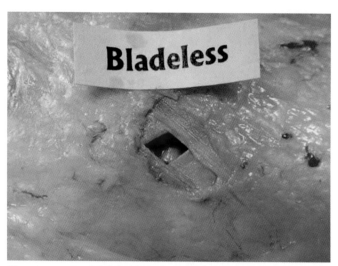

Figure 4.2.5. Fascial defect following placement of a bladeless trocar (Xcel, Ethicon Endo-Surgery).

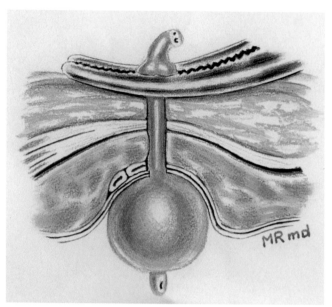

Figure 4.2.7. Placement of Foley catheter to tamponade laceration of the inferior epigastric vessels. From Nezhat et al.[22]

Perhaps the most common complication of trocar placement is laceration of abdominal wall vessels, particularly the deep inferior epigastric vessels. Although these should always be identified before port placement, occasionally they are lacerated by a medially directed path of trocar placement, even though the skin incision is properly placed. Several techniques have been advocated for control of this complication. In the author's experience, the simplest is passage of a 12F Foley catheter through the port, inflation of the balloon, and tamponade of bleeding by pulling back on the catheter. The catheter can then be secured by an umbilical cord clip and left in place for 12 hours. After deflation of the balloon and removal of the catheter, patients can be observed for intraperitoneal bleeding (Figure 4.2.7).

Others have described suture ligating the vessels above and below the point of laceration by an intraperitoneal approach [22] Although this is a reliable method, it can be time consuming and requires good laparoscopic suturing skills. External ligation under laparoscopic guidance is also an effective option as shown in Figure 4.2.8.

Electrodessication by bipolar forceps is also a technique that has been described; however, the resultant ischemic injury at the site may lead to adhesion formation, or even a larger defect in the fascia and subsequent hernia formation (Figure 4.2.9).

Small bowel or prepped large bowel perforations, when recognized, can be managed by primary repair (Figure 4.2.10). The site of perforation should be marked by grasping with a laparoscopic instrument and the loop of bowel then delivered through a small laparotomy incision. After controlling any bleeding in the mesentery, and ruling out a through-and-through perforation, the defect can be closed in two layers. Mesenteric bleeding or through-and-through lacerations should be managed by resection. Unfortunately, many bowel injuries are not recognized at the time of surgery. Delayed diagnosis is marked by intraperitoneal sepsis or obstruction. The morbidity and mortality are much higher with delayed diagnosis. Most prudent laparoscopic surgeons routinely administer a bowel preparation as used for colonoscopy. As a rule, any telephone complaints of abdominal distention, pain, nausea, vomiting, or fever should be immediately evaluated.

Retroperitoneal vascular injuries have the greatest morbidity and mortality. In our institution, the right common iliac vessels are the most commonly injured. This agrees with case reports from Dixon [23] showing the observed sites of injury in five cases (Figure 4.2.11).

Immediate steps are tamponade of the bleeding with a laparoscopic instrument if visualization permits. Injudicious use of energy sources should be avoided as the ureter may be at risk for electrosurgical injury and thrombosis of the distal external iliac or femoral vessels has been known to lead to amputation of the lower extremity on the affected side. Rapid laparotomy by vertical incision will allow adequate exposure for vessel repair or graft placement. While this is being done, the patient should be crossmatched for replacement blood components,

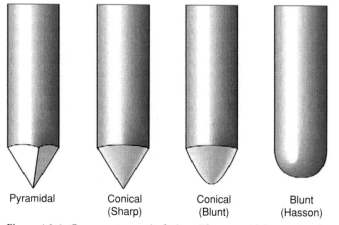

Pyramidal | Conical (Sharp) | Conical (Blunt) | Blunt (Hasson)

Figure 4.2.6. Common trocar tip designs. The pyramidal or cutting tip is associated with a larger fascial defect. From Fuller et al.[1]

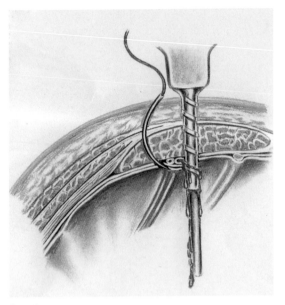

Step 1

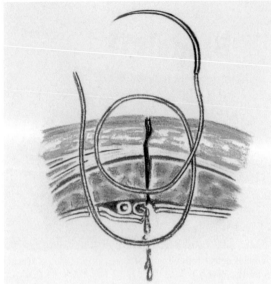

Step 2

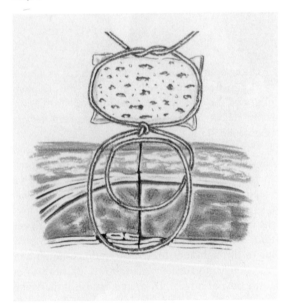

Step 3

Figure 4.2.8. Suture management of inferior epigastric vessel laceration. From Nezhat et al.[22]

vascular surgical consultation called for, and maximum supportive therapy by anesthesia started. After identification of the laceration site, gentle manual tamponade will stop the hemorrhage and allow time for assistance to arrive. One may consider heparinizing the distal vessel with 10,000 units of heparin in 20 mL of saline to avoid distal thrombosis. Delay in these steps will often lead to shock with subsequent adult respiratory distress syndrome, acute tubular necrosis, and prolonged ICU management. A plan with designation of vascular consultants, instrument sets, and coordination of nursing and anesthesia support should be established in any hospital performing laparoscopic surgery.

Other organs at risk include the uterus, adnexa, and urinary tract. If injured primarily, control bleeding. If expo-

sure is adequate and the operator's skills permit, laparoscopic suturing can be accomplished. Repair of cystotomy should be followed by catheter drainage for up to 7 days. Retrograde cystogram will confirm bladder closure after catheter removal.

Hernia formation at the trocar site has been reported with trocars as small as 5 mm.[23–26] Richter's hernias that incarcerate only part of the circumference of bowel are likely to occur at port site defect and are more difficult to diagnose because of the lack of complete bowel obstruction signs. Consequently, the prudent laparoscopic surgeon would elect to close all ports 10 mm or greater at the fascial level and all 5-mm ports that are subject to trocar reinsertion or excessive instrumentation during a major case.

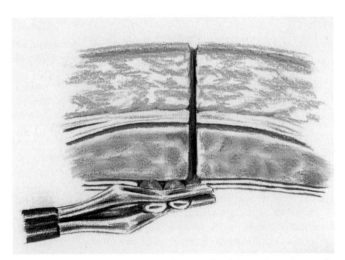

Figure 4.2.9. Electrodessication of lacerated inferior epigastric vessels. From Nezhat et al.[22]

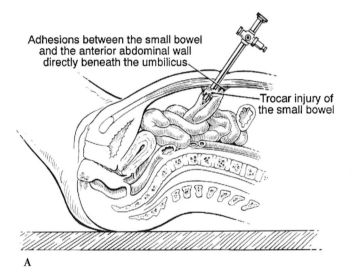

Adhesions between the small bowel and the anterior abdominal wall directly beneath the umbilicus

Trocar injury of the small bowel

A

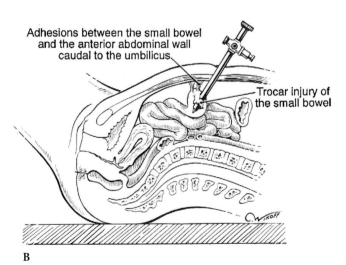

Adhesions between the small bowel and the anterior abdominal wall caudal to the umbilicus

Trocar injury of the small bowel

B

Figure 4.2.10. Bowel perforation at site of adhesions by primary trocar. From Nezhat et al.[22]

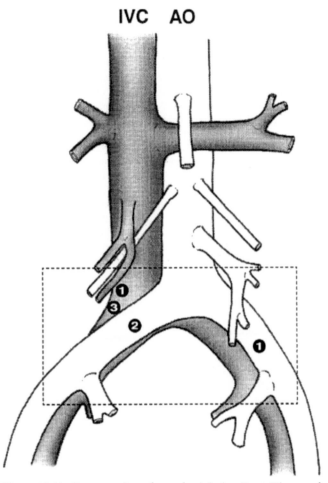

IVC AO

Figure 4.2.11. Common sites of vascular injuries. From Dixon and Carrillo.[23]

CONCLUSION

Proper technique of insertion and trocar placement is essential for successful laparoscopic surgery. Bladeless trocars or those that dilate rather than incise the fascia are less traumatic and may reduce the incidence of hernia formation. Major complications occur rarely but are of high morbidity and mortality. Complications should be promptly recognized and aggressively managed to avoid poor outcomes.

REFERENCES

1. Fuller J, Scott W, Ashar B, Corrado J. Laparoscopic trocar injuries: a report from a US FDA center for devices and radiological health systematic technology assessment of medical products committee. Report from the FDA November 2003. Available at: http://www.fda.gov/cdrh/medicaldevicesafety/ stamp/ trocar.html. Accessed February 2, 2007.
2. Hasson H. A modified instrument and method for laparoscopy. *Am J Obstet Gynecol.* 1971;110:886–887.
3. Molloy D, Kaloo P, Cooper M, Nguyen T. Laparoscopic entry: a literature review and analysis of techniques and complications of primary port entry. *Aust N Z J Obstet Gynaecol.* 2002;42:246–354.

4. Hanney R, Carmalt H, Merrett N, Tait N. Use of the Hasson cannula producing major vascular injury at laparoscopy. *Surg Endosc.* 1999;13:1238–1240.

5. Dingfelder J. Direct laparoscope trocar insertion without prior pneumoperitoneum. *Obstet Gynecol.* 1978;21:45–47.

6. Bonjer H, Hazebroek E, Kazemier G, Giuffrida M, Meijer W, Lange J. Open versus closed establishment of pneumoperitoneum in laparoscopic surgery. *Br J Surg.* 1997;84:599–602.

7. Brill A, Cohen B. Fundamentals of peritoneal access. *J Am Assoc Gynecol Laparosc.* 2003;10:286–297.

8. Jansen F, Kolkman W, Bakkum E, de Kroon C, Trimbos-Kemper T, Trimbos J. Complications of laparoscopy: an inquiry about closed- versus open-entry technique. *Am J Obstet Gynecol.* 2004;190:634–638.

9. Corson S, Batzer F, Gocial B, Maislin G. Measurement of the force necessary for laparoscopic trocar entry. *J Reprod Med* 1989;34:282–284.

10. Bhoyrul S, Vierra M, Nezhat C, Krummel T, Way L. Trocar injuries in laparoscopic surgery. *J Am Coll Surg.* 2001;192:677–683.

11. Corson S, Chandler J, Way L. Survey of laparoscopic entry injuries provoking litigation. *J Am Assoc Gynecol Laparosc.* 2001;8:341–347.

12. Kaali S. Complications associated with optical access laparoscopic trocars. *Obstet Gynecol.* 2002;100:614–615.

13. Sharpe H, Dodson M, Draper M, Watts D, Doucette R, Hurd W. Complications associated with optical access laparoscopic trocars. *Obstet Gynecol.* 2002;9:553–555.

14. Thomas M, Rha K, Ong A, et al. Optical access trocar injuries in urological laparoscopic surgery. *J Urol.* 2003;170:61–63.

15. U.S. Food and Drug Administration. *Manufacturer Device Report #18216.* 1994; Rockville, MD: U.S. Department of Health and Human Services.

16. McCarus SD, et al. Improving herniation outcomes without trocar site fascial closure: a multicenter trial. Presented at American College of Surgeons 90th Annual Clinical Congress, New Orleans, LA; October 10–14, 2004.

17. Turner DJ. A new radially expanding access system for laparoscopic procedures versus conventional cannulas. *J Am Assoc Gynecol Laparosc.* 1996;3:609–615.

18. Yim S, Yuen P. Randomized double-masked comparison of radially expanding access device and conventional cutting tip trocar in laparoscopy. *Obstet Gynecol.* 2001;97:435–438.

19. Harkki-Siren P, Kurki T. A nationwide analysis of laparoscopic complications. *Obstet Gynecol.* 1997;89:108–112.

20. Philips P, Amaral J. Abdominal access complications in laparoscopic surgery. *J Am Coll Surg.* 2001;192:525–536.

21. Schafer M, Lauper M, Krahenbuhl L. Trocar and Veress needle injuries during laparoscopy. *Surg Endosc.* 2001;15:275–280.

22. Nezhat C, Nezhat F, Luciano A, Siegler A, Metzger D, Nezhat C. In: *Operative Gynecologic Laparoscopy Principles and Techniques,* "Complications" New York: McGraw Hill; 1995:293, 295.

23. Dixon M, Carrillo E. Iliac vascular injuries during elective laparoscopic surgery. *Surg Endosc.* 1999;13:1230–1233.

24. Boughey J, Nottingham J, Walls A. Richter's hernia in the laparoscopic era: four case reports and review of the literature. *Surg Laparosc Endosc Percutan Tech.* 2003;13:55–58.

25. Nezhat C, Nezhat F, Seidman D, Nezhat C. Incisional hernias after operative laparoscopy. *J Laparoendosc Adv Surg Tech A.* 1997;7:111–115.

26. Nezhat F, Nezhat C, Seidman D. Incisional hernias after advanced laparoscopic surgery. *J Am Assoc Gynecol Laparosc.* 1996:3(4 suppl):S34–S35.

SUGGESTED READING

Bhoyrul S, Payne J, Steffes B, Swanstrom L, Way L. A randomized prospective study of radially expanding trocars in laparoscopic surgery. *J Gastrointest Surg.* 2000;4:392–397.

Chapron C, Cravello L, Chopin N, Krieker G, Blanc B, Dubuisson J. Complications during set-up procedures for laparoscopy in gynecology: open laparoscopy does not reduce the risk of major complications. *Acta Obstet Gynecol Scand.* 2003;82:1125–1129.

Chapron C, Dubuisson J, Bernard H, Feldman S. Predicting risk of complications with gynecologic laparoscopic surgery. *Obstet Gynecol.* 1999;93:318–319.

Hasson H, Galanopoulos C, Langerman A. Ischemic necrosis of small bowel following laparoscopic surgery. *JSLS.* 2004;8:159–163.

Jacobson M, Oesterling S, Milki A, Nezhat C. Laparoscopic control of a leaking mestenteric vessel secondary to trocar injury. *JSLS.* 2002;6:389–391.

Jugool S, McKain E, Swarnkar K, Vellacott K, Stephenson B. Randomized clinical trial of the effect of pneumoperitoneum on cardiac function and haemodynamics during laparoscopic cholecystectomy. *Br J Surg.* 2004;91:1527. Comment on: *Br J Surg.* 2004;91:848–854.

McKernan J, Finley C. Experience with optical trocar in performing laparoscopic procedures. *Surg Laparosc Endosc Percutan Tech.* 2002;12:96–99.

Merlin T, Hiller J, Maddern G, Jamieson G, Brown A, Kolbe A. Systematic review of the safety and effectiveness of methods used to establish pneumoperitoneum in laparoscopic surgery. *Br J Surg.* 2003;90:668–679.

Nezhat C, Childers J, Nezhat F, Nezhat CH, Seidman D. Major retroperitoneal vascular injury during laparoscopic surgery. *Hum Reprod.* 1997;12:480–483.

Nezhat F, Silfen S, Evans D, Nezhat C. Comparison of direct insertion of disposable and standard reusable laparoscopic trocars and previous pneumoperitoneum with Veress needle. *Obstet Gynecol.* 1991;78:148–150.

Nuzzo G, Giuliante F, Tebala G, Vellone M, Cavicchioni C. Routine use of open techniques in laparoscopic operations. *J Am Coll Surg.* 1997;184:58–62.

Orlando R, Palatini P, Lirussi F. Needle and trocar injuries in diagnostic laparoscopy under local anesthesia: what is the true incidence of these complications? *J Laparoendosc Adv Surg Tech A.* 2003;13:181–184.

Rosen D, Lam A, Chapman M, Carlton M, Cario G. Methods of creating pneumoperitoneum: a review of techniques and complications. *Obstet Gynecol Surv.* 1998;53:167–174.

Rubenstein J, Blunt L Jr, Lin W, User H, Nadler R, Gonzalez C. Safety and efficacy of 12-mm radial dilating ports for laparoscopic access. *BJU Int.* 2003;92:327–329.

Saber A, Boros M. Chilaiditi's syndrome: what should every surgeon know? *Am Surg.* 2005;71:261–263.

Seidman D, Nasserbakht F, Nezhat F, Nezhat C. Delayed recognition of iliac artery injury during laparoscopic surgery. *Surg Endosc.* 1996;10:1099–1101.

Shah P, Ramakantan R. Pneumoperitoneum and pneumomediastinum: unusual complications of laparoscopy. *J Postgrad Med.* 1990;36:31–32.

Siqueira T Jr, Paterson R, Kuo R, Stevens L, Lingeman J, Shalhav A. The use of blunt-tipped 12-mm trocars without fascial closure in laparoscopic live donor nephrectomy. *JSLS.* 2004;8:47–50.

Swank D, Bonjer H, Jeekel J. Safe laparoscopic adhesiolysis with optical access trocar and ultrasonic dissection. A prospective study. *Surg Endosc.* 2002;16:1796–1801.

Tarik A, Fehmi C. Complications of gynaecological laparoscopy – a retrospective analysis of 3572 cases from a single institute. *J Obstet Gynaecol*. 2004;24:813–816.

Teoh B, Sen R, Abbott J. An evaluation of four tests used to ascertain Veres needle placement at closed laparoscopy. *J Minim Invasive Gynecol*. 2005;12:153–158.

Ternamian A. A trocarless, reusable, visual-access cannula for safer lap-aroscopy; an update. *J Am Assoc Gynecol Laparosc*. 1998;5:197–201.

Thomson A, Abbott J, Lenart M, Willison F, Vancaillie T, Bennett M. Assessment of a method to expel intraperitoneal gas after gyneco-logic laparoscopy. *J Minim Invasive Gynecol*. 2005;12:125–129.

Vilos G, Vilos A. Safe laparoscopic entry guided by Veress needle CO_2 insufflation pressure. *J Am Assoc Gynecol Laparosc*. 2003;10:415–420.

5 | LAPAROSCOPIC SUTURING

Camran Nezhat, Ceana Nezhat, and Farr Nezhat

The ability to suture laparoscopically increases a laparoscopist's versatility. Suturing is used for hemostasis and to oppose tissues during reconstructive procedures. Different types of sutures are available for endoscopic use. The Endoloop (Ethicon) suture, a preformed slipknot attached to a rigid, disposable 5-mm applicator, is available in 0-chromic gut, polyglactin, polydioxanone, and polypropylene (Figure 5.1). The loop is positioned around the pedicle by grasping the structure to be removed and pulling it through the loop. The loop is tightened against the applicator, and the suture is cut with scissors or the laser beam against a backstop.

Suture material is available with a straight or curved swaged needle specifically designed for laparoscopic use. It is available in 0-chromic catgut, 4-0 polydioxanone with a swaged ST-4 needle (PDS, Ethicon), and polyglactin. The suture is grasped with forceps several centimeters from the needle. The grasper with suture is inserted intra-abdominally through the 5-mm accessory trocar sleeve.

To place the needle intra-abdominally, the grasper or needle driver is removed along with the trocar sleeve, which remains around the grasper's shaft. The suture is grasped about 5 cm from the needle, and the grasper is reintroduced with the trocar sleeve into the suprapubic incision site. The needle follows the grasper into the abdominal cavity. A needle larger than a CT-1 is awkward to use intra-abdominally. Once the suture is placed, several techniques can be used to secure the knot. An Endoloop with a pre-made knot is tightened around the pedicle with the plastic knot pusher. Other types of extracorporeal knots are the Duncan [1] and clinch knots, but their closure depends on a single knot that may slip. The knot may not slide because of suture friction. Tissue trauma may result from the suture being pulled in opposite directions through transfixed tissue as the needle is withdrawn from the abdomen when a sliding knot is applied.

Intracorporeal knotting is difficult and requires practice. An instrument-tying method employed within the abdomen uses two forceps and suture material. The suture may get caught in the articulation point of the forceps and break. However, variations of the fisherman's clinch knot prevent some difficulties. The use of the knot pusher was described originally in 1972.[2] The principles of this instrument do not differ from those of tying sutures deep in the pelvis, where the surgeon uses a finger to push and secure the knot. Length of sutures used in intracorporeal and extracorporeal suturing differs, with about 13 cm and 90–100 cm, respectively.[3]

Extracorporeal knot tying simplifies laparoscopic suturing. Instruments that help this process include a needle holder, needle driver, suture introducer, and scissors. A suture is loaded into the needle holder, holding the suture below the swage point so that the needle will collapse into the introducer. The needle holder is inserted into the introducer (Figure 5.2). The introducer is placed into a 5-mm trocar, and the needle driver is placed into a contralateral trocar. A needle is advanced into the abdominal cavity and passed from the holder to the driver. While the needle is steadied with the driver, the holder is repositioned to the desired location. The needle is tapped with the driver to lock it into a right-angle position. The needle is rearmed with the driver. A driver is used to pass the needle through the tissue, and then grasp the tip and pass the needle to the holder (Figure 5.3). To reduce the risk of pulling the suture out of the tissue, tension on the suture line is kept to a minimum. The holder, needle, and excess suture line are withdrawn from the abdominal cavity through the introducer. An assistant covers the introducer channel to maintain a pneumoperitoneum (Figure 5.4). The surgeon cuts the suture below the swage point and makes a single-throw knot with the two suture ends. The knot is held securely with the thumb and third finger while three revolutions are made around both suture strands with the free end of the suture (Figure 5.5). The tail of the suture is inserted through the first loop directly above the assistant's hand. After the tail is passed through the loop, the operator pulls up on the tail to form the knot and cuts the tail approximately 0.6 cm above the knot. The end of the Endoknot (Johnson & Johnson) shaft is snapped off at the colored band, allowing the shaft to slide the knot downward (Figure 5.6). Placing the shaft perpendicular to the knot reduces suture breakage and ensures knot security. The Endoknot cannula is placed in the introducer (Figure 5.7). When the surgeon pulls back on the small end piece of the Endoknot shaft while sliding the plastic shaft forward, the knot is allowed to move forward as the loop decreases in size. The Endoknot cannula acts as an integral knot pusher for placement of the formed knot. Scissors inserted through the contralateral trocar are used to cut the excess suture. The procedure for pre-tied knot is similar to the technique described above except for forming the knot (Figures 5.7 through 5.12).

Intracorporeal knot tying is used during microsurgery and fine suturing. It is more difficult and time consuming than extracorporeal knot tying. The instructions for introducing the needle and suture into the abdomen are the same as those for extracorporeal knot tying. The needle and the entire suture are placed in the abdominal cavity. After the needle is positioned, it is grasped with the needle holder (Figure 5.13). While the grasping forceps apply pressure to the tissue being sutured, the suture is inserted through the tissue (Figure 5.14). Graspers hold the needle, and the needle holder applies counterpressure to the tissue (Figure 5.15). The needle is removed from the tissue. Enough suture to

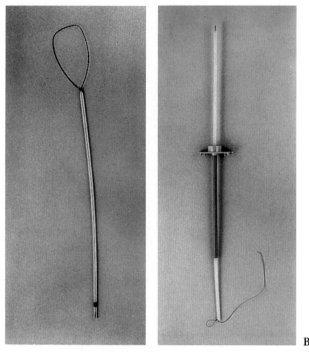

Figure 5.1. (**A**) Endoloop suture, a pretied slipknot, is attached to a rigid disposable applicator. (**B**) It is inserted into the trocar sleeve.

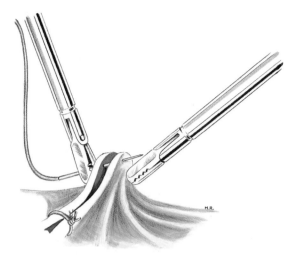

Figure 5.3. The needle driver was placed into a contralateral sleeve. The needle was advanced into the abdominal cavity and passed from the holder to the driver. While the needle was steadied with the driver, the holder was repositioned to the desired location. The needle was tapped with the driver to lock it into a right-angle position. The needle is rearmed with the driver. The driver is used to pass the needle through the tissue and then grasp the tip and pass the needle to the holder.

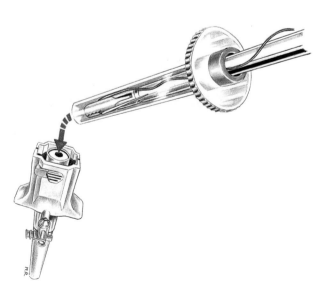

Figure 5.2. The needle holder is inserted into the introducer. The introducer is placed into a 5-mm sleeve.

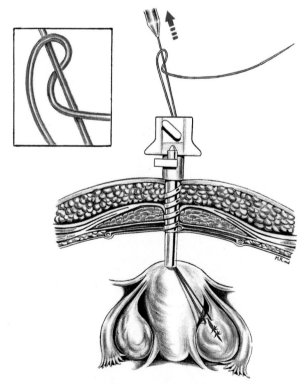

Figure 5.4. The needle holder and excess suture lines were withdrawn from the abdominal cavity through the introducer. (An assistant covers the introducer channel to prevent the loss of pnuemoperitoneum.) After the surgeon cuts the suture beneath the swage point, a single throw knot is made with the two suture ends (inset).

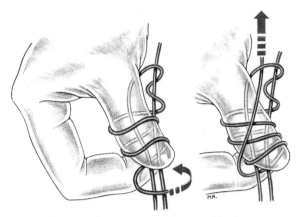

Figure 5.5. Three revolutions are made around both suture strands with the free end of the suture (left). The tail of the suture is inserted through the first loop (right). The tail of the suture is inserted through the first loop directly above the surgeon's thumb.

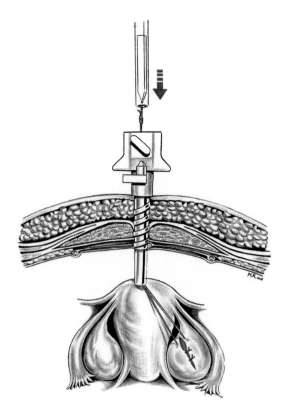

Figure 5.7. The Endoknot cannula acts as an integral knot pusher for placement of the formed knot.

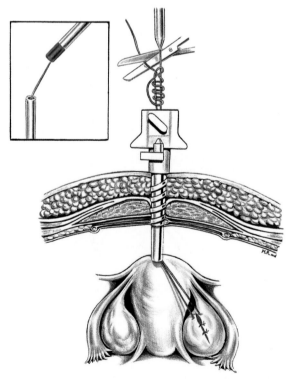

Figure 5.6. The suture tail is cut about 0.6 cm above the knot. The end of the Endoknot shaft is snapped out at the colored band (inset), allowing the shaft to slide the knot downward. Placing the shaft perpendicular to the knot lessens suture breakage and ensures knot security.

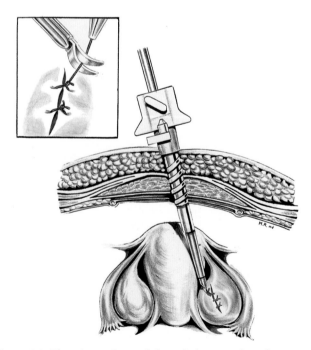

Figure 5.8. The scissors, inserted through the contralateral trocar, are used to cut the knot (inset). The pretied Endoknot consists of synthetic absorbable suture material with a hollow plastic tube that is narrowed at one end and scored at the other. The center of the plastic tube has a 4-0 stainless steel suture that is looped at the narrow end and swaged at the surgical needle. The scored end of the device serves as the handle. The primary advantage of this device is that the knot is preformed and does not have to be made manually by the surgeon.

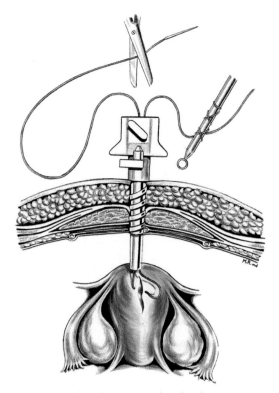

Figure 5.9. The needle and suture are placed in the 3-mm suture intro-ducer. After the needle is passed through the tissue, the needle and suture are brought out of the cannula and the suture is cut.

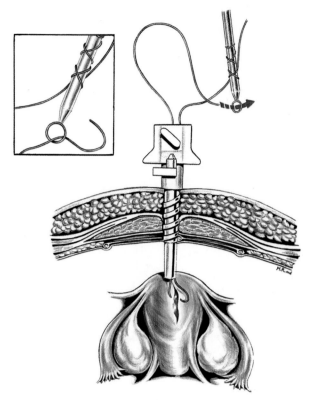

Figure 5.10. About 5 cm of the longest end of the suture is pushed through the wire loop near the tapered end of the cannula. The inset shows a close-up of this process.

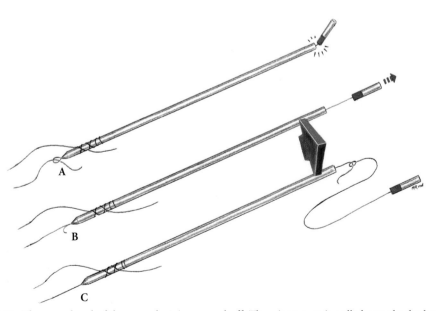

Figure 5.11. The scored end of the cannula A is snapped off. The wire suture is pulled completely through B. The scored end is discarded C.

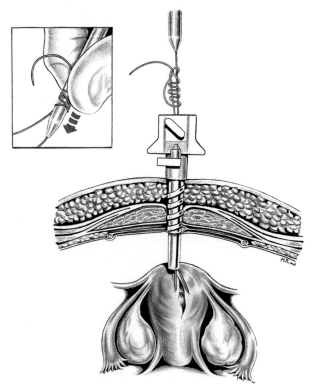

Figure 5.12. The pretied slipknot is pushed off the conical end of the cannula (inset). The excess suture is trimmed at the end of the slipknot. The slipknot is pushed into the trocar and onto the tissue to be sutured.

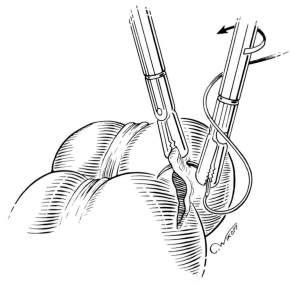

Figure 5.14. While grasping forceps hold the tissue being sutured, the suture is inserted through the tissue.

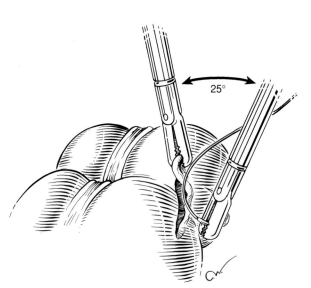

Figure 5.13. After the needle is positioned, it is grasped with the needle holder.

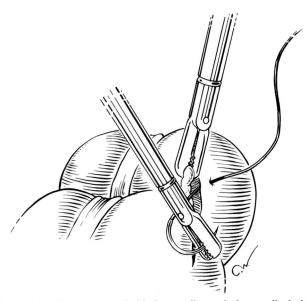

Figure 5.15. The graspers hold the needle, and the needle holder applies counterpressure on the tissue.

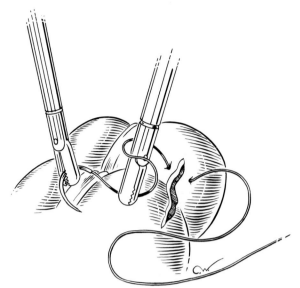

Figure 5.16. The needle is removed from the tissue. Enough suture is pulled through to form a knot, leaving a sufficient tail.

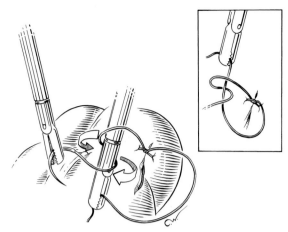

Figure 5.17. The needle is grasped with a grasping forceps, and two or three loops are made around the needle holder. The free end of the suture is grasped with the needle holder and brought inside the formed loops (inset).

knots are applied over the suture, reversing the direction of the sutures with each successive knot.

form a knot is pulled through, leaving a sufficient tail (Figure 5.16). The needle is grasped with a grasping forceps, and two or three loops are made around the needle holder. The free end of the suture is grasped with the needle holder and brought inside the formed loops (Figure 5.17), and using both grasping forceps and the needle holder, the suture is tied over the tissue. Additional

REFERENCES

1. Weston PV. A new clinch knot. *Obstet Gynecol* 1991;78:144.
2. Clarke HC. Laparoscopy—new instruments for suturing and ligation. *Fertil Steril* 1972; 23:274.
3. Desai PJ, Moran ME, Calvano CJ, Parelch AR. Running suture: the ideal length facilitates this task. *J Endourol* 2000; 14:191–194.

6 | INTRAPERITONEAL AND RETROPERITONEAL ANATOMY

Jyoti Yadav, M. Shoma Datta, Ceana Nezhat, Camran Nezhat, and Farr Nezhat

Sound surgical technique, whether during laparotomy or laparoscopy, is based on accurate anatomic knowledge. Laparoscopic surgeons must adapt to the altered appearance of anatomy due to the effects of pneumoperitoneum, Trendelenburg positioning, and traction from a uterine manipulator. There are inherent limitations of laparoscopy related to the fixed visual axis, loss of depth of field, and magnification. Furthermore, laparoscopes with different angles of view make orientation more challenging.

Because a three-dimensional field is projected to video monitors as a two-dimensional image, it is imperative for the endoscopic surgeon to understand that the anatomic structures appearing superior on the monitor are actually anterior and those inferior are posterior.

In this chapter, we describe some important anatomic relations that are critical during laparoscopic procedures.

SUPERFICIAL INTRAPERITONEAL ANATOMY (LANDMARKS TO RETROPERITONEAL STRUCTURES)

Superficial intraperitoneal landmarks within the pelvis alert the operator to key anatomic structures in the retroperitoneal space (Figure 6.1A–C).

The umbilicus is located at the level of L3–L4, although the location varies with the patient's weight, the presence of abdominal panniculus, and the position of the patient on the operating table (supine vs. Trendelenburg). The abdominal aorta bifurcates at L4–L5 in 80% of cases.[1]

The parietal peritoneum over the anterior abdominal wall is raised at five sites, representing the five umbilical folds. The median umbilical fold, running from the dome of the bladder to the umbilicus, covers the obliterated urachus. Lateral to the urachus, on either side, are the medial umbilical folds, overlying the obliterated umbilical arteries. Just lateral to each medial umbilical fold is the lateral umbilical ligament (fold), formed by the peritoneum overlying the inferior epigastric vessels before their entry into the rectus sheath as they course cephalad to join the superior epigastric artery. In most cases, their location may be visually confirmed through the laparoscope, avoiding injury to them during the placement of accessory trocars.

On either side of the rectouterine pouch, the peritoneum reflects over the uterosacral ligaments, forming the uterosacral folds. Slightly lateral and superior to the uterosacral fold is often another fold of peritoneum, the ureteric fold, which covers the ureter.

Many additional key structures can be identified transperitoneally before any dissection. The internal iliac artery travels parallel and just posterior to the ureter. The external iliac artery is several centimeters anterior to it on the psoas muscle. The external and internal iliac arteries may then be followed superiorly to find the bifurcation of the common iliac arteries at the pelvic brim overlying the sacroiliac joint. This is an ideal location to identify the ureter traversing the point of bifurcation as it enters the pelvis. The right common iliac artery may then be followed superiorly to the bifurcation of the aorta, above the presacral space at approximately the fourth lumbar vertebra. The left common iliac artery is more difficult to identify because of the overlying mesentery of the sigmoid colon. The left common iliac vein is located just medial and inferior to the left common iliac artery in the presacral space. At times it covers the entire space between the common iliac arteries.

PELVIC BRIM

Multiple important structures enter the pelvic cavity at the pelvic brim and can be appreciated layer by layer (Figure 6.2A–D). Starting superficially from the peritoneal surface toward the sacroiliac joint, the following structures are found in close proximity to each other and can be recognized laparoscopically as superficial peritoneal landmarks: the peritoneum, the ovarian vessels in the infundibulopelvic ligament, the ureter, the bifurcation of the common iliac artery, and the common iliac vein. Dissecting deeper layers, the medial edge of the psoas muscle, the obturator nerve, and the parietal fascia overlying the capsule of the sacroiliac joint will be exposed. The lumbosacral trunk lies medial to the obturator nerve.

PELVIC SIDEWALL

The pelvic sidewall is entered by opening the peritoneal reflection bordered by the round ligament anteriorly, the infundibulopelvic ligament medially, and the external iliac artery laterally (Figures 6.3A–G and 6.4B). Based on avascular planes, there are three surgical layers.

First Layer of the Pelvic Sidewall

Medially, the first layer is the parietal peritoneum with the ureter attached to it in its own fascial sheath. The ureter can be retracted

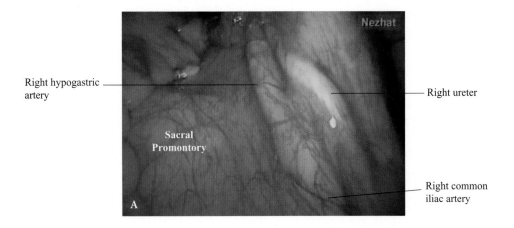

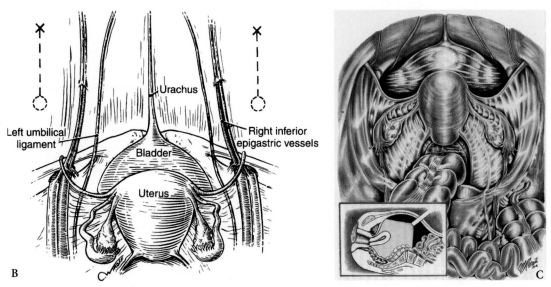

Figure 6.1. (**A**) View of the right pelvic brim. (**B**) Deep inferior epigastric vessels run lateral to the umbilical ligament. (**C**) A laparoscopic view of the pelvis. The inset shows the effect of the Trendelenburg position.

medially by incising this peritoneum, or it can be separated by blunt or hydrodissection.

Second Layer of the Pelvic Side Wall

The second surgical layer consists of the internal iliac vessels and their visceral anterior branches: uterine, superior vesical leading to the obliterated umbilical, inferior vesical, vaginal, and the middle rectal arteries.

Third Layer of the Pelvic Side Wall

From anterior to posterior lie the (i) psoas muscle with the external iliac artery on its medial aspect, (ii) external iliac vein just medial and posterior to it, and (iii) external iliac vein beneath the obturator internus muscle with the obturator nerve and vessels coursing along its anterior border toward the obturator canal.

PELVIC LYMPH NODES

The external pelvic nodes are found along the external iliac artery and vein from the bifurcation of the common iliac vessels to the deep circumflex iliac veins caudally. The obturator nodes are found in the obturator fossa, which is bordered medially by the hypogastric artery; laterally by the external iliac vein, the obturator internus muscle, and its fascia; and anteriorly by the obturator nerve and vessels. The nodes along the hypogastric vessels up to the bifurcation of the common iliac artery and vein comprise the hypogastric group.

BASE OF THE BROAD LIGAMENT

The base of the broad ligament (Figures 6.4A,B) comprises the cardinal ligament, also known as the ligament of Mackenrodt. Dissection of the pelvic sidewall will lead into this

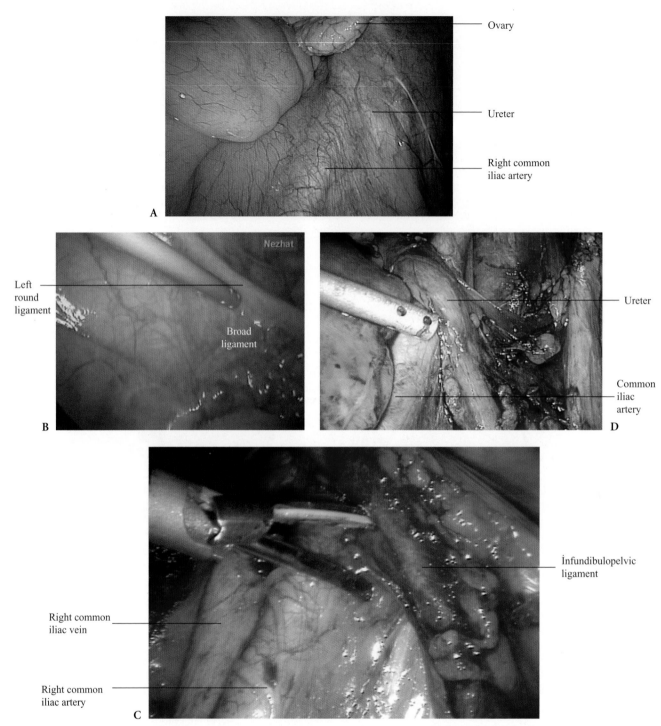

Figure 6.2. (**A**) The laparoscopic view of the pelvic brim before the incision. (**B**) A view of left broad ligament. (**C**) Right pelvic wall dissection during pelvic lymphadenectomy. (**D**) The dissection of right pelvic sidewall is completed and the crossing of the ureter on common iliac vessels at the pelvic brim is clearly seen.

region. It is important to comprehend that the internal iliac artery continues into the superior vesical artery and then into the obliterated umbilical artery. Traction on the medial umbilical fold will help identify the internal iliac artery, and the medial branch passing superior to the ureter can then be identified as the uterine artery. The upper portion of the cardinal ligament is penetrated by the ureter as it travels into the tunnel of Wertheim just beneath the uterine artery, 1 to 2 cm lateral to the isthmus of the uterus, immediately lateral to the uterosacral ligament. This is one of the most common sites of ureteric injury in gynecologic procedures.

The base of the broad ligaments delineates two important spaces: Anteriorly is the paravesical space and just posterior, toward the sacrum, is the pararectal space. The extent of lateral dissection toward the pelvic sidewall and consequently excision of the ligament of Mackenrodt determines the class of radical hysterectomy.

AVASCULAR SPACES OF THE PELVIS

Three pairs of ligaments divide the pelvis into eight avascular spaces (Figure 6.5A,B).

Prevesical (Retropubic) Space of Retzius

The space of Retzius, or the *retropubic space*, is a potential avascular space with vascular borders between the back of the pubic bone and the anterior wall of the bladder (Figure 6.6).

The retropubic space is bounded anteriorly by the transversalis fascia, which inserts on the posterior surface of the pubic symphysis. The urethra, the paraurethral (pubourethral) ligaments, and the urethrovesical junction (bladder neck) form the floor of this space. The pubic symphysis and the adjacent superior pubic rami with Cooper's ligament represent the inferior limit.

Paravesical Space

Laterally, the retropubic space is contiguous with the *paravesical* spaces (Figure 6.7A,B), their point of separation being the medial umbilical ligaments (obliterated umbilical arteries). The paired paravesical space is bound laterally by the obturator internus muscle and the obturator nerve, artery, and vein, just beneath the bony arcuate ridge of the ileum. The posterior border (toward the sacrum) is the endopelvic fascial sheath around the internal iliac artery and vein and its anterior branches, as they course toward the ischial spine. The pubocervical fascia forms the floor of this lateral compartment as it inserts into the arcus tendineus fasciae pelvis (fascial white line). The muscular white line (arcus tendineus levator ani), which is the origin of the levator ani muscles, is just above the level of the fascial white line. Accessory obturator arteries and veins are often present and course from the inferior epigastric vessels and drape across the pectineal (Cooper's) ligament on their way to anastomose with the obturator vessels in the obturator canal. The surgeon must always look for them, such as in the case of a retropubic colposuspension, because they are present in approximately 40% of patients.

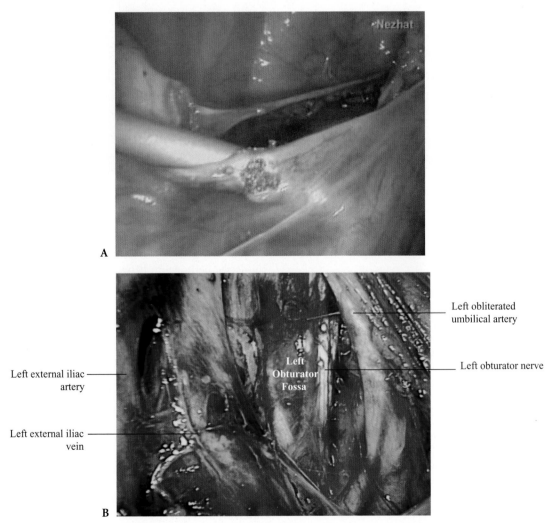

A

B

Left external iliac artery

Left external iliac vein

Left Obturator Fossa

Left obliterated umbilical artery

Left obturator nerve

Figure 6.3. (**A**) An incision is made in the left broad ligament lateral or parallel to the infundibulopelvic ligament to develop the paravesical space. The round ligament can be divide either before or after this space is developed. This incision can be made by the scissors, the harmonic shear, or by the CO_2 laser. (**B**) A view of the left obturator fossa. *(Continued)*

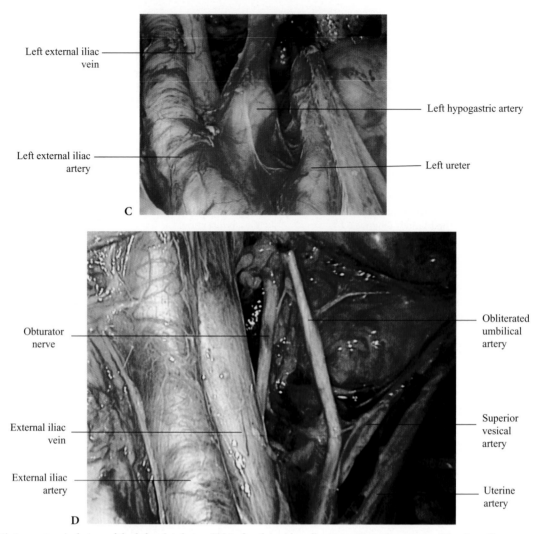

Figure 6.3. (**C**) An anatomical view of the left pelvic brim. (**D**) Left pelvic sidewall retroperitoneal anatomy. *(Continued)*

Pararectal Space

The pararectal space is triangular, with the base of the cardinal ligament representing the anterior border (Figure 6.7C,D). The medial border is the ureter and the lateral border is the internal iliac artery. This space can be easily developed by bluntly dissecting posterior to the origin of the uterine artery and lateral to the ureter.

Vesicovaginal and Rectovaginal Spaces

The *vesicovaginal* space is a potential avascular space between the anterior surface of the vagina and the posterior aspect of the bladder, bordered laterally by the bladder pillars or the vesicouterine/vesicocervical ligaments (Figure 6.8A–C). Entry to this space can be accomplished by incising the vesicouterine fold of peritoneum.

The *rectovaginal* space is bounded by the vagina anteriorly, the rectum posteriorly, and the perineal body inferiorly and laterally (Figure 6.9A–C). The space is entered by incising the posterior cul-de-sac peritoneum between the two uterosacral ligaments, which lies superiorly.

Presacral (Retro-rectal) Space

The retro-rectal space is between the rectum anteriorly and the sacrum posteriorly (Figure 6.10). This space is entered abdominally by dividing the mesentery of sigmoid colon or through the pararectal spaces. Inferiorly this space terminates at the level of the levator muscle and laterally continues as the pararectal fossae. The middle sacral artery and a plexus of veins are attached superficial to the anterior longitudinal ligament of the sacrum. The endopelvic fascia in this space envelops the visceral nerves of the superior hypogastric plexus and the lymphatic tissue. The lateral boundary of the presacral space is formed by the common iliac artery, ureter, and inferior mesenteric artery traversing through the mesentery of the sigmoid colon on the left side.

Lateral and inferior dissection in the presacral space leads to the structures entering the pelvis over the pelvic brim.

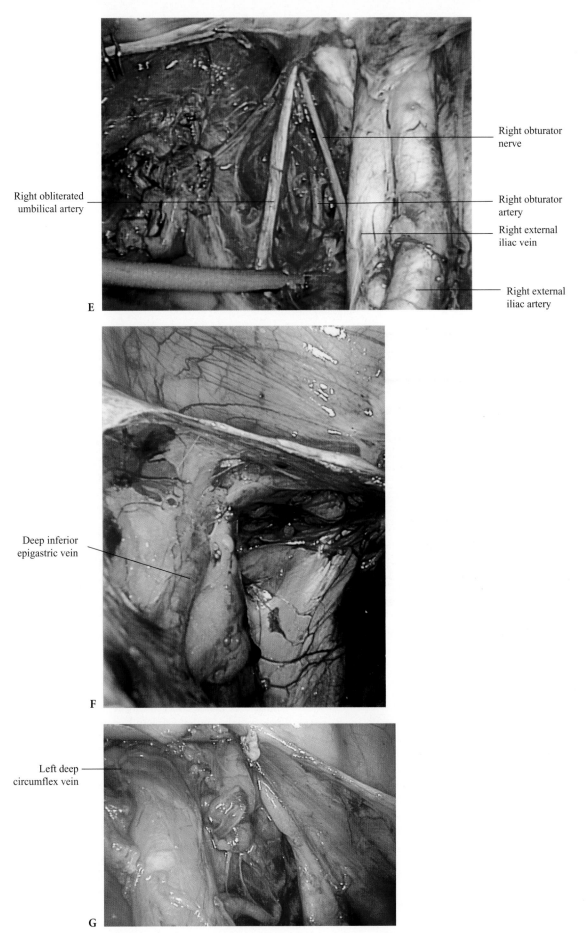

Right obturator
nerve

Right obliterated
umbilical artery

Right obturator
artery

Right external
iliac vein

Right external
iliac artery

E

Deep inferior
epigastric vein

F

Left deep
circumflex vein

G

Figure 6.3. *(Continued)* (**E**) Right pelvic sidewall retroperitoneal anatomy. (**F**) The course of deep inferior epigastric vein from its origin. (**G**) The deep circumflex vein is identified during pelvic lymphadenectomy.

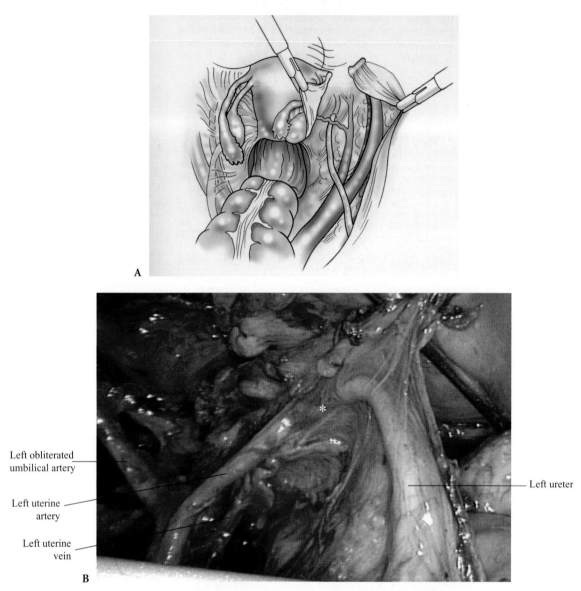

Figure 6.4. (**A**) Right pelvic side-wall exposure. (**B**) To prevent injuries, the ureter must be identified before irreversible action is taken. Here is one of the most vulnerable sites of ureteral injury and the anatomy of water under the bridge is clearly seen.

THE PARA-AORTIC REGION

The para-aortic region is the anatomic area from the renal vessels down to the bifurcation of the common iliac arteries in the posterior abdominal retroperitoneum (Figure 6.11A-E). For practical purposes, this region is divided into two areas.

The lower para-aortic area is bounded by the bifurcation of the aorta up to the level of the inferior mesenteric artery superiorly, the psoas muscles laterally, and the bifurcation of the common iliacs inferiorly. Dissections for lymphatic tissue for uterine or cervical cancer involve this area.

The infrarenal area (upper para-aortic area) extends from the level of the inferior mesenteric artery up to the left renal vein. Usually the ovarian arteries exit the anterior aspect of the aorta in the midportion of this area. The right ovarian vein travels next to the right ureter and empties into the vena cava. The left ovarian vein travels with the left ureter but empties into the left renal vein. These structures lie on the anterior surface of the psoas

muscle. A major concern on the left side is injury to the renal vein and the lumbar veins and arteries arising from the posterior aspect of the aorta and vena cava. The inferior extension of this region is the "presacral" space.

The landmarks, which should be kept in mind for para-aortic lymphadenectomies, from right to left are the psoas muscle; ovarian vessels; right ureter, medial to the psoas muscle and lateral to the inferior vena cava; vena cava to the right lateral of the aorta; and aorta and both common iliac arteries. Below the bifurcation of the aorta superficially is the superior hypogastric nerve plexus and the presacral nodes, and beneath them, the left common iliac vein crossing from the left to the right. On the left side of the aorta are the inferior mesenteric artery, the sigmoid colon, and its mesentery. On a deeper plane are the lumbar veins and artery medially and the left ureter laterally, which can be seen after left lymphadenectomy. On the far left is the left psoas muscle (Figure 6.11C).

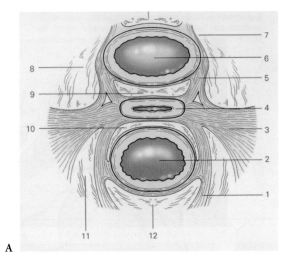

1- Uterosacral ligament
2- Rectum
3- Cardinal ligament
4- Vagina
5- Bladder pillar
6- Urinary bladder
7- Prevesical space
8- Paravesical space
9- Vesicovaginal space
10- Rectovaginal space
11- Pararectal space
12- Retrorectal space

A

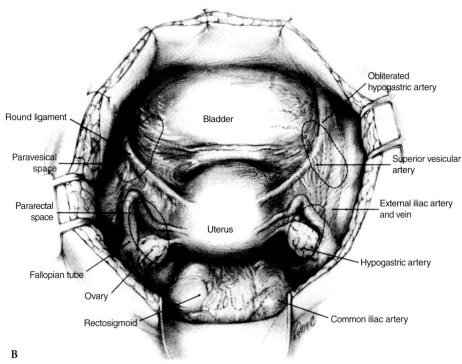

Obliterated
hypogastric artery

Round ligament

Bladder

Paravesical
space

Superior vesicular
artery

Pararectal
space

External iliac artery
and vein

Uterus

Hypogastric artery

Fallopian tube

Ovary

Common iliac artery

Rectosigmoid

B

Figure 6.5. (**A**) Avascular spaces and their ligamental boundries. (**B**) Illustrated are the eight avascular spaces and their anatomic relationship during the laparatomy.

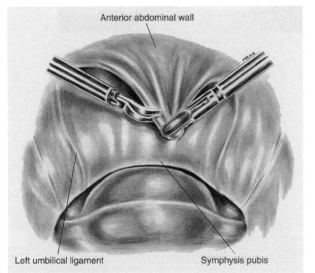

Anterior abdominal wall

Left umbilical ligament   Symphysis pubis

A

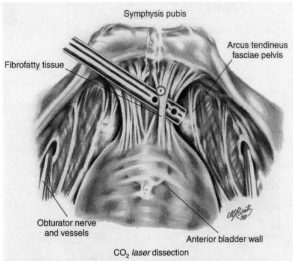

Symphysis pubis

Fibrofatty tissue

Arcus tendineus
fasciae pelvis

Obturator nerve
and vessels

Anterior bladder wall

CO_2 *laser* dissection

B

Figure 6.6. (**A**) A posterior view of the anterior abdominal wall during the Retzius space development (**B**) The space of Retzius is developed with blunt and sharp dissection of fibrofatty tissue. Care is taken to avoid periurethral neurovascular injury.

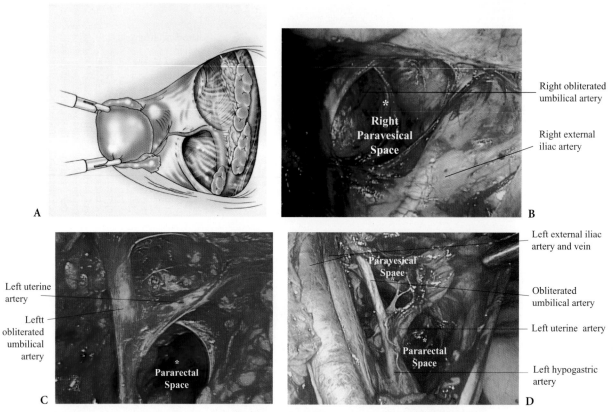

Figure 6.7. (**A**) The right paravesical space is developed. (**B**) The paravesical spaces limited by obturator internus muscle and the pelvic diaphragm laterally, the bladder pillar medially, the endopelvic fascia inferiorly, uterine artery posteriorly, and the medial umbilical ligaments superiorly. (**C**) The pararectal spaces are limited by the levator ani laterally, by the rectal pillars medially, by the anterolateral aspect of sacrum posteriorly, and uterine and cardinal complex anteriorly. (**D**) The relationship of pararectal and paravaginal spaces with the uterine artery.

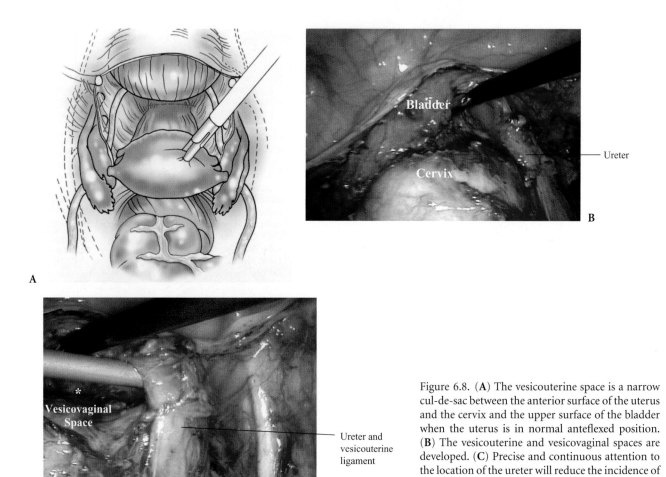

Figure 6.8. (**A**) The vesicouterine space is a narrow cul-de-sac between the anterior surface of the uterus and the cervix and the upper surface of the bladder when the uterus is in normal anteflexed position. (**B**) The vesicouterine and vesicovaginal spaces are developed. (**C**) Precise and continuous attention to the location of the ureter will reduce the incidence of complications.

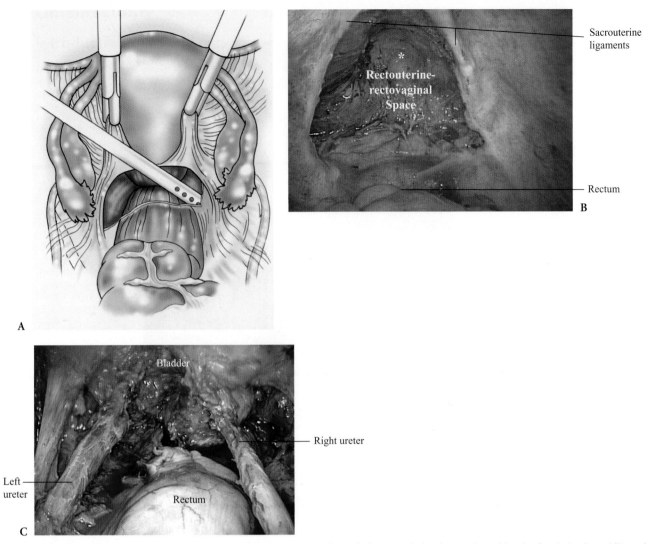

Figure 6.9. (**A**) The rectouterine (rectovaginal) space. The entire space, bounded anteriorly by the cervix and by the fornix in the midline, the uterosacral folds laterally, and the rectum posteriorly. (**B**) The rectovaginal space is completely developed. (**C**) Once all ligaments are dissected, all the spaces open to each other.

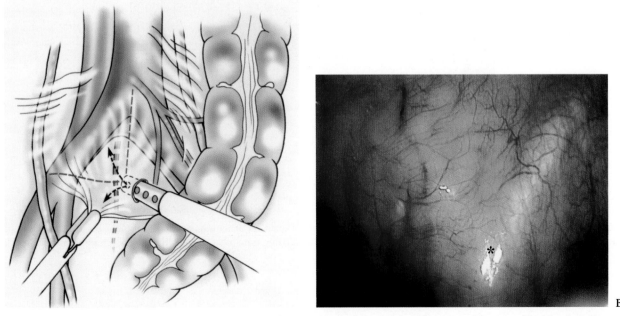

Figure 6.10. (**A**) Exposure of aortic caval bifurcation. (**B**) Intraperitoneal view of the bifurcation of the aorta (*). *(Continued)*

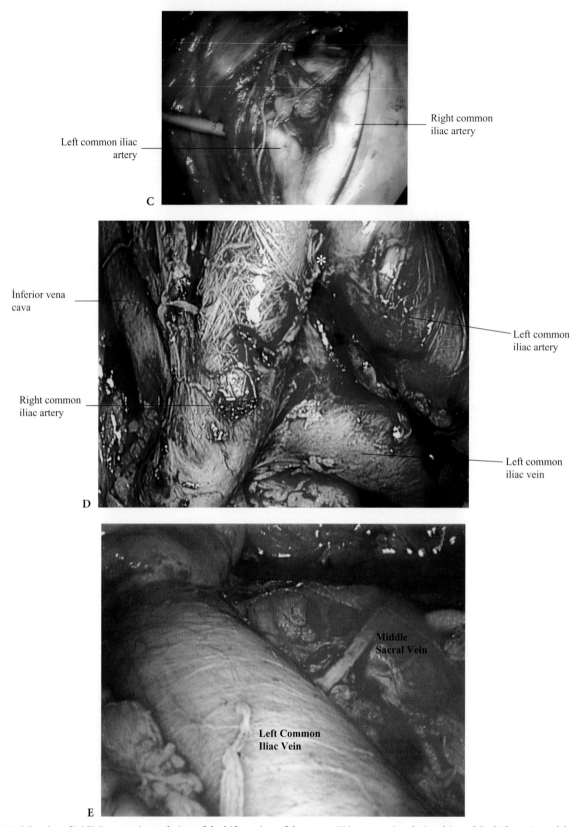

Figure 6.10. (*Continued*) (**C**) Retroperitoneal view of the bifurcation of the aorta. (**D**) Anatomic relationships of the bifurcation of the aorta and inferior vena cava. (**E**) The middle sacral vessels are in the midline on the sacrum. Care must be taken during dissection of this region.

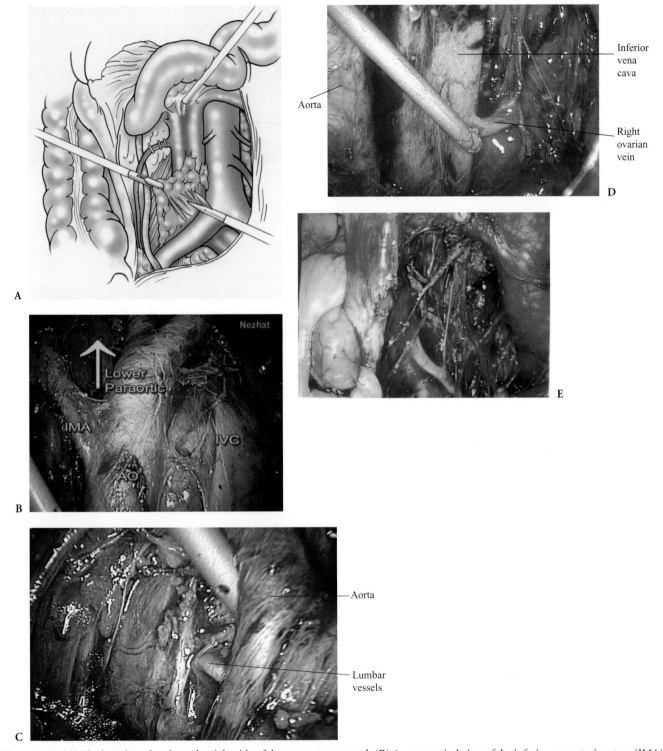

Figure 6.11. (**A**) The lymph nodes along the right side of the aorta are removed. (**B**) An anatomical view of the inferior mesenteric artery (IMA) and its origin from the aorta. (**C**) Anatomic relationships of the lumbar vessels to the aorta. (**D**) Anatomic relationships of the drainage of the right gonadal vein to I.V.C. (**E**) Anatomic view of the left upper para-aortic area after the lymphadenectomy.

THE URETER

The lumbar ureter lies on the psoas muscle medial to the ovarian vessels (Figures 6.2D,E, 6.4B, and 6.11A,B). It enters the pelvic cavity just superficial to the bifurcation of the common iliac artery and just deep to the ovarian vessels, which lie in the infundibulop-elvic ligament at the pelvic brim. It lies in the anterior medial leaf of the broad ligament as it courses toward the bladder and can be recognized by its characteristic peristaltic motion. The ureter then passes just lateral to the uterosacral ligament, approximately 2 cm medial to the ischial spine through the upper part of the cardinal ligament at the base of the broad ligament. Here it lies just beneath the uterine artery, approximately 1.5 to 2 cm lateral to the side of the cervix. The ureter forms a "knee" turn at this point and travels medially and anteriorly to pass on the anterolateral aspect of the upper third of the vagina toward the bladder (Figure 6.4 A,B and 6.9C).

REFERENCES

1. Nezhat F, Brill AI, Nezhat CH, et al. Laparoscopic appraisal of the anatomic relationship of the umbilicus to the aortic bifurcation. *J Am Assoc Gynecol Laparosc.* 1998;5:135.

SUGGESTED READING

Morrow CP, Curtin JP. Surgical anatomy. In: *Gynaecologic Cancer Surgery*. New York: Churchill Livingstone; 1996:67–139.

Nezhat CR, Siegler AM, Nezhat F, Nezhat C, Seidman DS, Luciano A. *Operative Gynecologic Laparoscopy*. 2nd ed. New York: McGraw Hill; 2000.

Pasic RP, Levine RL. *A Practical Manual of Laparoscopy: A Clinical Cookbook*. Lancashire, UK: Parthenon Publishing Group; 2002.

Rogers RM Jr, Childers JM. *Laparoscopic Gynecologic Anatomy: The Surgical Essentials.*

Smith JR, Del Priore G, Curtin J, Monaghan JM. *An Atlas of Gynecologic Oncology*. London: Martin Dunitz; 2001.

7 | FERTILITY

Section 7.1. Frontiers in Fertility

Kutluk Oktay and Amr M.A. Azim

The field of reproductive medicine is evolving rapidly. We are living in an era in which what was seemingly impossible a decade ago is being made possible, and century-old dogmas are being challenged. Thanks to new cryopreservation technologies, infertility and premature ovarian failure, especially when induced by medical treatments, are no longer unavoidable consequences. Whereas success with oocyte cryopreservation is gradually approaching acceptable levels for use in patients who face the risk of ovarian failure due to medical treatments or to create "egg banks" for oocyte donation, ovarian tissue cryopreservation and transplantation promise to be a way to reverse menopause and restore fertility. Yet, the recently proposed possibility of the presence of germ stem cells in human bone marrow is even more intriguing. Whereas bone marrow and peripheral blood transplants result in repopulation of chemotherapy-treated ovaries with primordial follicles in rodents, germ stem cell markers are already shown in human bone marrow and peripheral blood.[1] According to this theory, the ovaries provide signals to the germ stem cells residing in the bone marrow and recruit new follicles via the bloodstream "on demand." Although shocking and contrary to the preexisting dogma that the ovarian reserve is predetermined before birth, this hypothesis is not without supporting evidence in humans and nonhuman primates, as illustrated by the following case study.

AN OVARIAN TRANSPLANT CASE IN SUPPORT OF THE GERM STEM CELL HYPOTHESIS

One ovary was removed and cryopreserved in a 29-year-old patient with recurrent Hodgkin's lymphoma before preconditioning chemotherapy for autologous hematopoietic stem cell transplantation. The preconditioning chemotherapy containing a high-dose alkylating agent put the patient in menopause immediately. The patient remained in menopause for 2.5 years, until her ovarian tissue was thawed and transplanted subcutaneously to her lower abdominal area, as described later. Two months after the transplantation, the patient felt follicle growth underneath her skin and conceived spontaneously. Three weeks after the termination of this abnormal pregnancy, the patient felt follicle growth in her graft and had a spontaneous menstruation a week later. In the next cycle, ovulation was detected by a luteinizing hormone (LH) surge, contemporaneously with follicle growth in the graft, at which time the patient had intercourse. The patient conceived immediately and delivered a healthy female child at term.

Although it is theoretically possible that these pregnancies following ovarian transplantation could represent a rare event of ovarian recovery after chemotherapy, occurrence of two preg-

nancies in the 3 months immediately following ovarian transplantation is highly intriguing, especially given the fact that this patient did not conceive during the previous 2.5 years, when she appeared to be in menopause. Is it possible that the chemotherapy damages the ability of the ovary to recruit germ stem cells from the bone marrow rather than damaging a preexisting stockpile of follicles? Could recovery of ovarian function and fertility after receiving sterilizing chemotherapy be the result of resumption of de novo production of primordial follicles? Could the transplanted ovary provide signals on behalf of the menopausal ovary to begin producing primordial follicles or for the bone marrow to provide germ stem cells to that ovary? Although only future translational laboratory experiments will determine whether this mechanism is operational in humans and can be responsible for ovarian transplant pregnancies, supporting evidence for germ cell renewal was provided from human and nonhuman primate studies published more than 50 years ago. Based on histologic data, Schwarz et al. [2] suggested the continuation of oogenesis in adult ovaries as early as in 1949. A study by Vermande-Van Eck [3] put forward a stronger argument for the production of primordial follicles in nonhuman primate ovaries. In that study, based on the incidence of atresia and the time it would take for atretic follicles to be cleared from the ovaries, it was estimated that the 90% of ovarian reserve would be depleted within the first 2 years of life. Considering the fact that the monkeys used in that study did not even experience puberty until the age of 4, and they remained fertile for 20 years, primordial follicles, neo-oogenesis remains a real possibility in postnatal ovaries.

The field of reproductive medicine is embracing an exciting future, and in the opinion of the senior author (K.O.), only by keeping an open mind for alternative explanations for previously dogmatized concepts can we support progress. A perfect example of this is the evolution, under pioneering leaders such as Dr. Nezhat, of laparoscopic techniques that were considered "shocking" a decade ago but are now the standard of care. The following gives only glimpse of what the future may hold for our field.

OOCYTE CRYOPRESERVATION

Oocyte cryopreservation has the potential to preserve fertility in females at risk of losing ovarian function due to medical/surgical treatments or at constitutionally high risk for early ovarian failure. This technique may also bypass some of the ethical concerns and legislative restrictions regarding embryo freezing. An oocyte bank system could be established to make oocyte donation more practical. Oocyte banking may also become a strategy to circumvent

Table 7.1.1: Slow Freezing of Human Mature Oocytes

Study	No. of Oocytes Thawed	Cumulus	Cryoprotectant	Survival,%	Fertlization,%	Cleavage,%	IVF/ICSI	PR/oocyte,%
Chen (1986, 1988) [9,13]	50	Partial	DMSO	76	71	60	IVF	6
van Uem (1997) [14]	4	No	DMSO	100	50	—	IVF	25
Al-Hasani (1987) [15]	205	Partial	DMSO/PROH	25	56/75	—	IVF	1
Tucker (1996) [16]	81	No	PROH	25	65	100	ICSI	3.7
Porcu (1997, 1998) [10,17]	709	No	PROH	56	63	90	ICSI	1.3
Porcu (1998) [18]	1502	No	PROH	54	57	91	ICSI	1.1
Borini (1998) [19]	129	No	PROH	31	51	94	ICSI	2.3
Tucker (1998) [20]	241	No	PROH	31	51	74	ICSI	2.1
Polack de Fried (1998) [21]	10	No	PROH	30	66	100	ICSI	0.2
Young (1998) [22]	9		PROH	89	100	62	ICSI	1.1
Winslow (2001) [23]	324	No	PROH	68	81	95	ICSI	5.3
Quintans (2002) [24]	109	No	PROH	63	59	100	ICSI	5.5
Fosas (2003) [25]	88	No	PROH	90	73	—	ICSI	4.6
Boldt (2003) [26]	90	No	PROH	74	59	85	ICSI	7.8

DMSO, dimethylsulfoxide; PR, pregnancies; PROH, 1,2 propanediol.

age-related decline in oocyte reserve and quality. Oocyte freezing may also be used if no sperm can be collected or retrieved (e.g., nonretrieval of sperm during testicular sperm extraction) during an in vitro fertilization (IVF) cycle.

The potential problems with oocyte freezing are freeze–thaw-induced hardening of zona pellucida, cytoskeleton damage, alteration of cortical granules, damage to meiotic spindle, increased incidence of polyploidy and aneuploidy, and parthenogenetic activation of oocytes. The different variables that may influence successful oocyte freezing include oocyte quality and age, maturation stage, presence of cumulus mass, type of cryoprotectant, and cryopreservation protocol (slow freeze–rapid thaw, vitrification).[4–6] The rate of abnormal fertilization after oocyte cryopreservation ranges from 5% to 15%. Finally, preimplantation genetic diagnosis (PGD) or at least prenatal determination of karyotype is advisable until long-term safety data are available.

History

The discovery by Polge, Smith, and Parks [7] in 1948 that fowl spermatozoa can survive freezing at −70°C in the presence of glycerol marks the onset of cryopreservation of reproductive cells and tissues. The first success with oocyte freezing was achieved in mouse in 1977, followed by other animals. In 1983, Trounson and Mohr [8] demonstrated that human embryos can be thawed after freezing with subsequent development and pregnancy. Two main methods of oocyte freezing have emerged, slow freezing and vitrification. The first human pregnancy from fertilization of slow-frozen mature oocyte was reported by Chen [9] in 1986.

In 1997, Porcu et al. [10] reported the first human live birth after thawing of mature human oocyte and intracytoplasmic sperm injection (ICSI). Cha et al. [11] in 1999 reported on a pregnancy from vitrified immature oocyte and IVF using 5.5 mol/L ethylene glycol as a cryoprotectant.

Slow Freezing of Mature Human Oocytes

Oocytes should be frozen shortly after harvesting, about 38 to 40 hours after human chorionic gonadotropin (hCG) injection. Most protocols employ slow freeze–rapid thaw using 1,2-propanediol (PROH) and sucrose as cryoprotectants. Sodium-depleted media were recently introduced.

There is considerable variation in the literature concerning survival after thawing, fertilization, cleavage, and pregnancy after cryopreservation of mature oocytes.

Oocyte cyopreservation is still not as efficient as embryo cryopreservation. Per oocyte live birth rates average around 1.7% to 2.0% compared with approximately 7% with fresh oocytes; this corresponds to 20% versus 60% live births per embryo transfer, respectively.[12] Some of the main oocyte cryopreservation reports are summarized in Table 7.1.1.

Vitrification of Mature Human Oocytes

Vitrification is defined as solidification of solution into a glassy state without ice formation. High concentrations of cryoprotectants and a very rapid cooling rate are used. The most commonly used cryoprotectant is ethylene glycol because of its relatively low toxicity and high permeability through zona and the cellular

Table 7.1.2: Vitrification of Human Mature Oocytes

Reference	No. of Oocytes	Cumulus	Cryoprotectant	Survival, %	Fertilization, %	Cleavage, %	IVF/ICSI	PR/oocyte, %
Kuleshova (1999) [28]	17	?	EG/S/straw	65	46%	60	ICSI	5.9
Yoon (2000) [29]	90	Yes	EG/S/grid	63	68	89	ICSI	3.3
Chen (2000) [30]	198	No	EG/S/straw	91	51	80	ICSI	No ET
Katayama (2003) [31]	46	?	EG/DMSO/Cryotop	94	91	90	ICSI	4.3
Yoon (2003) [32]	474	Yes	EG/S/grid	69	72	95	ICSI	1.3

EG, ethylene glycol; ET, embryo transfer; S, sucrose.

membrane. Some authorities suggest that vitrification is more suitable than slow freezing for oocyte cryopreservation because of control of solute concentration/dehydration, short duration outside the incubator, brief temperature shock, and preservation of zona pellucida. Results of vitrification of human oocytes are presented in Table 7.1.2. Modifications that may improve results of vitrification include addition of synthetic macromolecules, microinjection of sugars, use of different cryocontainers (pulled straws, cryoloops, grids), and cytoskeleton stabilizers (taxanes). Recently, Liebermann et al. [27] achieved over 80% survival of 1120 mature human oocytes after vitrification using a mixture of ethylene glycol, dimethylsulfoxide (DMSO), polymer macromolecules, sucrose, and synthetic serum substitute. However, there have been only 10 deliveries from this procedure and its true potential remains to be determined. Moreover, because oocytes are vitrified in an open system, viral cross-contamination in liquid nitrogen is a possibility.

Cryopreservation of Immature Oocytes

Immature human oocytes can survive cryopreservation, with subsequent maturation to metaphase II oocytes.[33] Chromosomes in prophase oocytes are not aligned along the equator plate, and they may be theoretically less susceptible to spindle damage during the freeze–thaw cycle. Immature oocytes can be obtained during an unstimulated cycle (e.g., during gynecologic surgery) (Table 7.1.3). Patients with polycystic ovarian disease may particularly benefit from this technology as they tend to produce a large number of immature oocytes. In addition, freezing immature oocytes has the potential to avoid ovarian hyperstimulation in patients at risk for ovarian hyperstimulation syndrome or when increased estrogen levels are considered hazardous (e.g., in breast cancer patients or patients at risk for thromboembolism). This method may also help cancer patients who do not have sufficient time to undergo ovarian stimulation before chemotherapy. Nevertheless, there have been very few reports and live births with cryopreserved immature oocytes, and the efficiency of this approach remains to be determined.

IN VITRO MATURATION OF OOCYTES

Retrieving immature oocytes and maturing them in vitro has the potential to avoid prolonged and expensive controlled ovar-

ian hyperstimulation, ovarian hyperstimulation syndrome, and exposure to high levels of estrogen when a high-risk condition exists.

History

Gregory Pincus [41] in 1935 and Roger Edwards [42] in 1965 showed that oocytes may spontaneously resume meiosis when removed from antral follicles. Research in 1970s and 1980s probed many of the steps involved in oocyte maturation, including the need for cumulus cells, the importance of follicular and oocyte size, molecular mechanisms involved in resumption of meiosis, culture conditions, protein synthesis and gene expression during oocyte maturation, and the effect of priming with follicle-stimulating hormone (FSH) and hCG. Although pregnancies from in vitro maturation (IVM) of immature oocytes obtained during conventional ovarian stimulation for IVF were reported in 1983, the first human pregnancy from an immature oocyte obtained during an unstimulated cycle was reported by Cha et al. [43] in 1991. In 1994, Trounson et al. [44] reported the first pregnancy after IVM of oocytes from a polycystic ovarian syndrome (PCOS) patient.

In Vitro Maturation of Oocytes from Antral Follicles

Oocytes for IVM can be obtained during a cesarean section delivery [43,45], during different phases of the ovarian cycle, from PCOS patients, and after ovarian stimulation.[44,46,47]

Luteal phase oocytes may display significantly higher maturation rates than those obtained during follicular phase, although this has not been a consistent finding in all studies.[48] The presence of a dominant follicle does not affect developmental competence of immature oocytes from antral follicles as they do not undergo atresia.[49]

Increased age and high day 3 levels of FSH, estradiol (≥ 200 pmol/L), and inhibin A (≥ 10 pg/mL) were associated with reduced immature oocyte recovery and pregnancy rate.[50]

The ability to resume meiosis after retrieval is largely dependent on follicular and oocyte size. Developmental competence increases as oocyte diameter increases from 90 to 120 μm.[51,52] Follicles with a minimum diameter of 5 mm can provide oocytes that can be matured in vitro, irrespective of exposure to gonadotropin stimulation.[53] Fertilization rate increases progressively in oocytes from follicles 10 mm or greater.

Table 7.1.3: Freezing of Human Immature Oocytes

Reference	No./Cycle/ Stage	Cumulus	Protocol	Survival, %	Maturation, %	Fertilization, %; Method	Cleavage, %	Result
Toth (1994) [33]	123 Stim MI	?	PROH Slow freeze–rapid thaw	59	83	62 IVF	58	3 blast
Baka (1995) [34]*	98 Stim GV-MI	Yes	PROH Slow freeze–rapid thaw	63	68	—	—	—
Tucker (1998) [35]	13 Stim GV		PROH Slow freeze–rapid thaw	23	67	100 ICSI	100	1 live birth
Son (1996) [36]	98 Unstim GV-MI	Yes	PROH Slow freeze Rapid thaw	55	59	43 IVF	17	No ET
Park (1997) [37]†	128 Unstim GV	Yes	PROH Slow freeze–rapid thaw	60	61	—	—	—
Cha (2000) [38]	301 Unstim/Stim GV (PCOD)	Yes	EG/S/grid vitrification	83	68	68 ICSI	90	ET, no pregnancy
Wu (2001) [39]‡	78 Unstim GV-MI	Yes	EG/S/grid vitrification	59	64	70 IVF	71	20 embryo 2 blast (7%) 1 biochem
Fuchinoue (2004) [40]§	137 Stim GV	Partial/No	EG+DMSO/S/F/ HTF/SSS/Cryotoop vitrification	79–90	58–85	62–78 ICSI	38–82	1 blast (0.7%)

F, Ficoll (Spectrum Medical Industries); HTF, human tubal fluid; SSS, synthetic serum substitute; GV, germinal vesicle; MI, metaphase I oocyte; PCOD, polycystic ovarian disease; Stim, stimulated; blast, blastocyst; biochem, biochemical pregnancy; Unstim, unstimulated.
*Oocytes matured before freezing had significant spindle abnormalities.
†High incidence of chromosomal abnormalities in oocytes thawed. No attempt at fertilization.
‡Oocytes aspirated from 4- to 11-mm follicles during chocolate cyst removal on days 9 to 12 of menstrual cycle.
§Best result when cumulus is present and Taxol (Bristol-Myers Squibb) was used.

The concept of short-course FSH stimulation before in vitro maturation was first introduced by the senior author in 1995 while working in Roger Gosden's laboratory. However, the effect of a short (truncated) course of FSH priming (75 to 150 IU/day for 3 to 6 days) on immature oocyte recovery and developmental capacity is undetermined. Although some researchers [50,53] reported at least doubling of the number of oocytes reaching metaphase II oocytes (MII) stage, others reported no benefit for such treatment on oocyte recovery and maturation.[54]

On the other hand, the exposure of immature oocytes to an ovulating dose of hCG 36 hours before retrieval appears to confer significant benefit on their development. The percentage of immature oocytes exhibiting germinal vesicle breakdown and reaching MII stage are increased. In addition, the time required for in vitro maturation is shortened (24 vs. 48 hours). Synchronization of follicular maturation after hCG assists in timing of in vitro fertilization by insemination or ICSI.[54,55] Although denuded oocytes can be matured to MII, their early embryonic development is questionable. The presence of cumulus cells appears to provide or mediate the action of several hormones/factors needed for IVM.[56]

About 5% to 7% of oocytes retrieved from IVF patients after ovarian hyperstimulation are immature (germinal vesicle [GV] stage). A fraction of these oocytes may mature in vitro spontaneously after removal of cumulus cells or by in vitro culture techniques. The developmental capacity of these "leftover" oocytes is generally low.[49] However, we find this technique most useful for cancer patients who are undergoing ovarian stimulation for oocyte or embryo freezing before chemotherapy. In our hands, IVM with second-day ICSI increases mature oocyte and embryo yield by at least 20% to 25% (unpublished data, Oktay K). Immature oocytes can also be obtained from ovaries removed for gynecologic conditions as well as from ovarian tissue removed for cryopreservation.[43,57]

Finally, a futuristic use of immature oocytes is for somatic cell nuclear transfer, and production of customized embryonic stem cells that are patient compatible for use by the donor of nuclear material (therapeutic cloning [58]). This concept was proved in mouse.[59] The erasure of somatic memory is essential for nuclear reprogramming (de-differentiation). This is usually incomplete after nuclear transfer and may lead to severe developmental abnormalities and poor implantation of cloned embryos.

IN VITRO MATURATION OF PREANTRAL AND PRIMORDIAL OOCYTES

Growth and maturation of primordial and preantral follicles is a major technical challenge for reproductive science. Primordial follicles (35 μm) are primary oocytes surrounded by one layer of flattened pregranulosa cells and constitute the ovarian reserve.

Preantral follicles (100 to 150 μm) are growing primary oocytes surrounded by several (up to six) layers of cuboidal granulosa cells. Theca cells are recruited from surrounding stroma around the basement membrane of the follicle.[60]

Primordial follicles can be isolated by partial enzymatic disaggregation followed by mechanical dissection [61] or can be kept in organ culture until they have grown to a stage where they can be more easily isolated. After isolation, follicles can be grown on collagen membrane, laminin, plastic culture plate, or under mineral oil.[62] They can also be grown in three-dimensional extracellular matrix environment.

Several culture systems were developed to support growth of preantral and primordial follicles (for review [60]).

To date, live offspring were produced by in vitro growth of primordial follicles only in the mouse [63], but this has not been possible with human primordial or preantral follicles.

The factors that control primordial and preantral follicle growth in vivo and in vitro are under extensive investigation at this time.

OVARIAN TISSUE CRYOPRESERVATION AND TRANSPLANTATION

History

The birth of a mammalian offspring after orthotopic transplantation of cryopreserved ovarian tissue was reported by Parrott in 1960 in mice.[63] Gosden in 1994 [64] reported on the delivery of two lambs after orthotopic transplantation of fresh and frozen–thawed ovarian grafts. Oktay (2000) [65] reported the first case of orthotopic transplantation of thawed ovarian cortical strips with return of ovarian function for a brief period. The first human embryo produced from heterotopic transplant of thawed ovarian cortical strips was reported by Oktay et al. in 2004. In the same year, delivery of a monkey after heterotopic transplantation of fresh ovarian tissue was reported.[66] Donnez and coworkers in 2004 reported on the occurrence of pregnancy and delivery following orthotopic transplantation of ovarian cortical pieces [67]; however, questions were raised regarding the source of the oocyte that resulted in the pregnancy as this patient still had occasional ovulation from her remaining ovaries.

Fertility preservation involves a number of procedures other than ovarian cryopreservation. Our algorithmic approach is summarized below. The most common indication for ovarian tissue freezing is a malignant disease requiring gonadotoxic chemotherapy.

The gonadotoxic effects of chemotherapeutic agents on steroid-producing cells as well as the oocytes are variable (Table 7.1.4). Alkylating agents are the most gonadotoxic. Cyclophosphamide-induced follicular damage is dose dependent. The mechanism of gonadotoxicity is probably through interference with cell cycle progression and induction of apoptosis. Older women are more susceptible to premature ovarian failure because of smaller primordial follicle pool size. Even after resumption of menses in younger patients, premature menopause may develop later in their reproductive life.[68] The use of symptoms (e.g., menses, hot flashes, chronologic age) to assess ovarian reserve after chemotherapy is unreliable. There are several established and developing means of ovarian reserve assessment. These include biochemical markers (baseline and stimulated FSH, LH, estradiol, inhibin-B, antimullerian hormone), biophysical markers (antral follicle count, ovarian volume, ovarian stromal blood flow), or dynamic testing (clomiphene citrate challenge test, gonadotropin-releasing hormone (GnRH) agonist stimulation test, and exogenous FSH ovarian reserve test).[69] Antimullerian hormone measurements appear to have strong promise in assessing ovarian reserve as this hormone is produced from very early-stage preantral follicles and the expression of its protein can be found in as early as primordial follicles.

Pharmacologic Ovarian Protection

Ovarian suppression by GnRH agonist does not seem to offer gonadal protection in men or women. It may, however, be possible to protect ovarian reserve by pharmacologic treatments. For example, rodent studies have shown that oocyte apoptosis can be suppressed during chemotherapy and radiation by the disruption of acid sphingomyelinase gene and this apoptotic pathway by sphingosine-1-phosphate treatment.[70,71]

IVF with Antiestrogen Compounds

Breast cancer is the most common malignant disease in reproductive-age women. Although its incidence has increased over the last several decades, the mortality of breast cancer has declined. Fifteen percent of breast cancer cases occur in women 40 years or younger.

During treatment, a hiatus of up to 6 weeks exists between surgery and chemotherapy. During that time, oocyte, embryo, or ovarian tissue cryopreservation can be performed.[72] Because controlled ovarian hyperstimulation using conventional regimens causes marked elevation in estrogen levels, alternative ovarian stimulation agents such as tamoxifen and aromatase inhibitors are used in combination with FSH.[72,73] When used

Table 7.1.4: Gonadotoxicity of Chemotherapeutic Agents

High risk
- Cyclophosphamide
- Chlorambucil
- Melphalan
- Procarbazine

Intermediate risk
- Cisplatinum
- Adriamycin
- Paclitaxel?

Low risk
- Methotrexat
- 5-Fluorouracil
- Vincristine
- Bleomycin
- Actinomycin D

Table 7.1.5: Major Reports of Ovarian Cortical Strip Transplantation in Humans

Study	Age, years	Indication	Cryoprotectant	Graft Site	Results	Onset, weeks[†]	Duration, months[‡]
Heterotopic							
Oktay (2001, 2003) [75,76]	35	Cervical cancer IIIb before chemoradiation	DMSO	Forearm	Follicular growth, oocyte retrieval	10	21
	37	BSO for benign disease	DMSO	Forearm	Follicular growth, menses, ovulation	24	≥24
Oktay (2004) [77]	30	Breast cancer IIb before chemotherapy	DMSO	Abdominal wall	Follicular growth, oocyte retrieval, IVM fertilization, ET	12	?
Kim (2004) [78]	37	Cervical cancer Ib at time of radical hysterectomy	DMSO	Abdominal and chest walls	Follicular growth, ovulation	14	7
Wolner-Hanssen (2005) [79]	37	Sjögren syndrome, pure red cell aplasia before HSCT	PROH	Forearm	Follicular growth	18	8
Orthotopic							
Oktay (2000, 2001) [80,81]	29	BSO for benign disease	PROH	Pelvic peritoneum	Follicular growth, ovulation, menses	15	≥10
Radford (2001) [82]	36	Hodgkin's after third relapse, before HSCT	PROH	ovary/peritoneum	Menses (×1)	28	9
Donnez (2004) [67]	25	Hodgkin's before chemotherapy	DMSO	Pelvic peritoneum	Follicular growth, menses, spontaneous conception, live birth*	20	?
Meirow (2005) [83]	28	NHL, relapse after chemotherapy	CS, small pieces	Right ovary/left ovary	Menses, follicular growth, natural cycle IVF, live birth*	32	≥9

BSO, bilateral salpingoophorectomy; CS, cortical strips; HSCT, hematopoietic stem cell transplantation; NHL, non-Hodgkin's lymphoma.
*Source of oocyte leading to pregnancy could be the native ovary rather than transplanted tissue.
†Weeks between transplantation and hormonal and/or clinical activity of the graft.
‡Months of hormonal activity or ovulation after grafting.

for this purpose, tamoxifen nearly doubles the number of oocytes retrieved and is associated with less cycle cancellation when compared with natural cycles.[72]

A recent prospective comparison between induction of ovulation with tamoxifen and letrozole in combination with low-dose FSH stimulation indicated no significant increase in the incidence of short-term cancer recurrence compared with non-IVF breast cancer controls. The letrozole–FSH protocol resulted in lower estradiol levels compared with tamoxifen–FSH and resulted in a larger number of oocytes with a trend toward a higher number of embryos.[73]

Letrozole, alone or in combination with FSH, may also be used to cryopreserve oocytes and embryos in endometrial cancer patients.[74]

Human Trials and Techniques

Main trials of ovarian tissue transplantation with or without cryopreservation are summarized in Table 7.1.5. This procedure has the most potential when ovarian tissue is cryopreserved before 40 years of age.[68] Ovarian transplantation techniques may be summarized as follows.

Orthotopic Ovarian Cortical Strip Transplantation

Oktay et al. 2001 [81]: Ovarian cortical pieces are strung using 6-0 Vicryl sutures (Ethicon) under a microsurgical microscope. Those are then anchored to a triangular biodegradable polycellulose membrane (Surgicel, Johnson & Johnson). The membrane is tagged by a suture at its apex and laparoscopically

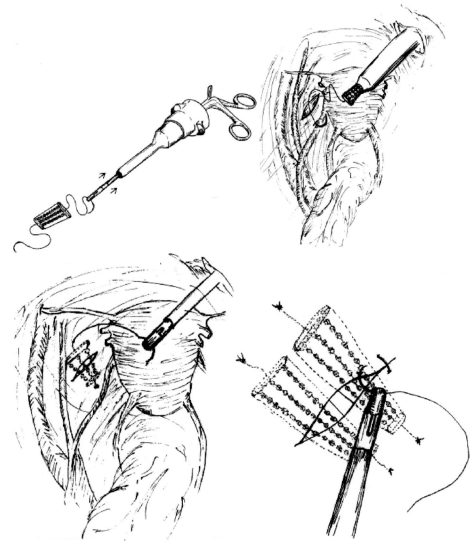

Figure 7.1.1. Technique of orthotopic ovarian transplant. See text for more details. From Oktay et al. [76], with permission from the American Society for Reproductive Medicine (ASRM).

inserted in a peritoneal pocket on the pelvic sidewall. The needle is passed through the peritoneum to wedge the graft in place. The peritoneum is then closed with laparoscopic suturing (Figure 7.1.1).

Meirow et al. 2005 [83]: Implantation of frozen-thawed ovarian cortical pieces in the menopausal ovary was first proposed by Oktay et al. In the Meirow group's report, three pairs of 5-mm transverse incisions were made in the ovary through the tunica albuginea. With blunt dissection, cavities were formed beneath the cortex for each of the three strips. Each piece of thawed ovarian tissue (1.5×0.5 cm in area and 0.1 to 0.2 cm in thickness) was gently placed in each cavity, and the incisions were closed with 4-0 Vicryl sutures (Figure 7.1.2).

Heterotopic Ovarian Cortical Strip Transplantation

Oktay et al. 2003 [76]: Each piece is tagged with 4-0 Vicryl by passing the needle between stroma and cortex under an operating microscope. The needle is then cut. A 1.5-cm transverse incision is made over the brachioradialis muscle, 5 to 10 cm below the antecubital fossa. Using blunt dissection, a pocket is created between

the fascia and the subcutaneous tissue. Attention is given to avoid injuring the larger veins and arteries. It is not desirable to perform extensive cauterization. Once the dissection is completed, the free end of the suture is threaded onto a reusable half-circle cutting

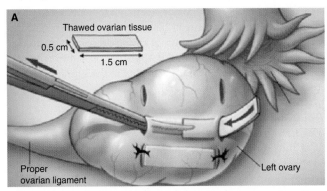

Figure 7.1.2. Technique of orthotopic ovarian transplantation. From Meirow et al. 2005 [77], with permission from *New England Journal of Medicine* and the author.

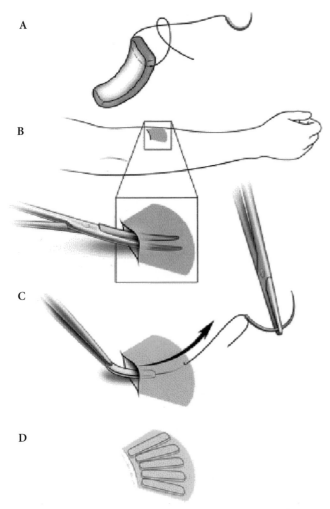

Figure 7.1.3. Technique of subcutaneous transplantation of ovarian cortical strips. From Oktay et al. 2003 [76], with permission from ASRM.

needle. This needle is inserted in the subcutaneous space as far as possible and passed through the skin, and the cortical piece is wedged into the subcutaneous pocket by pulling on the suture. The transplanted strips are inserted with the cortical side facing up. The needle is then removed, and the free end of the suture is held with a mosquito clamp. The purpose of this suture pull-through technique is to guide the tissue placement and to avoid overlapping the strips, instead of anchoring them. The sutures are cut and the skin is closed using an intradermal/subcuticular suture. A nonpressure dressing is applied. The same technique applies when the tissues are transplanted in the suprapubic subcutaneous location (Figure 7.1.3).

Transplantation of an Intact Human Ovary with Its Vascular Pedicle

Although this technique had partial success in sheep, it has not been possible to cryopreserve whole human ovaries. This is mainly because of the larger size of human ovaries and the inability to efficiently cryopreserve both the oocytes and the vascular pedicle. Nevertheless, this is an active research area in the cryopreservation field. [84]

Table 7.1.6: Risk of Ovarian Metastases According to Cancer Type

Low risk (≤1%)
  Breast cancer stage I–III
  Hodgkin's lymphoma
  Non-Hodgkin's lymphoma
  Wilm's tumor
  Ewing sarcoma
  Nongenital rhabdomyosarcoma
  Osteosarcoma
  Squamous cell carcinoma of the cervix

Moderate risk (1% to 10%)
  Breast cancer stage IV
  Adeno/adenosquamous carcinoma of the cervix
  Colon cancer

High risk (≥10%)
  Leukemia
  Neuroblastoma
  Burkitt lymphoma

Safety of Ovarian Transplantation; Transmission of Cancer Cells

The risk of cancer metastases from various sites to the ovary depends on type and stage of cancer (Table 7.1.6).[85]

Animal experiments involving mice (leukemia) and human ovaries (Hodgkin's lymphoma) yielded variable results. No case of transmission of malignant cells after cure and transplantation has been reported in human studies so far. Development of reliable methods for detection of malignant cells in ovarian grafts is essential. Candidate methods, in addition to light microscopy, include polymerase chain reaction assays and Northern blot and immunohistochemistry for myeloperoxidase expression in acute myeloid leukemia.

Other strategies include purging of tumor cells from the graft using specific antibodies [86], in vitro growth and maturation of preantral follicles [60], and xenografting (Figure 7.1.4).[87]

HUMAN EMBRYONIC STEM CELLS AND REPRODUCTION

Embryonic stem cells (ESCs) are clonogenic immortal pluripotent cells capable of differentiation into all three germ layers and germ cells. Adult stem cells (ASCs) are unipotent or multipotent mortal cells that form cells of lineage of tissue they originate from. Some ASCs may retain the plasticity to colonize a variety of tissues under certain conditions; for example, bone marrow–derived stem cells can demonstrate multiplicity of linear differentiation (multipotent adult progenitor cells). The *niche* is a microenvironment composed of support cells and associated signals for controlling stem cell self-renewal and proliferation.

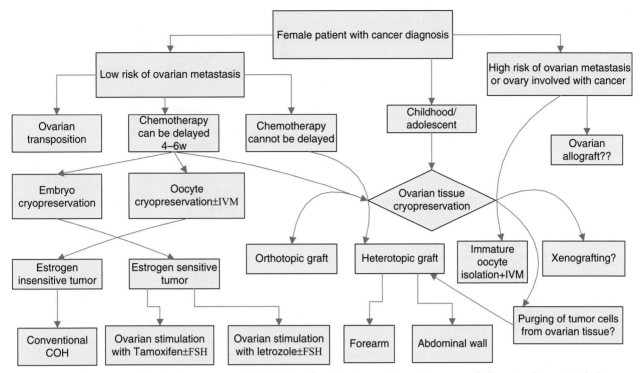

Figure 7.1.4. Proposed fertility preservation algorithm for a female cancer patient. COH, controlled ovarian hyperstimulation.

Totipotency of ESCs

Totipotent cells are capable of differentiating to extraembryonic and embryonic tissue and are derived from early zygote. Pluripotent cells can differentiate to germ layers only and are generally derived from inner cell mass (ICM) of blastocyst. Totipotential differentiation of mouse ESCs is supported by their ability to generate primordial germ cells that can develop into male and female gametes and form a blastocyst-like structure that can give rise to embryonic layers and trophectoderm.[88–91] Moreover, haploid male gametes derived from ESCs were capable of fertilizing mouse oocytes with formation of blastocysts.

Derivation of Human ESCs

Human embryonic stem cells can be derived from:

1. Inner cell mass (ICM) of blastocyst.[92] Blastocysts can be obtained by IVF or nuclear transfer to oocytes.
2. Morula.[93,94]
3. Single blastomere of eight-cell stage preimplantation embryo.[95]

The most common method is to derive ESC lines from ICM obtained by immunosurgery. Blastocysts are typically donated by women undergoing IVF. Zonae are removed. Blastocysts are exposed to rabbit antisera then transferred to guinea pig complement to kill trophectoderm cells.[96] Cells are co-cultured on meiotically inactivated embryonic feeder cells to form colonies. Cultures are supplemented by leukemia inhibitory factor, other growth factors, and protein source. Colonies are passaged weekly until a cell line is established.[97] Cells can then attach or take the

form of hanging drop (embryoid bodies). These cells can differentiate spontaneously after prolonged culture to all three germ layers and also to primordial germ cells (PGCs) as described by Clark et al. [98] in 2004.

Formation of Primordial Germ Cells from ESCs

ESCs are capable of formation of male gametes in EB [88] and female gametes in attached monolayer cultures.[90]

ESCs tagged by special reporter system (knock-in of green fluorescent protein (*GFP*) or B-D-galactosidase (*LacZ*) genes in octamer-4 homeodomain transcription factor of POU family or mouse vasa homologue (mvh) loci) have been cultured without feeder cells or growth factors. BMP4 (bone morphometric protein 4) or retinoic acid is added because of its mitogenic effect on PGCs. Cultures are arranged to form colonies or EBs. Cells develop in these culture systems within 7 days and express genes specific for PGCs.

Detection of Primordial Germ Cell Formation In Vitro

Analysis of germ cell–specific markers can be used to detect the differentiation of PGCs from ESCs (Figure 7.1.5). Because of significant overlap between markers expressed in somatic cells, ESCs, and PGCs, a combination approach includes sequential analysis of markers, morphologic studies, histochemical methods, and analysis of steroidogenic enzyme gene expression.[90,98]

Generating Oocytes from ESCs

By days 8 to 12 in culture, aggregates of cells containing putative PGCs (mvh+) and somatic cells separate from the rest of

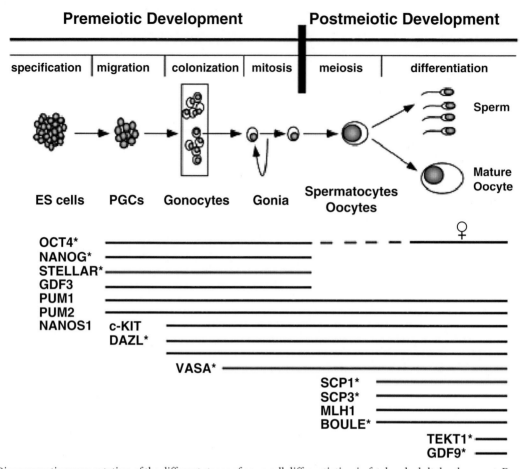

Figure 7.1.5. Diagrammatic representation of the different stages of germ cell differentiation in fetal and adult development. Expected expression patterns of genes used to predict each stage of germ cell development are shown by the name of the gene together with the *black bars* extending to the right of each gene name. All genes shown are enriched in germ cells relative to somatic cells; those that are expressed only in germ cells following gastrulation in vivo are indicated by an *asterisk*. Thus, genes known to be expressed in undifferentiated human embryonic stem cells include *OCT4*, *GDF3* (growth and differentiation factor 3), *NANOG*, *STELLAR*, *PUM1*, *PUMILIO 1*, *PUM2*, *PUMILIO 2*, and *NANOS 1*. Genes known to be expressed in PGC development through to later stages of germ cell differentiation include *DAZL* (deleted in azoospermia-like), *c-kit*, *stella*, and *Nanos*. Genes known to be expressed from gonocyte formation include *VASA*. Genes expressed during meiosis include *SCP1* (synaptonemal complex protein 1 and 3), *MLH1*, *Mut-L Homolog 1*, and *BOULE*. Adult oocyte-specific marker: *Gdf9*. Adult spermatid-specific marker: *TEKT1*, *Tektin1*.

the colonies. These are removed and cultured in a medium that supports IVM. Overnight these cells expand and organize into a follicle-like structure. By day 16 in culture, these structures express markers of entry into meiosis (DMC1, SCPs) as well as morphologic evidence of nuclear change (chromatin decondensation). On the other hand, surrounding somatic cells start to express granulosa cell markers (GDF9, steroidogenic enzymes, and estrogen production). By days 23 to 25 in culture, oocyte-like cells in these structures express markers of MII oocytes (zona pellucida proteins, polar body, spindle). On days 42 to 45, blastocyst-like structures are found floating in culture. These expressed markers of preimplantation embryos are probably formed by parthenogenetic activation of oocytes.[90]

Similar experiments have confirmed the formation of haploid male gametes from ESCs in EB by 20 days in culture. After transfer to recipient testis, they were able to complete spermatogenesis and the resultant spermatozoa were able to fertilize oocytes after ICSI.[88,89]

Although the technology is in its infancy, the spontaneous initiation of germ cell development from ESCs in vitro carries profound implications for both reproductive biology and reproductive medicine.

CONCLUSIONS

This century holds great promise for exciting developments in our field. The advent of molecular and cryopreservation techniques and stem cell technology is likely to change the way we look at the limits of the reproductive life span. As geriatrics has become one of the most prominent subspecialties of medicine because of the aging population, fertility preservation will become one of the most important aspects of our field given the increasing desire to delay childbearing. The trend for delaying childbearing is not only influenced by social reasons but also by increased life span and improved odds of surviving malignant and other chronic debilitating illnesses. An open-minded approach will facilitate the progress and better enable us to help our patients improve their quality of life.

REFERENCES

1. Johnson J, Bagley J, Skaznik-Wikiel M, et al. Oocyte generation in adult mammalian ovaries by putative germ cells in bone marrow and peripheral blood. *Cell*. 2005;122(2):303–315.

2. Schwarz OH, Young CC, Crouse JC. Ovogenesis in the adult human ovary. *Am J Obstet Gynecol*. 1949;58:54–64.

3. Vermande-Van Eck GJ. Neo-ovogenesis in the adult monkey. *Anat Rec*. 1956;125:207–224.

4. Porcu E. Oocyte freezing. *Sem Reprod Biol*. 2001;19(3):221–230.

5. Van der Elst J. Oocyte freezing: here to stay? *Hum Reprod*. 2003;9:463–470.

6. Chen S, Lien K, Chao H, Ho Y, Yang T. Effects of cryopreservation on meiotic spindle of oocytes and its dynamics after thawing: clinical implication in oocyte freezing – a review article. *Mol Cell Endocrinol*. 2003;202:101–107.

7. Polge C, Smith AU, Parks AS. Revival of spermatozoa after vitrification and dehydration at low temperature. *Nature (Lond)*. 1949;164:666.

8. Trounson A, Mohr L. Human pregnancy following cryopreservation, thawing and transfer of an eight cell embryo. *Nature*. 1983;305:707–709.

9. Chen C. Pregnancy after human oocyte cryopreservation. *Lancet*. 1986;884–886.

10. Porcu E, Fabbri R, Seracchioli R, et al. Birth of healthy female after intracytoplasmic sperm injection of cryopreserved human oocyte. *Fertil Steril*. 1997;68:724–730.

11. Cha KY, Hong SW, Chung HM, et al. Pregnancy and implantation from vitrified oocytes following in vitro fertilization (IVF) and in vitro culture (IVC). *Fertil Steril*. 1999;72(suppl 1):S2.

12. Oktay K, Cil A, Veek L, Bang H. Comparative efficiency of IVF between frozen-thawed oocytes and fresh oocytes. *Fertil Steril*. 2005;84(suppl 1):S37.

13. Chen C. Pregnancies after human oocyte cryopreservation. *Ann N Y Acad Sci*. 1987;541:541–549.

14. van Uem JF, Siebzehnrubl ER, Schuh B, Koch R, Trotnow S, Lang N. Birth after cryopreservation of unfertilized oocytes. *Lancet*. 1987;1:752–753.

15. Al-Hasani S, Diedrich K, van der Ven H, Reinecke A, Hartje M, Krebs D. Cryopreservation of human oocytes. *Hum Reprod*. 1987;2:695–700.

16. Tucker M, Wright G, Morton P, Shanguo L, Massey J, Kort H. Preliminary experience with human oocyte cryopreservation using 1,2-propanediol and sucrose. *Hum Reprod*. 1996;11(7):1513–1515.

17. Porcu E, Fabbri R, Seracchioli R, et al. Birth of six healthy children after intracytoplasmic sperm injection of cryopreserved human oocyte [abstract]. *Hum Reprod*. 1998;13(suppl 1):124.

18. Porcu E, Fabbri R, Ciotti P, et al. Cycles of human oocyte cryopreservation and intracytoplasmic sperm injection: results of 112 cycles [abstract]. *Fertil Steril*. 1998;72(suppl.1):S2.

19. Borini A, Bafaro M, Bonu M, at al. Pregnancy after oocyte freezing and thawing, preliminary data [abstract]. *Hum Reprod*. 1998;13(suppl 1):124–125.

20. Tucker M, Morton E, Wright G, Switzer C, Massey J. Clinical application of human egg cryopreservation. *Hum Reprod*. 1998;13:3156–3159.

21. Polak de Fried E, Notrica J, Rubinstein M, Marazzi A, Gomez Gonzalez M. Pregnancy after human donor oocyte cryopreservation and thawing in association with intracytoplasmic sperm injection in a patient with ovarian failure. *Fertil Steril*. 1998;69:555–557.

22. Young E, Kenny A, Puigdomenech E, Van Thillo G, Tiveron M, Piazza A. Triplet pregnancy after intracytoplasmic sperm injection of cryopreserved oocytes: case report. *Fertil Steril*. 1998;70(2):360–361.

23. Winslow K, Yang D, Blohm P, Brown S, Josim P, Nguyen K. Oocyte cryopreservation: a follow-up of sixteen births [abstract]. *Fertil Steril*. 2001;76(suppl 1):S120.

24. Quintans C, Donaldson M, Bertolino V, Pasqualini R. Birth of two babies using oocytes that were cryopreserved in a choline-based freezing medium. *Hum Reprod*. 2002;17(12):3149–3152.

25. Fosas N, Marina F, Torres P, et al. The births of five Spanish babies from cryopreserved donated oocytes. *Hum Reprod*. 2003;18(7):1417–1421.

26. Boldt J, Cline D, McLaughlin D. Human oocyte cryopreservation as an adjunct to IVF–embryo transfer cycles. *Hum Reprod*. 2003;18:1250–1255.

27. Liebermann J, Tucker M, Sills E. Cryoloop vitrification in assisted reproduction: analysis of survival rates in ≥1000 human oocytes after ultra-rapid cooling with polymer augmented cryoprotectant. *Clin Exp Obstet Gynecol*. 2003;30:125–129.

28. Kuleshova L, Gianaroli L, Magli C, Ferraretti A, Trounson A. Birth following vitrification of a small number of human oocytes: case report. *Hum Reprod*. 1999;14:3077–3079.

29. Yoon T, Chung H, Lim J, Han S, Ko J, and Cha KY. Pregnancy and delivery of healthy infants developed from vitrified oocytes in a stimulated in vitro fertilization–embryo transfer program. *Fertil Steril*. 2000;74:180–181.

30. Chen S, Lien Y, Chao K, Lu H, Ho H, Yang Y. Cryopreservation of mature human oocytes by vitrification with ethylene glycol in straws. *Fertil Steril*. 2000;74(4):804–808.

31. Katayama K, Stehlik J, Kuwayama M, Kato O, Stehlik E. High survival rate of vitrified human oocytes results in clinical pregnancy. *Fertil Steril*. 2003;80(1):223–224.

32. Yoon T, Kim T, Park S, et al. Live births after vitrification of oocytes in a stimulated in vitro fertilization-embryo transfer program. *Fertil Steril*. 2003;79(6):1323–1326.

33. Toth T, Baka S, Veek L, Jones H, Mausher S, Lanzendorf S. Fertilization and in vitro development of cryopreserved human prophase I oocytes. *Fertil Steril*. 1994;61:891–894.

34. Baka S, Toth T, Veeck L, Jones H Jr, Muasher S, Lanzendorf S. Evaluation of the spindle apparatus of in-vitro matured human oocytes following cryopreservation. *Hum Reprod*. 1995;10(7):1816–1820.

35. Tucker M, Wright G, Morton P, Massey J. Birth after cryopreservation of immature oocytes with subsequent in vitro maturation. *Fertil Steril*. 1998;70(3):578–579.

36. Son W, Park S, Lee K, et al. Effects of 1,2-propanediol and freezing-thawing on the in vitro developmental capacity of human immature oocytes. *Fertil Steril*. 1996;66:995–999.

37. Park S, Son W, Lee S, Lee K, Ko J, Cha K. Chromosome and spindle configurations of human oocytes matured in vitro after cryopreservation at the germinal vesicle stage. *Fertil Steril*. 1997;68(5):920–926.

38. Cha KY, Chung HM, Lim JM, Ko JJ, Han SY, Choi DH, Yoon TK. Freezing immature oocytes. *Molec Cell Endocrinol*. 2000;169(1-2):43–47.

39. Wu J, Zhang L, Wang X. In vitro maturation, fertilization and embryo development after ultrarapid freezing of immature human oocytes. *Reproduction*. 2001;121:389–393.

40. Fuchinoue K, Fukunaga N, Chiba S, Nakajo Y, Yagi A, Kyono K. Freezing of human immature oocytes using cryoloops and Taxol in vitrification solution. *J Assist Reprod Genet*. 2004;21(5):307–309.

41. Pincus G, Enzmann E. The comparative behavior of mammalian eggs in vivo and in vitro. The activation of ovarian eggs. *J Exp Med*. 1935;62:655.

42. Edwards R. Maturation in vitro of mouse, cheep, cow, pig, Rhesus monkey and human ovarian oocytes. *Nature (Lond)*. 1965;208:349–351.

43. Cha K, Koo J, Ko J, Choi D, Han S, Yoon T. Pregnancy after in vitro fertilization of human follicular oocytes collected from

nonstimulated cycles, their culture in vitro and their transfer in a donor oocyte program. *Fertil Steril.* 1991;55(1):109–113.

44. Trounson A, Wood C, Kausche A. In vitro fertilization and the fertilization and developmental competence of oocytes recovered from the untreated polycystic ovarian patients. *Fertil Steril.* 1994;62:353–362.

45. Hwang J, Lin Y, Tsai YL. In vitro maturation and fertilization of immature oocytes: a comparative study of fertilization techniques. *J Assist Reprod Genet.* 2000;17:39–43.

46. Barnes F, Kausche A, Tiglias J, Wood C, Wilton L, Trounson A. Production of embryos from in vitro matured primary human oocytes. *Fertil Steril.* 1996;65:1151–1156.

47. Mikkelsen A, Smith S, Lindenberg S. In-vitro maturation of human oocytes from regularly menstruating women may be successful without follicle stimulating hormone priming. *Hum Reprod.* 1999;14(7):1847–1851.

48. Whitacre K, Seifer D, Friedman C, et al. Effects of ovarian source, patient age, and menstrual cycle phase on in vitro maturation of immature human oocytes. *Fertil Steril.* 1998;70(6):1015–1021.

49. Trounson A, Anderiesz C, Jones G. Maturation of human oocytes in vitro and their developmental competence. *Reproduction.* 2001;121(1):51–75.

50. Mikkelsen A, Lindenberg S. Benefit of FSH priming of women with PCOS to the in vitro maturation procedure and the outcome: a randomized prospective study. *Reproduction.* 2001;122(4):587–592.

51. Eppig J, Schroeder A, O'Brien M. Developmental capacity of mouse oocytes matured in vitro: effects of gonadotrophic stimulation, follicular origin and oocyte size. *J Reprod Fertil.* 1992;95(1):119–127.

52. Durinzi K, Saniga E, Lanzendorf S. The relationship between size and maturation in vitro in the unstimulated human oocyte. *Fertil Steril.* 1995;63(2):404–406.

53. Wynn P, Picton H, Krapez J, Rutherford A, Balen A, Gosden R. Pretreatment with follicle stimulating hormone promotes the number of human oocytes reaching metaphase II by in-vitro maturation. *Hum Reprod.* 1998;13:3132–3138.

54. Lin Y, Hwang J, Huang L, et al. Combination of FSH priming and hCG priming for in-vitro maturation of human oocytes. *Hum Reprod.* 2003;18(8):1632–1636.

55. Chian R, Buckett W, Tulandi T, Tan S. Prospective randomized study of human chorionic gonadotropin priming before immature oocyte retrieval from unstimulated women with polycystic ovarian syndrome. *Hum Reprod.* 2000;15:165–170.

56. Chian R, Tan S. Maturational and developmental competence of cumulus-free immature human oocytes derived from stimulated and intracytoplasmic sperm injection cycles. *Reprod Biomed Online.* 2002;5(2):125–132.

57. Hovatta O. Methods of cryopreservation of human ovarian tissue. *Reprod Biomed Online.* 2005;10(6):729–734.

58. Trounson A, Pera M. Human embryonic stem cells. *Fertil Steril.* 2001;76(4):660–661.

59. Wakayama S, Ohta H, Kishigami S, et al. Establishment of male and female nuclear transfer embryonic stem cell lines from different mouse strains and tissues. *Biol Reprod.* 2005;72(4):932–936.

60. Smitz J, Cortivrindt R. The earliest stages of folliculogenesis in vitro. *Reproduction.* 2002;123:185–202.

61. Gosden R, Mullan J, Picton H, Yin H, Tan S. Current perspective on primordial follicle cryopreservation and culture for reproductive medicine. *Hum Reprod Update.* 2002;8(2):105–110.

62. Eppig J, O'Brien M. Development in vitro of mouse oocytes from primordial follicles. *Biol Reprod.* 1996;54(1):197–207.

63. Parrott D. The fertility of mice with orthotopic ovarian grafts derived from frozen tissue. *J Reprod Fertil.* 1960;1:230–241.

64. Gosden RG, Baird DT, Wade JC, Webb R. Restoration of fertility to oophorectomized sheep by ovarian autografts stored at −196 degrees C. *Human Reproduction* 1994;9(4):597–603.

65. Oktay K, Karlikaya G. Ovarian function after transplantation of frozen, banked autologous ovarian tissue. *N Eng J Med.* 2000;342(25):1919.

66. Lee DM, Yeoman RR, Battaglia DE, Stouffer RL, Zelinski-Wooten MB, Fanton JW, Wolf DP. Live birth after ovarian tissue transplant. *Nature* 2004;428:137–138.

67. Donnez J, Dolmans M, Demylle D, et al. Live birth after orthotopic transplantation of cryopreserved ovarian tissue. *Lancet.* 2004;364(9443):1405–1410.

68. Oktay K, Yih M. Preliminary experience with orthotopic and heterotopic transplantation of ovarian cortical strips. *Sem Reprod Biol.* 2002;20(1):63–73.

69. Singh K, Davies M, Catterjiee R. Fertility in female cancer survivors: Pathophysiology, preservation, and ovarian reserve testing. *Human Reproduction* 2005;11(1):69–89.

70. Tilly J, Kolesnick R. Sphingolipids, apoptosis, cancer treatments and the ovary: investigating a crime against female fertility. *Biochim Biophys Acta.* 2002;1585(2–3):135–138.

71. Morita Y, Perez GI, Paris F, et al. Oocyte apoptosis is suppressed by disruption of the acid sphingomyelinase gene or by sphingosine-1-phosphate therapy. *Nat Med.* 2000;6(10):1109–1114.

72. Oktay K, Buyuk E, Davis O, et al. Fertility preservation in breast cancer patients: in vitro fertilization and embryo cryopreservation after ovarian stimulation with tamoxifen. *Hum Reprod.* 2003;18:90–95.

73. Oktay K, Buyuk E, Libertella N, Akar M, Rosenwaks Z. Fertility preservation in breast cancer patients: a prospective controlled comparison of ovarian stimulation with tamoxifen and letrozole for embryo cryopreservation. *J Clin Oncol.* 2005;23(19):4347–4353.

74. Oktay K, Buyuk E, Rosenwaks Z. Novel use of aromatase inhibitor for fertility preservation via embryo cryopreservation in endometrial cancer. *Fertil Steril.* 2003;80(suppl 3):S144.

75. Oktay K, Economos K, Kan M, Rucinski J, Veeck L, Rosenwaks Z. Endocrine function and oocyte retrieval after autologous transplantation of ovarian cortical strips to the forearm. *JAMA.* 2001;286(12):1490–1493.

76. Oktay K, Buyuk E, Rosenwaks Z, Rucinski J. A technique for transplantation of ovarian cortical strips to the forearm. *Fertil Steril.* 2003;80(1):193–198.

77. Oktay K, Buyuk E, Veeck L, et al. Embryo development after heterotopic transplantation of cryopreserved ovarian tissue. *Lancet.* 2004;363(9412):837–840.

78. Kim S, Hwang I, Lee H. Heterotopic autotransplantation of cryobanked human ovarian tissue as a strategy to restore ovarian function. *Fertil Steril.* 2004;82(4):930–932.

79. Wolner-Hanssen P, Hagglund L, Ploman F, Ramirez A, Manthorpe R, Thuring A. Autotransplantation of cryopreserved ovarian tissue to the right forearm 4(1/2) years after autologous stem cell transplantation. *Acta Obstet Gynecol Scand.* 2005;84(7):695–698.

80. Oktay K, Karlikaya G. Ovarian function after transplantation of frozen, banked autologous ovarian tissue. *N Eng J Med.* 2000;342(25):1919.

81. Oktay K, Aydin B, Karlikaya G. A technique for laparoscopic transplantation of frozen-banked ovarian tissue. *Fertil Steril.* 2001;75(6):1212–1216.

82. Radford J, Lieberman B, Brison D, et al. Orthotopic reimplantation of cryopreserved ovarian cortical strips after high-dose chemotherapy for Hodgkin's lymphoma. *Lancet.* 2001;357(9263):1172–1175.

83. Meirow D, Levron J, Eldar-Geva T, et al. Pregnancy after transplantation of cryopreserved ovarian tissue in a patient with ovarian failure after chemotherapy. *N Eng J Med.* 2005;353(3):318–321.

84. Revel A, Elami A, Bor A, Yavin S, Natan Y, Arav A. Whole sheep ovary cryopreservation and transplantation. *Fertil Steril*. 2004;82 (6):1714–1715.

85. Ayhan A, Guvenal T, Salman M, Ozyuncu O, Sakinci M, Basaran M. The role of cytoreductive surgery in nongenital cancers metastatic to the ovaries. *Gynecol Oncol*. 2005;98(2):235–241.

86. Schroder C, Timmer-Bosscha H, Wijchman J, et al. An in vivo model for purging of tumor cells from ovarian tissue. *Hum Reprod*. 2004;19(5):1096–1075.

87. Aubard Y. Ovarian tissue xenografting. *Eur J Obstet Gynecol Reprod Biol*. 2003;108(1):14–18.

88. Geijsen N, Horoschak M, Kim K, Gribnau J, Eggan K, Daley G. Derivation of embryonic germ cells and male gametes from embryonic stem cells. *Nature*. 2004;427(6970):148–154.

89. Toyooka Y, Tsunekawa N, Akasu R, Noce T. Embryonic stem cells can form germ cells in vitro. *Proc Natl Acad Sci U S A*. 2003;100(20):11457–11462.

90. Hubner K, Fuhrmann G, Christenson L, et al. Derivation of oocytes from mouse embryonic stem cells. *Science*. 2003;300(5623):1251–1256.

91. Lacham-Kaplan O, Chy H, Trounson A. Testicular cell conditioned medium supports differentiation of embryonic stem (ES) cells into ovarian structures containing oocytes. *Stem Cell*. 2006;24:266–273.

92. Trounson A. Human embryonic stem cell derivation and directed differentiation. *Ernst Schering Res Found Workshop*. 2005;(54):27–44.

93. Strelchenko N, Verlinsky O, Kukharenko V, Verlinsky Y. Morula-derived human embryonic stem cells. *Reprod Biomed Online*. 2004;9(6):623–629.

94. Tesar PJ. Derivation of germ-line-competent embryonic stem cell lines from preblastocyst mouse embryos. *Proc Natl Acad Sci U S A*. 2005;102(23):8239–8244.

95. Chung Y, Klimanskaya I, Becker S, et al. Embryonic and extraembryonic stem cell lines derived from single mouse blastomeres. *Nature*. 2006;439:216–219.

96. Solter D, Knowles B. Immunosurgery of mouse blastocyst. *Proc Natl Acad Sci U S A*. 1975;72(12):5099–5102.

97. Cowan C, Klimanskaya I, McMahon J, et al. Derivation of embryonic stem-cell lines from human blastocysts. *N Eng J Med*. 2004;350(13):1353–1356.

98. Clark A, Bodnar M, Fox M, et al. Spontaneous differentiation of germ cells from human embryonic stem cells in vitro. *Hum Mol Genet*. 2004;13(7):727–739.

Section 7.2. Assessment of the Endometrial Cavity in the Patient with Infertility

Richard O. Burney and Amin A. Milki

The prevalence of uterine abnormalities in patients presenting with infertility is as high as 50% [1–3], and these are believed to play a major role among the 30% of couples who undergo advanced reproductive treatment for multifactorial infertility.[4] For patients undergoing in vitro fertilization, lower pregnancy rates are observed in the setting of uterine cavity anomalies.[5–7] The role of uterine pathology is a key factor in discordant pregnancy outcomes among recipients of shared oocytes in an ovum donation program.[8] Importantly, the correction of these anomalies has been associated with improved pregnancy rates.[3] Therefore, the evaluation of the couple with infertility should include an assessment of the endometrial cavity. Traditionally, the basic infertility work-up has included a hysterosalpingogram to evaluate both the uterine cavity as well as the patency of the fallopian tubes. Other modalities to assess the endometrial cavity have subsequently developed. These include transvaginal sonography and sonohysterography and hysteroscopy. A variety of endometrial pathologies may prove deleterious to fertility. These include endometrial polyps, leiomyomata, intrauterine adhesions, mullerian anomalies, and prior exposure to diethylstilbestrol (DES). In this chapter, we review the various imaging modalities. Additionally, we review the perturbations of normal endometrial anatomy that these modalities can discern.

DIAGNOSTIC MODALITIES

Hysterosalpingography

Allowing assessment of both tubal and uterine pathology, hysterosalpingography (HSG) has become a basic component of the initial infertility evaluation. HSG is reliable and well tolerated. In addition to diagnostic yield, the study is potentially therapeutic. A randomized controlled clinical trial comparing oil versus water-soluble contrast at HSG in infertile patients showed a 33% pregnancy rate with oil and a 17% pregnancy rate with water-based contrast within nine ovulatory cycles after HSG.[9] Most pregnancies occurred within 7 months of the imaging study. These substantial cumulative pregnancy rates may have been secondary to the flushing of inspissated mucus and debris from the lumen of the tube(s) to recreate patency. Inhibition of peritoneal fluid immune cell function by oil-based contrast has been demonstrated in tissue culture studies, and this may explain the significantly higher pregnancy rates observed with oil versus water-soluble dye.[10]

The HSG study is ideally timed after the cessation of menses and before ovulation. The dilated periuterine venous architecture during the menses increases the incidence of vascular intravasation of contrast, and should be avoided. The risk of infectious sequelae after HSG is 0.3% to 1.3%.[11] A potential prophylactic strategy is 100 mg of doxycycline taken twice daily for 5 days, starting 2 days before the procedure in patients testing positive for *Chlamydia* serum antibody or with a history of prior pelvic inflammatory disease.[12] To ease cramping associated with the procedure, the patient is asked to take a nonsteroidal anti-inflammatory medication approximately 1 hour before the study. The ability to appreciate subtle abnormalities of the reproductive tract is best garnered in real time, and this is the basis for recommending the attendance of the gynecologist at fluoroscopy. A reusable (Jarcho) cannula or disposable balloon–catheter system attached to a syringe containing contrast is used for the procedure. Before insertion, the system should be adequately flushed to minimize artifact associated with air bubbles. After a sterile preparation of the cervix and vaginal vault, the instillation cannula or catheter is placed intracervically. Gentle pressure is used to inject approximately 3 to 5 mL of contrast. The optimal time to appreciate abnormalities of the endometrial cavity is during the early filling phase of the study, as these defects may be concealed by overdistending the uterus with contrast agent. Lesions of the endometrial cavity appear as areas of low contrast at HSG because of the space-filling effect of the pathologic entity (Figure 7.2.1). Within the cavity, polyps, fibroids, synechiae, mullerian anomalies, and the architectural sequelae of intrauterine DES exposure can be appreciated. If a balloon–catheter system is used, it is important to deflate the balloon at the conclusion of the study to fully evaluate the lowermost portion of the endometrial cavity.

Complications associated with HSG are possible. In addition to infection, vasovagal reaction and allergic reaction to contrast have been reported. Vasovagal reaction is exemplified by nausea and/or lightheadedness and is transient. The radiation exposure, when radiation time is limited and equipment properly calibrated, is well within established margins of safety.[13] Calculated at 3.7 milligrays, the radiation exposure during HSG is thought to impart low teratogenic risk to an unsuspected pregnancy.[14] Because very few pregnancies exposed to HSG have been reported, conclusions regarding actual risks are difficult to make. Consequently, every precaution to exclude the possibility of pregnancy should be taken before the study.

The sensitivity and specificity of HSG vary with the particular abnormality noted. Although HSG has 85% to 100% sensitivity for detecting tubal pathology [15,16], it is only 75% sensitive in documenting intrauterine adhesions.[17] HSG has a sensitivity as low as 50% in the detection of intrauterine filling defects and cannot reliably differentiate polyps from submucosal leiomyomata.[17,18] As compared with subsequent hysteroscopy, HSG evidenced a 37% false-negative rate in patients scheduled for IVF treatment.[5]

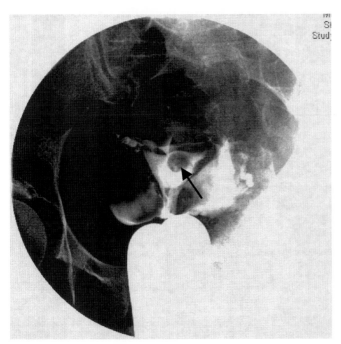

Figure 7.2.1. Hysterosalpingogram demonstrating a filling defect (*arrow*). Subsequent hysteroscopy revealed a 1 × 2 cm endometrial polyp.

Transvaginal Sonography

Transvaginal sonography (TVS) is safe, relatively noninvasive, and readily available in most clinics. Because of these features, sonography has been advocated as an initial screening modality in patients with infertility. In addition to screening for uterine pathology, the position of the uterus and angle of the uterocervical canal can be recorded for optimization of future intrauterine catheterization. The phase of the menstrual cycle affects the appearance of the endometrial echo. In the late proliferative phase, a trilaminar appearance is appreciated (Figure 7.2.2). Following ovulation, the endometrial echo in the secretory phase is more homogeneous and opaque.

With the use of a high-resolution transducer, TVS is capable of detecting endometrial polyps (Figure 7.2.3), leiomyomata and

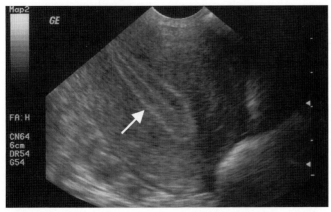

Figure 7.2.2. Transvaginal ultrasound of the uterus demonstrating a normal trilaminar image of the endometrium (*arrow*).

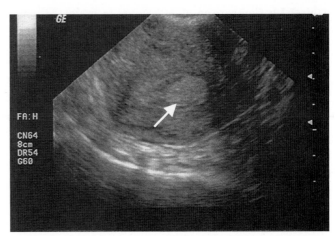

Figure 7.2.3. Transvaginal ultrasound demonstrating an endometrial polyp (*arrow*). The patient also had an HSG performed, which is depicted in Figure 7.2.1.

at times intrauterine synechiae (see Figure 7.2.6), and mullerian abnormalities such as bicornuate or septate uteri.[19]

TVS is limited by an inability to precisely localize intrauterine lesions and by the difficulty in delineating intramural from submucosal leiomyomata. Additionally, the phase of the menstrual cycle may pose a challenge in the diagnosis of more subtle intrauterine lesions. These limitations served as the impetus for the development of sonohysterography, a technique that combines sonography with distention of the endometrial cavity.

Sonohysterography

Sonohysterography, or saline infusion sonography (SIS), involves the instillation of saline into the uterine cavity during ultrasound. This technique combines the advantages of TVS with a high level of diagnostic accuracy, and is easily performed in the office setting.

As with HSG, sonohysterography is ideally performed in the follicular phase after the cessation of menses. An insemination catheter without an anchoring balloon can be successfully used in the nulliparous patient. However, for the patient with a patulous cervix, a balloon catheter system is recommended. A prospective study of six different catheter systems found no significant differences among them in terms of reliability and ease of use.[20] Using sterile technique, intracervical placement of a primed balloon catheter is performed. Warmed saline or Ringer's lactated solution is slowly infused and the cavity scanned in both longitudinal and transverse planes. If a balloon catheter is used, the balloon should be deflated at the conclusion of the procedure to allow for assessment of the lower uterine segment. Complications are rare. Cramping and/or vasovagal symptoms occur in less than 9% of patients.[21] The risk of infection is reported to be less than 1%.[22]

Sonohysterography appears to be superior to HSG in the detection of intrauterine pathology, correctly identifying 90% of abnormalities among infertile patients.[23] These data are consistent with those observed in patients with abnormal uterine bleeding in the general gynecologic setting, where sonohysterography has sensitivities of 87% and 93% in the detection of intrauterine pathology and endometrial polyps, respectively.[24,25]

Table 7.2.1: Comparison of Techniques to Evaluate the Endometrial Cavity in an Infertile Population (as Compared with Hysteroscopy)

Diagnostic Method	Patients, no.	Sensitivity, %	Specificity, %	Study
HSG	106	79	60	Raziel et al. (1994) [26]
HSG	464	98	15	Golan et al. (1996) [27]
HSG	216	80	70	Wang et al. (1996) [28]
HSG	62	73	100	Alatas et al. (1997) [23]
TVS	62	36	100	Alatas et al. (1997) [23]
TVS	38	81	95	Ayida et al. (1997) [29]
TVS	98	91	83	Ragni et al. (2005) [30]
Sonohysterography	62	91	100	Alatas et al. (1997) [23]
Sonohysterography	38	88	100	Ayida et al. (1997) [29]
Sonohysterography	98	98	94	Ragni et al. (2005) [30]

Compared with conventional transvaginal ultrasound, sonohysterography has both higher sensitivity (93% vs. 65%) and specificity (94% vs. 76%) for the detection of endometrial polyps in the patient with abnormal bleeding.[25]

Hysteroscopy

Hysteroscopy is regarded as the gold standard against which other imaging modalities are compared (Table 7.2.1).

Office hysteroscopy has become increasingly popular in the assessment of the endometrial cavity. The ability to perform this procedure in the office setting is a consequence of several advancements. First, the development of small, 3.1- to 3.5-mm flexible and 3- to 5-mm rigid hysteroscopes has obviated extensive cervical dilation beyond 5 mm. Second, advancement in anesthetic medication has facilitated patient tolerance of the procedure. Finally, the development of a coaxial bipolar electrode system for use with crystalloid distention media has improved both the tolerance and safety of the procedure.

The preoperative assessment of the patient undergoing hysteroscopy should include a transvaginal ultrasound in the office. This affords high-resolution screening of the uterus for large uterine abnormalities. Patients with submucosal fibroids greater than 1.5 cm or major uterine malformations should be triaged to operative management in an operating room rather than an office setting. Additionally, transvaginal ultrasound allows assessment of uterine position. An anteverted uterine position is found in approximately 74% to 90% of nulliparous women, demonstrated in studies using either ultrasound [31] or magnetic resonance imaging [32] of uterine position. Advising the patient with an anteverted uterus to present with a full bladder at the time of hysteroscopy serves to straighten the cervicouterine canal and facilitates cervical dilation and subsequent placement of the hysteroscope. Contraindications are similar to those for HSG. Patients suspected of having an active pelvic infection should not undergo hysteroscopic evaluation until the infection has completely resolved.

To optimize visualization of the endometrial cavity during hysteroscopy, the procedure should be performed during the early to mid-follicular phase of the cycle. This also minimizes the possibility of pregnancy. Pharmacologic treatments to minimize endometrial interference with the procedure include oral contraceptives and GnRH agonists. These pretreatments serve to further minimize endometrial thickness at the time of anticipated hysteroscopy. The hysteroscopy is then optimally timed 4 to 5 weeks after administration of the GnRH agonist. In patients for whom a nonelectrolyte distending medium is planned, a GnRH agonist for endometrial preparation may also reduce the cerebral risks associated with dilutional hyponatremia.[33] For patients undergoing IVF, the procedure can be conveniently scheduled during the oral contraceptive phase before controlled ovarian hyperstimulation (COH). Such timing has been associated with a significantly improved pregnancy rate when compared with a longer interval between office hysteroscopy and IVF cycle start.[3]

Patient tolerance of office hysteroscopy has been optimized by advancements in pain control medication regimens. Excellent acceptance of diagnostic hysteroscopy using a 5-mm scope without analgesia has been reported.[34] However, when the possibility of an operative component to the office hysteroscopy exists, pain medications should be considered. A regimen that includes a benzodiazepine such as diazepam, a narcotic such as acetaminophen with hydrocodone, and a nonsteroidal anti-inflammatory medication such as intramuscular ketorolac provides excellent pain control when coupled with a paracervical block. Alternatively, conscious sedation with intravenous fentanyl and midazolam can be coupled with the paracervical block. Typically, patients receiving conscious sedation require no more than 1 mg of midazolam and 100 μg of fentanyl for excellent analgesia. The paracervical block consists of a local anesthetic such as 1% lidocaine without epinephrine in the amount of 5 to 7 mL each injected at the 4 and 8 o'clock positions of the cervix.

Hysteroscopes for office use are currently manufactured in both rigid and flexible forms. Those suitable for office hysteroscopy are typically 5 mm or less in outer diameter, thereby requiring minimal cervical dilation. Importantly, these scopes still allow an operative channel. The viewing angle may range from 0° to 70° from the horizontal. Though rigid hysteroscopes are more commonly used, the flexible hysteroscopes provide an advantage in accessing the cavity of patients with difficult cervicouterine junctions and in visualizing the tubal ostia of patients with

Table 7.2.2: Comparison of Distending Media

Factor	Hyskon	Sorbitol	Saline	CO$_2$
Availability	Worst	Intermediate	Best	Intermediate
Maintenance of distention	Best	Intermediate	Worst	Intermediate
Cleanliness	Worst	Intermediate	Intermediate	Best
Office use	Worst	Intermediate	Best	Best
Miscibility with blood	Best	Best	Intermediate	Worst
Ability to aspirate	Best	Intermediate	Intermediate	Worst
Flushing capability	Intermediate	Intermediate	Best	Worst
Operative capability	Best	Best	Intermediate	Worst
Complications	Intermediate	Intermediate	Low	Low
Maximum deficit		1500 mL*	2500 mL*	

*Maximum fluid deficits per Committee on Hysteroscopic Fluid Guidelines of the American Association of Gynecologic Laparoscopists.[39]
Modified from Baggish MS, Barbot J, Valle R, eds. *Diagnostic and Operative Hysteroscopy: A Text and Atlas.* New York: Mosby-Year Book; 1989.

funneling of the cornua. Yet these situations are atypical, and the choice of hysteroscope remains one of personal preference and convenience.

The choice of distending media for use during office hysteroscopy includes both gas and liquid types (Table 7.2.2). Carbon dioxide gas is the only gas currently used as a distending medium. This medium must be introduced with an insufflator specifically designed for hysteroscopic insufflation, with a maximal flow of 100 mL/minute and a maximum pressure of 100 mm Hg.[35] In the past, the substitution of laparoscopic insufflators for hysteroscopic use resulted in cases of gas embolism. Fluid distending media consist of both low-viscosity and high-viscosity subtypes. Hyskon (32% dextran 70 and 10% dextrose in water; Pharmacia) represents a high-viscosity agent. Immiscible with blood, Hyskon provides the advantage of clear visualization during operative hysteroscopy involving resection of vascular endometrial pathology. However, the thick consistency of this medium renders it somewhat difficult to clean. Low-viscosity agents consist of nonelectrolyte solutions, such as glycine, sorbitol, and mannitol, and electrolyte solutions. The nonelectrolytes are ideally suited to operative hysteroscopic techniques in which monopolar electric current is planned. With the exception of mannitol, these media are hypo-osmolar, and therefore require careful surveillance of fluid status to minimize complications of hyponatremia and decreased serum osmolality, such as cerebral edema. On the other hand, mannitol 5% is iso-osmolar and has the advantage of diuretic activity. Though fluid overload and attendant risk of pulmonary edema are possible with electrolyte media, the risk of hyponatremia is much less than that associated with nonelectrolytes. For diagnostic purposes, electrolyte media represent a popular choice. Typically, less than 1 L of crystalloid such as normal saline or lactated Ringer's is sufficient for the procedure. The development of the coaxial bipolar electrode surgical system has made current-based operative hysteroscopy possible using electrolyte as the distending medium. Several studies have demonstrated excellent patient tolerance of the bipolar electrosurgical approach.[36–38]

The technique of office hysteroscopy is prefaced by adequate patient counseling, which serves to minimize patient anxiety and optimize tolerance of the procedure. After a sterile prep of the vaginal vault, the cervix is gently dilated to sufficient diameter to admit the hysteroscope. The scope can be advanced under direct visualization. For difficult cervicouterine junctions, abdominal ultrasound guidance may be used to help advance the hysteroscope safely. An easy passage of cervical dilators and hysteroscope is critical, as this is the stage of the procedure at which most uterine perforations occur. The rate of uterine perforation with the procedure is 0.1% to 1.4%.[40] However, with a full bladder in the patient with an anteverted uterus, ultrasound guidance, and hysteroscopic visualization of the cervical canal, this complication can be significantly minimized if not eliminated. Once the hysteroscope is advanced into the uterine cavity, patient discomfort can be reduced by adjusting the rate of distention media inflow to a level that provides adequate visualization of the cavity. A thorough evaluation of the cavity is performed. With oblique scopes, the posterior segment of the cavity is readily visualized. The scope must be angled to afford visualization of the lateral and anterior aspects. Finally, the cornual regions and tubal ostia are inspected. The availability of video monitoring systems enhances the patient experience by providing real-time feedback. This in turn facilitates the postprocedural counseling of the patient.

The most important benefit of hysteroscopy is the ability to immediately treat most pathology that is encountered (Table 7.2.3). Many hysteroscopes used in the office setting have an operative channel through which various instruments can be introduced. The targeted removal of endometrial polyps is afforded by grasping forceps. Scissors can be used for the resection of intrauterine synechiae and septi. The removal of submucosal fibroids is conducted with the coaxial bipolar electrode. A variety of tips allows the operator to tailor the instrument for the particular task. Significantly, all of these operative procedures can be performed using electrolyte distention media. Studies have demonstrated excellent surgical results with office hysteroscopic procedures, with success rates of 98% to 100%.[41–43]

Table 7.2.3: Findings of 1000 Office Hysteroscopies before In Vitro Fertilization

Findings	Cases, no. (%)
Normal findings	618 (62)
Endometrial polyps	323 (32)
Submucous fibroids	27 (3)
Intrauterine adhesions	25 (3)
Polypoid endometrium	9 (0.9)
Septum	5 (0.5)
Bicornuate uterus	3 (0.3)
Retained products of conception	3 (0.3)

Taken with permission from Hinckley and Milki.[43]

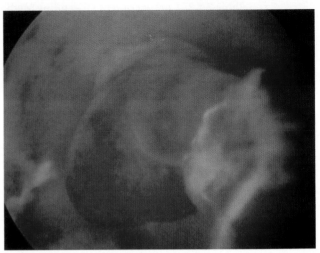

Figure 7.2.4. Hysteroscopy demonstrating an endometrial polyp.

Complications associated with office hysteroscopy are rare, with a reported rate of 0.28% to 2.7%.[44,45] The rate of complication has been associated with the type of hysteroscopic procedure performed. Infection, bleeding, sequelae of fluid overload, cervical laceration, and uterine perforation are possible. A very large retrospective survey of operative hysteroscopies performed at multiple centers demonstrated an infection rate of 0.01%.[46] However, the investigators acknowledge uncertainty as to whether antibiotic prophylaxis was used in a number of these procedures. For patients deemed to be at risk for endomyometritis, perioperative prophylaxis with an outpatient antibiotic such as doxycycline is advisable.

Bleeding sufficient to require intervention has been reported to occur at a rate of 0.5% to 1.9% of operative hysteroscopic cases. This is less common in office hysteroscopic cases. Tamponade with the intrauterine placement of a Foley catheter 30-mL balloon or with dilute vasopressin-treated uterine packing has been described.[47,48] It is imperative to determine with certainty whether the bleeding is consequent to uterine perforation. Lateral uterine or cervical perforations may result in significant hemorrhage. Finally, fluid overload is a complication that is best avoided by limiting excess fluid absorption. Guidelines for monitoring have been previously published.[39] Though patient size and health status are important variables to consider in establishing a fluid deficit threshold, the procedure should be discontinued if the fluid deficit reaches 1500 mL of a nonelectrolyte solution or 2500 mL of an electrolyte medium. In the office setting, electrolyte solutions are the medium of choice. Though not associated with hyponatremic sequelae, excessive absorption of electrolyte solutions during hysteroscopy has led to pulmonary edema. Consequently, prophylactic fluid monitoring is essential.

PATHOLOGY AFFECTING THE ENDOMETRIAL CAVITY

Uterine pathologies that have been demonstrated to adversely affect embryo implantation include endometrial polyps, leiomyomata, uterine septation, intrauterine synechiae, and DES. There-

fore, the pathogenesis and management of each of these conditions deserves review.

Endometrial Polyps

Endometrial polyps represent the most common intracavitary finding in the infertile patient population (Figure 7.2.4). Even in the absence of abnormal uterine bleeding, endometrial polyps may be discovered in women with infertility. The incidence of asymptomatic endometrial polyps in women with infertility has been reported to range from 10% to 32%.[43,49]

The influence of circulating estrogen on the development of endometrial polyps is well documented. In the context of patients undergoing hysteroscopy before in vitro fertilization, the high incidence of endometrial polyps may be secondary to the hyperestrogenemia associated with prior gonadotropin cycles. Additionally, polyps tend to be increasingly common with patient age. Polyps may be asymptomatic or associated with abnormal uterine bleeding. Grossly, endometrial polyps are pink–gray to white with smooth, glistening surfaces. The tip or the entire polyp may be hemorrhagic. Found most commonly in the uterine fundus and cornual regions, polyps range from lesions millimeters in size to those that occupy the entire endometrial cavity. A number of other entities, including endometrial hyperplasia and carcinoma and sarcoma, may have a polypoid appearance. Hence, it is important to obtain pathologic review of polyps, particularly large or unusual appearing forms.

A comparison of imaging modalities in the detection of endometrial polyps in the infertile population is presented in Table 7.2.4.

Though the incidence of endometrial polyps in the infertile population is well defined, the etiologic significance of this finding is more recently elucidated. In a retrospective study of patients diagnosed with a polyp during COH, a trend toward higher spontaneous abortion rates was observed.[50] A prospective study of 224 infertile women who underwent hysteroscopy suggested a 50% pregnancy rate achieved with polypectomy.[51] Finally, a randomized prospective study of 215 infertile patients with sonographic diagnosis of endometrial polyps was conducted to evaluate the impact of polypectomy on fertility.[18] Subjects

Table 7.2.4: Comparison of Techniques to Detect Endometrial Polyps in an Infertile Population (as Compared with Hysteroscopy)

Diagnostic Method	Patients, no.	Sensitivity, %	Specificity, %	Study
HSG	65	50	83	Soares et al. (2000) [17]
TVS	74	71	100	Shalev et al. (2000) [49]
TVS	65	75	97	Soares et al. (2000) [17]
TVS	98	81	92	Ragni et al. (2005) [30]
Sonohysterography	65	100	100	Soares et al. (2000) [17]
Sonohysterography	98	100	98	Ragni et al. (2005) [30]

were randomized to either hysteroscopic polypectomy or diagnostic hysteroscopy with polyp biopsy. The mean polyp size in both groups was 16 mm. Patients in the polypectomy arm evidenced a relative risk of 2.1 (95% CI, 1.5–2.9) of achieving pregnancy as compared with patients in the polyp biopsy arm, with 65% of pregnancies in the polypectomy group achieved spontaneously. Interestingly, the authors did not find a significant relationship between polyp size and pregnancy outcome, suggesting a possible biochemical interference with implantation posed by the presence of an endometrial polyp. In sum, the evidence to date supports the targeted removal of endometrial polyps in the optimization of fertility outcomes.

Leiomyomata

Leiomyomata are the most common tumors of the uterus, occurring most commonly in women of reproductive age, particularly in the 30s and 40s. The impact of fibroids on fertility depends on the parameters of location, number, and size. Types of leiomyomata include subserosal, intramural, and submucosal varieties. Submucous myomas, by virtue of their mass effect and inhospitable surface area for nidation, have been clearly associated with infertility and with pregnancy loss. These myomas appear as rounded masses that bulge to varying extents into the endometrial cavity, and the overlying endometrium may be atrophic, congested, ulcerated, or hemorrhagic. Because of their intracavitary location, submucosal fibroids may be effectively removed via a hysteroscopic approach (Figure 7.2.5).

A comparison of imaging modalities for the detection of submucosal leiomyomata is provided in Table 7.2.5. Sonohysterography and hysteroscopy are equivalent in the detection of submucosal myomas. Whereas SIS offers the advantage of allowing measurement of the overall dimensions of the lesion, office hysteroscopy may afford the removal of small submucous lesions in the same setting.

The impact of intramural (defined as greater than 50% volume within the myometrium) myomas upon fertility remains controversial. Although some studies showed reduced implantation and conception rates in women with intramural fibroids [53,54], others have not demonstrated an adverse effect.[55,56] One study demonstrated a size-dependent impact of intramural myomas, with those measuring greater than 4 cm associated with lower pregnancy rates following IVF/ICSI treatment.[57] The mechanism by which intramural lesions may impair fertility is unproven. Alterations in uterine artery blood flow, local cytokine

release, and/or gene expression profiles have been purported. Insofar as leiomyomata cluster with other estrogen-dependent disorders, such as endometriosis, adenomyosis, and endometrial polyps, their role in infertility may be purely associative. Nonetheless, an in-depth review of six previously published trials concluded that only intramural fibroids that resulted in cavity distortion or impingement were deleterious to fertility.[58] The beneficial effect of removing such cavity-distorting lesions was validated in a recent case-controlled study.[59]

Finally, studies have consistently failed to find an impact of subserosal leiomyomata (defined as ≥50% volume projecting beyond the *outer* uterine contour) upon fertility.

Uterine Septation

With an incidence of 2% to 3%, uterine septation represents the most common mullerian fusion defect.[60] Clinical sequelae of the septated uterus may include infertility, spontaneous pregnancy loss in the first or second trimester, or late-trimester pregnancy complications. However, pregnancy outcome in the presence of a uterine anomaly may depend on the location of blastocyst implantation in a particular cycle, and this may explain the situation in which a woman with a septate uterus might

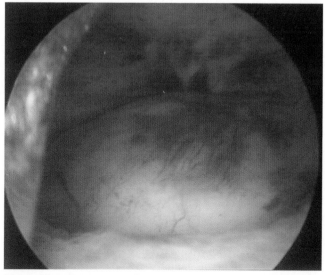

Figure 7.2.5. Hysteroscopy demonstrating a submucosal leiomyoma.

Table 7.2.5: Comparison of Techniques to Detect Submucosal Myomas (as Compared with Findings at Hysterectomy)

Diagnostic Method	Patients, no.	Sensitivity,%	Specificity,%	Study
TVS	52	90	98	Cicinelli et al. (1995) [52]
Sonohysterography	52	100	100	Cicinelli et al. (1995) [52]
Hysteroscopy	52	100	100	Cicinelli et al. (1995) [52]

encounter recurrent pregnancy loss even after having delivered a term infant.

Hysteroscopic septoplasty has been demonstrated to decrease significantly the risk for spontaneous abortion in women with septate uteri, and surgical therapy is indicated in patients with known uterine septi and a history of recurrent spontaneous abortion.[61] Indications for surgical correction of septation when the presenting complaint is infertility are less obvious. Among seven series of hysteroscopic metroplasties performed for infertility, the overall pregnancy rate after treatment was 48%.[61] It is still reasonable to consider surgical management in some infertile patients with uterine septi because septoplasty may maximize the chance of having a live birth by decreasing the associated risks for spontaneous abortion and preterm labor.

The hysteroscopic approach to septum resection is often performed with microscissors, the resectoscope, or laser. The coaxial bipolar electrode surgical system, providing the advantage of operating in a crystalloid distention medium, has been successfully applied toward hysteroscopic septum resection.[62]

Intrauterine Synechiae

About 13.5% of 74 infertile women scheduled for IVF treatment were found to have intrauterine adhesions when evaluated with diagnostic hysteroscopy.[49] Causes of intrauterine adhesions are often iatrogenic, with patient histories typically involving intraoperative or postoperative complications of uterine evacuations for menorrhagia, pregnancy termination, or postpartum hemorrhage. Other causes of intrauterine synechiae include intrauterine infection with pathogens such as *Schistosoma* and mycobacteria. In some third-world countries, tuberculous endometritis may be an important cause of uterine factor infertility.[63] Tuberculous endometritis differs from most other types of endometrial infection, and uterine scarring and infertility are significant sequelae even after treatment.[64] Severe forms of Asherman's syndrome have been associated with amenorrhea, menstrual irregularity, spontaneous abortion, and recurrent pregnancy loss.

Ultrasound can detect the presence of synechiae (Figure 7.2.6). The performance of TVS at midcycle (trilaminar endometrium) rather than after menstrual cessation provides better imaging of small intrauterine adhesions.[40]

Hysteroscopic resection is the method of choice for the management of intrauterine synechiae (Figure 7.2.7).

Postoperative prevention of reformation of adhesive disease may involve estrogen therapy alone or in combination with intraoperative placement of an intrauterine device, such as a pediatric Foley catheter, for 7 days. It is thought that estrogen rapidly rebuilds the endometrial lining after surgery and thereby prevents the development of scar tissue. A typical regimen consists of conjugated estrogen at a dosage of 2.5 to 5 mg/day for 1 to 2 months. The surgical management of intrauterine adhesions is reported to be very effective, with pregnancy rates above 80% among patients treated for mild to moderate disease.[65]

DES Exposure

Exposure to DES in utero increases a woman's risk for congenital reproductive tract malformations and obstetric complications, including preterm labor and cervical incompetence.[66] In one study, almost 70% of women exposed to DES in utero were noted to have uterine malformations on HSG. The most common finding was the T-shaped uterus.[67] Whether DES-exposed women also have higher rates of infertility remains unclear.[68] One investigator reported that decreased fertility in these women was particularly prevalent when constriction of the upper segment of the uterus was present.[69] This question is difficult to study, however, because there is great variation in the degree of congenital uterine, tubal, and cervical anomalies associated with exposure. Furthermore, some abnormalities may promote other infertility factors. For instance, cervical anomalies may promote production of suboptimal cervical mucus, or cervical stenosis may promote retrograde menstruation and the subsequent development of endometriosis. Indeed, a recent large prospective cohort study of patients with laparoscopically confirmed disease identified a significantly elevated risk (RR 1.8, CI 1.2–2.8) of endometriosis among women exposed to DES.[70]

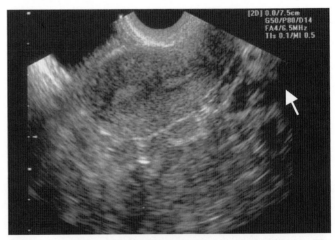

Figure 7.2.6. Ultrasound demonstrating intrauterine adhesion. The uterus is imaged in the longitudinal plane. Note the break in the endometrial echo (*arrow*) consistent with an adhesion. The patient subsequently underwent hysteroscopic lysis of the adhesional band.

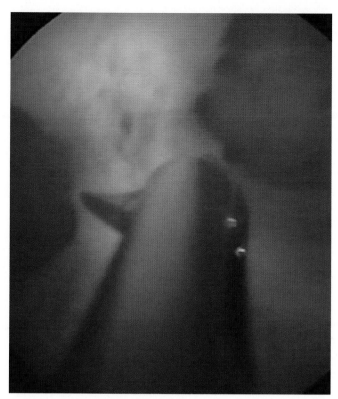

Figure 7.2.7. Lysis of central intrauterine adhesion (imaged in Figure 7.2.6) during office hysteroscopy.

Overall, when a DES-exposed woman has uterine anomalies on HSG and greater than 1 to 2 years of primary infertility, her prognosis for future pregnancy is extremely poor.[71] Metroplasty for correction of T-shaped and hypoplastic DES-exposed uteri has unproven value and is not routinely recommended. Results of IVF treatment are somewhat compromised in infertile DES-exposed women. Although ovarian response rates to COH are comparable in DES-exposed women and nonexposed women with unexplained infertility, DES exposure is associated with significantly lower implantation rates in IVF.[72] In the United States, DES was banned in 1971, and the identification of the aforementioned sequelae is becoming increasingly rare as affected women advance beyond reproductive age.

CONCLUSIONS

Given the prevalence of intrauterine abnormalities, the accurate assessment of the endometrial cavity is of vital importance in the work-up of the patient with infertility. The clinician's armamentarium of approaches to this assessment includes both radiologic and endoscopic studies. The choice of which modality to employ is dependent on several variables, including accessibility, reliability, and cost. The patient history may provide information that heightens the probability of a particular type of lesion, and the sensitivity profile of the various imaging modalities for this type of lesion may favor a particular approach. Transvaginal ultrasound provides a readily available initial screening of the uterus and ovaries. HSG affords visualization of intracavitary lesions

as well as functional assessment of the fallopian tubes. Sonohysterography and hysteroscopy provide excellent visualization of endometrial pathology, with office hysteroscopy allowing intervention for some types of lesions in the same setting. A thorough understanding of the endometrial pathologies that can impair fertility can optimize the approach to the patient presenting with infertility.

REFERENCES

1. Romano F, Cicinelli E, Anastasio PS, Epifani S, Fanelli F, Galantino P. Sonohysterography versus hysteroscopy for diagnosing endouterine abnormalities in fertile women. *Int J Gynaecol Obstet.* 1994;45:253–260.
2. Brown SE, Coddington CC, Schnorr J, Toner JP, Gibbons W, Oehninger S. Evaluation of outpatient hysteroscopy, saline infusion hysterosonography, and hysterosalpingography in infertile women: a prospective, randomized study. *Fertil Steril.* 2000;74:1029–1034.
3. Mooney SB, Milki AA. Effect of hysteroscopy performed in the cycle preceding controlled ovarian hyperstimulation on the outcome of in vitro fertilization. *Fertil Steril.* 2003;79:637–638.
4. Centers for Disease Control and Prevention. *2000 Assisted Reproductive Technology Success Rates: National Summary and Fertility Clinic Reports.* Atlanta, GA: Centers for Disease Control and Prevention; December 2001.
5. Shamma FN, Lee G, Gutmann JN, Lavy G. The role of office hysteroscopy in in vitro fertilization. *Fertil Steril.* 1992;58:1237–1239.
6. Narayan R, Rajat, Goswamy K. Treatment of submucous fibroids, and outcome of assisted conception. *J Am Assoc Gynecol Laparosc.* 1994;1:307–311.
7. Kupesic S, Kurjak A, Skenderovic S, Bjelos D. Screening for uterine abnormalities by three-dimensional ultrasound improves perinatal outcome. *J Perinat Med.* 2002;30:9–17.
8. Zenke U, Chetkowski RJ. Transfer and uterine factors are the major recipient-related determinants of success with donor eggs. *Fertil Steril.* 2004;82:850–856.
9. Rasmussen F, Lindequist J, Larsen C, Justesen P. Therapeutic effect of hysterosalpingography: oil versus water soluble contrast media: a randomized, prospective study. *J Radiol.* 1991;179:75–78.
10. Goodman SB, Rain MS, Hill JA. Hysterosalpingography contrast media and chromotubation dye inhibit peritoneal lymphocyte and macrophage function in vitro: a potential mechanism for fertility enhancement. *Fertil Steril.* 1993;59:1022–1027.
11. Pittaway DE, Winfield AC, Maxson W, et al. Prevention of acute pelvic inflammatory disease after hysterosalpingography: efficacy of doxycycline prophylaxis. *Am J Obstet Gynecol.* 1983;147:623–626.
12. Glatstein IZ, Sleeper LA, Lavy Y, et al. Observer variability in the diagnosis and management of the hysterosalpingogram. *Fertil Steril.* 1997;67:233–237.
13. Karande VC, Pratt DE, Balin MS, et al. What is radiation exposure to patients during a gynecoradiologic procedure? *Fertil Steril.* 1997;67:401–403.
14. Jongen VH, Collins JM, Lubbers JA, Van Selm M. Unsuspected early pregnancy at hysterosalpingography. *Fertil Steril.* 2001;76:610–611.
15. Krynicki E, Kaminski P, Szymanski R, et al. Comparison of hysterosalpingography with laparoscopy and chromopertubation. *J Am Assoc Gynecol Laparosc.* 1996;3:S22–S23.
16. Reis MM, Soares SR, Cancado ML, et al. Hysterosalpingo contrast sonography (HyCoSy) with SH U 454 (Echovist) for the assessment of tubal patency. *Hum Reprod.* 1998;13:3049–3052.

17. Soares SR, Barbosa dos Reis MM, Camargos AF. Diagnostic accuracy of sonohysterography, transvaginal sonography, and hysterosalpingography in patients with uterine cavity diseases. *Fertil Steril.* 2000;73:406–411.

18. Perez-Medina T, Bajo-Arenas J, Salazar F, et al. Endometrial polyps and their implication in the pregnancy rates of patients undergoing intrauterine insemination: a prospective, randomized study. *Hum Reprod.* 2005;20:1632–1635.

19. Dijkhuizen FP, Brolmann HA, Potters AE, et al. The accuracy of transvaginal ultrasonography in the diagnosis of endometrial abnormalities. *Obstet Gynecol.* 1996;87:345–349.

20. Dessole S, Farina M, Capobianco G, et al. Determining the best catheter for sonohysterography. *Fertil Steril.* 2001;76:605–609.

21. Dessole S, Farina M, Rubattu G, et al. Side effects and complications of sonohysterosalpingography. *Fertil Steril.* 2003;80:620–624.

22. Bonnamy L, Marret H, Perrotin F, et al. Sonohysterography: a prospective survey of results and complications in 81 patients. *Eur J Obstet Gynecol Reprod Biol.* 2002;102:42.

23. Alatas C, Aksoy E, Akarsu C, et al. Evaluation of intrauterine abnormalities in infertile patients by sonohysterography. *Hum Reprod.* 1997;12:487–490.

24. Schwarzler P, Concin H, Bosch H, et al. An evaluation of sonohysterography and diagnostic hysteroscopy for the assessment of intrauterine pathology. *Ultrasound Obstet Gynecol.* 1998;11:337–342.

25. Kamel HS, Darwish AM, Mohamed SA. Comparison of transvaginal ultrasonography and vaginal sonohysterography in the detection of endometrial polyps. *Acta Obstet Gynecol Scand.* 2000;79:60–64.

26. Raziel A, Arieli S, Bukovsky I, Caspi E, Golan A. Investigation of the uterine cavity in recurrent aborters. *Fertil Steril.* 1994;62:1080–1082.

27. Golan A, Eilat E, Herman A, et al. Hysteroscopy is superior to hysterosalpingography in infertility investigation. *Acta Obstet Gynecol Scand.* 1996;75:654–656.

28. Wang CW, Lee CL, Lai YM, et al. Comparison of hysterosalpingography and hysteroscopy in female infertility. *J Am Assoc Gynecol Laparosc.* 1996;3:581–584.

29. Ayida G, Chamberlain P, Barlow D, et al. Uterine cavity assessment prior to in vitro fertilization: comparison of transvaginal scanning, saline contrast hysterosonography and hysteroscopy. *Ultrasound Obstet Gynecol.* 1997;10:59–62.

30. Ragni G, Diaferia D, Vegetti W, et al. Effectiveness of sonohysterography in infertile patient work-up: a comparison with transvaginal ultrasonography and hysteroscopy. *Gynecol Obstet Invest.* 2005;59:184–188.

31. Henne MB, Milki AA. Uterine position at real embryo transfer compared to mock embryo transfer. *Hum Reprod.* 2004;19:570–572.

32. Rizk DE, Czechowski J, Ekelund L. Magnetic resonance imaging of uterine version in a multiethnic, nulliparous, healthy female population. *J Reprod Med.* 2005;50:81–83.

33. Taskin O, Buhur A, Birincioglu M, et al. Endometrial Na+, K+-ATPase pump function and vasopressin levels during hysteroscopic surgery in patients pretreated with GnRH agonist. *J Am Assoc Gynecol Laparosc.* 1998;5:119–124.

34. Wong AY, Wong K, Tang LC. Stepwise pain score analysis of the effect of local on outpatient hysteroscopy: a randomized double-blind, placebo-controlled trial. *Fertil Steril.* 2000;73:1234–1237.

35. American College of Obstetricians and Gynecologists Technology Assessment. Hysteroscopy. *Obstet Gynecol.* 2005;106:439–442.

36. Fernandez H, Gervaise A, de Tayrac R. Operative hysteroscopy for infertility using normal saline solution and a coaxial bipolar electrode: a pilot study. *Hum Reprod.* 2000;15:1773–1775.

37. Bettocchi S, Ceci O, Di Venere R, et al. Advanced operative office hysteroscopy without anaesthesia: analysis of 501 cases treated with a 5 Fr. bipolar electrode. *Hum Reprod.* 2002;17:2435–2438.

38. Guida M, Pellicano M, Zullo F, et al. Outpatient operative hysteroscopy with bipolar electrode: a prospective multicentre randomized study between local anaesthesia and conscious sedation. *Hum Reprod.* 2003;18:840–843.

39. Loffer FD, Bradley LD, Brill AI, et al. Hysteroscopic fluid monitoring guidelines: from the Ad Hoc Committee on Hysteroscopic Fluid Guidelines of the American Association of Gynecologic Laparoscopists. *J Am Assoc Gynecol Laparosc.* 2000;7:167–168.

40. Hulka JF, Peterson HA, Phillips JM, Surrey MW. Operative hysteroscopy: American Association of Gynecologic Laparoscopists' 1993 Member Survey. *J Am Assoc Gynecol Laparosc.* 1995;2:131–132.

41. Nagele F, O'Connor H, Davies A, Badawy A, Mohamed H, Magos A. 2500 outpatient diagnostic hysteroscopies. *Obstet Gynecol.* 1996;88:87–92.

42. Vercellini P, Cortesi I, Oldani S, Moschetta M, De Giorgi O, Crosignani PG. The role for transvaginal ultrasonography and outpatient diagnostic hysteroscopy in the evaluation of patients with menorrhagia. *Hum Reprod.* 1997;12:1768–1771.

43. Hinckley MD, Milki AA. 1000 office-based hysteroscopies prior to in vitro fertilization: feasibility and findings. *JSLS.* 2004;8:103–107.

44. Jansen FW, Vredevoogd CB, van Ulzen K, Hermans J, Trimbos JB, Trimbos-Kemper TC. Complications of hysteroscopy: a prospective, multicenter study. *Obstet Gynecol.* 2000;96:266–270.

45. Propst AM, Liberman RF, Harlow BL, Ginsburg ES. Complications of hysteroscopic surgery: predicting patients at risk. *Obstet Gynecol.* 2000;96:517–520.

46. Aydeniz B, Gruber IV, Schauf B, Kurek R, Meyer A, Wallwiener D. A multicenter survey of complications associated with 21,676 operative hysteroscopies. *Eur J Obstet Gynecol Reprod Biol.* 2002;104:160–164.

47. Goldrath MH. Uterine tamponade for the control of acute uterine bleeding. *Am J Obstet Gynecol.* 1983;147:869–872.

48. Townsend DE. Vasopressin pack for treatment of bleeding after myoma resection. *Am J Obstet Gynecol.* 1991;165:1405–1407.

49. Shalev J, Meizner I, Bar-Hava I, et al. Predictive value of transvaginal sonography performed before routine diagnostic hysteroscopy for evaluation of infertility. *Fertil Steril.* 2000;73:412–417.

50. Lass A, Williams G, Abusheikha N, et al. The effect of endometrial polyps on outcomes of in vitro fertilization (IVF) cycles. *J Assist Reprod Genet.* 1999;16:410–415.

51. Shokeir TA, Shalan HM, El-Shafei MM. Significance of endometrial polyps detected hysteroscopically in eumenorrheic infertile women. *J Obstet Gynaecol Res.* 2004;30:84–89.

52. Cicinelli E, Romano F, Anastasio PS, et al. Transabdominal sonohysterography, transvaginal sonography, and hysteroscopy in the evaluation of submucous myomas. *Obstet Gynecol.* 1995;85:42–47.

53. Eldar-Geva T, Meagher S, Healy DL, et al. Effect of intramural, subserosal, and submucosal uterine fibroids on the outcome of assisted reproductive technology treatment. *Fertil Steril.* 1998;70:687–691.

54. Hart R, Khalaf Y, Yeong C-T, et al. A prospective controlled study of the effect of intramural uterine fibroids on the outcome of assisted conception. *Hum Reprod.* 2001;16:2411–2417.

55. Jun S, Ginsburg E, Racowsky C, Wise L, Hornstein M. Uterine leiomyomas and their effect on in vitro fertilization outcome: a retrospective study. *J Assist Reprod Genet.* 2001;13:139–143.

56. Yarali H, Bukulmez O. The effect of intramural and subserous uterine fibroids on implantation and clinical pregnancy rates in patients having intracytoplasmic sperm injection. *Arch Gynecol Obstet.* 2002;266:30–33.

57. Oliveira FG, Abdelmassih VG, Diamond MP, et al. Impact of subserosal and intramural uterine fibroids that do not distort

the endometrial cavity on the outcome of in vitro fertilization-intracytoplasmic sperm injection. *Fertil Steril.* 2004;81:582–587.

58. Donnez J, Jadoul P. What are the implications of myomas on fertility? *Hum Reprod.* 2002;17:1424–1430.

59. Surrey ES, Minjarez DA, Stevens JM, et al. Effect of myomectomy on the outcome of assisted reproductive technologies. *Fertil Steril.* 2005;83:1473–1479.

60. Asthon D, Amin HK, Richart RM, et al. The incidence of asymptomatic uterine anomalies in women undergoing transcervical sterilization. *Obstet Gynecol.* 1988;72:28–30.

61. Homer HA, Li TC, Cooke ID. The septate uterus: a review of management and reproductive outcome. *Fertil Steril.* 2000;73:1–14.

62. Zikopoulos K. Hysteroscopic septum resection using the Versapoint system in subfertile women. *Reprod Biomed Online.* 2003;7:365–367.

63. Oosthuizen AP, Wessels PH, Hefer JN. Tuberculosis of the female genital tract in patients attending an infertility clinic. *S Afr Med J.* 1990;77:562–564.

64. Varma TR. Genital tuberculosis and subsequent fertility. *Int J Gynaecol Obstet.* 1991;35:1–11.

65. Ismajovich B, Lidor A, Confino E, et al. Treatment of minimal and moderate intrauterine adhesions (Asherman's syndrome). *J Reprod Med.* 1985;30:769–772.

66. Goldberg JM, Falcone T. Effect of diethylstilbestrol on reproductive function. *Fertil Steril.* 1999;72:1–7.

67. Kaufman RH, Adam E, Binder GL, et al. Upper genital tract changes and pregnancy outcome in offspring exposed in utero to diethylstilbestrol. *Am J Obstet Gynecol.* 1980;137:299–308.

68. Berger MJ, Goldstein DP. Impaired reproductive performance in DES-exposed women. *Obstet Gynecol.* 1980;55:25–27.

69. Senekjian EK, Potkul RK, Frey K, et al. Infertility among daughters either exposed or not exposed to diethylstilbestrol. *Am J Obstet Gynecol.* 1988;158:493–498.

70. Missmer SA, Hankinson SE, Spiegelman D, et al. In utero exposures and the incidence of endometriosis. *Fertil Steril.* 2004;82:1501–1508.

71. Berger MJ, Alper MM. Intractable primary infertility in women exposed to diethylstilbestrol in utero. *J Reprod Med.* 1986;31:231–235.

72. Pal L, Shifren JL, Isaacson KB, et al. Outcome of IVF in DES-exposed daughters: experience in the 90s. *J Assist Reprod Genet.* 1997;14:513–517.

Section 7.3. Ultrasound Oocyte Retrieval

Rosa Moghadam and Salli Tazuke

Since the birth of the first IVF baby in 1978 [1], IVF and related assisted reproductive technologies (ARTs) are increasingly used to overcome all types of infertility disorders. More than 48,000 infants were born from ART treatments in 2003, representing more than 1% of the U.S. birth cohort.[2] With steady improvements in outcomes, ART has become the primary treatment modality for several clinical diagnoses, such as tubal factor and severe male factor infertility. Furthermore, ART has become an excellent option for any patient who has exhausted less complex treatment modalities and who has competent oocytes, spermatozoa, and a normal uterine cavity.

HISTORY

The history of IVF/ART actually dates back to 1890, when Schenck achieved fertilization of donor rabbit oocytes in vitro and then Heape transferred the embryos to a recipient rabbit.[3] Success in other mammalian models was not reported further until 1969, when Chang reported a successful in vitro fertilization and intrauterine embryo transfer in mouse.[4] The application in humans was first reported by Edwards in 1966 when oocytes were successfully retrieved by mini-laparotomy and matured in vitro.[5,6] As oocyte yield during the natural cycle was low, initially the focus was on developing the retrieval procedures via operative laparoscopy. During the 1970s, because of the ability to obtain a magnified view of the ovary, laparoscopic egg recovery had higher recovery rates, up to 33% to 45% [7,8], and finally culminated in in vitro fertilization of human oocytes and pregnancy in 1978 by Steptoe and Edwards.[1] Successful laparoscopic oocyte harvest, however, requires visual access to the majority of the ovarian surface area and could not be used in the setting of significant pelvic or ovarian adhesions. The ultrasound-guided method of oocyte retrieval was developed by Lenz and Lauritsen [9] from Denmark in 1981 for patients whose ovaries were inaccessible by the laparoscopic approach. The success rate, however, was much lower than that of the laparoscopic method initially.[10] Initially, transabdominal or endovaginal ultrasound was performed while the aspirating needle was introduced into the ovary via the percutaneous–transvesical, transurethral–transvesical, or transvaginal route. Subsequent to the development of the modern-day endovaginal transducer, which allowed clear visualization of the ovarian follicles, transvaginal oocyte retrieval by inserting a needle through the vaginal fornices into the pelvic cavity has become the dominant approach since the initial report in 1983 by Gleicher.[11,12] Transvaginal ultrasound–guided oocyte harvest is not only less invasive compared with the laparoscopic approach but also has been associated with a higher IVF rate, possibly by limiting exposure to the toxic effect of general anesthesia or carbon dioxide pneumoperitoneum on the ova.[13,14] On the other hand, the reproductive endocrinology and infertility (REI) physician should be familiar with the laparoscopic approach to oocyte harvest so that even patients with ovaries in an unusual position can have optimal oocyte recovery.

In this section, we first present an overview of indications, patient assessment, and ovarian stimulation protocols for IVF and then follow with a detailed description of the transvaginal oocyte retrieval procedure.

Patient Assessment and Ovarian Stimulation for ART

Once the decision to move to ART treatment has been made, another decision needs to be made regarding how the patient's cycle will be best managed: what dose of gonadotropin will be given and how premature LH surges will be prevented. Pretreatment assessment of ovarian reserve and gonadotropin responsiveness, together with the patient's age, provides a basis for deciding on a stimulation protocol.[15] The most commonly used biochemical marker for ovarian function testing has been the basal serum FSH on cycle day 2 or 3. Basal FSH level is an indirect estimate of ovarian reserve and depends on an intact hypothalamic–pituitary axis. However, a recent meta-analysis on the performance of basal FSH level in the prediction of poor ovarian response and failure to become pregnant after IVF concluded that clinical application of basal FSH is appropriate only in patients with very elevated FSH.[16,17] Inhibin B is another marker, secreted mainly by granulosa cells of the preantral ovarian follicles, and is thought to reflect the size of the ovarian follicular pool.[18] During the menopausal transition, women with elevated levels of FSH have significantly lower levels of inhibin B compared with those with normal levels of FSH.[19,20] Decreased inhibin B was also found in women with normal FSH levels, suggesting that changes in inhibin B levels may precede elevation in FSH levels.[21] Antimullerian hormone (AMH), a member of the transforming growth factor-β family, is a newer biomarker produced by granulosa cells from primordial follicles. The function of AMH in adult ovaries is hypothesized to inhibit the recruitment of primordial follicles into the pool of growing follicles.[22] AMH levels show a progressive decrease with age [23], supporting the notion that AMH levels correlate directly with the size of the available follicle pool in the ovary. Serum AMH levels fluctuate minimally during the menstrual cycle [23,24], which makes it more convenient to be used as a biomarker of ovarian reserve. Use of serum AMH levels to predict success with IVF treatments needs further validation. Ultrasound-based measurement of ovarian size has been shown to decrease in women aged 40 years and older and may be an earlier indicator of menopausal status than menstrual history.[25–28] A correlation between ovarian volume and reproductive outcome in IVF cycles has been shown [27], and this test is inexpensive and relatively easy to perform, with minimal intra- and interobserver variations. [25]

Antral follicle count (AFC), defined as the number of follicles 10 mm or less in diameter detected by ultrasound in the early follicular phase of the menstrual cycle, is another parameter found to correlate with age.[29] A recent meta-analysis comparing basal FSH levels and AFC revealed that AFC is more predictive of ovarian response to infertility treatments [17] and an estimate of the size of the cohort of follicles available for stimulation in a given cycle may be made. A normal basal antral follicle count (BAF) between 8 and 18 typically will produce 8 to 20 oocytes at the time of retrieval following intermediate-dose stimulation with 225 to 300 IU of gonadotropin in women under 35 years of age. For women over 35, consideration for receiving 450 IU of gonadotropin may be given based on their age.

Patients with a high BAF (≥18) tend to have a polycystic ovary–like appearance with multiple follicles in the periphery of the ovary with an exaggerated stromal component. Low-dose stimulation following GnRH agonist down-regulation is typically chosen and carefully monitored by serial ultrasound and estradiol levels to decrease the risk of severe ovarian hyperstimulation syndrome. Patient with a low BAF (≤8) tend to be low responders who are resistant to stimulation and require more aggressive protocols. These patients will benefit from avoiding oversuppression of the pituitary gland as well as use of 450 IU of gonadotropin per day during the stimulation phase.

Stimulation of multiple follicle growth can induce a premature LH surge in the absence of strategies to suppress the pituitary gonadotrope. Before the availability of GnRH analogues, as many as one in seven cycles was canceled because of premature ovulation. Desensitization of gonadotrope is typically accomplished by administering GnRH analogues starting up to 10 days preceding the intended stimulation.[30] The GnRH agonist down-regulation is sometimes associated with failure to respond to subsequent stimulation with gonadotropins. This may occur even in women who have regular cycles on their own and are receiving supraphysiologic doses of gonadotropin. Women who are at highest risk for poor response subsequent to GnRH agonist down-regulation of gonadotrope are those who have low BAF counts, have a history of poor responsiveness to gonadotropin, are greater or equal to 40 years of age, and have unexplained infertility. In such patients, alternative stimulation using GnRH antagonists or GnRH agonist flare cycles may be used. GnRH antagonists became clinically available in 1999 and are now widely used for stimulation protocols. As the gonadotropes are not suppressed at the onset of ovarian stimulation, patients typically receive similar or lower doses of gonadotropins. The GnRH antagonist is administered when the leading follicle size reaches 12 to 14 mm, at which point an LH-containing gonadotropin or low-dose hCG is supplemented in addition to the gonadotropin doses.

Another alternative protocol that allows prevention of premature LH surge is the use of microdose GnRH analogues to induce endogenous gonadotropin flare to augment the exogenous gonadotropin doses.[31] Premature LH surges have been reported but are very rare. Ovarian stimulation is followed by serial ultrasounds and estradiol levels, initially after 4 days of stimulation and then every 1 to 2 days until at least two follicles reach 16 to 18 mm in average diameter. hCG 5000 or 10,000 IU is administered 35 hours before the transvaginal oocyte retrieval schedule.

TRANSVAGINAL OOCYTE RETRIEVAL PROCEDURE

Proper room and equipment setup is crucial for successful recovery of oocytes with high fertilization and development potential.

Room Setup

An ambulatory suite is useful for this procedure. Equipment includes an operating table with lithotomy position, an ultrasound machine (Figure 7.3.1) with a transvaginal transducer and needle guide (Figure 7.3.2), heating blocks, test tubes (Figure 7.3.3), a syringe with a blunt needle, a single- or double-lumen echo-tipped 16- to 18-gauge needle (Figure 7.3.4), a suction pump, anesthetic equipment (Figure 7.3.5), and a well-equipped IVF lab (Figures 7.3.6, 7.3.7). The ultrasound transducer is typically of high frequency (6.5 MHz) and the endovaginal probe may be equipped with a needle guide for the oocyte retrieval. The IVF lab should be in close proximity to the procedure room (Figure 7.3.8), which will prevent the adverse effects of room temperature on the oocytes. The temperature of the heating block and all the lab tables are set up at 37°C. If there is no heating block available in the operating room, retrieval should be done as quickly as an embryologist can examine the specimens. During egg retrieval, follicular aspirates and all flushes are maintained at 37°C ± 0.5°C and a pH of 7.4 ± 0.1.

Vacuum and Needle Setup

Two different types of needles (single- and double-lumen) are available (Figure 7.3.4) with sufficient diameter (16- to 18-gauge) to prevent cumulous oophorous disruption during aspiration.[32] If flushing is done, a double-lumen needle is preferred.[33,34] Needles are echo-tipped and as a result are readily visualized with ultrasound during aspiration. Recovery rate and quality of the oocytes are influenced by the suction pressure applied to the needle. A negative pressure between 100 and 120 mm Hg is applied to the needle at the instant of follicular puncture and stopped after needle withdrawal. Higher pressures may lead to damaged and fractured oocytes.[33,34]

Anesthesia

Transvaginal ultrasound–guided oocyte retrieval is typically done as an outpatient procedure under conscious sedation. Patients need to have fasted for at least 6 hours before the procedure. A combination of hypnotics such as propofol or a sedative hypnotic such as midazolam and/or intravenous (IV) opioids are used to achieve adequate relaxation and anesthesia. Multiple studies indicate a steady rise in the level of anesthetic agents in follicular fluid shortly after starting the procedure. The effect of these anesthetics on oocyte fertilization is not clear, but some report dose- and

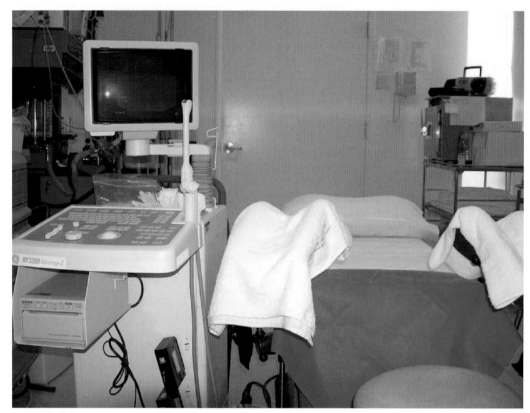

Figure 7.3.1. An operating table with lithotomy position and ultrasound with a transvaginal transducer.

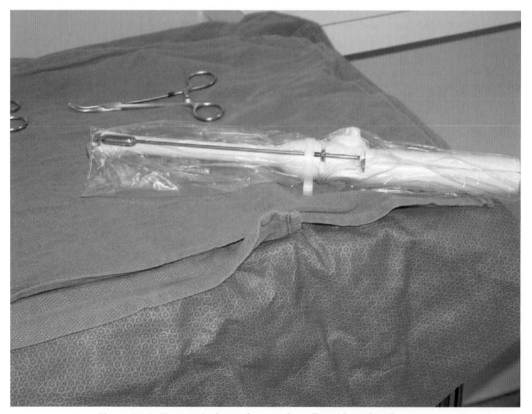

Figure 7.3.2. Transvaginal transducer and needle guide and probe cover.

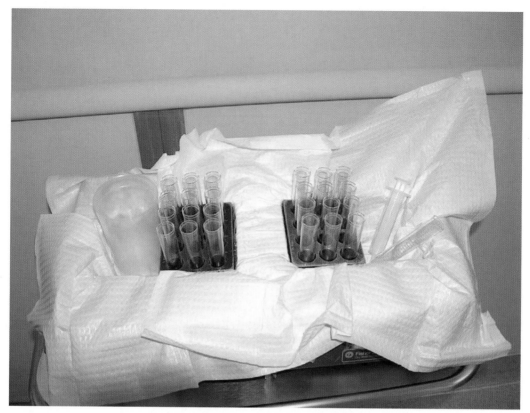

Figure 7.3.3. Heating blocks and test tubes.

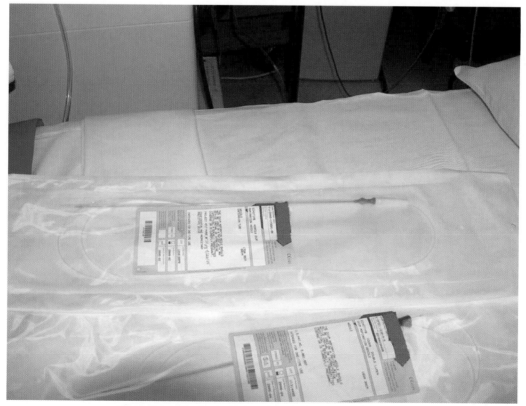

Figure 7.3.4. Single- (*upper*) and double-lumen needle (*lower*).

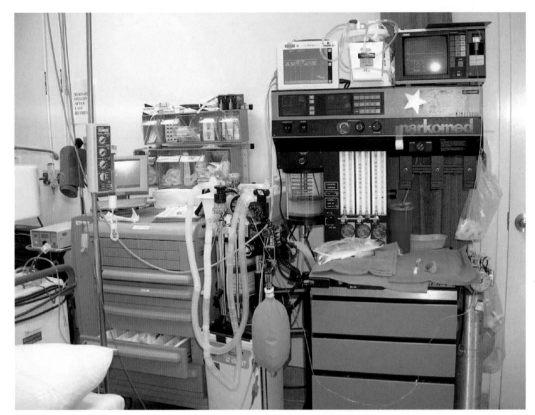

Figure 7.3.5. Anesthetic equipment.

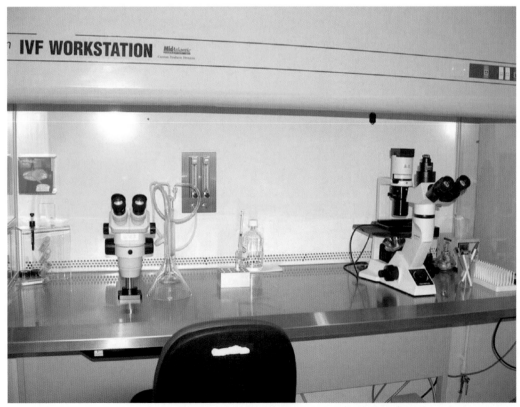

Figure 7.3.6. IVF lab: microscopes. All the tables are set at 37°C.

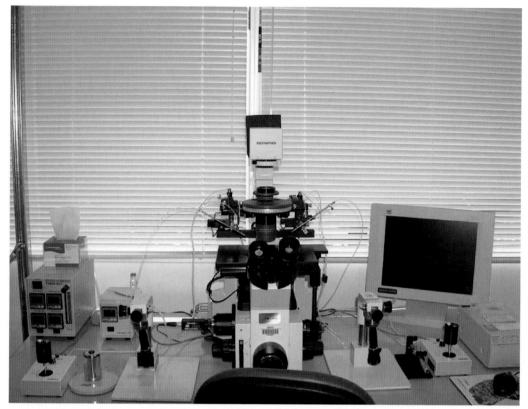

Figure 7.3.7. IVF lab: microinjection device.

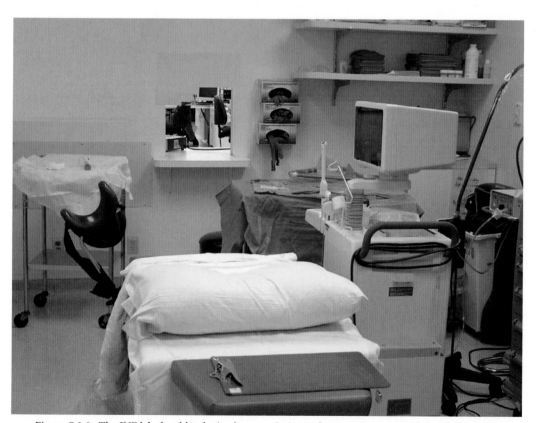

Figure 7.3.8. The IVF lab should to be in close proximity to the operating room. Notice the window.

time-dependent decreases in fertilization rate.[35,36,37] In general, it is prudent to minimize anesthesia exposure, but the duration of the procedure may vary from 10 to 30 minutes depending on the operator's skill, number of follicles, evacuation pressure set up, and the flushing technology.

Procedure Description

The patient is placed in the dorsal lithotomy position and after achieving sufficient sedation, the vagina is prepared either with saline lavage alone or a wash with an antiseptic cleanser. If Betadine (Purdue) is used, the vagina should be irrigated copiously with normal saline to minimize oocyte toxicity. Today, most centers use normal saline alone, and there appears to be no increase in postprocedure infection [38], particularly when a prophylactic antibiotic such as doxycycline is used around the time of the procedure. A high-frequency endovaginal probe covered with a conducting jelly and a sterile latex cover or condom is introduced into the vagina with its affixed needle guide (Figure 7.3.2). The ovaries are located, and each follicle is in turn aligned with the puncture line on the monitor. The needle is inserted into the closest follicle in the plane of its largest diameter visualized by ultrasound. The tip of the aspirating needle is then advanced into the center of the follicle along the shortest path. As negative pressure is applied, collapse of the follicle is readily visualized and the needle tip may be manipulated to curette the follicle. The follicular content is collected in a tube and transferred to a heating block maintained at 37°C until the assistant hand delivers the sample to the embryologist in the adjoining IVF laboratory. If all the follicles in each ovary can be aspirated through a single puncture site, the number of separate needle punctures through the vaginal wall and into the ovary will be minimized. Care must be taken to identify the location of hypogastric vessels to prevent inadvertent puncture and serious intra-abdominal bleeding. When the needle is withdrawn from one ovary, it should be flushed with culture medium to clear any retained oocytes from the line. During the procedure, if the aspirates are found not to contain oocytes by the embryologist, or if the patient has only a few follicles, flushing may maximize the oocyte recovery rate and absolute number of oocytes. The use of flushing during oocyte retrieval, however, is somewhat controversial. Multiple follicle flushes are time-consuming procedures, and several prospective studies have reported possible detrimental effects of flushing on oocyte quality and fertilization rates.[33,34] If flushing is done, the number of flushings should be limited to two (4 mL). Flushing may be done with two types of media, a commercially available prepared media or heparinized buffered saline prepared by the embryologist. No difference in oocyte recovery, fertilization, or cleavage rate between the two flushing media has been found.[39]

Transvaginal ultrasound–guided oocyte retrieval has a number of advantages over the laparoscopic approach: (1) oocytes can be recovered in case of severe pelvic adhesions, (2) general anesthesia is not necessary, (3) transvaginal follicular puncture has lower potential morbidity, (4) the operative and recovery times are reduced, and (5) oocytes are not exposed to carbon dioxide pneumoperitoneum, which may acidify the follicular fluid. Complications from the oocyte retrieval procedure include infection, bleeding, and trauma to the adjacent organs. According to some reports, the incidence of postprocedure infection ranges from 0.2% to 0.58%, including a high rate of tubo-ovarian abscess for-

mation in up to 0.24% of the cases.[40–42] Abscess formation occurs between 1 and 6 weeks following retrieval. Predisposing factors for infection include a past history of pelvic inflammatory disease, puncture of an endometriotic cyst, puncture of the hydrosalpinx, and incidental bowel penetration during egg recovery. Puncture of an endometriotic cyst, in particular, may be associated with chemical peritonitis or postoperative abscess formation.[43,44] To reduce these risks, the cyst should be irrigated with the flushing media and intraoperative prophylactic IV antibiotics are recommended. The endometrioma contents are also considered to be toxic to the oocytes, and care must be taken to flush the needles and use new Petri dishes in the lab. Any pelvic infections post retrieval will likely lead to a lower implantation rate.[42]

Multiple puncture sites in the vaginal vault and/or inappropriate handling of the vaginal probe will increase the risk of bleeding. The risk of vaginal bleeding has been reported to be as high as 0.09%.[45,47] Bleeding from the vaginal puncture site frequently will stop with pressure applied to the site with the vaginal probe during the procedure. Rarely, there is a need to suture the puncture sites after withdrawing the needle at the end of the procedure. Aspiration of blood from the needle signifies injury to the follicular wall or ovarian blood vessels. Keeping the needle in the center of the follicle minimizes injury to the follicular wall. If a retroperitoneal hematoma or internal bleeding is suspected, observation with pelvic ultrasound to ascertain persistent bleeding should be done after the procedure and prompt intervention and emergency laparotomy should be done to prevent significant blood loss. Ultrasound-guided oocyte retrieval is rarely associated with injury to neighboring organs, such as the bladder, intestines, ureters, and appendix. Although anesthetic complications are also rare, vagovagal reaction leading to severe bradycardia and cardiac arrhythmia and asystole following deep abdominal pressure on very high ovaries has been reported.[45]

Embryo Transfer

Embryos are transferred in most centers at either the third or fifth day after oocyte retrieval, depending on the experience of the embryology lab. The placement of the embryos into the endometrial cavity is a critical step that affects the overall success. Echo-tip Teflon-coated embryo transfer catheters have permitted optimization of this step under abdominal ultrasound guidance.[48] A trial of mapping for determining the optimal technique for intrauterine catheter placement noted in the cycle before the stimulation would allow smooth embryo transfer.

Luteal Support

Oocyte retrieval by aspiration of follicles also results in removal of a substantial portion of the granulosa cells. Combined with suppression of the gonadotropes, some patients will have greatly reduced progesterone production in the luteal phase. Luteal support should be done with either exogenous progesterone or additional hCG injections during the luteal phase. Several formulations of progesterone are commercially available: intramuscular progesterone in oil, vaginal micronized progesterone capsules, vaginal suppositories, and vaginal gel. Studies comparing them have not found any to be superior over others [49], but none of the studies has been large enough to have sufficient power. Progesterone supplementation is continued until the luteal–placental shift that occurs during the 10th to 12th weeks of gestational age.

REFERENCES

1. Steptoe PC, Edwards RG. Birth after re-implantation of a human embryo. *Lancet.* 1978;2:366.

2. Centers for Disease Control and Prevention. 2003 Assisted Reproductive Technology Success Report. Available at: http://www.cdc.gov/ART/ART2003/nation.htm.

3. Heape W. Preliminary note on the transplantation and growth of mammalian ova within a uterine foster mother. *Proc R Soc.* 1890;48:457–458.

4. Iwamatsu T, Chang MC. In vitro fertilization of mouse eggs in the presence of bovine follicular fluid. *Nature.* 1969;224:919–920.

5. Edwards RG. Maturation in vitro of human ovarian oocytes. *Lancet.* 1965;ii:926–929.

6. Edwards RG, Donahue RP, Baramki TA, Jones HW. Preliminary attempts to fertilize human oocyte matured in vitro. *Am J Obstet Gynecol.* 1966;96:192.

7. Steptoe PC, Edwards RG. Laparoscopic recovering of preovulatory human oocytes after priming of ovaries with gonadotropins. *Lancet.* 1970; ii:683–689.

8. Lopata A, Johnstone IWH, Leeton JF, Muchnicki D, Talbot TM, Wood C. Collection of human oocytes at laparoscopy and laparotomy. *Fertil Steril.* 1974;25:1030.

9. Lenz S, Lauritsen JG, Kjellow M. Collection of oocytes for IVF by ultrasonically guided follicular puncture. *Lancet.* 1981;1:1163.

10. Robertson R, Picker R, O'Neill C, Ferrier A, Saunders D. An experience of laparoscopic and trans-vesicle oocyte retrievals in an IVF program. *Fertil Steril.* 1986;45:88.

11. Gleicher N, Friberg J, Fullan N, et al. Egg retrieval for in-vitro fertilization by sonographically controlled vaginal culdocentesis. *Lancet.* 1983;2:508.

12. Russell J, Decherney AH, Hobbins J. A new trans-vaginal probe and biopsy guide for oocyte retrieval. *Fertil Steril.* 1987;47:350.

13. Lavy G, Restropo-Candelo J, Diamond M, Shapiro B, Grumbeld L, Decherney AH. Laparoscopic and transvaginal ova recovery: the effect on ova quality. *Fertil Steril.* 1988;49:1002.

14. Marrs R. Does the method of oocyte collection have a major influence on IVF? *Fertil Steril.* 1986;46:193.

15. Scott RT Jr, Hofmann GE. Prognostic assessment of ovarian reserve. *Fertil Steril.* 1995;63:1–11.

16. Bancsi LF, Broekmans FJ, Mol BW, Habema JD, te Velde ER. Performance of basal follicle-stimulating hormone in the prediction of poor ovarian response and failure to become pregnant after in vitro fertilization: a meta-analysis. *Fertil Steril.* 2003;79:1091–1100.

17. Hendriks DJ, Mol BW, Bancsi LF, te Velde ER, Broekmans FJ. Antral follicle count in the prediction of poor ovarian response and pregnancy after in vitro fertilization; a meta-analysis and comparison with basal follicle-stimulating hormone level. *Fertil Steril.* 2005;83:291–301.

18. Lockwood GM, Mutuukrishna S, Ledger WL. Inhibins and activins in human ovulation, conception and pregnancy. *Hum Reprod Update.* 1998;4:284–295.

19. Klein NA, Illingworth PJ, Groome NP, McNeilly AS, Battaglia DE, Soules MR. Decreased inhibin B secretion is associated with the monotropic FSH rise in older, ovulatory women: a study of serum and follicular fluid levels of dimeric inhibin A and B in spontaneous menstrual cycles. *J Clin Endocrinol Metab.* 1996;81:2742–2745.

20. Muttukrishna S, Child T, Lockwood GM, Groome NP, Barlow DH, Ledger WL. Serum concentrations of dimeric inhibins, activin A,

gonadotrophins and ovarian steroids during the menstrual cycle in older women. *Hum Reprod.* 2000;15:549–556.

21. Seifer DB, Scott RT Jr, Bergh PA, et al. Women with declining ovarian reserve may demonstrate a decrease in day 3 serum inhibin B before a rise in day 3 follicle-stimulating hormone. *Fertil Steril.* 1999;72:63–65.

22. Durlinger AL, Visser JA, Themmen AP. Regulation of ovarian function: the role of anti-Mullerian hormone. *Reproduction.* 2002;124:601–609.

23. de Vet A, Laven JS, de Jong FH, Themmen AP, Fauser BC. Anti-mullerian hormone serum levels: a putative marker for ovarian aging. *Fertil Steril.* 2002;77:357–362.

24. Cook CL, Siow Y, Taylor S, Fallat ME. Serum mullerian-inhibiting substance levels during normal menstrual cycles. *Fertil Steril.* 2000;73:859–861.

25. Higgins RV, van Nagell JR Jr, Woods CH, Thompson EA, Kryscio RJ. Interobserver variation in ovarian measurements using transvaginal sonography. *Gynecol Oncol.* 1990;39:69–71.

26. Syrop CH, Willhoite A, Van Voorhis BJ. Ovarian volume: a novel outcome predictor for assisted reproduction. *Fertil Steril.* 1995;64:1167–1171.

27. Lass A, Skull J, McVeigh E, Margara R, Winston RM. Measurement of ovarian volume by transvaginal sonography before ovulation induction with human menopausal gonadotrophin for in-vitro fertilization can predict poor response. *Hum Reprod.* 1997;12:294–297.

28. Sharara FI, McClamrock HD. The effect of aging on ovarian volume measurements in infertile women. *Obstet Gynecol.* 1999;94:57–60.

29. Ruess ML, Kline J, Santos R, Levin B, Timor-Tritsch I. Age and the ovarian follicle pool assessed with transvaginal ultrasonography. *Am J Obstet Gynecol.* 1996;174:624–627.

30. Meldrum DR, Wisot A, Hamilton F, Gulary AL, Huynh D, Kempton W. Timing of initiation and dose schedule of leuprolide influences the time course of ovarian suppression. *Fertil Steril.* 1988;50:400–402.

31. Scott RT, Navot D. Enhancement of ovarian responsiveness with micro-doses of GnRH agonist during ovulation induction for in vitro fertilization. *Fertil Steril.* 1994;61:880–885.

32. Scott RT, Hofmann GE, Muasher SJ, Acosta AA, Kreiner DK, Rosenwaks Z. A prospective randomized comparison of single and double lumen needles for transvaginal follicular aspiration. *J In Vitro Fert Embryo Transfer.* 1989;6:98–101.

33. Kingsland CR, Taylor CT, Aziz N, Biskerton N. Is follicular flushing necessary for oocyte retrieval? A randomized trial. *Hum Reprod.* 1991;6:382.

34. Tan SL, Waterstone J, Wren M, Parsons J. A prospective randomized study comparing aspiration only with aspiration and flushing for transvaginal ultrasound directed oocyte recovery. *Fertil Steril.* 1992;58:356–360.

35. Hayes MF, Succo AG, Savoy-Moore RT, Magyar DM, Endler GC, Moghissi KS. Effect of general anesthesia on fertilization and cleavage of oocytes in vitro. *Fertil Steril.* 1987;48:975–981.

36. Soussis I, Boyd O, Paraschos T, Duffy S, Bower S, Troughton P, Lowe J, Grounds R. Follicular fluid levels of midazolam, fentanyl and alfetanyl during transvagianl oocyte retrieval. *Fertil Steril* 1995;64:1003–1007.

37. Coetsier T, Dhont M, DeSutter P, Merchiers E, Versichelen L, Rosseel MT. Propofol anesthesia for ultrasound guided oocyte retrieval: accumulation of the anesthetic agent in follicular fluid. *Hum Reprod* 1992;7:1422.

38. Van Os HC, Roozenburg BJ, Janssen-Caspers HA, Leerentveld RA, Scholtes MC, Zeilmaker GH, Alberda AT. Vaginal disinfection with povidone iodine and the outcome of in-vitro fertilization. *Hum Reprod* 1992;7:349–350.

39. Biljan MM, Dean N, Hemmings R, Bissonnette F, Tan SL. Prospective randomized trial of the effect of two flushing media on oocyte collection and fertilization rates after in vitro fertilization. *Fertil Steril.* 1997;68:1132–1134.

40. Howe RS, Wheeler C, Mastroianni L Jr, Blasco L, Tureck R. Pelvic infection after transvaginal ultrasound-guided ovum retrieval. *Fertil Steril* 1988;49:726–728.

41. Curtis P, Amso N, Keith E, Bernard A, Shaw RW. Evaluation of the risk of pelvic infection following transvaginal oocyte recovery. *Hum Reprod* 1992;7:625–626.

42. Ashkenazi J, Farhi J, Dicker D, Feldberg D, Shalev J, Ben-Rafael Z. Acute pelvic inflammatory disease after oocyte retrieval: adverse effects on the results of implantation. *Fertil Steril* 1994;61:526–528.

43. Yaron Y, Peyser MR, Samuel D, Amit A, Lessing JB. Infected endometriotic cysts secondary to oocyte aspiration for in vitro fertilization. *Hum Reprod* 1994;9:1759–1760.

44. Nargund G, Parsons J. Infected endometriotic cysts secondary to oocyte aspiration for in vitro fertilization. *Hum Reprod* 1995; 10:1555.

45. Bennett SJ, Waterstone JJ, Cheng WC, Parsons J. Complication of transvaginal ultrasound-directed follicle Aspiration. A review of 2670 consecutive procedure. *J Assist Reprod Genet* 1993;10:72.

46. Dicker D, Ashkenazi J, Feldberg D, Levy T, Dekel A, Ben-Rafael Z. Severe abdominal complication after transvaginal ultrasonographically guided retrieval of oocytes for in vitro fertilization and embryo transfer. *Fertil Steril* 1993;59:1313–1315.

47. Serour GI, Aboulghar M, Mansour R, Sattar MA, Amin Y, Aboulghar H. Complications of medically assisted conception in 3500 cycles. *Fertil Steril* 1998;70:638–642.

48. Hurley V, Osborn J, Leoni M, Leeton J. Ultrasound-guided embryo transfer: a controlled trial. *Fertil Steril* 1991;55: 559–562.

49. Soliman S, Daya S, Collins J, Hughes EG. The role of luteal phase support in infertility treatment: a meta-analysis of randomized trials. *Fertil Steril.* 1994;61:1068–1076.

Section 7.4. Ultrasonography and the Embryo Transfer

Eric Flisser and Jamie A. Grifo

The original description of the "clinical touch" transfer technique described advancing the embryo transfer catheter tip until contact was made with the uterine fundus and subsequently withdrawing the catheter 5 to 10 mm before expelling the embryos. However, as follow-up studies on transfer technique have demonstrated the toxic consequences of provoking intrauterine bleeding and the effect of induced uterine contractions, increased emphasis has been placed on atraumatic technique. Because contact with the uterine fundus is now avoided, the definition of clinical touch transfer has subsequently evolved to include transfers in which contact with the uterine fundus is avoided, but additional machinations to identify catheter position, namely ultrasonography, is not performed. This technique, sometimes described as "blind" because visual confirmation of the location of catheter tip is not made, relies on the operator's subjective sense of catheter placement and other visual cues, such as depth markings placed at regular intervals along the catheter, for successful execution.

Ultrasonography as an adjunct to embryo transfer was employed early in the experience of human IVF, but this aspect of assisted reproductive technology did not garner much interest until vast improvements in other aspects of IVF, such as culture techniques, were made. The possibility that this seemingly innocuous step could undermine the complex process that preceded it had been noted, but efforts to assess the utility of ultrasonography during embryo transfer were lacking. The first study to illuminate the possibilities of ultrasonography and highlight the pitfalls of blind embryo transfer techniques compared 12 transfers performed by clinical touch to 16 using transabdominal ultrasonography.[1] When ultrasonography was performed, the catheter was introduced into the uterine cavity until it was seen curling as a result of contact with the fundus, and then it was withdrawn slightly. In three of 16 transfers guided by ultrasonography (18.8%), the catheter was observed abutting the posterior wall of the uterus after the operator had deemed the placement satisfactory. The practitioner was unaware of the poorly positioned catheter until alerted by the ultrasound findings, which suggested that clinical cues to catheter position might be insufficient. Ultrasound-assisted transfer was subjectively easier to perform, though this might have stemmed from operator bias, and less blood or catheter distortion was observed. The authors noted that they did not have statistical proof that this was a superior method of embryo transfer in the small number of subjects studied, but they recognized further investigation was needed.

The unreliable nature of traditional catheter placement was also revealed in a transvaginal ultrasonography study that demonstrated transfer catheters abutting the fundus in 17.4% and adjacent to a tubal ostium in 7.4% of 121 consecutive transfers.[2] Whether complex manipulations required to place the transfer catheter, remove the speculum, and introduce the vaginal probe played a role in the final catheter location is a possibility, nevertheless, the practitioner was unaware of the catheter's location relative to anatomic landmarks.

ALTERNATE USE OF TRANSABDOMINAL ULTRASONOGRAPHY (NOT ONLY FOR EMBRYO TRANSFER)

The use of ultrasound has typically been to confirm the correct placement of the transfer catheter tip, yet other applications are available. One study assessed whether pretransfer measurement of the uterocervical angle, an angle defined by a line aligning the external and internal cervical os and another line extending from the internal os through the fundus, would have an effect on transfer outcome.[3] This quasi-randomized study allocated patients on an alternating basis to ultrasound-assisted or "clinical feel" embryo transfer. Transfers done without ultrasonography were done with straight catheters; those performed after ultrasound assessment of the uterocervical angle had the transfer catheter bent to mimic the degree of flexion. A Frydman TDT catheter was used in all cases by first placing the rigid outer sheath with its obturator, then replacing the obturator with the flexible inner catheter for embryo transfer.

A marked improvement in pregnancy rate was demonstrated when the angle was measured and the outer sheath molded to mimic the degree of bend before transfer (26.3 vs. 18.4%, $P \leq 0.02$). The study observed a significant decrease in the presence of blood in the transfer catheter in the ultrasound group (26.3% vs. 33.4%, $P \leq 0.05$) as well as proportionally fewer difficult transfers (8.4% vs. 26.8%, $P \leq 0.00001$). However, whether this result arose from the use of ultrasonography or from bending the transfer catheter is unclear, and whether the difficulty of transfer was a preexisting characteristic of these patients, because allocation was not truly random, remains a possibility. It is possible that placing a bend in the transfer catheter permits it to more easily seek a path of least resistance, self-guiding its trajectory through the cervical canal. Without a bend, the straight catheter might resist conforming to the contour of the canal, abrading the endocervix and initiating bleeding. Because the uterocervical angle was not measured in the control group, it is unclear whether these patients had a higher proportion of steep uterocervical angles and if they would have benefited from a molded catheter by comparison.

A significantly higher rate of volsellum forceps use was observed in the control group (9.7% vs. 1.6%, $P \leq 0.00001$), which might have contributed to the study outcome, given the possibility of induced uterine contractions. The authors demonstrated that a wider uterocervical angle was associated with a decreased chance of pregnancy. If ultrasound had been performed in both groups, measurement of the uterocervical angle and the consequence of pretransfer catheter preparation could have been more clearly assessed. The study authors, however, did not compare an association with degree of difficulty and the uterocervical angle, though difficult transfers alone were not more likely to lead to pregnancy failure. The presence of blood in the catheter was associated with decreased pregnancy rates, as in other studies (OR 0.54; 95% CI, 0.35–0.84). The study suggests that placing a bend in the transfer catheter may facilitate its ease of placement, particularly in cases in which a significant degree of anteflexion or retroversion is suspected or has been previously observed.

The Catheter

Many studies have attempted to determine the optimal embryo transfer catheter.[4–8] Data have been conflicting, though transfer techniques now favor use of flexible catheters and minimizing cervical manipulation. Atraumatic transfer includes avoidance of contact with the uterine fundus that might provoke uterine contractions. The optimal catheter is one that can be reliably and accurately placed with a minimum of tissue trauma.

Ultrasonography has been used as an adjunct in some of these studies. A comparison of the Wallace and Frydman catheters demonstrated no significant difference between catheters when the choice of catheter was initially selected based on trial transfer before the start of ovarian stimulation.[8] During the trial transfer, Wallace catheters were used and if successfully placed, slated for use at the time of embryo transfer; if the catheter could not be passed easily, the Frydman catheter was selected. At the time of transfer, 6.5% of patients in the Wallace transfer group were switched to the Frydman catheter because of difficulty at transfer. The clinical pregnancy rates (41.6% vs. 36%) and implantation rates (16% vs. 14.4%) were not significantly different between groups, but showed a trend favoring transfer with the Wallace catheter, which might be more clearly revealed in a larger study. Blood, however, was seen on the catheter more frequently with the Frydman catheter (7.9% vs. 12.6%, $P = 0.02$). All transfers were done under ultrasound guidance. Because this study was not randomized and results not analyzed on an intention-to-treat basis, it cannot directly compare whether these catheters yield equivalent results or whether prestimulation trial transfer can improve ease of transfer, but suggests that Wallace catheters may be superior, and that additional manipulations to assist transfer with this catheter, such as having the patient maintain a full bladder or using a tenaculum to straighten the uterocervical angle, may be warranted.

In a quasi-randomized study of transabdominal ultrasound-guided embryo transfer, the Wallace and Frydman transfer catheters were compared; randomization for the use of ultrasound was done by availability of the ultrasonographer, and the transfer catheter was chosen by the embryologist.[9] The Wallace and the Frydman catheters yielded similar pregnancy rates (30.3% and 30.7%, respectively).

As technical improvements such as the introduction of "soft" embryo catheters have added to improved outcomes, changes in design, such as improved echogenicity of these catheters, may also

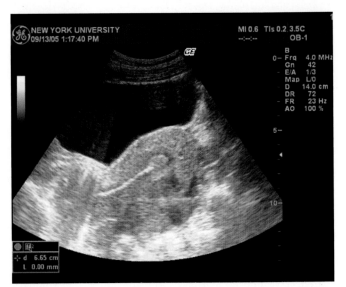

Figure 7.4.1. Sureview catheter visualized on transabdominal ultrasonography.

enhance their utility (Figure 7.4.1). Whether these design changes improve outcomes, or simply provide additional reassurance for the operator, has yet to be conclusively demonstrated.

One observational study anecdotally reported subjective improvement in visualization of a specially designed flexible coaxial catheter, the Cook Echo-Tip catheter, in 20 embryo transfers.[10] However, no comparisons were made during the study, and whether improved ultrasound visualization would lead to improved transfer outcomes was not investigated. The specially designed catheter used an echogenic, stainless steel ring imbedded in the distal tip of the inner catheter. The authors postulated that decreased manipulation of the inner catheter in attempts to visualize the catheter during ultrasonography would cause less disruption and trauma to the endometrium and might subsequently lead to improved outcomes. The sawing motion, they reported, variously employed to identify traditional catheters, might promote endometrial trauma. The authors also suggested that this back-and-forth technique used to assist visualization of the standard catheter might nullify gains achieved by employing ultrasound guidance, and might account for studies demonstrating equivalence in outcomes when ultrasound guidance is tested against blind transfer techniques. However, although vigorous catheter movements might traumatize the endometrial lining, slight to-and-fro movements of the catheter may not be any more damaging than complete withdrawal and replacement of the catheter, as performed in the case of retained embryos.

A quasi-randomized comparison study of 251 patients comparing ultrasound assistance using either the Wallace catheter or the Cook Echo-Tip catheter demonstrated no difference in implantation rates (30% vs. 35%) and clinical pregnancy rates (57% vs. 55%).[11] Although the authors reported improved visualization of the specially designed catheter, it was not statistically more conspicuous than the standard catheter (100% vs. 95%), though it was subjectively easier to identify during transfers with obese patients or when the bladder was insufficiently full. No improvement in outcomes was noted when analysis by degree of technical difficulty was performed. Although no difference was seen, a power calculation was not reported; additionally, patients in the study were not truly randomized: subjects were assigned to treatment and control groups on an alternating basis, and even though the compared characteristics of the two groups showed no significant difference, the scheduling order of patient transfers could have introduced bias, which could have resulted in failure to reject the null hypothesis. Additional study of these newer catheters may be justified.

Alternate Techniques to Improve Transfer; Confounding Variables on Ultrasonographically Guided Transfer

Mock transfer to facilitate actual embryo transfer is a frequently employed technique. However, the optimal timing and method for performing mock transfer are not clear. Some practitioners prefer to perform mock transfer in the cycle preceding transfer, at the start of stimulation or immediately before the true embryo transfer. Concerns regarding timing the trial transfer center on possible trauma to the endometrium immediately before embryo transfer, which could lower success rates. However, the uterus is not rigidly fixed within the pelvis and performance of mock transfer weeks before transfer may not accurately present the clinical situation at time of transfer. An algorithm for mock transfer permits selection of an appropriate catheter by using progressively more rigid catheters.

Difficult embryo transfers were associated with a statistically lower pregnancy rate in a study comparing outcomes in cases where a mock transfer had been performed.[12] Patients having a difficult transfer, characterized by degree of effort required to place the catheter successfully, had a statistically lower implantation rate than easy transfers (4% vs. 20.4%, $P = 0.005$), and patients having mock transfers before transfer had a higher pregnancy rate (22.8% vs. 13.1%, $P = 0.02$) and implantation rate (7.2% vs. 4.2%, $P = 0.03$) than those who did not. At time of embryo transfer, there were no difficult transfers in patients who had a prior mock transfer, whereas 37.6% of the control group had difficult transfers.

One descriptive study of mock transfer performed immediately before embryo transfer showed that difficulty of transfer, scored separately from the type of catheter required, was associated with transfer outcome. Those requiring "strong manipulation and pressure" were significantly less likely to achieve pregnancy.[13] Twenty of the 113 transfers performed (17.7%) were noted to have blood on the catheter tip, though in this study a difference in pregnancy outcome for these cases was not seen.

Additional techniques, like having the patient maintain a full bladder before transfer, may facilitate the ease of transfer in a patient with an anteverted uterus by straightening the uterocervical angle. A full bladder will also improve visualization when concurrent transabdominal ultrasonography is performed during transfer.

Whether ultrasound improves the ease of transfer, however, is unclear. Although the position of the catheter within the uterus and its relationship to the uterine fundus or other landmarks can be measured, the introduction of the catheter to the cervical canal may not be facilitated because the images may not reveal small details of the canal. With two-dimensional (2-D) imaging, the full length of the canal and endometrial stripe may not be visible in a single plane. Resolution maximums, related to the frequency of sound wave and the resulting echotexture of the tissue, may further limit visual information gained by the scan. Finally, the vaginal speculum may block much of the electromagnetic signal, interfering with visualization of the catheter as it passes through the cervix.

In a prospective, randomized trial of Frydman, Wallace, and TDT catheters, although outperformed by the other catheters, pregnancy rates using the TDT catheter were significantly improved with the application of ultrasonography (19.4 vs. 9.2%, $P \leq 0.05$).[14] The effect of ultrasonography was not assessed with the competing catheters. The metal mandrel of the TDT catheter improved visualization of its placement, and this characteristic was thought to be the cause of improved pregnancy rates when ultrasonography was employed during these transfers. However, whether this characteristic is correlated with an improved result has not yet been determined with specially designed, echogenic, soft catheters.

When performing transabdominal ultrasonography, having the patient maintain a full bladder may facilitate image resolution by providing a medium for the propagation of sound waves, and may also serve to straighten the cervical canal of an anteverted uterus, facilitating transfer. This clinical pearl may not improve performance related to the use of the ultrasound, but to manipulation of existing anatomic relationships. Conversely, a full bladder in the case of a retroverted uterus may only exacerbate uterocervical angle deflection.

Possibly, mechanical effects associated with performing transabdominal ultrasonography are at the root of improvements in transfer, such as pressure against the anterior abdominal wall with the transducer and distention of the bladder, which can straighten the uterocervical angle.

However, in a randomized study, no difference in clinical pregnancy rates was noted among patients receiving clinical touch transfer (35.7%) or transabdominal ultrasound-assisted embryo transfer with or without a distended bladder (39% and 38.7%, respectively).[15] When the bladder was full, the requirement for using an obturator was less often necessary (13.4%) than when ultrasonography was performed without a full bladder (32.8%) and when ultrasonography was not used (32.5%, $P \leq 0.02$). Similarly, a full bladder was associated with a decreased need for a tenaculum (8.9% vs. 26.5% vs. 25%, $P \leq 0.002$) or the use of a hysterometer (1.5% vs. 14% vs. 15%, $P \leq 0.002$).

In a randomized study of 100 patients with a history of "easy" mock embryo transfers, investigators examined whether the use of transabdominal ultrasonography enhanced IVF outcome in these cases.[16] Easy mock transfers, performed before controlled ovarian hyperstimulation, were defined as those in which a Frydman catheter was placed without effort and without cervical manipulation. All patients underwent ICSI after a standardized stimulation protocol. After stimulation, embryo transfer was performed to within 0.5 to 1 cm of the uterine fundus confirmed with ultrasound guidance or, in controls, based on the prior uterine cavity measurement. Treatment characteristics between groups were similar. As compared with the control group, there was no advantage to ultrasound guidance in the resulting implantation (19.6% vs. 16.3%), pregnancy (42.0% vs. 30.0%), or miscarriage rates (4.7% vs. 13.3%), though the study was underpowered to eliminate the possibility of a type II statistical error (failing to reject the null hypothesis when the alternate hypothesis is true) with the highest confidence ($\alpha = 0.05$, $\beta = 0.80$), which would have required 267 subjects, assuming the pregnancy rates held constant.

A study of recipients of donated oocytes demonstrated an increase in pregnancy rate, defined by detection of hCG, and implantation rate in transfers guided by ultrasound compared with historical controls.[17] Although this study eliminated some issues of confounding by using an oocyte donation model, the modality of ultrasound employed varied (transvaginal, $n = 75$; transabdominal, $n = 20$) and patients having transfers without ultrasound guidance had uterine depth measured immediately before transfer by direct contact with the uterine fundus using a Tom Cat catheter (Kendall), whereas in the ultrasound-assisted cases, the uterine fundus was avoided and no mock transfer was performed. Improvement in outcomes was seen only in easy transfers: pregnancy rate (63.1% vs. 36.1%) and implantation rate (28.8% vs. 18.4%).

REPEAT TRANSFERS AND VISUALIZATION OF THE CATHETER

Repeat placement of transfer catheters has no effect on outcome. No significant difference in pregnancy rates was observed in a retrospective analysis of embryo transfers between 1135 successful first attempts and 69 transfers requiring additional attempts (24.7% vs. 23.2%).[18] In addition, the distribution of multiple pregnancies was similar between groups. Factors contributing to retained embryos were difficult transfer and blood or mucus contamination of the catheter. No difference was seen in the rate of retained embryos when Wallace (2.3%), Embryon (6.3%), or other catheters (7.1%) were used. The authors of this study did not aspirate cervical mucus before transfer. Multiple attempts to place transfer catheters were not associated with a decrease in presence of a gestational sac when the cause was retained embryos or when imposed time restrictions on the duration of transfer lapsed.[4]

When ultrasonography is used, the to-and-fro movement used to identify poorly visualized transfer catheters because of patient characteristics, such as obesity or significant uterine retroflexion, may have the same effect on the endometrium as complete withdrawal and reinsertion of the catheter. This suggests that the advantages of echogenic catheters, specifically designed for use in ultrasound-assisted transfer, might not confer additional benefits, except as a tool to teach embryo transfer technique or for quality assurance and retraining if one operator's results deviated from practice norms of a group. However, no conclusive trials using these catheters have been reported.

Additional benefits to using a specially designed echogenic catheter include providing reassurance to the operator, confirming catheter placement, and, when the ultrasound image is visible to the patient, providing distraction during the transfer process.

OPERATOR AT TRANSFER

The operator performing the transfer can have profound effects on the cycle outcome: In a program with a 46% clinical pregnancy rate, the success rate of cycles stratified according to the provider performing the embryo transfer ranged from 17.0% to 54.3%.[19] With this in mind, it becomes difficult to assess how the addition of any technique or protocol can improve outcomes, given the number of possible confounding influences.

The embryo transfer is a critical and highly sensitive component of the IVF cycle. Even when techniques are standardized, outcomes are uncertain. When instituted, some techniques may require a "learning curve" before equivalency among all operators is achieved.[20] This may apply not only to performing embryo transfer but also to improvement when adjunct techniques are incorporated, such as the addition of visual feedback using ultrasound images.

As has been shown, embryo transfer technique can be taught. An evaluation of nurses trained to perform transfer showed no difference compared with physicians.[7] The use of ultrasonography may serve to assist training protocols, providing confirmation and confidence for operators learning the technique.

Just as experience can affect the outcome of embryo transfer, it is likely that experience with performing ultrasound-guided transfers affects its utility as an adjunct technique. Identification of the endometrial cavity, the transfer catheter, and other pelvic structures requires practice, as does optimization of acquired images and correlation between visual and tactile feedback. Because of anatomic differences among patients, the scanning parameters can be adjusted to improve image quality; however, changes in scale alter the corresponding visual and physical depth ratio, so care must be taken when advancing the catheter. The ability to individualize image acquisition will permit transfer of any advantages using this technique to all patients.

Outcomes have improved by previous performance of a mock embryo transfer to assess the difficulty of catheter placement and to provide guidelines for transfer, by permitting notations about the direction of the cervical canal, the length of the uterus, and potential obstructions or hazards. The timing of mock transfer has varied among practitioners: before the IVF stimulation, during stimulation, and immediately before embryo transfer.

TRANSABDOMINAL ULTRASONOGRAPHY

The advantages of routine ultrasonography at embryo transfer appear clear; however, because of design limitations, many studies showing an improvement in outcome are less than ideal and may overstate the contribution of ultrasound to the desired effect. Despite findings that did not reach statistical significance, a trend toward improved pregnancy outcome encouraged the authors of one study to recommend the use of ultrasound in all difficult transfers and in older women.[21] Comparing 93 patients who underwent transabdominal ultrasound–assisted transfer when an ultrasonographer was available to 94 patients who received clinical touch transfer showed a trend toward increasing pregnancy rates, defined by the presence of a gestational sac (37.8% vs. 28.9%), though the increase was not significant. A trend toward improvement was also noted in difficult transfers (54.5% vs. 10.0%). Clinical touch transfer was performed by placing the catheter as close as possible to the uterine fundus without touching it; embryos were deposited within 1 cm of the fundus in the intervention group. No prior uterine sounding or measurements were reported. This study was limited by lack of true randomization and unreliable technique. Because the length of the uterine cavity is not standardized among patients, subjective placement of the catheter to within 10 mm of the fundus without specific data on each patient and without coming in contact with the fundus is a challenging task. Under these conditions, ultrasound guidance would be expected to improve pregnancy rates, and although it is interesting to note that no statistical difference was noted, this was likely because of the sample size. If clinical touch transfer patients are systematically disadvantaged compared with patients receiving ultrasound-assisted embryo transfer, ultrasound guidance for all cases would be appropriate.

A retrospective study showing improvement in clinical outcomes when transabdominal ultrasound was performed (38.4% vs. 25.4%) was similarly complicated by comparing the performance of true clinical touch transfers with ultrasound-guided transfers that avoided contact with the uterine fundus.[22] An additional confounding factor was a concurrent increase in the use of soft transfer catheters over the study period; the independent effects of ultrasound guidance, avoidance of the fundus, and employing flexible catheters cannot be easily disassociated, though in regression analysis, the catheter choice, but not use of ultrasound, was associated with significant differences in outcome.

Another controlled, randomized study of 330 subjects demonstrated an increase in implantation rates (19.6% vs. 12.6%) and clinical pregnancy rates (37.1% vs. 25.0%) when transabdominal ultrasound guidance was used.[23] The authors touted the use of ultrasound in its ability to permit assessment of the uterocervical angle and therefore to permit pretransfer catheter preparation to accommodate this variable. Presumably, this improved the ease of transfer, but the authors did not compare this variable between groups. In addition, the ability to assess uterine cavity position and depth was lauded because it permitted individualization of transfer depth. However, patients in the control group all received transfer to a fixed distance (6 cm), and this may have contributed to the study result because transfer depth was not individualized. A prior sounding might have minimized differences for both of these variables: pretransfer assessment of the uterocervical angle and embryo transfer depth.

A quasi-randomized study of transabdominal ultrasound guidance was performed applying ultrasound based on the availability of the ultrasonographer.[9] Neither pregnancy rates (29% vs. 30.3%) nor implantation rates (15.5% vs. 14.2%) were different in the presence or absence of the ultrasound machine in the 178 transfers performed.

In a randomized, controlled study, transabdominal ultrasonography was demonstrated to increase implantation and clinical pregnancy rates, the presence of a gestational sac, compared with clinical touch transfer.[24] Mock transfer was performed in all patients before ovarian hyperstimulation and notations made regarding the position of the uterus and direction of the cervical canal so that transfers performed without ultrasound could avoid touching the uterine fundus using these records as a guide. However, although a Frydman catheter was used in all transfers, in the ultrasound group, its outer guide was not employed, whereas it was routinely used in the control group. By protocol, a degree of difficulty was assigned, depending on the need for a tenaculum, metal sound, or additional maneuvers, such as cervical dilation. A statistically higher proportion of transfers were technically easy compared with controls, and a trend toward higher pregnancy rates was seen with easy transfers, although not statistically significant.

In a prospective, quasi-randomized study, 1069 embryo transfers were split between ultrasound guidance and clinical touch transfer according to room assignment for embryo transfer (an ultrasound machine was available in only one of the two operating rooms used).[25] Patients in this study received embryo transfer 3, 4, or 5 days following oocyte retrieval, according to the number and quality of embryos available. Patients lacking at least one good-quality embryo were excluded from the study. Although differences in characteristics between the transfer subgroups were not observed, a statistical difference in pregnancy rate was seen between the patients undergoing ultrasound-guided embryo transfer on days 3 (45.9 vs. 31.7%, $P = 0.001$) and 4 (43.5% vs. 27.0%, $P = 0.035$), but not day 5 (56.3% vs. 45.7%).

The authors postulated that changes in endometrial receptivity can be provoked by traumatic embryo transfer, resulting in advancement of the putative "window of receptivity," causing premature decidualization and disrupting synchrony between embryo developmental stage and the endometrium; once a specific developmental stage has been achieved, external influences cannot disrupt the timeline and are less likely to influence implantation. This would account for the decreasing strength of difference in outcome on subsequent transfer days. An additional explanation offered suggested that the number of patients receiving day 5 transfer were not sufficient to demonstrate a statistical difference. The authors did not, however, report whether use of ultrasound was correlated with ease of transfer, decreased blood in the catheter, number of attempts, time required to perform the transfer, additional maneuvers, such as tenaculum or volsellum use, or other parameters that might correlate with less traumatic embryo delivery, because the expert gynecologist performing the transfer presumably minimized confounding that might otherwise be caused by multiple or inexperienced operators. Why ultrasound guidance would improve transfer only on days 3 and 4 remains unclear, especially given the conflicting results seen in other studies.

A prospective, randomized study of 800 embryo transfers was designed to detect an 8% increase in pregnancy rate with 80% power at 5% significance based on an average 17% pregnancy rate in the clinic in which it was performed.[26] Both fresh and frozen transfers were included. No differences in patient characteristics, including the distribution of fresh and frozen transfers, were observed. Despite use of ultrasonography, no significant difference was observed between the treatment and control groups (26.0% vs. 22.5%), although a statistically significant difference in implantation rate was observed (15.3% vs. 12.0%, $P = 0.048$.) The relatively low pregnancy rate, compared with more recent studies, may be its own confounding variable. Although the study was appropriately designed based on a historical average, other factors, such as lab conditions, not correctable by ultrasound transfer may limit the study results. In addition, fixed distance of transfer (6 cm) may be suboptimal for a large subpopulation of patients; it does not take advantage of the individualization that ultrasound transfer or clinical touch transfer based on prior sounding permits, which may be the critical factor accounting for observed improvements in pregnancy rates seen by some authors.

Two studies assessing the use of transabdominal ultrasound showed significant increases in outcome variables when the technique was employed. In a prospectively randomized study, 362 subjects undergoing fresh embryo transfer on postretrieval days 2, 3, 5, and 6 were assigned to clinical touch transfer or transabdominal ultrasound–guided transfer.[27] A statistical increase in implantation was noted (25.3% vs. 18.1%, $P \leq 0.01$), as was an increase in the pregnancy rate (50.0% vs. 33.9%, $P \leq 0.002$). Ultrasound-guided transfer was performed by watching the catheter advance until it was approximately 15 to 20 mm from the uterine fundus; clinical touch transfer was performed by subjective assessment of the operator, trying to place the embryos as close to the fundus as possible without touching it. The comparison is imperfect because the depth of transfer was not individualized in the clinical touch group, touching the fundus might have occurred by error (establishing a cause for the increased pregnancy rates in the treatment group), and differences existed in the location of embryo deposition: 15 to 20 mm in the treatment group and as close as possible to the fundus without touching in the control group. No difference was seen in the ease of transfer between groups.

In the second study, frozen–thawed embryo transfers were examined.[28] One hundred eighty-four patients undergoing frozen embryo cycles were randomized to clinical touch and ultrasound-assisted transfer. Again, a statistical increase in implantation (19.1% vs. 11.7%, $P \leq 0.05$) and clinical pregnancy (34.4% vs. 19.8%, $P \leq 0.05$) was observed. Clinical touch transfer in these cases was performed by attempting to place the embryos 15 to 20 mm from the fundus, as with the ultrasound-assisted transfers, using prior ultrasound measurement of uterine cavity length, performed within the 3 months preceding the transfer, to assist correct catheter placement. Although this technique likely improved the clinical transfer, use of ultrasound to measure uterine cavity length may not provide a reliable estimate and may have disadvantaged subjects in the control group.[29]

The advantages of transabdominal ultrasonography demonstrated in these studies might stem from avoidance of contact with the uterine fundus, minimizing uterine contractions and endometrial trauma, and by consistency in depositing transferred embryos to an optimal implantation site, 15 to 20 mm from the fundus. However, these methods may be employed without the use of ultrasonography by using prior uterine sounding measurements to guide catheter placement.

An excellent randomized, controlled trial of transabdominal ultrasound–assisted embryo transfer in recipients of donated oocytes failed to demonstrate a difference in IVF outcome between groups.[30] The study was designed to detect a 15% difference in pregnancy rates, defined by the visualization of fetal cardiac activity, with $\beta = 0.8$ and $\alpha = 0.05$. Characteristics of the two groups were not different, and preparation for embryo transfer, including instructing all patients to have a full bladder regardless of group assignment, was the same. Embryo transfer differed only in that the catheter was advanced to within 1 to 1.5 cm of the fundus in the ultrasound group and as close as possible to the fundus without touching in the control group. No uterine sounding prior to cycle start was reported. Statistical analysis demonstrated no differences in pregnancy rates (59.9% vs. 55.1%), implantation rates, or multiple pregnancy rates. No difference was noted in ease of transfer or presence of blood in the catheter. Additional catheter movement in the ultrasound group used infrequently to help visualize the catheter when ultrasound images were suboptimal could add a confounding variable, but increased trauma, evidenced by bloodied catheters, was not present. Although it is possible that a smaller difference in pregnancy rates exists, this study presents the best evidence against improvement in IVF outcomes when experienced providers perform embryo transfer without ultrasound guidance.

Our quasi-randomized, retrospective comparison of 249 patients supports this conclusion: Outcomes of IVF cycles in which all embryo transfers were performed by one physician (JG) with or without transabdominal ultrasound guidance dependent on the availability of the ultrasonographer (EF) were compared.[31] No patient characteristics studied were significantly different, and no differences in clinical pregnancy rates were observed (46.2% vs. 46.2%).

A retrospective study comparing 823 embryo transfers raised important issues when considering the validity of studies comparing outcomes.[32] In this study, no difference was seen in pregnancy between the transabdominal ultrasound–guided group (48%) and the clinical touch group (44%). Before transfer, a mock transfer was attempted first with a soft catheter; if it could not be passed, a more rigid catheter was used. Following transfer, the difficulty of transfer was rated using a protocol, according to maneuvers performed by the physician performing the transfer. In the first year of the study, only clinical touch transfers were performed. In the second year, all transfers were done under ultrasound guidance.

The frequency of difficult transfer varies in each study, and the effect of an intervention is dependent on the frequency of a condition's occurrence; overall, the rate of difficult transfer is low, so detecting improvement may be difficult to demonstrate. Factors that have been negatively associated with transfer outcome were diminished in the ultrasound-guided group (presence of blood, $P = 0.01$, or mucus, $P = 0.04$ in the catheter), though these characteristics were not associated with differences in pregnancy rates between groups in the study when logistic regression was performed. No differences were observed when the number of embryos transferred was analyzed or when the analysis was performed according to the clinician performing or the embryologist assisting the transfer.

The only factor determined to have prognostic significance in this study was use of a soft-pass catheter, though choice of catheter was determined before employing ultrasonography. The use of the soft catheter was statistically more frequent (98% vs. 95%, $P = 0.02$) in the ultrasound group, which suggests that the characteristics of the patients were not entirely similar and that a more exaggerated result of the use of ultrasound (assuming that it has a positive effect on establishing pregnancy) would result, yet no statistical difference in outcomes was seen, despite this bias. The authors noted that placement of the mock transfer catheter could influence outcome in an unpredictable fashion; it follows that additional manipulation to place a more rigid catheter, in addition to use of the more rigid catheter for transfer, would disadvantage the clinical touch group. Though graded according to guidelines, the clinician's opinion of difficulty of transfer could have in part been subjectively biased by the presence of the ultrasound machine. A significantly higher distribution of easy transfers was noted in the ultrasound group ($P = 0.01$).

The authors commented that the decreased frequency of negative factors associated with pregnancy outcome, such as blood or mucus in the catheter or the use of a tenaculum, made transabominal ultrasound guidance a useful adjunct to embryo transfer. Given the low prevalence of complicated transfers, statistical evidence justifying its use may be obscured.

One meta-analysis that combined eight prospective, controlled trials of transabdominal ultrasound–assisted transfer calculated a significant improvement in pregnancy rate and embryo implantation when all of these studies (OR 1.51; 95%CI, 1.32–1.73) or when only the subset of truly randomized studies (OR 1.44; 95% CI, 1.18–1.74) was examined.[33] However, meta-analysis is limited by the quality and design of the studies evaluated, and the possible confounding issues and technical flaws of these studies have been detailed. The most important contribution of this analysis was the calculation that demonstrating a 5% improvement in pregnancy rate with 80% power would have required a 2500-patient study, assuming a pregnancy rate of 25%. Higher pregnancy rates would necessitate larger studies, as do smaller differences in outcomes. When overall pregnancy rates are low, confounding factors, including steps preceding transfer, such as embryo culture, may contribute to outcome and may make the observed improvements less likely to represent real effects of the planned intervention. When study conditions are suboptimal, calculating the contribution of an intervention can be difficult. Conversely, under optimal conditions, a small contribution may be more difficult to detect without an impractically large study population. A second meta-analysis of these randomized, controlled trials analyzed additional outcome parameters, but was inconclusive as to why ultrasound guidance might improve outcomes.[34] The multiple pregnancy rate, the miscarriage rate, and the ectopic pregnancy rate were not significantly different. Additionally, differences in study design made analysis of the effect on the ease of transfer impossible to determine.

Although the utility of ultrasound guidance can be hotly debated, the most important central tenet in the practice of medicine holds: No study has demonstrated an adverse effect of performing ultrasound-guided embryo transfer, meeting an important primary objective: *primum non nocere.*

ECTOPIC PREGNANCY

Ectopic pregnancy is a well-documented complication of IVF. Embryo transfer technique may play a role in its occurrence, especially if embryos are transferred directly to damaged fallopian tubes. In a nonrandomized comparison, two embryo transfer techniques were compared: fixed transfer distance to true clinical touch technique.[35] Because the measured maximal length of the uterocervical canal was 68 mm and the maximal depth performed by clinical touch was 90 mm, the dangers of ignoring clinical data are demonstrated. The rate of ectopic pregnancy was significantly higher when the clinical touch technique was employed ($P \leq 0.05$), all were at depths exceeding 60 mm, but a fixed depth did not prevent ectopic pregnancy from occurring in the comparison group. The disparities in insertion distance and measured depth by ultrasound can only be explained by kinking of the transfer catheter or by placement of the catheter through the tubal ostium, which could facilitate tubal implantation. In another study, when the length of catheter inserted into the uterus was subtracted from the ultrasonographically measured depth of the uterine cavity, although not statistically significant, a trend toward increasing ectopic pregnancy occurred with lower and negative values.[36]

With transabominal ultrasound guidance, one group observed a 6.3% rate of ectopic pregnancy in patients with a history of tubal infertility and a 3.3% rate when all 3543 guided embryo transfers were examined.[37]

Ectopic pregnancy may also be associated with the size of the uterine cavity. When all patients received transfer of embryos to a distance of 5 mm from the uterine fundus, as determined by prior uterine sounding, those with uterine depth of 7 cm or less had a significantly higher rate of ectopic pregnancy ($P \leq 0.0005$) compared with patients with uterine depth of 7 to 9 cm; the frequency of tubal disease and the number of embryos transferred were not different between groups.[38]

The site of transfer has been shown to be a risk factor for ectopic pregnancy. When a quasi-randomized study was performed comparing deep transfer (≤ 5 mm from the fundus) to midfundal transfer (≥ 15 mm) based on prior uterine measurement, a significant increase in the proportion of ectopic pregnancies was seen when deep transfer was performed (1.5% vs. 0.4%, $P = 0.029$) without a difference in pregnancy rate (14.2% vs. 12.2%).[39]

Performing true clinical touch transfers was associated with higher ectopic pregnancy rates compared with when embryos were transferred to a fixed distance into the uterine cavity (≤ 55 mm from the external cervical os).[40] When clinical touch was performed, catheters were threaded to between 55 mm and 90 mm from the external os. By ultrasonography, the uterine depth in all study patients was 59.3 $\pm$ 4.2 mm (mean $\pm$ SD). Patients were quasi-randomized into each arm of the study, which demonstrated a significantly higher rate of ectopic pregnancy when true clinical touch transfer was performed (16.7% vs. 1.8%, $P \leq 0.05$), though pregnancy rates between groups were not significantly different.

An analysis of ectopic pregnancy and intrauterine pregnancy in one IVF program revealed that ectopic pregnancies were more likely to be associated with difficult transfers (OR 3.91; 95% CI, 1.49–10.23).[41] These transfers were performed using the true clinical touch technique, which by possibly provoking uterine contractions, may have contributed to the overall ectopic pregnancy rate.

Although elevated compared with the general population, the relatively low incidence of ectopic pregnancy in the IVF population may hinder attempts to prove whether ultrasound-assisted transfer can reduce the occurrence of ectopic pregnancy. To establish a statistical difference, a large sample size must be accumulated. Most studies have shown no significant difference in ectopic pregnancy between treatment and control groups. Currently, ultrasound guidance does not seem to prevent ectopic implantations from occurring or to reduce its incidence. Three-dimensional (3-D) ultrasonography, which permits visualization of the depth of the catheter and its deviation from the midline, may help prevent placing the embryo transfer catheter near the tubal opening.[42]

TRANSVAGINAL ULTRASONOGRAPHY

Transvaginal ultrasound–guided embryo transfer has not been assessed as frequently as the technically easier transabdominal ultrasonography. Because of closer proximity to pelvic organs, the resolution and detail of transvaginal ultrasonography are often superior to transabdominal scanning, and it does not require having a distended bladder to improve visualization. Although it does not require having a separate ultrasonographer, intravaginal placement of the ultrasound probe, speculum, and transfer catheter may be cumbersome because of performance of simultaneous, semi-independent tasks, though practice certainly decreases the task complexity.

An initial quasi-randomized study of transvaginal ultrasound–guided embryo transfer that compared 94 cases to 246 matched controls noted no significant improvement in pregnancy outcome compared with the control group (20.2% vs. 17.5%).[43] Randomization was performed based on the availability of transfer personnel. Anecdotally, the authors preferred ultrasound guidance because of successful catheter placement in patients with complicated anatomy.

A retrospective comparison demonstrated improvement when transvaginal ultrasound–assisted transfer was performed in 402 subjects compared with 444 historical clinical touch controls.[44] Patient characteristics were similar (age, number of oocytes retrieved, number of embryos transferred, and difficulty of transfer), but the resulting pregnancy rate was significantly different (28.9% vs. 13.1%, $P \leq 0.01$). However, the study compared true clinical touch transfers, in which the outer catheter was placed in physical contact with the fundus and then withdrawn, to a technique in which the catheter did not touch the fundus. The authors did not comment on the presence of blood in the transfer catheter, so this confounding variable might have contributed to the treatment outcome. The ectopic pregnancy rates were similar between groups.

Another transvaginal ultrasound–assisted embryo transfer study retrospectively compared patients who had previously failed IVF to a subsequent cycle in which transvaginal ultrasonography was performed.[45] Twenty-three subjects were identified that could be paired with previous cycle failures when transvaginal ultrasound was not performed. No significant difference in patient characteristics from the two attempts was noted, including patient age and cycle characteristics.

Because these cycle characteristics were the same, the authors concluded that the use of ultrasound guidance was the key factor for the difference in outcome. However, because the study was retrospective and historical control cases were collected over the preceding 3 years, unaccounted and possibly subtle confounding variables may have played a role in the outcome, such as changes in lab technique. Additionally, the comparison to previous cycle failure is suboptimal: Even despite optimal stimulation and lab conditions, with a large cohort of high-quality embryos to select from for transfer, some patients inexplicably fail to become pregnant; a patient not pregnant from one cycle may achieve pregnancy in the next under identical conditions. The cause of the first failure cannot be definitively identified, so a subsequent intervention may not be responsible for a successful outcome. Though a statistical increase in the pregnancy rate was seen for all patients 40 years and younger during the 9-month study period compared with the preceding 3 years, the absence of analysis for other variables undermines the strength of the association.

THREE- AND FOUR-DIMENSIONAL ULTRASONOGRAPHY

The role of 3-D and "real-time" 3-D or "four-dimensional" (4-D) imaging in embryo transfer is still under investigation. Naturally,

the development of this modality and its clinical application, investigation, and publication add to the lag time in the implementation of the new technology.

An early study in the use of this modality was performed to assess the accuracy of traditional 2-D ultrasound-guided transfer. Following transfer, the position of the transfer catheter was maintained and 3-D volumetric image scanning, using either a transabdominal or transvaginal probe, was performed; the resulting images were retrospectively compared with the 2-D technique.[46] In four of the 21 cases in which sufficient images were obtained for analysis, 3-D modeling was assessed as demonstrating a significant deviation in catheter localization compared with placement determined by 2-D images viewed at the time of actual transfer. Catheter placement was thought to deviate in an anterior–posterior or lateral direction, deflecting away from the ideal, midline position in these cases, including in one case in which placement of the catheter tip was shown localized to the cornual region of the uterus.

However, although this study demonstrated that obtaining 3-D images of intrauterine catheters is feasible, it did not address the impact or utility of using this technique. Because no clinical decisions were made on images created using 3-D technology, no comparative conclusions can be drawn. Additionally, because outcome measures were not reported for these embryo transfers, the consequence of seeing a misplaced catheter on 3-D images when correct placement was believed to be obtained from 2-D scan cannot be evaluated. Without outcomes data, the 3-D data's value cannot be assessed.

Three-dimensional images were postulated to improve upon 2-D images by identifying cases in which migration of the catheter, directed by a path of least resistance, led to malposition within the cavity. However, the acceptable degree of variance from the midline is still unknown; therefore, the contribution of this information has uncertain utility. Additionally, it is not known how far embryos migrate after transfer, either by physiologic interactions with endometrial cells or uterine contractility, or by the fluid dynamics of the transfer droplet. The precision of embryo placement may always be susceptible to factors not controlled by clinical technique.

An observational study using 3-D ultrasonography demonstrated that 81% (26/32) of embryos that implanted successfully did so at the area of initial transfer, suggesting that in cases in which uterine contraction–associated movement of the embryo does not occur, the air bubble serves as an appropriate proxy for the location of transferred embryos and that implantation location can be biased by the transfer technique.[42] Because ectopic pregnancies in this study were located on the ipsilateral side to the location of the air bubble at time of transfer, and because no ectopic pregnancy occurred when the air bubble remained in the midfundal area, deviation of the catheter from the midline may play a role in creating ectopic pregnancy even when the catheter remains in the uterus, though prevention of ectopic pregnancy by monitoring catheter alignment to the midline has not been studied.

Limitations of this equipment include higher complexity of image acquisition and subsequent interpretation of the acquired images. Real-time 3-D imaging, like all procedures, will require experience for optimal use.

Another descriptive study of 1222 consecutive patients undergoing embryo transfer using concurrent 4-D ultrasound imaging demonstrated the ease of use of this equipment.[47] The authors used a putative "maximal implantation potential point" as a target for the embryo catheter tip, a point at the intersection of two lines bisecting the uterine cornua at the junction with the fallopian tubes. Use of this calculated point personalizes the transfer target to the contour of each patient's uterus, tailoring the transfer to the idiosyncrasies of the patient's anatomy. The authors recognize, however, that the utility of identifying this point accurately is debatable because of uncertainty regarding the degree of decrement in implantation potential as a function of the distance from this "point of maximal implantation." Ultimately, this target may represent not a highly discriminate point of maximal implantation, but a broader implantation zone, which would deemphasize such a specific target, though it may continue to be a useful guidepost. For acceptability of use, there were no measured outcome variables recorded regarding the ease of transfer and the degree of effort or of accuracy at reaching the specified target point.

AIR IN THE UTERINE CAVITY; LOCATION OF TRANSFER; ACTIVITY FOLLOWING TRANSFER

Catheter loading, using varying amounts of transfer media or including air in the catheter, is not a standardized technique. Air bubbles, frequently included in transfer catheters to assist visualization of the transfer droplet, can be observed ultrasonographically. Air pockets are not normally present in the uterine cavity, though transferring air along with the media drop does not appear to have a negative effect on transfer or implantation. A mock transfer study using equivalent volumes of methylene blue dye demonstrated that air in the catheter had no effect on dye expulsion through the cervix.[48] A randomized study of transfer including or excluding air in the catheter was performed in 196 patients and demonstrated no difference in establishing pregnancy when air was included in the catheter.[49]

Movement of the air bubble toward the fundus can be seen even when the uterus is retroverted, suggesting that an active transport mechanism exists within the uterus.[50] In one analysis, movement of the transfer-associated air bubble was associated with an increase in the pregnancy rate compared with transfers in which the bubble remained stationary (45.4% vs. 15.6%, $P \leq 0.001$), which the authors suggested is a sign of endometrial receptivity.[51] In few cases in the same series (5.0%), the bubble moved in the direction of the cervix during catheter withdrawal, all 5 mm or less. In all but one case in this series, the observed movement ranged from 2 to 5 mm, and although ultrasonography was continued until the transfer-associated bubble became stationary, it is possible that movement resumed after ultrasonography was discontinued.

In analysis of the effect of the presence of air in the transfer catheter, no differences in pregnancy rates were seen when the group was subdivided by the final location of the transfer bubble as identified by ultrasound, whether in the upper, mid-third, or lower uterus, although a comparison of the quality and number of the embryos among these subdivisions was not reported.[49] However, failure to visualize the air bubble following transfer is ominous; in cases in which the air bubble from the transfer could not be located, no pregnancy was established.[44]

The role of providing ultrasound guidance is to verify the proper location of the catheter. Whether clinical transfer or ultrasound-guided transfer is performed, the optimal location for embryo placement must be considered. The use of ultrasonography is not simply limited to evaluating the location of the catheter with a simple binary result; it also permits the operator to judge specific distances to anatomic landmarks, and in 3-D ultrasonography, the degree of deviation from the midline may be simultaneously assessed. However, despite this ability, there is still debate as to the best location to deposit embryos. Although early studies of embryo transfer observed by ultrasonography suggested that there was no association between the catheter tip location and establishment of pregnancy [52], more recent literature suggests that the catheter location plays an important role.

In a descriptive study of 3-D ultrasonography, the location of the gestational sac following transfer showed that in cases in which pregnancy was established, the implantation site was biased toward the location of the embryo transfer–associated air bubble at the time of transfer.[42]

In one randomized study, patients were selected to undergo embryo transfer at the top half or bottom half of the endometrial cavity.[53] The endometrial cavity length was calculated by transvaginal ultrasound exam performed preretrieval, during ovarian stimulation, by measuring the distance from the internal os to the uterine fundus. All transfers were performed by the same provider using one type of catheter, only transfers in which the catheter could be visualized were included in the final analysis, and all transfers were done on the same postretrieval day using a standard protocol. No difference in outcomes, including implantation rate, clinical pregnancy rate, ectopic pregnancy rate, and spontaneous loss rate, was observed. A power calculation before the study was designed to detect a 15% difference in resulting pregnancy rates. Although this study leaves open the possibility that a smaller difference in outcomes may exist by choice of transfer site, the similar rate of spontaneous abortion suggests that site of transfer may not play as significant a role as other factors.

One study of ultrasound-guided transfer randomized 180 subjects according to transfer distance from the uterine fundus, as measured by transabdominal ultrasonography.[54] Patients having transfers at 15 ± 1.5 mm and 20 ± 1.5 mm from the fundus had significantly higher implantation rates (31.3% and 33.3%, respectively) than patients receiving transfers at 10 ± 1.5 mm (20.6%). Because of the possibility of post-transfer embryo movement, the middle depth may be the optimal locale. The authors noted that no pregnancies occurred in the few patients whose transfer depth exceeded 20 mm from the fundus (18 cases). If the transfer droplet can migrate or be transported 2 to 5 mm from its transfer location, as observed in a prior study [2], the middle depth (15 mm) would seem most appropriate because it would keep the majority of embryos within acceptable boundaries (≤20 mm and ≥10 mm) from the fundus, even after factoring in embryo drift or transport.

In one evaluation of the transfer depth, blind uterine sounding performed before stimulation was characterized as an unreliable measure of uterine depth; the transfer distance from the fundus, as calculated by the difference between the ultrasound estimates of uterine depth, measured from the endometrial fundus to the external cervical os, and the length of the catheter inserted into the uterus were correlated with pregnancy outcome.[36] Catheter placement was guided to a "suitable point" near the fundus using ultrasound guidance, though this location was undefined. When depth was categorized, patients receiving transfers to a calculated depth that was less than 0 mm from the measured length of the cavity to the external os (i.e., the length of catheter inserted from external os to its tip exceeded the ultrasound measure of the distance from the external os to the fundal endometrium) had significantly worse outcomes. However, for this calculated difference to be negative, the catheter tip would have to be located in the fallopian tube, in the myometrium, or in an unknown location, possibly curled within the cavity. A negative calculated value occurred in 18% of transfers. If the catheter tip was well visualized at transfer, this suggests that the assessment of uterine depth by ultrasound was unreliable and any formula using this value, such as the calculated depth of transfer, was also inaccurate.

Excellent pregnancy rates were demonstrated when the target of ultrasound-guided embryo transfer was placed in the thickest portion of the endometrial cavity.[55]

Ultrasound guidance may permit more precise placement of the transfer catheter. An analysis of transfer depth performed by standardized measurements relative to the size of the uterine cavity demonstrated improved implantation and pregnancy rates when embryos were placed in an area bounded by the lower third and midpoint of the endometrial cavity.[56] The catheter depth was standardized using a mathematical formula to compensate for variations in size of the human uterus. Patients receiving transfer to the low to mid-cavity area were noted to have a significantly higher live birth rate (RR = 1.48; 95% CI, 1.08–2.02; P = 0.02) and pregnancy rate (RR = 1.44; 95% CI, 1.09–1.91; P = 0.01), and a higher implantation rate (RR = 1.59; 95% CI, 1.23–2.05; $P \leq$ 0.001) when compared with patients receiving transfer between 0.5 cm and 1.0 cm.

Despite coordinating transfer droplet placement to a specific site, active and passive transport mechanisms may alter the final location of the embryos, in addition to complex fluid interactions among the transfer droplet, the catheter, and endometrial tissue.

Fluoroscopic imaging of radiopaque dye demonstrated that a transferred bolus of fluid dynamically moves following transfer.[57] Almost half the patients studied showed fluid movement immediately after injection, and only 68% of subjects had all or part of the fluid bolus remaining in the uterus during the observation period. Although dye differs from transfer medium in density and viscosity and the quantity used in the study was greater than typically used at transfer, studies of uterine contraction frequency have demonstrated transfer droplet–associated movement. Uterine contractions, stimulated by manipulation of the cervix or by touching the uterine fundus, may play a role in decreasing implantation. Supraphysiologic levels of hormones may also contribute to this phenomenon.

Touching the uterine fundus is associated with increased uterine contraction activity and may interfere with implantation by relocating embryos to suboptimal sites or expelling the embryos from the cavity entirely. Using contrast material to mimic transfer medium, an increased contraction rate was seen in oocyte donors following retrieval 45 minutes following mock transfer after the fundus was deliberately touched with the transfer catheter.[58] No increase in activity was seen when contact with the fundus was avoided. Additionally, use of a tenaculum to assist transfer has been associated with an increase in contraction activity.[59]

Uterine contractions measured immediately before embryo transfer were inversely correlated to clinical pregnancy rates ($P \leq$ 0.001), though the direction of the contraction wave was not. Plasma progesterone was negatively correlated with uterine contraction rates ($P \leq$ 0.001).[60]

Patients are frequently concerned about embryos "falling out" of the uterus and are often fearful that they will disrupt the process by moving. Bed rest has traditionally had a role in the care of patients. In natural conception, bed rest is not necessary, though the manipulations required for transcervical embryo transfer may change this requirement. From a theoretical view, the varying interval from replacement of embryos to implantation suggests that ambulation should have no effect on outcome.

The persistence of a "catheter track," a channel created by placing and removing a catheter in a previously potential space in the uterus, was observed via ultrasonography to remain for at least 30 minutes.[1] Whether this artifact of transfer was clinically important was unknown, and so, empirically, patients have typically been left supine with varying degrees of leg elevation or in Trendelenburg position for an arbitrary interval following embryo transfer. Without definitive evidence for its utility, the rest period has varied substantially, including periods such as 3 to 4 hours [61] and up to 6 hours [1] or longer.

Observational study of the transfer-associated air bubble following the embryo transfer suggests that prolonged (or possibly any) period of bed rest is unnecessary.[62] In 101 transvaginal ultrasound–guided embryo transfers, no movement of the bubble occurred in 95 subjects (94.1%) when patients were reassessed via ultrasound after immediately standing following the transfer procedure. In four patients (4.0%), air bubble movement was limited to 1 cm or less, and only in two (2.0%) was movement between 1 cm and 5 cm. Because the embryos are not directly observed, the significance of air bubble movement is an imperfect proxy: Embryos may move with or independently from this transfer marker.

Whether promoting prolonged bed rest in patients following embryo transfer can improve implantation has been tested by several investigators. To test the hypothesis, 182 patients were randomized to 20 minutes of bed rest versus 24 hours of bed rest following embryo transfer.[63] Patients in the long-stay group were transferred to a stretcher and brought to a clinic for prolonged rest. In the short-stay group, no instructions regarding restriction of activity were given following discharge. No differences were seen in the establishment of pregnancy (24.1% vs. 23.6%), spontaneous abortion rate (19% vs. 14.2%), or multiple gestation (18.1% vs. 13.6%). The method of randomization was not reported, and the patient was randomized one time, though some underwent multiple cycles, which suggests that other factors may have affected the study outcome. The power of the study may also have been insufficient to detect differences in outcomes.

In a randomized comparison of 424 patients randomized to 1 hour of bed rest or 24 hours rest, no difference was seen in clinical pregnancy rates between groups (22% vs. 18%), though a higher implantation rate was observed in the group with limited rest (14.4 vs. 9%), which was reflected in a significant difference in the multiple gestation rate, despite similarities in the age of patients, infertility diagnosis, and the quality and number of embryos transferred.[64] The difference in implantation rates is exceptional and the cause uncertain, though the authors postulated a role for the potential psychologic consequences of restrictions in activity.

One IVF program that does not employ bed rest after embryo transfer compared its results with historical controls from a national database.[65] The clinic demonstrated a statistically greater clinical pregnancy rate compared with the database, which suggests that a variable bed rest interval might not play a role in embryo implantation 1 or more days following transfer. However, differences in an individual clinic's protocols and results compared with a national amalgam might have been great enough to obscure the detrimental effect of immediate ambulation, if present. The study demonstrates that pregnancy is not excluded by immediate ambulation.

To assess the effect of immediate ambulation, 406 patients undergoing fresh IVF cycles were given the option of ambulation or bed rest.[66] Although not randomized, patient characteristics such as age, number of retrieved oocytes, quality of embryos, and number of embryos transferred were not different. Between the 167 patients who opted for immediate ambulation and the 239 patients who chose 1 hour of bed rest, no difference in pregnancy rates was observed (24.6% vs. 21.3%). The study was underpowered to detect a difference in the observed pregnancy rates with $\beta = 0.8$ and $\alpha = 0.05$, but 4400 subjects per group would have been required to achieve this level of significance. This study gives some evidence that any differences, if present, will likely be small.

Optimal placement of embryos is still the subject of debate. However, following transfer movement of the transfer droplet suggests that there are limitations to the utility of accurate placement, given passive movement of the transfer droplet, from catheter withdrawal, and active transport, from uterine contractions. Despite the precision afforded by catheter markings, uterine sounding, and visualization by ultrasound guidance, not all factors can be controlled. After transfer of the embryos into the uterus, even the most precise of transfers can be altered.

The effect of fluid dynamics in the uterine microenvironment attributable to transfer failure has not been quantified. However, a number of observed phenomena have been reported. Following expulsion into the uterine cavity, reversal of flow of transfer medium toward the lower uterine segment along the sides of the catheter has been termed "capillary flowback".[61] Capillary flowback presumably results from the adhesive and cohesive properties of the medium, the catheter, and the endometrium. Too rapid withdrawal of the embryo transfer catheter may create negative pressure within the cavity or leave a void, encouraging the transfer medium (and embryos) to migrate. Surface tension and the complex interaction of solid and liquid physics, coupled with possible electromagnetic forces from charged surface proteins, makes prediction of embryo movement impossible.

The proper amount of pressure placed on the plunger has also never been assessed except in subjective terms: "moderately rapid" [61], "avoid white-knuckling the fingers" [11], "gently expelled" [44], "avoid turbulent flow around the catheter tip." [1]

Certain stimuli can provoke uterine contractions, including manipulation of the cervix. The waves of uterine contractions can cause the embryos to be transported to a suboptimal implantation site or may expel the embryos from the uterus completely, resulting in failed cycles or in ectopic pregnancy, if the embryos are transported retrograde to a fallopian tube. Placement of the catheter through the cervix may be a sufficient stimulus to induce contractions, and whether the duration of the

catheter's placement has any effect on outcome was examined in a prospective, randomized trial of 100 subjects. [67]. Patients were randomized to either immediate removal of the catheter or to a 30-second delay after the embryos were expelled before the catheter was removed. Characteristics of the patients were not different, including the distribution of day of transfer (day 3 or day 5 post retrieval), the age of the patients, the number and quality of embryos transferred, the cause of infertility, and stimulation parameters. All the transfers were defined as "easy" because none required use of extensive cervical manipulation or the use of a tenaculum. There was no significant difference in implantation rates between immediate withdrawal and the 30-second wait (60.8% vs. 69.4%).

The authors concluded that no benefit was achieved from waiting to withdraw the catheter, though they acknowledged that the result may have been from lack of statistical power or insufficient delay. However, the authors pointed out that uterine contractions may persist for 45 minutes following embryo transfer, so longer waiting periods are not realistically employable. The authors postulated that the act of placing the catheter through the cervix is the causative event in initiating uterine contractions via prostaglandin release. Although no transfer was deemed "difficult," the total time required to position the transfer catheter once contact was made with the cervix was not examined as an additional potential determinant of outcome.

Although a prolonged wait following expulsion of the embryos does not appear necessary, it would be prudent to remove the catheter slowly to minimize disruption of the endometrium and to avoid drawing the transfer droplet toward the lower uterine segment. Additionally, pressure should be applied continuously to the plunger until the catheter is completely removed from the uterus to prevent creating negative pressure in the syringe, which could inadvertently withdraw the droplet and embryos.

ULTRASONOGRAPHY FOR NONCERVICAL TRANSFER

When transcervical embryo transfer has proven difficult or impossible, surgical embryo transfer under ultrasound guidance has been attempted. This technique has been used infrequently. Early attempts to perform this procedure were unsuccessful [68]; however, transvaginal ultrasound–guided transmyometrial embryo transfer and transabdominal ultrasound–assisted transurethral embryo transfer successes have been reported.[69] One case series reported good pregnancy rates (36.5%) with a vaginal approach [70], and a small, independent trial found similar pregnancy rates.[71] A prospective, randomized study failed to demonstrate a difference in outcome between transmyometrial and transcervical embryo transfer in patients with cervical stenosis, because none of the 15 patients with this diagnosis achieved pregnancy during the study. [72]

CONCLUSION

There are various determinants that can complicate the success of an embryo transfer. Each factor contributing to the probability of successful outcome may have a critical threshold that irrevocably causes IVF cycle failure. Failure to deliver embryos to the endometrial cavity, directly or indirectly, will never result in a viable pregnancy, but the critical factor is rarely so conspicuous. Studying subtle influences is challenging, given the number of confounding variables.

The benefit of ultrasonography may exist for only a very small subset of patients in whom an inappropriate transfer site would have been chosen without visual confirmation. Unfortunately, identification of these cases is difficult, so physicians will need to decide whether routine ultrasound guidance is feasible or if it should be employed only in cases in which difficulty is anticipated, using a protocol to select cases for ultrasound guidance.

Despite the increasing use of ultrasound assistance, however, clinical touch transfer may be more practical for some; the added benefit of ultrasound guidance in individual cases must always be considered.[73] Recommending universal adoption of this technique is premature; improved outcomes have not been conclusively established. However, ultrasonography has never been demonstrated to detract from IVF success, and it may safely be used for all transfers. Because of its noninvasive nature and because performance of transabdominal ultrasound at transfer can frequently be done with little or no added cost, ultrasound guidance may become routine.

REFERENCES

1. Strickler RC, Christianson C, Crane JP, Curato A, Knight AB, Yang V. Ultrasound guidance for human embryo transfer. *Fertil Steril.* 1985;43:54–61.

2. Woolcott R, Stanger J. Potentially important variables identified by transvaginal ultrasound-guided embryo transfer. *Hum Reprod.* 1997;12:963–966.

3. Sallam HN, Agameya AF, Rahman AF, Ezzeldin F, Sallam AN. Ultrasound measurement of the uterocervical angle before embryo transfer: a prospective controlled study. *Hum Reprod.* 2002;17:1767–1772.

4. Goudas VT, Hammitt DG, Damario MA, Session DR, Singh AP, Dumesic DA. Blood on the embryo transfer catheter is associated with decreased rates of embryo implantation and clinical pregnancy with the use of in vitro fertilization-embryo transfer. *Fertil Steril.* 1998;70:878–882.

5. Ghazzawi IM, Al-Hasani S, Karaki R, Souso S. Transfer technique and catheter choice influence the incidence of transcervical embryo expulsion and the outcome of IVF. *Hum Reprod.* 1999;14:677–682.

6. Gonen Y, Dirnfeld M, Goldman S, Koifman M, Abramovici H. Does the choice of catheter for embryo transfer influence the success rate of in-vitro fertilization? *Hum Reprod.* 1991;6:1092–1094.

7. Barber D, Egan D, Ross C, Evans B, Barlow D. Nurses performing embryo transfer: successful outcome of in-vitro fertilization. *Hum Reprod.* 1996;11:105–108.

8. Urman B, Aksoy S, Alatas C, et al. Comparing two embryo transfer catheters. *J Reprod Med.* 2000;45:135–138.

9. Al-Shawaf T, Dave R, Harper J, Linehan D, Riley P, Craft I. Transfer of embryos into the uterus: how much do technical factors affect pregnancy rates? *J Assist Reprod Genet.* 1993;10:31–36.

10. Letterie GS, Marshall L, Angle M. A new coaxial catheter system with an echodense tip for ultrasonographically guided embryo transfer. *Fertil Steril.* 1999;72:266–268.

11. Karande V, Hazlett D, Vietzke M, Gleicher N. A prospective randomized comparison of the Wallace catheter and the Cook Echo-tip® catheter for ultrasound-guided embryo transfer. *Fertil Steril.* 2002;77:826–830.

12. Mansour R, Aboulghar M, Serour G. Dummy embryo transfer: a technique that minimizes the problems of embryo transfer and improves the pregnancy rate in human in vitro fertilization. *Fertil Steril.* 1999;54:678–681.

13. Sharif K, Afnan M, Lenton W. Mock embryo transfer with a full bladder immediately before the real transfer for in-vitro fertilization treatment: the Birmingham experience of 113 cases. *Hum Reprod.* 1995;10:1715–1718.

14. Wisanto A, Janssens R, Deschacht J, Camus M, Devroey P, Van Steirteghem AC. Performance of different embryo transfer catheters in a human in vitro fertilization program. *Fertil Steril.* 1989;52:79–84.

15. Lorusso F, Depalo R, Bettocchi S, Vacca M, Vimercati A, Selvaggi L. Outcome of in vitro fertilization after transabdominal ultrasound-assisted embryo transfer with a full or empty bladder. *Fertil Steril.* 2005;84:1046–1048.

16. de Camargo Martins AMV, Baruffi RLR, Mauri AL, et al. Ultrasound guidance is not necessary during easy transfers. *J Assist Reprod Genet.* 2004;21:421–425.

17. Lindheim SR, Cohen MA, Sauer MV. Ultrasound guided embryo transfer significantly improves pregnancy rates in women undergoing oocyte donation. *Int J Gynaecol Obstet.* 1999;66:281–284.

18. Nabi A, Awonuga A, Birch H, Barlow S, Stewart B. Multiple attempts at embryo transfer: does this affect in-vitro fertilization treatment outcome? *Hum Reprod.* 1997;12:1188–1190.

19. Hearns-Stokes RM, Miller BT, Scott L, Creuss D, Chakraborty PK, Segars JH. Pregnancy rates after embryo transfer depend on the provider at embryo transfer. *Fertil Steril.* 2000;74:80–86.

20. Papageorgiou TC, Hearns-Stokes RM, Leondires MP, et al. Training of providers in embryo transfer: what is the minimum number of transfers required for proficiency? *Hum Reprod.* 2001;16:1415–1419.

21. Kan AKS, Abdalla HI, Gafar AH, et al. Embryo transfer: ultrasound-guided versus clinical touch. *Hum Reprod.* 1999;14:1259–1261.

22. Wood EG, Batzer FR, Go KJ, Gutmann JN, Corson SL. Ultrasound-guided soft catheter embryo transfers will improve pregnancy rates in in-vitro fertilization. *Hum Reprod.* 2000;15:107–112.

23. Li R, Lu L, Hao G, Zhong K, Cai Z, Wang W. Abdominal ultrasound-guided embryo transfer improves clinical pregnancy rates after in vitro fertilization: experiences from 330 clinical investigations. *J Assist Reprod Genet.* 2005;22:3–8.

24. Matorras R, Urquijo E, Mendoza R, Corcóstegui B, Expósito A, Rodríguez-Escudero FJ. Ultrasound-guided embryo transfer improves pregnancy rates and increases the frequency of easy transfers. *Hum Reprod.* 2002;17:1762–1766.

25. Prapas Y, Prapas N, Hatziparasidou A, et al. Ultrasound-guided embryo transfer maximizes the IVF results on day 3 and day 4 embryo transfer but has no impact on day 5. *Hum Reprod.* 2001;16:1904–1908.

26. Tang OS, Ng EHY, So WWK, Ho PC. Ultrasound-guided embryo transfer: a prospective randomized controlled trial. *Hum Reprod.* 2001;16:2310–2315.

27. Coroleu B, Carreras O, Veiga A, et al. Embryo transfer under ultrasound guidance improves pregnancy rates after in-vitro fertilization. *Hum Reprod.* 2000;15:616–620.

28. Coroleu B, Barri PN, Carreras O, Martínez F, Veiga A, Balasch J. The usefulness of ultrasound guidance in frozen-thawed embryo transfer: a prospective randomized clinical trial. *Hum Reprod.* 2002;17:2885–2890.

29. Sher G, Fisch JD. Measuring uterine depth with colpohydrosonography. *J Reprod Med.* 2003;48:325–329.

30. García-Velasco JA, Isaza V, Martinez-Salazar J, et al. Transabdominal ultrasound-guided embryo transfer does not increase pregnancy rates in oocyte recipients. *Fertil Steril*. 2002;78:534–539.

31. Flisser E, Grifo JA, Krey LC, Noyes N. Transabdominal ultrasound-assisted embryo transfer and pregnancy outcome. *Fertil Steril*. In press.

32. Mirkin S, Jones EL, Mayer JF, Stadtmauer L, Gibbons WE, Oehninger S. Impact of transabdominal ultrasound guidance on performance and outcome of transcervical uterine embryo transfer. *J Assist Reprod Genet*. 2003;20:318–322.

33. Buckett WM. A meta-analysis of ultrasound-guided versus clinical touch embryo transfer. *Fertil Steril*. 2003;80:1037–1041.

34. Sallam HN, Sadek SS. Ultrasound-guided embryo transfer: a meta-analysis of randomized controlled trials. *Fertil Steril*. 2003;80:1042–1046.

35. Yovich JL, Turner SR, Murphy AJ. Embryo transfer technique as a cause of ectopic pregnancies in in vitro fertilization. *Fertil Steril*. 1985;44:318–321.

36. Pope CS, Cook EKD, Arny M, Novak A, Grow DR. Influence of embryo transfer depth on in vitro fertilization and embryo transfer outcomes. *Fertil Steril*. 2004;81:51–58.

37. Sieck UV, Jaroudi KA, Hollanders JMG. Ultrasound guided embryo transfer does not prevent ectopic pregnancies after in-vitro fertilization. *Hum Reprod*. 1997;12:2081–2085.

38. Egbase PE, Al-Sharhan M, Grudzinskas JG. Influence of position and length of uterus on implantation and clinical pregnancy rates in IVF and embryo transfer treatment cycles. *Hum Reprod*. 2000;15:1943–1946.

39. Nazari A, Askari HA, Check JH, O'Shaughnessy A. Embryo transfer technique as a cause of ectopic pregnancy in in vitro fertilization. *Fertil Steril*. 1993;60:919–921.

40. Yovich JL, Turner SR, Murphy AJ. Embryo transfer technique as a cause of ectopic pregnancies in in vitro fertilization. *Fertil Steril*. 1985;44:318–321.

41. Lesny P, Killick SR, Robinson J, Maguiness SD. Transcervical embryo transfer as a risk factor for ectopic pregnancy. *Fertil Steril*. 1999;72:305–309.

42. Baba K, Ishihara O, Hayashi N, Saitoh M, Taya J, Kinoshita K. Where does the embryo implant after embryo transfer in humans? *Fertil Steril*. 2000;73:123–125.

43. Hurley VA, Osborn JC, Leoni MA, Leeton J. Ultrasound-guided embryo transfer: a controlled trial. *Fertil Steril*. 1991;55:559–562.

44. Kojima K, Nomiyama M, Kumamoto T, Matsumoto Y, Iwasaka T. Transvaginal ultrasound-guided embryo transfer improves pregnancy and implantation rates after IVF. *Hum Reprod*. 2001;16:2578–2582.

45. Anderson RE, Nugent NL, Gregg AT, Nunn SL, Behr BR. Transvaginal ultrasound-guided embryo transfer improves outcome in patients with previous failed in vitro fertilization cycles. *Fertil Steril*. 2002;77:769–775.

46. Letterie GS. Three-dimensional ultrasound-guided embryo transfer: a preliminary study. *Am J Obstet Gynecol*. 2005;192:1983–1988.

47. Gergely RZ, DeUgarte CM, Danzer H, Surrey M, Hill D, DeCherney AH. Three dimensional/four dimensional ultrasound-guided embryo transfer using the maximal implantation potential point. *Fertil Steril*. 2005;84:500–503.

48. Mansour RT, Aboulghar MA, Serour GI, Amin TM. Dummy embryo transfer using methylene blue dye. *Hum Reprod*. 1994;9:1257–1259.

49. Krampl E, Zegermacher G, Eichler C, Obruca A, Strohmer H, Feichtinger W. Air in the uterine cavity after embryo transfer. *Fertil Steril*. 1995;63:366–370.

50. Sieck UV, Jaroudi KA, Hollaners JMG. Ultrasound guided embryo transfer does not prevent ectopic pregnancies after in-vitro fertilization. *Hum Reprod*. 1997;12:2081–2085.

51. Woolcott R, Stanger J. Potentially important variables identified by transvaginal ultrasound-guided embryo transfer. *Hum Reprod*. 1997;12:963–966.

52. Rosenlund B, Sjöblom P, Hillensjö T. Pregnancy outcome related to the site of embryo deposition in the uterus. *J Assist Reprod Genet*. 1996;13:511–513.

53. Franco JG Jr, Martins AM, Baruffi RL, et al. Best site for embryo transfer: the upper of lower half of endometrial cavity? *Hum Reprod*. 2004;19:1785–1790.

54. Coroleu B, Barri PN, Carreras O, et al. The influence of the depth of embryo replacement into the uterine cavity on implantation rates after IVF: a controlled, ultrasound-guided study. *Hum Reprod*. 2002;17:341–346.

55. Prapas Y, Prapas N, Hatziparasidou A, et al. Ultrasound-guided embryo transfer maximizes the IVF results on day 3 and day 4 embryo transfer but has no impact on day 5. *Hum Reprod*. 2001;16:1904–1908.

56. Frankfurter D, Trimarchi JB, Silva CP, Keefe DL. Middle to lower uterine segment embryo transfer improves implantation and pregnancy rates compared with fundal embryo transfer. *Fertil Steril*. 2004;81:1273–1277.

57. Knutsen V, Stratton CJ, Sher G, McNamee PI, Huang TT, Soto-Albors C. Mock embryo transfer in early luteal phase, the cycle before in vitro fertilization and embryo transfer: a descriptive study. *Fertil Steril*. 1992;57:156–162.

58. Lesny P, Killick SR, Tetlow RL, Robinson J, Maguiness SD. Embryo transfer – can we learn anything new from the observation of junctional zone contractions? *Hum Reprod*. 1998;13:1540–1546.

59. Lesny P, Killick SR, Robinson J, Raven G, Maguiness SD. Junctional zone contractions and embryo transfer: it is safe to use a tenaculum? *Hum Reprod*. 1999;14:2367–2370.

60. Fanchin R, Righini C, Olivennes F, Taylor S, de Ziegler D, Frydman R. Uterine contractions at the time of embryo transfer alter pregnancy rates after in-vitro fertilization. *Hum Reprod*. 1998;13:1968–1974.

61. Leong M, Leung C, Tucker M, Wong C, Chan H. Ultrasound-assisted embryo transfer. *J In Vitro Fert Embryo Transf*. 1986;3:383–385.

62. Woolcott R, Stanger J. Ultrasound tracking of the movement of embryo-associated air bubbles on standing after transfer. *Hum Reprod*. 1998;13:2107–2109.

63. Botta G, Grudzinskas G. Is a prolonged bed rest following embryo transfer useful? *Hum Reprod*. 1997;12:2489–2492.

64. Amarin ZO, Obeidat BR. Bed rest versus free mobilization following embryo transfer: a prospective randomized study. *BJOG*. 2004;111:1273–1276.

65. Sharif K, Afnan M, Lashen H, Elgendy M, Morgan C, Sinclair L. Is bed rest following embryo transfer necessary? *Fertil Steril*. 1998;69:478–481.

66. Bar-Hava I, Kerner R, Yoeli R, Ashkenazi J, Shalev Y, Orvieto R. Immediate ambulation after embryo transfer: a prospective study. *Fertil Steril*. 2005;83:594–597.

67. Martínez F, Coroleu B, Parriego M, et al. Ultrasound-guided embryo transfer: immediate withdrawal of the catheter versus a 30 second wait. *Hum Reprod*. 2001;16:871–874.

68. Lenz S, Leeton J. Evaluating the possibility of uterine transfer by ultrasonically guided transabdominal puncture. *J In Vitro Fert Embryo Transf*. 1987;4:18–422.

69. Parsons JH, Bolton VN, Wilson L, Campbell S. Pregnancies following in vitro fertilization and ultrasound-directed surgical embryo transfer by periurethral and transvaginal techniques. *Fertil Steril*. 1987;48:691–693.

70. Kato O, Takatska R, Asch RH. Transvaginal-transmyometrial embryo transfer: the Towako method; experiences of 104 cases. *Fertil Steril*. 1993;59:51–53.

71. Sharif K, Afnan M, Lenton W, Bilalis D, Hunjan M, Khalaf Y. Transmyometrial embryo transfer after difficult immediate mock transcervical transfer. *Fertil Steril*. 1996;65:1071–1074.

72. Groutz A, Lessing JB, Wolf Y, Azem F, Yovel I, Amit A. Comparison of transmyometrial and transcervical embryo transfer in patients with previously failed in vitro fertilization-embryo transfer cycles and/or cervical stenosis. *Fertil Steril*. 1997;67:1073–1076.

73. Sohan K, Woodward B, Ramsewak SS. Successful use of transrectal ultrasound for embryo transfer in obese women. *J Obstet Gynaecol*. 2004;24:839–840.

Section 7.5. Salpingostomy and Salpingectomy

Jaime Ocampo, Mary Jacobson, Mario Nutis, and Camran Nezhat

Approximately 25% to 35% of women's infertility is caused by tubal disease.[1] The most common cause of tubal disorder is pelvic inflammatory disease; other causes include endometriosis, salpingitis isthmica nodosa, complicated appendicitis, and surgery.

Because the fallopian tube may be affected at different sites, tubal damage is categorized into proximal or distal tubal disease. Proximal tubal disease accounts for 10% to 25% of tubal infertility. The most common etiology of proximal tubal disease is salpingitis isthmica nodosa. Other causes of proximal obstruction may be mucus plugs, cornual synechiae, polyps, and tubal endometriosis. Distal tubal disease commonly refers to the development of hydrosalpinges; however, other anatomic abnormalities, such as fimbrial phimosis or tubal adhesions, may constitute distal tubal disease. Distal tubal disease may account for up to 85% of tubal infertility.[1]

Surgical treatment for tubal disease waned after the advent of IVF. However, in recent years it has become evident that for specific tubal pathologies, specifically hydrosalpinges, surgical intervention needs to be considered, even in patients undergoing IVF.[2,3]

SURGICAL TREATMENT OF HYDROSALPINGES

A hydrosalpinx, or fluid-filled tube, occurs after an inflammatory process damages the serosa and mucosa of the fallopian tube, creating an occlusion in the distal part of the tube. As a result, normal and pathologic secretions may accumulate in the tube. The frequency of hydrosalpinges in distal tubal disease is approximately 10% to 30%.[4]

Hydrosalpinges have been shown to have a negative effect on pregnancy rates. In 1998, Zeyneloglu et al. [5] presented a meta-analysis of 23 studies that looked at the relation of hydrosalpinges and IVF outcome. They suggested that the existence of hydrosalpinges reduced the implantation rate and increased the risk of loss in patients undergoing IVF. Similar findings were presented in a Cochrane review done in 2004 by Johnson et al.[3] They were able to find only three randomized controlled studies that looked at surgical treatment of hydrosalpinges. The pooled results of these studies showed that the odds for pregnancy and live birth were increased with laparoscopic salpingectomy for hydrosalpinges before IVF. This prompted the authors to conclude that "the option of laparoscopic salpingectomy should be considered for all women with hydrosalpinges who are due to undergo IVF."[3]

Although the actual mechanism by which hydrosalpinges decrease pregnancy rates is unknown, there are several proposed theories. In the murine model, multiple studies have documented that hydrosalpinx fluid is embryotoxic. However, similar studies have failed to show toxicity in human embryos.[6] Mansour et al. [7] proposed that a mechanical interference with implantation occurred as the hydrosalpinx fluid leaked into the uterine cavity. In this study, the presence of fluid in the endometrial cavity reduced pregnancy rates and most women with fluid in the endometrial cavity had a hydrosalpinx at the time of IVF. Other studies have shown that the endometrium may become less receptive to embryo implantation when exposed to hydrosalpinx fluid. Meyer et al. [8] studied the expression of endometrial integrins in women with hydrosalpinges. They found a significant decrease in the integrin marker $\alpha v \beta 3$. Deficiency in this marker and two others ($\alpha 1 \beta 1$, $\alpha 4 \beta 1$) has been shown to have a deleterious effect on endometrial receptivity to embryo implantation.

CHOICE OF SURGICAL PROCEDURE

There has been considerable controversy as to the best and most appropriate surgical intervention for hydrosalpinges. Less invasive procedures like needle aspiration of hydrosalpinx fluid, salpingostomy, fimbriolysis, and proximal tubal occlusion have been proposed.

The success of these treatments is closely related to the severity of tubal disease. There have been several grading systems for assessing tubal damage. Tubal factors that affect the success of tubal surgery include thickness of the fallopian tube wall, adhesions of the tubal mucosa, and in some classifications, serosal adhesions.[9] In general, tubes classified with mild tubal disease have conception rates of 60% with fimbrioplasty and 81% with salpingostomy.[1] This is likely the result of an intact tubal mucosa – there is evidence that a healthy mucosa has a much better prognosis of success with fimbrioplasty and salpingostomy because the tube's ability to retrieve and transport ooctyes is usually preserved.[9]

Although the proposed systems for assessing tubal disease and choosing the adequate surgical procedure seem feasible, in practice they are difficult to carry out because most grading systems require the ability to perform a salpingoscopy to adequately grade the extent of tubal disease. These procedures can be carried out in tertiary centers with surgeons that have extensive experience with this type of procedure; however, this makes access much more difficult for the general infertility population.

Other issues to keep in mind are the high risk of ectopic pregnancy – up to 20% with salpingostomy – with tubal surgery done on inadequately assessed tubal disease.[9] In a review article on the management of hydrosalpinges, Sabatini et al. [9]

suggested that tubes with bipolar damage, mucosal adhesions, dense serosal adhesions, or thick walls as well as any tubes larger than 3 cm are unsuitable for tubal surgery, and salpingectomy should be the procedure of choice.

Recently there has been considerable debate over the use of proximal tubal occlusion for treatment of hydrosalpinges in infertility patients. The most recent study to compare this procedure with salpingectomy was done by Kontoravdis et al.[10] This study found similar improvement in implantation rates and pregnancy rates with tubal occlusion. There was a trend toward better outcomes with salpingectomy, but these numbers did not reach statistical significance.

Ultrasound-guided aspiration of hydrosalpinx fluid has also been proposed. Some researchers have performed this procedure just before an IVF cycle is done. This procedure, however, has a high rate of recurrence, with some reporting reaccumulation of the hydrosalpinx fluid within 2 days after the procedure.[11]

SALPINGECTOMY

Salpingectomy is the most widely used method for treatment of hydrosalpinges in infertility patients. The evidence for use of this procedure is based on two small randomized controlled studies and multiple retrospective studies. Critics of this procedure claim that the indiscriminate use of salpingectomy for hydrosalpinges should not be adopted because corrective surgery may be just as successful in adequately assessed tubal disease. However, adequate assessment of tubal disease requires salpingoscopy, a procedure

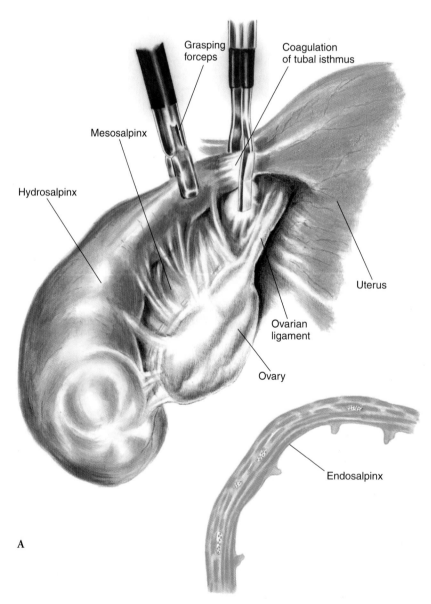

Figure 7.5.1. Salpingectomy is done with bipolar electrocoagulation for hemostasis. (**A**) The isthmic portion of the tube is coagulated and cut close to the uterus. *(Continued)*

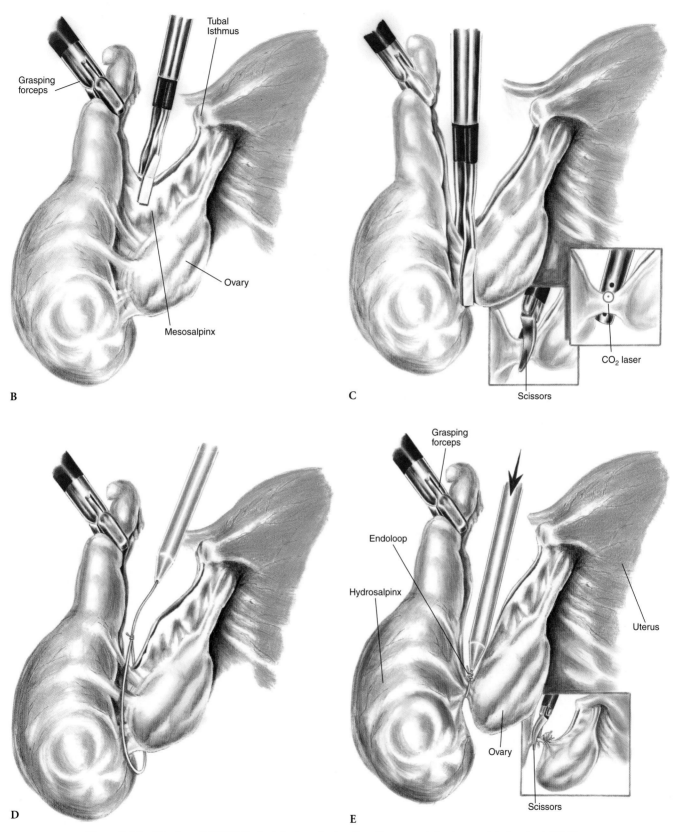

Figure 7.5.1. *(Continued)* (**B**) While the tube is under traction, the mesosalpinx is coagulated and cut. (**C**) Sharp scissors (*inset*) or the ultra-pulse CO_2 laser are used for cutting. (**D**) The Endoloop is passed around the tube and the mesosalpinx is ligated with one suture. (**E**) The mesosalpinx is cut above the tube. An adequate stump remains to prevent the ligature from slipping (*inset*).

not widely taught or performed. Without assessment of the tubal mucosa, it would be very difficult to accurately predict the success of salpingostomy or fimbriolysis. The possible impairment of ovarian blood supply after salpingectomy has been proposed, raising the possibility of decreased ovarian response undergoing hyperstimulation for IVF cycles. This theory was proposed after studies done on women who underwent salpingectomy after an ectopic pregnancy showed a decrease in follicle formation. However, subsequent studies have shown no impairment in ovarian response to IVF treatment.[12] Proximal tubal occlusion may represent another option in the treatment of hydrosalpinges in infertility patients. However, evidence for adoption of this procedure in place of salpingectomy is still fairly scant.

TECHNIQUE FOR SALPINGECTOMY

Salpingectomy is an easy procedure that requires instruments commonly used to do tubal electrocoagulation for sterilization. [13] The necessary instruments are a bipolar electrocoagulator, grasping forceps, scissors, and a laparoscope. A CO_2 laser also may be used. The laparoscope and 5-mm suprapubic trocars are placed, through which the graspers and bipolar electrocoagulator are inserted. Peritubal adhesions are lysed, and the tube is grasped at the isthmic portion. The proximal portion of the isthmus is coagulated and cut, using either scissors or laser (Figure 7.5.1A–C). If scissors are used, the bipolar electrocoagulator must be removed and replaced with the scissors through the same secondary trocar, or a third accessory trocar may be placed. The laser is faster and more precise than the scissors. Cutting is done in layers so that there is less chance to overshoot the coagulated area and get into an area beyond the coagulated tissue. Once the tubal isthmus is transected, the mesosalpinx is coagulated alternately and cut at intervals of 1 to 2 cm in the direction of the tubo-ovarian ligament.

Alternatives to bipolar electrocoagulation of the mesosalpinx are the Endoloop sutures (Ethicon) and automated stapling device (Endopath ELC 35, Ethicon). Before the Endoloop ligature is used, both the proximal portion of the tube and its distal attachment to the ovary (fimbria ovarica) are coagulated and cut. The Endoloop is passed around the tube, and the mesosalpinx is ligated with one Endoloop and removed. The mesosalpinx is cut above the ligature. An adequate stump is left to prevent the ligature from slipping (Figure 7.5.1D,E). The stapling device is introduced through a 12-mm trocar incision. After adhesions are lysed and the tube is mobilized, it is pulled up and put under traction. The stapler is used from the proximal to the distal end to staple and cut the tube. One or two applications are sufficient

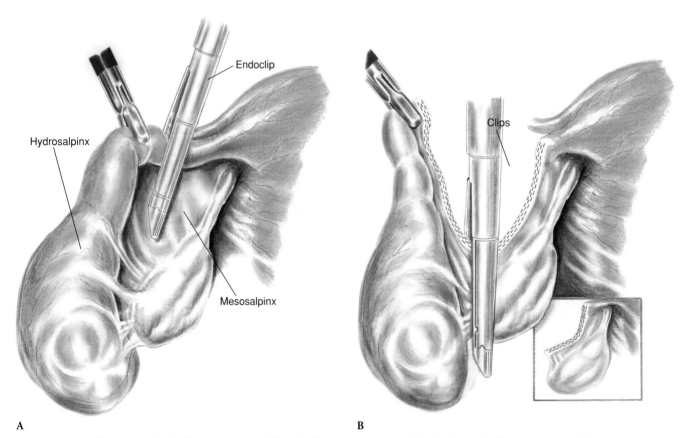

A   **B**

Figure 7.5.2. (**A**) Salpingectomy is achieved with an automatic stapling device. The first application of the stapling device is to the proximal portion of the tube across the mesosalpinx. The tube is under traction. (**B**) The second application completes the salpingectomy (*inset*). A view of the mesosalpinx after the tube has been removed.

for the entire tube (Figure 7.5.2A,B). Once detached, the tube is removed from the pelvis through a suprapubic trocar sleeve or the operating channel of the laparoscope. Removal of a larger tube (a ruptured tubal pregnancy or hydrosalpinx) requires an Endopouch (Ethicon) or another method of removal. The pelvic cavity is irrigated. The intra-abdominal pressure is decreased to reveal bleeding temporarily controlled by a pneumoperitoneum. This is especially important when one is using a stapling device.

REFERENCES

1. Kodaman PH, Arici A, Seli E. Evidence-based diagnosis and management of tubal factor infertility. *Curr Opin Obstet Gynecol*. 2004; 16(3):221–229.

2. Mansour R, Aboulghar M, Serour GI. Controversies in the surgical management of hydrosalpinx. *Curr Opin Obstet Gynecol*. 2000;12:297–301.

3. Johnson NP, Mak W, Sowter MC. Surgical treatment for tubal disease in women due to undergo in vitro fertilisation. *Cochrane Database Syst Rev*. 2004;(3):CD002125.

4. Hull MG, Glazener CM, Kelly NJ, et al. Population study of causes, treatment and outcome of infertility. *Br Med J (Clin Res Ed)*. 1985;291:1693–1697.

5. Zeyneloglu HB, Arici A, Olive DL. Adverse effects of hydrosalpinx on pregnancy rates after in vitro fertilization embryo transfer. *Fertil Steril*. 1998;70:492.

6. Chen CD, Yang JH, Lin KC, Chao KH, Ho HN, Yang YS. The significance of cytokines, chemical composition, and murine embryo development in hydrosalpinx fluid for predicting the IVF outcome in women with hydrosalpinx. *Hum Reprod*. 2002;17(1):128–133.

7. Mansour RT, Aboulghar MA, Serour GI, Riad R. Fluid accumulation of the uterine cavity before embryo transfer: a possible hindrance for implantation. *J In Vitro Fert Embryo Transf*. 1991;8(3):157–159.

8. Meyer WR, Castelbaum AJ, Somkuti S, et al. Hydrosalpinges adversely affect markers of endometrial receptivity. *Hum Reprod*. 1997;12(7):1393–1398.

9. Sabatini L, Colin D. The management of hydrosalpinges: tubal surgery or salpingectomy? *Curr Opin Obstet Gynecol*. 2005;17:323–328.

10. Kontoravdis A, Makrakis E, Pantos K, et al. Proximal tubal occlusion and salpingectomy result in similar improvement in in vitro fertilization outcome in patients with hydrosalpinx. *Fertil Steril*. 2006;86(6):1642–1649.

11. Bloechle M, Schreiner T, Lisse K. Recurrence of hydrosalpinges after transvaginal aspiration of tubal fluid in an IVF cycle with development of a serometra. *Hum Reprod*. 1997;12(4):703–705.

12. Sacks G, Trew G. Reconstruction, destruction and IVF: dilemmas in the art of tubal surgery. *BJOG*. 2004;111(11):1174–1181.

13. Nezhat C, Nezhat F, Winer W. Salpingectomy via laparoscopy: a new surgical approach. *J Laparosc Surg*. 1991;1:91.

HYSTEROSCOPY

Section 8.1. Evaluation and Management of the Uterine Septum

Eric J. Bieber and Edie L. Derian

Uterine anomalies are a relatively common congenital abnormality, with uterine septum being the most common (Table 8.1.1).[1] This is even truer in patients with recurrent pregnancy loss, in whom rates of uterine abnormalities may approach 15% to 27%. Historically, the uterine septum has been approached via laparotomy through either a Tompkins or Jones procedure. These successful but highly morbid procedures required laparotomy, significant hospital stays, and subsequent cesarean delivery and had a high risk of adhesion formation. More recently, this surgery has been supplanted by hysteroscopic or other minimally invasive methodologies for treatment. This section focuses on the embryologic development of the genital tract that may lead to mullerian abnormalities, discusses the work-up of patients before treatment, evaluates the appropriate candidates for surgical procedures, and discusses the technical aspects of the procedure itself, postoperative recommendations, and results of various modalities of treatment. In addition, complications specific to these procedures are reviewed.

EMBRYOLOGY

It is unclear what the exact rate of mullerian abnormalities is in the general population as there have been no good cross-sectional studies of normal patients. It is believed that the incidence is in the range of 1% to 6%, and there are numerous variations. The American Fertility Society (now the American Society for Reproductive Medicine) has published a classification system to standardize the nomenclature among surgeons (Tables 8.1.1, 8.1.2).[2] Women with recurrent pregnancy loss (RPL) appear to have a much higher incidence of anomalies relative to the general population. Salim et al. [3] in evaluating patients with and without RPL noted an anomaly rate of 1.7% in patients without RPL and a rate of 6.9% in those with three or more losses. Several hypotheses have been proposed to explain the wide range of abnormalities that may occur. The most prominent theory suggests the mullerian ducts initially fuse together as one structure and that this begins caudally at the mullerian tubercle and proceeds unidirectionally in a cephalad manner. The ultimate result is one cavity that is divided in the midline by a septum, which is then reabsorbed. Given the wide range of abnormalities, early in the century it was suggested that resorption of the septum may begin anywhere within the septum and proceed in either or both directions. Uterine anomalies were thus attributed to either failures of the mullerian elongation process, abnormal fusion, canalization, or resorption. More recently, several case reports of patients with a uterine septum and cervical duplication with a vaginal septum have been published – cases that would be inconsistent with the aforementioned

hypothesis.[4,5] Muller et al. [6] proposed an alternate theory suggesting that at the beginning of the 10th week, the lowermost portions of the mullerian ducts (between the isthmus cranially and the urogenital sinus caudally) fuse at the medial aspects. This creates a single cavity that comprises the upper vagina, cervix, and isthmus. Interestingly, they suggest that at the upper aspects there is not true fusion, but rather at the triangular junction between the two mullerian ducts, there is rapid division of cells that then connects the two ducts and converges with the lower septum. Like the original hypothesis, resorption then follows. In this model, if the initial fusion did not occur correctly but the upper fusion did occur, a patient might have both a vaginal septum and two cervices but a unified cavity separated by a septum, as the prior case reports suggest.

Patients with uterine anomalies may also have associated anomalies of the urogenital tract. It has been estimated that in the case of a unicornuate uterus, up to 40% of patients may have renal anomalies. These are generally noted on the side of the remnant uterine horn.[7] In an early report, Valle and Sciarra [8] found two of 12 patients with a uterine septum to have a urologic abnormality. More recently, Heinonen [9], in evaluating patients with a complete septum and vaginal septum, found 11 of 55 patients (20%) had genitourinary abnormalities, with five patients who had ipsilateral renal agenesis and six with a double ureter.

MORPHOLOGY

The actual morphology of the uterine septum has been suggested as the reason for poor reproductive function in patients with this abnormality. The most common hypothesis suggests a decrease in vascularity to the septum that may decrease the likelihood of implantation and functional placentation. Several groups have investigated these tenets to ascertain if differences exist within the structure of the septum versus normal uterine tissue that might lead to reproductive loss. Sparac et al. [10] performed resectoscopic biopsy of septa in 63 women undergoing metroplasty. They noted preoperatively that evaluation of the uterine septum with transvaginal color Doppler imaging demonstrated vascularity consistent with radial arteries. Histopathology of the septum specimens demonstrated both connective tissue and myometrial tissue. They proposed that the muscular tissue within the septum might create irregular contractile patterns that may increase the risk of abortion. Fedele et al. [11] evaluated the ultrastructural aspects of the uterine septum by discretely sampling endometrium overlying the septum as well as endometrium from the nonseptal lateral wall. Using scanning electron microscopy, they demonstrated the following changes in the tissue overlying

Table 8.1.1: Incidence of Uterine Anomalies

Anomaly	Incidence, %
Septate uterus	55
Unicornuate uterus	20
Bicornuate uterus	10
Uterus didelphys	5–7

Data from Troiano RN.[1]

Table 8.1.2: American Society for Reproductive Medicine Classification of Mullerian Anomalies

Class	Anomaly
I	Mullerian agenesis or hypoplasia
II	Unicornuate uterus
III	Didelphys uterus
IV	Bicornuate uterus
V	Septate uterus
VI	Arcuate uterus
VII	Diethylstilbestrol (DES)-exposed uterus

From The American Fertility Society.[2]

the septum: reduced number of glandular ostia, irregular non-ciliated cells with rare microvilli, incomplete ciliogenesis on ciliated cells, and a decrease in the ciliated/nonciliated ratio. They believe these changes represent a decrease in the sensitivity of the endometrial cells overlying the uterine septum, which might have an impact on the receptivity to embryos.

WORK-UP

Many individuals will have a uterine septum diagnosed as part of an evaluation for repetitive loss. In these settings, a complete work-up and evaluation for the underlying issues of reproductive loss should be performed.

Hysterosalpingography (HSG) is one technique used for identifying a uterine/mullerian abnormality. The test is relatively easy to perform, with low cost compared with surgery. Uterine sub-cavities generally are well visualized, and often the extent of the uterine septum may be estimated (Figure 8.1.1).[12] Unfortunately, the radiographic appearance of the uterine septum is not significantly different from a bicornuate uterus, which is managed in a much different fashion. One study found only 55% accuracy in differentiating these entities via HSG, with the difficulty being that the uterine fundus cannot be evaluated to assess whether an indentation exists.[13] In addition, smaller uterine septa may also be missed if a significantly anteverted or retro-verted uterus is not brought into an axial plane or if medium is injected too quickly to outline the uterine cavity. The advantage of HSG besides simplicity is the ability to concomitantly evaluate the fallopian tubes. HSG has also been used in the postoperative evaluation after septoplasty to evaluate if a residual septum is still present.

Ultrasonography is the simplest and least invasive methodology for evaluating the uterus as well as other pelvic structures. More recently, the addition of saline infusion sonohysterography (SHG) has also been used to aid in further evaluating the uterine cavity. Transvaginal ultrasound may be superior to transabdominal ultrasound, although both have been effectively used. The ultrasound appearance of a septate uterus demonstrates little or no indentation at the fundus as one scans from one cornual region to the next. The septum itself appears as a different echogenic area within the endometrium and extending cephalad. Pellerito et al. [14] noted 100% sensitivity and 80% specificity for diagnosing a uterine septum. Alborzi et al. [15] performed a small prospective trial and noted the ability of SHG to differentiate a bicornuate from a septate uterus. They questioned if laparoscopy would be necessary given these findings. Most recently,

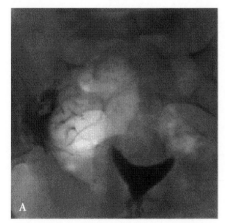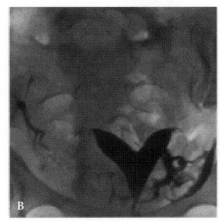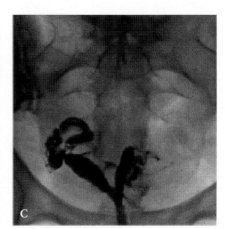

Figure 8.1.1. Hysterosalpinographic (HSG) images from three patients with recurrent early pregnancy loss. The three images show varying degrees of division of the uterine cavity. (**A**) HSG diagnosis: normal uterus; surgical diagnosis: uterine septum extending one third the length of uterine cavity. (**B**) HSG diagnosis: septum versus bicornuate uterus; operative diagnosis: uterine septum extending three quarters the length of the uterine cavity. (**C**) HSG diagnosis: septum versus bicornuate uterus; operative diagnosis: long uterine septum. From Proctor JA and Haney AF.[12]

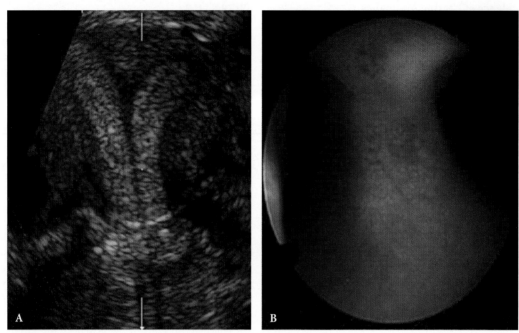

Figure 8.1.2. (**A**) Three-dimensional ultrasound longitudinal view of the uterus demonstrating a complete uterine septum. (**B**) Hysteroscopic view of the uterus demonstrating a uterine septum reaching approximately 40% of the uterine cavity. From Weissman A et al.[16]

three-dimensional ultrasound has been suggested as an improved tool for accessing mullerian abnormalities (Figure 8.1.2).[16] Raga et al. [17] evaluated three-dimensional ultrasound and found a 91.6% correlation with laparoscopic findings. Other studies are less compelling regarding three-dimensional ultrasound in adding additional information above and beyond that noted with standard two-dimensional imaging.[18] Given the high sensitivity and specificity as well as the relative ease to perform SHG, it may be difficult to ascertain that the further expense and lack of wide availability of this newer technology are justifiable.

Magnetic resonance imaging (MRI) is yet one more imaging modality available for evaluating mullerian abnormalities

(Figures 8.1.3, 8.1.4).[4] Several studies have suggested that MRI has a high ability to noninvasively differentiate uterine anomalies, especially in complex anatomic situations.[19,20] Fedele et al. [21] suggested that uterine septa have MRI findings of maximal fundal indentation of 10 mm or less and an angle of 60° or less between the medial margins of the hemicavities. Doyle [22] evaluated ultrasound, HSG, and MRI for diagnosing mullerian abnormalities and noted the correct anatomic

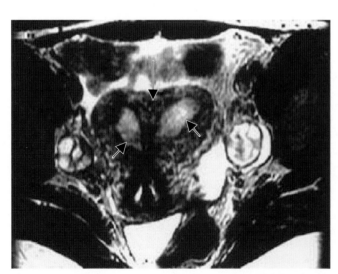

Figure 8.1.3. Axial magnetic resonance image demonstrating double uterine cavities (*white arrows*) and uterine septum (*black arrow*). The ovaries are the circular structures on either side of the uterine cavities. From Hundley AF et al.[4]

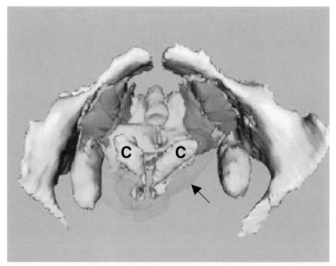

Figure 8.1.4. Magnetic resonance–based three-dimensional image of the uterus and pelvic organs (superior view). The double cavities are labeled *C*, and the dimmed-out uterine muscle outline is shown with the *black arrow*. Color legend: pale yellow, ovaries; brown, levator ani; beige-pink, vagina; white, pelvic bones; yellow, urethra; pink-brown, obturator internus. From Hundley AF et al. [4] and Scott P and Magos A.[23]

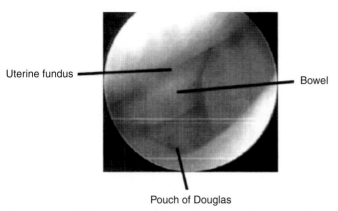

Figure 8.1.5. Culdoscopic view of posterior aspect of the uterus showing a normal fundal outline consistent with a nonbicornuate uterus.

diagnosis 96%, 85%, and 6% of the time, respectively. Given the expense of MRI, its use might be most appropriate for situations that are complicated or in which multiple anomalies may concomitantly exist.

Hysteroscopy remains the standard for evaluation of intracavitary abnormalities. It additionally offers the opportunity for treatment as further discussed. Unfortunately, hysteroscopy does not allow evaluation of the external uterine contour, and thus a firm diagnosis of septate versus bicornuate uterus cannot be established simply by hysteroscopy alone. Culdoscopy has also been suggested as an alternative to laparoscopy or other imaging technologies as a means of directly inspecting the uterine contour. Scott and Magos [23] reported a case in which ultrasound could not rule out a bicornuate uterus but on culdoscopy a normal uterine contour was demonstrated and allowed a hysteroscopic septoplasty to then be performed in real time (Figure 8.1.5). Laparoscopy remains the gold standard for evaluation of the uterus and the adnexa and also provides opportunity for concomitant visualization during the operative hysteroscopic procedure.

PROCEDURE

Preoperative

Once the work-up has been completed and a decision made to proceed with surgery, consideration as to the timing of surgery should occur. Generally, we prefer to perform surgery in the follicular phase as early as possible after the patient has finished menses. At this point, there is minimal endometrial tissue present to obscure visualization during hysteroscopy as well as limited vascularity. Cervical cultures may be performed on patients who might be at higher risk, and a pregnancy test should be performed if there is any possibility of pregnancy.

An alternative to performance of the surgery during the follicular phase that has been proposed by some is the use of gonadotropin-releasing hormone (GnRH) agonist or agents such as danazol before surgery. Results have been mixed with some of these interventions, especially as they relate to metroplasty. Perino et al. [24] compared the GnRH agonist leuprolide with no treatment preoperatively in patients undergoing septoplasty and noted no difference in operative time, intraoperative bleed-

ing, or use of media between the groups. In contrast, Fedele et al. [25] compared GnRH agonist with danazol as pretreatment and noted that use of danazol made the procedure simpler and also allowed easier introduction of the resectoscope. Although we did use these agents earlier in our experience, most recently for simple uterine septum cases, we prefer not to have patients endure the side effects of these agents, as the net gain appears negligible, and instead proceed more expediently to surgical correction. There may, however, be unique situations in which pretreatment might still be considered appropriate.

Surgery

The surgical technique for metroplasty has evolved profoundly since the time when the Tompkins or Jones procedure was standard treatment. Currently, hysteroscopic techniques have supplanted open techniques unless other pathology dictates a laparotomy. However, even in this setting, hysteroscopic treatment of the uterine septum would still be recommended secondary to the decrease in potential subsequent risk.

Multiple methodologies exist for the actual performance of the surgery, including operative hysteroscopy with scissors, resectoscopic incision, laser metroplasty, and bipolar needle electrodes. Not one of these techniques has been demonstrated to be superior to another. There were early discussions that with the use of electrosurgery or laser, there might be lateral thermal damage, which might decrease healing or increase the likelihood of subsequent adhesion formation. Fortunately, the uterus and the endometrium in particular appear to have a high inherent ability to heal, making these concerns largely unfounded. Advantages of the use of scissors (or laser) include the ability to use isotonic solutions such as normal saline or lactated Ringer's, which are electrolyte containing, because electrosurgery is not being used. In addition, scissors may often be introduced through a relatively small operative hysteroscope versus the larger caliber of the resectoscope. Alternatively, the 180° loop may be used with the resectoscope, and given the larger diameter, it may be easier to have greater movement of fluids within the cavity, thus improving visualization.

Although data suggest it is possible to perform metroplasty without a laparoscopy in patients in whom the diagnosis of a uterine septum is assured, many surgeons still prefer to have a laparoscope in place to guide the procedure. Initially, it must be ascertained if the patient also has a concomitant vaginal septum. This may be removed in the same setting, allowing easier access to the subcavities (Figure 8.1.6).[19] Assessment should have already been performed to evaluate if the patient has one or two cervices. Diagnostic evaluation may then be performed to evaluate the extent of the septum, thickness of the septum, position of the ostia, and relative size of the two subcavities, and whether other concomitant pathologies, such as polyps, leiomyomata, or intrauterine adhesions, exists. Depending on their position within the cavity, it might be necessary to first deal with these issues before beginning the septoplasty. It is important to both understand the position of the uterus and, preferably through the use of a tenaculum, to bring the uterus into a midaxial position. Once the anatomy has been well defined, incision of the septum may be started. Historically, it was believed that the septum would need to be resected. It is now apparent that in almost all cases, even with thick septum, removal is rarely required. As the septum

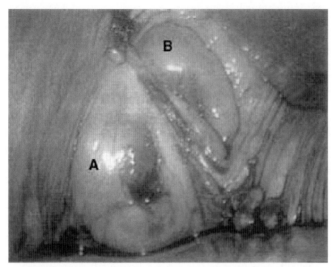

Figure 8.1.6. View of double cervix after resection of longitudinal septum. Double cervices are labeled *A* and *B*. From Hundley AF et al.[4]

is slowly incised, the tissues will retract anteriorly and posteriorly and thus obviate the need for resection or removal. It is crucial to stay in the midsection of the septum as the incision proceeds. It is relatively easy to begin incising ever more posteriorly and eventually into the endo- or myometrium. By making slow progress with the incision and continuously backing away from the septum and reassessing progress, it may be easier to maintain the correct area of incision. It is also critical as the procedure progresses to continuously monitor the position of the ostia to best appreciate how far cephalad to carry the incision. Some authors have suggested that most uterine septa are relatively avascular and thus at a point where bleeding is seen, the upper margin of the incision may be reached. Unfortunately, the previously presented data regarding the morphology of uterine septa do not exactly correlate with the clinical picture of little bleeding and avascularity. If a laparoscope is in place, this may also help to elucidate the breadth of the incision. Occasional transillumination will demonstrate the relative thickness of the remaining myometrium. Unfortunately, there is no foolproof method for gauging if the incision is not far enough and whether a residual septum will result, possibly requiring additional surgery, versus extending the incision too far into the myometrium and increasing the risk of subsequent uterine rupture. Allowing the intrauterine pressure to decrease will also allow the surgeon a further assessment of need for additional incision and whether there are bleeding points that need to be controlled.

In the case of a complete septum, with or without duplicated cervices, it will be more difficult to begin the procedure. In these situations, a Foley catheter bulb may be placed in one of the subcavities and an incision will be required from one subcavity to the other through the septum (Figure 8.1.7).[26] Although some authors have advocated avoiding incisions to unify cervices, more recent data have suggested this is unnecessary and may increase the duration of procedures as well as difficulty, without a substantive change in outcome.[27]

It is critical during septolysis that fluid input and output be continuously measured. This is true for all cases, but is especially true if using electrosurgery and hypotonic media such as glycine or sorbitol. Although most metroplasty procedures will be of relatively short duration, if a venous sinus is entered, fluid may be lost at a much quicker pace.

Intravenous antibiotics may be used during metroplasty, although little good evidence exists to support this practice in patients who have negative cervical cultures. However, as most patients undergoing these procedures are desirous of subsequent fertility, risk of subacute infection may cause many surgeons to treat with a broad-spectrum antibiotic during surgery as well as for a period of time postoperatively.

Gynecoradiologic Procedures

Karande and Gleicher [28] reported an alternate method of treatment of the uterine septum using fluoroscopic techniques. They reported on 14 patients who underwent incision of their septa using hysteroscopic scissors and a special balloon cannula or microlaparoscopy scissors and a cervical cannula. They were able to successfully complete these procedures in the ambulatory setting. Unfortunately, long-term results are not known and this is a small case series. The advantage of avoidance of anesthesia and complications of fluid media must be weighed against the exposure to ionizing radiation and the limited experience.

Postoperative Management

Postoperatively, patients may require little if any specific treatment. Historically, balloon catheters or occasionally inert intrauterine devices (IUDs) were placed within the uterine cavity in an effort to keep the denuded areas where the septal incision was performed from adhering together. Limited specific data exist to support or refute these practices. Fortunately, in the majority of cases, few adhesions will exist postoperatively and rarely will the walls fuse together.

Estrogen has also been administered after septoplasty in an effort to promote endometrial regrowth into the denuded areas. Typically, in patients who did not otherwise have a contraindication to estrogen, a relatively high dose of daily conjugated estrogen 1.25 to 5.0 mg would be prescribed for 1 to 2 months, followed by progestin on the last 10 days. More recently, Dabirashrafi et al. [29] evaluated this practice by performing a randomized prospective trial on 50 patients undergoing septoplasty. At follow-up postoperative exam, no patients in either the estrogen treatment group or the no-treatment group were noted to have intrauterine adhesions or septal fusion. Nawroth et al. [30] similarly retrospectively evaluated postoperative treatment via either cyclical hormone replacement therapy (HRT) and an IUD, HRT alone, or no treatment. Similar subsequent ongoing pregnancy rates were seen between the groups, and the authors suggest no need for specific postoperative treatment.

After several months, patients may be reevaluated with HSG or hysteroscopy to assess completeness of septal removal. It has generally been believed that a small residual septum 1 cm or less may have a negligible impact on subsequent reproductive outcome. Fedele et al. [31] evaluated this issue studying subsequent reproductive history in patients with a residual septum between 0.5 and 1 cm in size. In this trial, they noted no difference in outcome between the groups with a normal cavity versus a larger defect. Kormanyos et al. [32] evaluated this issue prospectively by studying 94 patients who had two or more miscarriages and

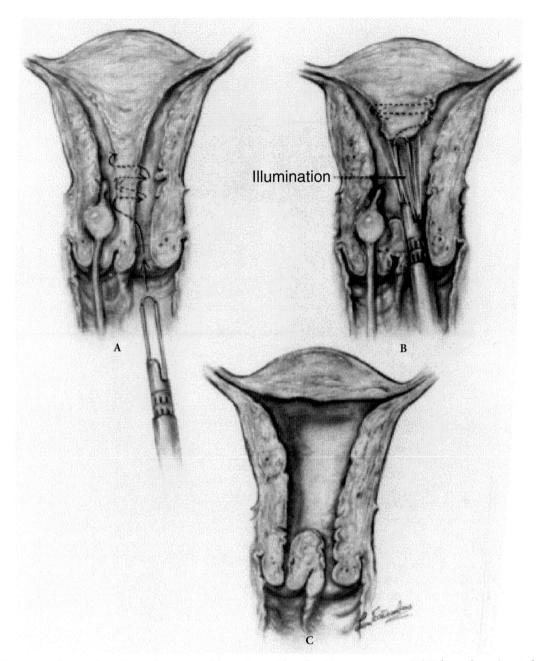

Figure 8.1.7. Hysteroscopic resection of a uterine septum in a patient with a class Va septate uterus. (**A**) Foley catheter inserted into the right cervix. The septum is incised until the bulb is identified. (**B**) The remaining septum is cut with electrocautery. (**C**) The septum has been cut and the cavities are united. From Rock et al.[26]

were undergoing hysteroscopic metroplasty. In 62%, the septum could be removed in its entirety with the initial surgery. Follow-up of the group of patients with normalized cavities versus those with a residual septum demonstrated a significant difference in reproductive loss in the residual group. Given these numbers, it is worthwhile to make patients aware that more then one procedure may be required to completely restore the cavity to normal.

Results

Multiple studies have retrospectively evaluated the impact of sep-tolysis on reproductive outcome. Unfortunately, no prospective, randomized trials exist to help better define if there is a group of patients who should not be treated. Many of these trials contain a cornucopia of patients ranging from primary infertility to multiple pregnancy losses. One of the largest reported trials evaluated 10 years of an Italian experience.[33] They noted that in the late 1980s, procedures were evenly divided between use of scissors and the resectoscope. Since then, the majority of procedures have been performed resectoscopically. In reporting on pregnancy outcome after metroplasty, they note 78% of patients reached term, 14% had miscarriages at 12 weeks or earlier, and 4% had miscarriages after 12 weeks gestation. Of interest, 88 of 808 patients had a postoperative evaluation that demonstrated a fundal notch 1 cm or greater in size. Valle [34] reported on 124 patients with uterine septa (115 of whom had reproductive loss and nine of whom had infertility) who underwent hysteroscopic treatment. Preoperatively, pregnancy results were poor, with 258 prior miscarriages (86.6%) and 28 preterm births (9.6%). After hysteroscopic treatment, results were markedly improved, with 81% of patients achieving pregnancy; of these, 83% were term, 7% were preterm but viable, and only 12% ended in first-trimester losses. Valle also reported favorable results in a small subset of patients who had a septum that continued through the cervix. Homer et al. [35] reported on an analysis of multiple studies published in the literature and found a miscarriage rate of 88% in 658 patients prior to septoplasty with a term delivery rate of only 3%. After surgery, this improved to a term delivery rate of 80%, with 14% miscarriages and 6% preterm. These results are typical of the many smaller trials that are reported throughout the literature.[36–40]

Most recently, Parsanezhad et al. [27] performed a randomized trial in patients with a complete septum extending to the cervix, comparing incision versus preservation of the cervical septum. They noted that preservation of the cervical septum was associated with longer operating times, greater fluid loss during surgery, and several cases of significant bleeding and pulmonary edema that were not seen in the group that had the cervical septum removed. Additionally, no differences were subsequently seen in reproductive function.

What remains unclear is the need for surgery in a nulligravid patient who is considering pregnancy and has been diagnosed with a uterine septum. Undoubtedly, many such patients are never diagnosed with an abnormality and carry their pregnancies uneventfully. Unfortunately, there again are no good data on how to best manage this scenario. When treatment required a laparotomy, and even early on in the hysteroscopic experience, many investigators recommended that patients have at least three miscarriages before entertaining treatment. As the technique has evolved, with excellent results and low morbidity, the prior recommendations have decreased to the present time, when some would advocate for the patient mentioned previously to undergo surgery as a means for decreasing the potential risk of miscarriage. Contrary to this opinion, investigators in Finland retrospectively evaluated 67 patients with a complete septate uterus and longitudinal vaginal septum.[9] In this cohort, only 36 of the patients had their vaginal septum incised and only four underwent metroplasty. Eight of 51 women (15.7%) attempting conception were diagnosed with nonuterine infertility, whereas 49 women who did not undergo metroplasty had 115 pregnancies (live birth, 72%; preterm, 12%; and miscarriages, 27%). Figure 8.1.8 demonstrates an ultrasound in a pregnant patient with a displaced uterine septum.[9] In an in vitro fertilization (IVF) unit in Israel, a 29-year-old patient with a complete uterine septum had one embryo replaced in each subcavity, with subsequent pregnancies in both.[16] Interestingly, at the time of cesarean delivery, metroplasty was attempted but subsequent evaluation demonstrated a residual septum through 40% of the cavity (Figure 8.1.2).

Although there is reasonable agreement that uterine septa increase pregnancy wastage, there remain questions regarding the impact of a septum on fertility itself. Pabuccu and Gomel [41] evaluated this issue in a prospective observational study on the impact of hysteroscopic metroplasty in 61 patients with primary unexplained infertility. They reported that after surgery, 41% conceived within 8 to 14 months, with 29.5% of the group

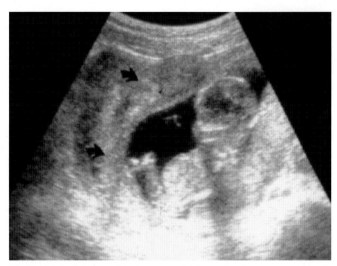

Figure 8.1.8. Sonographic image at 13th week of pregnancy reveals lateral displacement of the uterine septum (*arrows*) in a woman with a complete uterine septum and a longitudinal vaginal septum. From Heinonen PK.[9]

having live births. They concluded that surgery might benefit this cohort of patients.

A further question is the issue of management before assisted reproductive technology (ART) treatments. Dicker et al. [42] studied 144 women who had elevations in human chorionic gonadotropin-beta (hCG-β) after treatment but no other clinical evidence of pregnancy, that is, preclinical spontaneous abortions. Hysteroscopy demonstrated that 14 of 144 of these patients (9.7%) had at least small uterine septa. Lavergne et al. [43] evaluated the pregnancy rates in patients undergoing ART treatments who had been noted to have congenital uterine anomalies. They found that compared with a control group with a normal uterus, the pregnancy rate per embryo transfer was decreased from 24.9% to 13.6% and implantation rate decreased from 11.7% to 5.8%. They note that implantation rates increased when the underlying anomaly could be surgically treated. These data might support intervention before attempted ART in this higher-risk group.

Complications

Complications for hysteroscopic metroplasty include general complications of hysteroscopy that are detailed elsewhere throughout the text and include those of fluid media as alluded to previously as well as traumatic and hemorrhagic complications. Kazer et al. [44] reported on two cases of late hemorrhage after metroplasty, an uncommon complication. In one of the larger series to be published on operative hysteroscopic complications, Propst et al. [45] noted a complication rate of 9.5% for uterine septum resection. Unfortunately, there were only 21 metroplasties in this case series, two of which had complications.

One recognized complication of septoplasty is subsequent uterine rupture. It is felt that the general risk of this complication is low given that the active myometrium is likely minimally disrupted. For this reason, cesarean section is not usually recommended unless an obstetric indication exists. However, there are now several case reports of uterine rupture after prior

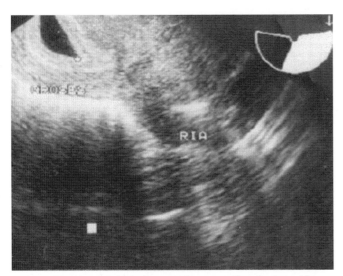

Figure 8.1.9. Transvaginal ultrasound: one uterine fundus with two uterine cavities. A gestational sac approximately 20 mm was seen in the right portion of the cavity, and an intrauterine device was seen in the left portion of the cavity. [48]

hysteroscopic resection. Interestingly, they include cases in which no electrosurgery was used and there was no evidence of uterine perforation at the time of surgery. Conturso et al. [46] reported on a patient who had undergone a hysteroscopic resection of a septum that was complicated by a fundal perforation. In the subsequent pregnancy, the patient was noted at 28 weeks to have a uterine rupture with protrusion of the amniotic sac. In another report, Angell [47] described a patient who underwent an uncomplicated hysteroscopic metroplasty with scissors. Subsequent evaluation demonstrated a residual septum, suggesting that the procedure did not involve active entry into the myometrium. During the patient's subsequent pregnancy, a perforation of the fundus from cornua to cornua was noted, causing exteriorization of the fetus and placenta. Given these reports, it is advisable to monitor patients who have undergone prior uterine surgery with a heightened sense during labor. Should there be abnormalities in fetal heart patterns or maternal abdominal pelvic pain, consideration should be given to the possibility of uterine rupture, with appropriate intervention if necessary.

The potential risk of a uterine septum must also be considered in cases of intrauterine contraception. If the diagnosis has not been previously made, an IUD may be placed into one subcavity. Dikensoy et al. [48] reported on a pregnant patient in whom the IUD was readily visible in the one subcavity while the pregnancy was visible in the other (Figure 8.1.9).

CONCLUSION

The management of the uterine septum has changed dramatically in the last quarter-century, and patients have certainly benefited from the evolution of minimally invasive techniques. In spite of these advances, many questions remain to be answered regarding which patients should undergo treatment and at what point. Recent case reports have generated questions regarding the applicability of prior hypotheses on embryogenesis that have caused

reevaluation of these older theories. Given the wide variety of manifestations that may be seen with urogenital anomalies, the astute clinician will need to continually readdress his or her thinking on these relatively common entities.

REFERENCES

1. Troiano RN. Magnetic resonance imaging of mullerian duct anomalies of the uterus. *Top Magn Reson Imaging*. 2003;14:269–279.
2. The American Fertility Society. Classifications of adnexal adhesions, distal tubal occlusion, tubal occlusion secondary to tubal ligation, tubal pregnancies, mullerian anomalies and intrauterine adhesions. *Fertil Steril*. 1988;49:944–955.
3. Salim R, Regan L, Woelfer B, Backos M, Jurkovic D. A comparative study of the morphology of congenital uterine anomalies in women with and without a history of recurrent first trimester miscarriage. *Hum Reprod*. 2003;18:162–166.
4. Hundley AF, Fielding JR, Hoyte L. Double cervix and vagina with septate uterus: an uncommon mullerian malformation. *Obstet Gynecol*. 2001;98:982–985.
5. Chang AS, Siegel CL, Moley KH, Ratts VS, Odem RR. Septate uterus with cervical duplication and longitudinal vaginal septum: a report of five new cases. *Fertil Steril*. 2004;81:1133–1136.
6. Muller P, Musset R, Netter A, Solal R, Vinourd JC, Gillet JY. [State of the upper urinary tract in patients with uterine malformations. Study of 133 cases.] *Presse Medicale*. 1967;75(26):1331–1336.
7. Fedele L, Bianchi S, Agnoli B, Tozzi L, Vignali M. Urinary tract anomalies associated with unicornuate uterus. *J Urol*. 1996;155:847–848.
8. Valle RF, Sciarra JJ. Hysteroscopic treatment of the septate uterus. *Obstet Gynecol*. 1986;67:253–257.
9. Heinonen PK. Complete septate uterus with longitudinal vaginal septum. *Fertil Steril*. 2006;85:700–705.
10. Sparac V, Kupesic S, Ilijas M, Zodan T, Kurjak A. Histologic architecture and vascularization of hysteroscopically excised intrauterine septa. *J Am Assoc Gynecol Laparosc*. 2001;8:111–116.
11. Fedele L, Bianchi S, Marchini M, Franchi D, Tozzi L, Dorta M. Ultrastructural aspects of endometrium in infertile women with septate uterus. *Fertil Steril*. 1996;65:750–752.
12. Proctor JA, Haney AF. Recurrent first trimester pregnancy loss is associated with uterine septum but not with bicornuate uterus. *Fertil Steril*. 2003;80:1212–1215.
13. Reuter KL, Daly DC, Cohen SM. Septate versus bicornuate uteri: errors in imaging diagnosis. *Radiology*. 1989;172:749–752.
14. Pellerito JS, McCarthy SM, Doyle MB, Glickman MG, DeCherney AH. Diagnosis of uterine anomalies: relative accuracy of MR imaging, endovaginal sonography, and hysterosalpingography. *Radiology*. 1992;183:795–800.
15. Alborzi S, Dehbashi S, Parsanezhad ME. Differential diagnosis of septate and bicornuate uterus by sonohysterography eliminates the need for laparoscopy. *Fertil Steril*. 2002;78:176–178.
16. Weissman A, Eldar I, Malinger G, Sadan O, Glezerman M, Levran D. Successful twin pregnancy in a patient with complete uterine septum corrected during cesarean section. *Fertil Steril*. 2006;85(2):494.e11–4.
17. Raga F, Bonilla-Musoles F, Blanes J, Osborne NG. Congenital mullerian anomalies: diagnostic accuracy of three-dimensional ultrasound. *Fertil Steril*. 1996;65(3):523–528.
18. Ayida G, Harris P, Kennedy S, Seif M, Barlow D, Chamberlain P. Hysterosalpingo-contrast sonography (HyCoSy) using Echovist-200 in the outpatient investigation of infertility patients. *Br J Radiol*. 1996;69:910–913.

19. Carrington BM, Hricak H, Nuruddin RN, Secaf E, Laros RK Jr, Hill EC. Mullerian duct anomalies: MR imaging evaluation. *Radiology.* 1990;176:715–720.

20. Patton PE, Novy MJ, Lee DM, Hickok LR. The diagnosis and reproductive outcome after surgical treatment of the complete septate uterus, duplicated cervix and vaginal septum. *Am J Obstet Gynecol.* 2004;190:1669–1675.

21. Fedele L, Dorta M, Brioschi D, Massari C, Candiani GB. Magnetic resonance evaluation of double uteri. *Obstet Gynecol.* 1989;74:844–847.

22. Doyle MB. Magnetic resonance imaging in mullerian fusion defects. *J Reprod Med.* 1992;37:33–38.

23. Scott P, Magos A. Culdoscopy to examine the contour of the uterus before hysteroscopic metroplasty for uterine septum. *BJOG.* 2002;109:591–592.

24. Perino A, Chianchiano N, Petronio M, Cittadini E. Role of leuprolide acetate depot in hysteroscopic surgery: a controlled study. *Fertil Steril.* 1993;59:507–510.

25. Fedele L, Bianchi S, Gruft L, Bigatti G, Busacca M. Danazol versus a gonadotropin-releasing hormone agonist as preoperative preparation for hysteroscopic metroplasty. *Fertil Steril.* 1996;65:186–188.

26. Rock JA, Roberts CP, Hesla JS. Hysteroscopic metroplasty of the Class Va uterus with preservation of the cervical septum. *Fertil Steril.* 1999;72:942–945.

27. Parsanezhad ME, Alborzi S, Zarei A, et al. Hysteroscopic metroplasty of the complete uterine septum, duplicate cervix, and vaginal septum. *Fertil Steril.* 2006;85:1473–1477.

28. Karande VC, Gleicher N. Resection of uterine septum using gynaecoradiological techniques. *Hum Reprod.* 1999;14:1226–1229.

29. Dabirashrafi H, Mohammad K, Moghadami-Tabrizi N, Zandinejad K, Moghadami-Tabrizi M. Is estrogen necessary after hysteroscopic incision of the uterine septum? *J Am Assoc Gynecol Laparosc.* 1996;3:623–625.

30. Nawroth F, Schmidt T, Freise C, Foth D, Romer T. Is it possible to recommend an "optimal" postoperative management after hysteroscopic metroplasty? A retrospective study with 52 infertile patients showing a septate uterus. *Acta Obstet Gynecol Scand.* 2002;81:55–57.

31. Fedele L, Bianchi S, Marchini M, Mezzopane R, Di Nola G, Tozzi L. Residual uterine septum of less than 1 cm after hysteroscopic metroplasty does not impair reproductive outcome. *Hum Reprod.* 1996;11:727–729.

32. Kormanyos Z, Molnar BG, Pal A. Removal of a residual portion of a uterine septum in women of advanced reproductive age: obstetric outcome. *Hum Reprod.* 2006;21:1047–1051.

33. Colacurci N, De Placido G, Perino A, Mencaglia L, Gubbini G. Hysteroscopic metroplasty. *J Am Assoc Gynecol Laparosc.* 1998;5:171–174.

34. Valle RF. Hysteroscopic treatment of partial and complete uterine septum. *Int J Fertil Menopausal Stud.* 1996;41:310–315.

35. Homer HA, Li TC, Cooke ID. The septate uterus: a review of management and reproductive outcome. *Fertil Steril.* 2000;73:1–14.

36. Saygili-Yilmaz E, Yildiz S, Erman-Akar M, Akyuz G, Yilmaz Z. Reproductive outcome of septate uterus after hysteroscopic metroplasty. *Arch Gynecol Obstet.* 2003;268:289–292.

37. Valli E, Vaquero E, Lazzarin N, Caserta D, Marconi D, Zupi E. Hysteroscopic metroplasty improves gestational outcome in women with recurrent spontaneous abortion. *J Am Assoc Gynecol Laparosc.* 2004;11:240–244.

38. Venturoli S, Colombo FM, Vianello F, Seracchioli R, Possati G, Paradisi R. A study of hysteroscopic metroplasty in 141 women with a septate uterus. *Arch Gynecol Obstet.* 2002;266:157–159.

39. Grimbizis G, Camus M, Clasen K, Tournaye H, De Munck L, Devroey P. Hysteroscopic septum resection in patients with recurrent abortions or infertility. *Hum Reprod.* 1998;13:1188–1193.

40. Litta P, Pozzan C, Merlin F, et al. Hysteroscopic metroplasty under laparoscopic guidance in infertile women with septate uteri: follow-up of reproductive outcome. *J Reprod Med.* 2004;49:274–278.

41. Pabuccu R, Gomel V. Reproductive outcome after hysteroscopic metroplasty in women with septate uterus and otherwise unexplained infertility. *Fertil Steril.* 2004;81:1675–1678.

42. Dicker D, Ashkenazi J, Dekel A, et al. The value of hysteroscopic evaluation in patients with preclinical in-vitro fertilization abortions. *Hum Reprod.* 1996;11:730–731.

43. Lavergne N, Aristizabal J, Zarka V, Erny R, Hedon B. Uterine anomalies and in vitro fertilization: what are the results? *Eur J Obstet Gynecol Reprod Biol.* 1996;68:29–34.

44. Kazer RR, Meyer K, Valle RF. Late hemorrhage after transcervical division of a uterine septum: a report of two cases. *Fertil Steril.* 1992;57:930–932.

45. Propst AM, Liberman RF, Harlow BL, Ginsburg ES. Complications of hysteroscopic surgery: predicting patients at risk. *Obstet Gynecol.* 2000;96:517–520.

46. Conturso R, Redaelli L, Pasini A, Tenore A. Spontaneous uterine rupture with amniotic sac protrusion at 28 weeks subsequent to previous hysteroscopic metroplasty. *Eur J Obstet Gynecol Reprod Biol.* 2003;107:98–100.

47. Angell NF, Tan Domingo J, Siddiqi N. Uterine rupture at term after uncomplicated hysteroscopic metroplasty. *Obstet Gynecol.* 2002;100:1098–1099.

48. Dikensoy E, Kutlar I, Gocmen A, Graves CR. Two cases of uterine septum with intrauterine device. *Br J Radiol.* 2005;78:952–953.

Section 8.2. Intrauterine Adhesions: Hysteroscopic Evaluation and Treatment

Rafael F. Valle

Intrauterine adhesions may interfere with both normal reproduction and menstrual patterns. When surgical treatment is undertaken under direct visualization using a hysteroscope, the altered menstrual patterns and the impaired reproductive function are markedly improved.

ETIOLOGY AND PATHOPHYSIOLOGY

Intrauterine adhesions are scars that result from trauma to a recently pregnant uterus. In over 90% of the cases, they are caused by curettage.[1–3] Usually, the trauma has occurred because of excessive bleeding requiring curettage 1 to 4 weeks after a delivery of a term or preterm pregnancy or after an induced abortion. During this vulnerable phase of the endometrium, any trauma may denude or remove the basalis endometrium, causing the uterine walls to adhere to each other and form a permanent bridge, distorting the symmetry of the uterine cavity. In rare circumstances, conditions such as abdominal metroplasties or myomectomies may cause intrauterine adhesions, but these adhesions are usually the result of misplaced sutures rather than the true coaptation of denuded areas of myometrium that occurs following postpartum or postabortal curettage.[3]

The type and consistency of these adhesions vary: Some are focal, some extensive, some mild, and some thickened and dense, with extensive fibromuscular or connective tissue components. The extent and type of uterine cavity occlusion correlate well with the extent of trauma during the vulnerable phase of the endometrium following a recent pregnancy. Some adhesions are focal; others completely occlude the uterine cavity. Consistency usually follows the longevity and duration of these adhesions, the older ones being thickened and dense and formed by connective tissue.[4–7]

Reproductive outcome seems to correlate well with the type of adhesions and the extent of uterine cavity occlusion. Therefore, it is useful to have a way of classifying these adhesions as filmy and composed of endometrial tissue, fibromuscular, or composed of connective tissue. The degree of uterine cavity occlusion is also important. Attempts to classify intrauterine adhesions by hysterosalpingography (HSG) give a good appraisal of the extent of uterine cavity occlusion, but it is impossible to determine by HSG the type of adhesions that are present. When using hysteroscopy alone, it is difficult to assess the extent of uterine cavity occlusion by visualization because the axis to the hysteroscopist is from the cervix to the fundus and not perpendicular to the uterine body as hysterography is, outlining the uterine cavity from a different axis. For this reason, the combination of HSG and hysteroscopy has been used most commonly to assess not only the extent of uterine cavity occlusion, but also the type of adhesions found by hysteroscopy at the time of treatment. Valle and Sciarra [3] used a three-stage classification of the extent and severity of intrauterine adhesions (mild, moderate, and severe) based on the degree of involvement shown on HSG and the extent and type of adhesions found on hysteroscopy. Three stages of intrauterine adhesions are defined as follows [3]:

Mild adhesions: filmy adhesions composed of basalis endometrial tissue producing partial or complete uterine cavity occlusion.

Moderate adhesions: fibromuscular adhesions – characteristically thick and still covered with endometrium that may bleed upon division – that partially or totally occlude the uterine cavity.

Severe adhesions: adhesions composed of connective tissue only, lacking any endometrial lining, and not likely to bleed upon division. These adhesions may partially or totally occlude the uterine cavity.

Recently, the American Fertility Society (now the American Society of Reproductive Medicine) proposed a classification of intrauterine adhesions based on the findings at HSG and hysteroscopy and their correlation with menstrual patterns.[8] Using a uniform classification for intrauterine adhesions greatly enhances our ability to evaluate, report, and compare results of different treatments of intrauterine adhesions, particularly when using these modalities following the hysteroscopic approach.

DIAGNOSIS AND INDICATIONS FOR TREATMENT

Intrauterine adhesions frequently result in menstrual abnormalities, such as hypomenorrhea or even amenorrhea, depending on the extent of uterine cavity occlusion. Patients with long-standing intrauterine adhesions may also develop dysmenorrhea. Over 75% of women with moderate or severe adhesions will have either amenorrhea or hypomenorrhea. Patients with significant uterine cavity occlusion secondary to intrauterine adhesions experience menstrual abnormalities more frequently, particularly amenorrhea (37%) and hypomenorrhea (31%). Patients with minimal or focal intrauterine adhesions may not demonstrate obvious menstrual abnormalities and may continue to have normal menses.[9]

Patients may also exhibit problems in reproduction, particularly pregnancy wastage, should the adhesions not totally occlude the uterine cavity. When total amenorrhea and total uterine cavity occlusion exist, the patient will generally be infertile. Other problems associated with intrauterine adhesions are premature labor, fetal demise, and ectopic pregnancy. When pregnancy is carried to term, placental insertion abnormalities, such as placenta accreta, percreta, or increta, may occur. Schenker and Margalioth [9] evaluated 292 patients who did not receive treatment for intrauterine adhesions. Of these, 133 women (45.5%) conceived, and of these, only 50 (30%) achieved a term pregnancy; 38 (23%) had preterm labor, and 66 patients had a spontaneous abortion (40%). In 21 patients (13%), placenta previa, ectopic pregnancy, and abnormal placental insertions, such as placenta accreta, were diagnosed.

The most important clue to the diagnosis of intrauterine adhesions is a history of trauma to the endometrial cavity, particularly following delivery or abortion. Secondary to that is a history of amenorrhea or hypomenorrhea. Because intrauterine adhesions are not related to hormonal events, an intact hypothalamic–pituitary–ovarian axis should result in a biphasic basal body temperature curve demonstrating ovulation; failure to withdraw from a progesterone challenge test in a patient who has a history of postpartum or postabortion intrauterine manipulation and who is amenorrheic will strengthen the diagnosis. Uterine sounding has been used to ascertain obstruction of the internal cervical os, but this test should be abandoned because of an increased danger of uterine perforation as well as inaccuracy of diagnosis. The most useful screening test for intrauterine adhesions is a hysterosalpingogram. It provides evaluation of the internal cervical os and uterine cavity, delineation of the adhesions, and information about the condition of the rest of the uterine cavity if adhesions do not completely occlude this area. About 1.5% of hysterosalpingograms performed for infertility evaluation demonstrate intrauterine adhesions.[10] When hysterosalpingograms are performed for repeated abortions, about 5% demonstrate intrauterine adhesions.[9] A history compatible with intrauterine adhesions will increase the yield of HSG for intrauterine adhesions in about 39% of patients.[11] These adhesions are stellate, irregular-shaped filling defects with ragged contours and variable locations in the uterine cavity. They are most commonly found in the central corporeal cavity and, less frequently, at the uterotubal cones and lower uterine segment.

Despite the usefulness of HSG as a screening method for patients suspected of having intrauterine adhesions, the final diagnosis is determined only by direct visualization with hysteroscopy because about 30% of abnormal hysterosalpingograms may be excluded and corrected by hysteroscopy.[12] The diagnosis can be confirmed by visualization, and the appropriate treatment can be provided once the adhesions are observed endoscopically.

HSG is useful in determining the extent of uterine cavity occlusion, but it cannot provide an appraisal of the consistency and type of intrauterine adhesions. For this reason, hysteroscopy becomes a useful adjunct to HSG by confirming the extent and type of intrauterine adhesions.

Other techniques, such as ultrasonography and MRI, have been used to make this diagnosis, but their accuracy is not well determined, and not enough experience exists with these techniques to supplant HSG and hysteroscopy.[13,14] Furthermore, the cost of MRI may be prohibitive.

METHODS OF TREATMENT

Treatment of intrauterine adhesions is surgical, consisting of removing those adhesions by division. In the past, blind methods of division were used with curettes, probes or dilators, or hysterotomy-assisted division of these adhesions under direct vision, but these techniques have failed to produce acceptable results and largely have been abandoned. Introduction of modern hysteroscopy has permitted transcervical division of adhesions under visual guidance; hysteroscopic methods have used mechanical means, such as hysteroscopic scissors, the resectoscope, and fiberoptic lasers.

Treatment of intrauterine adhesions with hysteroscopic scissors is the most common method employed. Because intrauterine adhesions, in general, are avascular, they may be divided (not removed); the treatment has been similar to that for division of a uterine septum. The adhesions are divided centrally, allowing the uterine cavity to expand upon division of the adhesions. This is performed using flexible, semirigid, and, occasionally, rigid or optical scissors. The most commonly used method is the semirigid hysteroscopic scissors because of the increased facility in manipulating the scissors, selectively dividing these adhesions when they retract upon cutting. Occasionally, thick connective tissue adhesions are present that form very thick stumps and benefit not only from division but also from removal. To achieve this effect, a sharp punch-biopsy forceps becomes most useful when lateral thick adhesions are present and the technique involves not only division of the adhesions but also removal. It is important to use a sharp biopsy forceps to selectively sculpture the uterine cavity to achieve a uniform symmetry. This technique is also useful at the uterotubal cones, particularly at the junction of the tubal openings and the uterus.

Although the semirigid and flexible scissors are most useful for the division of adhesions by hysteroscopy, the rigid optical scissors are less helpful in this endeavor. Because of the thick, sturdy configuration of these adhesions, when the uterine wall is thin and sclerotic, there is greater chance of uterine perforation, particularly because a panoramic view is impaired. Targeted dissection, which is easily obtained with the flexible and semirigid scissors, is hampered and difficult with optical scissors (Figures 8.2.1–8.2.8).

Fluids with electrolytes should be used when dividing these adhesions mechanically with scissors, because the adhesions are cut close to the myometrial tissue and the extensive area of denudation may predispose to fluid intravasation. Normal saline, dextrose 5% in half normal saline, and Ringer's lactate are most appropriate. Care must be taken to measure the amount of fluid used and the amount recovered when using the hysteroscope, particularly if the instrument has inflow and outflow, permitting an estimate of the amount of fluid that has not been recovered. Care also must be taken to measure the total inflow and outflow of fluids and ascertain that the intrauterine pressure does not exceed the mean arterial pressure of about 100 mm Hg. These procedures must be expedited to avoid excessive intravasation of fluid.

Depending on the extent of uterine cavity occlusion, division is done under visual control by cutting the adhesions in the middle to avoid uterine damage at the level of the uterine wall. When there is total uterine cavity occlusion, selective dissection of adhesions begins at the internal cervical os until a neocavity is created, then

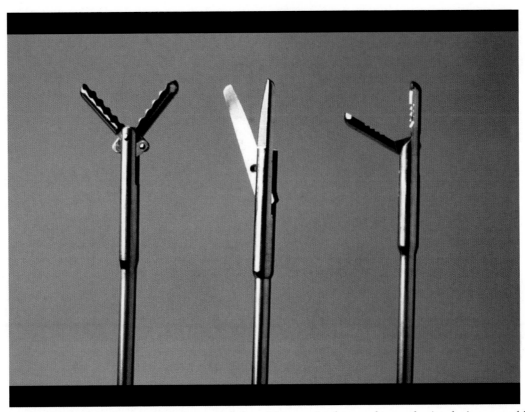

Figure 8.2.1. Semirigid 7F hysteroscopic operative instruments (left to right: grasping forceps, sharp and pointed scissors, cup biopsy forceps).

the dissection progresses until the uterotubal cones are free. When extensive adhesions are present, the hysteroscopist should be alert to perforation. Concomitant laparoscopy or sonography should be considered in all cases. Upon completion of the procedure, indigo carmine is injected transcervically to test for tubal patency.

The procedure is performed by systematically dividing the adhesions and cutting as much as feasible, particularly when there is total uterine cavity occlusion.[3,15]

The advantages of using hysteroscopic scissors for the division of intrauterine adhesions are those of mechanical

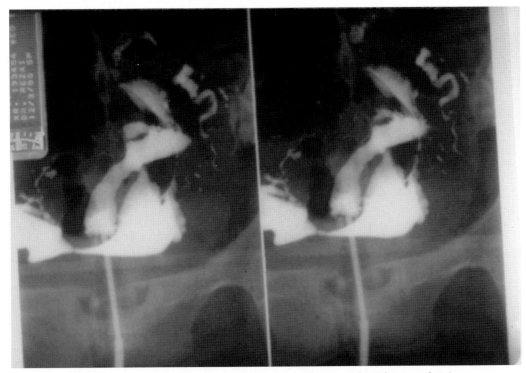

Figure 8.2.2. Hysterosalpingogram showing focal adhesion at the right cornual region.

146 — **Rafael F. Valle**

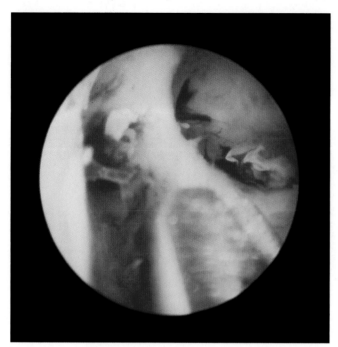

Figure 8.2.3. Hysteroscopic view of the tip of scissors approaching the adhesion for division.

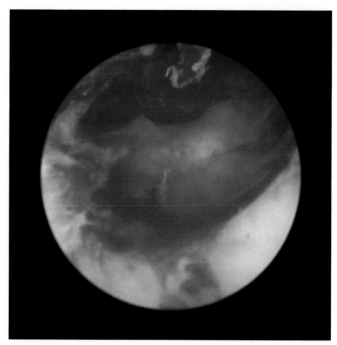

Figure 8.2.5. Hysteroscopic view of the resultant symmetric uterine cavity following division of the adhesion.

methods. Mechanical tools provide excellent landmarks when dividing these adhesions, particularly when approaching the juxtaposed myometrium. Bleeding may be observed at the myometrium, and this warns the hysteroscopist to stop the dissection so as to avoid perforation. No scattering of energies is produced to damage the small areas of healthy endometrium, which are the reservoir for future reepithelialization. This is an important consideration because no extensive healthy endometrium can be found when extensive intrauterine adhesions are present.

The disadvantages are that it may sometimes be difficult to manipulate semirigid instrumentation, particularly to the lateral walls of the uterine cavity. Scissors may not provide the sharpness or mechanism to cut these adhesions, as the scissors do not close well distally and need to be readjusted and sharpened frequently.

Treatment of intrauterine adhesions using the resectoscope is an alternative to mechanical tools. The resectoscope can be used to divide intrauterine adhesions either with a resetting loop, a loop bent forward, or specifically designed electrodes that can be directly applied to the adhesions, dividing them easily. These are in the form of knives or wires that must be specifically and selectively directed to the adhesions, particularly those in the lateral portion of the uterus or at the uterotubal cones. When using the resectoscope, fluids without electrolytes must be used – for example, dextrose 5% in water, glycine 1.5%, sorbitol

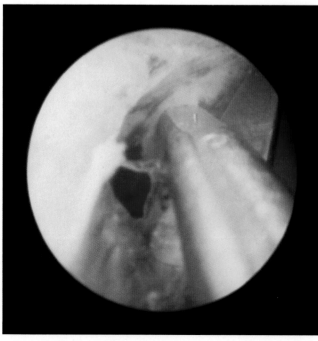

Figure 8.2.4. Hysteroscopic division of the adhesion.

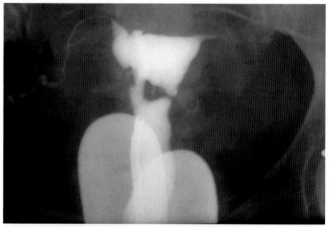

Figure 8.2.6. Hysterosalpingogram showing focal adhesions in the lower portion of the uterus.

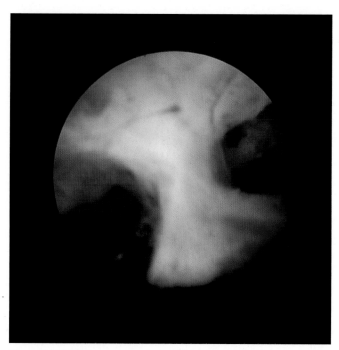

Figure 8.2.7. Hysteroscopic view of the central adhesion connecting the uterine walls.

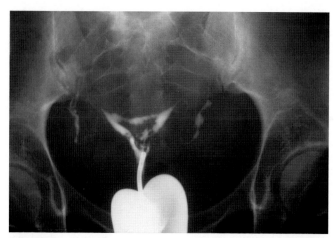

Figure 8.2.9. Extensive central intrauterine adhesions on hysterosalpingogram.

3.5%, mannitol 5% – which provide excellent visualization and are useful distending media. When dividing these adhesions, the resectoscopic loop may not be the appropriate electrode to use because it is designed to resect rather than to selectively divide the adhesions centrally. When the resectoscopic loop has been used for this purpose, several complications have occurred, particularly as a result of future sacculations of the uterus, dehiscences, and perforations. Ascertaining where the adhesions fin-

ish and where the normal myometrium begins is difficult, and the resections may be so deep that a portion of the myometrium may be shaved during division of the adhesions. Electrodes, such as the knife or wire types that can selectively be directed to the adhesions and divide them systematically, have been specifically designed for this purpose. Nonetheless, concern remains about scattering the energy and damaging the peripheral healthy endometrium. With the use of specific electrodes, this effect may be somewhat decreased. It is important to monitor the operation with concomitant laparoscopy or sonography because the landmarks of junction between adhesions and myometrium may be lost, and the coagulating effect this energy may produce in the myometrium may obscure a view of small vessels that, when bleeding, warn the hysteroscopist to stop further dissection (Figures 8.2.9–8.2.15).

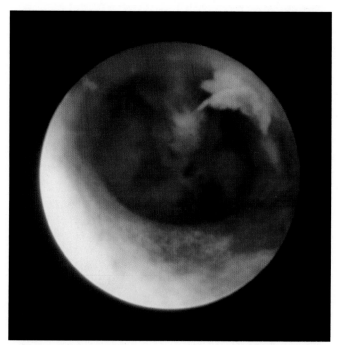

Figure 8.2.8. Following treatment, the uterine cavity achieves symmetry.

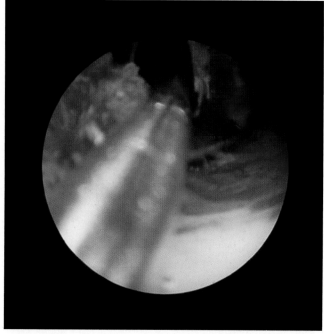

Figure 8.2.10. Systemic hysteroscopic division of adhesions with semirigid scissors.

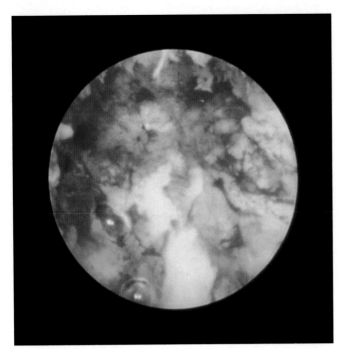

Figure 8.2.11. Complete division of the adhesions results in a symmetric uterine cavity.

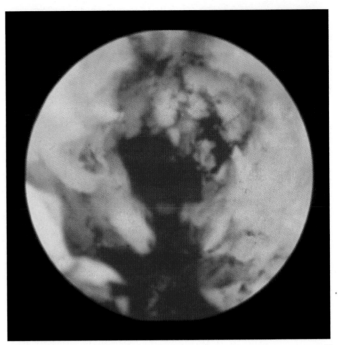

Figure 8.2.13. Following the initial hysteroscopic treatment, a small neocavity is obtained with remaining thick fibrotic stumps.

Use of the resectoscope has few advantages. Bleeding is decreased during dissection because of the electrical coagulating effect. The resectoscopic continuous flow system allows estimation of the deficit of fluid, thus decreasing the chances of fluid overload.

There are also disadvantages. Monopolar energy must be used. Only fluids devoid of electrolytes can be used. Additionally, electrosurgical damage of peripheral healthy endometrium and the loss of landmarks may occur while coagulating close to the myometrium, resulting in inadvertent invasion of this area. Finally, electrical damage to surrounding organs with or without perforation is a risk.[16]

Treatment of intrauterine adhesions with fiberoptic lasers, such as the neodymium: yttrium–aluminum–garnet (Nd:YAG),

argon, and KTP/532, may also be used to divide intrauterine adhesions. However, their application has been somewhat limited. The Nd:YAG laser with sculptured or extruded fibers may be a useful tool to selectively divide intrauterine adhesions, particularly those that are lateral and fundal.[15] Care must be taken to use these fibers by contact and selectively be aware of the overall symmetry of the uterine cavity, because the coagulating power of the laser may cause an effect similar to that of electrosurgery – that

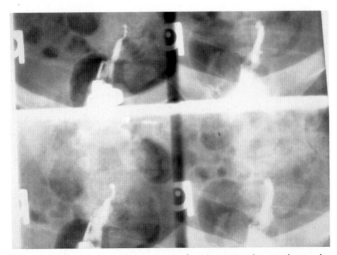

Figure 8.2.12. Hysterosalpingogram showing extensive uterine cavity occlusion and deformity with a small central tract made by uterine sounding.

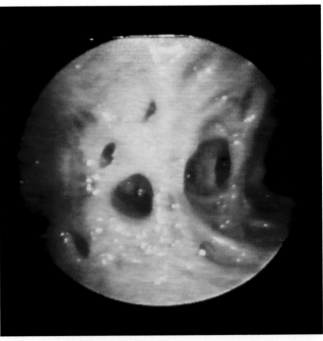

Figure 8.2.14. Extensive fibrotic adhesions involving a large portion of the uterine cavity.

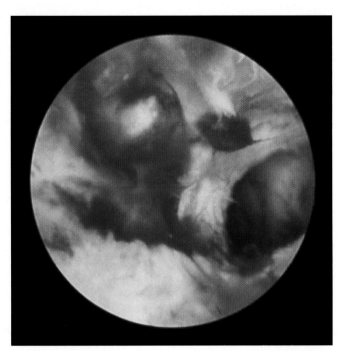

Figure 8.2.15. Extensive occlusion of the uterine cavity with fibrotic adhesions. A small island of the uterine cavity at 3 to 4 o'clock is free of adhesions.

is, coagulation and cutting – and the landmarks of the juxtaposed myometrium may be lost while performing division of the adhesions. Small arteries that cross the myometrium may not bleed, so dissection may proceed further than necessary. The hysteroscopic manipulation of the fiberoptic lasers is very easy and is facilitated by the use of oblique telescopes. The argon and KTP/532 lasers use the sharpest fibers to cut rather than to coagulate.[17]

Because lasers are not conductive, fluids with electrolytes should be used. Normal saline, dextrose 5% in half normal saline, and Ringer's lactate provide excellent visualization and contain sodium if excessive fluids are absorbed. The use of these electrolyte-containing fluids will not prevent pulmonary edema but will decrease the risk of hyponatremia; therefore, more fluid may be used than when using fluids devoid of electrolytes. Ideally, a hysteroscope with a continuous-flow system – or one with true inflow and outflow – should be used to monitor the injected fluid and keep a perfect account of the deficit or nonrecovered fluid.

Use of the laser is attractive and has the benefit of easy manipulation, but requires more time than use of mechanical tools, such as hysteroscopic scissors. It is important, therefore, when using this type of energy to expedite the procedure as much as possible so as to prevent excessive fluid from being intravasated.

Of late, vaporizing electrodes have been introduced in an attempt to use them with electrolytic solution distending the uterus. Concerns similar to those with electrosurgery apply, particularly without evaluation of the penetration and scattering these electrodes produce when applied to tissues.

The treatment of severe intrauterine adhesions remains a challenge, and other methods have been suggested to simplify the treatment, such as concomitant fluoroscopy or sonography, transfundal uterine injection of dyes, coaxial injection of radiopaque material, vital dyes to distinguish fibrous adhesions from residual endometrium, endometrial electrosurgical scoring, blind lateral sounding of the uterine cavity, and hysterotomy for transfundal dissection of the adhesions. However, all these methods have been used in a limited fashion and have not consistently proved their efficacy.[18]

INTRA- AND POSTOPERATIVE MANAGEMENT

The principal goal of therapy is to remove the adhesions surgically. Because most of these patients have a sclerotic or destroyed endometrium, they need other adjunctive therapy to promote reepithelialization and a mechanical separation of the uterine walls to prevent the reformation of adhesions. These adjuncts are intrauterine splints, prophylactic antibiotics, and estrogens, to promote reepithelialization.

Prophylactic antibiotics are used routinely in these patients in view of a traumatized endometrium and the extensive manipulation these patients usually require. The antibiotics used are in the form of cephalosporins: cefazolin, 1 g intravenous (IV) piggyback 1 half-hour before the procedure, followed by cephalexin, 500 mg four times daily by mouth (PO) for a week, should an intrauterine splint be placed. Additionally, in patients with extensive intrauterine adhesions, an indwelling 8F pediatric Foley catheter is inserted and 3.0 to 3.5 mL of a sterile solution instilled. The catheter is left in place for a week to prevent reformation of adhesions. Adjunctive hormonal therapy consists of conjugated estrogens in the form of Premarin (Wyeth Pharmaceuticals), 2.5 mg twice daily for 30 or 40 days, depending on the extent of uterine cavity occlusion and the type of adhesions found. The more extensive and old the adhesions, the more prolonged the hormonal treatment must be. In the last 10 days of this artificial cycle, medroxyprogesterone acetate (Provera, Pfizer), 10 mg a day, is given PO for 10 days, to induce withdrawal bleeding. Upon completion of the hormonal treatment, and once withdrawal bleeding has ceased, a hysterosalpingogram is performed to assess the results of the operation and decide on further therapy or initiation of attempts at conception. Patients with filmy, focal adhesions may not require HSG, but may need an office hysteroscopy to assess uterine cavity symmetry.[3,19]

RESULTS OF TREATMENT

The results of hysteroscopic treatment of intrauterine adhesions have correlated well with the extent of uterine cavity occlusion and the type of adhesions present. Normal menstruation is restored in over 90% of the patients.[3,19] The reproductive outcome correlates well with the type of adhesions and the extent of uterine cavity occlusion. Of 187 patients treated hysteroscopically by Valle and Sciarra [3], removal of mild, filmy adhesions in 43 cases gave the best result, with 35 (81%) term pregnancies. In 97 moderate cases of fibromuscular adhesions, 64 (66%) term pregnancies occurred; and in 47 severe cases of connective tissue adhesions, 15 (32%) term pregnancies occurred. Overall restoration of menses occurred in 90% of the patients, and the overall term pregnancy rate was 79.7%. These results demonstrate a much better reproductive outcome than was previously obtained with blind methods of therapy (Table 8.2.1).

Table 8.2.1: Hysteroscopic Lysis of Intrauterine Adhesions

Study	Patients, no.	IUD	E/P	Antibiotics	NL Menses (%)	Pregnant (%)	Term (%)
			Results			Reproductive Outcome	
Edstrom (1974)	9	+	−	−	2	1	1
March and Israel (1981) [19]	38	+	+	+	38 (100)	38 (100)	34 (79.1)
Neuwirth et al. (1982) [15]	27	+	+	+	20 (74)	4 (51.8)	13 (48.1)
Sanfilippo et al. (1982)	26	+	+	−	26 (100)	6 (100)	3 (50)
Siegler and Kontopoulos (1981) [5]	25	Foley catheter	+	−	13 (52)	11 (44)	6 (24)
Hamou et al. (1983)	69	+	+	−	59 (85.5)	20 (51.3)	15 (38.4)
Sugimoto et al. (1984)	258	+	+	−	180 (69.7)	107 (41.4)	64 (24.8)
Wamsteker (1984)	36	+	+	+	34 (94.4)	17 (62.9)	12 (44.4)
Friedman et al. (1986) [16]	30	−	+	−	27 (90)	24 (80)	23 (76.6)
Valle and Sciarra (1988) [3]	187	+Foley catheter	+	+	167 (89.3)	143 (76.4)	114 (60.9)
Zuanchong and Yulian (1986) [see 18]	70	+	+	+	64 (84.3)	30 (85.7)	17 (48.5)
Lancet and Kessler (1988) [21]	98	Hyskon	Flexible scissors, electrosurgery		98 (100)	86 (87.8)	77 (89.5)
Pabuccu et al. (1997) [22]	40	Glycerin	Murphy probe scissors		33 (82.5)	27 (67.5)	23 (57.5)
Feng et al. (1999) [23]	365	Dextrose 5%	Biopsy forceps/scissors		294 (83.7)	*156 (83.8)	145 (92.9)
Totals	1298				1060 (87.5)	718 (72.3)	603 (87.2)

*, of 186 desiring pregnancy; −, xxx; E/P, estrogen/progesterone; NL, normal; +, positive; −, negative.
Modified from Siegler AM Valle RF, Lindemann HJ, Mencaglia L. *Therapeutic Hysteroscopy: Indications and Techniques.* St. Louis: CV Mosby; 1990:103.

Results following treatment of intrauterine adhesions using the resectoscope have been similar; nonetheless, the reported postoperative complications may be serious and should be kept in mind when using this type of instrument. A few series reported lysis of adhesions with fiberoptic lasers, but when the lasers are used appropriately, results should not vary much from those reported with electrosurgery.[16,20]

SUMMARY AND CONCLUSIONS

The introduction of hysteroscopy has provided gynecologists with a simplified and less invasive method of treatment for many conditions affecting the uterine cavity that in the past required major surgery. Undoubtedly, one of the conditions that has benefited from the hysteroscopic approach is the management of intrauterine adhesions. This approach has offered a more accurate evaluation and more refined treatment, with

markedly improved surgical results. The hysteroscopic treatment of intrauterine adhesions provides the opportunity for restoration of the uterine cavity's symmetry, which resolves menstrual abnormalities, and leads to improvement of reproductive function with the removal of the causes of repetitive abortions and infertility. All these salutary effects greatly support the hysteroscopic approach for women affected with intrauterine adhesions as the method of choice in their management. The treatment of intrauterine adhesions can be accomplished by four different techniques: scissors, resectoscope, fiberoptic lasers, and vaporizing bipolar electrodes. All have advantages and disadvantages and must be used with knowledge of each particular technology and its drawbacks. Each technique should be tailored not only to the anatomy, embryology, and etiology of each process but also to the experience and knowledge of the operator. The operator should select the appropriate method and technique for each patient. In the treatment of intrauterine adhesions, the semirigid scissors guided by the hysteroscope offer the best alternative for treatment of this condition. The goals of therapy should be a successful pregnancy for those patients with impaired reproduction, keeping in mind the safety of the patient, with the least morbidity possible, the absence of complications, the overall effectiveness, and diminution of unnecessary cost. [8] Versatility plays a significant role in the selection of therapeutic alternatives; the surgeon has to intelligently select the best method for each individual patient.

REFERENCES

1. Asherman JG. Amenorrhea traumatica (atretica). *J Obset Gynaecol Br Emp.* 1948;55:23–30.
2. Asherman JG. Traumatic intrauterine adhesions. *J Obstet Gynaecol Br Emp.* 1950;57:892–896.
3. Valle RF, Sciarra JJ. Intrauterine adhesions: hysteroscopic diagnosis, classification, treatment, and reproductive outcome. *Am J Obstet Gynecol.* 1988;158:1459–1470.
4. Foix A, Bruno RO, Davidson T, Lema B. The pathology of postcurettage intrauterine adhesions. *Am J Obstet Gynecol.* 1966;96:1027–1033.
5. Siegler AM, Kontopoulos VG. Lysis of intrauterine adhesions under hysteroscopic control: a report of 25 operations. *J Reprod Med.* 1981;26:372–374.
6. March CM, Israel R, March AD. Hysteroscopic management of intrauterine adhesions. *Am J Obstet Gynecol.* 1978;130:653.
7. Siegler AM, Valle RF. Therapeutic hysteroscopic procedures. *Fertil Steril.* 1988;50:685–701.
8. The American Fertility Society. Classifications of adnexal adhesions, distal tubal occlusion, tubal occlusion secondary to tubal ligation, tubal pregnancies, mullerian anomalies, and intrauterine adhesions. *Fertil Steril.* 1988;49:944–955.
9. Schenker JG, Margalioth EJ. Intrauterine adhesions: an updated appraisal. *Fertil Steril.* 1982;37:593–610.
10. Dmowski WP, Greenblatt RB. Asherman's syndrome and risk of placenta accreta. *Obstet Gynecol.* 1969;34:288–299.
11. Klein SM, Garcia CR. Asherman's syndrome: a critique and current review. *Fertil Steril.* 1973;24:722–735.
12. Valle RF, Sciarra JJ. Current status of hysteroscopy in gynecologic practice. *Fertil Steril.* 1979;32:619–632.
13. Confino E, Friberg J, Giglia RV, Gleicher N. Sonographic imaging of intrauterine adhesions. *Obstet Gynecol.* 1985;66:596–598.
14. Vartiainen J, Kajanoja P, Ylostalo PR. Ultrasonography in extended placental retention and intrauterine adhesions: a case report. *Eur J Obstet Gynecol Reprod Biol.* 1989;30:89–93.
15. Neuwirth RS, Hussein AR, Schiffman BM, Amin HK. Hysteroscopic resection of intrauterine scars using a new technique. *Obstet Gynecol.* 1982;60:111–113.
16. Friedman A, Defazio J, DeCherney AH. Severe obstetric complications following hysteroscopic lysis of adhesions. *Obstet Gynecol.* 1986;67:864–867.
17. Newton JR, Mackenzie WE, Emens MJ, Jordan JA. Division of uterine adhesions (Asherman's syndrome) with the Nd-YAG laser. *Br J Obstet Gynaecol.* 1989;96:102–104.
18. Valle RF. Intrauterine adhesions (Asherman's syndrome). In: Marty R, Blanc B, deMontgolfier R, eds. *Office and Operative Hysteroscopy.* New York: Springer-Verlag; 2002:229–242.
19. March CM, Israel R. Gestational outcome following hysteroscopic lysis of adhesions. *Fertil Steril.* 1981;36:455.
20. Intrauterine adhesions. In: Siegler AM, Valle RF, Lindemann HJ, Mencaglia L. *Therapeutic Hysteroscopy: Indications and Techniques.* St. Louis: CV Mosby; 1990:82–105.
21. Lancet M, Kessler I. A review of Asherman's syndrome, and results of modern treatment. *Int J Fertil.* 1988;33:14–24.
22. Pabuccu R, Atay V, Orhon E, et al. Hysteroscopic treatment of intrauterine adhesions is safe and effective in the restoration of normal menstruation and fertility. *Fertil Steril.* 1997;68:1141–1143.
23. Feng ZC, Yang B, Shoo J, Liu S. Diagnostic and therapeutic hysteroscopy for traumatic intrauterine adhesions after induced abortions: a clinical analysis of 365 cases. *Gynaecol Endosc.* 1999;8:95–98.

Section 8.3. Hysteroscopic Myomectomy

Charles J. Ascher-Walsh and Michael Brodman

The introduction of the hysteroscopic myomectomy represented a revolution in the treatment of uterine fibroids. Thousands of women worldwide have avoided more invasive surgical treatment in the form of a hysterectomy by using the hysteroscope to treat relatively minor problems, such as submucosal myomas and endometrial polyps. The combination of technologic advances in luminescence, electrosurgery, and metalwork has allowed surgeons to diagnose and treat intrauterine pathology in ways that greatly decrease patient discomfort and risk and minimize the number of lost productive days. The resectoscope is an essential tool for the gynecologist desiring to provide his or her patient with the best available options.

HISTORY

Hysteroscopic myomectomy has classically been performed with an instrument called a resectoscope. Newer therapies use other instrumentation and are discussed in a later section; however, the bulk of hysteroscopic myomectomies performed today continue to be done using the resectoscope. Gynecology borrowed this technology from urology. Before Neuwirth and Amin [1] reported the first case of using a resectoscope for the treatment of a submucosal myoma in 1976, urologists had been using the device for decades.

The development of the resectoscope resulted from scientific advancements in a variety of fields. Current resectoscopes require a light source to be able to see the pathology, a fenestrated sheath to reach the pathology both visually and with instrumentation, and an electric cutting source to resect the pathology. After Thomas Edison invented the incandescent lamp in 1879, it was just over 20 years before Reinhold Wappler and William Otis presented the first American-made cystoscope to the American Association for Genito-Urinary Surgeons in 1900.[2]

By 1926, advances in technology allowed Bumpus to describe what could be seen as the earliest predecessor to our current resectoscope. He combined a cylindrical knife attached to a high-frequency current designed for coagulation with a fenestrated sheath and light source. The combination of these components for transurethral resection of the hypertrophied prostate was the basis for all future designs. In that same year, the first reported case describing the use of a device described as a "resectoscope" was published by Maximilian Stern.[3] His device consisted of an insulated shaft in which was placed a 0.5-cm tungsten cutting loop attached to an electrical current. The loop was situated at a right angle to the shaft and placed over a defect in the shaft at the distal end. This end was placed over the prostate, and the loop was moved away from and toward the viewer to cut the hypertrophied tissue.

The first report of the use of electrosurgery in humans came from the French physicist d'Arsonval.[4] He demonstrated in 1893 that using alternating currents of 2 kHz to 2 MHz caused tissue heating and cutting without muscle or nerve stimulation. Surgeons began to use electrosurgical techniques while performing a variety of surgeries. At the same time Stern was developing his resectoscope, William T. Bovie developed an electrosurgical unit for tissue cautery that was first used by Harvey Cushing on October 1, 1926, at the Peter Bent Brigham Hospital in Boston to remove a vascular myeloma.[5] Joseph McCarthy took advantage of this new technology by modifying the resectoscope to include a magnifying lens and improved insulation of the sheath. He reported these advances and the instrument's use in the *New England Journal of Medicine* in 1932.[6]

Iglesias and his colleagues [7] further modified the resectoscope to a model that urologists and gynecologists continue to use today. They added a second sheath around the current design that allowed for a separate outflow tract. This allowed for continuous irrigation, which allowed the procedure to be performed with less bladder pressure. The constant flow also resulted in better visualization. They reported on this in 1975, and within a year, Neuwirth and Amin [1] were reporting on its use for resecting a submucosal myoma. It was the addition of the outflow tract that allowed its use for this purpose and brought on a revolution in gynecologic surgery.

INSTRUMENTATION

The gynecologic resectoscope used today is a modification of the urologic resectoscope. The primary difference is a blunter distal end. The instrumentation is similar to that found in operative hysteroscopy, with the addition of an electrode and electrosurgical device. Standard equipment of hysteroscopy includes the hysteroscope, a light source, a video camera, and a medium for distention.

The standard resectoscope comes in a variety of sizes, typically between 24F and 28F. These resectoscopes all use a 4-mm telescope and have separated inflow and outflow sheaths. There are smaller resectoscopes with 3-mm telescopes, but these are not well suited for resecting submucosal myomas and are more appropriate for polyps or intrauterine adhesions. The telescopes vary from 0° to 30°, depending on operator preference. The 12° telescope seems to be best suited for resection of a myoma as it allows for best, continuous visualization of the electrode. In the 0° scope, the electrode may impair a significant part of the visual field; in the 30° scope, the electrode may extend beyond the visual field. The 12° telescope allows for complete visualization of the electrode through its entire range of motion while having only a small amount of visual field obstruction. Depending on the brand, the telescopes have a panoramic field of vision between 70° and 120°. The focus is set on infinity, which magnifies objects more the closer they are to the lens. The telescopes are designed to provide the best visualization 30 to 35 mm from the lens. Operators should try a variety of instruments to determine which one they find most appropriate for each situation.

The sheaths have fenestrations to allow for different tracts for the camera, electrode, inflow distention medium, and outflow medium. The distention medium flows in through the inner sheath. On some devices, this is the port most proximal to the eyepiece. Others have the inflow and outflow at the same distance from the eyepiece. For these devices, the inflow is found on the same side of the device as the attachment for the electric cable. It is important to attach the inflow and the outflow correctly as there is more resistance in the outflow sheath. This increased resistance allows for the distention of the uterine cavity. The increased pressure from the distended uterine cavity results in an equilibrium between the inflow and outflow tracts. The open cavity and continuous movement of fluid allow for better visualization of the uterine cavity and potential pathology within it.

Although the distention fluid is discussed in the next section, the devices used to instill and monitor the fluid are equally important. There are a variety of devices available, from those as simple as a hand pump to provide enough force to push the fluid into and distend the cavity, to complex pressure devices that vary inflow to maintain specific intrauterine pressures and collect the outflow fluid to monitor fluid deficits. The hand pump is typically much less expensive than the fluid monitoring units. It allows the surgeon to control the inflow of fluid, allowing for a rapid change in flow to correct poor visibility due to a lack of distention or to fluid clouded by blood. However, use of a hand pump relies on the surgeon to not overdistend the cavity, which may lead to a more rapid absorption of the distention medium. Because hypotonic distention medium is the most common type of medium used, a fluid imbalance may lead to serious sequelae from hyponatremia, including death. Hysteroscopic myomectomy will frequently require a significant amount of time to complete, making fluid balance an important issue. Surgeons considering new equipment for hysteroscopy should seriously consider some of the newer devices that allow closer monitoring of fluid deficits so as to decrease the risks to their patients. Surgeons using older devices need to be aware of these risks and to adjust their setup and techniques to minimize these risks. Using drapes that have fluid-collecting pockets that are placed under the buttocks so that fluid is not lost onto the floor or using floor suction devices can minimize the amount of fluid that is not accounted for during the procedure.

The electrode most frequently used for hysteroscopic myomectomies is the loop electrode. Electrodes also come in other types, including the roller ball, barrel, and point electrodes used for a variety of procedures, including endometrial ablation, removal of adhesions or polyps, and resection of a uterine septum. The loop electrodes have versions in which the loop is situated at angles of 0°, 45°, 90°, and 120° from the shaft. The most commonly used electrode for myomectomies is the 90° loop.

The electrodes are attached to a high-frequency electrosurgical unit preferably with a digital wattage indicator, such as the commonly used unit from Valleylab called the Valleylab Return

Electrode Monitoring Circuit. The most commonly used current for hysteroscopic myomectomy is monopolar. The VersaPoint unit by Gynecare is a bipolar unit and is discussed in the section on newer devices. A monopolar current in electrosurgery is an alternating radiofrequency current that runs from the generator through the electrode to the surgical site. Because the surgical site does not conduct the current as well as the electrode, it is rapidly heated, and cutting and coagulation are accomplished by this method. The current is then dispersed throughout the body so that it loses any power within a few millimeters of the electrode. It is again collected at the grounding pad and returned to the generator, which completes the electrical circuit. Most electrical units offer a cutting or coagulation current or a blend of the two. The electrical current is represented by a sinusoidal waveform. A cutting wave is a continuous wave, whereas a coagulation wave is made up of intermittent bursts. The power of the waveform, measured in watts, is determined by the voltage and the time delivered. Because coagulation waveforms are intermittent and hence have an actual current only 25% of the time, equal voltage peaks in cutting and coagulation currents result in a lower wattage for the coagulation current. To achieve equal wattage – that is, setting the generator on equal settings for both cutting and coagulation currents – the voltage peaks must be significantly higher in the coagulation current. With higher voltage peaks, the force behind the flow of electrons, although intermittent in the case of coagulation, is higher and the electrons can be driven deeper into the tissue. This makes the use of the coagulation current slightly more dangerous as the thermal spread of tissue destruction is greater.

Tissue is cut by the intracellular fluid being rapidly heated to the point at which the cell is literally vaporized. As the cell is torn apart by vaporization, the tissue is cut. The continuous waveform is better at creating this vaporization than is the intermittent coagulation waveform. The intermittent current results in a slower heating of cells. Depending on the type of cell being treated, the coagulation waveform may still be used to cut tissue, especially if it is moved quickly through the tissue, although it is more likely to slowly desiccate and fulgurate the tissue, eventually leading to carbonization. Intracellular fluid is a good medium for conducting electricity, so when the fluid is vaporized by the cutting current, the low peak voltage is not able to drive the current further into the tissue. The intermittent coagulation current heats the cells more slowly, so the water in the cells does not flash into steam. The cells are dehydrated more slowly. The higher peak current of the coagulation current allows it to be driven further into the tissue, continuing to heat the tissue until only the carbon is remaining. It is for this reason that a cutting current allows for an easier and safer removal of submucosal myomas. The electrode tends to pass through the tissue with less resistance, and there is less risk of thermal spread, which is important as one approaches the uterine serosa during the removal of larger myomas.

DISTENTION MEDIA

The uterine cavity is a potential space and hence requires some type of medium to distend it so that surgery can be performed. Because of the vascular nature of the uterus, the media used to distend the cavity may be absorbed. The higher the pressure used for distention, the greater the media absorption. It is therefore important to choose the best medium for the job at hand. The perfect substance would be isotonic and have little impact on fluid volumes in the body. Its absorption would not cause electrolyte abnormalities. It would allow for good visualization. It would not cause hemolysis and would not conduct electricity. It would also allow for easy cleaning of the instruments after use, and the fluid itself would be inexpensive to use. This perfect medium does not exist, however, and one must weigh the risks and benefits of available media when choosing which one to use for each procedure.

The following media have been used for uterine distention: carbon dioxide, Hyskon, Ringer's lactate (RL), normal saline (NS) and half normal saline, glycine, sorbitol, mannitol, cytal (sorbitol and mannitol), and dextrose 5% in water (D_5W). For our purposes, the discussion is limited to fluid that is suited for the resectoscope. RL and NS contain electrolytes and are conductive. The current diffuses in every direction away from the electrode, and no cutting effect is found. They are therefore not suited for the resectoscope. D_5W and water are nonconductive; however, they are rapidly absorbed and can lead quickly to a dangerous state of hyponatremia. Hyskon is an electrolyte-free solution with extremely high viscosity. It is composed of dextran 70 in 10% dextrose. It is very thick and slowly absorbed. The high viscosity makes it very difficult to use in the continuous-flow resectoscopes currently available. More importantly, unless meticulously cared for, Hyskon left in hysteroscopes and resectoscopes can quickly ruin the equipment. Because of this latter problem, most surgeons have found it too costly to continue its use.

Glycine is the fluid most commonly used in resectoscopic surgery today. It has also been the most commonly used fluid by urologists. The fluid is 1.5% of the amino acid in water. It is a hypotonic fluid, having an osmolality of 200 mOsm/L.[8] This osmolality causes minimal hemolysis but may cause significant hyponatremia and fluid overload. Glycine is metabolized to ammonia and glyoxylic acid in the liver and kidney. The ammonia is excreted as urea, and the glyoxylic acid is further reduced to oxalate and excreted by the kidney. Glycine's plasma half-life is approximately 85 minutes. Surgeons frequently check intraoperative or immediately postoperative serum sodium levels for confirmation of hyponatremia. This problem will worsen, however, as the glycine is metabolized and should therefore be rechecked at least an hour after the procedure to be sure that the problem is not worsening.

Sorbitol and mannitol are sugar solutions with similar chemical characteristics, although they are broken down in different ways. They both are nonconducting fluids that are good for visualization and use in continuous-flow devices. Both are hypotonic and, like glycine, may cause fluid overload and hyponatremia with excessive absorption. Whereas sorbitol is broken down to glucose and fructose, mannitol remains mostly unmetabolized. Mannitol is excreted quickly by the kidney and acts as a diuretic, counteracting the hyponatremia and fluid overload. As a medium, it may be the best suited for the resectoscope, although mannitol alone has a higher viscosity so may be slightly more difficult to work with.

Most resectoscope cases use glycine as the distention fluid. Given the risks of hyponatremia and fluid overload, it is important to understand the mechanisms of distention as well as the complications that are caused by hyponatremia and the ways in which it is treated. Fluid absorption is related to a number of factors within the uterus. Fluid is absorbed through the vascularity of the uterus. The greater the uterine pressure, the higher the rate of fluid absorption. Visualization adequate for surgery can usually be achieved with pressures between 75 mm Hg and 100 mm Hg. Any amount of pressure over this will usually not add to visibility but will only increase the rate of fluid absorption. In low-tech units that do not incorporate the monitoring of fluid pressure, placing a bag of low-viscosity fluid 1 m above the supine patient will result in a pressure of 73 mm Hg whereas placing it 1.5 m above the patient will increase the pressure to 110 mm Hg.[9] Hand pumps can significantly increase the pressure to values far in excess of what is necessary for appropriate visualization. The best units are those that closely monitor the pressure necessary to inject the fluid and maintain this pressure at levels less than 100 mm Hg. These units should also involve an under-buttock drape to assure total outflow collection and a return system that correctly determines the fluid deficit in a continuous fashion.

Absorption of hypo-osmolar low-viscosity fluids such as glycine may lead to fluid overload and hyponatremia, which can potentially result in the death of the patient. Continuous monitoring should occur during the case. Once a deficit of 1 L is reached, the surgeon should begin to conclude the procedure. The deficit should not surpass 1.5 L, and once this deficit is approached, the procedure should come to an immediate conclusion. If greater than 1 L is lost, the patient should be monitored in the recovery room and serial serum sodium levels should be checked. As glycine or sorbitol is metabolized, serum sodium may continue to rise, even after the completion of the procedure. If the serum sodium level increases after an initial period of observation of at least 30 minutes, and the initial serum sodium was at least 125 mmol/L, it is safe to discharge the patient. The highest reported serum sodium that still resulted in cerebellar herniation and death was 121 mmol/L, reported by Baggish et al.[8] The signs and symptoms of hyponatremia include an initial bradycardia and hypertension. The patient may then develop nausea, vomiting, seizures, pulmonary edema, and cardiac abnormalities. Without correction, the final stage is coma and death, usually caused by cerebral edema due to the hypo-osmolar state leading to cerebral herniation through the brainstem.

Treatment of hyponatremia should be instituted as soon as it is recognized. Frequently, this simply means stopping the procedure. If significant hyponatremia is suspected, a diuretic such as furosemide should be given immediately. Although chronic hyponatremia is expressly not treated with diuretics, acute hyponatremia, especially in this setting, is. Electrolytes should be monitored serially. In the setting of severe hyponatremia – that is, serum sodium levels less than 120 mOsm/L – central monitoring may be considered to assess the complex changes in hemodynamics that may ensue. Normal saline should be given instead of hypertonic solutions to prevent ensuing hypernatremia. Serum sodium may be increased up to 2 mEq/L per hour. Too rapid correction of hyponatremia may lead to central pontine myelinolysis. Although it is more likely to occur in the correction of chronic hyponatremia, it still is a risk in the acute surgical setting and can be avoided by not using hypertonic solution or the rapid infusion of normal saline.

PATIENT EVALUATION AND PREPARATION

Fibroids are one of a number of structural abnormalities in the uterus that may cause abnormal bleeding. The list also includes endometrial polyps, endometrial hyperplasia or cancer, and ade-nomyosis. Numerous studies are available that attempt to differ-entiate among the possible causes. The most important first step is a thorough history and physical. A postmenopausal woman or teenager with abnormal bleeding is much less likely to have fibroids as a cause than is a 45-year-old woman with excessive menstruation. The teenager should be evaluated for anovulatory or other hormonal causes of abnormal bleeding, whereas the post-menopausal woman should be evaluated to rule out endometrial cancer. A long history of irregular menses, every 3 to 4 months, that are frequently excessive is more likely to point to a hormonal cause of abnormal bleeding compared with a recent, progres-sive increase in the volume of menstruation in a woman with an enlarged uterus on exam, which more likely indicates myomas as the cause. Although the history and physical may not give an absolute diagnosis for the abnormal uterine bleeding, they often point to the direction of focus to achieve this diagnosis and, hence, the appropriate treatment.

If a structural abnormality is suspected, ultrasound is usu-ally the modality of choice for the initial evaluation. Ultrasound is very sensitive for the detection of uterine myoma. With the addition of sterile saline injected into the uterine cavity, the pos-itive predictive value (PPV) for the detection of a submucosal lesion is very high. Cepni et al. [10] found a PPV of 78% to 81%, depending on menstrual status, for submucosal myoma using a saline-infused sonogram (SIS). De Vries et al. [11] demonstrated an increase in sensitivity in diagnosing intracavitary lesions from regular vaginal sonogram to SIS from 60% to 88%. Using an SIS, ultrasound can usually differentiate between polyps, myomas, and carcinoma. Ultrasound can also be used to diagnose adeno-myosis, although the sensitivity and specificity are not as high. If the diagnosis is in doubt, MRI, although more costly, can bet-ter differentiate adenomyosis from other uterine pathology. In addition, it is very useful in determining the size, number, and location of uterine fibroids in preparation for surgery.

Three-dimensional sonography has shown some promise in the diagnosis of submucosal myomas. Salim et al. [12] demons-trated a 75% to 95% specificity in determining the level of involve-ment in the myometrium. This could aid surgeons in determining whether a patient is a candidate for hysteroscopic resection.

Hysteroscopy is considered the gold standard for diagnosis. It is redundant and adds unnecessary risks to take a patient to the operating room simply to diagnose a submucosal myoma with no immediate plans to resect it. However, the ability to perform in-office, diagnostic hysteroscopy significantly decreases these risks. CO_2 is frequently used as the distending medium, and, with min-imal discomfort, a diagnosis can be made. Because of the sig-nificant effort, on the part of both the surgeon's office and the patient, to schedule a case for the operating room and perform the preoperative evaluation required by many hospitals, an in-office hysteroscopy may occasionally save much unnecessary effort and lost time.

HSG was frequently used in the past to diagnose myomas. Although it is still useful in infertility evaluation and often leads to further work-up for myomas, it is not as sensitive or specific as SIS. It is also more invasive, with a higher risk of salpingitis/pelvic inflammatory disease, so is no longer as commonly used to eval-uate fibroids alone.

A hysteroscopic myomectomy is most likely to be performed in cases of abnormal uterine bleeding or infertility. Although

myomas generally may cause a myriad of symptoms, unless the myoma is causing abnormal bleeding or affecting fertility, a sur-geon usually is not justified in performing a procedure that has potential surgical and anesthetic complications. Performing a hysteroscopic resection of a myoma will typically not resolve symptoms related to the bulk of a uterus secondary to myomas. Therefore, an appropriate work-up of abnormal uterine bleeding and infertility is necessary before proceeding to surgery.

Abnormal uterine bleeding is a very common problem with a great variety of causes. Before operating for a submucosal myoma, other causes of bleeding must first be explored. Anovulatory bleeding is a common cause of abnormal uterine bleeding. It is frequently found in the perimenarcheal and perimenopausal age groups. Whereas fibroids are extremely unlikely in the for-mer, they are very common in the latter. In fact, the period of most rapid fibroid growth is often during the few years pre-ceding menopause because of the hormonal changes that occur around this time. Without the progestin withdrawal from ovu-lation, the continuously stimulated endometrium can randomly bleed, occasionally quite excessively. Women with polycystic ovar-ian syndrome also frequently have abnormal bleeding due to anovulation. Not all submucosal myomas cause abnormal uter-ine bleeding. In addition, not all submucosal myomas require surgical management. Hence, working up and medically treat-ing other causes are prudent first steps before proceeding to surgery. The complete evaluation for abnormal uterine bleeding is beyond the scope of this section. Causes to assess, other than structural ones, include bleeding disorders; hormonal causes, such as anovulation; thyroid disease; hypothalamic dysfunction from excessive weight loss, stress, and exercise; and foreign bod-ies, such as an IUD. Patients over 40 years of age or with a history of untreated abnormal uterine bleeding for a period greater than 1 year should have an endometrial biopsy to rule out cancer.

Medical treatment for abnormal uterine bleeding, including that caused by a submucosal myoma, should be considered. Oral contraceptive use typically decreases blood loss during menses by 50%.[13] Taking oral contraceptives in a continuous fash-ion frequently may stop menses altogether. Cyclic and continu-ous progestins may also be used in a similar fashion to decrease menstruation. A progestin-containing IUD usually results in a decrease in menstruation and frequently results in amenorrhea. Unfortunately, however, abnormal bleeding caused by structural defects such as submucosal myomas frequently do not respond to medical therapy and require surgery.

Before gynecologists adopted the use of the resectoscope, the vast majority of patients treated surgically for abnormal uter-ine bleeding proceeded to hysterectomy, usually via laparotomy. They would be subjected to all the potential complications associ-ated with this procedure, including prolonged pain, long hospital stay, and loss of work. The use of the resectoscope changed this significantly for patients with abnormal bleeding due to a sub-mucosal myoma. They are now able to have their problem dealt with in an outpatient setting, with significantly less anesthesia and decreased surgical risks. To maximize the chances of success with the procedure, however, the patient and her uterus must be optimized before the procedure.

The general principles of patient optimization before surgery apply to patients who are undergoing resection of a submucosal myoma. Significant anemia should be corrected if possible before proceeding to the operating room to decrease the intraoperative risk of heart attack and stroke and to decrease the need for transfusion and its associated risks. Hormonal therapies such as oral contraceptives and progestins alone may decrease the bleeding enough so that the patient may increase her hemoglobin with supplemental iron therapy alone. GnRH agonists are sometimes necessary to stop the menstrual cycle altogether to enable the woman to establish a surgically safe hemoglobin level.

Patients with concomitant medical conditions, such as diabetes or thyroid disease, should be maximally managed medically to decrease the risk of perioperative complications. Patients should be well nourished, well rested, and relatively free of stress when entering any surgical procedure.

The endometrium should preferentially be in the early proliferative phase for any hysteroscopy. The endometrium is thinnest at this point and less likely to hide small lesions. However, it is not always possible to schedule this naturally. Because of the availability of the surgeon and irregular menstrual cycles, it is often necessary to manipulate the menstrual cycle, either with oral contraceptives or progestins, to schedule the procedure with the endometrium in the appropriate state. Prolonged progestin treatment, as found in depomedroxyprogesterone acetate, frequently leads to endometrial atrophy, which allows for greater visualization during the procedure. However, the effect is variable and frequently outweighed by the side effects that may coincide with this type of treatment, such as irregular bleeding, bloating, weight gain, decreased libido, and headaches. Oral continuous progestins, such as medroxyprogesterone acetate and norethindrone acetate, also may be used. Although they must be taken on a daily basis, they have the benefit of being able to be stopped at any time if the symptoms become unbearable for the patient.

Because the surgical removal of submucosal myomas is limited by the amount of distention fluid absorbed, it is especially important for patients with larger myomas, who may take more time to resect, to be optimally prepared for surgery. This frequently involves the use of GnRH agonists. After administration, there is a brief period of stimulation over the first few days and then a decrease in action of the hypothalamic–pituitary–ovarian axis to a point of senescence. This results in a reversible pseudomenopausal state with very low levels of both circulating estrogens and progestins. This has multiple effects on the patient and the uterus specifically. First, it stops menstruation, which allows time for the anemic patient to increase her hemoglobin.

GnRH agonists are best given just before the proliferative phase, preferably from the middle to the end of menstruation. During this period, the initial stimulation has less of a chance to result in an increase in bleeding. If the GnRH agonist is used later in the cycle, it should be given with 7 days of a concomitant progestin to stabilize the endometrium and inhibit further proliferation and potential bleeding secondary to the initial stimulation.[14] If the agent is given during menses, by the end of the next cycle, the endometrium should be atrophic. If the agent is given midcycle to late in the cycle, the surgeon needs to wait until the completion of the following menstrual cycle.

In addition to thinning the endometrium, GnRH agonists also have other effects in preparation for a hysteroscopic myomectomy, such as causing myomas to shrink. Studies differ on the amount, but the decrease is in the range of 30% to 50% by the second to third month of treatment.[15,16] Most studies do not demonstrate significantly more shrinking after the third month,

so using the medication for more than 3 months for this purpose alone has little benefit. Shrinking the myoma should allow for a quicker removal and therefore less time for absorption of distention media. In large myomas, it may make the difference between completing the procedure in one step versus having to stage the removal secondary to fluid and electrolyte risks.

GnRH agonists also cause a contraction of the uterine vessels to approximately one half their initial diameter, which results in decreased bleeding from exposed vessels during resection. Therefore, less infusion of the distention fluid is required to clear the blood. Perino et al. [17] demonstrated that by giving leuprolide acetate preoperatively to patients undergoing hysteroscopic myomectomy, there was a significant decrease in operative time, intraoperative bleeding, volume of distention fluid infused, and persistence of fibroids 2 months postoperatively.

Patients should be warned about the potential side effects of GnRH agonists before use. Most patients experience symptoms similar to those felt in early menopause, including hot flushes and vaginal dryness. Many have severe mood swings and changes in weight. Rare problems such as bone pain may also occur, so surgeons should not use the medication longer than is thought necessary to best prepare the patient for surgery.

A few reports have been written on using suction curettage as a way to optimize the cavity before hysteroscopy.[18,19] The claimed advantage is decreased cost because time is saved and it is easier to schedule the procedure, not just at the follicular stage; there is less use of medications, therefore, less risk for ensuing complications; and tissue from the entire cavity is sent for evaluation, not just tissue from the fibroid. Cases of hyperplasia that are not readily visually apparent would therefore not be missed. However, many of these patients will have had an endometrial biopsy before going to the operating room, decreasing the chance of missing other pathology. By curetting the cavity in a premenopausal woman with the intention of removing the entire endometrium, the risk for intrauterine adhesions that could affect fertility is theoretically higher. In addition, by disrupting the entire cavity, there is significantly more intrauterine bleeding, increasing the amount of distention fluid to clear and the risk of fluid imbalance. Although it is helpful to have some data supporting this technique when one finds oneself in the operating room with an unprepared endometrium for whatever reason, it is not the ideal method of uterine preparation for hysteroscopic myomectomy.

Cervical preparation can aid in the procedure as well. A postmenopausal and nulliparous woman may have a cervix that is difficult to dilate. The use of preoperative laminaria or intravaginal dinoprostone may help soften the cervix and allow for dilatation appropriate for the resectoscope. Although it is rare for this to actually be necessary for cervical dilatation, the less difficult the surgeon finds each step of the procedure, the less likely he or she is to experience any complications.

THE PROCEDURE

Although newer techniques are available for the resection of submucosal myomas, they are discussed in a later section. Here we focus on the use of the resectoscope with a loop electrode.

The procedure begins with the selection of equipment. As previously discussed, the resectoscope comes in different sizes on the French (F) scale, the most common of which are 24F to

28F, and the loop electrode comes with different angles. The telescopes also come with angles from 0° to 30°. Most surgeons are limited to whatever their operating room has available to them; however, if there is a choice, the surgeon should try different sizes to determine the one with which he or she is most comfortable. With the current use of saline-infused ultrasound and MRI, in most cases, the surgeon can be fairly certain that he or she is dealing with a submucosal myoma. In these cases, it is best to go directly into the cavity with the resectoscope and not use the diagnostic scope first. The main reason is that there is only so much fluid that the patient can absorb before the case must be stopped. It is useless to waste this time on an initial survey with the diagnostic hysteroscope. The extremely rare risk of cervical damage is far outweighed by the increased risk of fluid overload.

The next important step is cervical dilatation. It is important to not overdilate the cervix as this may lead to the loss of distention fluid around the resectoscope and difficulty in distending the cavity to appropriately see the myoma. This may be a problem in the case of a prolapsing myoma, in which the cervix is already significantly dilated before starting the procedure. In a case in which the cervix has been overdilated either by surgical error or by a prolapsing myoma, the surgeon can try to occlude the cervix by placing towel clamps either unilaterally or bilaterally on the cervix. Another option that is typically more successful in achieving the appropriate occlusion but takes more time involves placing a cerclage-like stitch around the cervix that can be tied around the resectoscope. The stitch can then be removed at the end of the procedure. It is also important not to underdilate the cervix as larger myomas often require forward-and-back movement of the entire resectoscope. This movement may be limited if the cervix is not sufficiently dilated, leading to possible complications.

The typical procedure is performed with a 12° telescope and a 90° loop. The resectoscope is designed so that the electrode has a spring that brings it back to the sheath, which is insulated at the end to protect the patient from inadvertent bleeding. The electrode should be maximally extended to give the best visualization of the pathology during resection. The movement of the electrode during resection should always be toward the operator. Movement away from the operator is more likely to result in uterine perforation and potential serious injury to the patient. There likely will be times when the loop is not visible as it should be on the far side of the myoma to resect it toward the operator; however, energy should be used only as the electrode is moved toward the operator. For larger myomas, the entire resectoscope must occasionally be moved with the electrode to shave off the entire length.

While shaving the myoma, difficulties often occur with the pieces. Occasionally, they get trapped between the electrode and the lens. This can usually be corrected by separating the electrode from the lens and making sure the flow of the distention medium is working. A piece of the myoma may also become attached to the electrode. Surgeons often struggle in vain to remove these pieces. If the surgeon simply continues the procedure, the piece will typically come off with the next cut. Occasionally, the surgeon may find it difficult to cut through the myoma with the electrode. This is typically because the power is set at too low a wattage or the surgeon is using a coagulation current instead of a cutting current. A cutting current wattage of 80 to 100 W is typically adequate for smoothly slicing the myoma. The current

works better by arcing it toward the tissue, so it is best to start the current just before the electrode actually makes contact with the tissue and to continue the movement smoothly. Moving too slowly may result in a coagulation of the tissue and a sticking of the electrode. Moving too quickly may lodge the electrode into tissue that has not yet been cut. Using the coagulation current at a setting between 30 and 40 W is appropriate for stopping bleeding from any significant vessels from the myoma. It is not useful for shaving the myoma as the peak voltage that is required makes this more dangerous to peripheral tissue both in and outside the uterus. Also, the intermittent current makes the cells less likely to desiccate and therefore cut the tissue, and more likely to char the tissue.

Bubbles may occur during cutting, as a result either of gas forming during the cutting itself or of air in the inflow tubing. These can be visually distracting to the operator. It is important to maintain a good seal throughout the circuit of distention fluid. When bubbles form in the cavity, placing the end of the resectoscope directly into the bubble and making sure that the outflow is turned on will usually eliminate the problem.

With regard to removing the myoma, there is debate as to how aggressive the surgeon should be. Many surgeons believe that for maximal safety, an operator should not resect below the endometrial surface. One would automatically believe that this may leave a significant part of the myoma behind. However, when the myoma is shaved from the cavity, surgeons will find that the normal contractile nature of the uterus tends to force the intramural portion of the myoma into the cavity. It is frequently possible to remove the entire myoma in this fashion without actually having to dissect below the endometrial surface. For this technique to be successful, it is necessary to have at least 40% to 50% of the myoma protruding into the cavity when starting the procedure.

Some surgeons insist that it is prudent to remove the entire myoma regardless of the depth in which it is situated in the myometrium. Although it is true that the procedure is more likely to achieve long-term success when the entire myoma is removed, the risks of perforation and subsequent injury to bowel or vascular structures increase significantly as one dissects deeper into the myometrium. Ultrasound guidance occasionally has been used to determine depth and distance from the serosa, but it does not eliminate the potential risks. Indman [20] proposed injecting carboprost, a methyl analogue of prostaglandin $F_{2\alpha}$, into the cervix. He reported on a series of 13 patients with a significant amount of the submucosal myoma intramural. He found that the carboprost caused uterine contraction, allowing 11 of the 13 myomas to be completely excised. No randomized study has been performed, and as this frequently happens without any injection, it is unclear whether carboprost truly makes any difference. As a general rule, a surgeon should proceed with extreme caution when dissecting below the endometrium.

Although it is a relatively safe procedure compared with abdominal myomectomy, hysteroscopic myomectomy has potential risks as well. The risks of fluid overload and hyponatremia are discussed earlier in this section. The risk of uterine perforation is higher in resectoscope cases. The cervix must be dilated to a greater amount to accommodate the large instrument, which may lead to perforation during dilatation. This is usually recognized once the scope is place, either because it goes directly into the abdominal cavity or because there is an immediate fluid

Table 8.3.1: Hysteroscopic Myomectomy for Abnormal Uterine Bleeding

Study	Cases, no.	Follow-up, %	Average Follow-up Time, months	Success (No Further Surgery), %
Polena et al. [21]	235	84	40	94.4
Wamsteker et al. [22]	51	93.3	20	93.3
Emanuel et al. [23]	285	94	46	85.5
Cravello et al. [24]	196	86.2	73	82.2
Marziani et al. [25]	84	97	36	80.9
Kuzel et al. [26]	45	100	48	100
Hart et al. [27]	194	100	27	79
Munoz et al. [28]	120	100	36	88.5
Brooks et al. [29]	90	100	6	91
Derman et al. [30]	177	100	108	83.9

imbalance. If the perforation occurs before the use of the electrode, the procedure must be stopped; however, the patient usually may simply be monitored in the recovery room for signs of intra-abdominal bleeding. Stable serial hemoglobin levels are reassuring, and the patient can be sent home and the procedure reattempted another day.

If the perforation occurs with the resectoscope while the electrode is charged, the potential for serious injury exists. The patient must have a thorough evaluation of the abdomen and pelvis, typically via laparoscopy, to determine the presence and extent of any injury. Unfortunately, thermal injuries to the intestine are not always readily apparent. If the bowel has been burned but not incised, the defect may only become apparent after a few days. Patients discharged home after this type of complication should be advised to monitor their temperature and report any gastrointestinal symptoms, specifically nausea and vomiting.

Another possible complication after this procedure, especially in patients with a desire for future fertility, is intrauterine adhesions. These are more likely if two opposing fibroids have been resected so that the surfaces are juxtaposed after the procedure is completed. Although this is rare, should it occur, the surgeon has the option of giving the patient supplemental estrogen immediately postoperatively, with the goal of rapidly developing the endometrium to prevent adhesions. Another method attempted in the past was the placement of an intrauterine Foley catheter to keep the opposing surfaces away from one another until estrogen formed spontaneously.

The immediate postoperative care of patients having undergone hysteroscopic myomectomy is generally not complicated. If an imbalance of fluid was noted during the procedure, the recovery room nurse should monitor the patient for signs and symptoms of fluid overload and hyponatremia, including bradycardia, hypertension, nausea, vomiting, seizures, pulmonary edema, and cardiac abnormalities. The management of these problems has been previously discussed. There is typically not much pain after this procedure. At our institution, we find that ketorolac 30 mg given IV soluset at the completion of the procedure is usually adequate anesthesia; our patients are not sent home with narcotics but are told to use an anti-inflammatory medication such

as ibuprofen. The need for more significant pain control can be an indication of a more serious injury during the surgery and should be evaluated appropriately.

Patients should be told to expect per vaginal bleeding for approximately 1 week after the surgery. The duration of bleeding may vary from a few days to 2 weeks, but the flow usually is very light. Patients should also be warned that their cycle may be abnormal for the next month or two and a heavy menses following the procedure is not indicative of what their usual menses will be like once they return to a regular cycle.

LONG-TERM RESULTS: MENORRHAGIA AND FERTILITY

Most studies evaluating the results of hysteroscopic myomectomies specifically focus on subsequent fertility and menorrhagia. The only true cure for uterine myomas is a total hysterectomy. Even women undergoing a supracervical hysterectomy for myomas should be advised that there is a very small risk of developing a cervical myoma in the future. It is therefore inherent in the hysteroscopic myomectomy procedure that a success rate of 100% should not be expected. Some surgeons argue that the immediate, postoperative results should be close to 100% of the time. However, many women have anatomically normal uteruses with menorrhagia, dysfunctional uterine bleeding. It is impossible to know whether a woman with a submucosal myoma is bleeding irregularly solely because of the myoma or because of some other undetectable problem in her uterus. Only by removing the myoma would this be found; however, its presence would be considered a surgical failure, even though the goal of removing the myoma may have been completely successful. We know from data on abdominal myomectomies that up to 30% of women who undergo the procedure will require an intervention for myomas in the future. There is no reason to believe that this should not be the case for patients with submucosal myomas as well.

Studies now exist looking at the 1- to 9-year follow-up of hysteroscopic myomectomies. Table 8.3.1 exhibits the results for patients treated specifically for abnormal bleeding. Hysteroscopic

Table 8.3.2: Fertility Rates after Hysteroscopic Myomectomy

Study	Patients, no.	Follow-up Period, months	% Followed	% with Pregnancies
Ubaldi et al. [31]	134	NA	NA	58.9
Goldenberg et al. [32]	15	12	100	47
Shokeir [33]	29	24	100	72.4
Bernard et al. [34]	31	24	100	35.5
Giatras et al. [35]	41	24	100	60.9

myomectomy has at least an 80% success rate for up to 9 years after surgery. Although it may seem that a failure rate of 20% is significantly high for any procedure, it is important to remember that the alternative would have been for the patients to have undergone a hysterectomy, with its associated increase in complications, pain, and lost productive time. In these studies, approximately half the patients who failed the procedure required a hysterectomy subsequently and the others had other forms of intervention, usually another hysteroscopy. At least 90% of these patients were able to avoid a hysterectomy by undergoing a minimally invasive outpatient procedure that has considerably fewer risks.

Infertility is another common reason for undergoing hysteroscopic myomectomy. Again, infertility is multifactorial, and many patients who are infertile will not be found to have any apparent problems. It is very possible that a woman may have infertility from an unknown source and have a submucosal myoma as well, so fertility rates after resection of myomas should be evaluated with this information in mind. Table 8.3.2 reports the findings from a number of studies designed to evaluate fertility after hysteroscopic myomectomy. Pregnancy rates vary from 35% to 70%, representing a dramatic increase in fertility after hysteroscopic myomectomy in patients having infertility and a submucous myoma. Given that these women typically would have had limited options – a myomectomy, with its associated morbidity, or a hysterectomy, which clearly eliminates any chance of fertility in the future – hysteroscopic myomectomy represents a great advancement.

NEW TECHNIQUES

Surgeons are always trying to improve on current techniques in an attempt to decrease operative risks and improve outcomes. The development of the hysteroscopic myomectomy is an example of this, and within the context of the hysteroscopic myomectomy, advances continue. Because of the fluid balance risks, better fluid management systems have emerged over the last few years that greatly enhance the surgeon's ability to closely monitor the fluid balance to significantly decrease the risk of the patient ever developing hyponatremia or general fluid overload. The most advanced system would monitor input and output, maintain a hysteroscopic intrauterine pressure sufficient to distend the cavity but not excessive, present all these data on the video screen used for the procedure, and have alarms to alert the surgeon when any parameters reached levels of increased risk. Surgeons would have to consciously choose to ignore the warnings to cause harm. As with any device, there is always the risk of instrument error,

so the surgeon should not have a complete sense of security with this instrumentation. Having the equipment decreases the risks but does not excuse the surgeon from monitoring all aspects of the surgery closely so as to catch equipment errors if they arise. Although there is no correction for poor surgical technique or judgment on the part of the surgeon, new devices limit the risk as much as possible.

Because a monopolar electric current is somewhat uncontrolled once it leaves the electrode, many surgeons believe a bipolar device is safer. With the standard monopolar electrode, the current has its greatest effect within millimeters from the electrode. It is then dispersed in all directions and is reaccumulated at the grounding pad and returned to the generator. The dispersed current is usually too weak to cause harm. The current will flow in a path of least resistance. In the setting of a hysteroscopic myomectomy, the myoma and the tissue surrounding it generally have a uniform resistance, so the current flows in all directions. If there is aberrant anatomy, it is possible that a channel of less resistance might exist, concentrating the current and potentially harming the patient. This is the reason the grounding pads are wide: if they were attached at a single point, the entire current would accumulate at that point and cause injury.

Bipolar instruments have opposing electrodes that are positive and negative, so the current flows only between the electrodes and is not dispersed throughout the patient. This more-controlled current should be safer as it is not dispersed through the patient. The VersaPoint system by Gynecare is an example of a system with this design. Clark et al. [36] performed a feasibility study on this technique, which they reported in 2002. Using the bipolar device, they operated on 37 women with a submucous myoma. They found that 92% of the patients were satisfied with the procedure, although only 78% reported improvement in bleeding. There were no operative complications, and the authors considered this technique to be an improvement over the standard monopolar technique.

In addition to the increased safety of the better-controlled current, bipolar techniques offer other advantages. Using a bipolar electrode allows the surgeon to use normal saline as the distending fluid. Although this does not eliminate the risks of fluid overload, it greatly decreases the risk of hyponatremia. This does not eliminate the need for close fluid monitoring, as at least one death has occurred as a result of fluid overload using this system. However, it increases the amount of fluid that may be safely absorbed to 2000 to 2500 mL, which may give the surgeon valuable additional time to perform the procedure completely.

The bipolar technique also has improved with regard to the tissue affected by the current. In most cases, as the electrode is moved through the myoma, it completely vaporizes the tissue. This eliminates or greatly decreases the amount of floating pieces of myoma that obscure the operative field, which may both lengthen the procedure and increase operative errors due to the obstructed view. One negative would be that the tissue is not evaluated by a pathologist to assure that the treated lesion is indeed a simple myoma and not a more serious condition, such as a sarcoma. This is very rare, however, and may not outweigh the benefits offered by this technique.

Another new technique eliminates the risk of electrosurgery. The Smith & Nephew operative hysteroscopy system involves a rotating morcellating blade. The opening is on the side of the distal end of the hysteroscope. This opening is placed on the myoma, and the rotating blade shaves the myoma. The cutting is all sharp as no electric current is used. The shaved pieces are immediately suctioned out of the uterus through the scope and collected for pathologic review. This technique uses the normal contraction of the uterus that occurs during a hysteroscopic myomectomy to both force the myoma out of the myometrium and contract the vessels surrounding the myoma to decrease bleeding. This technique limits the surgeon's ability to dissect deeper into the uterine wall to remove the entire myoma if it is not expelled by uterine contraction, a limitation that is probably safer for the patient. The procedure, like the bipolar technique, may be performed with normal saline, with the same decreased risk of hyponatremia. Surgeons should have some type of electrosurgery device available to manage bleeding should it occur.

The opportunity to improve patient care drives those in the medical field to constantly search for new devices and techniques. With the adoption of the resectoscope, gynecologists have been able to save countless women from experiencing excessive pain, lost productive time, and unnecessary major surgery. Although risks exist in everything we do as surgeons, the resectoscope greatly reduces those involved in surgeries for uterine myomas. Advances continue to reduce these risks and make the options for treatment of uterine myoma safer for women suffering from the effects of this condition.

REFERENCES

1. Neuwirth RS, Amin HK. Excision of submucous fibroids with hysteroscopic control. *Am J Obstet Gynecol*. 1976;126:95–99.
2. Nesbit RM. A history of transurethral prostatic resection. In: Silber SJ, ed. *Transurethral Resection*. New York: Appleton-Century-Crofts; 1977:1–17.
3. Stern M. Resection of obstruction at the vesical orifice. *JAMA*. 1926;87:1726–1730.
4. d'Arsonval A. Action physiologique dex courants alternatifs a grand frequence. *Arch Physiol Norm Pathol*. 1893;5:401–408.
5. Goldwyn RM. Bovie: the man and the machine. *Ann Plast Surg*. 1979;2(2):135–153.
6. McCarthy JF. The management of prostatic obstruction by endoscopic revision. *N Engl J Med*. 1932;207(7):305–312.
7. Iglesias JJ, Sporer A, Gellman AC, Seebode JJ. New Iglesias resectoscope with continuous irrigation, simultaneous suction, and low intravesicle pressure. *J Urol*. 1975;114:929–933.
8. Baggish MS, Brill AI, Rosensweig B, Barbot JE, Indman P. Fatal acute glycine and sorbitol toxicity during operative hysteroscopy. *J Gynecol Surg*. 1993;9:137–143.
9. Loffer FD. Complications from uterine distention during hysteroscopy. In: Corfman KS, Diamond MP, DeCherney A, eds.

Complications in Laparoscopy and Hysteroscopy. Boston: Blackwell Scientific Publications; 1993:117–186.
10. Cepni I, Ocal P, Erkan S, et al. Comparison of transvaginal sonography, saline infusion sonography and hysteroscopy in the evaluation of the uterine cavity pathologies. *Aust N Z J Obstet Gynaecol*. 2005;45(1):30–35.
11. de Vries LD, Dijkhuizen FP, Mol BW, Brolmann HA, Moret E, Heintz AP. Comparison of transvaginal sonography, saline infusion sonography, and hysteroscopy in premenopausal women with abnormal uterine bleeding. *J Clin Ultrasound*. 2000;28(5):217–223.
12. Salim R, Lee C, Davies A, Jolaoso B, Ofuasia E, Jurkovic D. A comparison study of three-dimensional saline infusion sonohysterography and diagnostic hysteroscopy for the classification of submucous fibroids. *Hum Reprod*. 2005;20:252–257.
13. Nilsson L, Rybo G. Treatment of menorrhagia. *Am J Obstet Gynecol*. 1971;110:713–720.
14. Brooks PG, Serden SP. Preparation of the endometrium for ablation with a single dose of leuprolide acetate depot. *J Reprod Med*. 1991;36:477–478.
15. Friedman AJ, Hoffman DI, Comite F, Browneller RW, Miller JD. Treatment of leiomyomata uteri with leuprolide acetate depot – a double blind, placebo controlled multicenter study. *Obstet Gynecol*. 1991;77:720–725.
16. Coddington CC, Brzyski R, Hansen KA, Corley DR, McIntyre-Seltman K, Jones HW. Short term treatment with leuprolide acetate is a successful adjunct to surgical therapy of leiomyomas of the uterus. *Surg Gynecol Obstet*. 1992;175:57–63.
17. Perino A, Chianchiano N, Petronio M, Cittadini E. Role of leuprolide acetate depot in hysteroscopic surgery: a controlled study. *Fertil Steril*. 1993;59:507–510.
18. Gimpelson RJ, Kaigh J. Mechanical preparation of the endometrium prior to endometrial ablation. *J Reprod Med*. 1992;37:691–694.
19. Lefler HT, Sullivan GH, Hulka JF. Modified endometrial ablation electrocoagulation with vasopressin and suction curettage preparation. *Obstet Gynecol*. 1991;77:949–953.
20. Indman P. Use of carboprost to facilitate hysteroscopic resection of submucous myomas. *J Am Assoc Gynecol Laparosc*. 2004, 11(1):68–72.
21. Polena V, Mergui JL, Perrot N, Poncelet C, Barranger E, Uzan S. Long-term results of hysteroscopic myomectomy in 235 patents. *Eur J Obstet Gynecol Reprod Biol*. 2007/Feb;130(2):272–7.
22. Wamsteker K, Emanuel MH, de Kruif JH. Transcervical hysteroscopic resection of submucous fibroids for abnormal uterine bleeding: results regarding the degree of intramural extension. *Obstet Gynecol*. 1993;82(5):736–740.
23. Emanuel MH, Wamsteker K, Hart AA, Metz R, Lammes FB. Long term results of hysteroscopic myomectomy for abnormal uterine bleeding. *Obstet Gynecol*. 1999;93(5 pt 1):743–748.
24. Cravello L, Farnarier J, Roger V, D'Ercole C, Blanc B. Hysteroscopic myomectomy. Functional results with an average follow-up of 6 years. *J Gynecol Obstet Biol Reprod*. 1998;27(6):593–597.
25. Marziani R, Mossa B, Ebano V, Perniola G, Mellusa J, Napolitano C. Transcervical hysteroscopic myomectomy: long term effects on abnormal uterine bleeding. *Clin Exp Obstet Gynecol*. 2005;32(1):23–26.
26. Kuzel D, Toth D, Fucikova Z, Cibula D, Hruskova H, Zivny. Hysteroscopic resection of submucosal myomas in abnormal uterine bleeding: results of a 4-year prospective study. *Ceska Gynecol*. 1999;64(6):363–367.
27. Hart R, Molnar BG, Magos A. Long term follow up of hysteroscopic myomectomy assessed by survival analysis. *Br J Obstet Gynaecol*. 1999;106(7):700–705.

28. Munoz JL, Jimenez JS, Hernandez C, et al. Hysteroscopic myomectomy: our experience and review. *JSLS*. 2003;7(1):39–48.

29. Brooks PG, Loffer FD, Serden SP. Resectoscopic removal of symptomatic intrauterine lesions. *J Reprod Med*. 1989;34(7):435–437.

30. Derman SG, Rehnstrom J, Neuwirth RS. The long-term effectiveness of hysteroscopic treatment of menorrhagia and leiomyomas. *Obstet Gynecol*. 1991;77(4):591–594.

31. Ubaldi F, Tournaye H, Camus M, Van der Pas H, Gepts E, Devroey P. Fertility after hysteroscopic myomectomy. *Hum Reprod Update*. 1995;1(1):81–90.

32. Goldenberg M, Sivan E, Sharabi Z, Bider D, Rabinovici J, Seidman DS. Outcome of hysteroscopic resection of submucous myomas for infertility. *Fertil Steril*. 1995;64(4):714–716.

33. Shokeir TA. Hysteroscopic management of submucous fibroids to improve fertility. *Arch Gynecol Obstet*. 2005;273(1):50–54.

34. Bernard G, Darai E, Poncelet C, Benifla JL, Madelenat P. Fertility after hysteroscopic myomectomy: effect of intramural myomas associated. *Eur J Obstet Gynecol Reprod Biol*. 2000;88(1):85–90.

35. Giatras K, Berkeley AS, Noyes N, Licciardi F, Lolis D, Grifo JA. Fertility after hysteroscopic resection of submucous myomas. *J Am Assoc Gynecol Laparosc*. 1999;6(2):155–158.

36. Clark TJ, Mahajan D, Sunder P, Gupta JK. Hysteroscopic treatment of symptomatic submucous fibroids using a bipolar intrauterine system: a feasibility study. *Eur J Obstet Gynecol Reprod Biol*. 2002;100(2):237–242.

Section 8.4. Hysteroscopic Tubal Cannulation

Tommaso Falcone and Jeffrey M. Goldberg

The concept of cannulating the intramural portion of the tube to relieve an obstruction in infertile patients has been around since the 19th century. Tubal cannulation is also performed for diagnostic assessment, transfer of gametes or embryos, and sterilization. The radiologic and hysteroscopic approaches to relieving obstruction were investigated in the mid-1980s and remain an integral part of infertility treatment.

DIAGNOSIS OF PROXIMAL TUBAL BLOCK

Approximately 25% to 30% of infertility in women is the result of tubal disease, with proximal tubal occlusion (PTO) accounting for the infertility in 10% to 25% of those patients.[1] Hysterosalpingogram (HSG) is the first-line technique for excluding anatomic defects in the uterine cavity and documenting tubal patency in infertility patients. It is part of the basic infertility work-up and is normally required in every patient.[2] PTO is found on 10% to 20% of hysterosalpingograms [1] and may be caused by obstruction due to tubal spasm or plugging by mucus and amorphous material or by occlusion from fibrosis or endometriosis. Infectious causes include salpingitis isthmica nodosa (SIN), pelvic inflammatory disease (PID), and tuberculosis. These infections may damage other areas of the tube, which will affect the prognosis of the treatment.

HSG is considered the standard test for assessment of the uterine tubes in patients with infertility. If HSG suggests patent tubes, tubal blockage is highly unlikely.[3] One study noted that 60% of patients with PTO on HSG were patent on repeat HSG 1 month later.[4] Similarly, tubal blockage on HSG is not confirmed by laparoscopy in up to 62% of patients.[3] It should be noted that laparoscopy is not the perfect gold standard as 2% of patients with bilateral tubal occlusion subsequently conceived spontaneously.[5] Also, Sulak et al. [6] reported that 11 of 18 patients with bilateral PTO on both HSG and laparoscopy were patent histologically.

Diagnostic laparoscopy and hysteroscopy to assess the uterus and tubes are probably more cost-effective than HSG in patients with pelvic pain, adnexal masses, or other indications for surgery as well as a history of PID or prior pelvic surgery. These patients are much more likely to have pelvic pathology requiring surgical treatment, regardless of the results of HSG.

MANAGEMENT OF PROXIMAL TUBAL BLOCKAGE

Historically, PTO was managed by coring out the uterine cornua and implanting the proximal fallopian tube within the endometrial cavity. The procedure was abandoned because of low pregnancy rates and increased risk for cornual rupture during pregnancy. It was replaced with microsurgical resection and anastomosis in the late 1970s. Transcervical tubal cannulation by fluoroscopic guidance was first reported in 1985 [7]; hysteroscopic tubal cannulation was reported 2 years later.[8]

As noted above, 60% of patients with PTO on HSG were shown to be patent on repeat HSG 1 month later.[4] Therefore, selective salpingography may be attempted if a repeat HSG at least 1 month later confirms persistent PTO. The repeat HSG is performed under intravenous conscious sedation using a balloon catheter with a 5F catheter advanced through it and wedged in the cornua under fluoroscopic guidance. Contrast is then injected, establishing patency in a third of the tubes.[9]

Tubal cannulation may be attempted in the two thirds of tubes that remained occluded during selective salpingography. A flexible guidewire is then passed through the tubal ostium and, if successful, a 3F catheter is advanced over the wire and contrast is injected (Figure 8.4.1). In one study, the procedure successfully established patency in more than 85% of cases.[1] After relieving the obstruction, distal tubal disease may be found (Figure 8.4.2).

Excision of the proximal tubes in cases of failed tubal cannulation revealed SIN, chronic salpingitis, or fibrosis in 93% of patients in one study.[10] About a third of the opened tubes reocclude.[1,9] Tubal perforation has been reported in 3% to 11% of cases but has always been innocuous.[11]

Laparoscopy with transcervical chromotubation with dilute indigo carmine should be performed to confirm PTO in infertility patients who have not had a diagnostic laparoscopy or in patients with known pelvic disease. Hysteroscopic cannulation may be attempted at that time if persistent PTO is noted. Success rates in terms of patency, reocclusion, and perforation are nearly identical to those for radiologic cannulation, but pregnancy rates are higher with the hysteroscopic approach.

Ongoing pregnancy rates following hysteroscopic tubal cannulation were similar to those for microsurgical resection and anastomosis of PTO: almost 50%. In this study report that analyzed several studies, the radiologic group was divided into "high-success" and "low-success." [1] However, the ongoing pregnancy rate after fluoroscopic canalization was significantly lower in the high-success group: 29%. The overall pregnancy rate in the low-success group was only 12.2%, with inadequate data to determine pregnancy outcomes. Unfortunately, there was no way to distinguish between these groups from the studies (Table 8.4.1).[1] The higher pregnancy rate with the hysteroscopic approach is likely the result of the fact that other pelvic pathology can be diagnosed and treated laparoscopically, whereas concurrent pelvic disease is unrecognized with fluoroscopic tubal cannulation.

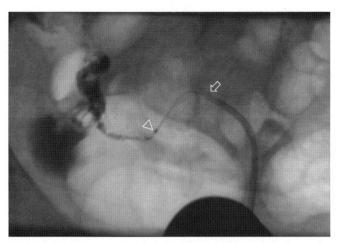

Figure 8.4.1. Fluoroscopic tubal cannulation. The *arrow* indicates the end of the outer catheter in the cornua, and the *arrowhead* is the tip of the inner catheter within the proximal tube.

TECHNIQUE

The contraindications to hysteroscopic tubal cannulation include active infection, heavy uterine bleeding, potential pregnancy, and uterine malignancy. Patients with known allergy or adverse reaction to contrast dye used to establish patency should be appropriately counseled. The potential complications associated with the procedure are listed in Table 8.4.2. Reversal of the occlusion in the cornua may improve fertility sufficiently to result in an ectopic pregnancy. The catheter or wire guide may dissect or perforate the tubal wall. A dissection of the tubal wall may lead to extravasation of the contrast material or dye.

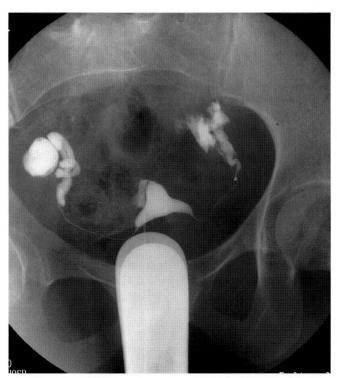

Figure 8.4.2. Appearance of the tube after successful cannulation of the tube shows distal tubal disease.

Table 8.4.1: Pregnancy Rates Following Treatment of Proximal Tubal Blockage

	Patients, no./ Studies, no.	Ongoing, no. (%) *	SAB, no. (%)	Ectopic, no. (%)
Microsurgery	175/5	83 (47.4)	7 (4)	13 (7.4)
Fluoroscopy†	163/4	47 (28.8)	11 (6.7)	4 (2.4)
Hysteroscopy	133/4	22 (48.9)	3 (6.7)	2 (4.4)

SAB, spontaneous abortion. See Honore et al. for source data. [1]
* ≥20 weeks gestation.
†High-success group.

Table 8.4.2: Adverse Effects of Hysteroscopic Tubal Cannulation

Damage to normal tube

    Dissection

    Perforation

Pain

Ectopic pregnancy

The standard cannulation set used is the Novy cornual cannulation set. The tubal cannulation technique was described by Novy and colleagues.[12] The procedure is carried out using a standard 5-mm hysteroscope with an operative channel. The procedure for fluoroscopic cannulation is accomplished using the same principle. The set has two separate catheter systems. The first is a 5F catheter, called the introducing catheter, with two ports: one for the introduction of the obturator and the other for the introduction of the second catheter, which is 3F.

Knowledge of the anatomy of the intramural portion of the tube is important to properly carry out the procedure. The intramural portion of the uterine tubes is typically 1 to 2 cm in length. Three patterns have been described.[13] The segment may be straight, curved, or tortuous. The course of the tube is not necessarily symmetrical in the patient, and each intramural portion may be different. The most frequent pattern is tortuous followed by straight and curved. The direction of the mucosal folds is toward the uterine tube. Introduction of the catheter should therefore follow this direction. There is a potential sphincter at this junction that is probably composed of the uterine smooth layers. This can close the tube, as evidenced by spasm during HSG.

Preoperatively, the patient may require something to facilitate cervical dilatation, such as the (off-label) use of misoprostol or insertion of laminaria tents. A preoperative antibiotic, such as a cephalosporin, should be given. A laparoscopy is performed simultaneously, and a "picture-in-picture" view is brought on the monitor so that the laparoscopic view of the fimbriated end of the tube and the hysteroscopic view of uterine cavity are simultaneously visualized (Figure 8.4.3). If the patient is shown to have distal tubal disease as well, the procedure is terminated.

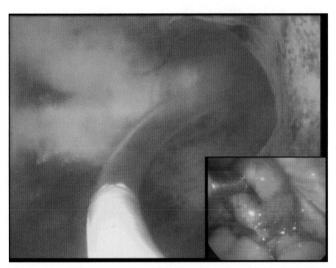

Figure 8.4.3. The outer catheter has been introduced through the hysteroscope into the uterine cavity. The distal transparent end is curved and is brought up to the tubal ostia.

Uterine tubes with proximal and distal disease should be referred for IVF. If the distal end of the tube is adequate, the next step is to inject dilute dye through a uterine manipulator to confirm the cornual obstruction. If confirmed, the hysteroscopic procedure can proceed.

The introducing catheter is inserted into the operating channel of the hysteroscope. An angled lens is typically used. The obturator is then removed and the catheter occluded. The tip of this catheter is curved and wedged against the tubal ostium (Figure 8.4.3). Dilute indigo carmine dye may be injected. If dye is seen coming from the tube, patency is confirmed and the procedure is finished. If no dye is seen, the inner catheter will be introduced to cannulate the tube.

The inner catheter has 1-cm markings. The guidewire is introduced through this catheter, which has a special adaptor for securing the wire. The wire is positioned at the tip of this catheter

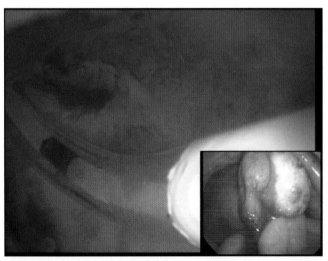

Figure 8.4.4. The inner catheter with markings is seen through the distal transparent sheath.

and the adaptor tightened. The catheter and wire are introduced through the side of the introducing catheter up to the tip. Both catheters and the guidewire should be flush. The cannulation of the tube occurs first with the guidewire, and then the inner catheter is brought over it. The guidewire is advanced slowly through the uterotubal junction into the intramural portion of the tube into the isthmic portion (Figure 8.4.4). This can be seen by laparoscopy. The catheter is then advanced over the guidewire. The distance into the tube can be measured by the markings on the catheter. The guidewire is removed and the dilute dye is injected under laparoscopic observation. If dye is observed, the procedure is terminated. If there is resistance to passage of the guidewire or catheter, an attempt is made to mobilize the tube laparoscopically. If unsuccessful, the procedure is terminated. If the cause of the obstruction is not apparent, the next step is to counsel the patient regarding tubal surgery or IVF.

REFERENCES

1. Honore GM, Holden AE, Schenken RS. Pathophysiology and management of proximal tubal blockage. *Fertil Steril.* 1999;71: 785–795.
2. Hedon B, Dechaud H, Boulot P, Laffargue F. Critical evaluation of the fallopian tube. In: Kempers RD, Cohen J, Haney AF, Younger BJ, eds. *Fertility and Reproductive Medicine.* Amsterdam: Elsevier Science; 1998:61–70.
3. Evers JL, Land JA, Mol BW. Evidence-based medicine for diagnostic questions. *Sem Reprod Med.* 2003;21:9–15.
4. Dessole S, Meloni GB, Capobianco G, Manzoni MA, Ambrosini G, Canalis GC. A second hysterosalpingography reduces the use of selective technique for treatment of a proximal tubal obstruction. *Fertil Steril.* 2000;73:1037–1039.
5. Mol BW, Collins JA, Burrows EA, Van DV, Bossuyt PM. Comparison of hysterosalpingography and laparoscopy in predicting fertility outcome. *Hum Reprod.* 1999;14:1237–1242.
6. Sulak PJ, Letterie GS, Coddington CC, Hayslip CC, Woodward JE, Klein TA. Histology of proximal tubal occlusion. *Fertil Steril.* 1987;48:437–440.
7. Platia MP, Krudy AG. Transvaginal fluoroscopic recanalization of a proximally occluded oviduct. *Fertil Steril.* 1985;44: 704–706.
8. Sulak PJ, Letterie GS, Hayslip CC, Coddington CC, Klein TA. Hysteroscopic cannulation and lavage in the treatment of proximal tubal occlusion. *Fertil Steril.* 1987;48:493–494.
9. Pinto AB, Hovsepian DM, Wattanakumtornkul S, Pilgram TK. Pregnancy outcomes after fallopian tube recanalization: oil-based versus water-soluble contrast agents. *J Vasc Intervent Radiol.* 2003;14:69–74.
10. Letterie GS, Sakas EL. Histology of proximal tubal obstruction in cases of unsuccessful tubal canalization. *Fertil Steril.* 1991;56:831–835.
11. Dessole S, Farina M, Rubattu G, Cosmi E, Ambrosini G, Battista NG. Side effects and complications of sonohysterosalpingography. *Fertil Steril.* 2003;80:620–624.
12. Novy MJ, Thurmond AS, Patton P, Uchida BT, Rosch J. Diagnosis of corneal obstruction by transcervical fallopian tube cannulation. *Fertil Steril.* 1988;50:434–440.
13. Rozewicki S, Radomska A, Kurzawa R. Relation between anatomical courses of the intramural portions of the uterine tubes and pelvic endometriosis. *Fertil Steril.* 2005;85:60–66.

Section 8.5. Hysteroscopic Sterilization

Stephanie N. Morris and Keith Isaacson

Tubal sterilization is the most common form of birth control used by women in the United States.[1] About half of all tubal sterilizations are performed as interval procedures (unrelated to pregnancy), the vast majority (89%) of which are completed laparoscopically.[1,2] Although laparoscopic tubal ligation is safe and effective, it requires general anesthesia and entry into the abdominal cavity, both of which are associated with rare but potentially serious complications.

Transcervical or hysteroscopic sterilization can offer patients an alternative option for permanent sterilization. Despite multiple efforts over the past 30 years, acceptable methods of transcervical permanent contraception have only recently been developed. Previous strategies for hysteroscopic sterilization have included mechanical tubal occlusive devices or plugs, intratubal or intrauterine sclerosing agents, and destruction of a portion of the fallopian tube with thermal energy.[3] Until recently, these attempts have been unsuccessful because of unacceptably high rates of pregnancy, ectopic pregnancy, expulsion of devices, infection, and perforation.

New hysteroscopic sterilization techniques offer effective permanent contraception without the discomfort, associated recovery time, and risks of a laparoscopic procedure with general anesthesia. Furthermore, hysteroscopic sterilization is an alternative for women in whom laparoscopy is especially difficult or contraindicated, such as women with severe cardiopulmonary disease, a history of prior abdominal or pelvic surgery with known extensive adhesions, or obesity.

Currently, there is only one hysteroscopic sterilization device approved by the U. S. Food and Drug Administration (FDA): Essure (Conceptus, San Carlos, CA). The Essure device has proved to be a highly effective permanent birth control option, with a low rate of associated adverse outcomes and high patient acceptance.[1,4–6] There are several other technologies currently undergoing initial clinical trials, including the Ovion system (American Medical Systems, Minnetonka, MN) and Adiana (Cytyc, Marlborough, MA).

ESSURE

Description and Mechanism of Action

The Essure system is the first hysteroscopic tubal sterilization device to be approved by the FDA, in 2002. Using a transvaginal approach, one micro-insert is placed in the proximal portion of each fallopian tube.[7] When the micro-insert is released, it expands and anchors itself in the fallopian tube. Over time, the micro-insert elicits a benign inflammatory response, which ultimately leads to tubal occlusion and permanent contraception.

As described in the package insert [7], the Essure micro-insert consists of a stainless steel inner coil and a nickel titanium (nitinol)-expanding outer coil. The inner coil attaches the device to the delivery wire that is used for placement of the device. The outer coil expands upon deployment and anchors the device in the fallopian tube. Polyethylene terephthalate (PET) fibers are wound in and around the inner coil. The PET fibers, which have been used in other medical devices, produce an immediate local inflammatory response characterized by macrophages, mononuclear cells, fibroblasts, foreign body giant cells, and plasma cells.[8,9] This inflammatory response peaks between 2 and 3 weeks and lasts approximately 10 weeks.[8,10] The resulting fibrosis causes occlusion of the fallopian tubes and results in permanent anchoring of the device and contraceptive effects.

During insertion, the micro-insert is maintained in the wound-down position through the use of a release catheter that is sheathed by a hydrophilic delivery catheter to help with tubal placement (Figure 8.5.1).[6] The outer coil expands from 4.0 cm in length and 0.8 mm in diameter in the wound-down position to 1.5 to 2.0 mm in diameter when released from the delivery wire, depending on the diameter and shape of the fallopian tube (Figure 8.5.2).[7]

Ideally, the micro-insert should span the uterotubal junction (UTJ), defined as the portion of the fallopian tube just as it exits the uterus (Figure 8.5.3). In this position, the springlike release of the device and expansion of the outer coil lead to anchoring during the acute phase of device implantation.[7] The PET fibers then elicit a chronic inflammatory and fibrotic response, leading to tissue ingrowth into the device and complete occlusion of the fallopian tube lumen, resulting in permanent retention of the micro-insert and the contraceptive effects.[9]

Clinical Use and Technique

There are several clinical considerations to keep in mind when performing an Essure placement. The Essure system is designed as an interval tubal sterilization technique. Therefore, the patient should be at least 6 weeks post delivery or termination.[7]

Ideally, the procedure should be timed with the patient's menstrual cycle. Insertion is recommended during the early proliferative phase of the menstrual cycle to improve visualization of the fallopian tube ostia and prevent placement in a luteal phase pregnancy.[7] Alternatively, the patient can be pretreated with oral contraceptive pills or Depo Provera (Pfizer) to help thin the endometrial lining and avoid placement in an undiagnosed pregnancy. As reported in a study by Kerin et al. [4], the time of the menstrual cycle during which the procedure was performed did not affect success rates of bilateral device placement. However, it

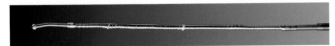

Figure 8.5.1. Essure micro-insert in wound-down configuration. The Essure micro-insert, when attached to the delivery wire in a wound-down configuration, is 4 cm in length and 0.8 mm in diameter. Used with permission from Conceptus.

was easier to see the tubal opening before ovulation, when the endometrial lining was thinner.[4]

Several measures should be taken to avoid placement during an undiagnosed pregnancy and to prevent unplanned pregnancy after insertion. First, a pregnancy test should be performed within 24 hours before the procedure. The combination of a pregnancy test and placement of the device during the first half of the cycle should help avoid an undetected luteal phase pregnancy. Finally, the patient should be advised to use contraception for 3 months after the procedure, until complete tubal occlusion and proper micro-insert placement can be verified by a hysterosalpingogram.[7]

Essure placement can be performed in the office or as outpatient surgery. The majority of these procedures can be performed with local anesthesia alone.[4,5,11] In a recent multicenter study of more than 100 women, 81% underwent the procedure with local paracervical block without additional intravenous sedation and tolerated the procedure well.[11] It is the decision of the patient and provider whether to use anesthesia, such as intravenous conscious sedation, in addition to a paracervical block. If only a paracervical block is used, an oral anxiolytic may be administered to the patient before the procedure. Our preferred technique for paracervical block involves injecting a total of 20 mL of 1% lidocaine without epinephrine, with 10 mL each at the 4 and 8 o'clock positions.[12] After the paracervical block is performed, it is important to wait several minutes before starting the procedure to give enough time for the anesthetic to take effect.

Regardless of the anesthetic choice, a nonsteroidal anti-inflammatory drug (NSAID) should be given 30 to 60 minutes before the procedure. Not only does this provide additional pain relief, but administration of NSAIDs before the procedure also increases the chance of successful cannulation of the fallopian tube and placement of the micro-inserts.[5] It is thought that preprocedural NSAIDs decrease the chance of tubal spasm, thus increasing the rate of successful placement.

To perform the insertion of the micro-inserts, the patient is placed in the semidorsal lithotomy position, using the exam table stirrups if the procedure is performed in the office. An open-sided speculum is placed in the vagina, the cervix is prepped with Betadine, and a paracervical block is performed. The micro-inserts are placed using the Essure delivery system through a small-caliber hysteroscope (usually 5-mm outer diameter) with

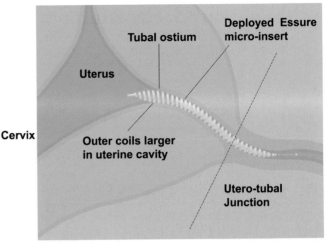

Figure 8.5.3. Diagram of the UTJ. The micro-insert should span the UTJ, defined as the portion of the fallopian tube just as it exits the uterus. In this location, the coils span the intramural and proximal isthmic portions of the fallopian tube. The device is placed far enough into the tube to prevent expulsion during uterine contractions during menses but still has a portion trailing into the uterine cavity. The outer diameter of the coils that trail into the uterus is larger than that of the coils in the fallopian tube, which helps anchor the device. The UTJ is most consistently the narrowest portion of the fallopian tube, which further aids in anchoring the device. Used with permission from Conceptus.

a continuous-flow system and an operating channel of at least 5F (1.7-mm internal diameter) (Figure 8.5.4). The hysteroscope is placed under direct visualization through the cervix and into the uterine cavity without prior cervical dilation. Normal saline is used during placement of the hysteroscope to aid in visualization as well as to gently dilate the cervical canal and uterus. An initial attempt to pass the hysteroscope may be made without the use of a tenaculum. If the hysteroscope is not passed easily, a tenaculum is placed to aid in the insertion, and if needed, cervical dilation may be performed.

Normal saline is used to distend the uterine cavity. Saline that is body temperature and introduced "under gravity" is recommended to help minimize patient discomfort. To achieve adequate distention, the saline bag must be approximately 120 to 140 cm above the uterus. Pressure bags may also be used to help maintain uterine distention if there is cervical leakage due to a patulous cervix.[7] Both tubal ostia should be visualized before placement of the device. A 12° or 30° hysteroscope may be used to help with visualization of the ostia as well as with cannulation of the fallopian tube (Figure 8.5.5). The 12° scope is helpful in cases of more-forward tubal ostia and in placement of the device,

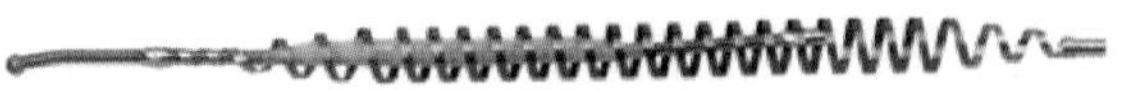

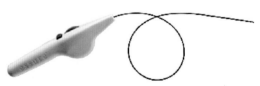

Figure 8.5.2. Expanded Essure device. The Essure micro-insert expands to a diameter of 1.5 to 2 mm, depending on the diameter and shape of the surrounding fallopian tube. Used with permission from Conceptus.

Figure 8.5.4. The Essure delivery system and hysteroscopic equipment. The Essure delivery system with the micro-insert attached to the delivery catheter. Used with permission from Conceptus.

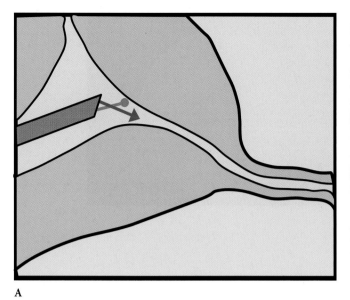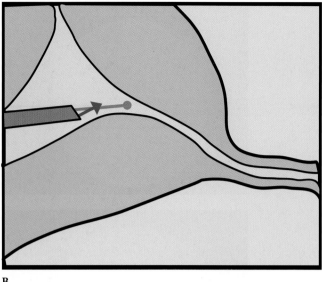

A   B

Figure 8.5.5. Use of a 30° hysteroscope lens can help with visualization or placement of the device. (**A**) Diagram of a 30° scope to help visualize ostia. By facing the lens of the 30° hysteroscope toward the ostia, the tubal ostia can be better visualized because of the optics. However, in this situation, the device protrudes through the operative channel parallel to the hysteroscope shaft, which may make placement more difficult. (**B**) Diagram of the scope turned the other way to help with placement. If the provider is having difficulty with placement of the device, the 30° hysteroscope can be turned to face away from the tubal ostia. This makes visualization of the ostia more difficult and often requires a more exaggerated angle to obtain visualization of the tubal opening. However, with this position, the delivery device exits the operative channel at an angle that can make entry into the tubal opening easier. *Blue arrow*, line of visualization through the 30° degree hysteroscope; *red ball*, path of the Essure delivery device after exiting the hysteroscope operative channel.

which exits the working channel at 0°. The 30° lens may help if the tubal ostia are at a difficult acute lateral angle. Once both ostia have been identified, the one that looks easier should be cannulated first, which will help prevent the endometrium from becoming edematous and obscuring the tubal ostium while the more difficult side is being cannulated.

The Essure delivery system is then passed though the introducer and down the working channel of the hysteroscope. With the tubal ostia in view, the Essure delivery system is advanced into the proximal fallopian tube with constant, gentle forward pressure, which helps prevent tubal spasm. When the black marker on the delivery catheter is at the ostia, the insert is in the ideal position spanning the intramural and proximal isthmic segments of the fallopian tube (Figure 8.5.6A). The micro-insert is now ready to be deployed. It is important that the handle of the delivery device is stabilized against the hysteroscope during retraction of the delivery catheter to prevent forward movement and displacement of the micro-insert. To deploy the insert, the thumbwheel on the Essure handle is rotated at one click per second, retracting the delivery catheter and exposing the wound-down micro-insert and its orange attachment to the delivery catheter (Figure 8.5.6B). Approximately 1 cm of the micro-insert's wound-down coils should be visible in the endometrial cavity; to confirm proper placement, the small notch in the wound-down insert should be located just outside the tubal ostium (Figure 8.5.6C). Once placement is verified, the button on the handle is depressed, enabling the thumbwheel to be further rotated. When the thumbwheel cannot be rotated any further, the withdrawal of the orange release catheter is complete, allowing the micro-insert to expand. Approximately 10 seconds are allowed for the outer coils to fully expand. With as few rotations as possible, the handle is rotated

counterclockwise until the delivery catheter has visibly disengaged from the micro-insert, and the delivery system is gently withdrawn from the insert.[7]

Once the delivery system has been withdrawn, the position of the micro-insert should be examined. Ideally, three to eight expanded outer coils should be trailing in the endometrial cavity (Figure 8.5.6C). If there are 18 or more coils seen in the endometrial cavity, the device should be removed; if fewer than 18 coils are identified in the cavity, the device should be left in place.[7] The procedure is then repeated on the contralateral side.

Essure placement is a relatively quick procedure to perform. During the pivotal, phase III trials, the mean hysteroscopy time was 13 minutes.[5] In this study, the procedure time decreased rapidly over the first five cases performed by a provider and slowly thereafter.[5] Since the pivotal trial, other studies have demonstrated even shorter average procedure times, ranging from 8 to 9 minutes.[11,13] In a study done by an independent group in Spain, the mean time for the procedure was 9 minutes; however, in the last 35 procedures (out of 85 total), the mean procedure time decreased to 4 minutes.[13]

Histologic Studies

To evaluate the histologic response to the Essure micro-inserts, a prehysterectomy study was performed. The Essure micro-inserts were placed in 33 women who subsequently underwent a hysterectomy between 24 hours and 12 weeks after device placement.[9]

The tissue response varied depending on the time elapsed since device placement. Initially, there was predominantly acute inflammation, followed by low-level chronic inflammation and

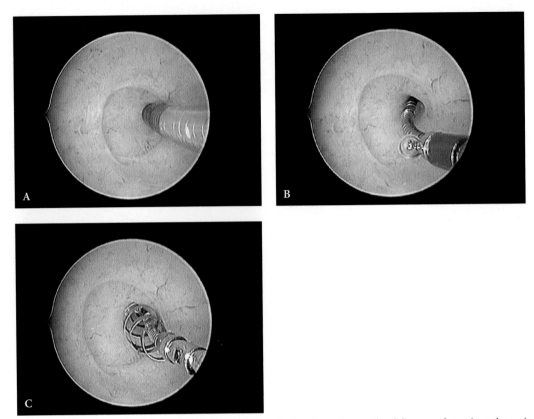

Figure 8.5.6. Steps for correct placement of the micro-insert. (**A**) When the black marker on the delivery catheter is at the ostia, the insert is in the ideal position spanning the intramural and proximal isthmic segments of the fallopian tube. (**B**) After retracting the delivery catheter and exposing the wound-down micro-insert, the orange attachment to the delivery catheter can be identified. To confirm proper placement, the small notch in the wound-down insert should be located just outside the tubal ostium before completing the deployment of the device. (**C**) Ideally, three to eight expanded outer coils should be trailing in the endometrial cavity. Here four coils are seen.

fibrosis (Figure 8.5.7).[9] The PET fibers elicited a strong fibrotic and inflammatory tissue response that extended into the space between the inner and outer coils of the micro-insert. The reaction was localized to the inner portion of the fallopian tube wall without evidence of fibrosis extending into the wall of the tube, peritubal adhesions, or serositis. Additionally, there was histologically normal tubal architecture within 5 mm of the distal end of the micro-insert.[9]

Rate of Bilateral Micro-insert Placement and Tubal Occlusion

The goal of the Essure procedure is to achieve successful placement of bilateral micro-inserts, which results in bilateral tubal occlusion. There does not appear to be an obvious relationship between successful placement of Essure micro-inserts and parity, obesity, history of prior surgery, mode of prior obstetric delivery (vaginal delivery or cesarean section), or time in the menstrual cycle during which the procedure was performed.[5,6] NSAIDs given before the procedure have been demonstrated to increase placement success rates.[5] According to one multicenter trial, placement success rates did not improve substantially in relation to increased surgeon experience with the device.[5] Depending on the study cited, successful bilateral placement rates range from 85% to 98%.[4–6,11,13] At 3 months after the procedure, HSG should be done to confirm correct device location and bilateral

tubal occlusion. Bilateral tubal occlusion rates have been reported to be between 96% and 99% in patients with successful bilateral placement.[4–6,11]

Failure of placement is often the result of tubal factors leading to increased resistance to advancement of the delivery catheter and micro-insert. If one micro-insert is placed and the contralateral one cannot be placed, the patient may undergo HSG. If the tube in which placement failed is patent, a repeat attempt at placement may be offered. If the tube is blocked, placement should not be attempted. If bilateral placement of the micro-inserts cannot be achieved, the patient is still a candidate for laparoscopic sterilization, or may consider vasectomy for her partner.

In the phase I clinical trial for Essure, 130 women between the ages of 21 and 43 seeking permanent birth control underwent device placement attempts at a single center.[6] Of these patients, 85% had successful placement of both micro-inserts and 3.6% had the micro-inserts in an unacceptable position on subsequent HSG; 98% of women with satisfactory placement of the micro-inserts had bilateral tubal occlusion demonstrated by HSG at 3 months (Figure 8.5.8).[6] Two women (2%) were found to have a small leakage past a correctly positioned micro-insert; on repeat HSG 3 months later, both had complete bilateral tubal occlusion.[6]

A multicenter phase II clinical trial revealed that 200 (88%) of the 227 women in whom the procedure was attempted had successful placement of bilateral devices.[4] Anatomic reasons, such

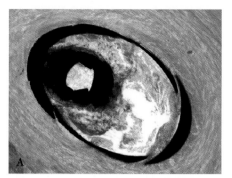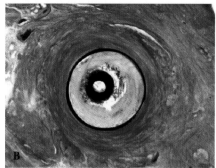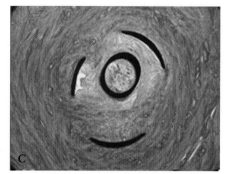

Figure 8.5.7. Histologic findings after Essure placement. (**A**) At 1 week, fibrosis and acute inflammatory cells can be seen infiltrating the device. (**B**) Four weeks after placement, both acute and chronic inflammatory cells are present and fibrosis is beginning to occlude the lumen. (**C**) At 10 weeks, dense fibrosis is filling the tubal lumen. Used with permission of Conceptus.

as tortuous variants of tubal anatomy, tubal spasm, occlusion, and stenosis, accounted for 48% of all placement failures. Procedure failures, such as the inability to cannulate or advance the catheter for unknown reasons, and device-related failure accounted for 22% and 19% of all placement failures, respectively. Of the 200 women with successful bilateral device placement, HSG 3 months after the initial procedure confirmed correct device placement in 191 patients (96%). Bilateral tubal occlusion was noted in 191 women (96%). Of the nine women who had evidence of dye passage past the micro-insert, seven had repeat HSG in 3 months that revealed bilateral tubal occlusion. Two women did not undergo repeat HSG; one patient expelled the device and the other had the device placed in the myometrium. Thus, 99% of the women with correct bilateral placement developed tubal occlusion and could rely on it for contraception by 6 months after placement. Four of the women with unsatisfactory device placement as iden-tified by HSG had bilateral tubal occlusion and thus could rely on these devices for contraception despite unsatisfactory placement as noted on HSG.

In a phase III multicenter clinical trial, 507 of the 518 women enrolled underwent an attempt at bilateral device placement.[5] In 11 women, micro-insert placement was not attempted because of endometrium or uterine polyps blocking the ostia, inability to visualize the ostia, or cervical stenosis. Bilateral placement of the micro-inserts was successful in 464 of the 507 women (92%); this was accomplished in one procedure in 446 women and in two procedures in 18 women. Of the remaining 8% of women with bilateral tubes in which bilateral placement was not achieved, most of the failures were attributed to anatomic abnormalities. Of the women with successful bilateral inserts, 96% had satisfac-torily located inserts on HSG and 92% had bilateral tubal occlu-sion. Repeat HSG in 3 more months (total of 6 months after the initial procedure) revealed bilateral occlusion in the women who had correct placement of the micro-inserts but not com-plete tubal occlusion at 3 months on HSG. Thus, ultimately, 98% of the women with successful bilateral micro-insert placement were found to have bilateral tubal occlusion. Overall, 89% of the women in whom micro-insert placement was attempted could rely on the device.

To overcome difficulty with cannulating tubes with anatomic abnormalities, Conceptus developed a new coil catheter to help cannulate areas of increased resistance.[11] The new design includes a hydrophilic coating, an improved flexible tip, a stream-lined profile, and proximal pushability. With this new delivery catheter, there was a 98% successful bilateral micro-insert place-ment rate; 99% of the patients who had successful bilateral device placement had complete tubal occlusion at 3 months on HSG.[11]

Given the high rate of tubal occlusion after correct bilateral placement of the Essure micro-inserts, eventually the 3-month postprocedure HSG may not be needed. This may help expand the use of hysteroscopic sterilization into communities and countries where resources and access to health care are limited or unavail-able. In other countries, such as Australia, the current recommen-dation by Conceptus is to check the location of the micro-inserts by an abdominal radiograph at 3 months post placement. Several studies support the use of ultrasound as a reliable method to con-firm micro-insert placement 3 months post procedure.[14,15] Ultrasound could verify micro-insert placement and possibly confirm tubal occlusion with the development of new echogenic contrast media.

Figure 8.5.8. Hysterosalpingogram 3 months after placement of Essure micro-inserts. HSG is performed 3 months post procedure to evaluate micro-insert location and bilateral tubal occlusion. On this radiograph, bilateral tubal occlusion is demonstrated.

Pregnancy Rates

In women who have had successful placement of the Essure device and a 3-month postprocedure hysterosalpingogram demonstrating bilateral tubal occlusion, there have been no reported intrauterine or ectopic pregnancies.[4–6] This 100% 1-year and 2-year effectiveness rate is encouraging. However long-term follow-up is needed and data are still being collected. It is important to note that although the contraceptive efficacy is extremely high if successful placement of the bilateral micro-inserts is achieved, a portion of the patients undergoing this procedure (2% to 15%) will not achieve successful bilateral placement and thus will need to use an alternative form of birth control.[4–6,11,13]

Patient Tolerance and Adverse Events

Overall, the placement of the Essure micro-inserts is well tolerated by patients and is associated with a low complication rate.[4,6,9,13] Patient satisfaction has been extremely high.[4,13] Patients have had rapid return to normal function, which was achieved by 60% of women within 1 day and by more than 75% of the women by day 2 after the procedure.[5] Discomfort and bleeding were two commonly associated symptoms.

In a large trial of more than 500 women, 65% of the study participants rated the pain as either mild or none during the procedure.[5] By discharge, 79% of the women rated the pain as either mild or none.[5] In women who reported postprocedure discomfort or pain, the pain was most commonly described as similar to menstrual cramps. Postprocedural pain resolved within 1 day, 3 days, and 1 week for 59%, 88%, and 99% of patients, respectively.[4]

Bleeding and spotting were also commonly associated symptoms. In one study, mild postprocedural spotting was noted in 34% of patients, but bleeding abated within 1 week for all patients.[9] Similarly, in the multicenter phase II clinical trials, 83% of women who had a device placed reported some bleeding after the procedure; almost all the patients (96%) stopped bleeding within 1 week.[4] The mean bleeding time was noted to be 3 days.[5]

The risk of other adverse outcomes, such as perforation, is quite low. The perforation risk has been reported to be around 1%.[4,5,11] In the first multicenter phase II clinical trial, there were six (3%) reported perforations of the uterine wall or tubal lumen. In four of these cases, the perforation was thought to be the result of a support catheter, which was subsequently discontinued. There were no significant complications from the perforations and no evidence of damage to the uterus or fallopian tubes, inflammation, or adhesion formation in the four patients who underwent a subsequent laparoscopic sterilization. In the phase III trials, an adverse outcome rate of 4.5% was reported.[5] More than two thirds of these "adverse outcomes" were the result of micro-insert expulsion. The perforation rate was 1%, with no clinical adverse events.

Other Considerations

Similar to any other sterilization procedure, the Essure micro-inserts cause permanent occlusion of the fallopian tubes. It is inevitable that some women who undergo the procedure will regret their decision later in life and wish to become pregnant. The only option for women who have undergone the Essure procedure is IVF. There is a theoretical concern that the portion of the device protruding into the uterine cavity could potentially interfere with implantation. Kerin et al. [4] argue that there is progressive tissue encapsulation of the device and that the device is made from inert, biocompatible materials, and thus the micro-insert is unlikely to interfere with embryo transfer and implantation. However, further studies will be needed to evaluate the impact of the Essure device on subsequent IVF.

OTHER PRODUCTS

Although Essure is the only FDA-approved hysteroscopic sterilization device, there are other products undergoing clinical trials for transcervical sterilization.

Ovion

At the time of this writing, the Ovion system has not been FDA-approved for use in the United States and is currently undergoing clinical trials. The Ovion system is 1 mm in outer diameter and can be placed through 3F working channels found in small rigid or flexible hysteroscopes (Figure 8.5.9A). The micro-insert is composed of a self-expanding nitinol frame embedded with PET fibers that support tissue ingrowth (Figure 8.5.9B). Similar to the Essure system, the nitinol frame acutely anchors the device in place, giving the PET fibers time to elicit the inflammatory response that leads to tissue ingrowth and subsequent tubal occlusion. The micro-insert is placed in the intramural portion of the fallopian tube. No portion of the device trails into the uterine cavity. Both micro-inserts are loaded into the delivery catheter at once, so they can be deployed one after the other without removal and replacement of the delivery catheter. Additionally, the micro-insert is released through a one-step push of a button once the correct location has been identified. This offers the benefit of

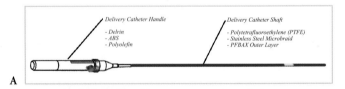

A

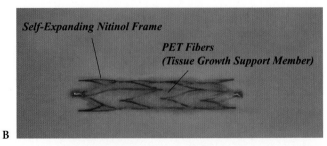

B

Figure 8.5.9. The Ovion system. (**A**) The Ovion system is 1 mm in outer diameter and can be placed through 3F working channels found in small rigid or flexible hysteroscopes. (**B**) The micro-insert is made up of a self-expanding nitinol frame embedded with PET fibers, which support tissue ingrowth.

a shorter procedure with fewer maneuvers. During the limited perihysterectomy studies, the procedure time was less than 5 minutes, with a successful placement rate of 94%.[16]

The Ovion system may have several potential advantages over the current available device. First, compatibility with the flexible hysteroscope allows for easier office use with less potential for patient discomfort and less need for anesthesia. In a small feasibility study, 14 of 15 women (93%) who had the Ovion system placed through a flexible hysteroscope did not require any anesthesia (local or intravenous). Additionally, the procedure may prove to be faster, given that both micro-inserts are loaded into the same delivery catheter and that the release mechanism involves only the push of a button. Finally, no portion of the device protrudes into the endometrial cavity. This could have potential benefits if pregnancy via IVF is desired later or if other hysteroscopic procedures, such as endometrial ablation, are desired at the time of or subsequent to device insertion.

Adiana

The Adiana transcervical sterilization system is currently undergoing clinical trials but is not yet approved by the FDA for clinical use at the time of this writing. This system uses a two-step approach to achieve tubal occlusion using an alternative technology.[17] First, a controlled thermal lesion is created with bipolar radiofrequency within the intramural portion of the fallopian tube. Next, a porous matrix about the size of a grain of rice is inserted within the tubal lumen, with no part protruding into the uterine cavity. The thermal injury to the endosalpinx removes the surface epithelium and stimulates healing, with ingrowth of healthy, vascularized tissue into the matrix pores. Tissue ingrowth both achieves occlusion of the tubal lumen and anchors the matrix.

The 5F catheter is placed down a continuous-flow hysteroscope that has a 6F working channel. An electrolyte-free distention medium is necessary for uterine distention. A black mark on the delivery catheter helps assure correct placement. Once the catheter is properly positioned, as indicated when the black marker is at the tubal ostia, the radiofrequency generator is activated. There is a position detection array and temperature sensors distal to the black mark to provide feedback to the generator as the tissues are heated (Figure 8.5.10). Once the tissue has been satisfactorily heated, the matrix is then released from the tip of the delivery catheter. Throughout the procedure, only the most proximal 12 mm are cannulated.[18] As the thermally damaged

fallopian tube heals, healthy, vascularized tissue grows into the porous matrix.

In one of the initial reports of the Adiana system, there was successful placement of the device in 94% of the 376 women undergoing attempt at placement.[19] In a more recent report of a multicenter trial of 500 women, there was a similar successful bilateral placement rate of 95%.[18] Of these 500 patients, 51% underwent the procedure with only local anesthesia; the remainder had additional sedation. The mean procedure time was 12 minutes. The pregnancy prevention rate was 99.7% at 1 year. There were no serious device-related adverse events noted.

CONCLUSION

Hysteroscopic sterilization offers patients an option for highly effective permanent contraception that avoids incisions and the need for general anesthesia and can be done in the office setting. It is well tolerated by the patient, affords rapid recovery and resumption of normal activities, and is associated with a low rate of adverse outcomes. Furthermore, hysteroscopic sterilization is a great alternative for women in whom laparoscopy is especially challenging and even contraindicated, such as those with obesity, severe cardiopulmonary disease, or a history of prior abdominal or pelvic surgery with known extensive adhesions.

REFERENCES

1. MacKay AP, Kieke BA Jr, Koonin LM, Beattie K. Tubal sterilization in the United States, 1994–1996. *Fam Plann Perspect.* 2001;33(4):161–165.
2. Westhoff C, Davis A. Tubal sterilization: focus on the U.S. experience. *Fertil Steril.* 2000;73(5):913–922.
3. Cooper JM. New approaches to hysteroscopic sterilization. *Contemp Ob Gyn.* 2003;48:8–20.
4. Kerin JF, Cooper JM, Price T, et al. Hysteroscopic sterilization using a micro-insert device: results of a multicentre phase II study. *Hum Reprod.* 2003;18:1223–1230.
5. Cooper JM, Carignan CS, Cher D, Kerin JF; Selective Tubal Occlusion Procedure 2000 Investigators Group. Microinsert nonincisional hysteroscopic sterilization. *Obstet Gynecol.* 2003;102(1):59–67.
6. Kerin JF, Carignan CS, Cher D. The safety and effectiveness of a new hysteroscopic method for permanent birth control: results of the first Essure pbc clinical study. *Aust N Z J Obstet Gynaecol.* 2001;41(4):364–370.
7. Essure [package insert]. San Carlos, CA: Conceptus Inc.; 2002.
8. Valle RF, van Herendael BJ. New indications for hysteroscopy: sterilization. In: van Herendael BJ, Valle R, Bettochi S, ed. *Ambulatory Hysteroscopy: Diagnosis and Treatment.* Chipping Norton, Oxfordshire, UK: Bladon Medical Publishing; 2004:143–151.
9. Valle RF, Carignan CS, Wright TC; STOP Prehysterectomy Investigation Group. Tissue response to the STOP microcoil transcervical permanent contraceptive device: results from a prehysterectomy study. *Fertil Steril.* 2001;76(5):974–980.
10. Estridge TD, Feldman DS. Quantification of vascular ingrowth into Dacron velour. *J Biomater Appl.* 1991;6(2):157–169.
11. Kerin JF, Munday DN, Ritossa MG, Pesce A, Rosen D. Essure hysteroscopic sterilization: results based on utilizing a new coil catheter delivery system. *J Am Assoc Gynecol Laparosc.* 2004;11(3):388–393.

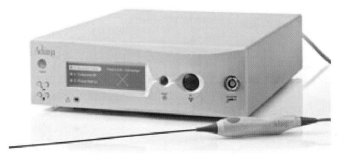

Figure 8.5.10. The Adiana system.

12. Glantz JC, Shomento S. Comparison of paracervical block techniques during first trimester pregnancy termination. *Int J Gynaecol Obstet.* 2001;72(2):171–178.

13. Ubeda A, Labastida R, Dexeus S. Essure: a new device for hysteroscopic tubal sterilization in an outpatient setting. *Fertil Steril.* 2004;82(1):196–199.

14. Kerin JF, Levy BS. Ultrasound: an effective method for localization of the echogenic Essure sterilization micro-insert: correlation with radiologic evaluations. *J Minim Invasive Gynecol.* 2005;12(1): 50–54.

15. Thiel JA, Suchet IB, Lortie K. Confirmation of Essure microinsert tubal coil placement with conventional and volume-contrast imaging three-dimensional ultrasound. *Fertil Steril.* 2005;84(2): 504–508.

16. Robles R, Isaacson K. Placement of a transcervical tubal occlusion device through a 3.5-mm O.D. flexible hysteroscope. *J Minim Invasive Gynecol.* 2005;12(5):S40.

17. Abbott J. Transcervical sterilization. *Best Pract Res Clin Obstet Gynaecol.* 2005;19(5):743–756.

18. Price T, Herbst S, Harris M, Prethus J, Anderson T, Garinger D. Permanent transcervical sterilization: the first 500 women treated in a multi-center trial. Presented at the American College of Obstetrics and Gynecology, 53rd Annual Meeting, San Francisco, CA, May 9–11, 2005.

19. Vancaillie T. Adiana hysteroscopic sterilization: interim results of the EASE clinical trial. Presented at the American Association of Gynecologic Laparoscopists Global Meeting; November 12, 2004; San Francisco, CA.

Section 8.6. Global Endometrial Ablation

Philip G. Brooks

In general, abnormal uterine bleeding has been recognized as a frequent and serious problem affecting women for hundreds of years. Its management has included attempts at destruction of the endometrium, especially for women who refuse hysterectomy or are poor candidates for major surgery. Previous methods of endometrial ablation included injection of sclerosing chemicals and drugs into the uterine cavity, delivery of ionizing radiation to the uterine cavity, and photoinactivation of the uterine lining, all of which were too toxic or too unsuccessful to be widely used. Prompted by the revolutionary miniaturization of hysteroscopes, the improvement in safety and effectiveness of distention media, and the successful development of cold light transmission, intrauterine exploration and surgical techniques developed rapidly and gave rise to investigation of ways to reduce the bleeding. The first breakthrough occurred in 1981 when Goldrath et al. [1] reported the development of hysteroscopically directed laser endometrial ablation, and the hope for effective, relatively safe, minimally invasive hysteroscopic ablation became reality.

This first technique used Nd:YAG laser energy delivered through the operative channel of the hysteroscope via a fiber. The results were very satisfactory, but because of the expense of the equipment and the fears of complications by less-skilled operators, the procedure was limited to a handful of well-trained hysteroscopists.

The next and most significant stimulus to the field of endometrial ablation for the conservative management of abnormal bleeding was the adaptation of the urologic resectoscope to gynecologic operative procedures. Hallez et al. [2], Neuwirth and Amin [3], and DeCherney and Polan [4] in the English-speaking literature and Lin [5] in the Japanese literature published reports on the successful management of such bleeding using electricity and resecting loops. As the number of cases accumulated, data presented to the U. S. Food and Drug Administration (FDA) were sufficient to warrant approval of the resectoscope for gynecologic indications in December 1989.[6] Subsequently, the lower cost, the equal effectiveness, and the greater ease of teaching and learning this technique resulted in the resectoscope becoming the gold standard for the management of abnormal uterine bleeding.

Despite intensive interest by both resectoscope manufacturers and teachers in training students and practicing physicians, the number of resectoscopic endometrial ablations grew slowly and the number of hysterectomies for abnormal uterine bleeding in the United States did not decrease. Complications due to electrical injuries of adjacent or adherent organs (bowel, bladder, or blood vessels) or due to excessive absorption (intravasation) of the sodium-free solutions required to complete these procedures have prompted the leaders in this field to seek other methods that ablate the endometrium and destroy the vascular supply to the underlying stroma in a more user-friendly, safe, and consistent manner.

The following text describes the new technologies approved by the FDA for endometrial ablation. Currently they include the Thermachoice (Gynecare), NovaSure (Cytyc), Cryogen HerOption™ (American Medical Systems), MEA (Microwave Endometrial Ablation, Microsulis Medical Limited), and HTA (HydroThermAblator, Boston Scientific) devices. FDA phase III studies required all these devices to be evaluated with standardized measuring of pre- and posttreatment blood loss, and to be compared with resectoscopic ablations in randomized, prospective trials. The presentation that follows attempts to describe the methodology, potential risks incurred in using the devices, complications reported to the FDA, and outcomes as reported to the FDA during the phase III studies and follow-up of the patients.

THERMACHOICE

Methodology

The Thermachoice system incorporates an intrauterine balloon (Figure 8.6.1) originally made of latex then changed to silicone to avoid the risk of latex allergy and to increase the pliability of the balloon to better conform to the configurations of the endometrial cavity and cornual areas. The balloon is inserted into the uterus via a 5-mm sheath. The balloon is then filled with saline solution, maintained at an intrauterine pressure of 160 to 180 mm Hg, and the liquid is heated to 87°C for 8 minutes.

Risk Factors

Because the device is inserted blindly into the endometrial cavity, there is a risk of partial or complete perforation of the uterus. A cavity integrity test, performed by injecting fluid through a channel in the inserter before heating the saline, attempts to avoid this risk. The device can be activated within a partial perforation of the uterine wall and with part of the balloon being in the cervical canal. The obvious fear of rupture of the balloons, with spill of hot saline into the vagina, has not been seen as the integrity of the balloons is tested before packaging. Through September 2004, 273 adverse events were reported to the MAUDE (Manufacturer and User Facility Device Experience) database of the FDA, including several deaths, 72 severe adverse events, and numerous bowel injuries.[7]

Outcomes

Thermachoice is the only device that has 5-year follow-up data: 23% of patients had amenorrhea, and overall success (as

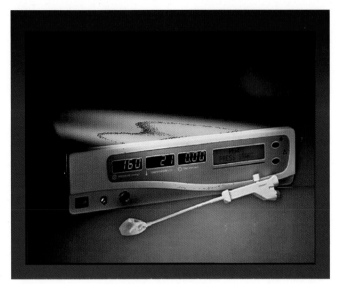

Figure 8.6.1. The Thermachoice™ system, showing console and disposable hand-piece with intrauterine balloon.

determined by menstrual scores and patient satisfaction, etc.) was reported as 68%. Hysterectomies were performed in 16% of the originally studied patients undergoing Thermachoice endometrial ablations, as noted in the 5-year follow-up report. The original FDA phase III studies required that all patients have a dilatation and curettage immediately before undergoing a Thermachoice endometrial ablation.

NOVASURE

Methodology

The NovaSure system is composed of an expandable wire mesh array (Figure 8.6.2) that is compressed into a 7.2-mm sheath when inserted into the uterus, then expands to fit the cavity. The semirigid mesh delivers bipolar electrical energy until electrical resistance (impedance) is complete, transmitting no more electrical energy through the electrically "dead" cells.

Risk Factors

Because the device also is inserted blindly into the endometrial cavity, there is a risk of partial or complete perforation of the uterus and a risk of extrusion or inadvertent placement into the upper cervical canal. A cavity integrity test, performed by injecting carbon dioxide through a channel in the sheath before activating the electricity, attempts to avoid this risk. Before activation, a negative pressure (suction) draws the uterine wall into closer apposition to the bipolar wand, and the negative pressure is maintained throughout the procedure. If the suction is broken (e.g., by an unrecognized perforation), the controller rapidly stops the flow of electricity. Despite these safety features, the FDA MAUDE database cites numerous serious adverse events, including bowel burns and uterine perforations. A recent modification to the system was instituted whereby once the system stops because of an alarm, the alarm and stoppage cannot be overridden. This modification was intended to prevent the alarm from being overridden, as occurred in the past, with very serious consequences.

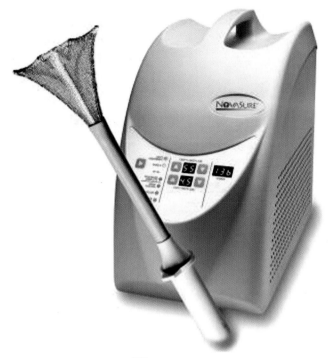

Figure 8.6.2. The NovaSure™ system showing console and disposable wand with expandable wire mesh array at distal end. (Courtesy of Cytyc Corporation and affiliates)

Unfortunately, according to the MAUDE database reports after the modification was instituted, there have been additional serious adverse events, including bowel burns.

Outcomes

Despite the number of complications reported to the FDA, NovaSure endometrial ablations are fast and effective. At the 24-month follow-up of the phase III study, amenorrhea was reported in 47% of patients, with a 92% satisfaction rate. The mean procedure time was 4.32 minutes, about one tenth as long as the resectoscopic ablation procedures. No pretreatment of the endometrium was required or provided in the FDA trials for this method.

CRYOGEN

Methodology

The Cryogen, or HerOption, system (Figure 8.6.3) uses a 5.5-mm metal-tipped probe inserted first into one cornu and then the other to deliver a liquid nitrogen coolant at −90°C to each area, generating a cytotoxic freeze zone. Treatment time is approximately 10 to 15 minutes, depending on the decision of the surgeon and the size of the uterine cavity. Requirements by the FDA include concomitant sonographic monitoring to ensure the uterine myometrial thickness is adequate to prevent transmural spread of damaging temperatures to adjacent or adherent bowel or bladder.

Risk Factors

In addition to the risk of inadvertent perforation due to blind insertion, the probe may be activated in a false passage or in

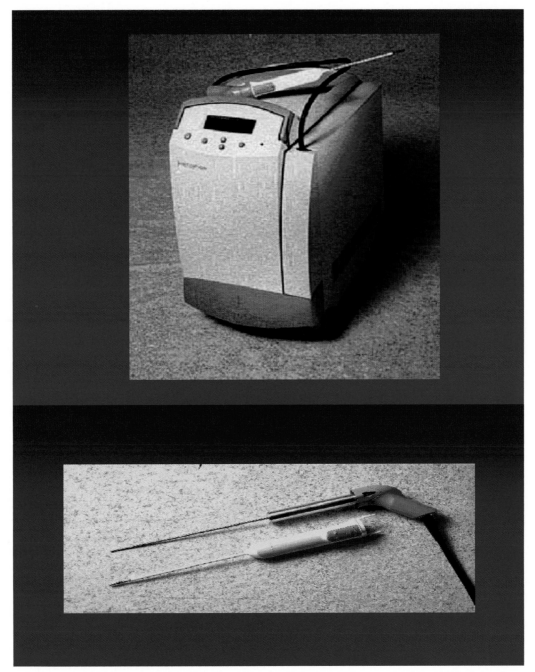

Figure 8.6.3. The Cryogen, or HerOption™, system, showing console (top) and disposable a 5.5-mm metal-tipped probe that is inserted into the uterus (bottom).

the endocervical canal. In addition, since 2002, despite a very small number of procedures performed in the United States, the MAUDE database has reported 11 serious adverse events, including six internal bowel injuries associated with the use of this device, some in the absence of documented uterine perforation.[7]

Outcomes

At 36 months, the amenorrhea rates are only 26% – among the lowest of all the global techniques. In addition, the hysterectomy and retreatment rates totaled 11%. Of special note is the fact that in the original 12-month FDA trial, over 25% of the procedures

had a mechanical failure at the time of the original procedure, resulting in the cancellation of the procedure or the need to open another kit.

MICROWAVE ENDOMETRIAL ABLATION

Methodology

The MEA system consists of a computerized controller and a 7-mm disposable probe (Figure 8.6.4) inserted blindly into the uterine cavity and then gradually withdrawn through the cavity with continued sweeping motions. The uterine temperature is monitored on a dial, and safety and efficacy are achieved by

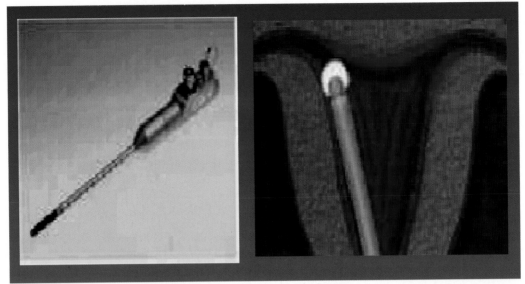

Figure 8.6.4. MEA™ system, showing a 7-mm disposable intrauterine probe, which is inserted and manipulated inside the uterine cavity (left), and the diagram of the action inside the uterus (right).

observing that the temperature remains in the prescribed zone. FDA phase III trials used GnRH agonists as pretreatment, but subsequent studies showed no difference in outcomes with or without pretreatment. The average treatment time is 11 minutes, including diagnostic hysteroscopy.

Risk Factors

Because the probe is inserted into the uterus and manipulated blindly, there are risks of perforation of the uterine wall and inadvertent damage to the endocervix. In addition, as a result of a number of bowel injuries in patients in whom no perforation was detected [7], the FDA approved the device with the mandate that uterine wall thickness must be ascertained by ultrasound before the procedure and diagnostic hysteroscopy must be performed after cervical dilatation but before the probe is placed inside the uterus.

Outcomes

Three-year results of the multicenter randomized FDA phase III trials demonstrated a very high amenorrhea rate.[8] Sixty percent of patients reported no menses, and overall success was reported to be 97%.

HYDROTHERMABLATOR

Methodology

The HTA system (Figure 8.6.5A) is the only system for global endometrial ablation that is performed under constant visualization – that is, it uses hysteroscopy to determine that the sheath is placed in the right spot and to make sure it stays there throughout the procedure. The telescope, any 3-mm hysteroscope, fits within a 7.8-mm polycarbonate sheath that allows the circulation of physiologic saline solution into the uterine cavity by gravity. The saline fluid bag is placed at a prescribed height to produce an intrauterine pressure to about 50 mm Hg. Initially the fluid is room temperature, and the computerized console monitors the volume to ascertain that a watertight seal exists. Once the computer confirms the seal, the operator activates the heating system and the fluid is heated to a temperature of 90°C for 10 minutes, resulting in the sealing of the vessels and the destruction of the surface epithelium. Because there is no rigid wand or confining balloon, the fluid can flow to all parts of the endometrial cavity, getting the destructive heat energy to a greater area than is achievable with probes, balloons, or wands. The original FDA study included preprocedure thinning of the endometrium with the use of an injectable GnRH agonist, Depo Lupron (TAP Pharmaceuticals), but recent reports confirm that this is unnecessary as it adds nothing to the success of the procedure in terms of control of the bleeding.

Risk Factors

Since the entire procedure is performed under direct visualization, the risk of perforation and internal organ damage is exceedingly low. The major risk appears to be the spill of hot saline into the vagina due to leakage through the cervix or from premature withdrawal of the sheath before adequate cooling of the liquid. Since 2002, the MAUDE database has reported only two internal injuries with the HTA procedure, one due to a known perforation – after which the procedure continued anyhow, against the manufacturer's instructions – and the other in a procedure wherein concomitant laparoscopy with intra-abdominal electrosurgery was performed, with no clear-cut definition as to which procedure caused the burn. A modification of the equipment recently was adopted by the manufacturer: the attachment of a tenaculum-stabilizing device (Figure 8.6.5B) that prevents inadvertent removal or slipping of the sheath through or out of the cervix before intended. Leakage of heated liquid through the oviducts has never been seen because intrauterine pressures is maintained at a level too low to overcome minimum cornual opening pressures.

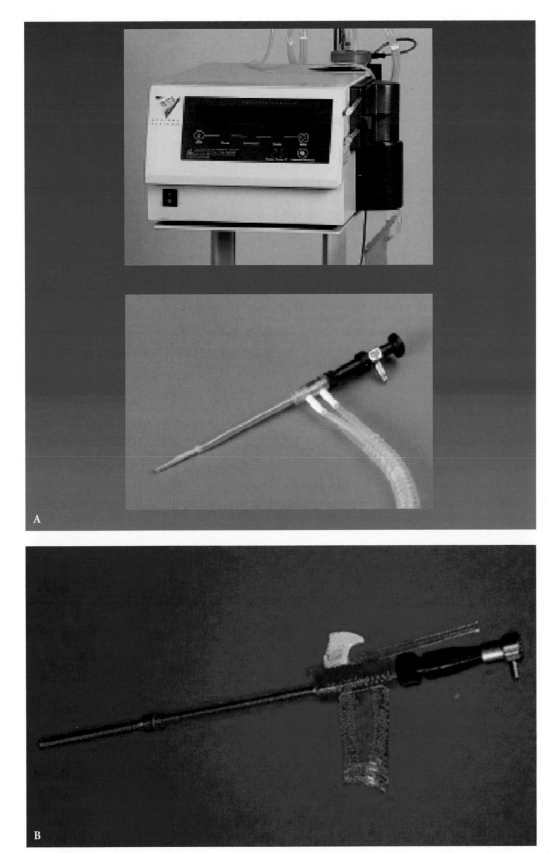

Figure 8.6.5. The HTA^{TM} system, showing the console (**A**, top) and the disposable sheath with a 3-mm hysteroscope attached (**A**, bottom); **B**. shows the new disposable sheath with the cervical stabilizer that reduces the risk of inadvertent withdrawal of sheath from uterus before cooling.

Outcomes

At 36 months, the amenorrhea rate for the patients in the FDA phase III trial was 53%. Success rate, as measured by patient satisfaction and reduction of bleeding, was reported to be 94%. Of interest are several reports describing the success of this system in the presence of submucous myomata, and the success of performing this procedure under local anesthesia.[9,10]

SUMMARY

As described above, there are five global ablation devices approved by the FDA for the management of abnormal uterine bleeding. Undoubtedly, more will be forthcoming, in an attempt to increase efficacy, improve outcomes, reduce the cost, and especially, improve safety. Regarding the latter, it should be obvious that the intent of all the devices is the destruction of the tissue that allows the excessive and unacceptable bleeding. If the destructive force is placed inadvertently in the wrong areas, there will be undesirable damage to tissue or organs not intended to be injured. There is ongoing development of the next generation of ablation devices that attempt to solve these problems in a faster, simpler, more consistent, and successful manner. It remains to be seen whether this will be accomplished.

Finally, there is a significant amount of effort being made to provide endometrial ablations as office procedures, using local instead of general anesthesia, thereby reducing one more area of increased cost and risk. Several studies have shown that pain from these procedures comes from high-pressure uterine distention and from movements and manipulations of devices inside the uterus. NovaSure and HTA are the only devices that do not distend the uterus under high pressures and are not manipulated inside the endometrial cavities during the active procedure. For many, the performance of the ablation blindly entertains too high a risk of perforation or partial uterine wall penetration, especially when performed as an office procedure. Only the HTA system is performed while viewing the cavity and the sheath placement hysteroscopically throughout the entire procedure.

Global endometrial ablation devices have been significantly and successfully added to the surgical armamentarium of practicing physicians for the management of abnormal uterine bleeding, in which hysterectomy for benign conditions can be safely avoided.

REFERENCES

1. Goldrath MH, Fuller T, Segal S. Laser photo vaporization of endometrium for the treatment of menorrhagia. *Am J Obstet Gynecol.* 1981;140:14–19.
2. Hallez JP, Netter A, Cartier R. Methodical intrauterine resection. *Am J Obstet Gynecol.* 1987;156:1080.
3. Neuwirth RS, Amin HK. Excision of submucous fibroids with hysteroscopic control. *Am J Obstet Gynecol.* 1983;131:95.
4. DeCherney A, Polan ML. Hysteroscopic management of intrauterine lesions and intractable uterine bleeding. *Obstet Gynecol.* 1983;61:392.
5. Lin B-L. The development of a new hysteroscopic resectoscope and its clinical applications for trans-cervical resection and endometrial ablation. *Jpn J Gynecol Obstet Endosc.* 1988;4:4–56.
6. Brooks PG, Loffer FD, Serden SP. Resectoscopic removal of symptomatic lesions. *J Reprod Med.* 1989;34:435.
7. U.S. Food and Drug Administration. MAUDE (Manufacturers and User Facility Device Experience) database. Available at: www.fda.gov/maude.
8. Harris M, Cooper JM. Microwave endometrial ablation: three-year outcomes of a multi-centered trial. *J Am Assoc Gynecol Laparosc.* 2005;12:125–128.
9. Glasser MH, Zimmerman JD. The HydroThermAblator system for management of menorrhagia in women with submucous myomas: 12- to 20-month follow-up. *J Am Assoc Gynecol Laparosc.* 2003;10:521–527.
10. Brooks PG. Endometrial ablation as an office procedure using local anesthesia. Presented at: American Association of Gynecologic Laparoscopists Annual Clinical Meeting; November 11, 2004; San Francisco, CA.

9 MANAGEMENT OF ADNEXAL MASSES
Section 9.1. The Adnexal Mass

Sophia Rothberger, Tanja Pejovic, and Farr Nezhat

The adnexa are in an anatomic region in the pelvis that includes the ovaries, the fallopian tubes, and the structures within the broad ligament. The differential diagnosis of an adnexal mass is complex because of the wide spectrum of disorders that involve the adnexa. Most frequently, adnexal masses involve the ovary itself because of its inherent growth properties through ovulation and thus its propensity for neoplasia.[1] During the evaluation of an adnexal mass, the picture may be further complicated as imaging does not always clearly delineate the adnexa from other nearby organs. An estimated 5% to 10% of women in the United States will undergo a surgical procedure for a suspected ovarian neoplasm during their lifetime.[2] Although the majority of adnexal masses are benign in nature, the primary goal of the diagnostic evaluation is the exclusion of malignancy.

ETIOLOGY

The differential diagnosis of the adnexal mass varies with age (Table 9.1.1). Age is also the most important factor in determining the potential for malignancy. In fact, the risk that an ovarian neoplasm is malignant increases 12-fold from ages 12 through 29 and 60 through 69.[3] Although there is emerging evidence that the presence of an adnexal mass in postmenopausal women is more common than once thought, masses found in premenarchal and postmenopausal women should be considered abnormal and must be promptly evaluated.

Premenarchal Patient

Because prepubertal girls are not under the influence of gonadotropic hormones, physiologic cysts are uncommon. Adnexal masses, therefore, have a higher rate of malignancy in girls than in women of reproductive age and require immediate surgical exploration. In the fetus and newborn, however, the influence of maternal hormones may cause follicular cysts. These regress on their own within 6 months of age.

Histologically, most prepubertal ovarian neoplasms are of germ cell origin. Abdominal pain is the most common presenting symptom and torsion is present in approximately 20% of cases. Ehren et al. [4] reported a series of 63 patients with ovarian tumors of different histology. The final diagnosis was benign teratoma in 65% of the cases. In 21% of the patients, the removed tumor was malignant. All patients younger than 12 years had germ cell tumors, whereas one patient, a 4-year-old girl, had an epithelial tumor. Appendicitis was the most common misdiagnosis. Rarer symptoms of adnexal mass include precocious puberty, hirsutism, urinary complaints, and primary or secondary amen-

orrhea. Other nongynecologic diagnoses may include Wilms' tumor, neuroblastomas, and gastrointestinal abnormalities.

Reproductive-Age Patient

The most common adnexal masses in reproductive-age women are benign functional cysts of the ovaries. These include follicular cysts, corpus luteum cysts, theca lutein cysts, and polycystic ovaries. Functional ovarian cysts are usually asymptomatic and tend to resolve spontaneously in 4 to 6 weeks. Occasionally they may be accompanied by some degree of pelvic discomfort, pain, or dyspareunia. In addition, the rupture of one of these cysts leads to peritoneal irritation and possibly hemoperitoneum. A functional cyst may also be complicated by torsion, resulting in severe pain. Other benign conditions include endometriosis (with ovarian endometriotic cysts), inflammatory enlargement of the fallopian tubes and ovaries (hydrosalpinges, tubo-ovarian abscess) due to pelvic infection, ectopic pregnancy, and trophoblastic disease.

Leiomyomata are common benign tumors of smooth muscle origin. They are found on 80% of surgically excised uteri and most frequently occur on the uterus and cervix; however, they may also be found on the broad ligament. Fibroids may resemble a suspicious ovarian mass on imaging when pedunculating into the posterior cul-de-sac or degenerated.

True benign ovarian neoplasms could also cause adnexal enlargement. These include most frequently serous or mucinous cystadenomas and benign cystic teratomas (Table 9.1.2). Cystic teratomas make up 70% of benign neoplasms in women younger than 30 and are made of the three germ cell layers. Mucinous and serous cystadenomas are usually multiloculated, with thin walls. It is unclear whether these are precursors of malignant neoplasms, although some changes may represent true ovarian intraepithelial neoplasia.

Other neoplastic processes include paraovarian cysts and ovarian and fallopian tube cancers. In certain instances, the mass is clinically indeterminate and may be the result of nongynecologic causes, such as full bladder, stool in the colon, distended cecum, peritoneal cyst, appendiceal abscess, diverticular abscess, Crohn's disease, ectopic kidney, urachal cyst, abdominal wall tumor, lymphoma, retroperitoneal sarcoma, metastatic tumor to the ovaries, and malignant diseases of the gastrointestinal system (Table 9.1.1).

Postmenopausal Patient

Any enlargement of the ovary is abnormal in the postmenopausal women and should be considered malignant until proven otherwise. The postmenopausal ovary atrophies to $1.5 \times 1.0 \times 0.5$ cm

Table 9.1.1: Differential Diagnosis of Adnexal Mass

Organ	Cystic	Solid

Ovary	Functional cyst
	Endometriosis
	Cystic neoplasm
	  Benign
	  Malignant
		Benign
		Malignant

Fallopian tube	Tubo-ovarian abscess or hydrosalpinx Paratubal cyst	Ectopic pregnancy Tubo-ovarian abscess Neoplasm
Uterus	Intrauterine pregnancy	Myoma
Bowel	Distended colon with gas and/or feces	Appendicitis Diverticulitis Diverticular abscess Colon cancer
Other	Distended bladder	Abdominal wall hematoma or abscess Pelvic kidney Retroperitoneal neoplasm

Table 9.1.2: Benign Ovarian Tumors

Non-neoplastic tumors
  Inclusion cyst
  Follicular cyst
  Corpus luteum cyst
  Pregnancy luteoma
  Theca lutein cyst
  Endometrioma

Neoplasm arising from the surface epithelium of the ovary
  Serous cystadenoma
  Mucinous cystadenoma
  Mixed forms

Neoplasms of stromal origin
  Fibroma (Meigs' syndrome*)
  Brenner tumor

Germ cell tumors
  Dermoid tumor (mature cystic teratoma)

* Meigs' syndrome: presence of ovarian fibroma and right-sided pleural effusion.

in size and should not be palpable on pelvic examination. Ovaries that are palpable must alert the physician to possible malignancy. The risk of malignancy in this age group is increased from 13% in premenopausal to 45% in postmenopausal women.[2] Still, 55% of postmenopausal women with palpable ovaries do have a benign tumor.

The most common ovarian tumors in this age group include epithelial ovarian tumors followed by stromal tumors and sex cord tumors. These are usually asymptomatic and diagnosed at late stages. Fallopian tube carcinoma is generally asymptomatic and may be found incidentally or at late stage of progression. Patients may experience a clear, watery discharge. Imaging may show a thickened tubular structure.

Table 9.1.3: Clinical Signs of a Malignant versus Benign Adnexal Mass

Malignant	Benign
Prepubertal or postmenopausal	Reproductive age
Personal history of nongynecologic cancer	
Family history of ovarian, breast, or colon cancer	
Rapid growth	No growth
Ascites	No ascites
Fixed	Mobile
Nodularity of rectovaginal septum	Smooth rectovaginal septum
Bilateral	Unilateral
Solid or complex	Cystic
Irregular	Smooth

Simple cysts are more common than once thought in this age group. Although devoid of gonadotropic stimulation, studies show that simple cysts exist in postmenopausal women. One Norwegian autopsy study by Dorum et al. [5] examined the adnexa of 234 postmenopausal women who died of nongynecologic causes, and 15% had ovarian cysts and 5% had paraovarian cysts. One cyst was a borderline cystadenoma and the rest were benign. Other studies have shown that the prevalence of asymptomatic simple cysts on ultrasound in postmenopausal women ranges from 3% to 15%.[6]

CLINICAL PRESENTATION AND EVALUATION

History and Physical Exam

Surgical exploration is the gold standard for diagnosis; however, much can be discerned about the diagnosis of an adnexal mass from a careful history, exam, and imaging. The majority of patients present with symptoms related to compression of the local pelvic organs due to the adnexal mass. Less commonly, an ovarian mass is discovered during a routine pelvic examination in an asymptomatic patient.

Once a mass is identified, onset and quality of pain, demographic considerations, menstrual associations, and bowel and bladder involvement may help develop an index of suspicion (Table 9.1.3). Patients with a personal or family history of colon, ovarian, or breast cancer are at higher risk for malignancy than others. The BRCA-1 and BRCA-2 genes are two of the known hereditary links for ovarian cancer, and testing is available.

In several surgical series, the reported incidence of ovarian malignancy in patients with a preoperative diagnosis of an ovarian mass ranged from 13% to 21%. In patients with a malignant process, the most common clinical symptom is abdominal discomfort due to ascites. Family and personal history raise the index of suspicion for cancer, and as previously mentioned, the most important predictor of malignancy is the age of the patient. However, even in postmenopausal women, the majority of adnexal masses (55%) are benign.[7]

The physical examination should include an abdominal, pelvic, rectovaginal, breast, and lymph node examination (Table 9.1.3). Although physical exam can identify new masses and help localize and characterize known masses, examination alone is often inaccurate in determining whether an adnexal mass is benign or malignant. Associated findings of disseminated disease help improve the accuracy of diagnosis. Imaging studies including ultrasound and/or computed tomography (CT) scans are usually required for further evaluation.

The Role of Pelvic Imaging

Pelvic ultrasound is currently the most useful technique for the diagnostic evaluation of an adnexal mass. Simple physiologic cysts, teratomas, and endometriomas have characteristic appearances on ultrasound and significantly lower the concern for malignancy when identified. The significant parameters for an ultrasonographic evaluation of the adnexal mass are the size, number of loculi, overall echo density, presence of septations with flow within, and presence of papillary or solid excrescences or nodules within the mass. There are no universally accepted criteria for the sonographic description of ovarian disease. However, the findings that suggest malignancy include size larger than 6 cm in postmenopausal women and larger than 8 cm in premenopausal women, presence of thick septations, papillary projections within the lumen of the cyst, complexity (cystic and solid areas) of the mass, and presence of nodules within the wall.

Various ultrasound techniques are available. Transvaginal ultrasound provides better resolution of the adnexa than does abdominal ultrasound.[8] Although most comparison studies have found gray-scale sonography to be superior to Doppler sonography, or that Doppler offers no significant improvement over gray-scale sonography, a minority of studies report Doppler features to be superior. Most authors prefer pulsatility index (PI) as a standard and consider a PI of 1.0 or less to be suggestive of malignancy; however, some authors use resistance index (RI), with values greater than 0.4 to 0.7 as indicators of malignancy.

A seminal work by Sassone et al. (1991) [9] evaluated an ultrasound scoring system to predict ovarian malignancy. Transvaginal sonographic pelvic images of 143 patients were correlated with surgicopathologic findings. The variables in the scoring system included the inner wall structure of the adnexal cyst, wall thickness, presence and thickness of septa, and echogenicity. The scoring system was useful in distinguishing benign from malignant masses, with a specificity of 83%, sensitivity of 100%, and positive and negative predictive values of 37% and 100%, respectively. Subsequently, Alcazar and Jurado [10] developed a logistic model to predict malignancy based on menopausal status, ultrasound morphology, and color Doppler findings in 79 adnexal masses. The authors derived a mathematical formula to estimate preoperatively the risk of malignancy (or benignity) of a given adnexal mass in a simple and reproducible way. When this formula was applied prospectively, 56 of 58 (96.5%) of adnexal masses were correctly classified. Although following a model would make management decisions more concrete, most clinicians base their decisions on the full clinical picture.

In general, CT is not routinely indicated for the evaluation of the adnexal mass, as it is not sensitive to lesions less than 2 cm in size. It is, therefore, not a good tool for the early detection of ovarian cancer. However, in cases in which malignancy is suspected, a CT scan may be used to further evaluate a patient with a hard fixed lateralized mass, ascites, abnormal liver function tests, or palpable abdominopelvic mass.

Magnetic resonance imaging (MRI) does not use ionizing radiation; therefore, it is useful in the evaluation of adnexal masses in pregnancy. It is also useful in further evaluation of adnexal masses detected by ultrasound and characterized as "intermediate" in nature. Grab et al. [11] investigated the accuracy of sonography versus MRI and positron emission tomography (PET) in 101 patients with asymptomatic adnexal masses detected who subsequently underwent laparoscopy. Ultrasonography established the correct diagnosis in 11 of the 12 ovarian malignancies (sensitivity, 92%), but the specificity was only 60%. With MRI and PET, specificity improved to 84% and 89%, but sensitivity declined. When all modalities were combined, specificity was 85%, sensitivity 92%, and accuracy 86%. However, because a negative MRI or PET does not rule out early ovarian cancer or borderline malignancy, ultrasound remains the most important tool in the evaluation of the adnexal mass.

Laboratory Studies

The most helpful laboratory studies in the evaluation of adnexal masses are the quantitative beta-human chorionic gonadotropin (β-hCG), complete blood count (CBC) with differential, and in selected cases, tumor markers. The quantitative β-hCG is essential in ruling out ectopic pregnancy. A CBC with differential is necessary when an infectious case is suspected. Serum tumor markers for malignant germ cell tumors, lactic dehydrogenase (LDH), β-hCG, and alpha-fetoprotein (AFP) should be obtained in the young patient with a cystic-solid or solid adnexal mass to evaluate the risk of a germ cell tumor (Table 9.1.4). A serum CA-125 level and carcinoembryonic antigen should also be obtained in patients with suspected gynecologic or gastrointestinal cancers respectively.

Although tempting, using CA-125 outside its clinical indications may cloud rather than clarify the differential diagnosis. CA-125 is elevated to levels greater than normal (35 IU/mL) in about 1% of healthy individuals. Also, in premenopausal women, CA-125 is elevated in a variety of benign conditions, including myoma, adenomyosis, benign ovarian tumors, pelvic inflammatory disease, liver disease, endometriosis, peritonitis, and pleural effusions. Normal pregnancy elevates CA-125 above normal, and hypothyroidism is associated with a slight elevation in CA-125. Serum CA-125 is elevated in 80% of all patients with serous

Table 9.1.4: Tumor Markers in Ovarian Neoplasms

Neoplasm	Marker
Epithelial ovarian cancer	CA-125
Mucinous epithelial ovarian tumors	CA-19-9
Dysgerminoma	LDH
Endodermal sinus tumor	AFP
Choriocarcinoma, placental site trophoblastic tumor	hCG, human placental lactogen
Granulosa cell tumor	Inhibin A

carcinoma of the ovary, but in only half of patients with stage I disease, making it a poor screening tool for detection of ovarian cancer.[12] As a diagnostic aid, CA-125 is most useful in post-menopausal women with a suspicious pelvic mass on ultrasound. In that subgroup of patients, a level greater that 65 IU/mL has been shown to have a positive predictive value of 97%.[13] The most reliable use of CA-125 is in the evaluation of patients with ovarian cancer to monitor treatment response or disease progression.[14]

MANAGEMENT

Indications for Surgery

The crucial decision regarding management of the reproductive-age woman with an adnexal mass is to observe the patient or proceed with surgical removal of the mass. Surgical removal of an adnexal mass is indicated when there is suspicion of malignancy, suspicion of torsion, or severe pain.[15] Surgical approach by laparotomy versus laparoscopy becomes the second question (Table 9.1.5).

Size may be an indication for removal because size is directly proportional to risk for malignancy and ovarian torsion. Simple cystic adnexal masses are rarely larger than 8 cm. During the reproductive years, simple cystic adnexal masses less than 8 cm in diameter could be followed expectantly in the asymptomatic

Table 9.1.5: Adnexal Mass: Indications for Surgery

Ovarian cystic structure ≥8 cm without regression for 6–8 weeks

Any cystic structure ≥10 cm

Any solid ovarian lesion

Ovarian lesion with papillary excrescences in the wall

Palpable adnexal mass in premenarchal or postmenopausal patient

Ascites

patient, as 70% of these masses will resolve spontaneously (Figure 9.1.1). The patient should undergo a repeat physical examination and pelvic ultrasound at a specified time interval. A common practice is to suppress ovulation with oral contraceptive pills, but the value of this strategy remains unproven.

Indications for surgery of a simple cyst include persistence of the mass, change in ultrasonic characteristics to a more complex appearance, solid enlargement, and evidence of ascites (Table 9.1.6). However, if the mass remains less than 8 cm, simple on ultrasound appearance, and asymptomatic, continued follow-up is a reasonable option. In the reproductive-age woman with an adnexal mass greater than 8 cm in diameter, solid appearance on ultrasound, bilaterality, and the presence of ascites, surgical

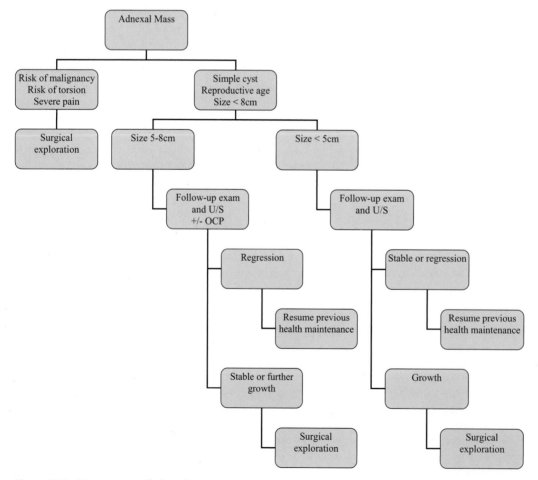

Figure 9.1.1. Management of adnexal mass.

Table 9.1.6: Histologic Classification of Malignant Ovarian Tumors

Epithelial ovarian cancer
- Serous
- Mucinous
- Endometrioid
- Clear cell
- Transitional cell carcinoma
- Undifferentiated carcinoma

Germ cell tumors
- Immature teratoma
- Malignant neoplasms arising within mature cystic teratoma
- Dysgerminoma
- Embryonal carcinoma
- Endodermal sinus tumor
- Choriocarcinoma
- Gonadoblastoma

Sex cord–stromal tumors
- Granulosa cell tumor (adult and juvenile types)
- Sertoli–Leydig tumor (arrhenoblastoma and Sertoli tumor)

Neoplasms derived from nonspecific mesenchyme
- Sarcoma
- Lymphoma

Metastatic tumors to the ovary
- Gastrointestinal tumor (Krukenberg)
- Breast
- Uterus

Table 9.1.7: Indications for Surgery with Functional Ovarian Cysts

Suspicion of malignancy

Symptoms evolve

Ascites

Change in ultrasound characteristic

Bilaterality

Suspicion of torsion

Size ≥8 cm

Severe pain

---

evaluation is indicated.[1] In premenarchal and postmenopausal patients, presence of an adnexal mass of any size is considered an indication for surgical removal of the mass. Classification of malignant ovarian tumors is given in Table 9.1.7.

Use of Laparoscopy

Once surgery is decided on, accurate diagnosis at surgery is essential in the management of adnexal masses. Many surgeons are now using the laparoscopic approach for the management of the adnexal mass in reproductive-age women when suspicion of malignancy is low. In a 1990 survey by the American Association of Gynecologic Laparoscopists, operative laparoscopy was accomplished in most patients and there were only 53 cases of unsuspected ovarian cancer in 13,739 cases (0.04%).[16] The benefits of laparoscopic surgery include shorter length of hospital stay, decreased postoperative pain and recovery time, and probably reduced cost.[17–20] However, there are understandable persisting concerns about the laparoscopic management of adnexal masses, including the failure to diagnose ovarian malignancies, tumor spillage, and inability to proceed immediately with a staging procedure and delay in therapy.

The ability to identify a malignancy during laparoscopy has been well studied. In the largest series of laparoscopically managed adnexal masses in reproductive-age women, Nezhat et al. [21] reported that the most reliable indicators of malignancy were the combination of laparoscopic visualization of the whole peritoneal cavity and frozen section analysis. Chapron et al. [22]

examined 26 patients with suspicious adnexal masses at the time of laparoscopy. In all 26 patients, frozen sections showed benign results, and in each case, definitive histologic diagnosis was confirmatory. Dottino et al. [23] found a discrepancy between the frozen section and final pathology in 3% of the cases. However, in a study of 149 patients with macroscopically suspicious ovarian masses, Canis et al. [24] found the frozen section to be accurate in 93% of the cases involving tumors smaller than 10 cm and in 74% of larger tumors. Intraoperative pathologic diagnosis was accurate in 77.8% of low malignant potential tumors.

Overall, the combined accuracy of laparoscopic visualization and intraoperative frozen section is good for the identification of malignancies. The two important exceptions are in very large tumors or tumors with borderline characteristics. The accuracy in these instances depends on the relative sample bias. The solution to this problem should be in removing the entire adnexa and allowing pathologic rather than surgical sampling. If a malignant ovarian neoplasm is discovered at the time of laparoscopy, the current standard of care is the performance of a comprehensive surgical staging procedure.

If a surgeon is prepared to convert to a laparotomy and an oncologist is available for surgical staging, laparoscopic surgery can be attempted for selected patients requiring operative treatment of an adnexal mass. Laparoscopy is inappropriate when there is metastatic disease, when frozen section diagnosis is not available, and when there is no preparation for staging and possible laparotomy. As with open cases, the patient should follow up with the physician postoperatively to determine the need for further therapy based on the results of full pathologic evaluation of the surgical specimen.

The standard operative approach to adnexal masses in postmenopausal women has been explorative laparotomy to ensure adequate exposure for the treatment of ovarian cancer. However, because the observation that even in this group of patients benign adnexal tumors are more frequent than malignant ones, some authors justify starting the surgical procedure laparoscopically. In the only prospective study, Dottino et al. [23] reported that nearly 90% of cases were managed laparoscopically. The same principles of carefully visualizing the entire peritoneal cavity and obtaining pelvic washings and biopsies for the diaphragm, paracolic gutters, and pelvis should be undertaken. Cystectomy is not recommended in postmenopausal women; removal of the entire adnexa with frozen section diagnosis is warranted.[25] Removal of a normal-appearing contralateral ovary should be performed according to preoperative consultation and past medical history.

In the premenarchal patient, the same laparoscopic principles for identifying a malignancy should be used. Performance of a careful inspection of the peritoneal cavity, sampling with generous biopsies, availability of frozen section, and use of the principles of cancer surgery are essential in the exclusion of germ cell malignancies in these young women.

Adnexal Mass in Pregnancy

Adnexal masses are frequently observed in gravid women, complicating as many as one in 190 pregnancies.[26] The risk of malignancy in the pregnant woman with an adnexal mass is 5%.[27] At least one third of adnexal masses discovered during pregnancy are found during routine obstetric ultrasonography, as both benign and malignant ovarian masses tend to be asymptomatic in pregnant women. Careful evaluation is necessary to differentiate between benign and malignant processes. In this regard, the sonographic appearance of the mass may be helpful. Simple cystic structures are most consistent with physiologic cysts. Most of the physiologic cysts resolve spontaneously by the end of the first trimester. Failure of a simple cyst to resolve by this time may be an indication for surgery. Other indications for surgery include tumor size greater than 6 cm, a solid or complex sonographic appearance of the mass, and the presence of bilateral abnormalities. Doppler ultrasound is potentially useful in differentiating high- and low-risk ovarian masses. Regardless of size, adnexal masses with blood flow characterized by a high resistive index appear to carry little risk, even when these masses fail to resolve by the second trimester. MRI may be helpful in situations in which ultrasound is equivocal or the mass cannot be distinguished from the uterine neoplasm.

Most ovarian cancers complicating pregnancy are either borderline malignant epithelial ovarian tumors or germ cell tumors.[1] The latter observation reflects the younger age of pregnant women when compared with the typical ovarian cancer patient. Dysgerminomas are the most common ovarian germ cell tumors complicating pregnancy, followed by endodermal sinus tumors. Sex cord or stromal tumors may also occur during pregnancy. Great care must be taken to differentiate sex cord–stromal tumors from a luteoma of pregnancy, ovarian decidualization, or benign granulosa cell tumor proliferations observed with the pregnancy. Although elevated levels of tumor markers are helpful in establishing a diagnosis in nonpregnant woman, elevations of these markers for reasons not related to malignancy reduce their diagnostic potential. For example, elevations of AFP and hCG may be effective markers for follow-up of endodermal sinus tumors and gestational trophoblastic tumors, respectively (Table 9.1.4). However, titers of all these markers as well as CA-125 are routinely elevated in pregnancy for reasons unrelated to malignancy. Their levels may be misleading, even when normalized as multiples of the mean for prenatal patients.

Only 3% to 5% of adnexal masses in pregnancy ultimately prove to be malignant. Thus, most may be managed conservatively, provided the patient's symptoms and the characteristics of the mass are consistent with benign etiology. Because adnexal masses are more likely to undergo torsion during pregnancy, explorative surgery may be necessary when a patient presents with symptoms and signs of torsion, such as severe or intermittent abdominal pain, nausea, and vomiting.

Surgery in pregnant patients is not without complications. Abdominal surgery in the first trimester is associated with a 12% spontaneous abortion rate, a number that is reduced to 0% in the third trimester. It also causes preterm labor in 30% to 40% of patients in the third trimester. The optimal time for surgery in pregnancy, therefore, is during the second trimester.[28] When first-trimester exploration and ovarian resection have been necessary, supplementary progesterone has been administered to decrease the likelihood of pregnancy loss. The efficacy of this treatment, however, remains unproven.

Laparoscopic surgery in pregnancy has been slow to gain popularity because of the potential risks of injury to the uterus and fetus. In fact, pregnancy formerly was a contraindication to laparoscopy. However, recent surgical studies of appendectomies and cholecystectomies have shown success with laparoscopy and similar outcomes with laparotomy, with decreased hospitalization and narcotic use.[28] Several reports have suggested the safe use of laparoscopy in the management of adnexal masses in the first and second trimesters. Laparoscopic management by an experienced team is a safe and effective procedure that allows for a reduced rate of postoperative complications and decreased maternal and fetal morbidity.[29,30] When performing laparoscopy in pregnant patients, special steps should be taken to protect the uterus while placing the trocars. Low-pressure pneumoperitoneum should be used, maternal end-tidal CO_2 gases should be monitored, the fetus should be monitored transvaginally, and the patient should be mobilized soon after surgery (Table 9.1.8).[28]

In the rare case of ovarian cancer, complete surgical staging should be performed in a manner similar to that in the nonpregnant woman. Although the gravid uterus makes the assessment of the retroperitoneum more difficult, every effort should be made to remove the tumor intact. The remaining ovary should be carefully inspected and biopsied if suspicious. Because germ cell tumors are almost invariably unilateral, it is not necessary to remove both ovaries. The exception is a dysgerminoma, which may be bilateral in 20% of cases and may be present in a grossly normal contralateral ovary. Even in this situation, it is not absolutely necessary to remove the entire ovary. However, if both ovaries are involved with malignancy and the gestation has reached the second trimester, both ovaries should be removed as the pregnancy no longer requires the hormonal support from the corpus luteum. Because dysgerminomas spread to para-aortic lymph nodes, every effort should be made to sample these nodes. An omentectomy and peritoneal biopsies along with

Table 9.1.8: Indications for Laparoscopy

Availability of intraoperative frozen section

Low suspicion of malignancy

No evidence of metastatic disease

Capability of converting to open

Experienced laparoscopic surgeon

cytologic assessment of the peritoneal cavity should routinely be performed.

Pregnant patients with stage IA or IB ovarian cancer may be managed conservatively with surgery and allowed to continue to term. Need for further chemotherapy is dictated by the histologic type of the tumor and the tumor's invasiveness. Cytotoxic chemotherapy should be avoided in the first trimester; however, it may be distributed in the second and third trimesters with little if any harm to the fetus. For this reason, women with stage IC or high-grade tumors should be given the opportunity to receive chemotherapy without terminating the pregnancy.

KEY POINTS

1. Five percent to 10% of women in the United States will undergo surgery for suspected ovarian neoplasm. Of these, 13% to 21% will be found to have ovarian cancer.

2. Age is the most important factor in determining the risk of malignancy.

3. In reproductive-age women, functional cysts are the most frequent finding. These may be managed conservatively as most disappear within 4 to 6 weeks.

4. Any cystic ovarian enlargement greater than 8 cm with a solid mass component is an indication for surgery in reproductive-age women.

5. Solid mass of any size is an indication for surgery in prepubertal girls. Abdominal pain and an abdominal mass are the two most frequent presenting symptoms in children. Malignant neoplasms are found in 8% of children undergoing surgery for an adnexal mass. Germ cell tumors are the most frequent malignant tumor in children.

6. Ovaries should not be palpable in postmenopausal women. Any ovarian enlargement in this age group is suggestive of malignancy until proven otherwise. Up to 40% to 45% of these patients who undergo surgery will have a malignant tumor. However, the most frequent finding is a benign ovarian neoplasm (fibroma or Brenner tumor).

7. Fibromas are benign and associated sometimes with a right-sided pleural effusion (Meigs' syndrome).

8. A combination of history, physical examination, tumor marker analysis, and pelvic ultrasound is used in the evaluation of an adnexal mass. Although pelvic ultrasound remains the best imaging tool for evaluation of ovarian pathology, MRI is useful in the diagnosis of endometriotic and hemorrhagic cysts. CT is useful in evaluating the extent of ovarian cancer.

9. The surgical approach to the adnexal mass has traditionally been via laparotomy. With the advancements in laparoscopy, more surgeons initially approach adnexal masses laparoscopically. Laparoscopy offers better visualization, shorter hospital stay, and lower rate of complications in comparison with laparotomy. The availability of frozen section diagnosis and ability to obtain immediate gynecologic oncology assistance in cases of malignant disease found are essential.

10. An adnexal mass is found in one in 190 pregnancies. The most frequent adnexal tumors in pregnancy are dysgerminomas and borderline ovarian tumors. The adnexal mass may be surgically removed safely during the second trimester of pregnancy. Surgeons with extensive laparoscopic experience can safely approach these masses laparoscopically.

REFERENCES

1. Disaia PJ, Creasman WT. The adnexal mass and early ovarian cancer. In: *Clinical Gynecologic Oncology*. 6th ed. St. Louis: Mosby; 2002:253–281.

2. Curtin JP. Management of the adnexal mass. *Gynecol Oncol*. 1994;55:S42–S46.

3. Koonings PP, Campbell DR, Mishell JR, Grimes DA. Relative frequency of primary ovarian neoplasms: a 10-year review. *Obstet Gynecol*. 1989;74:921–926.

4. Ehren IM, Mahour GH, Isaacs H. Benign and malignant ovarian tumors in children and adolescents. *Cancer*. 1984;147:339–343.

5. Dorum A, Blom GP, Ekerhovd E, et al. Prevalence and histologic diagnosis of adnexal cysts in postmenopausal women: an autopsy study. *Am J Obstet Gynecol*. 2005;192:48–54.

6. Oyelese Y, Kueck KS, Barter JF, et al. Asymptomatic postmenopausal simple ovarian cyst. *Obstet Gynecol Surv*. 2002;57:803–809.

7. Shalev E, Eliyahu S, Peleg D, Tsabari A. Laparoscopic management of adnexal cystic masses in postmenopausal women. *Obstet Gynecol*. 1994;83:594–596.

8. Kurjak A, Predanic M, Kupresic-Urek S, Jukic S. Transvaginal color and pulsed Doppler assessment of adnexal tumor vascularity. *Gynecol Oncol*. 1993;50:3–8.

9. Sassone A, Timor-Tritch I, Artner A, et al. Transvaginal sonographic characterization of ovarian disease: evaluation of a new scoring system to predict ovarian malignancy. *Obstet Gynecol*. 1991;78:7–11.

10. Alcazar JL, Jurado M. Prospective evaluation of a logistic model based on sonographic morphologic and color Doppler findings developed to predict adnexal malignancy. *J Ultrasound Med*. 1999; 18:837–843.

11. Grab D, Flock F, Stohr I. Classification of asymptomatic adnexal masses by ultrasound, magnetic resonance imaging, and positron emission tomography. *Gynecol Oncol*. 2000;77:454–459.

12. Jacobs I, Davies AP, Bridges J, et al. Prevalence screening for ovarian cancer in postmenopausal women by CA125 measurement and ultrasonography. *BMJ*. 1993;306:1030–1032.

13. Brooks SE. Preoperative evaluation of patients with suspicious ovarian cancer. *Gynecol Oncol*. 1994;55:80–90.

14. Meyer T, Rustin GSJ. Role of tumor markers in monitoring epithelial ovarian cancer. *Br J Cancer*. 2000;82:1535–1538.

15. Berek JS. Benign diseases of the female reproductive tract. In: *Novak's Gynecology*. 13th ed. Philadelphia: Lippincott Williams & Wilkins; 2002:396–399.

16. Hulka JF, Parker WH, Surrey MW, Phillips JM. Management of ovarian masses. AAGL 1990 survey. *J Reprod Med*. 1992;37:599–602.

17. Mais V, Ajossa S, Piras B, et al. Treatment of nonendometriotic benign adnexal cyst. A randomized trial to evaluate benefits in early outcome. *Am J Obstet Gynecol*. 1996;174:654–658.

18. Davison J, Park W, Penney L. Comparative study of operative laparoscopy vs. laparotomy: analysis of financial impact. *Reprod Med*. 1993;38:357–360.

19. Lundorff PJ, Thorburn J, Hahlin M, et al. Adhesion formation after laparoscopic surgery in tubal pregnancy: a randomized trial versus laparotomy. *Fertil Steril*. 1991;55:911–915.

20. Maruiri F, Azziz A. Laparoscopic surgery for ectopic pregnancies: technology assessment and public health implications. *Technol Steril*. 1993;59:487–498.

21. Nezhat FR, Nezhat CH, Welander CE, Benigno B. Four ovarian cancers diagnosed during laparoscopic management of 1011 women with adnexal masses. *Am J Obstet Gynecol.* 1992;167:790–796.

22. Chapron C, Dubuisson JB, Kadoch O, et al. Laparoscopic management of organic ovarian cysts: is there a place for frozen section in the diagnosis? *Hum Reprod.* 1998;13:324–329.

23. Dottino PR, Levine DA, Ripley DL, Cohen CJ. Laparoscopic management of adnexal masses in premenopausal and postmenopausal women. *Obstet Gynecol.* 1999;93:223–228.

24. Canis M, Mashiach R, Wattiez A, et al. Frozen section in laparoscopic management of macroscopically suspicious ovarian masses. *J Am Assoc Gynecol Laparosc.* 2004;11:365–369.

25. Pejovic T, Nezhat F. Laparoscopic management of adnexal masses. The opportunities and the risks. *Ann N Y Acad Sci.* 2003;943:255–268.

26. Whitecar MP, Turner S, Higby MK. Adnexal masses in pregnancy: a review of 130 cases undergoing surgical management. *Am J Obstet Gynecol.* 1999;181:19–24.

27. Schnee DM. The adnexal mass in pregnancy. *Mo Med.* 2004;101: 42–45.

28. Curet MJ, Allen D, Joskoff RK, Pitcher DE, Curet LB, Miscell BG, Zucker KA. Laparoscopy during pregnancy. *Arch Surg.* 1996;131: 5:546–550.

29. Mathevet P, Nessah K, Dargent D, Mellier G. Laparoscopic management of adnexal masses in pregnancy. A case series. *Eur J Obstet Gynecol Reprod Biol.* 2003;108:217–222.

30. Yen PM, Ng PS, Leung PL, Rogers MS. Outcome in laparoscopic management of persistent adnexal mass during the second trimester of pregnancy. *Surg Endosc.* 2004;18:1354–1357.

Section 9.2. Ovarian Cystectomy

Camran Nezhat, Ceana Nezhat, and Farr Nezhat

Evolving technology has made it possible to treat most persistent ovarian cysts laparoscopically. However, these operations must be done judiciously. Although the role of laparoscopy in the management of malignancy is expanding, laparotomy remains the procedure of choice when ovarian malignancy is encountered or strongly suspected.

INTRODUCTION

One percent to 2% of women develop ovarian cancer during their lifetime, and when the disease is detected, two thirds of them are in stage III or stage IV.[1] During laparoscopy, ovarian cancer can be discovered so that immediate laparotomy and appropriate staging are possible. Laparotomy may be required for optimal surgical therapy, and postoperative radiotherapy or chemotherapy is instituted as needed. A recent study suggested that a delay between laparoscopy and laparotomy may affect the distribution of disease stage adversely.[2] Whenever a malignant tumor has been missed at laparoscopy, restaging is required and should be considered an oncologic emergency.[3] Given the reduced morbidity, patient disability, and cost, having an oncologist available facilitates the safe treatment of adnexal masses by operative laparoscopy. Conversion from the laparoscopic approach rarely is required.[4]

A serious concern is that an ovarian cyst assumed to be benign subsequently may prove to be a stage I ovarian carcinoma. Even careful laparoscopic examination may underestimate early-stage ovarian cancer or borderline tumors.[5,6] If contents spill during their aspiration or with an ovarian cystectomy, the stage is upgraded from IA to IC. The risks associated with spillage of cystic contents have been evaluated.[7] In a multivariate analysis of stage I epithelial ovarian cancer, the factors that influenced the rate of relapse in 519 patients were the tumor grade, the presence of dense adhesions, and a large volume of ascites. Intraoperative spillage at laparotomy showed no adverse effect on the prognosis of stage I ovarian cancer.[8] The survival of women with borderline tumors who were managed initially by cystectomy, with or without spillage, was not decreased, and there was no evidence of disseminated disease an average of 7.5 years after diagnosis.[9] The laparoscopic approach to borderline ovarian tumors is possible in early-stage disease and does not seem to negatively affect long-term survival.[10]

The risk of spread remains questionable in patients who have the appropriate operation. In two large studies, the incidence of ovarian malignancy in patients with a known adnexal mass was between 1.2% [11] and 0.3%.[12] The results of a 1991 survey of the members of the American Association of Gyneco-logic Laparoscopists (AAGL) showed that laparoscopic excision of unsuspected invasive ovarian cancer was uncommon. Only 53 instances were reported among 13,739 laparoscopic ovarian cystectomies, an incidence of 0.4%.[13] Similar results were found in a countrywide survey undertaken in Austria, which included 16,601 laparoscopies on adnexal masses. Ovarian tumors subsequently were found to be malignant in 108 cases (0.65%).[14]

A laparotomy may be needed to ensure optimal staging and treatment in cases of malignancy. A survey of gynecologic oncologists revealed 12 borderline ovarian tumors and 30 invasive ovarian cancers initially managed by laparoscopic excision.[15] Most patients did not have a staging laparotomy for weeks after the cancer was found. These patients did not have careful preoperative screening, and appropriate surgical treatment was delayed.

PREOPERATIVE EVALUATION

Laparoscopic treatment of adnexal masses depends on the patient's age, findings on pelvic examination, imaging studies, and serum markers.

Physical Examination

A large, solid, fixed or irregular adnexal mass accompanied by ascites is suspicious for malignancy (Table 9.2.1). Cul-de-sac nodularity, ascites, cystic adnexal structures, and fixed adnexa occur with both endometriosis and ovarian malignancy.

Ultrasound

Transvaginal ultrasound is the primary imaging modality for evaluating adnexal masses.[16] Cystic, unilocular, unilateral masses less than 10 cm with regular borders are probably benign. Malignant ovarian cysts are associated with irregular borders, a size greater than 10 cm with papillations, solid areas, thick septa (≥ 2 mm), ascites, and a matted bowel. Using ultrasonographic criteria, accurate predictions of benign masses were made in 96% of patients.[16,17] Nezhat and coworkers [12] found that none of the four malignant cysts in their series had any ultrasound criteria for malignancy. However, laparoscopic diagnosis of adnexal masses that are suspicious at ultrasound prevents many laparotomies for the treatment of benign masses.[18]

The role of ultrasound screening in detecting ovarian cancer in asymptomatic women is still questionable. A systematic review of prospective screening studies found that the sensitivity of ultrasound screening at 1 year was around 100% (95% CI, 54–100).[19] However, false-positive rates ranged between 1.2%

Table 9.2.1: Malignant Potential of Ovarian Cysts by Physical Examination

Clinical Findings	Benign	Malignant
Size ≥7 cm	+ +	+ +
Size ≤7 cm	+ +	+ +
Unilateral	+ + + +	+
Bilateral	+ +	+ + + +
Cystic	+ + + +	+
Solid	+ +	+ + +
Solid and cystic	+	+ + + +
Mobile	+ + + +	+
Fixed	+	+ + + +
Irregular	+	+ + + +
Smooth	+ + + +	+
Ascites	+	+ + + +
Cul-de-sac nodules	+	+ + +

+, least probable; + + + +, most probable.

and 2.5% for gray-scale ultrasound, between 0.3% and 0.7% for ultrasound with color Doppler, and between 0.1% and 0.6% for CA-125 measurement followed by ultrasound screening. This implies that in an annual screening of a population with an incidence of 40 per 100,000, with no cancers missed, between 2.5 and 60 women would be operated on for every primary ovarian cancer detected.

Functional cysts gradually regress or resolve spontaneously or with hormonal suppressive therapy within 8 weeks (Figure 9.2.1). Persistent cysts that are functional or hemorrhagic on ultrasound should be removed.

Serum Markers

CA-125 is a tumor-associated antigen that is used to detect the nature of an ovarian cyst (Tables 9.2.2, 9.2.3). Levels below 35 U/mL are associated with benign tumors, but the sensitivity and specificity vary. The presence of other benign conditions can elevate CA-125 levels. In 80% of premenopausal women, elevated CA-125 levels were associated with pregnancy, endometriosis, fibroids, adenomyosis, cystic teratomas, and acute or chronic salpingitis. Only 50% of patients with stage I ovarian cancers had elevated CA-125 levels, compared with 90% of women with stage II.[20]

In 70 women with a history of endometriosis, serum CA-125 concentrations were not correlated with the persistence or resolution of ovarian cysts.[21]

Computed Tomography and Magnetic Resonance Imaging

The role of CT and MRI relative to ultrasound in evaluating an ovarian cyst is evolving. The resolution characteristics of CT depend on differences in x-ray attenuation between calcium, water, fat, and air. Soft tissue differences are enhanced with intravenous contrast. MRI relies on differences in the hydrogen content of fat and water, magnetic relaxation time, and blood flow, ultimately resulting in additional soft tissue contrast. In one study, MRI had a sensitivity of 95% and a specificity of 88% in distinguishing malignant from benign lesions, whereas transvaginal ultrasound had 75% sensitivity and 98% specificity.[22] MRI and the T_2 signal intensity were useful for detecting the presence of endometriomas based on evaluating the density of the cyst fluid and its iron concentration.[23] Unenhanced and contrast-enhanced MRI was shown to maximize the discrimination between benign and malignant masses in patients with sonographically indeterminate ovarian lesions.[24]

Serial turboFLASH (fast, low-angle shot) images with and without diffusion–perfusion (DP) gradients have been used to evaluate the contents of cystic ovarian lesions. When these images were used, the apparent diffusion coefficients were calculated within the cystic contents of these lesions. It was found that diffusion-weighted MRI could be used to differentiate between the cystic contents of benign and malignant ovarian lesions.[25]

Meticulous pretreatment evaluation remains basic to the successful management of suspected ovarian masses. The additional expense of CT and MRI seems justified only in selected patients in whom further characterization of the adnexal mass may influence directly the type of management selected.[26,27]

Cyst Aspiration

Cytologic examination of the cystic fluid does not provide an accurate diagnosis in many patients.[28] Ten percent to 65% of aspirates were interpreted as benign when malignancy was present.[12,29,30] In a review, the accuracy of transvaginal and transrectal fine-needle aspiration and ultrasound-guided punctures of ovarian cysts was disappointing.[31] The false-negative rate was especially high for nonfollicular cystic lesions.[32] This procedure is not suggested for treatment because of the high rate of recurrence.[33–35]

In a study, 278 women with simple ovarian cysts were allocated randomly to either simple observation or ultrasound-guided fine-needle aspiration. The rate of resolution was 46% with aspiration and 45% with observation. The authors concluded that expectant management for up to 6 months does not cause risks for the patients and that aspiration does not provide better results than does simple observation.[36]

Sonographically guided therapeutic aspiration of symptomatic ovarian cysts may alleviate symptoms.[37] However, this procedure, although more rapid than extirpation, may be associated with abscess formation.[38]

TREATMENT

Medical Treatment

Oral contraceptives have been prescribed for some cystic adnexal masses (≤6 cm) in reproductive-age women on the assumption that decreasing gonadotropin stimulation to a functional cyst will hasten its resolution. The results of one study failed to report any benefit from ovarian suppressive therapy.[39] However, the cysts were less than 5 cm, and the study included women who had

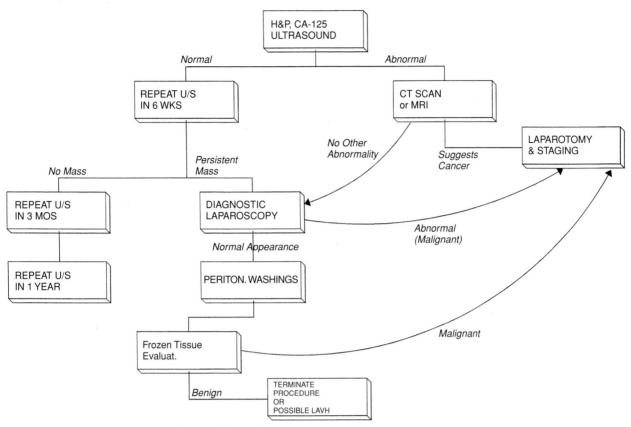

Figure 9.2.1. Evaluation of a postmenopausal ovarian cyst.

received ovulation induction medication. Two additional randomized trials have since shown that although oral contraceptive therapy is very effective in the management of functional ovarian cysts, expectant management achieves similar success rates.[40,41]

A randomized study evaluated the effectiveness of various hormonal regimens in treating 70 women who had unilateral or bilateral ovarian cysts assumed to be physiologic (functional) and a history of endometriosis.[21] The patients were assigned randomly to one of the following groups: group I (control), no treatment; group II, oral contraceptives (35 μg ethinyl estradiol and 1 mg norethindrone); group III, oral contraceptives (50 μg ethinyl estradiol and 1 mg norethindrone); group IV, danazol 800 mg/day. Serum CA-125 concentrations were measured in 32 women. At 6 weeks of follow-up, complete resolution of cysts was found in group I, 12 of 18 (66.7%); group II, five of nine (55.6%); group III, eight of 14 (57.1%); and group IV, seven of 13 (53.9%). Two of the 22 women with persistent cysts opted for 6 weeks of additional medical therapy and achieved complete resolution, 19 underwent laparoscopy, and one was lost to follow-up. All laparoscopic findings revealed benign masses. It was concluded that no statistically significant effect was found when hormonal treatment was compared with expectant management.[21]

Hormonal suppressive therapy may be prescribed during the follow-up of benign-appearing ovarian cysts, but there is little scientific evidence for its effectiveness compared with expectant management.

Recommended Approach

Attempts to remove ovarian cysts laparoscopically sometimes require conversion to laparotomy because cancer may be discovered and an immediate laparotomy then becomes necessary. Treatment of benign-appearing adnexal masses must follow a protocol of (1) cytologic examination of pelvic and cyst fluid, (2) frozen section of a biopsy specimen, and (3) removal of the mass for histologic examination. Aspirating a cyst and vaporizing or coagulating the capsule are not acceptable choices. The safe laparoscopic approach to ovarian cysts has been described by Mage and coworkers.[11] Those authors reported findings in 481 patients (ages 9 to 88) who had ovarian cysts, including 96 functional cysts, 100 endometriomas, 100 serous cysts, 91 teratomas, 51 mucinous cysts, and 58 paraovarian cysts. Among these patients, 19 underwent laparotomy for confirmed or suspected malignancy based only on laparoscopic evaluation, and 10 of them were benign. Five ovarian cancers and four borderline tumors were found and handled immediately by laparotomy. Dense pelvic adhesions or cysts larger than 10 cm were the indications for laparotomy in 42 women. Nezhat and colleagues [12] evaluated 1011 premenopausal women with ovarian cysts laparoscopically and found four ovarian cancers. Preoperative assessment included an initial pelvic exam, vaginal ultrasound, and the CA-125 level.[11] Three of the four unsuspected cancers were found on frozen or permanent sections of the cyst wall. One malignant tumor was 3 cm and grossly appeared to be an

Table 9.2.2: CA-125 Levels Correlated with Type of Cyst

Patients, no.	Cyst	No.	Size, cm	Age Range, years	CA-125 Level, U/mL Range	Mean	Cystic No.	%	Semicystic No.	%	Solid No.	%	Other No.	%
360	Endometrioma	162	2–5	16–54	≥2–212	45.7	123	68.9	22	22.8	14	7.5	3	0.8
		179	6–10		2–195	28.7	115		54		10		–	
		19	11–25		5–237	48.2	10		6		3		–	
219	Functional	172	2–5	11–47	≤2–135	15.7	98	58.0	40	25.1	6	3.7	28	13.2
		45	6–10		≤2–53	11.2	28		14		2		1	
		2	11–12		6	6.0	1		1		–		–	
34	Simple	13	2–5	23–47	5–76	7.0	10	76.5	–	8.8	–	5.9	3	8.8
		19	6–10		2–195	31.5	14		3		2		–	
		2	11–12		–	–	2		–		–		–	
30	Benign cystic teratoma	16	2–5	17–44	≤5–9	7.0	7	43.3	7	36.7	1	13.3	1	6.7
		12	6–10		5–29	14.9	6		3		2		1	
		2	11–14		12	12.0	–		1		1		–	
17	Serous	8	2–5	33–40	14–47	30.5	7	82.4	–	5.9	–	5.9	1	5.9
		7	6–10		10–42	23.7	6		1		–		–	
		2	11–15		47–51	49.0	1		–		1		–	
11	Mucinous	4	25	31–35	≤5	≤5.0	2	54.5	2	45.5	–	–	–	–
		5	6–10		≤5–30	10.6	2		3		–		–	
		2	11–25		9–11	10.0	2		–		–		–	
17	Hydrosalpinges	16	5–10	26–45	≤5–35	12.8	6	41.2	8	47.1	–	–	2	11.8
		1	11–12		≤5	≤5.0	1		–		–		–	
46	Miscellaneous	30	2–5	22–45	≤5–135	27.4	19	67.4	2	6.5	–	4.3	9	21.7
		15	6–10		≤5–10	5.5	11		1		2		1	
		1	11–17		36	36.0	1		–		–		–	

endometrioma; histologic examination revealed an endometrioid carcinoma (Table 9.2.4).[12] Preoperative examinations did not detect malignancy.

Although ovarian neoplasms may occur at any age, the risk of malignancy is highest during prepuberty and menopause. Ovarian activity is associated with an increased incidence of functional ovarian cysts and other benign pathologic conditions. These observations, combined with age differences in the sensitivity and specificity of clinical testing, have led to the following recommendations for evaluating and managing adnexal masses.

Although clinical examination and the results of the preoperative work-up often indicate the benign or malignant nature of cysts, only histology can provide the absolute diagnosis. The benefits of doing frozen sections during laparoscopic management of organic ovarian cysts were investigated in 228 patients who underwent adnexectomy for an ovarian mass.[42] After the preoperative work-up and the diagnostic phase of laparoscopy, 26 patients (11.4%) presented with suspected signs of malignancy restricted to the ovary. Those 26 patients underwent a laparoscopic adnexectomy with extraction of the excised tissues using an endoscopic bag, followed by frozen section. For all these patients, the results of the frozen section were that the lesion was benign. In every case, the definitive histologic results confirmed the frozen section findings. This strategy allowed the gynecologist to avoid laparotomy, especially in the nine postmenopausal patients whose adnexal masses appeared complex on ultrasound.

Malignancy is not the only concern in handling an ovarian cyst. If the risk of malignancy is relatively low, patients who wish to preserve their reproductive organs should have the least aggressive therapy. In premenopausal women, besides ascertaining the characteristics of the adnexal mass, resection of ovarian tissue may cause adhesions and should be minimized (Table 9.2.5).

In postmenopausal women, the incidental finding of adnexal masses will increase with the more frequent application of

Table 9.2.3: Sensitivity and Specificity of Diagnostic Tests

	Premenopausal		Postmenopausal	
	Sensitivity, %	Specificity, %	Sensitivity, %	Specificity, %
Specialist ultrasound	50	96	78	92
Clinical impression	17	92	68	85
CA-125	50	69	84	92

Modified from Finkler N, Benacerrat B, Lavin F. Comparison of serum CA-125, clinical impression and ultrasound in the preoperative evaluation of ovarian masses. *Obstet Gynecol.* 1988;72:659.

Table 9.2.4: Findings at Laparoscopy in Four Women Who Had Ovarian Cancer

	Case 1 Serous Cystadenocarcinoma	Case 2 Endometrioid Low-Malignant-Potential Tumor	Case 3 Papillary Mucinous Cystadenocarcinoma	Case 4 Clear Cell Carcinoma
Patient age, years	44	45	43	33
Stage	IIIC	IA	IIA	IA
Tumor size, cm	7	3	13	6
Serum CA-125 level, U/mL	N/A	7	17	2
Ultrasonographic finding	Septated semicystic	Cystic	Septated semicystic	Septated semicystic

diagnostic imaging. Although routine pelvic sonographic screening of asymptomatic postmenopausal women may find early ovarian cancer, the procedure is not cost-effective. Wolf and coworkers [43] screened 149 asymptomatic women more than 50 years of age and discovered cysts in 22 (14.8%), ranging in size from 0.4 to 4.7 cm. Two additional women had septated masses, but no ovarian cancers were detected. In a study that screened 5479 women age 45 or older, 6.1% had abnormal scans.[44] When the scans were repeated 2 to 8 weeks later, only 59% were persistently abnormal. Five ovarian cancers were found, two in the first screen and three in the follow-up screen; all were stage I.

The low prevalence of ovarian cancer in the population and its rate of progression may limit the potential cost-effectiveness of screening.[19] Current data do not seem to support the view that screening asymptomatic postmenopausal women who have a normal pelvic examination is justified. Although it is clear that ultrasound and multimodal screening can detect ovarian cancer in asymptomatic women, there is currently no evidence that screening improves the outcome for women in any risk group.

The preoperative evaluation for an ovarian cyst includes a history, pelvic examination, ultrasound, and serum CA-125. If any combinations of these tests are suggestive of malignancy, an abdominal and pelvic CT scan is done. If the scan shows signs of malignancy (ascites, omental cake, etc.), the patient undergoes a staging laparotomy or chemotherapy. When the CT is negative, a laparoscopy is planned and consent is obtained for laparotomy. Preoperatively, the patient has a mechanical and antibiotic bowel preparation and a chest radiograph and signs the appropriate consent.

Intraoperative Therapy

Intraoperative evaluation includes cell washings from the pelvis and upper abdomen to be saved for evaluation if a malignancy is found. The upper abdomen and pelvis are explored, and excrescences or suspicious areas are sampled and sent for frozen section.

After the pelvis and upper abdomen are examined, the cyst contents are aspirated. Once the capsule is opened, the interior of the capsule is examined and suspicious areas are biopsied, and then the tissue is sent for frozen section. The entire cyst capsule is removed to search for an early carcinoma that may escape gross detection.[12] Whether to do an oophorectomy or cystectomy depends on the patient's age and the characteristics of the mass.

Ovarian Cystectomy

An ideal ovarian cystectomy consists of the removal of the intact cyst with limited trauma to the residual ovarian tissue. Alternatively, the cyst fluid may be drained to minimize spillage and facilitate removal.

Three methods to manage ovarian cysts are drainage, excision, and thermal ablation or coagulation. When the cyst is excised, histopathologic examination is complete and the risk of recurrence is lessened. Aspiration is recommended for functional cysts detected laparoscopically and confirmed by frozen section. Postoperatively, hormonal suppressive therapy is advised. Because thermal ablation does not destroy the entire cyst wall and the underlying ovarian cortex may be damaged by the heat, excision is preferred.

Many cysts are ruptured during their manipulation despite the use of a delicate technique. The intact removal of a cyst 10 cm or larger is difficult laparoscopically. Aspiration before removal of large cysts is practical. It is accomplished with an 18-gauge laparoscopic needle passed through the suction–irrigator probe while the cyst is stabilized with suction applied over the cyst. The needle is inserted into the cyst, and the contents are aspirated (Figure 9.2.2). The suction–irrigator system reduces the spillage by applying suction at the cannula. Alternatively, a suction–irrigator probe may be inserted into the cyst (Figure 9.2.3 inset). Another

Table 9.2.5: Premenopausal Ovarian Cysts

Preoperative Evaluation	Intraoperative Evaluation
History and physical examination	Diagnostic laparoscopy examination
Transvaginal ultrasound	Peritoneal washing
Hormonal suppressive	Cyst aspiration; therapy if indicated
Informed consent	Evaluation of the cyst
Draw blood and save for possible tumor marker	Possible frozen section Cystectomy or oophorectomy

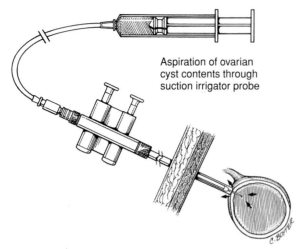

Aspiration of ovarian cyst contents through suction irrigator probe

Figure 9.2.2. For pure cysts larger than 2 cm, an 18-gauge laparoscopic needle is passed through the suction–irrigator probe. While the cyst is stabilized with suction applied over the cyst wall, the needle is inserted into the cyst and the contents are aspirated.

technique involves the passage of a 5-mm trocar and sleeve. The trocar is placed into the cyst and then removed, and then the suction–irrigator is inserted (Figure 9.2.3). This method works well for endometriomas and mucinous cystadenomas but is not advisable for benign teratomas that contain hair.

The aspirate is sent for cytologic examination, and the ovary is freed from adhesions to the lateral pelvic wall, uterus, or bowel. The cyst and pelvis are irrigated continuously, especially for benign cystic teratomas, mucinous cystadenomas, and endometriomas. The most dependent portion of the cyst wall is

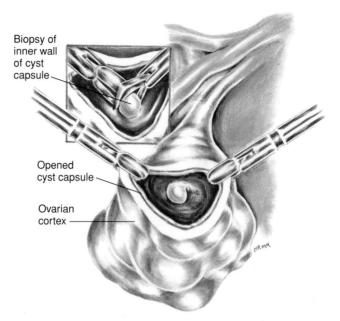

Biopsy of inner wall of cyst capsule

Opened cyst capsule

Ovarian cortex

Figure 9.2.4. The most dependent portion of the cyst wall is opened, and the internal surface is inspected. If excrescences or papillomas are found, a biopsy specimen (*inset*) is taken and sent for frozen section. The ovarian cortex is held apart with graspers.

opened, and the internal surface is inspected (Figure 9.2.4). If excrescences or papillae are found, a biopsy specimen is sent for frozen section (Figure 9.2.4 inset). Dilute vasopressin is injected between the capsule and the ovarian cortex to create a plane for hydrodissection and reduce oozing in the capsule (Figure 9.2.5A). The capsule is stripped from the ovarian stroma using two

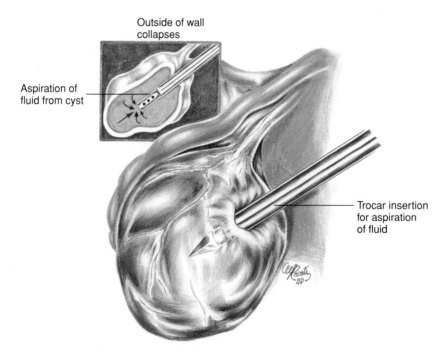

Outside of wall collapses

Aspiration of fluid from cyst

Trocar insertion for aspiration of fluid

Figure 9.2.3. The trocar is placed into the cyst and then removed, and the suction–irrigator (*inset*) is inserted. This method works well for endometriomas and mucinous cystadenomas but is not advisable for teratomas that contain hair. The aspirate is sent for cytologic examination. The cyst and pelvis are irrigated continuously.

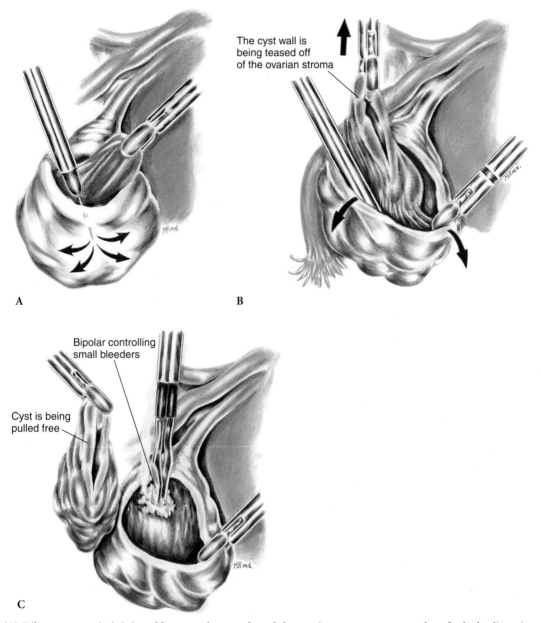

Figure 9.2.5. (**A**) Dilute vasopressin is injected between the capsule and the ovarian cortex to create a plane for hydrodissection and to reduce oozing in the capsule. Sometimes it is difficult to separate the cyst wall from the ovarian cortex, and so this injection technique facilitates the stripping procedure. (**B**) The capsule is stripped from the ovarian cortex by using two grasping forceps and the suction–irrigator probe for traction and countertraction. The specimen is sent for histologic examination. (**C**) Bipolar forceps can be used to control bleeding.

grasping forceps and the suction–irrigator probe for traction and countertraction (Figure 9.2.5B). It is sent for histologic examination. The laser is used at low power (10 to 20 W continuous) to seal blood vessels at the base of the capsule and at higher power to vaporize small remnants of capsule. Bipolar forceps are used to control bleeding (Figure 9.2.5C).

Sometimes it is difficult to remove the capsule from the ovarian cortex, and so injecting dilute vasopressin between the capsule and the cortex facilitates the stripping procedure (Figure 9.2.6). If the cyst wall cannot be identified, the edge of the ovarian incision can be "freshened" with scissors, and the resulting clean edge

reveals the different structures. If this does not free the capsule, the base of the cyst is grasped, and traction is applied to the cyst with countertraction to the ovary. The entire cyst or portions of the wall may be adherent to the ovary, requiring sharp or laser dissection to free it completely. Large cysts require partial oophorectomy, using a high-power laser or scissors to remove the distorted portion of the ovary. The remaining cyst wall is stripped from the ovarian stroma (Figure 9.2.7).

Teratomas often can be excised intact, but if the cyst ruptures, the resulting contamination will be greater than it would if the cyst were opened and aspirated. The atraumatic development of

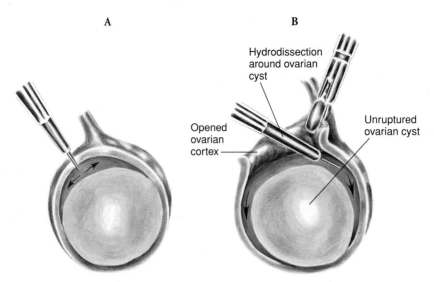

Figure 9.2.6. (**A**) A 16- or 20-gauge needle is introduced through an accessory trocar sleeve into the space between the cyst wall and the ovarian cortex. (**B**) A plane is developed using the suction–irrigator as a blunt probe.

the plane between the cyst wall and the ovarian tissue is an important first step that is accomplished by using hydrodissection. An 18- or 20-gauge needle is introduced through an accessory trocar sleeve, or a 7.5-inch spinal needle (American Hydro-Surgical Instruments) is inserted through the abdominal wall into the space between the cyst wall and the ovary. The plane is developed by using the suction–irrigator as a blunt probe. After removal of the cyst, the base of the capsule is irrigated and coagulation is achieved with a CO_2 laser or bipolar electrocoagulation. The edges of the ovarian cortex are connected with a low-power laser (10 to 20 W) or bipolar electrocoagulator. A grasping forceps helps merge the ovarian edges. If the ovarian edges overlap, the

defect is left to heal without suturing because adhesions are more likely after the use of sutures (Table 9.2.6).[45] If the edges of the ovarian capsule do not meet, a low-power laser applied to the inner surface will invert them. In rare instances, one or two fine absorbable monofilament sutures are needed to bring the ovarian edges together (Figure 9.2.8). Sutures are placed inside the ovary to decrease the formation of adhesions.

Tissue can be removed from the abdominal cavity by using one of the following techniques:

1. *Containment bags.* Excised tissue is placed into a small plastic prepared bag introduced into the pelvis through a 10-mm

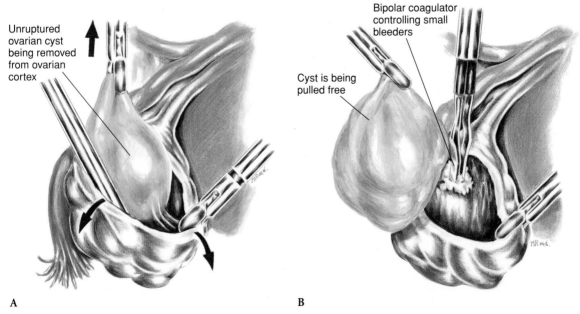

Figure 9.2.7. (**A**) The unruptured ovarian cyst is removed from the ovarian cortex. Irrigation helps in the hydrodissection as the ovarian cortex is held with graspers for countertraction. (**B**) As the cyst is enucleated, the base of the ovarian bed is coagulated with bipolar forceps to achieve hemostasis.

Table 9.2.6: Incidence of Adhesion Formation in Patients with and without Laparoscopic Ovarian Suturing

	Type of Cyst					Adhesions			
	Benign Cystic								
Suture	Endometrioma	Teratoma	Mucinous	Serous	Simple	None	Filmy/Minimal Vascularity	Dense/ Nonvascular	Dense/ Vascular
No	27	4	2	1	2	11	22	2	1
Yes	19	6	0	2	4	5	6	15	5

trocar (Endobag, Ethicon). The tissue is placed in the bag, traction is applied to the bag, and after the trocar sleeve is removed, it is pulled through a trocar incision to the anterior abdominal wall. The edges of the bag are pulled toward the anterior abdominal wall. Cystic contents are aspirated, and the deflated cyst is pulled out of the peritoneal cavity (Figure 9.2.9). A solid mass is morcellated inside the bag and removed. Attempting to pull the bag out of the abdomen before the cyst is collapsed or morcellated causes rupture of the bag and contamination of the abdominal cavity or anterior abdominal wall.

2. *Colpotomy.* Through a colpotomy, large pieces of solid tissue such as myomas and cystic masses can be removed. Some cystic masses are so fragile and large that it is impossible to remove them intact through a colpotomy. The tumor mass is brought to the vaginal incision and drained transvaginally (Figure 9.2.10). After the mass is removed, the pelvic cavity is irrigated and suctioned. The colpotomy is repaired vaginally or laparoscopically. Nezhat and colleagues [46] found that colpotomy is not associated with significant postoperative adhesions.

3. With another technique, the cystic mass is brought to the surface of the abdominal incision, drained, and extracted similarly to the method for removal by colpotomy.

No tissue should be left in the pelvic cavity or on the abdominal wall. Implantation of ovarian tissue in the abdominal and pelvic cavity may cause an ovarian remnant syndrome.[47] Contamination of the anterior abdominal wall should be avoided, and if this happens, all tissue must be removed and the incision must be irrigated copiously. Abdominal wall metastasis has been reported after contamination of the wall during laparoscopy for ovarian cancer.[48]

Benign Cystic Teratomas

Benign cystic teratomas are germ cell tumors that occur predominantly in young women. Laparoscopic removal may be technically difficult, but it can be done successfully. After laparoscopic excision and removal by a posterior colpotomy, normal ovaries and few adhesions were seen at a repeat laparoscopy.[49] If this is unsuccessful, one should go on to laparotomy to ensure complete excision of the tumor.

The suction–irrigator is placed in the cyst, the contents are aspirated, and the cavity is irrigated copiously. The interior of the cyst is inspected, and its lining is grasped and removed from the ovary. The lining is removed from the pelvis through a 10-mm accessory trocar, the operating channel of the laparoscope, a colpotomy, or an Endobag. The cyst wall is inspected and sent for

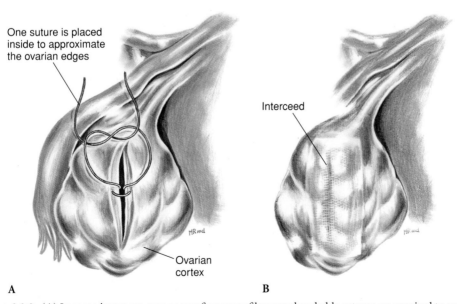

One suture is placed inside to approximate the ovarian edges

Ovarian cortex

Interceed

A   B

Figure 9.2.8. (**A**) In some instances, one or two fine monofilament absorbable sutures are required to approximate the edges of the ovarian cortex. The sutures are placed inside the ovary to lessen the formation of adhesions. (**B**) Interceed (Gynecare) may be placed over the sutured site.

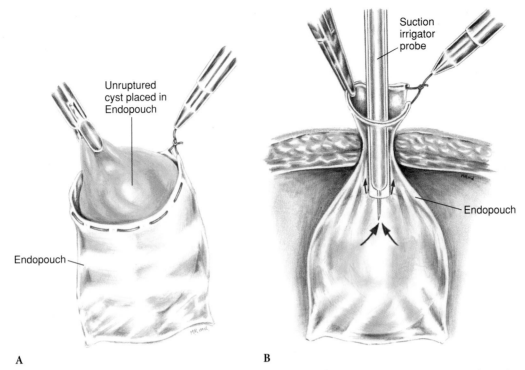

A   B

Figure 9.2.9. (**A**) The unruptured cyst is placed in an Endopouch introduced into the pelvic cavity through a 10-mm trocar sleeve. (**B**) The plastic containment bag is pulled to the level of the anterior abdominal wall. If the mass is cystic and too large to be pulled through the cannula, a suction–irrigator probe is used to aspirate the cystic fluid and reduce the size of the mass. If the excised tissue is solid, it can be cut into pieces or morcellated until the material can be pulled safely through a 10-mm trocar sleeve. Pulling the bag before the included tissue can be pulled through the sleeve can rupture the cyst and contaminate the anterior abdominal wall and peritoneal cavity.

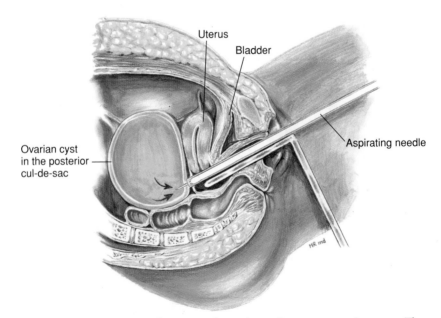

Figure 9.2.10. A colpotomy may be used to remove large pieces of myoma or cystic masses. The cystic mass is brought into the cul-de-sac and drained transvaginally. The culdotomy may be repaired either vaginally or laparoscopically. After the mass is removed, the pelvis is irrigated copiously and suctioned. Laparoscopic culdotomy has not been associated with significant pelvic adhesions.

frozen section. The pelvis is irrigated with lactated Ringer's solution until all evidence of sebaceous material is removed because incomplete removal may cause peritonitis. During irrigation, the ovarian stroma is inspected to verify hemostasis. Bleeding areas are coagulated with a defocused laser or bipolar forceps.

The ability to prevent rupture and spillage of teratomas using this laparoscopic technique has been demonstrated, but this approach may be time consuming and requires expert surgical technique.[50] During laparoscopic operative management, aquadissection compared with blunt dissection and scissors is associated with less intraoperative spillage, because with this method, it is easier to avoid cyst rupture.[51]

For large teratomas (≥8 cm); the ovary is placed in the cul-de-sac next to a colpotomy. Draining the cyst and removing its wall transvaginally lessen the risk of contamination and maintain a minimally invasive approach. The vagina is prepared with povidone–iodine (Betadine) before colpotomy.

Laparoscopically assisted vaginal removal of these cysts is an alternative to laparotomy when adnexal mobility is proven and vaginal extraction is feasible.[52] Laparoscopically assisted transvaginal ovarian cystectomy allows the removal of larger cystic teratomas. Compared with conventional laparoscopic cystectomy, there is less of a tendency to spill the contents and operative time is reduced.[53]

The outcome of conservative laparoscopic treatment of these cysts removed from the abdominal cavity without and with an Endobag was studied in a prospective, randomized trial in Rome.[54] In the 55 women studied, 58 cysts (mean diameter, 5.6 ± 2.03 cm) were enucleated and removed at operative laparoscopy through a 10- to 12-mm cannula sleeve without intraoperative or postoperative complications. Mean operating time was 73 minutes. When cysts were removed with an Endobag, operating time was reduced over removal without the Endobag (63 vs. 81 minutes, P 0.05). Obvious spillage of contents occurred in 13 patients (43.3%) when the Endobag was not used but occurred in only one patient in the study group because the bag ruptured (P 0.05). No signs or symptoms of peritonitis were observed in women with evident cystic spillage and patients in whom no bag was used when spillage was possible. It was concluded that removing cysts in an Endobag reduced both operating time and spillage. However, controlled intraperitoneal spillage of cyst contents did not increase postoperative morbidity as long as the peritoneal cavity was washed thoroughly. The observation that spillage of the contents of the cyst does not lead to complications was noted earlier and attributed to liberal irrigation of the peritoneal cavity.[55]

REFERENCES

1. Benjamin I, Rubin SC. Initial surgical management of advanced epithelial ovarian cancer. *Cancer Invest.* 1997;15:270.
2. Lehner R, Wenzl R, Heinzl H, et al. Influence of delayed staging laparotomy after laparoscopic removal of ovarian masses later found malignant. *Obstet Gynecol.* 1998;92:967.
3. Canis M, Botchorishvili R, Kouyate S, et al. Surgical management of adnexal tumors. *Ann Chir.* 1998;52:234.
4. Hidlebaugh DA, Vulgaropulos S, Orr RK. Treating adnexal masses: operative laparoscopy vs. laparotomy. *J Reprod Med.* 1997;42:551.
5. Guglielmina JN, Pennehouat G, Deval B, et al. Treatment of ovarian cysts by laparoscopy. *Contracept Fertil Sex.* 1997;25:218.
6. Malik E, Bohm W, Stoz F, et al. Laparoscopic management of ovarian tumors. *Surg Endosc.* 1998;12:1326.
7. Webb MJ, Decker DG, Mussey E, et al. Factors in influencing survival in stage I ovarian cancer. *Am J Obstet Gynecol.* 1973;116:222.
8. Dembo AJ, Davy M, Stenwick AE, et al. Prognostic factors in patients with stage I epithelial ovarian cancer. *Obstet Gynecol.* 1990;74:263.
9. Lim-Yan S, Cajigas H, Scully R. Ovarian cystectomy for serous borderline tumors: a follow-up study of 35 cases. *Obstet Gynecol.* 1998;72:775.
10. Cadron I, Amant F, VanGorp T, Neven P, Levnen K, Vergote I. The management of borderline tumors of the ovary. *Current Opinion in Oncology.* 2006;18(5):488–493.
11. Mage G, Canis M, Manhes H, et al. Laparoscopic management of adnexal cystic masses. *J Gynecol Surg.* 1990;6:71.
12. Nezhat C, Nezhat F, Welander CE, et al. Four ovarian cancers diagnosed during laparoscopic management of 1,011 adnexal masses. *Am J Obstet Gynecol.* 1992;167:790.
13. Hulka JF, Parker WH, Surrey M, et al. Management of ovarian masses: AAGL 1190 survey. *J Reprod Med.* 1992;37:599.
14. Wenzl R, Lehner R, Husslein P, Sevelda P. Laparoscopic surgery in cases of ovarian malignancies: an Austria-wide survey. *Gynecol Oncol.* 1996;63:57.
15. Maimon M, Seltzer V, Boyce J. Laparoscopic excision of ovarian neoplasms subsequently found to be malignant. *Obstet Gynecol.* 1991;77:653.
16. Herrmann U, Locher G, Goldhirsch A. Sonographic patterns of malignancy: prediction of malignancy. *Obstet Gynecol.* 1987;69:777.
17. Granberg S, Norstrom A, Wikland M. Comparison of endovaginal ultrasound and cytological evaluations of cystic ovarian tumors. *J Ultrasound Med.* 1991;10:9.
18. Canis M, Pouly JL, Wattiez A, et al. Laparoscopic management of adnexal masses suspicious at ultrasound. *Obstet Gynecol.* 1997;89:679.
19. Bell R, Petticrew M, Sheldon T. The performance of screening tests for ovarian cancer: results of a systematic review. *Br J Obstet Gynaecol.* 1998;105:1136.
20. Jacobs I, Bast R. The CA-125 tumor associated antigen: a review of the literature. *Hum Reprod.* 1989;4:1.
21. Nezhat CH, Nezhat F, Borhan S, et al. Is hormonal treatment efficacious in the management of ovarian cysts in women with histories of endometriosis? *Hum Reprod.* 1996;11:874.
22. Scoutt L, McCarthy SM, Lange R, et al. Evaluation of ovarian masses on MRI with ultrasound correlation. *Radiology.* 1990;177:242.
23. Takahashi K, Okada S, Okada M, et al. Magnetic resonance relaxation time in evaluating the cyst fluid characteristics of endometrioma. *Hum Reprod.* 1996;11:857.
24. Yamashita Y, Hatanaka Y, Torashima M, et al. Characterization of sonographically indeterminate ovarian tumors with MR imaging: a logistic regression analysis. *Acta Radiol.* 1997;38:572.
25. Moteki T, Ishizaka H. Evaluation of cystic ovarian lesions using apparent diffusion coefficient calculated from turboFLASH MR images. *Br J Radiol.* 1998;71:612.
26. Patel VH, Somers S. MR imaging of the female pelvis: current perspectives and review of genital tract congenital anomalies, and benign and malignant diseases. *Crit Rev Diagn Imaging.* 1997;38:417.
27. Woodward PJ, Gilfeather M. Magnetic resonance imaging of the female pelvis. *Semin Ultrasound CT MR.* 1998;19:90.
28. DeCrespigny L, Robinson HP, Daboren RAM, et al. The "simple" cyst: aspirate or operate? *Br J Obstet Gynecol.* 1989;96:1035.
29. Kjellgren RK. Ovarian cyst fenestration via laparoscopy. *J Reprod Med.* 1978;21:16.

30. Trope C. The preoperative diagnosis of malignancy of ovarian cysts. *Neoplasia*. 1981;28:117.

31. Hasson HM. Ovarian surgery. In: Sanfilippo JS, Levine RL, eds. *Operative Gynecological Endoscopy*. New York: Springer-Verlag; 1989.

32. Mulvany NJ. Aspiration cytology of ovarian cysts and cystic neoplasms: a study of 235 aspirates. *Acta Cytol*. 1996;40:911.

33. Lipitz S, Seidman DS, Menczer J, et al. Recurrence rate after fluid aspiration from sonographically benign-appearing ovarian cysts. *J Reprod Med*. 1992;37:845.

34. Larsen JF, Pedersen OD, Gregerson E. Ovarian cyst fenestration via the laparoscope. *Acta Obstet Gynecol Scand*. 1986;65:529.

35. Marana R, Caruana P, Muzii L, et al. Operative laparoscopy for ovarian cysts: excision vs. aspiration. *J Reprod Med*. 1996;41:435.

36. Zanetta G, Lissoni A, Torri V, et al. Role of puncture and aspiration in expectant management of simple ovarian cysts: a randomised study. *BMJ*. 1996;313:1110.

37. Troiano RN, Taylor KJ. Sonographically guided therapeutic aspiration of benign-appearing ovarian cysts and endometriomas. *AJR Am J Roentgenol*. 1998;171:1601.

38. Mikamo H, Kawazoe K, Sato Y, et al. Ovarian abscess caused by *Peptostreptococcus magnus* following transvaginal ultrasound-guided aspiration of ovarian endometrioma and fixation with pure ethanol. *Infect Dis Obstet Gynecol*. 1998;6:66.

39. Steinkampf MP, Hammond KR, Blackwell RE. Hormonal treatment of functional ovarian cysts: a randomized, prospective study. *Fertil Steril*. 1990;54:775.

40. Ben-Ami M, Geslevich Y, Battino S, et al. Management of functional ovarian cysts after induction of ovulation: a randomized prospective study. *Acta Obstet Gynecol Scand*. 1993;72:396.

41. Turan C, Zorlu CG, Ugur M, et al. Expectant management of functional ovarian cysts: an alternative to hormonal therapy. *Int J Gynaecol Obstet*. 1994;47:257.

42. Chapron C, Dubuisson JB, Kadoch O, et al. Laparoscopic management of organic ovarian cysts: is there a place for frozen section diagnosis? *Hum Reprod*. 1998;13:324.

43. Wolf SL, Gosnik BB, Feldesman MR, et al. Prevalence of simple adnexal cysts in postmenopausal women. *Radiology*. 1991;180:65.

44. Campbell S, Goessens L, Goswamy R, et al. Real-time ultrasonography for the determination of ovarian morphology and volume: a possible early screening test for ovarian cancer. *Lancet*. 1982;1:415.

45. Nezhat C, Nezhat F. Postoperative adhesion formation after ovarian cystectomy with and without ovarian reconstruction. Abstract presented at: American Fertility Society Annual Meeting; October 21, 1991; Orlando, FL.

46. Nezhat F, Brill AI, Nezhat CH, et al. Adhesion formation after endoscopic posterior colpotomy. *J Reprod Med*. 1993;38:534.

47. Nezhat C, Nezhat F. Operative laparoscopy for the management of ovarian remnant syndrome. *Fertil Steril*. 1992;57:1003.

48. Gleeson NC, Nicosia SV, Mark JE, et al. Abdominal wall metastases from ovarian cancer after laparoscopy. *Am J Obstet Gynecol*. 1993;169:522.

49. Nezhat C, Winer W, Nezhat F. Laparoscopic removal of dermoid cysts. *Obstet Gynecol*. 1989;73:278.

50. Remorgida V, Magnasco A, Pizzorno V, Anserini P. Four year experience in laparoscopic dissection of intact ovarian dermoid cysts. *J Am Coll Surg*. 1998;187:519.

51. Luxman D, Cohen JR, David MP. Laparoscopic conservative removal of ovarian dermoid cysts. *J Am Assoc Gynecol Laparosc*. 1996;3:409.

52. Pardi G, Carminati R, Ferrari MM, et al. Laparoscopically assisted vaginal removal of ovarian dermoid cysts. *Obstet Gynecol*. 1995;85:129.

53. Teng FY, Muzsnai D, Perez R, et al. A comparative study of laparoscopy and colpotomy for the removal of ovarian dermoid cysts. *Obstet Gynecol*. 1996;87:1009.

54. Campo S, Garcea N. Laparoscopic conservative excision of ovarian dermoid cysts with and without an Endobag. *J Am Assoc Gynecol Laparosc*. 1998;5:165.

55. Lin P, Falcone T, Tulandi T. Excision of ovarian dermoid cyst by laparoscopy and by laparotomy. *Am J Obstet Gynecol*. 1995;173:769.

Section 9.3. Laparoscopic Operations on the Ovary

Tanja Pejovic and Farr Nezhat

Although most benign ovarian tumors can be treated laparoscopically, observation of the adnexa enables a gynecologist to decide whether laparotomy is indicated.

OVARIAN BIOPSIES

It is often difficult to immobilize the ovary because of its smooth surface and firm texture. The uterine–ovarian ligament can be grasped to lift and rotate it, or the ovary can be wedged against the pelvic side wall by using the flattened edges of open or closed forceps. Sometimes Morgagni peritubal cysts can be used as a handle or the uterus can be manipulated under the ovary to provide a shelf (Figure 9.3.1). Overly aggressive manipulation may cause lacerations in the capsule and result in bleeding from follicles or cysts.

A punch biopsy specimen of a lesion from the antimesenteric border of the ovary is sufficient for most purposes. Palmer biopsy forceps can take tissue without penetrating the vascular medulla [1], although a small wedge resection yields the best histologic features of the ovarian stroma and cortex. Alternatively, tissue can be obtained by using toothed forceps and laparoscopic scissors or a laser (Figure 9.3.2). Bleeding is controlled with bipolar electrocoagulation; sutures should be avoided so that postoperative adhesions can be minimized.[2]

INDICATIONS FOR OOPHORECTOMY

In 1980, Semm [3] reported his experience with a laparoscopic approach to oophorectomy and salpingo-oophorectomy. Since then, several authors have described the efficacy and safety of these procedures using different techniques.[4–8] Laparoscopy may encourage ovarian conservation during hysterectomy and more conservative management of pain caused by adnexal disease. If necessary, oophorectomy may be done laparoscopically at a later date, with a short hospital stay and recovery period. The indications for oophorectomy are as follows:

1. Persistent localized pain despite previous lysis of adhesions or treatment of endometriosis
2. Residual ovary syndrome
3. Dysgenetic gonads
4. Ovarian cysts 5 cm or greater with ovarian damage, or when spillage of cystic contents increases the likelihood of complications (cystic teratomas, mucinous cystadenomas, malignancy)
5. Unilateral tubo-ovarian abscess

6. Prophylactic therapy for advanced breast cancer
7. Early ovarian cancer in young women (stage I)

A uterine manipulator is inserted for traction and countertraction to aid in the exposure and manipulation of the ovary. The pelvis and especially the adnexa are inspected to plan the surgical approach. Before starting the procedure, it is important to observe the course of the ureter as it crosses the external iliac artery near the bifurcation of the common iliac artery at the pelvic brim. The left ureter may be more difficult to find because the base of the sigmoid mesocolon often covers it. If the ureter cannot be seen through the intact peritoneum, it must be identified by retroperitoneal dissection. If the patient does not have a uterus, it is essential to insert a vaginal probe or sponge stick so that the surgeon can maintain orientation, particularly with procedures involving extensive adhesions. When anatomic landmarks are distorted by adhesions, endometriosis, or prior surgical extirpation, one should begin the procedure at the most normal area and work toward the more distorted parts of the operative field. The entire ovary must be removed to prevent ovarian remnant syndrome or tumor development in a dysgenetic gonad. At the conclusion, the operative field is inspected and clots are removed with a suction–irrigator or grasping forceps. Pedicles are inspected under water and with decreased pneumoperitoneum,[9] and hemostasis is obtained with bipolar electrocoagulation.

OOPHORECTOMY AND SALPINGO-OOPHORECTOMY

Management of the Infundibulopelvic Ligament

Three techniques have been described for managing the infundibulopelvic ligament: bipolar electrodesiccation, suture ligation with pre-tied sutures, and automatic stapling. Patient costs are approximately $600 for the linear stapler and $48 for each pre-tied ligature. There is no extra charge for bipolar electrocoagulation.

A bipolar forceps is preferable for hemostasis of the infundibulopelvic ligament.[4] Endoloop sutures (Ethicon) cannot be applied in the presence of adhesions that distort the anatomy, and it is difficult to place Endoloop sutures on large pedicles such as the mesovarium and infundibulopelvic ligament, even if the anatomy is normal. Once it is applied, the slipknot can loosen under the tension of the large pedicle, increasing the risk of intraoperative hemorrhage, or a piece of the ovary may be left in the pedicle, predisposing the patient to ovarian remnant syndrome.[10]

Aside from cost, there are several drawbacks to the stapling device. The instrument is bulky, and the operator must note its

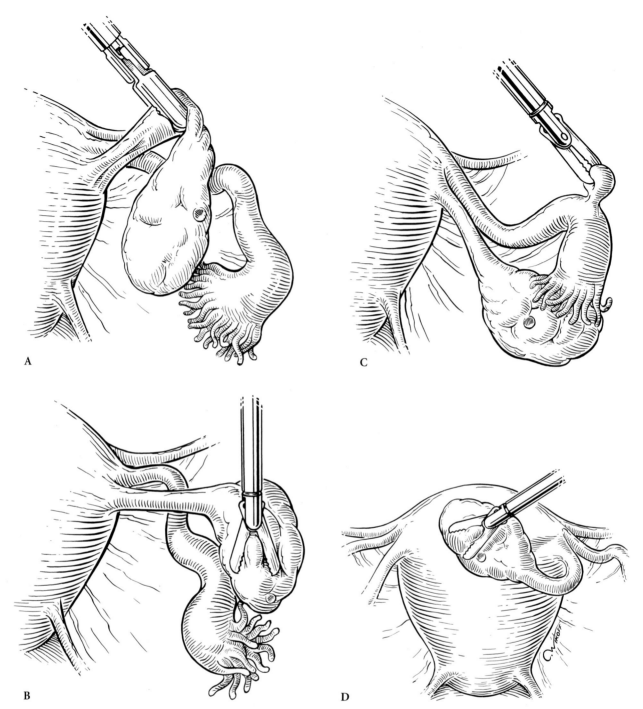

Figure 9.3.1. Different methods of immobilizing the ovary. (**A**) Grasping the utero-ovarian ligament. (**B**) Wedging the ovary against the pelvic side wall. (**C**) Grasping tubal or ovarian inclusion cysts. (**D**) Using the uterus as a platform.

proximity to the ureter, bowel, and bladder. Adequate desiccation of tissue with bipolar forceps by monitoring the flow of electrons on an ammeter has been suggested before transecting the pedicles. Excessive desiccation creates friable tissue and increases thermal damage, and the tissue may adhere to the forceps. A self-limiting bipolar electrocoagulator (Valleylab Force II series generator, Boulder, CO) provides controlled desiccation without charring the adjacent tissue. In this mode, the power peaks at 100 ohms instead of 300 to 500 ohms in typical generators.

The power then "rolls off" to provide the desired surgical effect without excess drying, blanching, or destruction of tissue.

The mechanism of closure of large blood vessels with high-frequency electrocoagulation was described by Sigel and Dunn.[11] Electrocoagulation begins with shrinkage of the vessel wall resulting from the denaturation of tissue proteins combined with the melting of the carbohydrate tissue components and the dehydration of tissue fluids. The resulting coagulum formed by this melting and fusion of the vessel wall obliterates

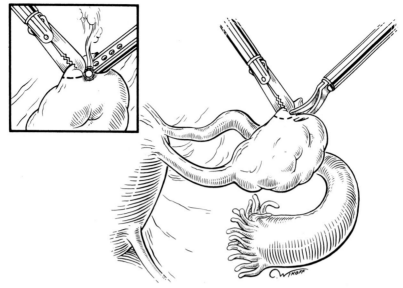

Figure 9.3.2. A small wedge biopsy specimen of the ovary is taken using a scissors or CO_2 laser (*inset*).

the lumen. The most successful closures are characterized by low levels of heating that end before char is formed, which preserve the inherent fibrillar structure of the connective tissue. Too much heating destroys the inherent fibrillar structure, forming a more amorphous coagulum that is poorly penetrated by fibroblasts and capillaries and characterized by an inflammatory-type reorganization and healing process that results in unsuccessful or weak closures. Further heating during electrocoagulation causes complete disintegration of the amorphous coagulum and carbonization.[11,12] Ammeters or flowmeters measure only the

flow of current in relation to tissue resistance and have no value in assuring hemostasis. Pedicles are reinspected after the intra-abdominal pressure has been lowered [9] because they can bleed again at the termination of a procedure once the hemostatic effects of the elevated abdominal pressures are lost.

The technique for oophorectomy is similar to that for salpingo-oophorectomy except that the tube must be protected from thermal damage. The procedure begins at the utero-ovarian ligament (Figure 9.3.3A). The pedicles are desiccated and cut.[4] The mesovarium is coagulated and cut into 2-cm bites, working

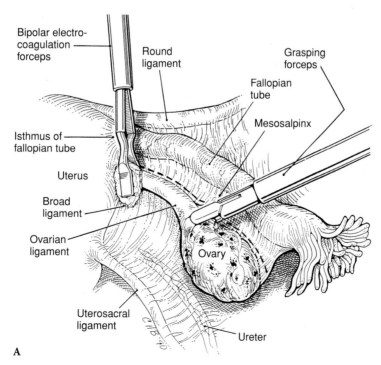

Figure 9.3.3. Oophorectomy is done by coagulating and cutting the mesovarium. (**A**) The procedure starts from the utero-ovarian ligament. (*Continued*)

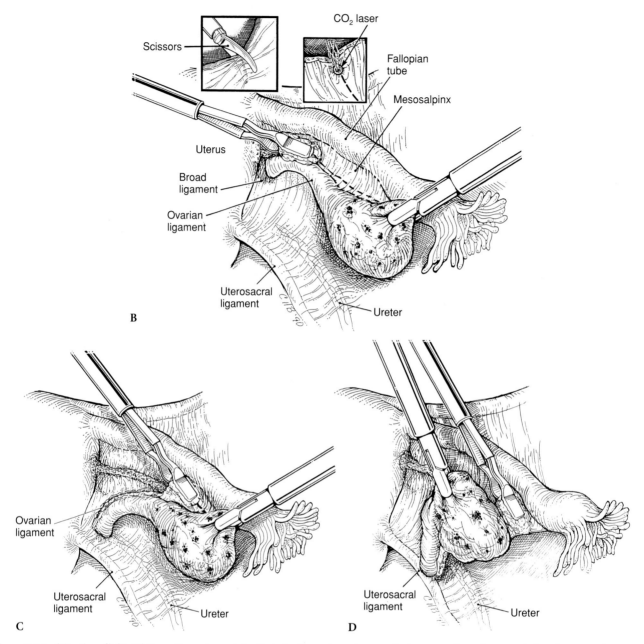

Figure 9.3.3. (*Continued*) (**B–D**) It continues toward the fimbria. *Insets* show the use of scissors or a laser for completing the reparation.

from the uterine side to the fimbria until the ovary is removed (Figure 9.3.3B–D). The latter step may jeopardize the fallopian tube if the mesovarium is overdesiccated. In some circumstances, it may be preferable to sharply incise the individual leaves of the mesovarium if the distance between the tube and the ovary is small. The underlying vascular tissue may be coagulated and divided to allow excision of the remaining ovary. Laparoscopic oophorectomy causes less morbidity than does oophorectomy by laparotomy, and the patient's recovery is shorter.[4]

An ovary and tube minimally involved with adhesions or endometriosis are approached from the infundibulopelvic ligament or the utero-ovarian ligament. Filmy adhesions that limit the mobility of the ovary are lysed. Ovarian cysts are aspirated and deflated, making removal of the ovary easier. The adnexa are removed by beginning with the infundibulopelvic ligament. This

approach is preferable if the uterus is to be removed or significant disease is found in the uterine–ovarian ligament, in patients with a prior hysterectomy, or if hemostasis of the ovarian vessels is necessary. The procedure begins with ureteral identification through the peritoneum as it enters the pelvic brim and travels parallel to the infundibulopelvic ligament.

The isthmic portion of the tube and the ovarian ligament are desiccated and cut (Figure 9.3.4). The ovary is held with a grasping forceps, and the infundibulopelvic ligament is put under traction by elevating it and pulling it medially. The infundibulopelvic ligament is desiccated with bipolar forceps and cut with a laser or scissors in 1- to 2-cm increments, working from lateral to medial until the adnexa are removed (Figures 9.3.5 through 9.3.8). To avoid damage to the lateral pelvic side wall, traction is used on the tube and ovary and excessive coagulation is avoided.

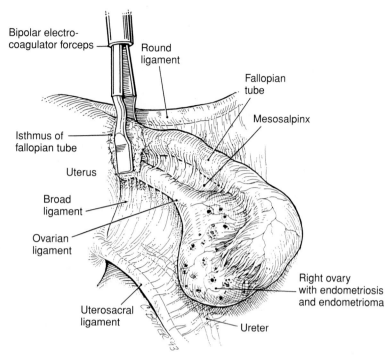

Figure 9.3.4. The procedure of salpingo-oophorectomy is begun by electrodesiccation and transection of the utero-ovarian ligament and the isthmic portion of the fallopian tube.

The Stapling Device

The laparoscopic linear stapling device used during gynecologic procedures is a modification of the stapling device used for bowel resection. The trocar site used to introduce the stapler is modified, depending on the specific adnexal disease. The trocar is introduced between the symphysis pubis and the umbilicus lateral to the rectus muscle and inferior epigastric vessels, although injury to inferior epigastric vessels is possible. At the end of the procedure, the fascia is closed to prevent a hernia. After the stapler is introduced, the adnexa are grasped with laparoscopic forceps and retracted medially and caudally to stretch

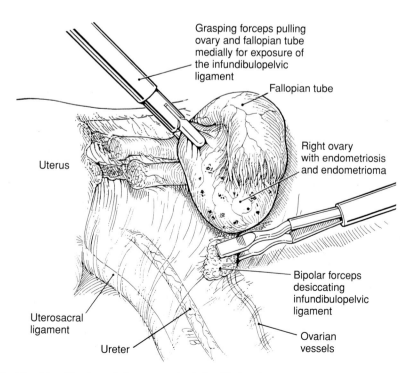

Figure 9.3.5. After identification of the ureter, the infundibulopelvic ligament is coagulated using a bipolar forceps while gentle traction is applied to the adnexa.

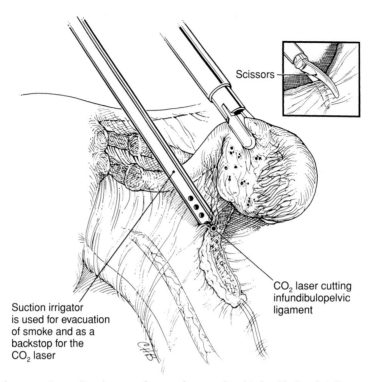

Figure 9.3.6. A laser or scissors (*inset*) are used to cut the coagulated infundibulopelvic ligament.

and outline the infundibulopelvic ligament. The ligament is grasped and secured with the stapler (Figures 9.3.9 and 9.3.10). The stapler is not fired until the contained tissue is identified and the ureter's safety is assured. Once transected, the staple line is examined for placement and hemostasis (Figure 9.3.11).

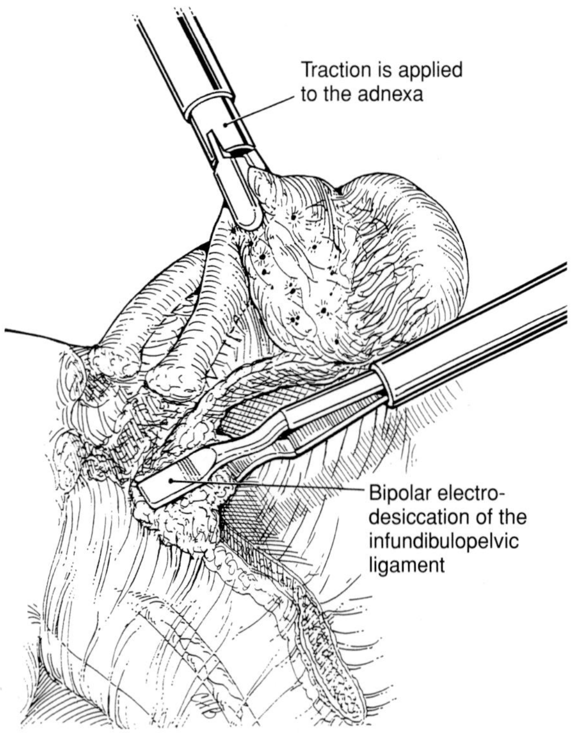

Usually one or two stapler applications are required for each adnexa.

The Endoligature

Pre-tied Endoloop sutures may be used in an oophorectomy or a salpingo-oophorectomy.[13] Peri-ovarian adhesions are lysed, and the ovary is freed. If a cyst is present, it is aspirated so that manipulation will be easier. The mesovarium and ovarian ligament are electrodesiccated and dissected to facilitate placement of the endoligature (Figure 9.3.12). The Endoloop (0 polydioxanone or polyglactin suture) is introduced into the abdominal

Figure 9.3.7. Coagulation and cutting of the infundibulopelvic ligament continue in 1- to 2-cm increments until it is removed completely.

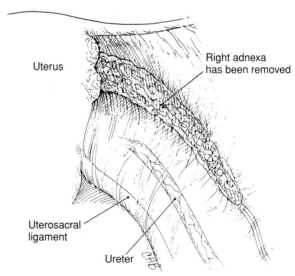

Figure 9.3.8. A view of the pelvic side wall after the adnexa is removed.

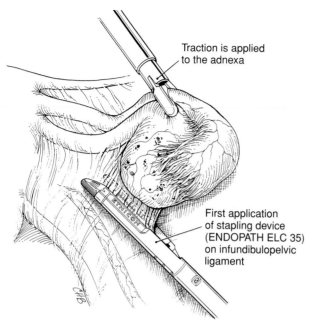

Traction is applied to the adnexa

First application of stapling device (ENDOPATH ELC 35) on infundibulopelvic ligament

Figure 9.3.9. A right salpingo-oophorectomy is done using a stapling device. The tube and ovary are under traction as the Endopath ELC 35 is applied across the infundibulopelvic ligament.

cavity through the mid-suprapubic trocar sleeve. Using forceps, the ovary is pulled through the Endoloop (Figure 9.3.12). Atraumatic forceps are used to assist in placement. The suture is pushed onto the mesovarium while a knot pusher is used on the opposite side to place the slipknot at the most lateral position on the mesosalpinx and mesovarium. The suture is tightened as the ovary is pulled toward the midline, and the tube is retracted with the atraumatic forceps. A second and, if necessary, a third Endoloop are placed, each successively closer to the pelvic wall so that the mesovarian pedicle will be long. The mesovarium is transected

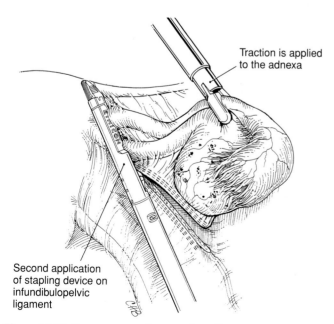

Traction is applied to the adnexa

Second application of stapling device on infundibulopelvic ligament

Figure 9.3.10. In most cases, the second application is necessary for complete removal of the adnexa.

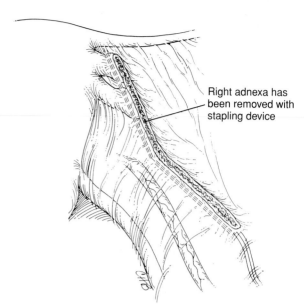

Right adnexa has been removed with stapling device

Figure 9.3.11. The pelvic side wall is seen after an adnexectomy with a stapling device.

with scissors. The pedicle is evaluated to confirm that the sutures have been placed beyond any ovarian tissue to avoid ovarian remnant syndrome (Figure 9.3.13).

For salpingo-oophorectomy, an Endoloop is placed over the adnexa after the ovarian ligament and tubal isthmus have been electrocoagulated and cut. The ovary and tube are grasped with forceps and pulled contralaterally. Simultaneously, the atraumatic forceps are used to push the Endoloop laterally, ensuring that the ligature is placed as far lateral as possible on the infundibulopelvic ligament. One or two additional sutures are placed progressively closer to the pelvic wall (at least 1 cm below the infundibulopelvic ligament) so that the pedicle will be long enough to prevent the sutures from slipping (Figure 9.3.14). The adnexal pedicle is transected with scissors. The ureter is evaluated at the pelvic brim to confirm that it is not damaged (Figure 9.3.15).

Dysgenetic Gonads

Individuals with androgen insensitivity syndrome have a high risk (20% to 30%) of developing malignancy in their gonads.[14] Phenotypic females with the XY karyotype require gonadectomy to protect them from developing gonadoblastoma. These gonads present as streaks, and the boundaries between the gonadal tissue and the peritoneum are not always clear. Because there is a chance that some of the dysgenetic gonadal tissue will be missed, the peritoneal borders must be kept wide. The laparoscopic approach for gonadectomy has been used in patients with male pseudohermaphroditism, including patients with pure gonadal dysgenesis, testicular feminization, and mixed gonadal dysgenesis and dysgenetic male pseudohermaphroditism.[14–16]

The laparoscopic procedure for removing a dysgenetic gonad is similar to that for removing an ovary that is densely adherent to the pelvic side wall.[17,18] Both the utero-ovarian and infundibulopelvic ligaments are electrocoagulated and cut. The mesovarium above and below is incised with scissors or the CO_2

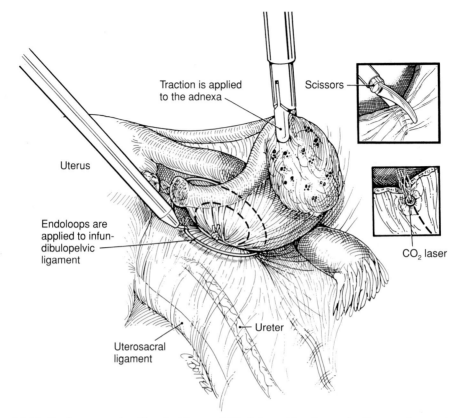

Figure 9.3.12. Oophorectomy is achieved with a partial Endoloop. After the ovarian ligament is coagulated and cut, two Endoloop sutures are passed over the ovary and mesovarium and tied beyond the ovarian tissue. *Insets* show the scissors (*top*) and laser (*bottom*) for the removal of the ligated mesovarium.

laser with hydrodissection (Figure 9.3.16). The loose areolar tissue immediately below the gonad is dissected away from the gonad.

Adherent Adnexa

Adhesions between the ovary and pelvic side wall, broad ligament, and bowel are lysed with the CO_2 laser or scissors until the ovary

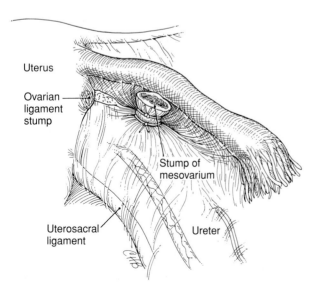

Figure 9.3.13. The right ovary is removed. An adequate stump should be left to prevent slippage of the ligature.

is freed. The ovary is grasped with a toothed forceps and elevated. It is put on stretch to create a plane between the ovary and the peritoneum. To avoid injury to ureters, blood vessels, and other underlying structures, the retroperitoneal area is entered and hydrodissection is carried out.[19] Using the suction–irrigator probe as a backstop, the adhesions are lysed close to the ovary. Removal of ovarian tissue may require excision of the peritoneum attached to the ovary.

The ovary may be enlarged, may be adherent to the pelvic side wall and broad ligament, or may contain endometriomas, so the surgeon may need to enter the retroperitoneal space (Figure 9.3.17). In this case, the ovary is removed by retroperitoneal dissection. After hydrodissection is done, an incision is made between the round and infundibulopelvic ligaments medial to the pelvic side wall (Figure 9.3.18). Blunt dissection, hydrodissection, and sharp dissection with the CO_2 laser are used to lyse adhesions and separate the adnexa and peritoneum, ureter, and blood vessels (Figure 9.3.19). Hemostasis is achieved with bipolar forceps. After dissection of the pelvic side wall, the remaining infundibulopelvic ligament, the ovarian ligament, and the proximal portion of the tube are coagulated and cut (Figure 9.3.20). The ureter is dissected from the ovary, and the adnexa are removed (Figure 9.3.21).

Residual Ovary

In patients who have had a previous hysterectomy, many of the usual landmarks in the pelvis are absent and extensive adhesions

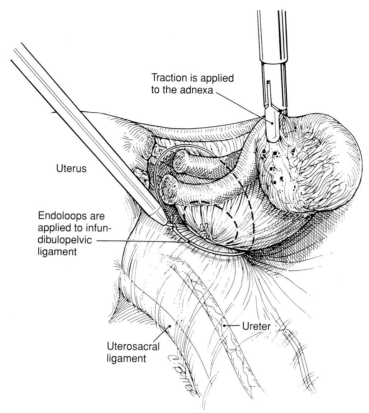

Figure 9.3.14. A right salpingo-oophorectomy is done using a pre-tied endoligature. After the ovarian ligament and tubouterine junction are coagulated and cut, the Endoloop is passed over the tube, ovary, and infundibulopelvic ligament and tied. One or two additional sutures may be necessary.

may involve the left ovary and descending colon. Lysis of adhesions is carried out cautiously to avoid damaging the bowel. If the ureter cannot be identified, it is necessary to open the retroperitoneal space. A sponge stick placed in the vagina aids in orientation.

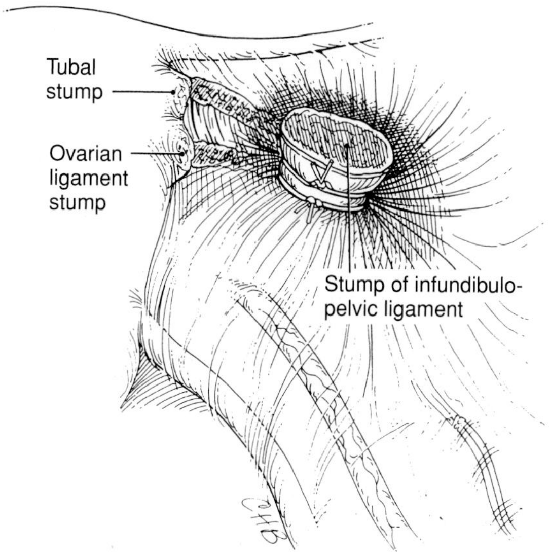

The ovary often is adherent to the vaginal cuff and is dissected from its attachment with scissors or the laser. The ureter is proximal to the lateral margins of the vaginal cuff, and its position can be altered from a previous operation. No ovarian fragments should remain on the pelvic side wall or vaginal cuff.

The ovary is immobilized with a grasping forceps and put on stretch, and the infundibulopelvic ligament is coagulated and transected in 1- to 2-cm increments until the ovary is removed. Depending on the pelvic anatomy, it is preferable to begin the

Figure 9.3.15. A view of the pelvic side wall after removal of the right adnexa.

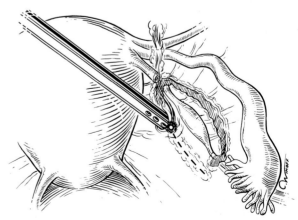

Figure 9.3.16. Excision of a streak ovary or dysgenetic gonad. The utero-ovarian and infundibulopelvic ligaments are electrocoagulated and cut. The mesovarium is incised with a CO_2 laser to free the tissue.

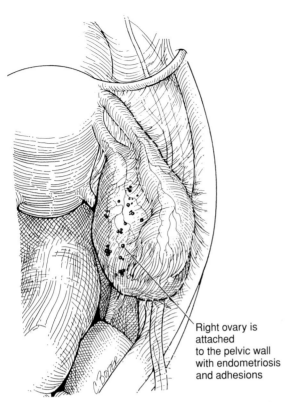

Figure 9.3.17. A large right endometrioma is attached to the pelvic side wall and ureter with fibrosis and adhesions.

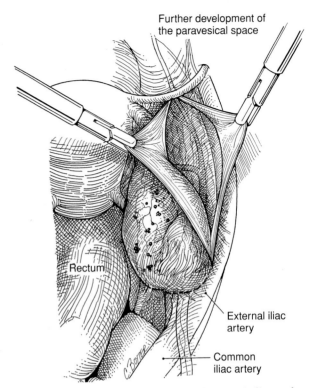

Figure 9.3.19. The peritoneum attached to the ovary is dissected medially from the retroperitoneal ureter and major pelvic side wall vessels.

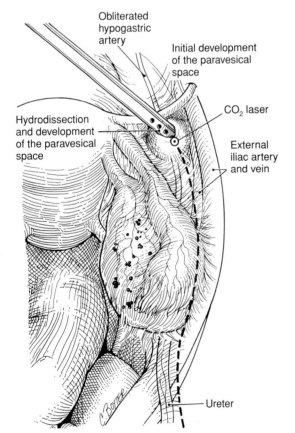

Figure 9.3.18. An incision is made with the CO_2 laser between the round ligament and the infundibulopelvic ligament to achieve an oophorectomy by retroperitoneal dissection. Hydrodissection and the suction–irrigator probe are used as a backstop for the laser.

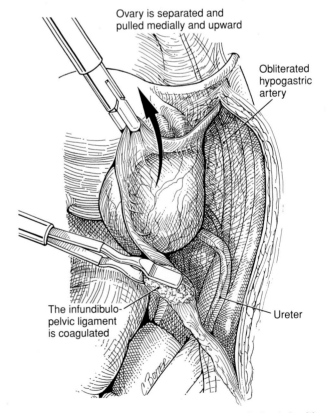

Figure 9.3.20. The adnexa are under traction, and the infundibulopelvic ligament is coagulated.

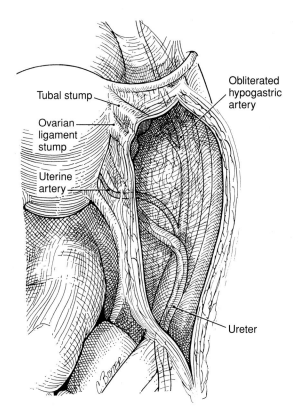

Figure 9.3.21. The pelvic side wall is observed after the right adnexa are removed with retroperitoneal dissection. The ureter and major retroperitoneal vessels can be seen.

Table 9.3.1: Results of Bilateral Ovarian Wedge Resection by Laparotomy

Author(s)	Patients, no.	Medical Failure	Ovulation, %	Conception, %
Adashi et al. [33]	90	Yes/no	64	48
Goldzieher and Green [56]	219	Yes/no	85	67
Buttram and Vaquero [57]	173	No	62	43
Lunde [58]	92	Yes	80	58
Hjortrup et al. [59]	29	No	86	77
Ronnberg et al. [60]	23	Yes	61	22

oophorectomy from the infundibulopelvic ligament to improve the anatomic relationships.

The ovary is removed through an abdominal incision as was described previously. If the ovary is large, it is cut into pieces. Colpotomy is done if the ovary is 5 cm or greater. However, colpotomy remote from a hysterectomy is technically difficult and is associated with significant risks if the bladder and rectosigmoid colon are adherent to the vaginal cuff.

Removal of Tissue

Removal of the ovary may be difficult if it is more than 5 cm in diameter. It can be removed through a 10-mm trocar sleeve placed in a suprapubic puncture, pulling the sleeve and forceps together and bringing the tissue to the incision. A Kelly or Kocher clamp is used to grasp the tissue to remove it from the abdomen. Alternatively, a long clamp is inserted through the accessory trocar incision and the tissue is grasped under direct observation and pulled from the abdomen through the trocar incision. The tube and ovary can be divided with scissors, a morcellator, or a laser and removed through trocar sleeves if fragmentation is not contraindicated by the characteristics of the cyst. If an open laparoscopy is required, the ovary is removed through an enlarged umbilical incision. After the ovary is removed, the pelvic cavity is irrigated and the pelvis is examined to assure hemostasis. For endometriomas and other cysts 5 cm or larger, the tissue is removed by posterior colpotomy. The cul-de-sac is identified by placing a sponge stick in the vagina and applying pressure to the posterior fornix between the uterosacral ligaments. An incision is

made between the uterosacral ligaments with a laser or unipolar knife electrode. Once the incision extends to the sponge stick, the ovary is brought to the incision and grasped vaginally with an Allis clamp. If a cyst is present, it is deflated with a large-bore needle or trocar while traction is applied to the ovary. As the ovary collapses, it is pulled into the vagina intact, with minimal spillage of its contents. The colpotomy is closed vaginally or laparoscopically, using two to three sutures. Removal of the ovary and vaginal closure of the colpotomy are facilitated by placing the patient's legs in the position for a vaginal hysterectomy.

If it is necessary to avoid spillage of the cyst contents, the ovary is removed in a specially designed laparoscopic bag (Endopouch, Ethicon).[20] The bag is removed through a posterior colpotomy incision [21] or an extended suprapubic incision. When the ovary is large and cystic, the bag is brought to the suprapubic or posterior colpotomy, the cyst is drained, and the deflated contained cyst is pulled from the abdominal cavity.

Ovarian Wedge Resection

Stein and Leventhal [22] described enlarged polycystic ovaries with the clinical features of menstrual aberrations, obesity, and hyperandrogenism. Although polycystic ovarian disease (PCOD) has variable manifestations, its hallmark is chronic anovulation. It was believed that the enlarged ovaries cause the condition, and so ovarian wedge resection was advocated. As ovulation induction agents were unavailable, ovarian wedge resection represented a major breakthrough, with ovulation and pregnancy rates of 80% and 50%, respectively. However, many patients who were initially ovulatory reverted to the previous anovulatory state after several months.[23] Although most had apparently normal ovulatory cycles, only 50% conceived (Table 9.3.1) because postoperative adhesions developed in many of these women (Table 9.3.2). The availability of ovulation-inducing medications in the 1960s and 1970s (clomiphene citrate [CC] and human menopausal gonadotropins [hMGs]) offered a nonsurgical approach to the treatment of anovulatory infertility that was safer than ovarian wedge resection. As a result, ovarian wedge resection was carried out rarely. CC therapy does not induce ovulation in all women. The alternative, hMG, is expensive, requires intensive monitoring, and may cause ovarian hyperstimulation. For

Table 9.3.2: Frequency of Adhesions after Wedge Resection by Laparotomy

Author(s)	Patients, no.	Percent with Adhesions
Adashi et al. [33]	7	100
Buttram and Vaquero [57]	40	100
Stein [61]	6	67
Weinstein and Polishuk [62]	19	42
Toaff et al. [63]	7	100
Portuondo et al. [64]	12	92
Total	91	85

Table 9.3.3: Results of Wedge Resection/Ovarian Drilling at Laparoscopy

Author(s)	Patients, no.	Ovulation, %	Conception, %
Gjonnaess [23]	62	92	69
Kojima [25]	12	83	58
Campo et al. [26]	12	45	41
Aakvag [27]	58	72	N/A
Kovacs et al. [29]	10	70	30
Keckstein et al. [30]	19	72	44
Daniell and Miller [31]	85	71	56
Greenblatt and Casper [65]	6	82	50
Armar et al. [66]	21	81	50
Gjonnaess [67]	252	92	84
Campo et al. [68]	23	56	56
Armar and Lachelin [69]	50	86	66
Gurgan et al. [70]	40	70	50
Naether et al. [71]	206	81	70

clomiphene-resistant patients, laparoscopic techniques have many advantages over gonadotropin therapy, including serial repetitive ovulation events, no increased risk of ovarian hyperstimulation or multiple pregnancies, and a lower incidence of spontaneous abortion. These procedures are not the first-line treatment for anovulatory patients with polycystic ovarian syndrome (PCOS), for whom CC remains the primary therapy.[24]

Some endoscopists have accomplished ovarian wedge resections laparoscopically [25], whereas others have reduced ovarian volume by taking multiple biopsies [23,26], coagulating with monopolar current [27–29], creating craters on the ovarian surface with lasers [30,31], or puncturing the small cysts on the ovarian surface.[32] Broadly similar results have been obtained using biopsy, multielectrocoagulation, and laser surgery: 50% or greater ovulation rate and a mean pregnancy rate of 50%.[24] Laparoscopic ovarian drilling appears to be associated with comparable rates of ovulation and conception (Table 9.3.3). Regardless of the method used to decrease ovarian mass, the hormonal changes observed with the laparoscopic procedures are similar to those observed after ovarian wedge resection by laparotomy.[24,33] Laparoscopic techniques offer cost savings and a lower risk of postoperative adhesions compared with wedge resection by laparotomy.[24] A disappointing finding is that the risk of postoperative adhesions is high (average, 30%) in women undergoing ovarian drilling (Table 9.3.4). Although adhesions were less common after laparoscopic multiple biopsies, they were observed in about 90% of patients after resection by laparotomy, 30% after laparoscopic electrocoagulation, and 50% after laparoscopic laser vaporization.[34] The possible effect of applying an oxidized regenerated cellulose (Interceed, Gynecare) barrier on postoperative surfaces after laparoscopic electrosurgical treatment for PCOS was studied in a prospective, randomized controlled study.[35] After bilateral ovarian treatment, one ovary was chosen randomly to have Interceed applied to its surface, using a specially designed applicator, with the other ovary serving as a control. Periadnexal adhesions of significant extent and severity developed in 57% of the women and 38% of the adnexa. The incidence of adhesions on the Interceed-treated side was 43%, whereas on the control side, it was 33%. In addition, the extent and severity of the adhesions appeared to be similar on the Interceed-treated and control sides. Larger numbers are required

Table 9.3.4: Frequency for Postoperative Adhesions after Laparoscopic Ovarian Drilling

Author(s)	Patients, no.	Percent with Adhesions
Portuondo et al. [64]	24	0
Greenblatt and Casper [65]	6	100
Gurgan et al. [72]	17	82
Dabirashrafi et al. [73]	43	16
Naether and Fischer [74]	62	19
Naether et al. [75]	26	27
Keckstein et al. [76]	11	27

to ascertain statistically the effects of Interceed on prevention of adhesions after laparoscopic electrosurgical treatment of PCOS.

Theoretically, wedge resection and ovarian drilling work by reducing androgen production in the ovarian stroma. Appropriate patients are women who fail to ovulate after 3 to 4 months on clomiphene and do not respond to hMG. The procedure is achieved by using a 10-mm videolaparoscope coupled to a CO_2 laser. A 5-mm second puncture is placed suprapubically in the midline and is used for a suction–irrigator or grasping instrument. Associated pelvic abnormalities are corrected before ovarian coagulation. Each ovary is fixed in the anterior cul-de-sac or held by the utero-ovarian ligament during treatment. The ultrapulse (40 to 80 W, 25 to 200 millijoules [mJ]) or superpulse (25 to 40 W) CO_2 laser is used. All visible subcapsular follicles are vaporized and drained, and randomly placed 2- to 4-mm–diameter craters are made in the ovarian stroma (Figure 9.3.22).

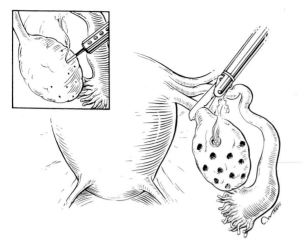

Figure 9.3.22. Ovarian drilling is used for PCOD. While the ovarian ligament is grasped and the ovary is held, multiple surface craters are created by the CO$_2$ laser, fiber laser, or needle electrode (*inset*).

Each ovary is treated symmetrically, and cysts are vaporized. The ovaries are irrigated, and hemostasis is obtained with bipolar forceps.

A potassium titanyl phosphate, neodymium: yttrium–aluminum–garnet (Nd:YAG), or argon laser can be used also.[30,31] The fiber is threaded through the central channel of a special 5-mm dual-channel suction–irrigation probe. When the dual-channel probe is used, it is possible to suction the smoke from vaporization at the site of occurrence. Holes are drilled in the ovary in a manner similar to that described for the CO$_2$ laser.

Ovarian coagulation has been done using unipolar punch biopsy forceps [23] or a needle electrode.[26–28] The power setting for the monopolar current is 20 to 30 W in a cutting mode to minimize thermal damage, and the power is activated just before the ovary is touched. The ovary is penetrated in approximately 10 to 15 sites at a depth of 3 to 5 mm.

Ovarian Torsion

Adnexal torsion is a surgical emergency. When this is diagnosed early, the adnexa can be unwound.[36,37] However, the diagnosis often is delayed because of the inconsistent presenting symptoms and signs and intermittent pain. When the diagnosis is delayed, the adnexa become congested, ischemic, hemorrhagic, and necrotic.[38] Gynecologists have been taught to remove tissue that has undergone torsion and ischemia because of the risk of thrombotic embolism arising from the ovarian vein. Way [39] reported successful conservative management of adnexal torsion. The affected structure was straightened to assess the viability, and even ovaries that appeared infarcted at laparotomy regained normal color after untwisting. No complications related to the procedure were reported. Because adnexal torsion produces no pathognomonic clinical findings, laparoscopy is used for diagnosis and treatment. Prompt laparoscopic examination is essential because delay is associated with gangrene.

A prospective, controlled follow-up study was designed to examine the effects of adnexal torsion on long-term ovarian histology and free radical scavenger (FRS) activity and subsequent viability after the detorsion of twisted ischemic adnexa. Adnexal

torsion was created by twisting the adnexa three times and fixing onto the side wall or by applying vascular clips in cycling female rats at 70 days of age. After an ischemic period of 4 to 36 hours, the twisted adnexa were removed and fixed. In the second group of rats, after the above ischemic periods, the torsions were relieved by untwisting or removing the vascular clips. Then the animals were perfused for a week, and adnexa were extirpated. After both ischemia and reperfusion, the removed adnexa were examined histologically and tissue concentrations of glutathione peroxidase, superoxide dismutase, catalase, and glutathione were ascertained. Regardless of the ischemic time, all the twisted adnexa were black–bluish. Despite the gross ischemic–hemorrhagic features, histologic sections revealed negligible changes, with intact ovarian structure similar to that of controls in 4- to 24-hour groups. Although decreased compared with controls, the change in tissue concentrations of FRS was not significant in the 4- to 24-hour groups. Only the 36-hour group showed prominent congestion on all sections and a significant decrease in all FRS concentrations studied. Although no long-term reperfusion injury was observed histologically in the 4- to 24-hour groups, the 36-hour group ended up with adnexal necrosis. These findings support the importance of early diagnosis and conservative surgical management (detorsion) in adnexal torsion. Lack of histologic changes and unimpaired FRS metabolism are consistent with recent data showing that vascular compromise is caused by venous or lymphatic stasis in early torsion; adnexal integrity is not correlated with gross ischemic appearance, thus providing evidence of adnexal resistance against ischemia.[40]

The causes of ovarian or adnexal torsion are paraovarian cysts, functional and pathologic ovarian cysts, ovarian hyperstimulation, tubal pregnancy, adhesions, and congenital malformation.[41,42] The ischemic structures are straightened gently with atraumatic forceps to avoid additional adnexal damage. In women with ovarian hyperstimulation, the functional cysts are drained before untwisting.[43] The abnormalities contributing to torsion should be treated. One should shorten the utero-ovarian ligament if its length may have contributed to ovarian torsion. A running suture of monofilament material is placed along the length of the utero-ovarian ligament (Figure 9.3.23) and tied to shorten it, limiting ovarian mobility.

Mage and associates [41], in a report of 35 patients, noted that 21 women showed no gross evidence of ischemia or mild changes, with immediate and complete recovery within 10 minutes of untwisting. In eight, the tube or ovary was dark red or black, but partial recovery was apparent after the pedicle was untwisted. Six had gangrenous adnexa that required salpingectomy or oophorectomy. The first two groups were managed conservatively; the third group underwent excision of the involved organ(s). The postoperative course in all patients was uneventful. Six of the eight women in the intermediate group underwent a second-look laparoscopy that showed complete recovery.

Ovarian Remnant Syndrome

In premenopausal women who have had a bilateral oophorectomy, a small piece of functional ovarian tissue may respond to hormonal stimulation with growth, cystic degeneration, or hemorrhage and produce pain.[44–46] In a rat model, Minke and colleagues [47] showed that devascularized ovarian tissue can

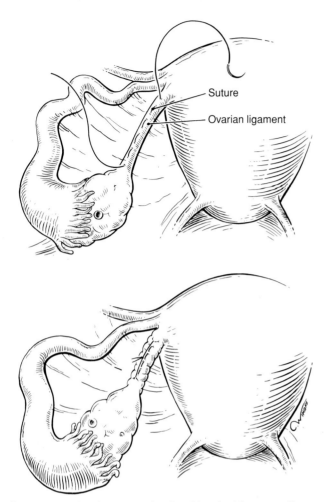

Figure 9.3.23. Ovarian suspension is achieved with a monofilament suture placed along the length of the utero-ovarian ligament and tied.

reimplant on intact or denuded peritoneal surfaces and that the revascularized tissue can become functional as evidenced by follicle formation and vaginal cornification.

Ovarian remnants remain because of dense adhesions, and distorted anatomic relationships invariably worsen with subsequent operations. It is not unusual for these patients to have had previous attempts to excise an ovarian remnant. Removal of the ovarian remnant is preferred, although the reported incidence of complications with laparotomy ranges from 16% to 30%.[48] The challenge and complications are related to the presence of extensive pelvic and abdominal adhesions from multiple previous operations, endometriosis, pelvic inflammatory disease, or ovarian cysts.

Diagnosis is based on history and localization of pelvic pain. Whereas some patients have cystic adnexal structures or ill-defined fixed masses, others have normal pelvic findings. Vaginal ultrasound can help locate the ovarian remnant.[49] Low or borderline levels of follicle-stimulating hormone in patients with documented bilateral oophorectomy are consistent with the presence of active ovarian tissue.[44] Hormonal suppression with oral contraceptives or a gonadotropin-releasing hormone agonist provides no relief in most patients.[10,50] CC or hMG is used to increase ovarian remnant size to confirm the diagnosis preoperatively or to aid in locating the tissue intraoperatively.[51]

Laparoscopic ultrasonography is used to detect ovarian remnants in patients in whom the pelvic anatomy is distorted by multiple adhesions.[52]

Past reviews have considered laparoscopy ineffective in the management of ovarian remnant syndrome because of the presence of dense pelvic adhesions.[48] However, the absence of complications in a series of 22 patients attests to the feasibility of the laparoscopic approach.[10]

Attention should be focused on prevention. Factors associated with ovarian remnant syndrome are the use of Endoloops for laparoscopic oophorectomy, multiple operative procedures with incomplete removal of pelvic organs, densely adherent ovaries, and multiple ovarian cystectomies for functional cysts.[10] When pre-tied sutures are used for the infundibulopelvic ligament, they should be placed below the ovarian tissue. Electrocoagulation and transection of the infundibulopelvic ligament or the application of clips is preferred. When the ovary is adherent to the pelvic side wall, retroperitoneal hydrodissection, meticulous adhesiolysis, and removal of the peritoneum underlying the ovary are essential in achieving a laparoscopic oophorectomy (Figure 9.3.20). The need for restraint in managing functional cysts is underscored by the fact that some patients in the author's [10] series had only a corpus luteum resected at first laparotomy.

A preoperative bowel preparation of GoLYTELY (Braintree Laboratories), enemas, and oral metronidazole is indicated. Anterior abdominal wall adhesions are probable after multiple laparotomies, and an open laparoscopy or mapping technique [53] is advisable. After all instruments are inserted, intra-abdominal adhesions are lysed and the ovarian remnants are dissected. Extensive and careful retroperitoneal dissection is required to facilitate identification and removal of the ovarian remnant tissue.[54,55] The anatomy of the retroperitoneal space is identified when the ovarian remnant is adherent to the lateral pelvic wall. The space beneath the peritoneum is injected with lactated Ringer's solution, and the peritoneum is opened to the infundibulopelvic ligament or its remnant. Adhesions are lysed until the course of the major pelvic blood vessels and the ureter can be traced and, if necessary, dissected. The ovarian blood supply is coagulated with bipolar forceps, and the ovarian tissue is excised and submitted for histologic examination.

When the remnant is adherent to the bowel, adhesions are lysed using hydrodissection and the CO_2 laser. Ovarian tissue embedded in the muscularis of the bowel is removed superficially, skinning the mucosa beneath it. The serosa and muscularis layers are imbricated with one to three interrupted 4-0 polydioxanone sutures in one layer. All remnant ovarian tissue should be removed. When the lesion is embedded in the bowel or bladder muscularis or when the ureter is involved or possibly obstructed, partial removal of the organ and repair are necessary.

REFERENCES

1. Yuzpe AA, Rioux JE. The value of laparoscopic ovarian biopsy. *J Reprod Med*. 1975;15:57.
2. Nezhat C, Nezhat F. Postoperative adhesion formation after ovarian cystectomy with and without ovarian reconstruction. Abstract presented at: American Fertility Society Annual Meeting; October 21, 1991; Orlando, FL.

3. Semm K. Course of endoscopic abdominal surgery. In: Friedrich E, ed. *Operative Manual for Endoscopic Abdominal Surgery*. Chicago: Year Book; 1984.

4. Nezhat F, Nezhat C, Silfen SL. Videolaseroscopy for oophorectomy. *Am J Obstet Gynecol*. 1991;165:1323.

5. Silva PD, Juffel ME, Beguin EA. Open laparoscopy simplifies instrumentation required for laparoscopic oophorectomy and salpingo-oophorectomy. *Obstet Gynecol*. 1991;77:482.

6. Russell JB. Laparoscopic oophorectomy. *Curr Opin Obstet Gynecol*. 1995;7:295.

7. Nezhat C, Nezhat F, Silfen SL. Laparoscopic hysterectomy and bilateral salpingo-oophorectomy using multifire GIA surgical stapler. *J Gynecol Surg*. 1990;6:287.

8. Daniell JF, Jurtz BR, Lee JY. Laparoscopic oophorectomy: comparative study of ligatures, bipolar coagulation and automatic stapling devices. *Obstet Gynecol*. 1992;80:325.

9. Nezhat C, Nezhat F, Winer W. Salpingectomy via laparoscopy: a new surgical approach. *J Laparosc Surg*. 1991;1:91.

10. Nezhat C, Nezhat F. Operative laparoscopy for the management of ovarian remnant syndrome. *Fertil Steril*. 1992;57:1003.

11. Sigel B, Dunn MR. The mechanism of blood vessel closure by high frequency electrocoagulation. *Surg Gynecol Obstet*. 1965;121(4):823.

12. Nezhat C, Nezhat F. Laparoscopic electrosurgical oophorectomy: risk of using "blanching" as the end point [letter to the editor]. *Am J Obstet Gynecol*. 1992;167:1151.

13. Semm K. *Operative Manual for Endoscopic Abdominal Surgery*. Chicago: Year Book; 1984.

14. Campo S, Garcia N. Laparoscopic gonadectomy in two patients with gonadal dysgenesis. *J Am Assoc Gynecol Laparosc*. 1998;5: 305.

15. Kriplani A, Abbi M, Ammini AC, et al. Laparoscopic gonadectomy in male pseudohermaphrodites. *Eur J Obstet Gynecol Reprod Biol*. 1998;81:37.

16. Ulrich U, Keckstein J, Buck G. Removal of gonads in Y-chromosome-bearing gonadal dysgenesis and in androgen insensitivity syndrome by laparoscopic surgery. *Surg Endosc*. 1996;10: 422.

17. Droesch K, Dorexch J, Chumas J, et al. Laparoscopic gonadectomy for gonadal dysgenesis. *Fertil Steril*. 1990;53:360.

18. Seifer DB. Laparoscopic adnexectomy in a prepubertal Turner mosaic female with isodicentric Y. *Hum Reprod*. 1991;6:566.

19. Nezhat C, Nezhat F. Safe laser excision or vaporization of peritoneal endometriosis. *Fertil Steril*. 1989;52:149.

20. Nezhat C, Nezhat F, Welander CE, et al. Four ovarian cancers diagnosed during laparoscopic management of 1,011 adnexal masses. *Am J Obstet Gynecol*. 1992;167:790.

21. Nezhat F, Brill AI, Nezhat CH, et al. Adhesion formation after endoscopic posterior colpotomy. *J Reprod Med*. 1993;38:534.

22. Stein IF, Leventhal ML. Amenorrhea associated with bilateral polycystic ovaries. *Am J Obstet Gynecol*. 1935;29:181.

23. Gjonnaess H. Polycystic ovarian syndrome treated by ovarian electrocautery through the laparoscope. *Fertil Steril*. 1984;41:20.

24. Judd HL, Rigg LA, Anderson DC, et al. The effects of ovarian wedge resection on circulating gonadotropin and ovarian steroid levels in patients with polycystic ovarian syndrome. *J Clin Endocrinol Metab*. 1976;43:347.

25. Kojima E. Ovarian wedge resection with contact Nd:YAG laser irradiation used laparoscopically. *J Reprod Med*. 1989;34:444.

26. Campo S, Garcia N, Caruso A, et al. Effect of celioscopy ovarian resection in patients with polycystic ovaries. *Gynecol Obstet Invest*. 1983;15:213.

27. Aakvaag A. Hormonal response to electrocautery of the ovary in patients with polycystic ovarian disease. *Br J Obstet Gynaecol*. 1985;92:1258.

28. Casper RF, Greenblatt EM. Laparoscopic ovarian cautery for induction of ovulation in women with polycystic ovary disease. *Semin Reprod Endocrinol*. 1990;8:209.

29. Kovacs G, Buckler H, Bangah M, et al. Treatment of anovulation due to polycystic ovarian syndrome by laparoscopic ovarian electrocautery. *Br J Obstet Gynaecol*. 1991;98:30.

30. Keckstein G, Rossmanith W, Spatzier K, et al. The effect of laparoscopic treatment of polycystic ovarian disease by CO_2 laser or ND-YAG laser. *Surg Endosc*. 1990;4:103.

31. Daniell JF, Miller W. Polycystic ovaries treated by laparoscopic laser vaporization. *Fertil Steril*. 1989;51(2):232.

32. Sumioki H, Utsunomyiya T, Matsuoka K, et al. The effect of laparoscopic multiple punch resection of the ovary on the hypothalamo-pituitary axis in polycystic ovary syndrome. *Fertil Steril*. 1988;50:567.

33. Adashi EY, Rock JA, Guzick D, et al. Fertility following bilateral ovarian wedge resection: a critical analysis of 90 consecutive cases of the polycystic ovary syndrome. *Fertil Steril*. 1981;36:320.

34. Campo S. Ovulatory cycles, pregnancy outcome and complications after surgical treatment of polycystic ovary syndrome. *Obstet Gynecol Surv*. 1998;53:297.

35. Saravelos H, Li TC. Post-operative adhesions after laparoscopic electrosurgical treatment for polycystic ovarian syndrome with the application of Interceed to one ovary: a prospective randomized controlled study. *Hum Reprod*. 1996;11:992.

36. Oelsner G, Bider D, Goldenberg M, et al. Long-term follow-up of the twisted ischemic adnexa managed by detorsion. *Fertil Steril*. 1993;60:976.

37. Shalev E, Bustan M, Yarom I, Peleg D. Recovery of ovarian function after laparoscopic detorsion. *Hum Reprod*. 1995;10:2965.

38. Steyaert H, Meynol F, Valla JS. Torsion of the adnexa in children: the value of laparoscopy. *Pediatr Surg Int*. 1998;13:384.

39. Way S. Ovarian cystectomy of twisted cysts. *Lancet*. 1946;2:47.

40. Taskin O, Birincioglu M, Aydin A, et al. The effects of twisted ischaemic adnexa managed by detorsion on ovarian viability and histology: an ischaemia-reperfusion rodent model. *Hum Reprod*. 1998;13:2823.

41. Mage G, Canis M, Manhes H, et al. Laparoscopic management of adnexal torsion. *J Reprod Med*. 1989;34:520.

42. Wagaman R, Williams RS. Conservative therapy for adnexal torsion. *J Reprod Med*. 1990;35:833.

43. Ben-Rafael Z, Bider D, Mashiach S. Laparoscopic unwinding of twisted ischemic hemorrhagic adnexum after in vitro fertilization. *Fertil Steril*. 1990;53:569.

44. Petit PD, Lee RA. Ovarian remnant syndrome: diagnostic dilemma and surgical challenge. *Obstet Gynecol*. 1988;71:580.

45. Siddall-Allum J, Rae T, Rogers V, et al. Chronic pelvic pain caused by residual ovaries and ovarian remnants. *Br J Obstet Gynaecol*. 1994;101:979.

46. Orford VP, Kuhn RJ. Management of ovarian remnant syndrome. *Aust N Z J Obstet Gynaecol*. 1996;36:468.

47. Minke T, DePond W, Winkelmann T, Blythe J. Ovarian remnant syndrome: study in laboratory rats. *Am J Obstet Gynecol*. 1994;171:1440.

48. Price FV, Edwards R, Buschsbaum HJ. Ovarian remnant syndrome: difficulties in diagnosis and management. *Obstet Gynecol Surv*. 1990;45:151.

49. Fleischer AC, Tait D, Mayo J, et al. Sonographic features of ovarian remnants. *J Ultrasound Med*. 1998;17:551.

50. Siddall-Allum J, Rae T, Rogers V, et al. Chronic pelvic pain caused by residual ovaries and ovarian remnants. *Br J Obstet Gynaecol*. 1994;101:979.

51. Kaminski PF, Sorosky JI, Mandell MJ, et al. Clomiphene citrate stimulation as an adjunct in locating ovarian tissue in ovarian remnant syndrome. *Obstet Gynecol*. 1990;76:924.

52. Nezhat F, Nezhat C, Nezhat CH, et al. Use of laparoscopic ultrasonography to detect ovarian remnants. *Am J Obstet Gynecol.* 1996;174:641.

53. Nezhat C, Nezhat F, Silfen SL. Videolaseroscopy: the CO_2 laser for advanced operative laparoscopy. *Obstet Gynecol Clin North Am.* 1991;18:3:585.

54. Lafferty HW, Angioli R, Rudolph J, Penalver MA. Ovarian remnant syndrome: experience at Jackson Memorial Hospital, University of Miami, 1985 through 1993. *Am J Obstet Gynecol.* 1996;174:641.

55. Kamprath S, Possover M, Schneider A. Description of a laparoscopic technique for treating patients with ovarian remnant syndrome. *Fertil Steril.* 1997;68:663.

56. Goldzieher JW, Green JA. The polycystic ovary: clinical and histological features. *J Clin Endocrinol Metab.* 1962;22:325.

57. Buttram VC, Vaquero C. Post-ovarian wedge resection adhesive disease. *Fertil Steril.* 1975;26:874.

58. Lunde O. Polycystic ovarian syndrome: a retrospective study of the therapeutic effect of ovarian wedge resection after unsuccessful treatment with clomiphene citrate. *Ann Chir Gynaecol.* 1982;71:330.

59. Hjortrup A, Kehlet H, Lockwood K, et al. Long term clinical effects of ovarian wedge resection in polycystic ovarian syndrome. *Acta Obstet Gynecol Scand.* 1983;62:55.

60. Ronnberg L, Ylostalo P, Ruokonen A. Hormonal parameters and conception rate during 5 different types of treatment of polycystic ovarian syndrome. *Int J Gynaecol Obstet.* 1985;23:177.

61. Stein IF. Wedge resection of the ovaries: the Stein Leventhal syndrome. In: Greenblatt RB, ed. *Ovulation.* Philadelphia: Lippincott; 1966.

62. Weinstein D, Polishuk WZ. The role of wedge resection of the ovary as a cause for mechanical sterility. *Surg Gynecol Obstet.* 1975;141:417.

63. Toaff R, Toaff ME, Peyser MR. Infertility following wedge resection of the ovaries. *Am J Obstet Gynecol.* 1976;124:92.

64. Portuondo JA, Melchor JC, Neyro JL, et al. Periovarian adhesions following ovarian wedge resection or laparoscopic biopsy. *Endoscopy.* 1984;16:143.

65. Greenblatt R, Casper RF. Endocrine changes after laparoscopic ovarian cautery in polycystic ovary syndrome. *Am J Obstet Gynecol.* 1987;156:279.

66. Armar NA, McGarrigle HHG, Honour J, et al. Laparoscopic ovarian diathermy in the management of ovulatory infertility in women with polycystic ovaries: endocrine changes and clinical outcome. *Fertil Steril.* 1990;53:45.

67. Gjonnaess H. Ovarian electrocautery in the treatment of women with polycystic ovary syndrome (PCOS): factors affecting the results. *Acta Obstet Gynecol Scand.* 1994;73:407.

68. Campo S, Felli A, Lamanna MA, et al. Endocrine changes and clinical outcome after laparoscopic ovarian resection in women with polycystic ovaries. *Hum Reprod.* 1993;8:359.

69. Armar NA, Lachelin GC. Laparoscopic ovarian diathermy: an effective treatment for anti-oestrogen resistant anovulatory infertility in women with the polycystic ovary syndrome. *Br J Obstet Gynaecol.* 1993;100:161.

70. Gurgan T, Urman B, Aksu T, et al. The effect of short-interval laparoscopic lysis of adhesions on pregnancy rates following Nd-YAG laser photocoagulation of polycystic ovaries. *Obstet Gynecol.* 1992;80:45.

71. Naether OG, Baukloh V, Fischer R, Kowalczyk T. Long-term follow-up in 206 infertility patients with polycystic ovarian syndrome after laparoscopic electrocautery of the ovarian surface. *Hum Reprod.* 1994;9:2342.

72. Gurgan T, Kisnisci H, Yarali H, et al. Evaluation of adhesion formation after laparoscopic treatment of polycystic ovarian disease. *Fertil Steril.* 1991;56:1176.

73. Dabirashrafi H, Mohamad K, Behjantia Y, et al. Adhesion formation after ovarian electrocauterization on patients with polycystic ovarian syndrome. *Fertil Steril.* 1991;55:1200.

74. Naether OG, Fischer R. Adhesion formation after laparoscopic electrocoagulation of the ovarian surface in polycystic ovary patients. *Fertil Steril.* 1993;60:95.

75. Naether OG, Fischer R, Weise HC, et al. Laparoscopic electrocoagulation of the ovarian surface in infertile patients with polycystic ovarian disease. *Fertil Steril.* 1993;60.

76. Keckstein G, Rossmanith W, Spatzier K, et al. The effect of laparoscopic treatment of polycystic ovarian disease by CO_2-laser or Nd:YAG laser. *Surg Endosc.* 1990;4:103.

Section 9.4. Management of the Ectopic Pregnancy

Bulent Berker, Ceana Nezhat, Farr Nezhat, and Camran Nezhat

Ectopic pregnancy, in which the gestational sac is outside the uterus, is the most common life-threatening emergency in early pregnancy. The first successful surgical treatment of ectopic pregnancy was described in 1883 by Tait. He performed salpingectomy on four women with ectopic pregnancy, and they all survived, an event that was extraordinary then. In 1973, Shapiro and Adler described treatment of ectopic pregnancy by laparoscopy, and today it is the standard surgical treatment of ectopic pregnancy.

A tubal pregnancy entails certain death of the gestation, a threat to the woman's life, and a subsequent successful pregnancy in less than 50% of patients. Until 1970, more than 80% of ectopic pregnancies were recognized after rupture. With the excellent resolution afforded by transvaginal sonography (TVS), the high sensitivity of radioimmunoassay of β-hCG, and the increased vigilance of clinicians, more than 80% of ectopic pregnancies now are detected before rupture.

INCIDENCE

Ectopic pregnancy is an important cause of maternal morbidity and occasionally mortality. Of all reported pregnancies, 1.3% to 2.0% are extrauterine. The incidence in the United States has increased greatly in the last few decades, from 4.5 per 1000 pregnancies in 1970 to an estimated 19.7 per 1000 pregnancies in 1992.[1] Of interest is the fact that unusual forms of ectopic pregnancy, such as interstitial and heterotopic pregnancies, are encountered more often. This is partly because of the more frequent use of assisted reproductive techniques.[2–5] In a series from Sweden [6], the incidence of ectopic pregnancy after in vitro fertilization was 4% and the most important risk factor was tubal disorder. Although the incidence of ectopic pregnancy in the general population is about 2%, the prevalence among pregnant patients presenting to an emergency department with first-trimester bleeding or pain, or both, is 6% to 16%.[7,8] Thus, greater suspicion and a lower threshold for investigation are justified.

Although earlier diagnosis has resulted in decreased maternal mortality and morbidity, hospitalizations for this condition increased from 17,800 in 1970 to 88,400 in 1989, representing a nearly fivefold rise.[9,10] Ranging in frequency from one in 250 to one in 87 live births, tubal pregnancy has emerged as a leading cause of maternal death, accounting for 10% of all maternal mortalities.[11]

From 1970 through 1989, more than 1 million ectopic pregnancies were estimated to have occurred among women in the United States.[12] The general trend was for the numbers and rates of ectopic pregnancy to increase over that 20-year period. The rate increased by almost fourfold, from 4.5 to 16.0 ectopic pregnancies per 1000 reported pregnancies. Although ectopic pregnancies accounted for less than 2% of all reported pregnancies during that period, complications of this condition were associated with approximately 13% of all pregnancy-related deaths.[12] However, during that period, the risk of death associated with ectopic pregnancy decreased 90%. The case fatality rate declined from 35.5 deaths per 10,000 ectopic pregnancies in 1970 to 3.8 in 1989.

There were 13 maternal deaths between 1997 and 1999 resulting from ectopic pregnancy in the United Kingdom and, despite falling mortality rates, ectopic pregnancy still accounts for 80% of first-trimester maternal deaths.[13] Nearly 32,000 ectopic pregnancies are diagnosed in the United Kingdom annually. The incidence in the United Kingdom appears to have changed little in the last decade, with 9.6 per 1000 pregnancies in 1991 to 1993 and 11.1 per 1000 pregnancies in 1997 to 1999. In other countries, however, the incidence of ectopic pregnancy appears to be decreasing. Between 1990 and 2001, Norway reported a fall in incidence from 17.2 to 9.5 per 10,000 women-years and a fall in the ratio of ectopic pregnancies to live births from 26.4 to 14.9 per 1000.[14] In the United States, estimated yearly numbers of ectopic pregnancies have fallen from 58,178 in 1992 to 35,382 in 1999.[15] It has been suggested that falling rates of pelvic inflammatory disease may be responsible for these changes in Norway.[14] In the United States, the increasing use of outpatient therapy for ectopic pregnancy has been shown to make incidence data increasingly unreliable [15] and this apparent fall in incidence may be an overestimate.

RISK FACTORS

Many studies have identified the risk factors for ectopic pregnancy.[16–18] A third of cases are associated with tubal damage caused by infection or surgery, and another third with smoking. No known cause can be established for the remaining third. Tubal infection contributes less to ectopic pregnancy risk than does smoking, though the risk of ectopic pregnancy increases with the number of pelvic infections.[19] Techniques of assisted reproduction increase the risk of ectopic pregnancy twofold to 4%.[18,19] The most frequent cause of tubal pregnancy is previous salpingitis, especially recurrent forms of the disease. Ascending pathogens, such as chlamydia, staphylococcus, and gonococcus (more rarely, tuberculosis), are liable to trigger subclinical infections that damage the tubal mucosa. The tubal mucosa may be destroyed, and the motility of the fallopian tube and the transport of oocytes may be impaired. Rare congenital anomalies of the proximal portion of the tube, such as rudimentary or extremely elongated tubes, may be associated with ectopic pregnancy. Intraluminal polyps could also influence the motility of the fallopian tube and thereby enhance the risk of ectopic pregnancy. Endometriosis may also damage or compromise tubal epithelium and motility and thus cause tubal pregnancy.

The risk of ectopic pregnancy is higher in nonwhite women (all races including African American, Asian, and American Indian women; relative risk is 1.6). Among inner-city African American women, cigarette smoking is an independent, dose-related risk factor for ectopic pregnancy.[20] The hazard is correlated with age; it increases three to four times in women between ages 35 and 44 compared with those 15 to 24.[21] The "epidemic" of tubal pregnancies in the 1970s and 1980s has been associated with the "baby boom" cohort (born 1945 to 1954), who were in their fertile period.[22]

About 61% of these women conceive subsequently, but only 38% of them deliver a living infant. The others either have a spontaneous abortion or suffer repeated extrauterine gestation.[23,24] About 95% of such pregnancies occur in the ampulla, where fertilization takes place, but they can develop elsewhere in the tube, cervix, ovary, or abdominal cavity (Figure 9.4.1). Risk factors for ectopic pregnancy in women who conceive after contraceptive failure are different from those for women trying to conceive. All contraceptives – hormonal and mechanical – protect against ectopic pregnancy. A higher risk of ovarian implantation exists in women who conceive while using intrauterine contraceptive devices.[25] A woman with an intrauterine device (IUD) in place who conceives is more likely to have an extrauterine pregnancy (EUP) than is a woman who conceives while using other contraceptive methods. Although an IUD is more effective in preventing an intrauterine pregnancy (IUP) than an EUP, women are not at

Table 9.4.1: Major Factors and Associated Relative Risks for Tubal Pregnancy

Risk Factors	Relative Risk, %
Current use of intrauterine devices	11.9
Use of clomiphene citrate	10.0
Prior tubal surgery	5.6
Pelvic inflammatory disease	4.0
Infertility	2.9
Induced abortion	2.5
Adhesions	2.4
Abdominal surgery	2.3
T-shaped uterus	2.0
Myomas	1.7
Progestin-only oral contraceptives	1.6

Source: Marchbanks et al.[25]

increased risk of developing an EUP compared with the general population solely because they are wearing an IUD.

The increase in tubal pregnancy also is attributed to a greater incidence of sexually transmitted diseases, previous tubal operations (either reconstruction or sterilization), delayed childbearing, and more successful clinical detection. Major risk factors for this life-threatening condition are listed in Table 9.4.1. Any condition that prevents or retards migration of the fertilized ovum to the uterine cavity predisposes a woman to an EUP.

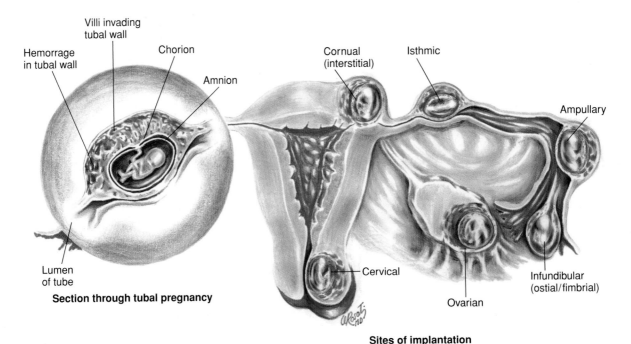

Figure 9.4.1. The sites of implantation of ectopic pregnancies, along with a section through an advanced tubal pregnancy. For all figures, please see reference [110].

Table 9.4.2: Symptoms and Signs Suggesting Tubal Pregnancy

Nausea, breast fullness, fatigue, interruption of menses

Lower abdominal pain, heavy cramping, shoulder pain

Uterine bleeding, spotting

Pelvic tenderness; enlarged, soft uterus

Adnexal mass, tenderness

Positive pregnancy test

Serum hCG levels $\leq$6000 IU/L at 6 weeks

Less than 66% increase in hCG titers in 48 hours

Positive culdocentesis (83%)

Absence of gestational sac in the uterus by TVS

Gestational sac outside the uterus by TVS

DIAGNOSIS

Symptoms

The usual pregnancy symptoms, including nausea, vomiting, breast fullness, fatigue, and interruption of the normal menstrual pattern, also occur with tubal pregnancies. Other symptoms more typical of EUP include lower abdominal pain of varying intensity and abnormal uterine bleeding ranging from amenorrhea to spotting or heavy bleeding. The presence of shoulder pain suggests possible rupture, with intraperitoneal blood flowing toward the diaphragm causing phrenic nerve irritation.

Physical Findings

Fever of more than 101°F is unusual. About one third of patients with ruptured tubal pregnancies experience syncope because of hypotension caused by hypovolemia. Signs of ectopic pregnancy, including lower abdominal tenderness with or without rebound, are more severe on the affected side. There may be tenderness with cervical motion. The uterus usually is enlarged and soft. An adnexal mass is present in 50% of these patients (Table 9.4.2).

Patients with abdominal peritoneal signs or definite cervical motion tenderness constitute a high-risk group, whereas patients with only midline menstrual-like cramping constitute a low-risk group.[26] Abdominal pain, rebound tenderness on abdominal examination, fluid in the pouch of Douglas at transvaginal ultrasound examination, and a low serum hemoglobin level are independent predictors of tubal rupture.[27] Another study discovered no constellation of physical examination findings that could confirm or exclude the diagnosis reliably.[28] Rebound tenderness and muscular rigidity were associated with a high likelihood of an EUP, whereas findings on speculum inspection and vaginal examination contributed little to confirm the diagnosis. Information provided by physical examination for the diagnosis is limited compared with that obtained from transvaginal sonogram (TVS) and serum hCG measurements. A pelvic digital examination for patients with a suspected EUP is of limited value.[29]

Laboratory Studies

The presence of a pregnancy can be discovered as early as 10 days after ovulation with sensitive serum assays for β-hCG. Isolated values of hCG can aid in the diagnosis only when used in combination with other diagnostic tests. It is the pattern of the rise and fall that is meaningful. Doubling of the hCG levels every 48 hours in the fifth gestational week is an indication of a normally growing IUP. However, using this criterion, 15% of normal IUPs could fall in the EUP category and 13% of EUPs would be missed. Besides having lower titers and slower increases in serum concentrations of hCG compared with normal pregnancies, ectopic pregnancies have slower declines in the hCG titers than do spontaneous abortions.

If a low serum hCG level ($\leq$1000 IU/L) is associated with a higher relative risk of ectopic pregnancy, then can very low levels predict a benign clinical course? In general, no. Although a single very low serum level ($\leq$100 IU/L) has been felt to be reassuring, in a review of 716 admitted patients with ectopic pregnancy, 29% of those with such a level were found to have tubal rupture at laparoscopy.[30] The risk of tubal rupture was similar across a wide range of hCG values. Another study identified 38 instances of rupture among women with serum levels ranging from 10 to 189,720 IU/L.[31]

Ultrasonographic identification of an intrauterine pregnancy (gestational sac plus yolk sac or other embryonic sign) rules out ectopic pregnancy in most patients.[32] The exception is in patients with ovulation induction and assisted conception, who are at risk of heterotopic pregnancy (dizygotic twins, one intrauterine and one extrauterine). Although this phenomenon is exceedingly rare in the general population (estimated frequency, one per 3889 to 30,000 pregnancies) [33], in the setting of assisted reproduction, it may occur in one in 100 pregnancies.[34] Kadar and colleagues [35] noted that the absence of an intrauterine gestational sac on abdominal ultrasound and serum β-hCG levels of 6000 to 6500 IU/L suggest an EUP. The presence of an apparent intrauterine gestational sac with levels below 6500 IU/L implies an EUP or a missed or spontaneous abortion. More accurate diagnostic studies are obtained with high-frequency vaginal transducers that can discover a normal gestational sac in 98% of women after the fifth week of pregnancy, when the hCG levels are between 1000 IU/L and 1500 IU/L, the so-called discriminatory zone.[36] In one study, the sensitivity of TVS for the prediction of EUP was 87% and the specificity was 94%.[37] The positive and negative predictive values were 92.5% and 90%, respectively. In the absence of an intrauterine sac, ectopic pregnancy is likely when a level of 1500 IU/L is associated with an adnexal mass or fluid in the pouch of Douglas or in patients without these clinical findings, with a level of at least 2000 IU/L.[38]

A single progesterone assay is predictive of an abnormal pregnancy but not specific for an extrauterine one. A value of 25 ng/mL or more suggests a normal IUP. Serum progesterone values of 15 ng/mL or less imply an abnormal pregnancy, ectopic pregnancy, or threatened abortion. A meta-analysis incorporating 26 studies evaluating one serum progesterone measurement for the diagnosis of EUP showed a good discriminative capacity for the diagnosis of pregnancy failure and that of a viable IUP. However, one measurement could not discriminate between an EUP and an IUP.[39]

Table 9.4.3: Comparative Results of Conservative Operations for Tubal Pregnancy by Laparotomy and Laparoscopy

Author(s)	Cases, no.	Intrauterine Pregnancy, %	Tubal Pregnancy, %
Laparotomy			
Vermesh et al. [41]*	30	42	16
DeCherney and Kase [44]	49	40	12
Stromme [47]	45	71	15
Timonen and Nieminen [48]	240	38	16
Total	364	47.75	14.75
Laparoscopy			
DeCherney and Diamond [43]	79	62	16
Pouly et al. [45]	118	64	22
Vermesh et al. [46]*	30	50	6
Total	227	58.67	14.67

*Controlled and prospectively randomized to laparotomy and laparoscopy.

The ideal marker for ectopic pregnancy would be specific for tubal damage or present only after endometrial implantation. Various markers have been assessed, including creatine kinase and fetal fibronectin, but none is sufficiently sensitive or specific for the diagnosis of ectopic pregnancy.[40] Culdocentesis revealing nonclotting blood is found in more than 50% of unruptured tubal pregnancies.[41] When it is used in combination with a positive pregnancy test, positive culdocentesis results suggest the presence of an EUP.

TREATMENT

Once the diagnosis is made, treatment choices include laparotomy, laparoscopy, chemotherapy, and expectant management. Hemodynamic instability previously was considered an indication for immediate laparotomy. The availability of optimal anesthesia and advanced cardiovascular monitoring and the ability to convert rapidly to laparotomy if required enable the safe performance of operative laparoscopy in most women with hypovolemic shock.[42] The superior exposure with laparoscopy provides the possibility of a rapid diagnosis and control of the bleeding, making laparoscopy a good choice.

Since 1970, a conservative approach to unruptured EUP has been advocated to preserve tubal function (Table 9.4.3). Several types of tubal operations have been done successfully.[43] These operations include linear salpingostomy, "milking" the pregnancy from the distal ampulla (Figure 9.4.2), and partial salpingectomy followed by anastomosis. Postoperative viable births or repeat EUPs are similar after salpingectomy with or without ipsilateral oophorectomy and salpingostomy.[44] In 321 tubal pregnancies treated conservatively by laparoscopy, it was reported that 15 (4.8%) required subsequent laparotomy or a second laparoscopic procedure as hCG levels failed to return to normal.[45]

The preferred operative approach is by laparoscopy.[46] This technique yields pregnancy rates comparable to those reported after laparotomy.[44–49] This laparoscopic procedure was proven in prospective randomized trials to be superior to laparotomy.[50] Vermesh and associates [46] prospectively randomized patients with unruptured EUP to either laparoscopy or laparotomy. Those authors analyzed postoperative morbidity, length of hospital stay, duration of convalescence, hospital cost, postoperative tubal patency by hysterosalpingography, and pregnancy rates. The two procedures were similarly safe and effective, but the laparoscopic approach was more cost-effective and required a shorter recovery period. The laparoscopic approach results in improved fertility rates because of reduced formation of postoperative adhesions.[51]

A systematic review [52] of three randomized controlled trials [53–55] showed that open salpingostomy when compared with laparoscopic salpingostomy increased rates of elimination of the tubal pregnancy (2.4% vs. 12.5%), mainly because of the higher persistent trophoblast rate with laparoscopic surgery. There was no difference in the subsequent tubal patency or in subsequent rate of intrauterine pregnancy or repeat ectopic pregnancy, but perioperative blood loss was higher with open surgery. Further studies are needed to establish whether the persistent trophoblast rate is as high as in the original studies.

Animal [56] and clinical [57] studies confirmed the impression that laparoscopic procedures were associated with reductions of new adhesions and re-formation of preexisting adhesions. Tubal healing and the extent of pelvic adhesions were assessed at repeat laparoscopy within 15 weeks of the initial operation.[58] Although tubal patency did not differ between the two groups, patients who were treated by laparotomy developed more adhesions. Brumsted and coworkers [59] reported a shorter convalescence of 8.7 ± 7.8 days in the laparoscopy group compared with 25.7 ± 16.2 days among the laparotomy patients ($P \leq 0.01$) and reduced postoperative analgesia requirements in the laparoscopy patients of 0.84 ± 2.3 doses compared with 4.64 ± 2.9 doses ($P \leq 0.01$) in the laparotomy group.

With adequate experience in operative endoscopy and with proper instruments, most patients with ectopic pregnancies can be treated successfully by laparoscopy, regardless of the gestation's size or location, the number of gestations, or the presence of tubal rupture.[60] At the initial exploratory procedure, both fallopian tubes are examined to avoid missing multiple ectopic pregnancies. Because of delayed childbearing and the expanded use of assisted reproductive technology, multiple EUPs may become more prevalent. After a nonstimulated menstrual cycle, three separate gestational sacs were identified in one woman at initial operative laparoscopy, one in the right tube and two in the left tube.[61]

Persistent ectopic pregnancy after laparoscopic salpingostomy arises in 4% to 15% of women.[40] Therefore, β-hCG concentrations should be followed until they are undetectable. Risk factors for persistent ectopic pregnancy are small ectopic pregnancies (≤ 2 cm), early surgical intervention (≤ 42 days from last menstrual period), and β-hCG values of 3000 IU/L or more. The rate of persistent ectopic pregnancy was reduced in one study from 14% to 2% with the use of prophylactic methotrexate, which also reduced the period of postoperative monitoring.[62]

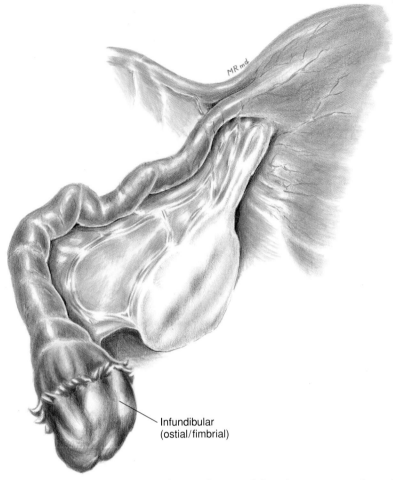

Figure 9.4.2. This infundibular pregnancy is about to be extruded. At laparoscopy, such conditions can be managed by grasping the tissue and completing the process. Bleeding usually is minimal.[110]

However, to avoid one additional case of persistent trophoblast after conservative surgery, eight women would need to be treated with methotrexate. Monitoring of the β-hCG concentrations would, therefore, seem to be a better option, provided that the woman is amenable to monitoring.

In the management of a tubal gestation, the gynecologist must consider the patient's desire for further childbearing. The patient is informed of the possibility of laparotomy with salpingectomy or more extirpative procedures because of uncontrollable bleeding or unexpected findings. If neither tube is salvageable, the uterus and at least one ovary is preserved to retain the possibility of in vitro fertilization.[63]

Laparoscopic Techniques

The location, size, and nature of the tubal pregnancy are established. Ruptured tubal pregnancies are treated successfully endoscopically if the bleeding has ceased or is stopped adequately. Once bleeding is controlled, the products of conception and blood clots are removed. A 10-mm suction instrument cleanses the abdominal cavity quickly. Forced irrigation with lactated Ringer's solution dislodges clots and trophoblastic tissue from the serosa of the peritoneal organs with minimal trauma to those structures.

Salpingotomy

For unruptured tubal pregnancies, the tube is identified and mobilized. To reduce bleeding, a 5- to 7-mL diluted solution containing 20 units of vasopressin (Pitressin, Monarch Pharmaceuticals) in 100 mL of normal saline is injected with a 20-gauge spinal or laparoscopic needle in the mesosalpinx just below the EUP and over the antimesenteric surface of the tubal segment containing the gestational products (Figure 9.4.3). The needle must not be within a blood vessel because intravascular injection of vasopressin solution can cause acute arterial hypertension, bradycardia, and death.[57]

Using a laser, microelectrode, or scissors, a linear incision is made on the antimesenteric surface extending 1 to 2 cm over the thinnest portion of the tube containing the pregnancy. The pregnancy usually protrudes through the incision and slowly slips out of the tube; it is removed by using hydrodissection or laparoscopic forceps (Figure 9.4.4). Forceful irrigation in the tube's opening can dislodge the gestation from its implantation. As the pregnancy is pulled out or extrudes from the tube, some products of conception may adhere to the implantation site by a ligamentous structure containing blood vessels. Using the electrocoagulator, this structure is coagulated before the tissue is removed. Oozing from the tube is common but usually ceases

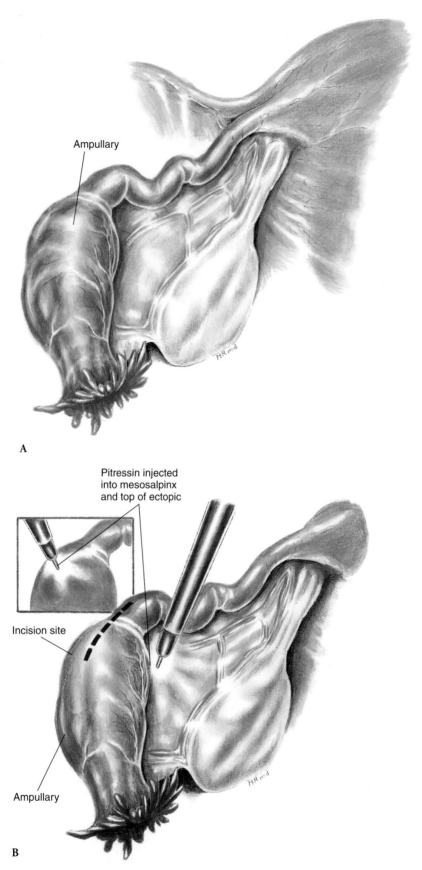

Figure 9.4.3. (**A**) An unruptured ampullary pregnancy. (**B**) Injection is done into the top of the tube (*inset*) and into the mesosalpinx with 5 to 7 mL of diluted Pitressin.

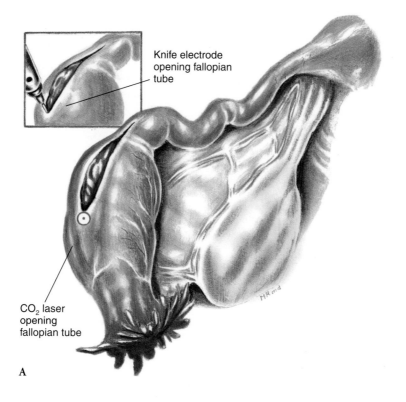

Knife electrode
opening fallopian
tube

CO_2 laser
opening
fallopian tube

A

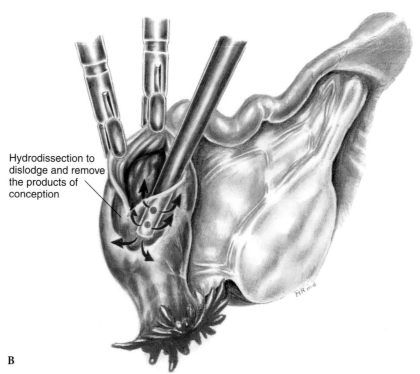

Hydrodissection to
dislodge and remove
the products of
conception

B

Figure 9.4.4. (**A**) The pregnancy is revealed by either a CO_2 laser or knife electrode (*inset*) after a tubal incision is made. (**B**) Products of conception are being separated from the tube. (*Continued*)

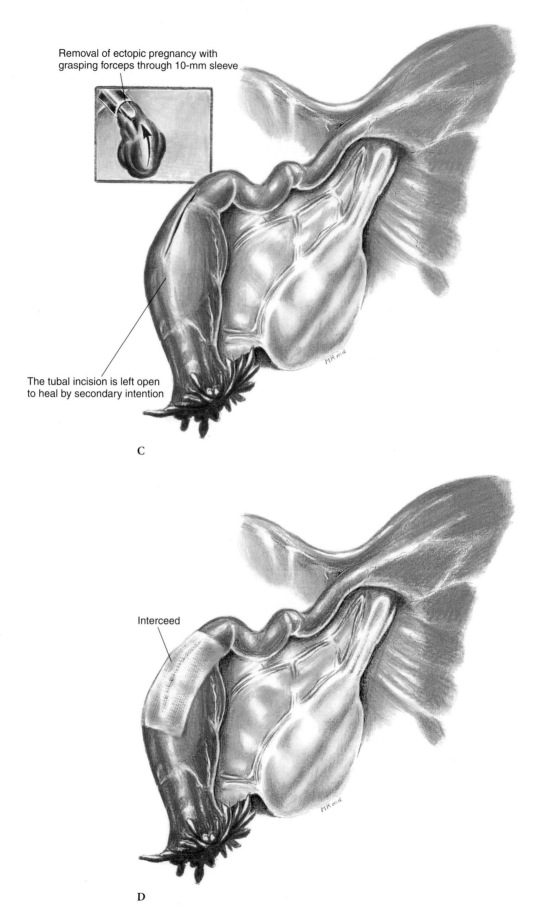

Removal of ectopic pregnancy with
grasping forceps through 10-mm sleeve

The tubal incision is left open
to heal by secondary intention

C

Interceed

D

Figure 9.4.4. (*Continued*) (**C**) Depending on the size of the pregnancy, the products of conception can be removed through a 5- or 10-mm trocar sleeve (*inset*). The tubal incision is not sutured and usually heals spontaneously. (**D**) In some instances, the incision may be covered with Interceed.

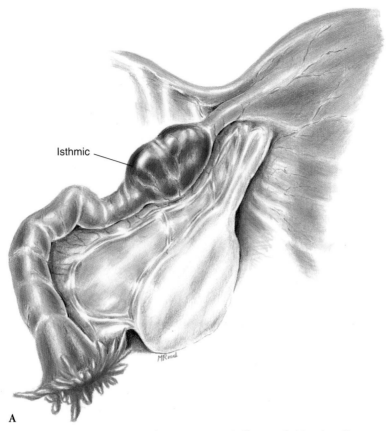

Figure 9.4.5. (**A**) An isthmic pregnancy is illustrated. (*Continued*)

spontaneously. Occasionally, coagulation is necessary with a defocused laser beam or an electrocoagulator. Depending on the size, the products of conception are removed through a 5- or 10-mm trocar sleeve.

Tubal Resection

Resection of the tubal segment that contains the gestation is preferable to salpingotomy for an isthmic pregnancy or a ruptured tube or if hemostasis is difficult to obtain. Segmental resection is done with bipolar electrosurgery, fiber lasers (potassium titanyl phosphate, argon, or Nd:YAG), CO_2 laser, sutures, or stapling devices.

Bloodless segmental resection is achieved by grasping the proximal and distal boundaries of the tubal segment containing the gestation with a Kleppinger forceps and coagulating them from the antimesenteric surface to the mesosalpinx. The segment is cut with laparoscopic scissors or a laser, with little risk of bleeding. The mesosalpinx under the pregnancy is coagulated, with particular attention given to the arcuate anastomosing branches of the ovarian and uterine vessels.[64] After coagulation, the mesosalpinx is cut (Figures 9.4.5 and 9.4.6).

Salpingectomy

Guidelines for choosing salpingectomy include the presence of uncontrolled bleeding, tubal destruction by the EUP, and a recurrent pregnancy in the same tube. Preoperative counseling should include the desire of the patient for future childbearing.

This operation is done by progressively coagulating and cutting the mesosalpinx, beginning with the proximal isthmic portion and progressing to the fimbriated end of the tube. It is separated from the uterus by using bipolar coagulation and scissors or a laser (Figure 9.4.7). A multifire stapling device for salpingectomy requires a 12-mm trocar and is expensive. Alternatively, one or two Endoloops (Ethicon) can be applied around the salpinx and then cut. The isolated segment containing the EUP is removed intact or in sectioned parts through the 10-mm trocar sleeve. Products of conception can be placed in a bag (Endopouch, Ethicon) and removed (Figure 9.4.8). Adhesions and other pathologic processes, such as endometriosis, are treated during removal of the EUP without prolonging the operation. Occasionally, a patient is admitted overnight to be observed for postoperative bleeding and to receive emotional support from the infertility team.

Salpingectomy or Salpingotomy

There has been considerable debate about whether salpingectomy or salpingostomy should be done at the time of surgery for an ectopic pregnancy. The possible advantages of removing the tube completely include almost entirely eliminating the risk of persistent trophoblast and that of a subsequent ectopic pregnancy, whereas the possible advantage of conserving the

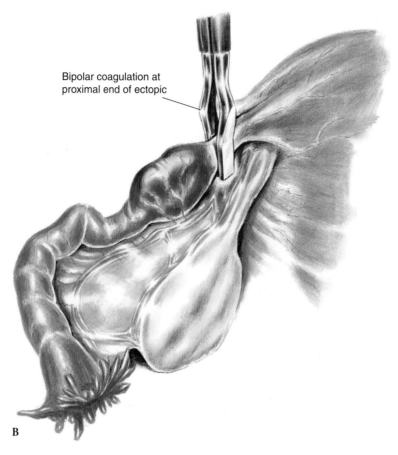

Bipolar coagulation at
proximal end of ectopic

B

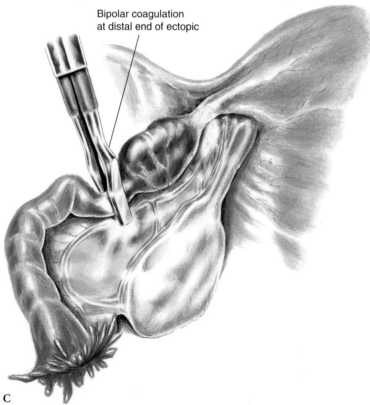

Bipolar coagulation
at distal end of ectopic

C

Figure 9.4.5. (*Continued*) (**B**) The bipolar forceps coagulates the proximal isthmic segment. (**C**) Electrocoagulation of the tube distal to the ectopic pregnancy.

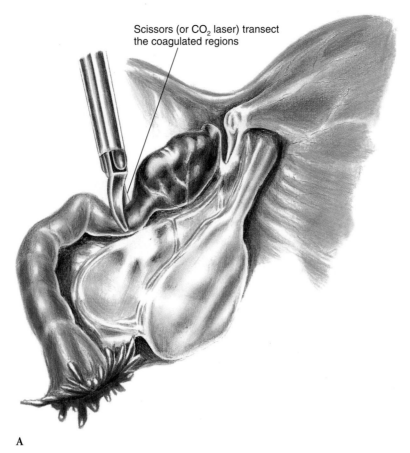

Scissors (or CO_2 laser) transect
the coagulated regions

A

Figure 9.4.6. (**A**) Either a scissors or a CO_2 laser is employed to transect the areas. (*Continued*)

fallopian tube is that future fertility is preserved.[40] There are no randomized controlled trials published that specifically compare laparoscopic or open salpingectomy and salpingotomy. Several reviewers suggest that subsequent intrauterine pregnancy rates are similar after both approaches. These data, however, must be interpreted with caution as the included studies are subject to a wide range of biases relating to patient selection, surgical procedures used, length of follow-up, and the proportion of patients lost to follow-up.[65,66]

There are four cohort studies that specifically compare laparoscopic tube-sparing and radical treatments of ectopic pregnancy.[67–70] Silva et al. [67] examined reproductive outcomes prospectively in 143 women undergoing laparoscopic salpingectomy or laparoscopic salpingotomy. The intrauterine pregnancy rates were similar when comparing the two groups (intrauterine pregnancy in 60% of subjects after salpingotomy versus 54% after salpingectomy; relative risk 1.11). In a study of 155 women, Job-Spira et al. [68] reported subsequent intrauterine pregnancy rates with salpingotomy that were comparable to those following salpingectomy (hazard ratio, 1.22). The cumulative pregnancy rates at 1 year were 72.4% after salpingotomy and 56.3% after salpingectomy. In a study by Mol et al. [69] of a cohort of 135 women, the fecundity rate ratio when comparing laparoscopic salpingotomy with salpingectomy during the 18-month

follow-up period was 1.4 for women with a healthy contralateral tube and 3.1 for women with contralateral tubal disease. The 3-year cumulative pregnancy rate was 62% after salpingotomy and 38% after salpingectomy. In a study by Bangsgaard et al. [70] reviewing a cohort of 276 women undergoing salpingotomy or salpingectomy, the subsequent cumulative pregnancy rate at 7 years was 89% following salpingotomy and 66% following salpingectomy. The hazard ratio for intrauterine pregnancy following salpingectomy was 0.63 when compared with salpingotomy. Regardless of the type of surgery, contralateral tubal abnormalities predispose the patient to recurrent ectopic pregnancy. There was no significant difference in the risk of repeat ectopic pregnancy (17% after conservative surgery and 16% after radical surgery).[70]

In summary, in the absence of a randomized study, salpingotomy remains the definitive and universal treatment for EUP in women who are hemodynamically stable and who wish to preserve their fertility.[1,2] The reproductive performance after salpingotomy appears to be equivalent to or better than that after salpingectomy, but the recurrent EUP rate may be slightly greater. Salpingectomy may be necessary for women with uncontrolled bleeding, recurrent ectopic pregnancy in the same tube, a severely damaged tube, or a tubal gestational sac greater than 5 cm in diameter.[1]

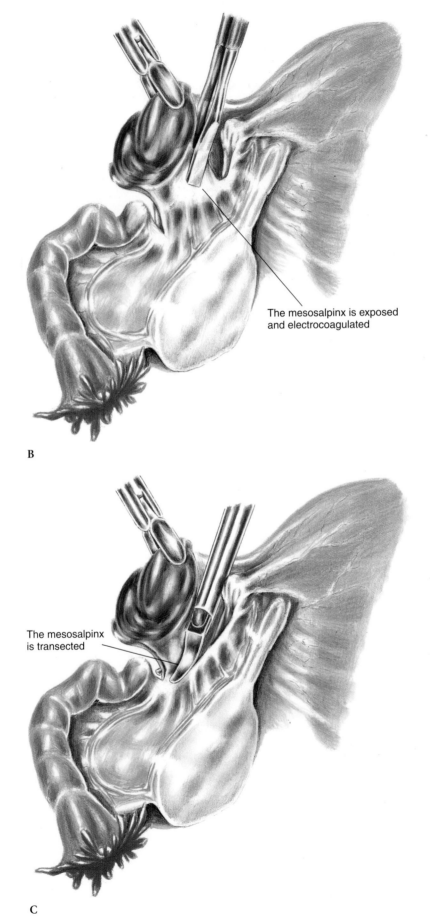

The mesosalpinx is exposed
and electrocoagulated

B

The mesosalpinx
is transected

C

Figure 9.4.6. (*Continued*) (**B**) The adjacent mesosalpinx is coagulated. (**C**) The isthmic ectopic pregnancy is removed. (*Continued*)

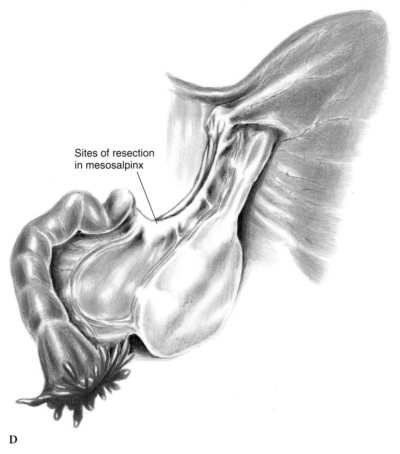

Sites of resection
in mesosalpinx

D

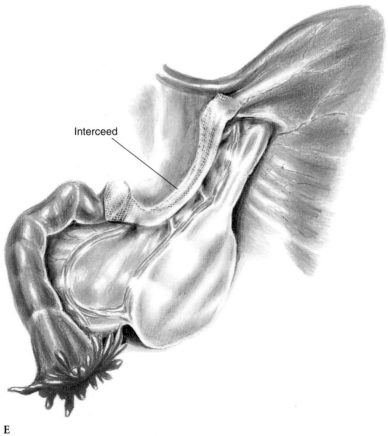

Interceed

E

Figure 9.4.6. (*Continued*) (**D**) The resected segments and mesosalpinx are seen. (**E**) Interceed is placed over the coagulated surfaces.

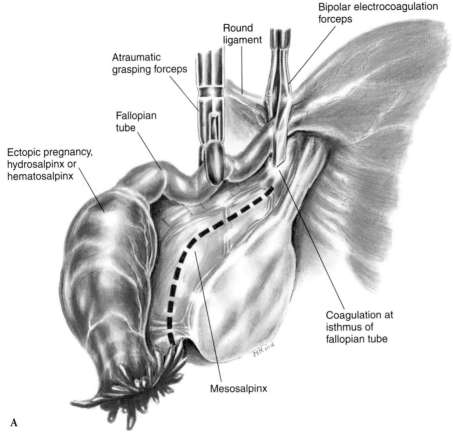

Figure 9.4.7. (**A**) Total salpingectomy is done by progressively coagulating and cutting the mesosalpinx, beginning with the isthmic segment. (*Continued*)

FOLLOW-UP

In 1 week, the patient returns for a serum hCG to ascertain resolution of the ectopic gestation. The hCG level should be undetectable or very low. If it is above 20 IU/L, a repeat blood test is ordered 1 to 2 weeks later, when the hCG should be undetectable.[71] If the levels persist, other treatment options must be considered.

INTERSTITIAL PREGNANCY

Interstitial (cornual) pregnancies occur rarely; the prevalence ranges from one in 2500 to one in 5000 live births. Because the morbidity and mortality are high, the correct diagnosis must be made and treatment must begin promptly. This type of EUP is associated with an increased risk of traumatic rupture and hemorrhagic shock, with a mortality rate of 2% to 2.5%. Later diagnosis and the increased vascularity of this area account for these increased risks. Two percent to 4% of ectopic gestations are interstitial. The anatomy favors the growing gestation, accounting for the late onset of symptoms and occasional reports of term interstitial pregnancies. The traditional management for interstitial

(cornual) pregnancy is salpingectomy with or without cornual resection and sometimes hysterectomy. In selected women, more conservative and less radical approaches are employed if the diagnosis is made early and the patient is stable. Other options include methotrexate (MTX) injections (local or systemic), potassium chloride injections (local), and prostaglandin administration. In a series of 15 patients, unruptured interstitial pregnancies were managed with local MTX administration of 1 mg/kg body weight under transvaginal ultrasound or laparoscopy.[72]

Interstitial pregnancy is suspected in women with an enlarged asymmetric uterus and an eccentrically placed gestational sac on sonography. Differential diagnoses include ovarian and abdominal pregnancy and a pregnancy in one horn of a bicornuate uterus. The diagnosis is confirmed by laparoscopy, and the treatment involves immediate laparotomy or a combined laparoscopic and hysteroscopic approach in certain patients.

At laparoscopy, the interstitial pregnancy is recognized as a cornual bulge stretching the myometrium and serosal surface (Figure 9.4.9). If the overlying myometrium is thick and intact, removal of the pregnancy by hysteroscopy is preferable. Early detection of an interstitial pregnancy can be managed by combining MTX and hysteroscopy.[73] A diagnostic laparoscopy is done to identify the location and accessibility of the gestation. If it is accessible by hysteroscopy, it is suctioned or resected using

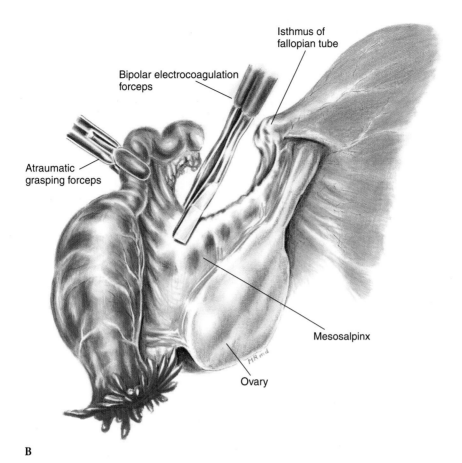

B

C

Figure 9.4.7. (*Continued*) (**B**) The mesosalpinx is coagulated with bipolar forceps. (**C**) The procedure is continued. (*Continued*)

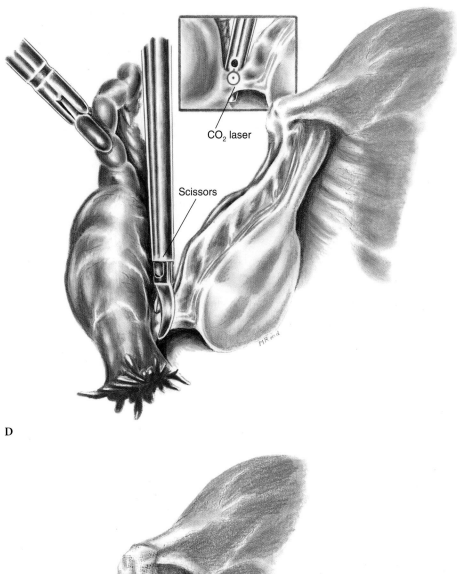

D

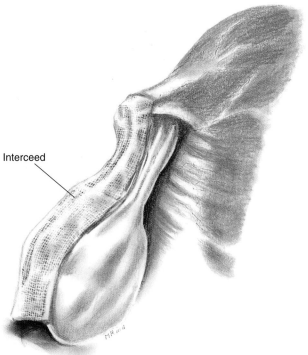

E

Figure 9.4.7. (*Continued*) (**D**) The tube is separated from the uterus by using bipolar coagulation and scissors or the laser (*inset*). The isolated tubal segment is removed intact or in sections through the 10-mm sleeve. (**E**) Interceed may be placed over the resected area to prevent postoperative adnexal adhesions.

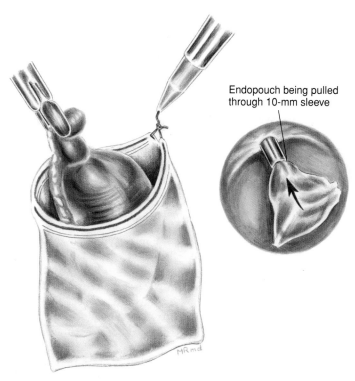

Figure 9.4.8. The resected tube containing the pregnancy is placed in an Endopouch. The *inset* shows removal through a 10-mm trocar sleeve.

forceps, scissors, or electrosurgery under hysteroscopic control. For larger pregnancies, it is better and faster to do a gentle curettage of the dilated interstitial–cornual area under laparoscopic control. To verify complete removal of the products of conception, hysteroscopic observation of the curetted cornu and the interstitial area is done.

If the pregnancy has eroded through the cornual myometrium, it is prudent to do a laparotomy to remove the pregnancy. In some patients, a laparoscopic approach is considered after the patient is counseled concerning the possibility of a laparotomy.[74–76] The cornu is vascular, and profuse bleeding may occur quickly..

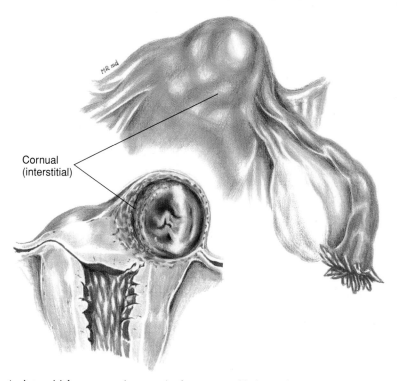

Figure 9.4.9. An interstitial pregnancy is recognized as a cornual bulge in the myometrium and serosal surface.

NONSURGICAL MANAGEMENT

Expectant Management

Other approaches to tubal pregnancy include expectant management and MTX. Because some tubal pregnancies end in tubal abortions or complete reabsorption, particular patients are monitored with repeated levels of hCG until tubal abortion or reabsorption occurs as suggested by falling hormonal levels.[77] With declining values and a starting hCG above 2000 IU/L, 93.3% failed on expectant management, whereas below 2000 IU/L, 60.0% succeeded.[78] This choice preserves tubal function and fertility, but tubal occlusion can result from retained products of conception.[79] Shalev and coworkers [78] found no difference in the resultant ipsilateral tubal patency or 1-year fertility rates of women succeeding or failing on expectant management. Rantala and Makinen [80] reported a pregnancy rate of 88% and a rate of repeat ectopic pregnancy of 4.2%. Patients who were treated expectantly had a good fertility outcome. Spontaneous regression of the EUP did not lead to increased tubal damage because of the risk for a repeat EUP.

Although ectopic pregnancy may resolve spontaneously through regression or tubal abortion, about 90% of women with ectopic pregnancy and serum β-hCG levels greater than 2000 IU/L require operative intervention owing to increasing symptoms or tubal rupture.[1] Tubal rupture also may occur when serum β-hCG levels are low or declining, or both. Expectant management should be offered only when transvaginal ultrasonography fails to show the location of the gestational sac and the serum levels of β-hCG and progesterone are low and declining. Because of the possibility of tubal rupture, these patients must be carefully monitored until the serum β-hCG concentration falls below 15 IU/L; at this point, almost all ectopic pregnancies resolve spontaneously, without rupture.

The overall efficacy of expectant management was 69.2% in 10 prospective studies.[2] Banerjee et al. [81] followed 135 women with an unknown location of their pregnancy. Complete data sets were obtained in 127 cases. These included 34 (27%) normal IUPs, 11 (9%) miscarriages, and 18 (14%) EUPs. A total of 64 pregnancies (50%) resolved spontaneously. These data show that most pregnancies of unknown location are abnormal and many resolve spontaneously. The role of expectant management in those with known EUP is limited because of its risks compared with the high efficacy and accessibility of MTX or surgical treatment.[2] The difficulty with such management lies in the selection of the proper patients. A patient with low or falling titers must understand the risks involved and have the ability to comply with instructions concerning follow-up.

Medical Treatment

Treatment with MTX is an alternative to surgery in up to a quarter of women with unruptured ectopic pregnancy. MTX has been recommended for women with a cornual pregnancy or an incomplete resolution of surgically treated ectopic gestation and for residual trophoblastic tissue. MTX, a folic acid antagonist, inhibits DNA synthesis in actively dividing cells, including trophoblasts. Patients who are poor risks because of induced ovarian hyperstimulation syndrome and those suspected of having extensive intraperitoneal abdominal adhesions may be treated medically if they are hemodynamically stable.

Two regimens are commonly used for the systemic administration of MTX. The first involves administration of MTX and leucovorin on alternate days until β-hCG concentrations begin to drop. This regimen has a success rate (defined as avoidance of surgery) of 93%.[82–84] The second regimen involves administration of a single dose of MTX, followed by repeated doses a week apart if β-hCG concentrations do not fall by 15% between days 4 and 7. As reported by Lipscomb et. al., more than 90% of women treated with the second regimen avoided surgery.[85] The criteria for MTX treatment of ectopic pregnancy are as follows: hemodynamic stability, ability and willingness of the patient to comply with posttreatment monitoring, pretreatment serum β-hCG concentration less than 5000 IU/L, and absence of ultrasound evidence of fetal cardiac activity.[1] In one study, patients were treated with MTX 1 mg/kg intravenously and leucovorin 0.1 mg/kg intramuscularly every other day for 4 days. These patients were admitted to the hospital and monitored during therapy with serum levels of aspartate aminotransferase, lactate dehydrogenase, hCG, and progesterone and with complete blood counts and platelet counts.[86] A single intramuscular injection of MTX (50 mg/m^2) without citrovorum rescue was used in 29 of 30 consecutive patients with unruptured ectopic pregnancies. Six patients experienced an increase in abdominal pain, and two were hospitalized for overnight observation.[87] This single-dose plan administered on an outpatient basis decreases the expense and lessens the side effects associated with the treatment of EUPs 3 to 5 cm or less in diameter.

One randomized controlled trial has been done to compare single-dose and multiple-dose regimens of MTX.[88] Fifty-one women with a presumed ectopic pregnancy were randomly assigned single-dose or multiple-dose MTX. The β-hCG concentration for inclusion was less than 10,000 IU/L. Single-dose MTX was successful in 90% and multiple-dose in 86% of women. There was no evidence of a difference in median time to resolution and no difference in adverse events between regimens. The efficacies of single- and multiple-dose regimens were recently compared in a meta-analysis of all available studies.[82] This meta-analysis of 26 studies included 267 women receiving a multiple-dose treatment and 1067 treated with single-dose therapy. The success rates (defined as not requiring surgery) were 88.1% for single-dose therapy and 92.7% for multiple-dose therapy, but the chances of failure were greater with single-dose therapy. Importantly, this difference was much more marked when results were adjusted for serum hCG values and the presence of fetal cardiac activity. Side effects were lower with single-dose therapy. Among women who were due to receive a single dose, 13.6% required two or more doses. These results suggest that it may be time to reevaluate the role of multiple-dose therapy in selected women.

Patients treated with MTX should be followed closely. The serum β-hCG concentration should be measured weekly. It is not unusual to see an increase in serum hCG levels in the following 3 days and mild abdominal pain of short duration (1 to 2 days). However, the pain may also be severe, perhaps as a result of tubal abortion or the formation of hematoma with tubal distention. Severe abdominal pain, however, may be a sign of actual or impending tubal rupture. If the serum β-hCG concentration has not declined by at least 25% 1 week after MTX administration, a second dose should be given. In general, a second dose is needed in 15% to 20% of patients.[82,89]

Use of mifepristone as an adjunctive treatment to MTX for ectopic pregnancy has been assessed in two randomized controlled trials. Although results of initial pilot studies seemed promising [90], those of a subsequent multicenter randomized trial noted no benefit of the combined regimen over MTX alone.[91] In the second trial [92], involving 50 women, both treatment approaches were successful, but only one of 25 women in the mifepristone and MTX group needed a second dose of MTX, whereas in the MTX-only group, four of 25 needed a second dose. The time to resolve the unruptured ectopic pregnancy was also significantly faster in the group who received combination mifepristone and MTX.[92] Further studies are needed to consider the role and cost of mifepristone in combination with MTX.

Injection of MTX into the gestational sac under ultrasound guidance or at laparoscopy is feasible, and 17 of 24 patients were treated successfully with this technique.[93] Seven of those patients required additional systemic injections, and one patient experienced tubal rupture 3 days after the initial injection. The tubal injection consisted of 10 to 20 mL of adrenaline 1:80,000 dilution injected into the mesosalpinx with a 22-gauge needle, followed by 100 mg MTX injected into the tubal gestation. Leucovorin 15 mg was given orally 30 hours after the administration of MTX. Subsequent systemic MTX injections were given intramuscularly, 50 mg every 2 to 4 days, according to the level of serum hCG. The relative efficacies of MTX and prostaglandin sulprostone (Nalador, Schering Laboratory, Lys-Lez-Lannoy, France) have been compared.[94] The medication was administered into the gestational sac and intramuscularly on days 3, 5, and 7 after the day of diagnosis in 21 patients with an unruptured tubal pregnancy. Both therapies were effective. However, 34% of patients underwent either laparotomy or laparoscopy for a ruptured tubal pregnancy or a persistent rise in hCG levels despite the treatment.

Local injection of MTX requires a sonographically visible EUP as well as technical skills and has less consistent success rates than does systemic MTX therapy.[95] Although local administration of MTX may be associated with a lower incidence of side effects, its administration is associated with more inconvenience to the patient and the medical staff.[96]

The route of MTX administration has also been recently revisited. Most recent case series have reported on intramuscular rather than local ultrasound-guided MTX administration, and there is a wide variation in reported success rates.[66,97] No randomized trial comparing route of administration has been undertaken, but in a review of 137 women treated by either intramuscular (50 mg/m^2) or local ultrasound-guided administration (1 mg/kg), the overall success rate was 67.1% and 92.5% in the two groups.[98] Multivariate analysis confirmed a higher success rate with locally administered MTX. The practicality of local treatment by laparoscopy is questionable. Local injection under laparoscopic guidance offers no advantage over ultrasound guidance because the women must undergo a laparoscopy if the medical treatment fails. It is more invasive than systemic MTX treatment, and the ectopic gestation can be removed easily during the laparoscopy.[65] Laparoscopy should now be performed to provide definitive treatment, which is removal of the ectopic pregnancy.

Outcomes of systemic MTX treatment have been similar to those of laparoscopic salpingotomy with respect to success rate, tubal patency, and the reproductive outcome. In a prospective randomized study of systemic MTX versus laparoscopic salpingostomy, Hajenius et al. [83] found a success rate of 82% after MTX treatment and 72% after salpingostomy. Unilateral tubal patency was 55% and 59%, respectively. It is important to note that the surgical approach can be done universally for all patients with ectopic pregnancy, whereas MTX treatment is given only to a selected group of patients. The two treatments can complement each other. The advantages of single systemic MTX compared with laparoscopic salpingostomy are noninvasiveness, avoidance of the risk of general anesthesia and surgery, shorter hospital stay, and lower cost.

Medical treatment of EUP with MTX has become the standard of care in many areas of the United States. However, patients with an EUP treated with MTX may require an emergency operation for rupture.[99] Systemic MTX therapy had a more negative impact on patients' health-related quality of life than did laparoscopic salpingostomy.[100] This negative impact on patients' health-related quality of life of systemic MTX therapy should be taken into account in deciding on the appropriate therapy for a tubal pregnancy. Systemic MTX therapy would be preferred by most patients as part of a completely nonsurgical management strategy.[95]

Laparoscopy was as effective as laparotomy in the treatment of tubal pregnancy and reduced the cost considerably.[101,102] Among stable patients, laparoscopic excision of EUPs saved nearly 25% of hospital cost per case compared with laparotomy.[103] Hemodynamic instability increased the cost of management because of the longer length of stay and higher laboratory costs. The cost savings may be lost if patients undergoing laparotomy are discharged on or before postoperative day 2 or if laparoscopic treatment of the EUP is not associated with rapid postoperative discharge.[104]

Medical treatment with MTX is supposed to offer cost savings by minimizing hospitalization.[105,106] Follow-up of patients receiving MTX often is prolonged, necessitating additional blood tests, repeat sonographic evaluations, and loss of days from work. However, a financial analysis of EUP management at a large health plan revealed that total charges were similar for laparotomy and laparoscopy ($6720 and $6840), whereas outpatient MTX therapy cost less than the two surgical procedures (average of $818 per case, $P \leq 0.001$).[107] Another economic analysis described the possible cost benefits of conservative tubal operations for EUP over salpingectomy.[108] In another study, Mol et al. [109] also found that systemic MTX was less costly than laparoscopy in women with initial serum hCG levels of less than 1500 IU/L. However, in women whose initial hCG levels were greater than 3000 IU/L, methotrexate treatment was more expensive.

REFERENCES

1. Murray H, Baakdah H, Bardell T, Tulandi T. Diagnosis and treatment of ectopic pregnancy. *CMAJ*. 2005;173(8):905–912.
2. Tulandi T, Sammour A. Evidence-based management of ectopic pregnancy. *Curr Opin Obstet Gynecol*. 2000;12(4):289–292.
3. Sowter MC, Farquhar CM. Ectopic pregnancy: an update. *Curr Opin Obstet Gynecol*. 2004;16(4):289–293.
4. National Center for Health Statistics. *Advanced Report of Final Mortality Statistics, 1992*. Hyattsville, MD: U.S. Department of Health and Human Services, Public Health Services, Centers for Disease Control and Prevention; 1994.

5. Goyaux N, Leke R, Keita N, et al. Ectopic pregnancy in African developing countries. *Acta Obstet Gynecol Scand.* 2003;82:305–312.

6. Strandell A, Thorburn J, Hamberger L. Risk factors for ectopic pregnancy in assisted reproduction. *Fertil Steril.* 1999;71:282.

7. Dart RG, Kaplan B, Varaklis K. Predictive value of history and physical examination in patients with suspected ectopic pregnancy. *Ann Emerg Med.* 1999;33:283–290.

8. Spandorfer SD, Barnhart KT. Role of previous ectopic pregnancy in altering the presentation of suspected ectopic pregnancy. *J Reprod Med.* 2003;48:133–136.

9. Rubin GL, Peterson HB, Dorfman SF, et al. Ectopic pregnancy in the United States: 1970 through 1978. *JAMA.* 1983;249:1725.

10. Ectopic pregnancy – United States, 1990–1992. *MMWR Morb Mortal Wkly Rep.* 1995;44:46.

11. Schneider J, Berger GJ, Gattell G. Maternal mortality due to ectopic pregnancy: a review of 102 deaths. *Obstet Gynecol.* 1977;49:557.

12. Goldner TE, Lawson HW, Xia Z, Atrash HK. Surveillance for ectopic pregnancy – United States, 1970–1989. *MMWR Morb Mortal Wkly Rep.* 1993;42:73.

13. Royal College of Obstetricians and Gynaecologists. *Why Mothers Die 1997–1999. The Fifth Report of the Confidential Enquiries into Maternal Deaths in the United Kingdom 1997–1999.* London: RCOG Press; 2001.

14. Bakken I, Skjeldestad F. Incidence and treatment of extrauterine pregnancies in Norway 1990–2001. *Tidssk Nor Laegeforen.* 2003;123:3016–3020.

15. Zane S, Kieke B, Kendrick J, Bruce C. Surveillance in a time of changing health care practices: estimating ectopic pregnancy incidence in the United States. *Matern Child Health J.* 2002;6:227–236.

16. Bouyer J, Coste J, Shojael T, et al. Risk factors for ectopic pregnancy: a comprehensive analysis based on a large case-control, population based study in France. *Am J Epidemiol.* 2003;157:185–194.

17. Bouyer J, Rachou E, Germain E, et al. Risk factors for extrauterine pregnancy in women using an intrauterine device. *Fertil Steril.* 2000;74: 899–908.

18. Fernandez H, Gerviase A. Ectopic pregnancies after infertility treatment: modern diagnosis and therapeutic strategy. *Hum Reprod.* 2004;10:503–513.

19. Hillis SD, Owens LM, Marchbanks PA, Amsterdam LF, MacKenzie WR. Recurrent chlamydial infections increase the risks of hospitalisation for ectopic pregnancy and pelvic inflammatory disease. *Am J Obstet Gynecol.* 1997;176:103–107.

20. Saraiya M, Berg GJ, Kendrick JS, et al. Cigarette smoking as a risk factor for ectopic pregnancy. *Am J Obstet Gynecol.* 1998;178(3):493.

21. Ectopic pregnancy – United States, 1986. *MMWR Morb Mortal Wkly Rep.* 1989;38:481.

22. Makinen J, Rantala M, Vanha-Kamppa O. A link between the epidemic of ectopic pregnancy and the "baby-boom" cohort. *Am J Epidemiol.* 1998;148:369.

23. Schoen JA, Nowak RJ. Repeat ectopic pregnancy: a 16-year clinical survey. *Obstet Gynecol.* 1975;45:542.

24. Sandvei R, Bergsio P, Ulstein M, et al. Repeat ectopic pregnancy – a twenty-year hospital survey. *Acta Obstet Gynecol Scand.* 1987;66:607.

25. Marchbanks PA, Annegers JF, Goulam GB, et al. Risk factors for ectopic pregnancy: a population based study. *JAMA.* 1988;259:1823.

26. Buckley RG, King KJ, Disney JD, et al. Derivation of a clinical prediction model for the emergency department diagnosis of ectopic pregnancy. *Acad Emerg Med.* 1998;5:951.

27. Mol BW, Ilajenius PJ, Engelsbel S, et al. Can noninvasive diagnostic tools predict tubal rupture or active bleeding in patients with tubal pregnancy? *Fertil Steril.* 1999;71:167.

28. Dart RG, Kaplan B, Varaklis K. Predictive value of history and physical examination in patients with suspected ectopic pregnancy. *Ann Emerg Med.* 1999;33:283.

29. Mol BW, Hajenius PJ, Engelsbel S, et al. Should patients who are suspected of having an ectopic pregnancy undergo physical examination? *Fertil Steril.* 1999;71:155.

30. Saxon D, Falcone T, Mascha EJ, Marino T, Yao M, Tulandi T. A study of ruptured tubal ectopic pregnancy. *Obstet Gynecol.* 1997;90:46–49. Comment in *Obstet Gynecol.* 1997;90:866–867.

31. Barnhart K, Mennuti MT, Benjamin I, Jacobson S, Goodman D, Coutifaris C. Prompt diagnosis of ectopic pregnancy in an emergency department setting. *Obstet Gynecol.* 1994;84:1010–1015.

32. Albayram F, Hamper UM. First-trimester obstetric emergencies: spectrum of sonographic findings. *J Clin Ultrasound.* 2002;30: 161–177.

33. Habana A, Dokras A, Giraldo JL, Jones EE. Cornual heterotopic pregnancy: contemporary management options. *Am J Obstet Gynecol.* 2000;182:1264–1270.

34. Tal J, Haddad S, Gordon N, Timor-Tritsch I. Heterotopic pregnancy after ovulation induction and assisted reproductive technologies: a literature review from 1971 to 1993. *Fertil Steril.* 1996;66:1–12.

35. Kadar N, DeVore G, Romero R. Discriminatory hCG zone: its use in the sonographic evaluation for ectopic pregnancy. *Obstet Gynecol.* 1981;58:156.

36. Goldstein SR, Snyder JR, Watson G, et al. Very early pregnancy detection with endovaginal ultrasound. *Obstet Gynecol.* 1988;72:200.

37. Shalev E, Yarom I, Bustan M, et al. Transvaginal sonography as the ultimate diagnostic tool for the management of ectopic pregnancy: experience with 840 cases. *Fertil Steril.* 1998;69:62.

38. Mol BW, Hajenius PJ, Engelsbel S, et al. Serum human chorionic gonadotropin measurement in the diagnosis of ectopic pregnancy when transvaginal sonography is inconclusive. *Fertil Steril.* 1998;70:972.

39. Mol BW, Lijmer JG, Ankum WM, et al. The accuracy of single serum progesterone measurement in the diagnosis of ectopic pregnancy: a meta-analysis. *Hum Reprod.* 1998;13:3220.

40. Farquhar CM. Ectopic pregnancy. *Lancet.* 2005;366(9485):583–591.

41. Vermesh M, Graczykowski JW, Sauer MV. Reevaluation of the role of culdocentesis in the management of ectopic pregnancy. *Am J Obstet Gynecol.* 1990;162:411.

42. Soriano D, Yefet Y, Oelsner G, et al. Operative laparoscopy for management of ectopic pregnancy in patients with hypovolemic shock. *J Am Assoc Gynecol Laparosc.* 1997;4:363.

43. DeCherney AH, Diamond MP. Laparoscopic salpingostomy for ectopic pregnancy. *Obstet Gynecol.* 1987;70:948.

44. DeCherney AH, Kase N. The conservative surgical management of unruptured ectopic pregnancy. *Obstet Gynecol.* 1979;54:451.

45. Pouly JL, Mahnes H, Mage G, et al. Conservative laparoscopic treatment of 321 ectopic pregnancies. *Fertil Steril.* 1986;46:1093.

46. Vermesh M, Silva PD, Rosen GF, et al. Management of unruptured ectopic gestation by linear salpingostomy: a prospective, randomized clinical trial of laparoscopy versus laparotomy. *Obstet Gynecol.* 1989;73:400.

47. Stromme WB. Conservative surgery for ectopic pregnancy: a 20-year review. *Obstet Gynecol.* 1973;41:215.

48. Timonen S, Nieminen U. Tubal pregnancy: choice of operative method of treatment. *Acta Obstet Gynecol Scand.* 1967;46:327.

49. Lundorff P, Thornburn J, Lindblom B. Fertility outcome after conservative surgical treatment of ectopic pregnancy evaluated in a randomized trial. *Fertil Steril.* 1992;57:998.

50. Nagele F, Molnar BG, O'Connor H, Magos AL. Randomized studies in endoscopic surgery – where is the proof? *Curr Opin Obstet Gynecol.* 1996;8:281.

51. Bruhat MA, Manhes H, Mage G, et al. Treatment of ectopic pregnancy by means of laparoscopy. *Fertil Steril.* 1980;33:411.

52. Hajenius PJ, Mol BWJ, Bossuyt PMM, Ankum WM, Van der Veen F. Interventions for tubal ectopic pregnancy. *Cochrane Database Syst Rev.* 2000;CD000324.

53. Lundorff P, Thorburn J, Hahlin M, Kallfelt B, Lindblom B. Laparoscopic surgery in ectopic pregnancy: a randomized trial versus laparotomy. *Acta Obstet Gynecol Scand.* 1991;70:343–348.

54. Murphy AA, Nager CW, Wujek JJ, Kettel LM, Torp VA, Chin HG. Operative laparoscopy versus laparotomy for the management of ectopic pregnancy: a prospective trial. *Fertil Steril.* 1992;57:1180–1185.

55. Vermesh M, Presser SC. Reproductive outcome after linear salpingostomy for ectopic gestation: a prospective 3 year follow up. *Fertil Steril.* 1992;57:682–684.

56. Luciano AA, Maier DB, Koch EI, et al. A comparative study of postoperative adhesions following laser surgery by laparoscopy versus laparotomy in the rabbit model. *Obstet Gynecol.* 1989;74:220.

57. Nezhat G, Metzger MD, Nezhat F, et al. Adhesion reformation after reproductive surgery by videolaseroscopy. *Fertil Steril.* 1990;53:1008.

58. Lundorff P, Hahlin M, Kallfelt B, et al. Adhesion formation after laparoscopic surgery in tubal pregnancy: a randomized trial versus laparotomy. *Fertil Steril.* 1991;55:911.

59. Brumsted J, Kessler G, Gibson G, et al. A comparison of laparoscopy and laparotomy for the treatment of ectopic pregnancy. *Obstet Gynecol.* 1988;71:889.

60. Nezhat G, Nezhat F. Conservative management of ectopic gestation (letter to the editor). *Fertil Steril.* 1990;53:382.

61. Frishman GN, Steinhoff MM, Luciano AA. Triplet tubal pregnancy treated by outpatient laparoscopic salpingostomy. *Fertil Steril.* 1990;54:934.

62. Graczykowski JW, Mishell DR Jr. Methotrexate prophylaxis for persistent ectopic pregnancy after conservative treatment by salpingostomy. *Obstet Gynecol.* 1997;89:118–122.

63. Luciano AA. Ectopic pregnancy. In: Quilling EJ, Zuspan FP, eds. *Current Therapy in Obstetrics and Gynecology.* Philadelphia: Saunders; 1990.

64. Nezhat F, Winer W, Nezhat C. Salpingectomy via laparoscopy: a new surgical approach. *J Laparoendosc Surg.* 1991;1:91.

65. Tulandi T, Saleh A. Surgical management of ectopic pregnancy. *Clin Obstet Gynecol.* 1999;42:31–38.

66. Sowter M, Frappell J. The role of laparoscopy in the management of ectopic pregnancy. *Rev Gynaecol Pract.* 2002;2:73–82.

67. Silva P, Schaper A, Rooney B. Reproductive outcome after 143 laparoscopic procedures for ectopic pregnancy. *Fertil Steril.* 1993;81:710–715.

68. Job-Spira N, Bouyer J, Pouly J. Fertility after ectopic pregnancy: first results of a population-based cohort study in France. *Hum Reprod.* 1996;11:99–104.

69. Mol B, Matthijsse H, Tinga D, et al. Fertility after conservative and radical surgery for tubal pregnancy. *Hum Reprod.* 1998;13:1804–1809.

70. Bangsgaard N, Lund C, Ottesen B, Nilas L. Improved fertility following conservative surgical treatment of ectopic pregnancy. *Br J Obstet Gynaecol.* 2003;110:765–770.

71. Jafri SZH, Loginsky JS, Bouffard JA, et al. Sonographic detection of interstitial pregnancy. *J Clin Ultrasound.* 1987;15:253.

72. Benifla JL, Fernandez H, Sebban E, et al. Alternative to surgery of treatment of unruptured interstitial pregnancy: 15 cases of medical treatment. *Eur J Obstet Gynecol Reprod Biol.* 1996;70:151.

73. Groutz A, Wolf Y, Gaspi B, et al. Successful treatment of advanced interstitial pregnancy with methotrexate and hysteroscopy: a case report. *J Reprod Med.* 1998;43:719.

74. Laury D. Laparoscopic treatment of an interstitial pregnancy. *J Am Assoc Gynecol Laparosc.* 1995;2:219.

75. Ostrzenski A. A new laparoscopic technique for interstitial pregnancy resection: a case report. *J Reprod Med.* 1997;42:363.

76. Grobman WA, Milad MP. Conservative laparoscopic management of a large cornual ectopic pregnancy. *Hum Reprod.* 1998;13:2002.

77. Kamreava MM, Taymor ML, Berger MJ, et al. Disappearance of human chorionic gonadotropin following removal of ectopic pregnancy. *Obstet Gynecol.* 1983;62:486.

78. Shalev E, Peleg D, Tsabari A, et al. Spontaneous resolution of ectopic tubal pregnancy: natural history. *Fertil Steril.* 1995;63:15.

79. Tulandi T, Ferenczy A, Berger E. Tubal occlusion as a result of retained ectopic pregnancy: a case report. *Am J Obstet Gynecol.* 1988;158:1116.

80. Rantala M, Makinen J. Tubal patency and fertility outcome after expectant management of ectopic pregnancy. *Fertil Steril.* 1997;68:1043.

81. Banerjee S, Aslam N, Zosmer N, et al. The expectant management of women with early pregnancy of unknown location. *Ultrasound Obstet Gynecol.* 1999;14:231.

82. Barnhart KT, Gosman G, Ashby R, Sammel M. The medical management of ectopic pregnancy: a meta-analysis comparing "single dose" and "multidose" regimens. *Obstet Gynecol.* 2003;101:778–784.

83. Hajenius PJ, Engelsbel S, Mol BWJ, et al. Systemic methotrexate versus laparoscopic salpingostomy in tubal pregnancy: a randomised clinical trial. *Lancet.* 1997;350:774–779.

84. Saraj A, Wilcox J, Najmabadi S, Stein S, Johnson M, Paulson R. Resolution of hormonal markers of ectopic gestation: a randomized trial comparing single-dose intramuscular methotrexate with salpingostomy. *Obstet Gynecol.* 1998;92:989–994.

85. Lipscomb GH, McCord ML, Stovall TG, Huff G, Portera SG, Ling FW. Predictors of success of methotrexate treatment in women with tubal ectopic pregnancies. *N Engl J Med.* 1999;341:1974–1978.

86. Fernandez H, Rainhorn JD, Papiernik E. Spontaneous resolution of ectopic pregnancy. *Obstet Gynecol.* 1988;71(2):171.

87. Stovall TG, Ling FW, Gray LA. Single doses of methotrexate for treatment of ectopic pregnancy. *Obstet Gynecol.* 1991;77:754.

88. Klauser CK, May WL, Johnson VK, Cowan BD, Hines RS. Methotrexate for ectopic pregnancy: a randomised "single dose" compared with "multidose" trial. *Obstet Gynecol.* 2005;105(suppl):64S.

89. Lipscomb GH, Bran D, McCord ML, Portera JC, Ling FW. Analysis of three hundred fifteen ectopic pregnancies treated with single-dose methotrexate. *Am J Obstet Gynecol.* 1998;178:1354–1358.

90. Perdu M, Camus E, Rozenberg P, et al. Treating ectopic pregnancy with the combination of mifepristone and methotrexate: a phase II nonrandomized study. *Am J Obstet Gynaecol.* 1998;179:640–643.

91. Rozenberg P, Chevret S, Camus E, et al. Medical treatment of ectopic pregnancies: a randomized clinical trial comparing methotrexate-mifepristone and methotrexate-placebo. *Hum Reprod.* 2003;18:1802–1808.

92. Gazvani MR, Baruah DN, Alfirevic Z, Emery SJ. Mifepristone in combination with methotrexate for the medical treatment of tubal pregnancy: a randomized, controlled trial. *Hum Reprod.* 1998;13:1987–1990.

93. Kooi S, Kock HC. Treatment of tubal pregnancy by local injection of methotrexate after adrenaline injection into the mesosalpinx: a report of 25 patients. *Fertil Steril*. 1990;54:580.

94. Fernandez H, Baton C, Lelaidier G, et al. Conservative management of ectopic pregnancy: prospective randomized clinical trial of methotrexate versus prostaglandin sulprostone by combined transvaginal and systemic administration. *Fertil Steril*. 1991;55:746.

95. Namnoum AB. Medical management of ectopic pregnancy. *Clin Obstet Gynecol*. 1998;41:382.

96. Parker J, Bisits A, Proietto AM. A systematic review of single-dose intramuscular methotrexate for the treatment of ectopic pregnancy. *Aust N Z J Obstet Gynaecol*. 1998;38:145.

97. Yao M, Tulandi T. Current status of surgical and nonsurgical management of ectopic pregnancy. *Fertil Steril*. 1997;67:421.

98. Nazac A, Gervaise A, Bouyer J, et al. Predictors of success in methotrexate treatment of women with unruptured tubal pregnancies. *Ultrasound Obstet Gynecol*. 2003;21:181–185.

99. Heard K, Kendall J, Abbott J. Rupture of ectopic pregnancy after medical therapy with methotrexate: a case series. *J Emerg Med*. 1998;16:857.

100. Nieuwkerk PT, Hajenius PJ, Ankum WM, et al. Systemic methotrexate therapy versus laparoscopic salpingostomy in patients with tubal pregnancy: I. Impact on patients' health-related quality of life. *Fertil Steril*. 1998;70:511.

101. Gray DT, Thornburn J, Lundorff P, et al. A cost-effectiveness study of a randomised trial of laparoscopy versus laparotomy for ectopic pregnancy. *Lancet*. 1995;345:1139.

102. Mol BW, Hajenius PJ, Engelsbel S, et al. An economic evaluation of laparoscopy and open surgery in the treatment of tubal pregnancy. *Acta Obstet Gynecol Scand*. 1997;76:596.

103. Foulk RA, Steiger RM. Operative management of ectopic pregnancy: a cost analysis. *Am J Obstet Gynecol*. 1996;175:90.

104. Learman LA, Grimes DA. Rapid hospital discharge following laparoscopy for ectopic pregnancy: a promise unfulfilled? *West J Med*. 1997;167:145.

105. Greinin MD, Washington AE. Cost of ectopic pregnancy management: surgery versus methotrexate. *Fertil Steril*. 1993;60:963.

106. Yao M, Tulandi T, Kaplow M, Smith AP. A comparison of methotrexate versus laparoscopic surgery for the treatment of ectopic pregnancy: a cost analysis. *Hum Reprod*. 1996;11:2762.

107. Hidlebaugh D, O'Mara P. Clinical and financial analyses of ectopic pregnancy management at a large health plan. *J Am Assoc Gynecol Laparosc*. 1997;4:207.

108. Mol BW, Hajenius PJ, Engelsbel S, et al. Is conservative surgery for tubal pregnancy preferable to salpingectomy? An economic analysis. *Br J Obstet Gynaecol*. 1997;104:834.

109. Mol BW, Hajenius PJ, Engelsbel S, et al. Treatment of tubal pregnancy in the Netherlands: an economic comparison of systemic methotrexate administration and laparoscopic salpingostomy. *Am J Obstet Gynecol*. 1999;181:945.

110. Nezhat C, Siegler A, Nezhat F, Nezhat C, Seidman D, Luciano A, *Operative Gynecologic Laparoscopy: Principles and Techniques*, 2nd ed. 2000. McGraw-Hill.

Section 9.5. Management of Tubo-ovarian Abcesses

Daniel S. Seidman, Bulent Berker, and Camran Nezhat

Tubo-ovarian abscess (TOA) is a severe sequela of pelvic inflammatory disease (PID) and occurs in almost one third of patients hospitalized with PID.[1] PID remains the most common gynecologic reason for admission to the hospital in the United States, accounting for 49 per 10,000 recorded hospital discharges. The exact incidence of PID, however, is unknown because the disease cannot be diagnosed reliably from clinical symptoms and signs.[2] Yet, it is estimated that PID affects at least once about 10% to 15% of young women in the United States. Moreover, because most PID is asymptomatic, this figure almost certainly underestimates the true prevalence among women of reproductive age.[3]

Tubo-ovarian abscess is part of a spectrum of inflammatory disorders of the upper female genital tract comprising PID that includes any combination of endometritis, salpingitis, pelvic peritonitis, and TOA.[4] Symptomatic or subclinical pelvic infections may progress rapidly into a TOA, which can rupture and cause peritonitis.[5]

Sexually transmitted organisms, especially *Neisseria gonorrhoeae* and *Chlamydia trachomatis*, are implicated in many cases of PID.[6] These microorganisms are rarely isolated from TOAs, but they are involved in the initiating event, that is, the invasion of the fallopian tube epithelium. This results in tissue damage and necrosis providing an ideal environment for subsequent anaerobic invasion and growth. Other microorganisms that comprise the vaginal flora, including anaerobes, *Gardnerella vaginalis*, *Haemophilus influenzae*, enteric gram-negative rods, and *Streptococcus agalactiae*, have also been associated with PID. In addition, cytomegalovirus, *Mycoplasma hominis*, and *Ureaplasma urealyticum* may be the etiologic agents in some cases of PID.[4]

Risk factors associated with the development of PID include inconsistent barrier contraception, possibly vaginal douching, and the use of oral contraceptive pills possibly masking the clinical severity of the disease. The small risk associated with the IUD is limited to the first few weeks after insertion.[1] Postpartum endometritis may also lead to PID.

The sequelae of PID may cause infertility, tubal pregnancy, chronic pelvic pain, and recurrent upper genital tract infection. The extent of tubal damage and pelvic adhesions depends on the severity of the infection, the number of PID episodes, and the etiology. Peritonitis is associated with a 17% risk of infertility compared with 3% for a mild infection. With each successive episode, the risk of infertility increases. The risk of ectopic pregnancy is six to 10 times higher in women who have had PID. Chronic pelvic pain occurs in 15% to 18% of patients after PID because of adhesions. About 25% of these patients will have at least one recurrent infection.[4]

DIAGNOSIS

Precise diagnosis of acute PID is the cornerstone of the treatment for the condition.[7] However, acute PID is difficult to diagnose because of the wide variation in the symptoms and signs.[4] Delay in diagnosis and effective treatment is of concern because it may contribute to inflammatory sequelae in the upper reproductive tract, including TOA. Among women with PID, many report subtle, nonspecific symptoms, such as dyspareunia, postcoital spotting, and abnormal uterine bleeding. In these situations, a bimanual examination could reveal cervical motion or adnexal tenderness. Even in the presence of "classic" symptoms and signs, such as lower abdominal pain, cervical motion and adnexal tenderness, elevated white cell count, fever, and a mass on ultrasound, other diseases are part of a differential diagnosis. The clinical diagnosis of acute PID is imprecise. Data indicate that a clinical diagnosis of symptomatic PID has a positive predictive value for salpingitis of 65% to 90% compared with laparoscopy.[3,4]

Additional criteria that support a diagnosis of PID include oral temperature above 101°F (38.3°C), abnormal cervical or vaginal discharge, elevated erythrocyte sedimentation rate and C-reactive protein, and laboratory documentation of cervical infection with *N. gonorrhoeae* or *C. trachomatis*.[4] However, recent critical review has suggested that there is insufficient evidence to support existing diagnostic criteria, which have been based on a combination of empirical data and expert opinion.[8] It has been suggested that a new evidence base is urgently needed, but this will require either a new investigation of the association between clinical presentation and PID based on a laparoscopic "gold standard" or the development of new diagnostic techniques.[8]

The most specific criteria for diagnosing PID are histopathologic evidence of endometritis on an endometrial biopsy specimen and laparoscopic abnormalities consistent with PID.[4] Laparoscopy, allowing direct visualization of the fallopian tubes, is usually considered the best single diagnostic test to obtain a more accurate diagnosis of salpingitis and a more complete bacteriologic diagnosis.[3] However, this diagnostic tool is invasive and often not readily available, and its use is not easy to justify when symptoms are mild or vague. Moreover, laparoscopy will not detect endometritis and may not detect subtle inflammation of the fallopian tubes. Consequently, a diagnosis of PID usually is based on clinical findings.

Laparoscopy is still considered a useful tool in selected cases, allowing rapid and precise identification of the infectious agent and extent of disease so that appropriate therapy can be instituted. Molander et al. [9] evaluated the efficacy of acute-phase operative laparoscopy in 33 women with clinically suspected PID. Laparoscopy confirmed the diagnosis of PID in 20 patients (61%);

11 women (33%) had other disease, and two (6%) had no evidence of disease. The authors concluded that acute-phase operative laparoscopy provided a final diagnosis in all but three of 33 patients (91%).[9]

In a subsequent study, these authors tried to assess the diagnostic accuracy of the laparoscopic diagnosis of PID.[10] They studied the observer agreement with laparoscopic diagnosis of PID using photographs among three senior consultants and three residents. The overall accuracy of the laparoscopic diagnosis of PID was 78%, the sensitivity was 27%, and the specificity was 92%. The overall intraobserver reproducibility of the diagnosis of PID was only fair, and it was clearly better among the consultants than among the residents. When specific diagnostic features (e.g., tubal erythema, edema, adhesions, cul-de-sac fluid) were separately analyzed, the results were no different, suggesting only poor to fair reproducibility. The investigators therefore concluded that based on photographic images, the observer reproducibility and the overall diagnostic accuracy of the laparoscopic diagnosis of PID are unsatisfactory when histopathologically proven PID is used as the gold standard.[10]

Imaging

Pelvic sonography is almost universally performed in patients with a clinical diagnosis of PID. Though the study may be normal or sometimes nonspecific, there are a variety of findings that are characteristic of this process. The experienced sonographer is able to evaluate the features of PID, salpingitis, pyosalpinx, tubo-ovarian complex, and TOAs.[11] Sonography may also help distinguish acute from chronic abnormalities in the fallopian tubes.[11] Transvaginal sonogram (TVS), showing thickened fluid-filled tubes with or without free pelvic fluid or a tubo-ovarian complex, is considered one of the most reliable criteria for diagnosing PID.[4] Newer diagnostic techniques that have been evaluated include Doppler ultrasound and MRI.[1]

Timor-Tritsch et al. [12] tried to identify sonographic markers of PID and to place these in a clinical context. They found that the best marker of tubal inflammatory disease, either acute or chronic, was the presence of an incomplete septum of the tubal wall, which was present in 92% of the total cases. A thick wall and the "cogwheel" sign were sensitive markers of acute disease, whereas a thin wall and "beads-on-a-string" sign were indicators of chronic disease. Palpable findings and surgical history were not discriminatory, but were present in three quarters and one third of their study population, respectively. Three false-positive cases were identified, including an ovarian cystadenoma, an appendiceal mucocele, and one case with peri-ovarian fluid accumulation. Timor-Tritsch and his colleagues [12] concluded that a tubo-ovarian complex and TOA should be considered separate entities that differ in their clinical implications. TVS allows one to distinguish between them. Furthermore, they found that distinguishing TVS characteristics are also of benefit for the diagnosis of acute versus chronic salpingitis.

The usefulness of power Doppler TVS in the diagnosis of PID was evaluated by Molander et al. [13]. Conventional TVS and power Doppler TVS were performed. All patients with suspected acute PID underwent laparoscopy to confirm the diagnosis. Power Doppler was used to assess the vascularity of any adnexal mass. The diagnosis of PID was confirmed by laparoscopy in 20 (67%) of the 30 women with clinically suspected acute PID. Specific TVS findings, including wall thickness 5 mm or greater, cogwheel sign, incomplete septa, and the presence of cul-de-sac fluid, discriminated women with acute PID from the control women with hydrosalpinx formation. Power Doppler TVS revealed hyperemia in all women with acute PID, but in only two women with hydrosalpinx, a statistically significant difference. Pulsatility indices were significantly lower in the acute PID group than in the control group. The authors concluded that power Doppler TVS was 100% sensitive and 80% specific in the diagnosis of PID, with an overall accuracy of 93%. Specific sonographic landmark findings and power Doppler findings were noted to augment the clinical diagnosis of PID and allow simple classification of the severity of the disease.[13]

Varras et al. [14] tried to identify the different sonographic markers on gray-scale and color Doppler sonography in TOA. They retrospectively analyzed the ultrasound records of a group of 25 women in whom the presence of TOA was confirmed by surgery and histopathology. A mass was found in all cases. The maximum diameter of the mass was 5 cm in two cases and between 5 cm and 10 cm in 23 cases. The mass was demonstrated at the anatomic position of the ovary in 21 cases (84%) and at the cul-de-sac in four cases (16%). The mass was a simple cyst in two cases (8%), in four cases it was cystic with diaphragms (16%), in four cases it was a thickened tube-shaped structure with multiple internal echoes (16%), and in 15 cases it was a mixture of cystic and solid elements (60%). Pyosalpinges with fluid–fluid levels were found in two cases. Fluid in the cul-de-sac was observed at a rate of 48%. Color Doppler sonography demonstrated abundant blood flow in the borders and the septa of the TOAs in 90% of the studied cases. Varras et al. [14] concluded that the ultrasonographic findings of TOAs are not specific. They suggested that the presence of a mass at the anatomic position of the ovary or at the cul-de-sac in combination with an increased number of white blood cells, elevated erythrocyte sedimentation rate, and clinical findings may be helpful for a correct diagnosis. In addition, they pointed out that color Doppler flow may help characterize the nature of the pelvic mass by detecting a significant rich blood flow in most cases of TOAs.[14]

CT is ordered with increasing frequency in patients with unexplained lower abdominal pain. It is important to correlate the TVS findings with those of the pelvic CT.[11] In cases of suspected TOA, CT and MRI findings may be helpful in demonstrating the extent of the disease, characterizing the lesions, and making a specific diagnosis.[15] These expensive imaging modalities may be of greatest value when used in cases of rare but specific causes of TOA, such as actinomycosis, tuberculosis, and xanthogranulomatous inflammation.[16]

TOA and Endometriosis

Women with stages III through IV endometriosis were observed to be more likely to develop TOAs compared with those without endometriosis.[17] This association was most strongly noted in nulliparous women or those who had delivered no more than two children. It was suggested that this association with parity may be related to endometriosis suppression, the prolonged duration of menstrual-free periods in multiparous women, or changes in the local immunity of the pelvic cavity.[17]

The presence of an ovarian endometrioma is a well-known risk factor for the development of a TOA or an ovarian abscess.[18] In a review of the medical records of 6557 gynecologic inpatients, the incidence of TOAs was found to be significantly higher in patients with endometrioma compared with patients without endometrioma (2.3% vs. 0.2%). The causes of the abscesses in the seven cases with endometrioma were contamination during surgery (one case), contamination during a transvaginal endometrioma aspiration (one case), an ascending infection (one case), and unknown in four cases.[18]

Tubo-ovarian abscess is a rare but well-recognized complication of in vitro fertilization (IVF) treatment.[19] The increased risk for TOA during IVF may occasionally be a result of reactivation of a latent pelvic infection, due to previous PID, following TVS-directed follicle aspiration and transcervical embryo transfer.[20] However, among women undergoing transvaginal oocyte pickup for IVF, when severe endometriosis or an ovarian endometrioma are present, there appears to be an increased risk for TOA. Late manifestation of pelvic abscess supports the notion that the presence of old blood in an endometrioma provides a culture medium for bacteria to grow slowly after transvaginal inoculation.[21] However, it is not yet clear whether more vigorous antibiotic prophylaxis and better vaginal preparation before oocyte pickup can prevent the risk of TOA developing after the procedure in patients with severe endometriosis and ovarian endometrioma.[22,23] It has been suggested that both the pseudocapsule of the endometrioma and the old blood inside it may prevent antibiotic prophylaxis from overcoming the transvaginal bacterial inoculation.[21] Small pools of old blood formed in the peritoneal cavity of patients with endometriosis may act as an isolated culture medium for the inoculated bacteria.

The altered immune system of patients with endometriosis may adversely affect the immune response to inoculated bacteria.[22] This altered immune response may explain the occurrence of PID in milder forms of endometriosis. It should be noted, however, that although it has long been hypothesized that dysregulation of the immune system plays a role in the pathogenesis of endometriosis, no report has so far linked the risk of infection in these patients to the altered immune system.[24]

TOA and Gynecologic Cancer in Postmenopausal Women

A significant association between TOAs in menopause and malignancy has been established.[25] Among postmenopausal women, Protopapas et al. [25] found a strong relationship between TOAs and concomitant gynecologic malignancy including a variety of cancers. The incidence of gynecologic cancer in postmenopausal patients who develop TOAs ranged from 25% to 47%.[25–27] The cases of gynecologic cancer included adenocarcinoma of the cervix, endometrial cancer, and epithelial ovarian cancer. Primary carcinoma of the fallopian tube may also present as TOA.[28,29]

TOAs represent a rather unusual entity in postmenopausal women when compared with those observed in women of reproductive age. A recent study has also suggested that there may be a new trend in the epidemiology of TOA occurring in older women, who do not present with the traditional risk factors for PID and TOA.[30] In postmenopausal women, the clinical picture is different from the typical occurrence of abdominal or pelvic pain, fever (temperature $\geq 38.5°C$), chills, and increased vaginal secretions. Postmenopausal women rarely report a history of acute PID, and many patients present with vague and nonspecific symptoms. Protopapas et al. [25] observed that moderate or severe abdominal pain was present in the majority of their patients, whereas pyrexia (temperature $\geq 38°C$) was absent in 59% of cases. Thus, in the postmenopausal patient, low abdominal pain accompanied by signs of peritoneal irritation, even when high fever is absent, may suggest serious acute surgical conditions.[25]

The existence of a gynecologic malignancy may predispose a patient to the development of a TOA for several reasons.[25] An advanced cervical or endometrial carcinoma may cause obstruction and subsequent entrapment of blood and upper genital tract secretions, creating an optimal anaerobic environment that may lead to the development of pyometra and/or a bilateral or unilateral TOA. A fallopian tube or ovarian carcinoma may cause excessive local destruction of normal anatomy, permitting anaerobic growth, which is optimized in conditions of low oxidation–reduction potential, low oxygen tension, and ample nutrient supply, all of which are provided by ischemic and necrotic neoplastic tissue.[25]

All postmenopausal women presenting with TOAs should therefore be thoroughly investigated to exclude a concomitant pelvic malignancy. Conservative treatment of TOAs has no place in menopause. Laparoscopy has a major role in investigating the nature of suspicious masses in postmenopausal women with PID.

It should be remembered that not only can the presentation of a carcinoma of the gynecologic tract mimic a TOA [29], but patients presenting with abdominal pain and a pelvic mass resembling an ovarian tumor may actually be found to suffer from a TOA. A pelvic TOA mimicking a pelvic malignancy may occur not only in postmenopausal women [31,32], but also in sexually inactive girls.[33]

TREATMENT

It is generally assumed that if PID is inadequately treated, this may lead to a complicated course occasionally involving the development of TOA. Moreover, because PID has high morbidity, management must be prompt to prevent long-term complications; about 20% of affected women become infertile, 20% develop chronic pelvic pain, and 10% of those who conceive have an ectopic pregnancy.[2] Repeated episodes of PID are associated with a four- to sixfold increase in the risk of permanent tubal damage.[2] Empirical treatment of PID with broad-spectrum antibiotics is thus always recommended in women who are at risk, if lower abdominal tenderness, adnexal tenderness, and cervical motion tenderness are present.[4] Initial treatment is provided on an outpatient basis. There are no apparent differences in clinical outcomes, whether a woman with PID is treated as an inpatient or an outpatient.[1] Combination drug regimens, including antibiotics against the most common factors underlying acute PID, seem to prevent most late sequelae in cases with mild or moderate salpingitis. However, this is not the case in women with a tubal or pelvic abscess.[4] Patients who do not improve under antibiotic therapy usually require hospitalization, additional diagnostic tests, and surgical intervention.[4]

The classic treatment of TOA used to be total abdominal hysterectomy with bilateral salpingo-oophorectomy, a procedure that promised rapid cure due to complete evacuation of infected tissue but had devastating consequences for young women.

Table 9.5.1: Management of Tubo-ovarian Abscess

Administration of broad-spectrum antibiotics

Transvaginal or percutaneous drainage

Ultrasound-guided intracavitary instillation of antibiotics

Laparoscopic draining and irrigation of abscess

Laparoscopic removal of infected tube or adnexa

With the advancement in broad-spectrum antibiotics and the availability of accurate imaging techniques, treatment of TOA has changed dramatically. Because most women with TOA are of reproductive age, the primary aim of management is to be as conservative as possible. Organ-preserving approaches are currently advocated for the management of TOA (Table 9.5.1).

Transvaginal ultrasound–guided aspiration combined with antibiotics is currently recommended as a first-line procedure for TOAs.[34] It has been shown to be an effective and safe treatment regimen. In a recent study from Norway, surgery was performed in only 20 women (6.6%) following 449 transvaginal aspirations performed on 302 women. The main indications for surgery were diagnostic or therapeutic uncertainty, such as suspected residual TOA abscess or pain. No procedure-related complications were diagnosed.[34]

In a randomized prospective study of 40 women diagnosed as suffering from TOA of less than 10 cm maximal diameter, intensive antibiotic therapy alone was compared with antibiotic therapy in association with early ultrasound-guided vaginal drainage.[35] Early transvaginal drainage of the abscess resulted in a favorable short-term response in 90% of the cases, whereas this was 65% in the control group.[35]

One-step sonographically guided aspiration of TOA followed by intracavitary antibiotic instillation has also been shown to offer an easy and safe alternative therapy in patients in whom treatment with systemic antibiotics has failed.[36]

Laparoscopic management of TOA was introduced almost three decades ago.[37,38] Laparoscopic procedures in women with TOA comprise pelvic irrigation in all patients and lysis of adhesions in most cases.[9] They usually also include laparoscopic draining and irrigation of the TOA or complete removal of the inflamed tube or adnexa.[9]

German investigators compared the outcome of operative laparoscopy for TOA with incision of the abscess cavity and lavage (organ-preserving treatment) only versus laparoscopic salpingectomy or salpingo-oophorectomy (ablative treatment).[39] In their retrospective analysis, 35 patients not wishing to have children underwent salpingectomy or salpingo-oophorectomy, whereas 25 patients wishing to remain fertile were treated by means of an organ-preserving procedure. Apart from one postoperative readmission because of lower pelvic pain in the organ-preserving group, there were no operative complications or serious systemic sequelae. In contrast, there was a significantly higher incidence of intraoperative and postoperative complications when ablative treatment was performed: one intestinal perforation requiring subsequent laparotomy, four serosal lesions, two lesions of the greater omentum, two lacerated collaterals of the internal iliac artery, one postoperative fever higher than

38°C for 2 days, two bowel obstructions, one thrombosis of the upper leg, and one thrombosis of the lower leg. The authors concluded that when laparoscopic treatment of TOA is performed, organ-preserving treatment should be chosen, irrespective of the patient's age or desire to have children, because of the risk of complications.[39]

Raiga and coauthors [40] studied 39 patients who were treated for adnexal abscesses. Those authors showed that laparoscopic surgery is a safe and efficient technique for treating this condition. No immediate reoperation was necessary within the first 2 months after the initial laparoscopic procedure. At a second-look laparoscopy, adhesiolysis was required in all of the patients. A salpingostomy was done in 17 women, and six others were referred for IVF. Subsequently, 12 of 19 patients who did not use any contraception became pregnant. Although laparoscopy remains the technique of choice in the initial management of adnexal abscesses, the anatomic results observed at second-look laparoscopy suggest that a second-look procedure should be considered for patients who desire future pregnancy, if they are not referred to IVF treatment. Moreover, laparoscopic removal of the tube may be warranted in some patients undergoing IVF treatment, as subsequent development of hydrosalpinges following inflammatory involvement of the tube may adversely affect the success of IVF.[41]

A recent retrospective study compared laparoscopic surgery in 19 women and conventional exploratory laparotomy in 37 women for managing patients with TOA.[42] Laparoscopic surgery was associated with a significantly decreased hospital stay, a lower percentage of wound infections, and a shorter time for fever to subside. Open laparoscopy thus seems to be a good alternative to traditional laparotomy in managing patients with TOA.

A laparoscopic study of acute PID was conducted in Nairobi, Kenya, among 133 patients with acute salpingitis.[43] TOAs were found significantly more frequently among HIV-1–infected compared with HIV-1–uninfected women (33% vs. 15%). TOAs were also significantly more common among women with low CD4 cell counts. Thus, in patients with laparoscopically verified acute salpingitis, the likelihood of TOA was related to HIV-1 infection and advanced immunosuppression.

THE LAPAROSCOPIC TECHNIQUE

The laparoscopic management of TOA as undertaken by Nezhat et al. [44] is performed in the following manner: Two 5-mm trocars are inserted in the lower quadrants, and a suction–irrigator probe and grasping forceps are inserted through the trocars. The pelvis, upper abdomen, and pelvic viscera are examined for free or loculated purulent material, and the course of both ureters is identified. Collections are dispersed gently with the suction–irrigator, and purulent fluid is aspirated. Cultures are taken from the inflammatory exudate. If necessary, the suction–irrigator is used to bluntly mobilize the omentum, small bowel, rectosigmoid, and tubo-ovarian adhesions (Figure 9.5.1).[45] After the abscess cavity is localized, it is drained and the suction–irrigator separates the bowel and omentum completely from the reproductive organs. TOAs are separated by using a combination of blunt lysis and hydrodissection. Adhesions caused by acute PID are soft and can be disrupted by gentle blunt dissection and hydrodissection. Hydrodissection is done by placing the tip of the

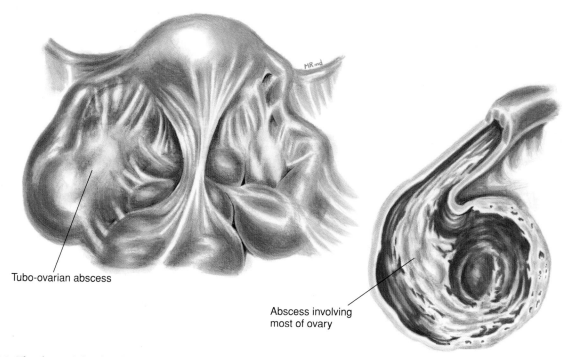

Figure 9.5.1. The abscess is localized and is exposed for drainage. The cut surface of the tubo-ovarian abscess is shown.

suction–irrigator between the tissues. The pressure of the fluid spray and the gentle force of the instrument create a plane for dissection (Figure 9.5.2). The 5-mm graspers provide traction and countertraction, improving observation of the affected area. After the abscess is mobilized, it is drained (Figure 9.5.3). Its walls are removed in sections by using the 5-mm graspers (Figure 9.5.4).

Though technically arduous, meticulous dissection of the abscess from the surrounding structures is important for success. Once the ovary is mobilized, rents or holes in it are irrigated copiously. Sutures are not required to repair the ovary. Graspers are inserted into the tubal ostium to spread it and free agglutinated fimbriae. Chromopertubation is not suggested because

edema in the interstitial tissue of the tube occludes the lumen. At the end of the procedure, the peritoneal cavity is irrigated with lactated Ringer's solution until the effluent is clear (Figure 9.5.5). The upper abdomen is irrigated also, and the remainder of the irrigation fluid is aspirated while the patient is in the reverse-Trendelenburg position. Between 300 mL and 400 mL of irrigation fluid is left in the pelvis to separate these organs during the early healing phase. Hydrodissection and gentle blunt dissection decrease the potential for intestinal injury; the laser and electrosurgery should be used sparingly.

In contrast to the adhesions associated with an acute abscess, chronic TOAs have dense walls. The bowel often adheres to pelvic

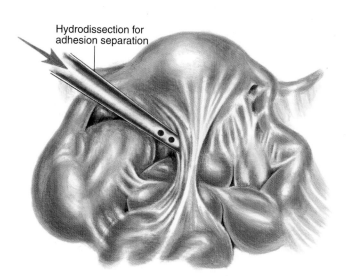

Figure 9.5.2. Hydrodissection and gentle blunt dissection reduce the potential for intestinal injury.

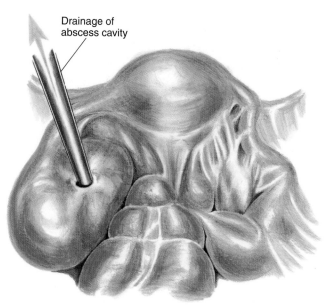

Figure 9.5.3. The abscess cavity is drained and irrigated.

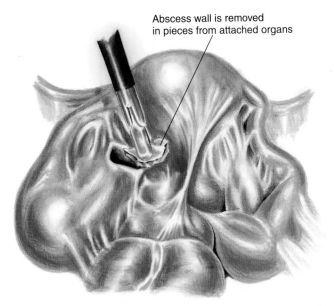

Abscess wall is removed
in pieces from attached organs

Figure 9.5.4. Sections of the abscess wall are removed in pieces using a 5-mm grasper.

organs and is dissected with difficulty; the adnexa appear as a dense mass, making it difficult to distinguish between the pyosalpinx and the ovary. Adhesiolysis technically is difficult and is associated with a high risk of complications.

SUMMARY

Recent epidemiologic studies indicate that the clinical panorama of PID is changing, with fewer patients hospitalized for PID but

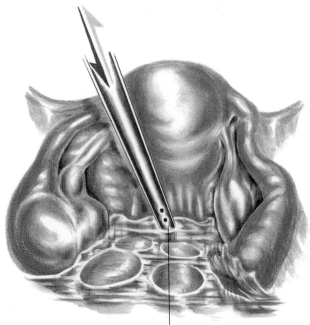

Copious lavage of both
the pelvis and abdomen

Figure 9.5.5. The pelvis is irrigated.

a higher percentage of patients developing TOA.[45] This may be attributed to changing risk factors, such as endometriosis, now recognized to influence the incidence of TOAs. Furthermore, although the direct medical costs of PID and its sequelae may be decreasing, they remain substantial.[46]

The initial management of TOA consists of conservative medical treatment with broad-spectrum antibiotics. However, it is now widely accepted that drainage of the abscess by transvaginal ultrasound or CT-guided aspiration or under direct laparoscopic guidance should be considered early after the diagnosis. Laparoscopic surgical intervention in selected cases allows for prompt management of TOAs and may prevent considerable short- and long-term morbidity.

All postmenopausal women presenting with a clinical picture suggestive of TOA should be thoroughly investigated to exclude a concomitant gynecologic or other pelvic malignancy. Even when such an association has not been confirmed after an extensive preoperative diagnostic work-up, conservative treatment has no place in such cases as it may lead to an unnecessary delay in the diagnosis of an occult cancer or of a life-threatening acute surgical condition.

REFERENCES

1. Barrett S, Taylor C. A review on pelvic inflammatory disease. *Int J STD AIDS*. 2005;16:715–720.
2. Ross J. Extracts from "Clinical Evidence": pelvic inflammatory disease. *BMJ*. 2001;322:658–659.
3. Morcos R, Frost N, Hnat M, Petrunak A, Caldito G. Laparoscopic versus clinical diagnosis of acute pelvic inflammatory disease. *J Reprod Med*. 1993;38:53–56.
4. Workowski KA, Levine WC. Centers for Disease Control: sexually transmitted diseases treatment guidelines. *MMWR Morb Mortal Wkly Rep*. 2002;51:1–80.
5. Walker CK, Landers DV. Pelvic abscesses: new trends in management. *Obstet Gynecol Surg*. 1991;46:615–624.
6. Miller WC, Ford CA, Morris M, et al. Prevalence of chlamydial and gonococcal infections among young adults in the United States. *JAMA*. 2004;291:2229–2236.
7. Heinonen PK, Leinonen M. Fecundity and morbidity following acute pelvic inflammatory disease treated with doxycycline and metronidazole. *Arch Gynecol Obstet*. 2003;268:284–288.
8. Simms I, Warburton F, Westrom L. Diagnosis of pelvic inflammatory disease: time for a rethink. *Sex Transm Infect*. 2003;79:491–494.
9. Molander P, Cacciatore B, Sjoberg J, Paavonen J. Laparoscopic management of suspected acute pelvic inflammatory disease. *J Am Assoc Gynecol Laparosc*. 2000;7:107–110.
10. Molander P, Finne P, Sjoberg J, Sellors J, Paavonen J. Observer agreement with laparoscopic diagnosis of pelvic inflammatory disease using photographs. *Obstet Gynecol*. 2003;101:875–880.
11. Horrow MM. Ultrasound of pelvic inflammatory disease. *Ultrasound Q*. 2004;20:171–179.
12. Timor-Tritsch IE, Lerner JP, Monteagudo A, Murphy KE, Heller DS. Transvaginal sonographic markers of tubal inflammatory disease. *Ultrasound Obstet Gynecol*. 1998;12:56–66.
13. Molander P, Sjoberg J, Paavonen J, Cacciatore B. Transvaginal power Doppler findings in laparoscopically proven acute pelvic inflammatory disease. *Ultrasound Obstet Gynecol*. 2001;17:233–238.
14. Varras M, Polyzos D, Perouli E, Noti P, Pantazis I, Akrivis CH. Tubo-ovarian abscesses: spectrum of sonographic findings with

surgical and pathological correlations. *Clin Exp Obstet Gynecol.* 2003;30:117–121.

15. Ha HK, Lim GY, Cha ES, et al. MR imaging of tubo-ovarian abscess. *Acta Radiol.* 1995;36:510–514.

16. Kim SH, Kim SH, Yang DM, Kim KA. Unusual causes of tubo-ovarian abscess: CT and MR imaging findings. *Radiographics.* 2004;24:1575–1589.

17. Chen MJ, Yang JH, Yang YS, Ho HN. Increased occurrence of tubo-ovarian abscesses in women with stage III and IV endometriosis. *Fertil Steril.* 2004;82:498–499.

18. Kubota T, Ishi K, Takeuchi H. A study of tubo-ovarian and ovarian abscesses, with a focus on cases with endometrioma. *J Obstet Gynaecol Res.* 1997;23:421–426.

19. Orvieto R. Bleeding and PID following ART. In: Allahbadia GN, Merchant R, eds. *Contemporary Perspectives on Assisted Reproductive Technology.* New Delhi: Elsevier; 2006:217–221.

20. Varras M, Polyzos D, Tsikini A, Antypa E, Apessou D, Tsouroulas M. Ruptured tubo-ovarian abscess as a complication of IVF treatment: clinical, ultrasonographic and histopathologic findings. A case report. *Clin Exp Obstet Gynecol.* 2003;30:164–168.

21. Younis JS, Ezra Y, Laufer N, Ohel G. Late manifestation of pelvic abscess following oocyte retrieval, for in vitro fertilization, in patients with severe endometriosis and ovarian endometriomata. *J Assist Reprod Genet.* 1997;14:343–346.

22. Moini A, Riazi K, Amid V, et al. Endometriosis may contribute to oocyte retrieval-induced pelvic inflammatory disease: report of eight cases. *J Assist Reprod Genet.* 2005;22:307–309.

23. Tsai YC, Lin MY, Chen SH, et al. Vaginal disinfection with povidone iodine immediately before oocyte retrieval is effective in preventing pelvic abscess formation without compromising the outcome of IVF-ET. *J Assist Reprod Genet.* 2005;22:173–175.

24. Dmowski PW, Braun DP. Immunology of endometriosis. *Best Pract Res Clin Obstet Gynaecol.* 2004;18:245–263.

25. Protopapas AG, Diakomanolis ES, Milingos SD, et al. Tubo-ovarian abscesses in postmenopausal women: gynecological malignancy until proven otherwise? *Eur J Obstet Gynecol Reprod Biol.* 2004;114:203–209.

26. Heaton FC, Ledger WJ. Postmenopausal tuboovarian abscess. *Obstet Gynecol.* 1976;47:90–94.

27. Hoffman M, Molpus K, Roberts WS, Lyman GH, Cavanagh D. Tuboovarian abscess in postmenopausal women. *J Reprod Med.* 1990;35:525–528.

28. Halperin R, Zehavi S, Gayer G, Herman A, Schneider D. Fallopian tube carcinoma presenting as tubo-ovarian abscess: a report of two cases with literature review. *Int J Gynecol Cancer.* 2005;15:1131–1134.

29. Verit FF, Kafali H. Primary carcinoma of the fallopian tube mimicking tubo-ovarian abscess. *Eur J Gynaecol Oncol.* 2005;26:225–226.

30. Halperin R, Levinson O, Yaron M, Bukovsky I, Schneider D. Tubo-ovarian abscess in older women: is the woman's age a risk factor for failed response to conservative treatment? *Gynecol Obstet Invest.* 2003;55:211–215.

31. Seoud MA, Kanj SS, Habli M, Araj GF, Khalil AM. Brucella pelvic tubo-ovarian abscess mimicking a pelvic malignancy. *Scand J Infect Dis.* 2003;35:277–278.

32. Gungor T, Parlakyigit EE, Dumanli H. Actinomycotic tubo-ovarian abscess mimicking pelvic malignancy. *Gynecol Obstet Invest.* 2002;54:119–121.

33. Dogan E, Altunyurt S, Altindag T, Onvural A. Tubo-ovarian abscess mimicking ovarian tumor in a sexually inactive girl. *J Pediatr Adolesc Gynecol.* 2004;17:351–352.

34. Gjelland K, Ekerhovd E, Granberg S. Transvaginal ultrasound-guided aspiration for treatment of tubo-ovarian abscess: a study of 302 cases. *Am J Obstet Gynecol.* 2005;193:1323–1330.

35. Perez-Medina T, Huertas MA, Bajo JM. Early ultrasound-guided transvaginal drainage of tubo-ovarian abscesses: a randomized study. *Ultrasound Obstet Gynecol.* 1996;7:435–438.

36. Caspi B, Zalel Y, Or Y, Bar Dayan Y, Appelman Z, Katz Z. Sonographically guided aspiration: an alternative therapy for tubo-ovarian abscess. *Ultrasound Obstet Gynecol.* 1996;7:439–442.

37. Anducci JE. Laparoscopy in the diagnosis and treatment of pelvic inflammatory disease with abscess formation. *Int Surg.* 1981;66:359.

38. Henry-Suchet J, Soler A, Loffredo V. Laparoscopic treatment of tubo-ovarian abscesses. *J Reprod Med.* 1984;8:579.

39. Buchweitz O, Malik E, Kressin P, Meyhoefer-Malik A, Diedrich K. Laparoscopic management of tubo-ovarian abscesses: retrospective analysis of 60 cases. *Surg Endosc.* 2000;14:948–950.

40. Raiga J, Canis M, Le Bouedec G, et al. Laparoscopic management of adnexal abscesses: consequences for fertility. *Fertil Steril.* 1996;66:712.

41. Johnson NP, Mak W, Sowter MC. Surgical treatment for tubal disease in women due to undergo in vitro fertilisation. *Cochrane Database Syst Rev.* 2004;CD002125.

42. Yang CC, Chen P, Tseng JY, Wang PH. Advantages of open laparoscopic surgery over exploratory laparotomy in patients with tubo-ovarian abscess. *J Am Assoc Gynecol Laparosc.* 2002;9:327–332.

43. Cohen CR, Sinei S, Reilly M, et al. Effect of human immunodeficiency virus type 1 infection upon acute salpingitis: a laparoscopic study. *J Infect Dis.* 1998;178:1352.

44. Nezhat F, Nezhat C, Silfen SL. Videolaseroscopy for oophorectomy. *Am J Obstet Gynecol.* 1991;165:1323–1330.

45. Nezhat C, Siegler A, Nezhat F, Nezhat C, Seidman D, Luciano A. Operations of the follopian tube. In *Operative Gynecological Laparoscopy: Principles and Techniques, 2nd ed.* 2000; McGraw-Hill.

46. Sorbye IK, Jerve F, Staff AC. Reduction in hospitalized women with pelvic inflammatory disease in Oslo over the past decade. *Acta Obstet Gynecol Scand.* 2005;84:290–296.

47. Rein DB, Kassler WJ, Irwin KL, Rabiee L. Direct medical cost of pelvic inflammatory disease and its sequelae: decreasing, but still substantial. *Obstet Gynecol.* 2000;95:397–402.

Section 9.6. Surgical Management of Polycystic Ovarian Syndrome

Michelle Tham and Alan B. Copperman

Polycystic ovarian syndrome (PCOS) is the most common manifestation of hormonal dysfunction in reproductive-age women today. The prevalence of PCOS is reported to be anywhere from 4% to 12%, with mild racial variations.[1] It is a complex disorder affecting multiple organ systems whose historical roots lie in Stein and Leventhal's 1935 case reports [2] describing seven women with a constellation of clinical symptoms including amenorrhea, infertility, obesity, hirsutism, and polycystic-appearing ovaries. What initially may have been considered primarily a reproductive disorder has since evolved into a disease entity that profoundly affects the cardiovascular, metabolic, and endocrine systems.

DIAGNOSIS

In 1990, the National Institutes of Health sponsored a conference to systematically describe polycystic ovarian syndrome, laying the foundation for a more dynamic definition by the 2003 Rotterdam European Society of Human Reproduction/American Society for Reproductive Medicine (ESHRE/ASRM) PCOS consensus workshop. Diagnostic criteria now include two of the following three cardinal features:

1. oligo- and/or anovulation
2. clinical and/or biochemical signs of hyperandrogenism
3. polycystic ovaries (via ultrasound)

The diagnosis is also contingent on ruling out other endocrinologic disorders, such as hyperprolactinemia, ovarian hyperthecosis, congenital adrenal hyperplasia (CAH), Cushing's syndrome, an androgen-secreting neoplasm, or acromegaly.[3] Initial laboratory assessment of the patient with suspected PCOS should serve to narrow the differential diagnosis and includes serum total testosterone, 17α-hydroxyprogesterone (to rule out CAH from 21-hydroxylase deficiency), and dehydroepiandrosterone (DHEA) levels. A 24-hour urine collection to measure free cortisol will assist in diagnosing Cushing's syndrome.

PCOS is associated with insulin resistance, and measurements of fasting glucose levels and insulin may also be performed, although the specificity of these tests tends to be poor. The gold standard of the hyperinsulinemic euglycemic clamp is not commonly used in clinical practice. Classically, PCOS has also been associated with an elevated luteinizing hormone (LH)–to–follicle-stimulating hormone (FSH) ratio; however, the actual levels of these pituitary peptides do not correlate with the severity of the disease and it is not mandatory to measure them to establish a clinical diagnosis.

PATHOGENESIS

At its core, PCOS is an ovarian dysfunction. The precise pathogenesis of this entity, however, involves far more than ovarian structure. The hyperandrogenic state seems to be the product of increased LH secretion in combination with enhanced ovarian theca cell responsiveness. The etiology of the increased LH levels has been purported to be secondary to increased pulse frequency of gonadotropin-releasing hormone (GnRH). This increased pulse frequency may be the result of an inherent defect in the GnRH pulse generator or of low circulating levels of progesterone from few ovulations leading to decreased negative feedback.[4]

In combination with elevated ovarian production of androgen, the amount of circulating sex hormone–binding globulin (SHBG) also plays a role in pathogenesis. There is an inverse relationship between insulin and SHBG. Insulin inhibits hepatic production of SHBG. Intuitively, in the hyperinsulinemic state of PCOS, SHBG is decreased and there are resultant higher levels of free testosterone. Adrenal androgen is also a contributing factor to PCOS, as approximately 50% of women will have enhanced production. It is unclear whether the adrenal dysfunction is critical to the progression of the disorder.

CLINICAL FEATURES

The characteristically androgen-dominated hormonal milieu of PCOS dictates clinical manifestations. Symptoms usually begin at menarche, and an early pubarche may in fact be a portent of PCOS in adulthood. Chronic anovulation and resultant lack of menses may lead to endometrial hyperplasia and in its worst consequence, carcinoma. Infertility is also common in PCOS patients because of the decreased frequency of ovulatory cycles. There have been recent associations among PCOS, insulin resistance, and recurrent early pregnancy loss, although the mechanism is unclear.

Hirsutism is another cardinal phenotypic feature of PCOS. Increased hair growth in PCOS patients is often found on the side of the face, upper lip, and chin. There may be a male pattern escutcheon and in severe cases, temporal balding and hair on the chest.

PCOS patients generally have enlarged ovaries with increased central stroma and an abundance of peripheral cystic follicles (see Figure 9.6.1). It is unclear whether there are simply a baseline elevated number of follicles or if the rate of their programmed cell death is retarded.[1] The hyperplastic ovarian stroma occupies approximately 25% of the medullary portion of the ovary.

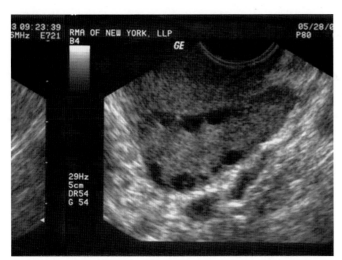

Figure 9.6.1. Typical appearance of an ovary in a woman with polycystic ovarian syndrome.

Ultrasound criteria have been defined and include 12 or more follicles 2 to 9 mm in diameter in each ovary and/or increased ovarian volume ($\geq$10 ml).[5]

Insulin resistance and a predisposition for type 2 diabetes are also part of the clinical syndrome. This may correlate with the approximately 50% of PCOS patients who are obese with the classic android pattern of increased waist-to-hip ratio and a higher proportion of visceral fat. Although clinically most PCOS patients do fall into a classic mold, there are always nonobese, fertile outliers who may have lesser manifestations of the disease process.

TREATMENT

Treatment of polycystic ovaries should be targeted toward the patient's primary complaint, be it infertility, clinical signs of hyperandrogenism, or prolonged amenorrhea. In a large percentage of cases, treatment is ultimately focused on balancing the elevated circulating androgens and restoring the normal endocrine axis either via weight reduction or pharmacologic assistance.

In the patient not desiring fertility, oral contraceptive agents assist in decreasing ovarian steroidogenesis and increasing SHBG. Clinically, oral contraceptive pills may diminish hirsutism and protect the endometrium by inducing regular shedding.

Oral antihyperglycemics such as metformin have also proven to be useful. Although there are conflicting data, most studies have shown associated decreased androgen levels, improvement in response to clomiphene citrate, and restoration of ovulation. One recent randomized, double-blinded placebo trial, however, failed to show effects of metformin on weight loss or menstrual frequency in obese PCOS patients and suggested that weight loss alone for that subset was the only successful factor.[6] Further efforts are being made to identify prognostic indicators to determine which modality is most likely to succeed in an individual patient.

The majority of women (70%) with PCOS who exhibit infertility as a result of chronic anovulation will respond to clomiphene citrate. Approximately 50% of these women will eventually then go on to conceive.[7] Gonadotropin therapy has traditionally been the next step in therapy for those who fail clomiphene; however, the ability to achieve monofollicular ovulation is challenging and there is considerable risk for ovarian hyperstimulation syndrome. In fact, recent data reported from our center comparing controlled ovarian hyperstimulation with IVF for patients with PCOS showed three times the pregnancy rate and less than one third the higher-order multiple gestation rate with IVF.[8] We concluded that though traditionally considered a more "aggressive" treatment of infertility, in patients with PCOS, IVF might actually be expensive and invasive but more "conservative."

Because of that increased risk, there have been some advocates for mechanical destruction of excess ovarian tissue. Decreasing functional ovarian mass may diminish intraovarian androgen production and possibly encourage increased FSH levels. This theory dates back to Stein and Leventhal's original work involving wedge resection of the ovary (though surgical management of this disease began to fall out of favor in the early 1980s). The technique, however, had been shown to be effective in as many as 90% of reported cases.[9] Unfortunately, although improving the hormonal milieu and often restoring ovulatory function, the technique often caused severe pelvic adhesions and subsequently resulted in mechanical infertility due to tubal disease.

Over the past two decades, laparotomy has largely been abandoned in these patients, and laparoscopy has taken its place. In fact, laparoscopic-assisted ovarian diathermy (most often via monopolar electrocautery) has been reported in more than 1000 patients, with variable success rates. Though too few to establish a consensus on the technique, the randomized trials that do exist comparing laparoscopic diathermy and gonadotropin therapy show similar rates of conception.[7] Laparoscopic ovarian drilling also offers the benefit of altering the hormonal composite of PCOS patients after surgery. There is often a reported decrease in serum LH, androgen concentration, and DHEA levels. This reduction in the intraovarian androgen levels allows for the development of functional follicles.[10] Inhibin levels also fall more permanently, but the overall improvement in hormonal status does not seem to affect the peripheral sensitivity to insulin. Although electrocautery is the most well studied, laser drilling and multiple biopsy technique have also been employed. In the electrocautery technique, the ovary is first isolated with laparoscopic grasping forceps. An insulated 8-mm monopolar needle is introduced at a 90° angle to the ovarian cortex and a series of puncture sites are created. A cutting current of 100 W is used to initially enter the cortex and is followed by 2 seconds of coagulation current at 40 W. The whole length of the needle may be placed into the ovary. Based on ovarian site, anywhere from 10 to 15 puncture sites may be made to adequately destroy ovarian tissue. The surface of the ovary is then irrigated with crystalloid before removing the trocars. Of note, the use of the laser has diminished secondary to anecdotal increases in adhesion formation and increased surface damage to the ovarian cortex.

Although laparoscopic ovarian drilling is efficacious and carries with it the benefit of multiple ovulatory cycles, relatively short operative time, a decrease in spontaneous abortions, and a lowered risk of multiple gestations, there may be disadvantages as well. A recent article suggested that bilateral ovarian drilling may result in diminished ovarian reserve. The authors suggested that unilateral drilling might have comparable results, without deleterious long-term effects.[11] Even with laparoscopy, however, significant postoperative tubo-ovarian adhesions, and thus compromised fertility, may result. With these potential iatrogenic effects on the patient, selection for this technique should be carefully assessed before proceeding.

Perhaps Stein and Leventhal's initial paper was our best clue for a cure. Wedge resection via laparotomy restored fertility in their case studies, corroborating their theory of mechanical crowding of the diseased ovary with follicles lacking the signal for programmed cell death. The true pathogenesis of PCOS, however, remains elusive. Whether a selection or combination of oral antihyperglycemics, selective estrogen receptor modulators, aromatase inhibitors, oral contraceptives, dietary modification, and/or mechanical ablation of excess ovarian tissue is the best treatment is still uncertain and must be individualized. What is clear is that a multisystem approach to this complex disease state must be employed for cardioprotection, optimal fertility, and long-term diminished risk for neoplastic processes.

REFERENCES

1. Chang RJ. Chapter 19. Polycystic ovarian syndrome and hyperandrogenic states. In: Strauss J, Barbieri R, eds. *Yen and Jaffe's Reproductive Endocrinology*. 5th ed. Philadelphia: Saunders; 2004:597–632.

2. Stein IF, Leventhal ML. Amenorrhea associated with bilateral polycystic ovaries. *Am J Obstet Gynecol*. 1935;29:181–191.

3. The Rotterdam ESHRE/ASRM-Sponsored PCOS Consensus Workshop Group. Revised 2003 consensus on diagnostic criteria and long-term health risks related to polycystic ovarian syndrome. *Hum Reprod*. 2004;19:41–47.

4. Ehrmann D. Polycystic ovarian syndrome. *N Engl J Med*. 2005;352:1223–1236.

5. Balen AH, Laven JS, Tan SL, Dewailly D. Ultrasound assessment of the polycystic ovary: international consensus definitions. *Hum Reprod Update*. 2003;9:505–514.

6. Tang T, Glanville J, Hayden CJ, White D, Barth JH, Balen AH. Combined lifestyle modification and metformin in obese patients with PCOS. A randomized, placebo-controlled, double-blind multicentre study. *Hum Reprod*. 2006;21:80–89.

7. Farquhar CM, Williamson K, Gudex G, Johnson NP, Garland J, Sadler L. A randomized controlled trial of laparoscopic ovarian diathermy versus gonadotropin therapy for women with clomiphene citrate-resistant polycystic ovarian syndrome. *Fertil Steril*. 2002;78:404–411.

8. Grunfeld L, Mukherjee T, Sandler B, Scott RT, Copperman AB. IVF, with a maximum of two embryo replacement is the treatment of choice for high responding patients. *Fertil Steril*, 80:101.

9. Adashi EY, Rock JA, Guzick D, Wentz AC, Jones GS, Jones HW Jr. Fertility following bilateral ovarian wedge resection. *Fertil Steril*. 1981;36:320–325.

10. Felemban A, Tan SL, Tulandi T. Laparoscopic treatment of polycystic ovaries with insulated needle cautery: a reappraisal. *Fertil Steril*. 2000;73:266–269.

11. Kandil M, Selim M. Hormonal and sonographic assessment of ovarian reserve before and after laparoscopic ovarian drilling in PCOS. *BJOG Int J Obstet Gynecol*. 2005;112:1427–1430.

Section 9.7. Ovarian Remnant

Ceana Nezhat

Ovarian remnants occur when ovarian tissue is inadvertently left in the pelvic cavity after oophorectomy. The remaining piece of functional ovarian tissue can respond to hormonal stimulation with growth, cystic degeneration, or hemorrhage and produce pain.[1–3] In the rat model, Minke and colleagues [4] showed that devascularized ovarian tissue can reimplant on intact or denuded peritoneal surfaces and the revascularized tissue can become functional as evidenced by follicle formation and vaginal cornification.

RISK FACTORS

Predisposing factors include increased vascularity causing difficult hemostasis, endometriosis, pelvic inflammatory disease, pelvic adhesions, and altered anatomy.[5,6] Because of preexisting conditions and prior surgeries, ovarian remnants are usually encased in adhesions (Figure 9.7.1) and are more likely to occur during oophorectomy when the ovary is densely adherent to adjacent structures. It is not unusual for these patients to have had previous attempts to excise the tissue.

DIAGNOSIS

Diagnosis is based on history and localization of pelvic pain. Symptoms of ovarian remnant usually occur within 5 years of oophorectomy.[5,7] The most frequent symptom is pelvic pain, which can present variably. Patient descriptions of pain may vary from cyclic to chronic pain, dull and aching to sharp and stabbing.[5] Patients may also experience low back pain, variable bowel symptoms, dyspareunia, pelvic mass, or ureteral compression.[7] Some patients have cystic adnexal structures or ill-defined fixed masses, whereas others have normal pelvic findings. Imaging studies, including vaginal ultrasound, CT, and MRI, are useful but not always indicative of ovarian remnant.[8] Preoperative follicle-stimulating hormone (FSH) levels can contribute to the diagnosis when found in the premenopausal range ($\leq$40) in patients who have undergone bilateral oophorectomy. However, the remaining ovarian tissue can produce estradiol levels incapable of suppressing gonadotropin; therefore, an FSH level of 40 mIU/mL or greater does not exclude the diagnosis.[1,9] In cases of unilateral oophorectomy, FSH levels are of no value. Hormonal suppression with oral contraceptives or GnRH agonist provides no relief in most patients.[2,10] Ovarian stimulation may be used to increase ovarian remnant size to confirm the diagnosis preoperatively or to aid in locating the tissue intraoperatively.[11] Laparoscopic ultrasonography may be helpful in detecting ovarian remnants in patients in whom the pelvic anatomy is distorted by multiple adhesions.[12]

TREATMENT

Surgical excision of the ovarian remnant is the best choice in the majority of cases. Past reviews considered laparoscopy ineffective in the management of ovarian remnant because of the presence of dense adhesions.[1,5,13,14] Since the publication of those reviews, there has been tremendous advancement in the field of operative laparoscopy, including improved instrumentation and training. Laparoscopy may offer additional benefits over laparotomy for treating ovarian remnants. The magnification provided by the laparoscope facilitates identification of the remnant tissue. Also, increased intra-abdominal pressure helps reduce blood loss, and the distention causes the retroperitoneal space to unfold, thus allowing for better visualization.[15] Laparoscopy is also less traumatic, which is a great benefit to these patients, who are likely to have undergone multiple prior surgeries.[10] A recent series showed that the number of recurrences of ovarian remnant and the number of conversions to laparotomy, along with postoperative complications, decreased as the surgeon's experience and technical advancements increased.[8]

It is imperative that the patient undergo thorough 1- or 2-day bowel prep (both mechanical and antibiotic). Before signing the consent form, the patient should be thoroughly counseled regarding the possibility of proctosigmoidoscopy, cystoscopy, or resection of portions of the bowel, bladder, or ureters, as well as the possibility of conversion to laparotomy, if indicated. With ovarian remnant, the patient must understand that the goal is complete resection of the ovarian tissue to prevent recurrence.

Anterior abdominal wall adhesions are probable after multiple prior surgeries, and an open laparoscopy, left upper quadrant entry, or mapping technique is advisable.[16] After all instruments are inserted, intra-abdominal adhesions are lysed and normal anatomy is restored as much as possible. The remnant tissue is identified and dissected. Extensive and careful retroperitoneal dissection is required to facilitate identification and removal of the ovarian remnant tissue.[6,15]

The anatomy of the retroperitoneal space is identified when the ovarian remnant is adherent to the lateral pelvic wall (Figure 9.7.2). The space beneath the peritoneum is injected with lactated Ringer's solution, and the peritoneum is opened to the infundibulopelvic ligament or its remnant. Adjustable pressure pumps for hydrodissection can be used to establish various pressures to assist in injecting physiologic solutions, such as lactated Ringer's, retroperitoneally to create a plane of dissection. Even in

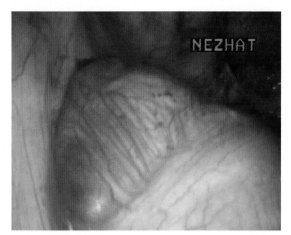

Figure 9.7.1. Ovarian remnant encased in adhesions.

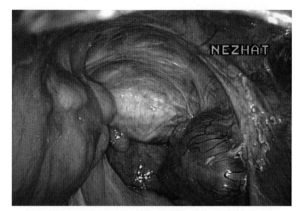

Figure 9.7.2. Ovarian remnant on the lateral pelvic side wall.

cases with retroperitoneal fibrosis, the combination of hydrodissection and sharp dissection with CO_2 laser is beneficial.[8] Adhesions are lysed until the course of the major pelvic blood vessels and the ureter can be traced and, if necessary, dissected. The ovarian blood supply is coagulated with bipolar forceps, and the ovarian tissue is excised and submitted for histologic examination. When the ovarian remnant is adhered to the vaginal cuff and bladder area (Figure 9.7.3A,B), deep dissection and extensive ureterolysis are not necessary; however, identification of the anatomy and a plane of dissection is essential.

When the remnant is adherent to the bowel (Figures 9.7.4, 9.7.5), adhesions are lysed using hydrodissection and the CO_2 laser or sharp dissection with harmonic devices or similar modalities. Ovarian tissue embedded in the superficial muscularis of the bowel is removed using a shaving technique. When the remnant is deeply embedded in the bowel or bladder muscularis or when the ureter is involved or possibly obstructed, partial resection of the invaded structure and repair are necessary. The serosa and muscularis layers are reinforced with one to three interrupted 4–0 polydioxanone or 0 polyglactin 910 sutures in one layer. Sigmoidoscopy and examination under water are used to confirm that the repair is airtight. Bipolar forceps or new sealing devices are used to desiccate the ovarian blood supply and the ovarian remnant, and the contiguous peritoneum and surrounding tissue are meticulously excised and submitted for histologic examination.

A variety of findings, including follicular cysts, endometriosis, corpus luteum, and ovarian cancer, have been revealed during histologic examination of ovarian remnant tissue. In fact, there are five documented cases of ovarian cancer developing in an ovarian remnant after total abdominal hysterectomy and bilateral salpingo-oophorectomy.[17]

The incidence of injury to the bladder, ureter, and bowel at laparotomy for ovarian remnant is estimated to be 3% to 33%, with injuries to the ureter significantly greater by laparotomy than by laparoscopy.[15] A recent study of ovarian remnant managed by laparoscopy reported the rate of intraoperative complications at 5.8%, with four intraoperative complications in 69 laparoscopies. However, there were no ureteral injuries.[8] This series and others have demonstrated that the rate of complications with laparoscopic treatment of ovarian remnant is comparable or lower when compared with those reported in laparotomy.[15,18]

The following are key steps to safe, complete resection of ovarian remnant. First, in those patients who have undergone prior bilateral salpingo-oophorectomy, the anatomy should be restored as completely as possible with bilateral side wall and cul-de-sac dissection. Any other pelvic pathology, such as endometriosis, should be treated. Second, the ureter should be identified and dissected completely, to the pelvic brim, if necessary. The utility of ureteral stents is controversial given reports in the literature of ureteral injury due to its rigidity.[1] Third, complete excision of the ovarian remnant, including a wide margin of healthy

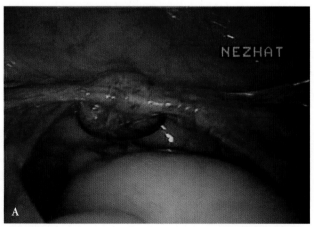

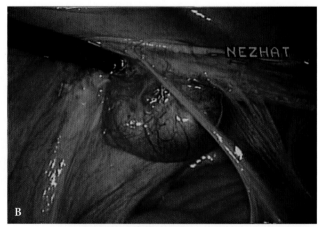

Figure 9.7.3. Ovarian remnant adherent to the vaginal cuff (**A**) and bladder (**B**).

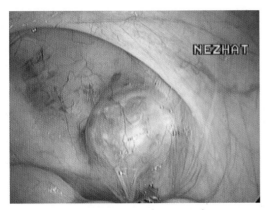

Figure 9.7.4. Retroperitoneal mass on the rectum.

tissue, must be executed. Resection of the adherent structures, such as portions of bowel or bladder, may be necessary to completely resect the tissue; however, this is necessary to prevent subsequent surgery due to recurrence. Fourth, the ovary should be removed in one piece, placed in a surgical specimen bag, and extracted from the abdominal cavity through an enlarged trocar site, posterior colpotomy, or large canula. However, in patients with severe endometriosis and para-ovarian adhesions, the ovary may be fragmented and removed in pieces, and great care must be taken to assure complete removal. The ability of devascularized ovarian tissue to reimplant on peritoneal surfaces has been shown in animal studies as well as the gynecologic population.[4,19] Wood et al. [20] described one case that required reoperation after laparoscopic adnexectomy to remove a small portion of ovary that had been left in the abdomen and apparently implanted on the bladder. Fragments of ovarian tissue left in the abdomen may implant and become hormonally active. Lastly, a complete and thorough examination of the abdominopelvic cavity should be performed before completing the procedure to identify any other possible sites of ovarian remnant.

PREVENTION

Attention should be focused on prevention. Factors associated with ovarian remnant are the use of Endoloops (Ethicon) for

laparoscopic oophorectomy, multiple operative procedures with incomplete removal of pelvic organs, densely adherent ovaries, and multiple ovarian cystectomies for functional cysts.[14] When pre-tied sutures or stapling devices are used for the infundibulopelvic ligament, they should be placed well below the ovarian tissue. As described by Semm [21], the infundibulopelvic ligament must be freely mobile if an Endoloop is used to ligate the ovarian blood vessels. Otherwise, the most proximal suture ligature may trap ovarian tissue on excision from this pedicle. Electrocoagulation and transection of the infundibulopelvic ligament or the application of clips is preferred. When the ovary is adherent to the pelvic side wall, retroperitoneal hydrodissection, meticulous adhesiolysis, and removal of the contiguous peritoneum underlying the ovary are essential for the prevention of this complication. The need for restraint in managing functional cysts is underscored by the fact that some patients in one series had only a corpus luteum resected at first laparotomy.[14]

CONCLUSION

In conclusion, despite the relative advantages of magnification and visual access to the deep recesses of the pelvis, laparoscopic removal of the ovary does not necessarily ensure its complete removal. Because of the complexity of the surgical management of ovarian remnant resulting in persistent pelvic pain and increasing risk of occurrence, it is advisable to decrease the chances of ovarian remnant using proper surgical techniques. In certain cases, ovarian remnant may not be preventable. When the ovary is densely adherent to adjacent visceral surfaces, the ability to differentiate ovarian tissue from surrounding structures based on color and consistency may be lost. In this case, the patient should be monitored for the development of symptomatic ovarian remnant.

REFERENCES

1. Pettit PD, Lee RA. Ovarian remnant syndrome: diagnostic dilemma and surgical challenge. *Obstet Gynecol.* 1988;71(4):580–583.
2. Siddall-Allum J, Rae T, Rogers V, et al. Chronic pelvic pain caused by residual ovaries and ovarian remnants. *Br J Obstet Gynaecol.* 1994;101:979.
3. Orford V, Kuhn R. Management of ovarian remnant syndrome. *Aust N Z J Obstet Gynaecol.* 1996;36(4):468–471.
4. Minke T, DePond W, Winkelmann T, Blythe J. Ovarian remnant syndrome: study in laboratory rats. *Am J Obstet Gynecol.* 1994;171:1440.
5. Symmonds RE, Pettit P. Ovarian remnant syndrome. *Obstet Gynecol.* 1979;54(2):174–177.
6. Lafferty HW, Angioli R, Rudolph J, Penalver MA. Ovarian remnant syndrome: experience at Jackson Memorial Hospital, University of Miami, 1985 through 1993. *Am J Obstet Gynecol.* 1996;174(2):641–645.
7. Johns DA, Diamond MP. Adequacy of laparoscopic oophorectomy. *J Am Assoc Gynecol Laparosc.* 1993;1(1):20–23.
8. Nezhat CH, Kearney S, Malik S, Nezhat C, Nezhat F. Laparoscopic management of ovarian remnant. *Fertil Steril.* 2005;83(4):973–978.
9. Scott RT, Beatse SN, Illions EH, Snyder RR. Use of GnRH agonist stimulation test in the diagnosis of ovarian remnant syndrome: a report of three cases. *J Reprod Med.* 1995;40(2):143–146.

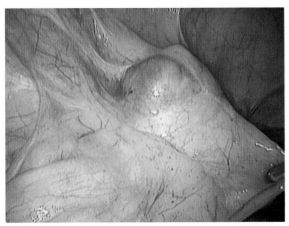

Figure 9.7.5. Ovarian remnant embedded in the sigmoid wall.

10. Nezhat F, Nezhat C. Operative laparoscopy for the treatment of ovarian remnant syndrome. *Fertil Steril.* 1992;57(5):1003–1007.

11. Kaminski PF, Sorosky JI, Mandell MJ, Broadstreet RP, Zaino RJ. Clomiphene citrate stimulation as an adjunct in locating ovarian tissue in ovarian remnant syndrome. *Obstet Gynecol.* 1990;76:924–926.

12. Nezhat F, Nezhat C, Nezhat CH, et al. Use of laparoscopic ultrasonography to detect ovarian remnants. *Am J Obstet Gynecol.* 1996;174:641.

13. Price FV, Edwards R, Buchsbaum HJ. Ovarian remnant syndrome: difficulties in diagnosis and management. *Obstet Gynecol Surv.* 1990;45:151.

14. Webb MJ. Ovarian remnant syndrome. *Aust N Z J Obstet Gynaecol.* 1989;29(4):433–435.

15. Kamprath S, Possover M, Schneider A. Description of a laparoscopic technique for treating patients with ovarian remnant syndrome. *Fertil Steril.* 1997;68(4):663–667.

16. Nezhat C, Nezhat F, Silfen SL. Videolaseroscopy: the CO_2 laser for advanced operative laparoscopy. *Obstet Gynecol Clin North Am.* 1991;18:3:585.

17. Narayansingh G, Cumming G, Parkin D, Miller I. Ovarian cancer developing in the ovarian remnant syndrome. A case report and literature review. *Aust N Z J Obstet Gynaecol.* 2000;40(2):221–223.

18. Abu-Rafeh B, Vilos GA, Misra M. Frequency and laparoscopic management of ovarian remnant syndrome. *J Am Assoc Gynecol Laparosc.* 2003;10(1):33–37.

19. Shemwell RE, Weed JC. Ovarian remnant syndrome. *Obstet Gynecol.* 1970;36:299–303.

20. Wood C, Hill D, Maher P, Lolatgis N. Laparoscopic adnexectomy: indications, technique and results. *Aust N Z J Obstet Gynaecol.* 1992;2:362–366.

21. Semm K. Tissue-puncher and loop-ligation – new aids for surgical therapeutic pelviscopy (laparoscopy) – endoscopic intra-abdominal surgery. *Endoscopy.* 1978;10:119–124.

10 | ENDOMETRIOSIS

Section 10.1. The Pathogenesis of Endometriosis

Richard O. Burney and Linda C. Giudice

Endometriosis is classically defined as the presence of endometrial glands and stroma in ectopic locations. Affecting from 6% to 10% of reproductive-aged women, endometriosis may result in dysmenorrhea, dyspareunia, chronic pelvic pain, and/or subfertility.[1] The prevalence of this condition in women experiencing pain, infertility, or both is as high as 50%. Endometriosis is a debilitating condition, posing quality-of-life issues for the individual patient. The disorder represents a major cause of gynecologic hospitalization in the United States, estimated to have exceeded $3 billion in inpatient health care costs in 2004 alone.[2,3] The significant individual and public health concerns associated with endometriosis underscore the importance of understanding its pathogenesis. The first recorded description of pathology consistent with endometriosis was provided by Shroen in 1690.[4,5] Despite the passage of time and extensive investigation, the exact pathogenesis of this enigmatic disorder remains unknown.

THEORIES REGARDING PATHOGENESIS

Numerous theories detailing the development of endometriosis have been described. For purposes of review, these theories can generally be classified into those that propose that implants arise from tissues other than the endometrium and those that propose that implants arise from uterine endometrium (Table 10.1.1).

Nonendometrial Origin

Metaplasia of coelomic epithelium represents a distinct pathogenic mechanism for the establishment of endometriotic implants. According to this theory, normal peritoneal tissue transforms via metaplastic transition to ectopic endometrial tissue.[6] The closely related induction theory holds that an endogenous inductive stimulus, such as a hormonal or immunologic factor, promotes the differentiation of undifferentiated cells in the peritoneal lining into endometrial cells.[7,8] The presence of incompletely differentiated cells in the lining of the peritoneal cavity that are capable of such transformation is implied by this theory, and is possibly supported by the finding of totipotent mesothelial serosal cells in the coelomic lining.[13] When ovarian surface epithelium is co-cultured with endometrial stromal cells in a collagen lattice and exposed to supraphysiologic levels of 17β-estradiol, endometriosis appears to arise via a metaplastic transformation of the mesothelium.[14] Finally, the theory of embryonic mullerian rests postulates that cells residual from embryologic mullerian duct migration maintain the capacity to develop into endometriotic lesions under the influence of estrogen.[9,10]

Support for these theories is found in clinical reports of histologically confirmed endometriotic tissue developing in patients without menstrual endometrium. Endometriosis has been documented in a patient with Rokitansky–Küster–Hauser syndrome, notable insofar as the patient did not have functioning endometrium.[15] Perhaps the most compelling evidence for a nonendometrial etiology comes from cases of men with prostate cancer undergoing high-dose estrogen treatment who were subsequently diagnosed with endometriosis.[16,17]

Endometrial Origin

Benign Metastasis

Originally proposed in the 1920s, the theory of benign metastasis holds that ectopic endometrial implants are the result of lymphatic or hematogenous dissemination of endometrial cells.[11,12,18] Evidence for this mechanism is substantial. Microvascular studies demonstrate the presence of lymph flow into the ovary from the uterine body, suggesting a possible role for the lymphatic system in the etiology of ovarian endometriosis.[19] In one study involving histologic examination of surgical specimens from 276 patients, the incidence of ovarian endometriosis and adenomyosis combination was 56%.[19] Endometriosis within lymph nodes has been documented in 6.5% of women at lymphadenectomy and 6.7% of women at autopsy.[20] The strongest evidence for the theory of benign metastasis is derived from reports of histologically proven endometriotic lesions occurring in sites distant from the uterus or pelvis, including bone, brain, and lung.[21]

Retrograde Menstruation

Initially proposed by Sampson [22,23] in the 1920s, the theory of retrograde menstruation is both intuitively attractive and supported by multiple lines of scientific evidence. According to this theory, eutopic endometrium is sloughed via patent fallopian tubes into the peritoneal cavity during menstruation. Indeed, the universality of this phenomenon is supported by the finding of menstrual blood in the peritoneal fluid of up to 90% of healthy women with patent fallopian tubes undergoing laparoscopy during the perimenstrual period of the cycle.[24] The incidence of bloody peritoneal fluid was only 15% in patients with bilaterally occluded tubes. Further support for this etiology is derived from studies of obstructed or compromised outflow tracts. In adolescent girls with congenital outflow obstruction, the prevalence of endometriosis is high.[25] Likewise, iatrogenic obstruction of the outflow tract in baboons resulted in endometriotic

Table 10.1.1: Classification of Theories Regarding the Pathogenesis of Endometriosis

Theory	Proponent(s)
Nonendometrial origin	
Coelomic metaplasia	Iwanoff, 1898 [6]
Induction	Levander and Normann, 1955 [7]; Merrill, 1966 [8]
Embryonic mullerian rests	Russell, 1899 [9]; Batt and Smith, 1989 [10]
Endometrial origin	
Benign metastasis	Halban, 1924 [11]
Retrograde menstruation/ implantation	Sampson, 1927 [12]

lesions within the peritoneal cavity in these animals.[26] Even subtle compromise of antegrade menstruation may predispose to formation of endometriosis, as evidenced by a recent study demonstrating a higher prevalence of endometriosis in women with a uterine septum.[27] The viability of the retrogradely menstruated endometrial cells is of paramount importance for the plausibility of the retrograde transplantation theory. This has been most elegantly addressed by the experiments of Ridley and Edwards [28], who injected menstrual effluent into the subcutaneous adipose layer of women scheduled to undergo laparotomy. At surgery, the site of injection was excised and histologic review demonstrated viable endometrial glands and stroma up to 180 days post injection.

The anatomic distribution of endometriotic lesions also favors the retrograde menstruation theory. Superficial implants are more often located in the posterior compartment of the pelvis [29] and in the left hemipelvis.[30] Primary and recurrent ovarian endometriomas are significantly more often located on the left ovary [31,32], in contrast to the distribution of nonendometriotic benign ovarian cysts, which do not display a predilection for sidedness.[33] Deeply infiltrating endometriosis also exhibits a double asymmetry, with lesions demonstrating a predilection for the posterior compartment and the left side of the pelvis in a large observational series.[34] The propensity for lesions to implant in the posterior cul-de-sac is explained by the accumulation of regurgitated menstrual effluent in this most dependent portion of the peritoneal cavity under the influence of gravity. The presence of a retroverted uterus, by allowing flow from the anterior to posterior compartment in the upright or supine position, is correlated with the finding of posterior deeply infiltrating lesions.[35] The propensity for the left hemipelvis to be affected by superficial, ovarian, and deeply infiltrating endometriosis is thought to be a function of the close anatomic relationship between the sigmoid colon and the left adnexa. By acting as an obstacle to the diffusion of menstrual effluent from the left fallopian tube, the sigmoid colon promotes stasis of this effluent, thereby extending the interval for regurgitated endometrial cells to implant to the left pelvic sidewall, the left uterosacral region, and the left ovary.

A murine model of endometriosis has provided new insight into the pathogenesis of peritoneal endometriosis.[36] The conditional activation of the *K-ras* oncogene in endometrial cells deposited into the peritoneum resulted in histologically confirmed peritoneal endometriotic implants in nearly 50% of mice within 8 months. On the other hand, similar activation of the *K-ras* oncogene in peritoneal cells showed no progression to endometriosis. These results in a mouse model would seem to support the theory of retrograde menstruation in the development of peritoneal endometriosis.

It follows that situations that decrease the available endometrium or that occlude the tubal conduit for retrograde deposition should evidence a reduced propensity for the establishment of endometriosis. Indeed, the rate of endometriosis recurrence is significantly reduced when endometrial ablation is coupled with the treatment of endometriosis.[37] In women with endometriosis who have undergone tubal sterilization, retrograde menstruation into the proximal tubal segment has been demonstrated to result in histopathologic implantation, which may result in tuboperitoneal fistulization [38] or severe dysmenorrhea.[39] The issue of whether tubal interruption can completely protect against the development of endometriosis is unknown.

Though retrograde menstruation explains the physical displacement of endometrial fragments into the peritoneal cavity, additional steps are necessary for the development of implants. Attachment of endometrial fragments to the epithelium of the peritoneum, invasion of the epithelium, establishment of a vascular supply, and circumvention of the immune response are necessary if endometriosis is to develop from retrograde passage of sloughed endometrium. It is the propensity for implantation that best accounts for the disparity between the 90% prevalence of retrograde menstruation and the nearly 10% prevalence of the disease. Hereditary or acquired properties of the endometrium, hereditary or acquired defects of the peritoneal epithelium, and/or defective immune clearance of sloughed endometrium are areas of active investigation in the search for the factor or factors that influence predisposition toward implantation of the displaced endometrial cells – a necessary correlate to theories proposing an endometrial origin to disease pathogenesis.

EVIDENCE FOR AN ENDOMETRIAL FACTOR IN THE PREDISPOSITION TO DISEASE

The evidence for an innate or acquired condition of the endometrial cells as the predisposing factor toward implantation is compelling. Endometrial stromal cells (ESCs) are the critical cells involved in implantation to the mesothelium. A recent study using ESCs and peritoneal mesothelial cells (PMCs) from a variety of sources in an in vitro binding assay demonstrated that the source of the ESCs rather than the source of the PMCs had the greatest impact on the rate of implantation.[40]

A genetic alteration of the endometrial cells influencing their tendency to implant may be hereditary, as a heritable component to the disease has been established. The risk for first-degree relatives of women with severe endometriosis is six times higher than for relatives of unaffected women.[41] Studies of monozygotic twins demonstrate high concordance rates for histologically confirmed endometriosis.[42,43] Familial aggregation implicating a genetic factor is further evidenced by population studies [44] and by a nonhuman primate model.[45] Linkage analysis has elucidated candidate genes with biologic plausibility. The largest

Table 10.1.2: Candidate Genes Implicated in the Pathogenesis of Endometriosis

Gene	Function	Reference(s)
MMP-3, -7	Matrix metalloproteinases	Bruner-Tran et al., 2002 [47]
KRAS	Oncogene	Dinulescu et al., 2005 [36]
PTEN	Tumor suppressor gene	Dinulescu et al., 2005 [36]
CYP19	Aromatase enzyme	Noble et al., 1996 [48]
17βHSD-2	Hydroxysteroid dehydrogenase	Zeitoun et al., 1998 [49]
BCL-2	Antiapoptosis	Jones et al., 1998 [50]

of these involved more than 1100 families with two or more affected sib-pairs, and established significance for a susceptibility locus in the region of chromosome 10q26.[46] Though a review of all the candidate genes and their possible associations with endometriosis is beyond the scope of this section, a partial list is provided in Table 10.1.2.

Microarray technology and other genomic approaches to evaluate global gene expression have provided novel insight into the pathogenesis of the condition.[51] This line of investigation holds great diagnostic promise, for if a fundamental difference in the endometrium is confirmed, then endometrial sampling may afford a nonsurgical approach to the diagnosis of the condition.

Alterations in hormonal responsiveness may influence the ability of endometrial cells to proliferate, attach to the mesothelium, and/or evade immune-mediated clearance. Though long appreciated clinically, the concept of endometriosis as an estrogen-dependent disorder is well supported by molecular evidence.[52] A striking finding in endometriotic (ectopic endometrial) tissue relative to eutopic endometrium is the increased expression of aromatase enzyme and decreased expression of 17β-hydroxysteroid dehydrogenase (17β-HSD) type 2.[48,49] The sum consequence of this differential expression profile is a marked increase in the locally bioavailable estradiol concentration. These findings provide molecular support to the clinically based description of endometriosis as an estrogen-dependent disease, and substantiate treatments aimed at promoting a hypoestrogenic peritoneal microenvironment. In addition to estrogen dependence, there is evidence to support the characterization of endometriosis as a progesterone-resistant condition.[53] Immunohistochemical studies demonstrate an overall reduction of progesterone receptors in endometriotic lesions relative to eutopic endometrium, and an absence of progesterone receptor-B (PR-B) in endometriotic lesions.[54] Additionally, endometrial expression profiling has documented dysregulation of progesterone-responsive genes in the luteal phase.[51,55]

Acquired aberrations of the endometrium have also been postulated to result in predisposition toward implantation of refluxed endometrial cells. The acquired aberration may be a random genetic event or consequent to an environmental exposure. Dioxin has received considerable attention as an environmental factor associated with endometriosis. Rhesus monkeys exposed to

daily dioxin (5 to 25 ppm) for 4 years developed endometriosis of dose-dependent severity.[56] Dioxin, also known as 2,3,7,8-tetrachlorodibenzo-p-dioxin (TCDD), is a ubiquitous environmental by-product of combustion.[57] Dietary or occupational exposure to this lipophilic compound may result in adipose accumulation. When bound to the aryl hydrocarbon receptor, the resulting complex may act as a transcription factor. Dioxin has been documented to exert carcinogenic and immunosuppressive effects in animal studies.[58] Though biologically plausible, a direct causal link between dioxin exposure and the development of endometriosis remains equivocal.[59] Interestingly, TCDD has been demonstrated to selectively down-regulate stromal PR-B expression and increase matrix metalloproteinase (MMP) expression in cultured endometrial cells, providing a potential mechanism for both predisposition to implantation and the observed progesterone resistance associated with this disorder.[60]

Finally, acquired genomic alterations represent a potential source for a conferred survival advantage to sloughed endometrial cells in the establishment of endometriotic implants. Such alterations may be consequent to environmental exposures or spontaneously occurring genetic events. Despite impressive power to detect linkage to loci with low effect sizes, only one region at 10q26 achieved modest significance ($P = 0.47$) in the recent genome-wide linkage study.[46] Importantly, the investigators used peripheral blood leukocytes as the source for the DNA in this disease association study. The absence of more associations in this study may be interpreted as evidence that the genetic predisposition to endometriosis owes more to genomic alterations in the uterine microenvironment than to heritable mutation. The endometrium is a setting of extraordinary cell turnover; consequently, it is vulnerable to errors of genetic recombination. The occurrence of genomic alteration in eutopic endometrium is well documented and may be consequent to epigenetic factors or oxidative stress.[61] If these genomic alterations result in loss or gain of function that results in a conferred survival advantage, then implantation of the cell(s) is favored. For example, a genomic alteration that results in the loss of a tumor suppressor gene may predispose the cell to proliferate, attach, or resist apoptosis. Loss of heterozygosity and somatic mutation of the tumor suppressor gene PTEN has been documented in 56% and 21% of solitary endometrial cysts of the ovary, respectively.[62] Genomic alterations within endometriotic implants have been described using the comparative genomic hybridization (CGH) microarrays.[63] Interestingly, the CGH profiles (chromosome loss or gain) clustered by anatomic location of the implant as peritoneal or ovarian. Though difficult to capture, genomic alterations common to both ectopic and eutopic endometrium from a given patient may hold promise in determining the genetic factor(s) that result in implantation of retrogradely sloughed endometrium.

EVIDENCE FOR A PERITONEAL FACTOR IN THE PREDISPOSITION TO DISEASE

A heritable or acquired condition of the peritoneal surface may predispose to the attachment and invasion of endometrial fragments. An intact mesothelium is likely to act as a protective barrier against the implantation of regurgitated endometrial tissue. Indeed, in vitro studies showed that endometrial fragments adhered to the peritoneum only at locations where the

Table 10.1.3: Immune Factors Implicated in the Pathogenesis of Endometriosis

Factor	Reference(s)
Increased activated macrophage fraction	Halme et al., 1984 [24]
Increased IL-8	Ryan et al., 1995 [76]
Increased RANTES	Khorram et al., 1993 [77]
Increased MCP-1	Akoum et al., 1996 [78]
Decreased NK cell activity	Oosterlynck et al., 1991 [68]
Increased TGF-β activity	Oosterlynck et al., 1994 [79]
Increased ICAM-1	Somigliana et al., 1996 [69]
Altered macrophage function–haptoglobin	Sharpe-Timms et al., 2002 [75]
Altered Th1: Th2 cell balance	Hsu et al., 1997 [80]
Increased IL-6 secretion	Tseng et al., 1996 [70]

basement membrane or extracellular matrix was exposed because of mesothelial layer damage.[64] Menstrual effluent has a harmful effect on the mesothelium and may autologously induce the local injury that promotes the implantation of endometrial cells.[65] However, the exact factors involved in mediating mesothelial damage are unknown.

More recently, gene expression profiling of the peritoneum from subjects with and without endometriosis demonstrated up-regulation of MMP-3 during the luteal phase and up-regulation of intracellular adhesion molecule-1 (ICAM-1), transforming growth factor-β (TGF-β), and interleukin-6 (IL-6) during the menstrual phase.[66] The differential expression of these cytokines and growth factors may create a microenvironment that encourages implantation of endometrial cells or protects them from immune-mediated clearance.

EVIDENCE FOR AN IMMUNE FACTOR IN THE PREDISPOSITION TO DISEASE

Normally, refluxed endometrial tissue is cleared from the peritoneum by the immune system, and the dysregulation of this clearance mechanism has been implicated in the predisposition to implantation and growth of endometrial cells (Table 10.1.3). Interestingly, larger tissue fragments as opposed to individual cells demonstrate an increased capacity to implant, presumably because of the protection from immune clearance afforded the cells residing on the inner aspects of such fragments.[67] Additionally, the eutopic endometrium from women with endometriosis was found to be more resistant to lysis by natural killer (NK) cells than was the eutopic endometrium from women without disease.[68] Subsequent studies identified the constitutive shedding of ICAM-1 by ESCs from patients with endometriosis as the potential mechanism by which these cells escape NK cell–mediated clearance.[69] Impaired NK cell function may confer a unique survival advantage to the regurgitated endometrial cells, thereby predisposing to the condition of endometriosis.

Gene expression profiling of menstrual phase endometrium in women with endometriosis demonstrated up-regulation of tumor necrosis factor-α (TNF-α), IL-8, and MMP-3 as compared with the corresponding profile in women without the condition.[66]. As IL-8 and TNF-α promote proliferation and adhesion of endometrial cells and angiogenesis, an overabundance of these cytokines may predispose to the development of endometriotic lesions. Compared with the disease-free controls, the eutopic endometrium of women with endometriosis showed an increased basal production of IL-6.[70] IL-6 plays a prominent role in many chronic inflammatory conditions and is secreted by macrophages as well as epithelial endometrial cells. Interestingly, IL-6 was shown to significantly stimulate aromatase expression in cultured endometriotic and adipocyte stromal cells.[71]

In addition to immunologic differences in the menstrual effluent, numerous studies have documented immune changes in the peritoneal microenvironment. Increasing evidence supports the conceptualization of endometriosis as a pelvic inflammatory condition. In women with endometriosis, the peritoneal fluid is remarkable for an increased number of activated macrophages and important differences in the cytokine/chemokine profile.[72,73] A proteomics approach identified a unique protein structurally similar to haptoglobin in the peritoneal fluid of patients with endometriosis.[74] This protein was subsequently found to bind to macrophages, reduce their phagocytic capacity, and increase their production of IL-6.[75] Other cytokines or chemokines expressed differentially in the peritoneal fluid of patients with endometriosis include IL-1; IL-8; regulated on activation, normal T expressed and secreted (RANTES); and monocyte chemoattractant protein-1 (MCP-1). [76–78] The latter three are chemoattractants that facilitate the recruitment of macrophages. Whether observed cytokine profiles are cause or consequence of endometriosis remains to be definitively determined. The development of nonhuman primate models of endometriosis may allow the delineation of the temporal relationship between lesions and cytokine profiles.

CONFOUNDERS IN ENDOMETRIOSIS RESEARCH

A major limitation to the progress of understanding the etiology of endometriosis is the clinical heterogeneity of the disease. Endometriosis may be asymptomatic, and the presence of endometrial tissue in the pelvis transiently does not appear to be necessarily pathologic.

Equally detrimental to progress in this field is the potential for inconsistency and inaccuracy in the laparoscopic diagnosis of endometriosis. Endometriotic lesions evidence variable characteristics at laparoscopy, rendering their visual diagnosis less certain. A recent study involving women with chronic pelvic pain undergoing laparoscopy determined laparoscopic visualization of lesions to be an inaccurate approach.[81] Of 122 excised peritoneal lesions from 54 patients, only 54% were confirmed to be endometriotic on histologic review. Consequently, 20 of the 54 patients who were surgically staged as having minimal to mild endometriosis at laparoscopy were misdiagnosed. This study highlights the value of histology of the lesion over macroscopic inspection as the gold standard in defining specimens in clinical and molecular studies. Biopsy from each affected area with detailed annotation of pathologic specimens is important in the prevention of false-negative histology for the patient and in the accuracy of reported results for the progress of endometriosis research.

RECONCILING THE DISPARITIES AMONG THEORIES: SUBCLASSIFICATION OF DISEASE

Though distinct in the description of pathogenesis, the theories of coelomic metaplasia, benign metastasis, and retrograde menstruation are not necessarily mutually exclusive. The disparity of the pathogenic theories may be reconciled by consideration of endometriosis as three separate entities: peritoneal, ovarian, and rectovaginal disease.[82] Each of these anatomic distributions of disease could arise by distinct mechanisms. Peritoneal endometriosis, by virtue of superficial and relatively transient localization, is best supported by retrograde menstruation with subsequent implantation. On the other hand, ovarian endometriosis may originate from coelomic metaplasia of included superficial epithelium contained in an estrogen-rich microenvironment, as evidenced by the previously described in vitro co-culture experiments conducted by Matsuura et al.[14] Finally, rectovaginal disease may represent direct extension from subserosal adenomyotic lesions of the lower uterine segment. Supporting this pathogenic mechanism is the observed anatomic coincidence of posterior subserosal adenomyosis with endometriosis.[83] Additionally, rectovaginal lesions are often characterized histologically by the presence of smooth muscle hyperplasia, resembling adenomyotic disease.

Preliminary results of experiments designed to explore the pathogenesis of endometriotic lesions in a mouse model contribute to the growing evidence for distinct etiologies of the peritoneal and ovarian types of endometriosis.[36] Conditional inactivation of the *K-ras* oncogene in the endometrium but not the pelvic peritoneum resulted in peritoneal endometriosis, with both endometrial glands and stroma present in the lesions. In a separate experiment, inactivation of *K-ras* oncogene in the ovarian surface epithelium of a donor mouse followed by transplantation of the ovary to a recipient mouse 5.5 months later showed only ovarian endometrioid lesions in the recipient. This series of experiments would suggest that the ovarian and peritoneal lesions in the mouse model have distinct origins, with the ovarian lesions arising from ovarian surface epithelium and the peritoneal lesions having a uterine or tubal origin.

Increasing molecular evidence supports these histopathologic findings. Both transcriptional and CGH studies of histologically confirmed lesions from patients with endometriosis revealed distinct profiles that correlate with anatomic localization.[63,84] These studies provide genotypic evidence for the classification of endometriosis as three separate phenotypes.

CONCLUSION

Since the original clinical description of endometriosis, much has been accomplished in furthering an understanding of this debilitating and burdensome disease. Several theories have developed to explain the pathogenesis of endometriosis, generally classified by the proposed origin of implants as endometrial or nonendometrial. Though no theory can account for all the described manifestations of endometriosis, the retrograde menstruation theory has gained widespread acceptance as an explanation for the dissemination of endometrial cells. The exact factor or factors that influence the survival and subsequent implantation of these cells remains equivocal. Innate or acquired properties of the endometrium, the peritoneum, and/or the immune system each represent plausible mechanisms to support the establishment of endometriotic implants. The molecular underpinnings for the observed clinical hallmarks of inflammation, estrogen dependence, and progesterone resistance are areas of active research. The heterogeneity of the disease requires adherence to histopathologic confirmation of implants in clinical and molecular research. Novel approaches to the conceptualization of endometriosis may prove necessary to reconcile discrepancies among the proposed theories of disease pathogenesis, although heterogeneity in pathogenesis appears the most likely explanation for disparate etiologies.

REFERENCES

1. Eskenazi B, Warner ML. Epidemiology of endometriosis. *Obstet Gynecol Clin North Am.* 1997;24:235–258.
2. Zhao SZ, Wong JM, Davis MB, Gersh GE, Johnson KE. The cost of inpatient endometriosis treatment: an analysis based on the Healthcare Cost and Utilization Project Nationwide Inpatient Sample. *Am J Manag Care.* 1998;4:1127–1134.
3. Barrier BF, Kendall BS, Ryan CE, Sharpe-Timms KL. HLA-G is expressed by the glandular epithelium of peritoneal endometriosis but not in eutopic endometrium. *Hum Reprod.* 2006;21:864–869.
4. Shroen D. *Disputatio inauguralis medica de ulceribus uteri.* Jena: Krebs; 1690:6–17.
5. Knapp VJ. How old is endometriosis? Late 17th- and 18th-century European descriptions of the disease. *Fertil Steril.* 1999;72:10–14.
6. Iwanoff NS. Dusiges cystenhaltiges uterusfibromyom compliciert durch sarcom und carcinom. (Adenofibromyoma cysticum sarcomatodes carcinomatosum). *Monatsch Geburtshilfe Gynakol.* 1898;7:295–300.
7. Levander G, Normann P. The pathogenesis of endometriosis. An experimental study. *Acta Obstet Gynecol Scand.* 1955;34:366–398.
8. Merrill JA. Endometrial induction of endometriosis across Millipore filters. *Am J Obstet Gynecol.* 1966;94:780–790.
9. Russell WW. Aberrant portions of the mullerian duct found in an ovary. Ovarian cysts of mullerian origin. *Bull Johns Hopkins Hosp.* 1899;10:8.
10. Batt RE, Smith RA. Embryologic theory of histogenesis of endometriosis in peritoneal pockets. *Obstet Gynecol Clin North Am.* 1989;16:15.
11. Halban J. Metastatic hysteroadenosis. *Wien Klin Wochenschr.* 1924;37:1205–1206.
12. Sampson JA. Metastatic or embolic endometriosis, due to menstrual dissemination of endometrial tissue into venous circulation. *Am J Pathol.* 1927;3:93.
13. Suginami H. A reappraisal of the coelomic metaplasia theory by reviewing endometriosis occurring in unusual sites and instances. *Am J Obstet Gynecol.* 1991;165:214–218.
14. Matsuura K, Ohtake H, Katabuchi H, Okamura H. Coelomic metaplasia theory of endometriosis: evidence from in vivo studies and

an in vitro experimental model. *Gynecol Obstet Invest*. 1999;47 (suppl, 1):18–22.

15. Rosenfeld DL, Lecher BD. Endometriosis in a patient with Rokitansky–Kuster–Hauser syndrome. *Am J Obstet Gynecol*. 1981; 139:105.

16. Oliker AJ, Harris AE. Endometriosis of the bladder in a male patient. *J Urol*. 1971;106:858–859.

17. Schrodt GR, Alcorn MO, Ibanez J. Endometriosis of the male urinary system: a case report. *J Urol*. 1980;124:722–723.

18. Javert CT. Observations on the pathology and spread of endometriosis based on the theory of benign metastasis. *Am J Obstet Gynecol*. 1951;62:477–487.

19. Ueki M. Histologic study of endometriosis and examination of lymphatic drainage in and from the uterus. *Am J Obstet Gynecol*. 1991;165:201–209.

20. Javert CT. The spread of benign and malignant endometrium in the lymphatic system with a note of coexisting vascular involvement. *Am J Obstet Gynecol*. 1952;64:780–806.

21. Jubanyik KJ, Comite F. Extrapelvic endometriosis. *Obstet Gynecol Clin North Am*. 1997;24:411–440.

22. Sampson JA. Perforating hemorrhagic (chocolate) cysts of the ovary; their importance and especially their relation to pelvic adenomas of endometrial type (adenomyoma of the uterus, rectovaginal septum, sigmoid, etc.). *Arch Surg*. 1921;3:245–323.

23. Sampson JA. Peritoneal endometriosis due to menstrual dissemination of endometrial tissue into the peritoneal cavity. *Am J Obstet Gynecol*. 1927;14:442–469.

24. Halme J, Hammond MG, Hulka JF, Raj SG, Talbert LM. Retrograde menstruation in healthy women and in patients with endometriosis. *Obstet Gynecol*. 1984;64:151–154.

25. Sanflilippo JS, Wakim NG, Schikler KN, Yussman MA. Endometriosis in association with uterine anomaly. *Am J Obstet Gynecol*. 1986;154:39–43.

26. D'Hooghe TM, Bambra CS, Suleman MA, et al. Development of a model of retrograde menstruation in baboons (*Papio anubis*). *Fertil Steril*. 1994;62:635–638.

27. Abuzeid M, Sakhel K, Ashraf M, Mitwally MF, Diamond MP. The association between uterine septum and infertility. *Fertil Steril*. 2005;84(suppl 1):S472.

28. Ridley JH, Edwards IK. Experimental endometriosis in the human. *Am J Obstet Gynecol*. 1958;76:783–790.

29. Dmowski WP, Radwanska E. Current concepts on pathology, histogenesis and etiology of endometriosis. *Acta Obstet Gynecol Scand*. 1984;123(suppl):29–33.

30. Al-Fozan H, Tulandi T. Left lateral predisposition of endometriosis and endometrioma. *Obstet Gynecol*. 2003;101:164–166.

31. Vercellini P, Aimi G, de Giorgi O, Maddalena S, Carinelli S, Crosignani PG. Is cystic ovarian endometriosis an asymmetric disease? *Br J Obstet Gynaecol*. 1998;105:1018–1021.

32. Vercellini P, Busaca M, Aimi G, Bianchi S, Frontino F, Crosignani PG. Lateral distribution of recurrent ovarian endometriotic cysts. *Fertil Steril*. 2002;77:848–849.

33. Vercellini P, Pisacreta A, Vicentini S, Stellato G, Pesole A, Crosignani PG. Lateral distribution of non endometriotic benign ovarian cysts. *Br J Obstet Gynaecol*. 2000;107:556–558.

34. Chapron C, Chopin N, Borghese B, et al. Deeply infiltrating endometriosis: pathogenetic implications of the anatomical distribution. *Hum Reprod*. 21:1839–1845.

35. Jenkins S, Olive DL, Haney AF. Endometriosis: pathogenetic implications of the anatomic distribution. *Obstet Gynecol*. 1986;67:335–338.

36. Dinulescu DM, Ince TA, Quade BJ, Shafer SA, Crowley D, Jacks T. Role of K-ras and Pten in the development of mouse models of endometriosis and endometrioid cancer. *Nat Med*. 2005;1:63–70.

37. Bulletti C, de Ziegler D, Stefanetti M, Cicinelli E, Pelosi E, Flamigni C. Endometriosis: absence of recurrence in patients after endometrial ablation. *Hum Reprod*. 2001;16:2676–2679.

38. Rock JA, Parmley TH, King TM, Laufe LE, Su BS. Endometriosis and the development of tuboperitoneal fistulas after tubal ligation. *Fertil Steril*. 1981;35:16–20.

39. Morrissey K, Idriss N, Nieman L, Winkel C, Stratton P. Dysmenorrhea after bilateral tubal ligation: a case of retrograde menstruation. *Obstet Gynecol*. 2002;100:1065–1067.

40. Lucidi RS, Witz CA, Chrisco MS, et al. A novel in vitro model of the early endometriotic lesion demonstrates that attachment of endometrial cells to mesothelial cells is dependent on the source of endometrial cells. *Fertil Steril*. 2005;84:16–21.

41. Simpson JL, Elias S, Malinak LR, Buttram VC Jr. Heritable aspects of endometriosis, I: genetic studies. *Am J Obstet Gynecol*. 1980; 137:327–331.

42. Hadfield RM, Mardon HJ, Barlow DH, Kennedy SH. Endometriosis in monozygotic twins. *Fertil Steril*. 1997;68:941–942.

43. Treloar SA, O'Connor DT, O'Connor VM, Martin NG. Genetic influences on endometriosis in an Australian twin sample. *Fertil Steril*. 1999;71:701–710.

44. Stefansson H, Geirsson RT, Steinthorsdottir V, et al. Genetic factors contribute to the risk of developing endometriosis. *Hum Reprod*. 2002;17:555–559.

45. Zondervan KT, Weeks DE, Colman R, et al. Familial aggregation of endometriosis in a large pedigree of rhesus macaques. *Hum Reprod*. 2004;19:448–455.

46. Treloar SA, Wicks J, Nyholt DR, et al. Genomewide linkage study in 1,176 affected sister pair families identifies a significant susceptibility locus for endometriosis on chromosome 10q26. *Am J Hum Genet*. 2005;77:365–376.

47. Bruner-Tran K, Eisenberg E, Yeaman G, et al. Steroid and cytokine regulation of matrix metalloproteinase expression in endometriosis and the establishment of experimental endometriosis in nude mice. *J Clin Endocrinol Metab*. 2002;87:4782–4791.

48. Noble A, Simpson SE, Johns A, Bulun SE. Aromatase expression in endometriosis. *J Clin Endocrinol Metab*. 1996;81:174–179.

49. Zeitoun K, Takayma K, Sasano H, et al. Deficient 17β-hydroxysteroid dehydrogenase type 2 expression in endometriosis-derived stromal cells. *J Clin Endocrinol Metab*. 1998;83:4474–4480.

50. Jones RK, Searle RF, Bulmer JN. Apoptosis and bcl-2 expression in normal human endometrium, endometriosis and adenomyosis. *Hum Reprod*. 1998;13:3496–3502.

51. Kao LC, Germeyer A, Tulac S, et al. Expression profiling of endometrium from women with endometriosis reveals candidate genes for disease-based implantation failure and infertility. *Endocrinology*. 2003;144:2870–2881.

52. Kitawaki J, Kado N, Ishihara H, Koshiba H, Kitaoka Y, Honjo H. Endometriosis: the pathophysiology as an estrogen-dependent disease. *J Steroid Biochem Mol Biol*. 2003;83:149–155.

53. Bulun SE, Cheng YH, Yin P, et al. Progesterone resistance in endometriosis: link to failure to metabolize estradiol. *Mol Cell Endocrinol*. 2006;248:94–103.

54. Attia GR, Zeitoun K, Edwards D, Johns A, Carr BR, Bulun SE. Progesterone receptor isoform A but not B is expressed in endometriosis. *J Clin Endocrinol Metab*. 2000;85:2897–2902.

55. Osteen KG, Bruner-Tran KL, Eisenberg E. Reduced progesterone action during endometrial maturation: a potential risk factor for the development of endometriosis. *Fertil Steril*. 2005;83:529–537.

56. Rier SE, Martin DC, Bowman RE, et al. Endometriosis in rhesus monkeys (*Maccaca mulatta*) following chronic exposure to 2,3,7,8-tetrachlorodibenzo-p-dioxin. *Fundam Appl Toxicol*. 1993;21:431–441.

57. Birnbaum LS. The mechanism of dioxin toxicity: relationship to risk assessment. *Environ Health Perspect*. 1994;102(suppl 9):157–167.

58. Hinsdill RD, Couch DL, Speirs RS. Immunosuppression in mice induced by dioxin (TCDD) in feed. *J Environ Pathol Toxicol*. 1980;4:401–425.

59. Guo SW. The link between exposure to dioxin and endometriosis: a critical reappraisal of primate data. *Gynecol Obstet Invest*. 2004;57:157–173.

60. Igarashi TM, Bruner-Tran KL, Yeaman GR, et al. Reduced expression of progesterone receptor-B in the endometrium of women with endometriosis and in cocultures of endometrial cells exposed to 2,3,7,8-tetrachlorodibenzo-p-dioxin. *Fertil Steril*. 2005;84:67–74.

61. Guo SW, Wu Y, Strawn E, et al. Genomic alterations in the endometrium may be a proximate cause for endometriosis. *Eur J Obstet Gynecol Reprod Biol*. 2004;116:89–99.

62. Sato N, Tsunoda H, Nishida M, et al. Loss of heterozygosity on 10q23.3 and mutation of the tumor suppressor gene PTEN in benign endometrial cyst of the ovary: possible sequence progression from benign endometrial cyst to endometrioid carcinoma and clear cell carcinoma of the ovary. *Cancer Res*. 2000;60:7052–7056.

63. Wu Y, Strawn E, Basir Z, et al. Genomic alterations in ectopic and eutopic endometrial of women with endometriosis. *Gynecol Obstet Invest*. 2006;62:148–159.

64. Groothuis PG, Koks CA, De Goeij AF, et al. Adhesion of human endometrial fragments to peritoneum in vitro. *Fertil Steril*. 1999;71:1119–1124.

65. Demir Weusten AY, Groothuis PG, Dunselman GA, et al. Morphological changes in mesothelial cells induced by shed menstrual endometrium in vitro are not primarily due to apoptosis or necrosis. *Hum Reprod*. 2000;15:1462–1468.

66. Kyama CM, Overbergh L, Debrock S, et al. Increased peritoneal and endometrial gene expression of biologically relevant cytokines and growth factors during the menstrual phase in women with endometriosis. *Fertil Steril*. 2006;85:1667–1675.

67. Nap AW, Groothuis PG, Demir AY, et al. Tissue integrity is essential for ectopic implantation of human endometrium in the chicken chorioallantoic membrane. *Hum Reprod*. 2003;18:30–34.

68. Oosterlynck DJ, Cornillie FJ, Waer M, et al. Women with endometriosis show a defect in natural killer activity resulting in a decreased cytotoxicity to autologous endometrium. *Fertil Steril*. 1991;56:45–51.

69. Somigliana S, Vigano P, Gaffuri B, Guarneri D, Busacca M, Vigbali M. Human endometrial stromal cells as a source of soluble intercellular adhesion molecule (ICAM)-1 molecules. *Hum Reprod*. 1996;11:1190–1194.

70. Tseng JF, Ryan IP, Milam TD, et al. Interleukin-6 secretion in vitro is up-regulated in ectopic and eutopic endometrial stromal cells from women with endometriosis. *J Clin Endocrinol Metab*. 1996;81:1118–1122.

71. Velasco I, Rueda J, Acien P. Aromatase expression in endometriotic tissues and cell cultures of patients with endometriosis. *Mol Hum Reprod*. 2006;12:377–381.

72. Halme J, Becker S, Wing R. Accentuated cyclic activation of peritoneal macrophages in patients with endometriosis. *Am J Obstet Gynecol*. 1984;148:85–90.

73. Rana N, Gebel H, Braun DP, Rotman C, House R, Dmowski WP. Basal and stimulated secretion of cytokines by peritoneal macrophages in women with endometriosis. *Fertil Steril*. 1996;65:925–930.

74. Sharpe-Timms KL, Piva M, Ricke EA, Surewicz K, Zhang YL, Zimmer RL. Endometriosis synthesizes and secretes a haptoglobin-like protein. *Biol Reprod*. 1998;58:988–994.

75. Sharpe-Timms KL, Zimmer RL, Ricke EA, Piva M, Horowitz GM. Endometriotic haptoglobin binds to peritoneal macrophages and alters their function in women with endometriosis. *Fertil Steril*. 2002;78:810–819.

76. Ryan IP, Tseng JF, Schriock ED, Khorram O, Landers DV, Taylor RN. Interleukin-8 concentrations are elevated in peritoneal fluid of women with endometriosis. *Fertil Steril*. 1995;63:929–932.

77. Khorram O, Taylor RN, Ryan IP, Schall TJ, Landers DV. Peritoneal fluid concentrations of the cytokine RANTES correlate with the severity of endometriosis. *Am J Obstet Gynecol*. 1993;169:1545–1549.

78. Akoum A, Lemay A, McColl S, Turcot Lemay L, Maheux R. Elevated concentration and biologic activity of monocyte chemotactic protein-1 in the peritoneal fluid of patients with endometriosis. *Fertil Steril*. 1996;66:17–23.

79. Oosterlynck D, Meuleman M, Waer M, Koninckx P. Transforming growth factor-B activity is increased in peritoneal fluid from women with endometriosis. *Obstet Gynecol*. 1994;83:287–292.

80. Hsu CC, Yang BC, Wu MH, Huang KE. Enhanced interleukin-4 expression in patients with endometriosis. *Fertil Steril*. 1997;67:1059–1064.

81. Marchino GL, Gennarelli G, Enria R, Bongioanni F, Lipari G, Massobrio M. Diagnosis of pelvic endometriosis with use of macroscopic versus histologic findings. *Fertil Steril*. 2005;82:12–15.

82. Nisolle M, Donnez J. Peritoneal endometriosis, ovarian endometriosis, and adenomyotic nodules of the rectovaginal septum are three different entities. *Fertil Steril*. 1997;68:585–596.

83. Sakamoto A. Subserosal adenomyosis: a possible variant of pelvic endometriosis. *Am J Obstet Gynecol*. 1991;165:198–201.

84. Wu Y, Kajdacsy-Balla A, Strawn E, et al. Transcriptional characterizations of differences between eutopic and ectopic endometrium. *Endocrinology*. 2006;147:232–246.

Section 10.2. Thoracic Endometriosis

Georgios E. Hilaris and Camran Nezhat

The purpose of this section is to provide practicing gynecologic endoscopic surgeons with up-to-date evidence on the etiopathogenesis, diagnosis, and treatment of thoracic endometriosis and to heighten the level of clinical suspicion of the syndrome. This syndrome possibly represents an underreported cause of catamenial spontaneous pneumothorax. A multidisciplinary approach by a thoracic and gynecologic surgical team offers the best chances for an accurate diagnosis and treatment of women with this syndrome.

INTRODUCTION

Endometriosis, defined as the presence of endometrial glands and stroma outside the endometrial cavity, is a common disease that affects approximately 2% to 15% of women of reproductive age.[1,2] Consequently, thoracic endometriosis is the presence of endometrial glands and stroma in the thoracic cavity.

Thoracic endometriosis syndrome (TES) encompasses mainly four clinical entities: catamenial pneumothorax (CP), catamenial hemothorax (CHt), catamenial hemoptysis (CH), and lung nodules, with the first being by far the most common clinical presentation.[3]

The diagnosis of thoracic endometriosis has improved substantially over the past two decades because of advances in endoscopic techniques (video-assisted thoracoscopic surgery [VATS] as well as laparoscopy) coupled with a higher level of clinical suspicion.

Its etiology and pathogenesis, however, are still not well understood. Hence, optimal management of thoracic endometriosis remains to be elucidated, with medical, surgical, or combined approaches being reported in the international literature thus far.

EPIDEMIOLOGY

The true incidence of TES remains unclear. Since Barnes [4] described the first case of thoracic endometriosis in 1953, there have been more than 250 cases of thoracic endometriosis and CP reported in the international literature.[5–13] In recent published series, however, up to one third (30%) of women hospitalized with a diagnosis of spontaneous pneumothorax had CP.[12,14] Thus, it is plausible that thoracic endometriosis is an underreported cause of secondary spontaneous pneumothorax in an age group of women in whom most cases of pneumothorax were so far thought to be primary.[15]

Like other sites of extragenital endometriosis, thoracic endometriosis seems to affect a slightly older population than does pelvic disease. The mean age at presentation of women with thoracic endometriosis is 35 ± 0.6 years, with a range from 15 to 54 years. Interestingly, pelvic endometriosis precedes thoracic endometriosis symptoms, occurring between 24 and 29 years – that is, approximately 5 to 7 years earlier.[3] Similar data come from a recent review of CP cases in 229 patients in whom the mean age at onset of symptoms was 34.2 ± 6.9 years, with a range from 15 to 47 years.[13]

Fifty percent to 84% of women diagnosed with thoracic endometriosis have associated pelvic endometriosis. The percentage, though, of women with pelvic disease who develop thoracic endometriosis is largely unknown.[3]

Most lesions are solitary, with the right hemithorax (mainly pleura and far less commonly the lung parenchyma) being involved in up to 92% of cases and the left hemithorax in 5% of cases; the remaining 3% have bilateral involvement.[13]

CP is the most frequent clinical presentation of patients with TES, occurring in approximately 80% of the cases; CHt occurs in 14% and CH in 5%. Least common are endometriotic nodules.[3,16]

ETIOLOGY AND PATHOGENESIS

Based on the anatomic location of the endometriotic lesions, thoracic endometriosis can be classified into pleural and bronchopulmonary (parenchymal). The former, which is the most common type, gives rise to CP and CHt, whereas the latter gives rise to CH and the exceedingly rare lung nodules.[16,17]

There is general agreement that thoracic endometriosis is the only cause of CHt, CH, and endometriotic lung nodules. Conversely, CP, although most frequently associated with thoracic endometriosis, may also have other etiologic mechanisms.[15]

Three theories have been proposed to explain the presence of thoracic endometriotic lesions: coelomic metaplasia, lymphatic or hematogenous embolization from the uterus or pelvis, and retrograde menstruation with subsequent transperitoneal–transdiaphragmatic migration of endometrial tissue.[3,14] The first theory cannot be supported by the almost 9:1 right-sided predominance of endometriotic pleural implants. On the other hand, the lymphovascular embolization theory could explain not only the parenchymal or bronchopulmonary endometriotic nodules but also other extrapelvic locations.[1,3] In fact, a review of autopsy data showed that cadavers with bronchopulmonary endometriosis usually had bilateral lesions whereas pleural and diaphragmatic lesions were almost always right sided.[18]

The theory of transdiaphragmatic passage of endometrial debris and/or air is now the most favored explanation for thoracic endometriosis. It best supports both the anatomic location of endometriotic lesions (found in the right pleura in more than 90% of the cases) and the exceedingly more common presentation of CP versus other, less common entities of TES.[19] This last theory is based on the concept that peritoneal fluid circulation within the abdomen follows a characteristic clockwise pattern that promotes flow of fluids (air, cell aggregates, pus) from the pelvis to the right subdiaphragmatic area through the right paracolic gutter. Transdiaphragmatic passage of peritoneal fluid into the right pleural cavity may occur through congenital or acquired defects and fenestrations [3,13,20] and may be the key pathognomonic feature of thoracic endometriosis. During menses, refluxed endometrial tissue or air may pass through these defects into the pleural space, favored by both the thoracoabdominal pressure gradient and the "piston-like" action of the solid liver bulk.[20]

As in the case of pelvic endometriosis, heterotopic endometrial implants adhere, proliferate, and follow hormonal cyclic changes. Recurrent bleeding and subsequent fibrosis may weaken the implantation site on visceral pleura that in subsequent cycles may rupture or bleed, causing pneumothorax or hemothorax, respectively. Bronchopulmonary implants, on the other hand, may erode the parenchyma or bronchi, causing hemoptysis and fibrosis, as in the case of lung nodules.

Based on the last two theories, it is not surprising that women with bronchopulmonary endometriosis tend to have a history of uterine manipulation or trauma (e.g., hysteroscopy, dilation and curettage); this supports the lymphovascular embolization theory, whereas those with pleural disease most often have a history of pelvic endometriosis.[16,17]

CLINICAL FEATURES

The most common presentation of TES is CP, which accounts for almost 80% of cases. Less frequent clinical entities include CHt (14% of cases), CH (5% of cases), and lung nodules.[3,16] CP is defined as a recurrent pneumothorax occurring within 72 hours from the onset of menstruation.[14] Though CP is typically cyclic, noncyclic recurrences occurring in the immediate premenstrual period [21,22] or ovulatory phase [23] have also been reported.

In most cases, CP is right sided [3,13], with the left side being rarely involved. Bilateral CP is possible but extremely rare.[24,25]

Patients with CP present with symptoms of spontaneous pneumothorax that are usually nonspecific, such as pleurisy, cough, and shortness of breath. Patients may also have referred peri-scapular or neck-irradiating pain due to diaphragmatic irritation. In most cases, symptoms are mild to moderate; severe presentations are rare.[15]

CHt is an uncommon manifestation of TES accounting for approximately 14% of cases. As with CP, CHt is almost always unilateral and right sided, although left-sided hemothorax has been reported.[26] Again, symptoms are nonspecific and include pleuritic pain, shortness of breath, and cough. The presence of bloody effusion is variable. Computed tomography (CT) of the chest may show multiloculated effusions, nodular lesions of the pleura, or bulky pleural masses.[6]

CH and lung nodules are both clinical entities of bronchopulmonary TES and very rare manifestations. Hemoptysis is a quite variable manifestation, with neither massive hemoptysis nor deaths being described so far. An association with menses may not always be appreciated, and diagnostic delays of up to 4 years from the onset of symptoms have been reported.[27] CH and lung nodules are interrelated entities. Thus, patients who present with CH frequently have associated lung nodules on imaging studies and vice versa.[15]

CP, CHt, CH, and lung nodules represent the main clinical entities in TES. However, they are not the only manifestations of TES. Specifically, in diaphragmatic-only endometriosis cases, catamenial phrenic nerve irritation causing a catamenial pain-only syndrome, namely cyclic shoulder, neck, epigastric, or right upper quadrant pain, may be the only presentation of TES.[28,29]

Overall, a high level of clinical suspicion is of paramount importance in TES. A detailed history might make the difference in promptly establishing a correct diagnosis and avoiding delays in treatment, which are commonly reported.

DIAGNOSIS

The most valuable tool in the diagnosis of thoracic endometriosis is a high level of clinical suspicion.[5] A cyclic (i.e., catamenial) constellation of symptoms can be considered pathognomonic for the disease. However, diagnosis is often delayed for more than 8 months from the onset of symptoms.[17].

Chest radiograph, CT, magnetic resonance imaging, thoracocentesis, and bronchoscopy are most useful in the differential diagnosis of the patient presenting with pneumothorax, hemothorax, hemoptysis, or lung nodules and help rule out malignancy, infection, and other pathologies. They all, however, have limited diagnostic yield in the diagnosis of TES per se, with variable and inconsistent findings.[5,17]. Interestingly, in the case of bronchopulmonary endometriosis, bronchoscopy-directed biopsies of suspected lesions usually fail to provide a tissue diagnosis, whereas brush cytology frequently shows distinctive features of endometrial cells.[30]

Performance of imaging studies or bronchoscopy during menses may assist in the diagnosis of pleural or bronchopulmonary disease. Repeat imaging studies or bronchoscopy during midcycle typically documents the disappearance of the previously reported findings, thus strengthening the clinical suspicion.[31]

VATS is at present the gold standard for both the definitive diagnosis and surgical treatment of CP.[5,12,13,15] In the largest review of CP cases, more than 50% (52.1%) of patients with CP assessed with VATS were diagnosed as having thoracic endometriosis. Diaphragmatic abnormalities (fenestrations or endometriosis, alone or combined) are nowadays the most commonly described lesions (38.8%), followed by endometriosis of the visceral pleura (29.6%). In the remainder of cases, discrete lesions, such as bullae, blebs, and scarring (23.1%), or no findings (8.5%) are noted.[13,14,21]

Diaphragmatic fenestrations range from a few millimeters to 2 cm.[14,32] Endometrial deposits in both the diaphragm and pleura have similar appearance and range from a few millimeters to 1 cm. Their color ranges from violet to brown, depending on the day of the menstrual cycle.[5,15,33]

Performance of a combined VATS and laparoscopy procedure in a single session is another diagnostic approach.[5] This way, the thoracic cavity as well as the pelvis and subdiaphragmatic region can be assessed. It may be particularly helpful in cases of inconclusive VATS, which may be the result of the presence of endometriosis in the abdominal-only aspect of the diaphragm, causing catamenial phrenic nerve irritation and pain.[29]

Although exploratory thoracotomy was performed extensively in the past, it is now reserved for select cases of prior thoracoscopic (VATS) failure or large lesions.

TREATMENT OPTIONS

Treatment of thoracic endometriosis can be medical, surgical, or a combination of both.

Medical Treatment

Medical treatment has long been considered the first step in the management of thoracic endometriosis. Danazol, progestational agents, oral contraceptive pills, and GnRH analogues have all been widely used.[15] All have equal effectiveness in alleviating symptoms, and the decision on which one to use is influenced by cost, compliance, and side effect profiles.[2] Among the agents studied however, GnRH agonists have been found to be more effective in controlling recurrences of CP, particularly when used for prolonged periods of as long as 1 year.[34–36]

Nevertheless, in the largest series of TES, which included 110 patients, medical treatment was far less effective than surgical treatment, with recurrence rates exceeding 50% regardless of the agent used. Specifically, recurrence rates at 6 and 12 months were 50% and 60% for medical and 5% and 25% for surgical treatment, respectively.[3] This is anticipated because at best, current agents can suppress endometriotic implant growth and activity only as long as they are being used.

Medical treatment often serves merely as a diagnostic tool. A positive response to medical treatment in women with suspected TES may be considered diagnostic, and surgical treatment may be sought.[31]

Surgical Treatment

Thoracentesis and chest tube placement are obviously first-step therapeutic interventions in the emergency room until further action is taken.

VATS is currently the gold standard for the surgical treatment of TES, especially CP. Laparoscopy aids in the surgical treatment of implants on the abdominal aspect of the diaphragm.

When endometriotic implants are the sole findings during VATS and are in the range of a few millimeters, they can be carefully fulgurated using bipolar diathermy or CO_2 laser, regardless of their location (i.e., parietal, visceral, or diaphragmatic pleura) (Figures 10.2.1 and 10.2.2). Larger endometriotic implants of the visceral pleura may be excised using sharp dissection.[5] Nonetheless, big lesions or deep parenchymal endometriotic nodules are best treated with parenchymal-sparing procedures, such as wedge resection [14] or subsegmentectomy [37], via a minithoracotomy. Occasionally, lobectomy may be required.[38]

Diaphragmatic lesions (endometriotic implants or perforations) are probably best treated by resection using endoscopic stapler devices, provided that the resected surface is relatively small.[14,20] Larger diaphragmatic perforations can be sutured,

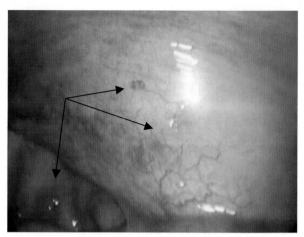

Figure 10.2.1. Endometriotic deposits in parietal and visceral pleura.

even though significant recurrences have been reported with the use of sutures.[39] The use of mesh to replace large diaphragmatic excisions has been described in three women who at 45 months' follow-up suffered no recurrences [21], although other authors have not confirmed these results.[40]

Another important therapeutic intervention is pleurodesis (mechanical, chemical, pleurectomy, or talcum). It can be performed alone or in conjunction with implant and/or perforation excision. In a literature review of 79 VATS-treated patients, 28 underwent pleurodesis alone, with a median recurrence-free interval of 61 months (10 days to 264 months).[13] Pleurodesis, especially in younger patients, should always be carried out concomitantly with VATS exploration. This way, an accurate diagnosis and treatment can be instituted and recurrences avoided. The pleural cavity and the diaphragm should be carefully explored. Otherwise, endometriotic implants or perforations may be overlooked.

If the abdominal aspect of the diaphragm is involved by endometriotic implants, an experienced team of gynecologic and thoracic surgeons can fulgurate or excise small lesions. Hydrodissection, laser fulguration, or excision can be carried out successfully.[29] However, if larger implants or defects are present, they should be approached via VATS, as the liver bulk

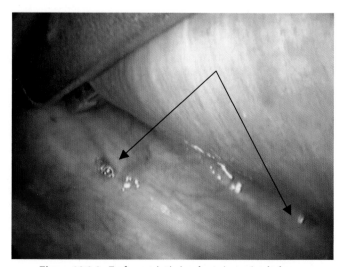

Figure 10.2.2. Endometriotic implants in parietal pleura.

and limited subdiaphragmatic space may not allow complete resection.[28]

There is limited information in the literature regarding surgical treatment of CHt and CH. Pleurectomy for CHt has been successfully reported in two cases.[6,41] A single case of CH, successfully treated with bronchoscopy-directed Nd:YAG laser destruction of an endobronchial implant, has also been reported.[42]

Finally, hysterectomy and BSO is the treatment of last resort when other options have failed. Nonetheless, TES may recur if the intrathoracic disease has not been properly addressed and hormone replacement treatment is initiated.[3]

Combined Treatment

Based on the suboptimal recurrence rates following either medical or surgical treatment, some investigators prefer surgical treatment followed by hormonal suppression in the postoperative period.[14,20,33,43]

CONCLUSION

TES is a challenging clinical entity. A high index of clinical suspicion is of paramount importance as both diagnosis and treatment may often be delayed for years. Endometriosis has variable and often subtle clinical and macroscopic features that can be best appreciated by experienced gynecologic endoscopic surgeons. Hence, a multidisciplinary approach from a thoracic and gynecologic surgical team carries the highest chance of making an accurate diagnosis and providing the appropriate treatment strategies.

REFERENCES

1. Olive DL, Schwartz LB. Endometriosis. *N Engl J Med.* 1993;328:1759–1769.
2. Hilaris GE, Nezhat CR. Endometriosis and pelvic pain. In: Wetter PA, Kavic MS, Levinson CJ, Kelley WE Jr, McDougall EM, Nezhat C, eds. *Prevention and Management of Laparoendoscopic Surgical Complications.* Miami: The Society of Laparoendoscopic Surgeons; 2005.
3. Joseph J, Sahn SA. Thoracic endometriosis syndrome: new observations from an analysis of 110 cases. *Am J Med.* 1996;100:164–170.
4. Barnes J. Endometriosis of the pleura and ovaries. *J Obstet Gynaecol Br Emp.* 1953;60:823.
5. Hilaris GE, Payne CK, Cannon W, Osias J, Nezhat CR. Synchronous rectovaginal, urinary bladder and pulmonary endometriosis. *JSLS.* 2005;9:78–82.
6. Ziedalski TM, Sankaranarayanan V, Chitkara RK. Thoracic endometriosis: a case report and literature review. *J Thorac Cardiovasc Surg.* 2004;127:1513–1514.
7. Poyraz AS, Kilic D, Hatipoglu A, Demirhan BA. A very rare entity: catamenial pneumothorax. *Asian Cardiovasc Thorac Ann.* 2005;13:271–273.
8. Peikert T, Gillespie DJ, Cassivi SD. Catamenial pneumothorax. *Mayo Clin Proc.* 2005;80:677–680.
9. Yoshioka H, Fukui T, Mori S, Usami N, Nagasaka T, Yokoi K. Catamenial pneumothorax in a pregnant patient. *Jpn J Thorac Cardiovasc Surg.* 2005;53:280–282.
10. Devue K, Coenye K, Verhaeghe W. A case of catamenial pneumothorax caused by thoracic endometriosis. *Eur J Emerg Med.* 2005;12:92–94.
11. Hiraoka N, Odama S, Unoura K, et al. Five cases of female pneumothorax with endometriosis on the blebs [in Japanese]. *Nihon Kokyuki Gakkai Zasshi.* 2005;43:53–58.
12. Marshall MB, Ahmed Z, Kucharczuk JC, Kaiser LR, Shrager JB. Catamenial pneumothorax: optimal hormonal and surgical management. *Eur J Cardiothorac Surg.* 2005;27:662–666.
13. Korom S, Canyurt H, Missbach A, et al. Catamenial pneumothorax revisited: clinical approach and systematic review of the literature. *J Thorac Cardiovasc Surg.* 2004;128:502–508.
14. Alifano M, Roth TH, Camilleri Broet S, Schussler O, Magdeleinat P, Regnard JF. Catamenial pneumothorax. A prospective study. *Chest.* 2003;124:1004–1008.
15. Alifano M, Trisolini R, Cancellieri A, Regnard JF. Thoracic endometriosis: current knowledge. *Ann Thorac Surg.* 2006;81:761–769.
16. Jubanyik KJ, Comite F. Extrapelvic endometriosis. *Obstet Gynecol Clin North Am.* 1997;24:411–440.
17. Nezhat CR, Berger GS, Nezhat F, Buttram VC Jr., Nezhat CH, eds. *Endometriosis: Advanced Management and Surgical Techniques.* New York: Springer-Verlag.
18. Kovaric JL, Toll GD. Thoracic endometriosis with recurrent spontaneous pneumothorax. *JAMA.* 1966;196:595.
19. Kirschner PA. Porous diaphragm syndromes. *Chest Surg Clin North Am.* 1998;8:449–472.
20. Alifano M, Cancellieri A, Fornelli A, Trisolini R, Boaron M. Endometriosis-related pneumothorax: clinico-pathological observations from a newly diagnosed case. *J Thorac Cardiovasc Surg.* 2004;127:1219–1221.
21. Bagan P, Le Pimpec Barthes F, Assouad J, Souilamas R, Riquet M. Catamenial pneumothorax: retrospective study of surgical treatment. *Ann Thorac Surg.* 2003;75:378–381.
22. Yamazaki S, Ogawa J, Koide S, Shohzu A, Osamura Y. Catamenial pneumothorax associated with endometriosis of the diaphragm. *Chest.* 1980;77:107–109.
23. Brown RC. A unique case of catamenial pneumothorax. *Chest.* 1989;95:1368.
24. Laws HL, Fox LS, Younger B. Bilateral catamenial pneumothorax. *Arch Surg.* 1977;112:627–628.
25. Wilhelm JL, Scommegna A. Catamenial pneumothorax: bilateral occurrence while on suppressive therapy. *Obstet Gynecol.* 1977;50:227–231.
26. Joseph J, Reed CE, Sahn SA. Thoracic endometriosis recurrence following hysterectomy with bilateral salpingo-oophorectomy and successful treatment with talc pleurodesis. *Chest.* 1994:106:1894–1896.
27. Cassina PC, Hauser M, Kacl G, Imthurn B, Schroder S, Weder W. Catamenial hemoptysis. Diagnosis with MRI. *Chest.* 1997;111:1447–1450.
28. Redwine DB. Diaphragmatic endometriosis: diagnosis, surgical management, and long-term results of treatment. *Fertil Steril.* 2002;77:288–296.
29. Nezhat C, Seidman DS, Nezhat F, Nezhat C. Laparoscopic surgical management of diaphragmatic endometriosis. *Fertil Steril.* 1998;69:1048–1055.
30. Kuo PH, Wang HC, Liaw YS, Kuo SH. Bronchoscopic and angiographic findings in tracheobronchial endometriosis. *Thorax.* 1996;51:1060–1061.
31. Hope-Gill B, Prathibha BV. Catamenial haemoptysis and clomiphene citrate therapy. *Thorax.* 2003;58:89–90.
32. Cowl CT, Dunn WF, Dechamp C. Visualization of diaphragmatic fenestration associated with catamenial pneumothorax. *Ann Thorac Surg.* 1999;68:1413–1414.
33. Alifano M, Venissac N, Mouroux J. Recurrent pneumothorax associated with thoracic endometriosis. *Surg Endosc.* 2000;14:680.

34. Tripp HF, Thomas LP, Obney JA. Current therapy of catamenial pneumothorax. *Heart Surg Forum*. 1998;1:146–149.

35. Tripp HF, Obney JA. Consideration of anatomic defects in the etiology of catamenial pneumothorax. *J Thorac Cardiovasc Surg*. 1999;117:632–633.

36. Slabbynck H, Laureys M, Impens N, De Vroey P, Schandevyl W. Recurring catamenial pneumothorax treated with a Gn-RH analogue. *Chest*. 1991;100:851–851.

37. Terada Y, Chen F, Shoji T, Itoh H, Wada H, Hitomi S. A case of endobronchial endometriosis treated by subsegmentectomy. *Chest*. 1999;115:1475–1478.

38. Kristianen K, Fjeld NB. Pulmonary endometriosis causing haemoptysis. Report of a case treated with lobectomy. *Scand J Thorac Cardiovasc Surg*. 1993;27:113–115.

39. Fonseca P. Catamenial pneumothorax: a multifactorial etiology. *J Thorac Cardiovasc Surg*. 1998;116:872–873.

40. Sakamoto K, Ohmori T, Takei H. Catamenial pneumothorax caused by endometriosis in the visceral pleura. *Ann Thorac Surg*. 2003;76:290–291.

41. Byanyima RK. Menstruation in an unusual place: a case of thoracic endometriosis in Kampala, Uganda. *Afr Health Sci*. 2001;1:97–98.

42. Puma F, Carloni A, Casucci G, Puligheddu C, Urbani M, Porcaro G. Successful endoscopic Nd-YAG laser treatment of endobronchial endometriosis. *Chest*. 2003;124:1168–1170.

43. Blanco S, Hernando F, Gomez A, Gonzalez MJ, Torres AJ, Balibrea JL. Catamenial pneumothorax caused by diaphragmatic endometriosis. *J Thorac Cardiovasc Surg*. 1998;116:179–180.

Section 10.3. Laparoscopic Treatment of Endometriosis

Bulent Berker, Thomas H. S. Hsu, Keith L. Lee, Ceana Nezhat, Farr Nezhat, and Camran Nezhat

Endometriosis is a common gynecologic condition found in women of reproductive age. The condition is associated with chronic pelvic pain and infertility, which may result in reduced quality of life, psychologic morbidity, and work absenteeism. It is characterized by the presence of uterine endometrial tissue outside the normal location – mainly on the pelvic peritoneum, but also on the ovaries and in the rectovaginal septum, and more rarely in the pericardium, pleura, and even the brain.[1,2] The prevalence of pelvic endometriosis approaches 6% to 10% in the general female population; in women with pain, infertility, or both, the frequency is 35% to 50%.[3] The disorder is most commonly diagnosed in women of reproductive age, although time to diagnosis may be very long because of variability in symptoms and signs and confusion with other disorders. Among gynecologic disorders, endometriosis is surpassed in frequency only by leiomyomas.[4]

The gold standard for diagnosis of pelvic disease is surgical assessment by laparoscopy or laparotomy, and many scoring systems have been developed to assess extent of disease. The American Society for Reproductive Medicine revised classification system for endometriosis (ASRM 1996) is the most widely accepted staging system.[5] Patients who have endometriosis present with different clinical complaints at various stages of the disease. Treatment depends on age of the patient, extent of the disease, severity of the symptoms, and desire for fertility. Intervention usually is indicated for pain, infertility, or impaired function of the bladder, ureter, or intestine. Medical and surgical forms of management are available.

HISTORICAL PERSPECTIVES

Rokitansky [6] described pelvic endometriosis of the fallopian tubes, ovaries, and uterus in 1860. Before 1960, therapy often required hysterectomy and bilateral salpingo-oophorectomy (BSO).[7] Conservative operations to relieve pain and preserve fertility have been modified significantly since the introduction of such therapy. After recognition of the negative impact of surgical trauma and postoperative adhesions on success rates, microsurgical techniques were developed and applied with improved results.[8] Nevertheless, recurrences were not eliminated.[9]

Recent advances in endoscopic surgical techniques and the increased sophistication of surgical instruments have offered new operative methods and techniques for the gynecologic surgeon.[10] The addition of a small video camera to the laparoscope (videolaparoscopy) greatly enhanced the popularity of operative endoscopy because of the possibility of operating in a

comfortable, upright position and using the magnification capabilities of the camera.[11,12] Nezhat et al. started performing laparoscopic GI and GU surgeries in the mid- to late 1980.[13] Currently, laparoscopy is perceived as a minimally invasive surgical technique that both provides a panoramic view of the pelvic organs and allows surgery at the time of diagnosis. Both laparotomy and operative laparoscopy are effective for the treatment of endometriosis in that they reduce the incidence of implants, relieve dysmenorrhea and pelvic pain, and improve fertility potential.[14–18] Unlike radical operations, conservative procedures frequently are not curative.[19,20]

CURRENT SURGICAL MANAGEMENT OF ENDOMETRIOSIS

The optimum management of endometriosis remains as problematic as ever. Endometriosis may be either asymptomatic or associated with minor symptoms and lesions that are sometimes self-limiting. It may also be associated with very severe symptoms and major pathologic lesions involving the vital structures of the pelvis. Different levels of symptomatology and pathology require different levels of therapeutic intervention.[21] The extent of surgery is dependent on the preoperative symptoms and the severity of disease. Most clinicians use the revised ASRM scoring system for endometriosis, which comprises four groups – minimal (stage I), mild (stage II), moderate (stage III), and severe (stage IV) – according to the operative findings.[22] Patients with minor disease may inadvertently be subjected to excessive investigations and invasive treatment, whereas those with major lesions might be underinvestigated such that appropriate treatment is delayed for years.

Since 1980, surgical instruments and techniques with varying degrees of efficacy have been introduced, including lasers, video cameras, monitors, electric generators, hydrodissection, microelectrodes, microsurgery, and operative laparoscopy.[23] The introduction of laser technologies revolutionized the surgical field of medicine. The combination of the cutting and hemostatic properties of lasers was useful for many surgical interventions, including laparoscopy and hysteroscopy, to improve their effectiveness and safety. However, application of surgical lasers (CO_2, argon, potassium titanyl phosphate [KTP], neodymium: yttrium–aluminum–garnet [Nd:YAG]) is limited by relatively high cost and the necessity for special training. There are definite advantages to using a high-powered CO_2 laser (especially the Ultrapulse 5000 L [Coherent Instruments]) as a long knife through the operative channel of the laparoscope. Because this laser does not penetrate water, it can be used with hydrodissection [23] to selectively treat sensitive areas in the bowel, bladder, ureters, and blood vessels. Laparoscopic diagnosis and excision of all forms of endometriosis are effective and may now be considered the "gold standard" of clinical care for women with endometriosis-related pain and infertility. The recognized advantages of operative laparoscopy include faster patient recovery and reduced cost.[24] Various treatment modalities are available for use at laparoscopic surgery. These include laser, scissors with monopolar electrocautery and bipolar coagulation, and harmonic scalpel, all of which allow resection and cauterization and vaporization of endometriosis. In a recent prospective study, laparoscopic excision of endometriosis significantly reduced pain and improved quality of life for up to 5 years.[25] Promising results have been obtained with more radical surgery, including extensive excision of deep disease and also removal of portions of bowel and bladder containing significant endometriosis. There may be a continuing role for hysterectomy in the management of endometriosis, but the evidence for concomitant oophorectomy is less convincing. In addition, as gynecologists become more proficient, pregnancy rates after operative laparoscopy should improve and surpass the results after laparotomy.

Laparoscopy versus Laparotomy

It is difficult to imagine any aspect of care for a gynecologic patient today – examination, surgical correction, monitoring of treatment efficacy – without endoscopy. The endoscopic approach is of vital importance for the differential diagnosis of gynecologic diseases, especially in unclear clinical situations in which other methods fail to reveal either the true diagnosis or extent of the pathology – for example, pelvic pain, adhesions, infertility, and endometriosis.[26] Indeed, it has been suggested that endoscopy be the approach of choice to all gynecologic conditions because of its acknowledged advantages, including minimal trauma, superb visualization, low incidence of complications, reduction of adhesion formation, and favorable postoperative course along with rapid recovery and cosmetic effect.[27,28]

The results of endoscopy and laparotomy are judged by many factors.[29] Three studies compared postoperative adhesion formation and re-formation after a standardized laser injury and laser adhesiolysis by both surgical approaches.[30–32] Laparoscopy caused fewer postoperative adhesions compared with laparotomy. After microsurgical salpingoplasty or adhesiolysis by laparotomy, adhesion recurrence rates were 40% to 72% and new adhesions occurred in more than 50% of patients.[33–37] However, when comparable operations are carried out laparoscopically, recurrence of postoperative adhesions appears to be less common [38] and new adhesions were either absent or less than 20%.[39] Lundorff and colleagues [36] evaluated the formation of adhesions after laparoscopy and laparotomy in patients treated for tubal pregnancy. Those authors stratified 105 women with tubal pregnancy by age and risk factors and prospectively randomized them to treatment by laparoscopy or laparotomy. Second-look laparoscopy revealed more adhesions in the laparotomy group.[36]

Data from animal [30–32] and clinical studies [33–37] suggest that laparoscopic operations are more effective for adhesiolysis, cause fewer new adhesions than does laparotomy, and reduce impairment of tubo-ovarian function.[36] The efficacy of laparotomy or laparoscopy has not been evaluated for restoring fertility or reducing pelvic pain. However, it has been reported that pain relief and pregnancy rates after operative laparoscopy are comparable to or better than those after laparotomy [9,13–17,24,29,36,40–42] for endometriosis (mild to severe), hydrosalpinges, and ectopic pregnancy.

Gomel [43] described the therapeutic efficacy of laparoscopic adhesiolysis in 1975. In a follow-up publication, he stated that "in trained hands, laparoscopic salpingo-ovariolysis is a low-risk procedure associated with a surprisingly good success rate." In his series of 92 patients with moderate to severe adnexal adhesive disease, the intrauterine pregnancy rate was 62.5%.[44] Subsequent studies confirmed that the results of laparoscopy were better than those obtained by laparotomy, especially in the case of severe endometriosis.[16,17,29,40–43] Even extensive endometriosis can be treated more effectively at laparoscopy and with better results than at laparotomy.[14,15]

Fayez and Collazo [41] noted pregnancy rates of 58% after laparoscopy and 36% after laparotomy. Chong and colleagues [45] assessed the relative efficacy of CO_2 laser surgery by laparoscopy and laparotomy in treating infertile patients with severe endometriosis; the mean revised American Fertility Society (rAFS) scores were 59 (laparoscopy) and 58 (laparotomy), with similar pregnancy rates. In two studies, CO_2 laser laparoscopy was compared with laparotomy as a treatment for all stages of endometriosis associated with infertility.[16,17] Operative laparoscopy was found to be safe and effective for all stages of endometriosis. The endoscopic approach should be considered only if the results with laparoscopy are equal to or better than those with laparotomy.[14,23,45] The reduced hospital cost and recovery period obtained with the laparoscopic approach cannot compensate for failure to achieve the optimal treatment.

The outcome of laparoscopy was compared with that of laparotomy in conservative surgical treatment for severe endometriosis.[46] A nonrandomized group of 216 patients underwent conservative surgical treatment for severe endometriosis by either laparoscopy ($n = 67$) or laparotomy ($n = 149$). The results from laparoscopy and laparotomy were equal for the treatment of infertility and chronic pelvic pain associated with severe endometriosis. However, a trend toward a higher pregnancy rate and less dyspareunia was observed after operations done for severe endometriosis by laparotomy compared with laparoscopy.

Laser laparoscopy was compared with traditional laparoscopy or laparotomy in the treatment of 309 infertile women with moderate or severe endometriosis.[47] These patients were treated with one of four options: operative laparoscopy with the CO_2 laser vaporization or resection, operative laparoscopy with electrocoagulation and sharp dissection, laparotomy with electrocoagulation and sharp dissection, and medical treatment with danazol. Pregnancy rates in the laparoscopy group were equal to or higher than those in the laparotomy group for both the entire population and the endometriosis-only subset. When the CO_2 laser was used as an adjuvant option, the rates were better, especially in patients with advanced disease and with endometriosis as the only infertility factor.

Operative laparoscopy is as efficacious in the treatment of recurrent endometriosis as it is in the treatment of the primary disease, and simplifies management of the disease for the clinician. It is currently believed that infertile women with recurrent endometriosis should be included in assisted reproduction programs. However, the poor results of these techniques and their cost make operative laparoscopy the treatment of choice in such women. Likewise, operative laparoscopy seems to offer notable advantages with respect to repeated courses of medical therapy, which are necessary for patients with pelvic pain associated with recurrent endometriosis. Busacca and colleagues [48] compared two consecutive surgical series for the cure of endometriosis. The patients were 81 women with recurrent endometriosis, 41 reoperated on at laparotomy from 1986 to 1991 and 40 reoperated on at laparoscopy from 1992 to 1996. The cumulative probability of recurrence of dysmenorrhea (34 and 43, respectively), and the frequency of recurrence of pelvic pain and dyspareunia and of clinical findings suggestive of the disease were not significantly different in the two groups. The rate of recurrence of dyspareunia was higher in the patients operated on at laparotomy as was the number requiring a third operation. However, this could be the result of the longer follow-up of this group. No significant difference was observed between the cumulative pregnancy rates at 24 months in the two groups (45 in the laparotomy and 54 in the laparoscopy group). The investigators concluded that operative laparoscopy seems as efficacious as conservative surgery at laparotomy in the treatment of recurrent endometriosis.

Conservative Operations

The goals of conservative operative procedures are to remove all implants, resect adhesions, relieve pain, reduce the risk of recurrence and postoperative adhesions, and restore the involved organs to a normal anatomic and physiologic condition. For infertile patients, restoration of the normal tubo-ovarian relationship is essential to enhance fertility. These goals may be achieved by using various surgical instruments (scalpel, scissors, lasers, or electrodes) and a variety of techniques (laparoscopy, laparotomy, combined endoscopy and minilaparotomy).

The usefulness of conservative surgery for pain relief is unclear, but it appears that immediate postoperative efficacy is at least as high as with medical treatment, and long-term outcomes may be considerably higher.[49] Women who desire pregnancy and whose disease is responsible for their symptoms of pain or infertility should have conservative operations. Although seldom curative, such procedures improve the likelihood of pregnancy and offer at least temporary pain relief. Approximately 25% of patients undergoing conservative operations will require a subsequent operation because of recurrence of endometriosis or progression of residual (microscopic) disease.[50] The rate of repeat interventions is related directly to the extent of disease and the ability to conceive postoperatively. Among those who achieve pregnancy after the initial operation, only 10% require another operation.[50,51] Conservative methods are cytoreductive, and recurrence of symptoms most likely is caused by the progression of existing microscopic disease that was not seen during the initial operation.[52–54]

Controversy remains regarding the benefit of surgical ablation of minimal-to-mild endometriosis at the time of laparoscopy. An extensive meta-analysis of published studies showed that either no treatment or surgery is superior to medical treatment for the management of minimal and mild endometriosis associated with infertility.[55] A randomized, controlled Canadian trial studied 341 infertile women to ascertain whether laparoscopic operations enhanced fecundity in infertile women with minimal or mild endometriosis.[56] The women were assigned randomly during diagnostic laparoscopy to undergo either resection or ablation of visible endometriosis or diagnostic laparoscopy only. Among the 172 women who had resection or ablation of endometriosis, 29% became pregnant 36 weeks after the laparoscopy and had pregnancies that continued for 20 weeks or longer, compared with 17.2% of the 169 women in the diagnostic laparoscopy group. Laparoscopic resection or ablation of minimal and mild endometriosis significantly improved fecundity in infertile women. Another randomized trial of laparoscopic ablation versus no treatment in 101 infertile women with minimal or mild disease demonstrated similar cumulative pregnancy rates during the first postoperative year (19.6% vs. 22.2%).[57] Another prospective study assessed the efficacy of CO_2 laser laparoscopy in treating 176 infertile women with minimal to mild endometriosis according to the ASRM classification in terms of pregnancy rates.[58] The patients were treated with one of four methods: 49 underwent operative laparoscopy with newly developed CO_2 laser vaporization or resection, 45 were treated by operative laparoscopy with simple monopolar electrocoagulation, 43 who had undergone only diagnostic laparoscopy did not receive any treatment, and 39 received danazol 800 mg/day for 3 months after diagnostic laparoscopy. Advanced laparoscopic operations with a laser were more efficient than were other modalities in treating infertile women with minimal to mild endometriosis in terms of pregnancy rates. Tulandi and al-Took [59] found no difference in the pregnancy rates of 101 infertile women with mild endometriosis treated laparoscopically either by excision or by electrocoagulation. The role of resection or ablation of moderate to severe disease is clear. Both fecundity and relief of pelvic pain are improved with surgery in patients with advanced-stage disease as compared with medical therapy or observation. One report suggested that fertility may be particularly improved with ablative procedures in patients with deep infiltrating endometriotic lesions.[60]

Radical Operations

Radical ablative surgery for endometriosis is indicated chiefly for symptoms of pain that fail to respond to conservative treatment. The sites of involvement must be carefully assessed and surgery planned taking account of the wishes of the patient concerning her fertility. Procedures include oophorectomy, salpingo-oophorectomy, hysterectomy, appendicectomy, and the excision of deeply infiltrating endometriosis possibly involving bowel resection. The most important arbiter of therapeutic success is the removal of the ovaries, hysterectomy and BSO offering the ultimate cure for this chronic condition.[61] Hysterectomy and BSO are indicated for patients with severe symptoms who have not responded to medical or conservative surgical treatment and are not interested in pregnancy. Fibrosis obliterates tissue planes and sometimes causes a suspicion of malignancy because of extensive involvement of the intestinal and urinary tracts. In advanced disease, the ovaries may be encased and densely adherent to the pelvic side wall. Ovarian dissection entails the risk of injury to the ureter, major blood vessels, and bowel. A retroperitoneal approach can isolate the ureter throughout its course to ensure complete removal of ovarian tissue and prevent ovarian remnant syndrome.[62] Bilateral oophorectomy is done for the purpose of the elimination of the estrogen that sustains and stimulates the ectopic endometrium.[63] Although conserving one ovary has resulted in reasonable cure rates [19,64,65], failure rates of 13% and 40% at 3 and 5 years, respectively, have been reported after laparotomy when ovarian function is preserved.[66]

Definitive surgery, which includes hysterectomy and BSO, is reserved for use in women with intractable pain who no longer desire pregnancy. In less severe cases, one ovary may be retained to preserve ovarian function, although improvement will be less definitive. The decision to perform bilateral oophorectomy at the time of surgery for endometriosis is dependent upon many factors, one of which is the opinion of the surgeon concerned. A postal survey performed in Australia revealed a conservative approach, with only 27.5% of surgeons electing to perform a hysterectomy in conjunction with bilateral oophorectomy.[67] Namnoum and colleagues [68] had determined the risk of reoperation and/or recurrence of symptoms after hysterectomy for the treatment of endometriosis. Among 138 women, 39 had a hysterectomy with ovarian preservation and 109 had all ovarian tissue removed. Of those whose ovaries were preserved, 62% had recurrent pain and 31% required intervention. The authors concluded that the women with ovarian preservation had six times the risk of developing recurrent pain and an eightfold greater risk of reoperation. At present, there is no consensus on this subject. Oophorectomy should be considered only once it is clear that the ovaries are a cause of the pelvic pain. To determine this, it is sometimes helpful to administer a 2-month course of gonadotropin-releasing hormone (GnRH) agonists to induce amenorrhea and a short-term cessation of ovarian function. Preoperative and postoperative medical therapy has a limited role in surgery, whereas women who have undergone oophorectomy should be treated with estrogen replacement, even at the risk of some recurrence.

HORMONE REPLACEMENT

Oophorectomy with or without hysterectomy is still a frequently chosen therapeutic option in women with extensive, infiltrating, or recurrent pelvic endometriosis who do not want children. In such patients, foci of endometriosis are often left in deep pelvic sites or on other organs, such as the bowel, ureters, and bladder. In fact, the difficulty of eradicating these lesions completely is the main reason for performing definitive surgery. Moreover, the women concerned are generally still far from physiologic menopause and therefore require hormone replacement therapy (HRT) for many years. In such cases, gynecologists often have reservations about instituting standard HRT because of the fear that the estrogens may induce a recurrence of the disease and its symptoms.[69] Although HRT involves some risks, after hysterectomy and BSO, patients often require HRT to relieve menopausal symptoms. Administering the minimal effective dose of estrogen is associated with only a small risk of recurrence.[66] The hormonal dependence of endometriosis is evident, as the disease is rarely found before menarche, after menopause, or during pregnancy, and it regresses during medical treatments that induce hypoestrogenemia. Endometriosis after menopause

is rare, although the influence of HRT in the pathogenesis of postmenopausal growth of endometriosis is still unclear. In the last 20 years, the recurrence of endometriosis in menopausal women has increased because of the use of HRT.[70] Several investigators advise against the use of HRT in patients with a history of endometriosis, a contraindication based on retrospective uncontrolled studies as well as theoretic and experimental considerations. No prospective controlled studies have been performed. Indeed, the majority of retrospective studies have employed types of HRT that are not presently in general use.

However, there is evidence that estrogen might stimulate the growth of endometriosis during menopause.[71,72] Studies concerning HRT after BSO or after total hysterectomy and BSO for endometriosis are scant. Most of them are retrospective, and the follow-up evaluations and diagnosis lack standardization. Most of them employ therapeutic regimes that are no longer used. The only randomized prospective study concerning HRT in endometriosis involved 21 women studied over 12 months, and the results suggested that tibolone may be a safe HRT in women with residual endometriosis.[69]

To estimate the risk of recurrence after administration of HRT in women who had endometriosis and who underwent BSO, Matorras et al. [73] conducted a prospective randomized trial. To circumvent the theoretical risk of malignancy, the HRT they used consisted of sequential administration of both estrogens and progesterone, even in patients without a uterus. Of the women with a histologic diagnosis of endometriosis in whom BSO was performed, 91.8% had a total hysterectomy. The authors observed a trend of a higher recurrence rate among patients receiving HRT versus controls. There was no recurrence among women who did not receive HRT, versus a 3.5% rate (four out of 115), or 0.9% per year, in women who received HRT. Among women receiving HRT, the following risk factors were detected: peritoneal involvement of 3 cm or greater (2.4% vs. 0.3% recurrence per year) and incomplete surgery (22.2% vs. 1.9% per patient). In their study, the Matorras group reported that patients with a history of endometriosis in whom total hysterectomy and BSO were performed had a low risk of recurrence when HRT was administered. In patients such as these, HRT is a reasonable option. However, in cases with peritoneal involvement of 3 cm or greater, the recurrence rate makes HRT a controversial option. If HRT is indicated, it should be monitored closely.

The recurrence rate with HRT in women who have had total hysterectomy and BSO is very low (0.5% per year); thus, HRT should not be contraindicated. Even so, these patients should be informed of and accept this recurrence rate. When a total hysterectomy has not been performed because of technical difficulties, the recurrence risk contraindicates the use of HRT. The beneficial effects of HRT do not compensate for the high recurrence rate of endometriosis. In cases with severe peritoneal involvement, although HRT is not totally contraindicated, the rate of recurrence is relatively high (9.1% per patient). If HRT is indicated, patients should be monitored closely, especially with vaginal ultrasound. If there is any suspicion of recurrence, HRT should be stopped.[73] The theoretic risks related to HRT in women with endometriosis are not limited to the possibility of disease recurrence. Although the likelihood may be only slight, there are reports of malignant change many years after surgery in women receiving HRT.[61] Extragonadal adenocarcinoma may develop after bilateral oophorectomy, even at sites far from the pelvis.[74] Unopposed estrogen stimulation may lead to premalignant or malignant transformation in the residual foci of endometriosis. Therefore, the addition of progestins to estrogen replacement therapy should be considered in women who have undergone hysterectomy with oophorectomy because of endometriosis, especially if they are known to have residual endometriosis.

APPEARANCES OF ENDOMETRIOSIS

Laparoscopic assessment in combination with histologic examination of the excised lesions remains the gold standard for diagnosis of endometriosis. Knowledge of the most common locations of endometriosis is required for accurate visual inspection of the pelvic and abdominal cavities. Three different forms of endometriosis must be considered during laparoscopic visualization: peritoneal implants, endometriomas, and deep infiltrating lesions of the rectovaginal septum. An increased awareness of the variations in the appearance of endometriotic lesions has resulted in an almost twofold increase in the diagnosis of endometriosis at laparoscopy.[75] Peritoneal implants are most commonly localized in the uterosacral ligaments, cul-de-sac, ovarian fossa, and adjacent pelvic side walls. Less frequently, implants may also be found in the upper abdomen as well as on the surface of the bladder and the bowel (predominantly rectum, sigmoid colon, appendix, and cecum). Hence, careful and close inspection of the entire peritoneal cavity should be performed. Magnification obtained during laparoscopy depends on the distance between the laparoscope and the area inspected; for example, the magnification rate is approximately 3.2 and 1.7 from a distance of 10 and 20 mm, respectively. Magnification allows the recognition of lesions as small as 400 μm for red and 180 μm for clear lesions.

Complete removal of endometriotic implants is difficult because of their variability in appearance and visibility. Powder burn lesions represent foci of inactive disease containing stroma and glands embedded in hemosiderin deposits.[76] These lesions are more common in older women and may not cause pain or infertility.[77] When implants involve the uterosacral ligaments, they are palpable as tender nodularities and can cause dysmenorrhea and dyspareunia. Atypical and nonpigmented lesions, which are seen as clear vesicles, pink vascular patterns, white scarred lesions, red lesions, yellow-brown patches, and peritoneal windows, represent active endometriosis and secrete prostaglandin in the peritoneal fluid.[78] The peritoneum must be examined from different angles and at different degrees of illumination to see vesicles or whitish lesions and the peritoneal folds must be stretched and searched for small, atypical lesions.

Deep nodular endometriosis is usually localized in the rectovaginal and uterovesical septum, in other fibromuscular pelvic structures (e.g., uterosacral ligaments), and in the muscular wall of pelvic structures. Rectovaginal nodules are histologically similar to an adenomyoma, being composed of smooth muscle, endometrial glands, and stroma. They probably constitute an entity distinct from peritoneal and ovarian endometriosis and are thought to originate from the mullerian rests present in

the rectovaginal septum.[79] Deep endometriotic lesions may be predominantly retroperitoneal, with little or no superficial peritoneal involvement. The depth of endometriotic implants may be related to the level of disease activity and symptoms (Figure 10.3.1). Cornillie and coworkers [80] reported that cellular activity of endometriosis was greater for both superficial and deep implants (58% and 68%, respectively) than for intermediate implants (25%). They postulated that early lesions result from proliferation of retrograde menstrual tissue and present as superficial implants. These lesions progress to an intermediate depth, where they either become inactive or progress and infiltrate deeper layers, usually more than 5 mm. Implants continue their biologic activity and proliferate, being stimulated by circulating steroid hormones because they are no longer dependent on the steroids in the peritoneal fluid.[78,81]

Microscopic endometriosis may be overlooked during surgical exploration but is identified by light and electron microscopy in normal-appearing peritoneum. This finding has been noted in patients with visible endometriosis in other areas of the pelvis [52,53] and patients with unexplained infertility in whom no endometriosis was seen at laparoscopy.[54,82] Microscopic presentation may preclude total resection, but two techniques can enhance visual detection. Near-contact laparoscopy magnifies the peritoneal area. In a series of 20 women with pelvic endometriosis, biopsy specimens were taken from peritoneum that appeared normal. The histologic studies of this tissue revealed only one case of microscopic endometriosis, and an additional two cases were suspicious for endometriosis.[53] The second technique for improved detection of microscopic endometriosis is "painting" the peritoneum and broad ligament with blood or serosanguineous fluid to render atypical lesions more evident.[83] Retroperitoneal hydrodissection of the anterior cul-de-sac, posterior broad ligaments, and pelvic side wall sometimes facilitates the identification of lesions (Figure 10.3.2).

At the time of laparoscopy, endometriomas may be identified as smooth-walled, dark-brownish cysts, usually strongly associated with the presence of adhesions. Upon incision, dense, brown, chocolate-like fluid is released. As reported by Vercellini et al. [84], careful visual inspection of the ovaries is usually highly reliable in identification of endometriomas, with 97% sensitivity and 95% specificity. Normal-appearing ovaries may contain endometriosis under an apparently normal cortex. By inserting a needle deep in the stroma and aspirating the ovary, Candiani and coworkers [85] identified small endometriomas in 48% of otherwise normal-appearing or slightly enlarged ovaries. They suggested that preoperative ultrasonographic evaluation is useful to screen for small subcortical ovarian cysts, which should be explored surgically with needle aspiration. The diagnosis of endometriosis is missed in at least 7% of patients and understaged in as many as 50%.[53] A careful examination of the pelvis is essential to diagnose and stage endometriosis and to be aware of its various appearances, including its presence as microscopic implants on visually normal peritoneal surfaces or as small, deep endometriomas within slightly enlarged but otherwise normal ovaries.

Using patient-assisted laparoscopy, Demco [86] studied the relationship of lesions of endometriosis to pelvic pain. He found that pain from endometriosis has little relationship to the location or color of lesions. However, red and vascular lesions were

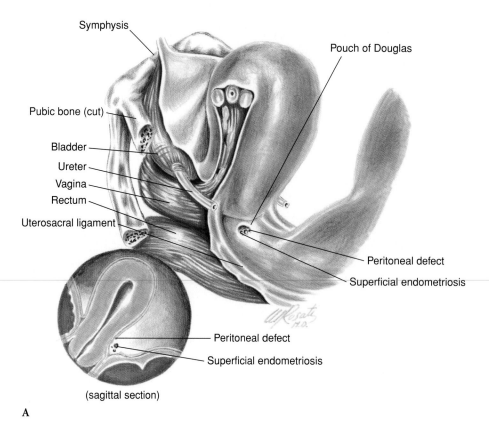

Symphysis

Pouch of Douglas

Pubic bone (cut)

Bladder

Ureter

Vagina

Rectum

Uterosacral ligament

Peritoneal defect

Superficial endometriosis

Peritoneal defect

Superficial endometriosis

(sagittal section)

A

Figure 10.3.1. (**A**) A peritoneal defect in the pouch of Douglas has an endometriotic implant at its base. The *inset* reveals a healed peritoneal defect with infiltrating endometriosis beneath it.

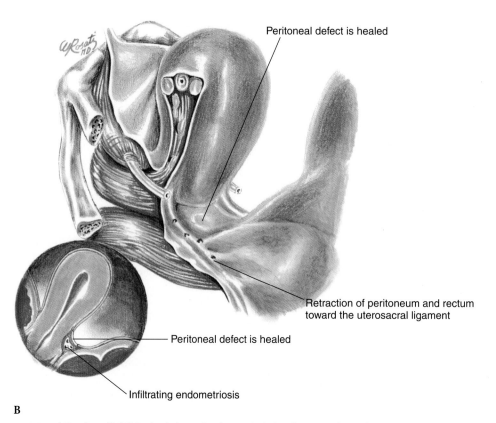

Peritoneal defect is healed

Retraction of peritoneum and rectum toward the uterosacral ligament

Peritoneal defect is healed

Infiltrating endometriosis

B

Figure 10.3.1. (*Continued*) (**B**) Sagittal view of endometriotic implants involving the uterosacral ligament. The *inset* shows infiltrating endometriosis beneath the peritoneum.

The bowel is retracted over the uterosacral ligaments

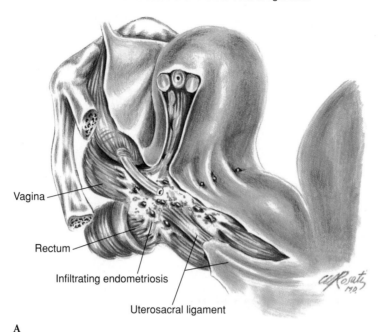

Vagina

Rectum

Infiltrating endometriosis

Uterosacral ligament

A

Figure 10.3.2. (**A**) Anatomic representation of the pelvic structures involved with implants of endometriosis. (*Continued*)

the most painful, followed by clear and white scar lesions. Least painful were black lesions. Pain extended beyond lesions to normal-looking peritoneum for up to 27 mm but was not consistent with respect to the type of lesion.

TREATMENT OF ENDOMETRIOTIC IMPLANTS

Diagnostic Laparoscopy

Initially, the surgeon explores the pelvic cavity to assess the extent of disease and identify abnormalities or distortions of the pelvic organs. Photographs and video recordings have been very useful for documenting the surgeon's findings. In a recent opinion statement, however, the American College of Obstetricians and Gynecologists' Committee on Professional Liability advised against physicians recording procedures because of a growing fear among clinicians that procedural tapes can be edited, enhanced, or otherwise manipulated for the purposes of winning liability suits against doctors.[87] The committee further cautioned that if a recording is made, the health care facility should keep the original tape and provide an exact copy to the patient. The location and boundaries of the bladder, ureter, colon, rectum, pelvic gutters, uterosacral ligaments, and major blood vessels are noted. The upper abdominal organs, abdominal walls, liver, and diaphragm should be evaluated for endometriosis or any other condition that may contribute to the patient's symptoms. The omentum and the small bowel are evaluated for disease and to ensure that they were not injured during insertion of the Veress needle or trocar. A rectovaginal examination is accomplished to evaluate deep and retroperitoneal endometriosis found in the lower pelvis at the rectovaginal septum, uterosacral ligament, lower colon, and

pararectal area. Deep retroperitoneal endometriosis is rare without a connection to the surface peritoneum.

In 15% of patients with endometriosis, the appendix is involved and should be examined.[88] An implant that has penetrated retroperitoneally several centimeters is called an "iceberg" lesion. It can be detected laparoscopically by palpating areas of the pelvis and bowel with the suction–irrigator probe. With the forceps or probe, endometriotic implants are examined to gauge size, depth, and proximity to normal pelvic structures. The diagnostic laparoscopy is extended to an operative procedure if the patient has been advised of this possibility.

Operative Laparoscopy

The operative procedure begins by lysing adhesions between the bowel and the pelvic organs to expose the pelvic cavity adequately. The ovaries are dissected from the cul-de-sac or pelvic side wall, and the tubes are freed from adhesions and chromopertubated. Endometrial implants and endometriomas are resected or vaporized, and if the patient has significant midline pelvic pain, uterosacral nerve ablation or presacral nerve resection is done.

Lysis of Bowel Adhesions

Bowel adhesions vary in thickness, vascularity, and cohesiveness. Some adhesions are stretched without tearing the tissue, excised with a laser harmonic scalpel or electrosurgery at the points of attachment to the pelvic organs, and removed. Dense adhesions are excised with scissors or any other cutting instrument. The CO_2 laser has more controlled penetration than do electrosurgery and fiber lasers. The structures requiring separation are pulled apart with forceps, and a cleavage plane is formed.

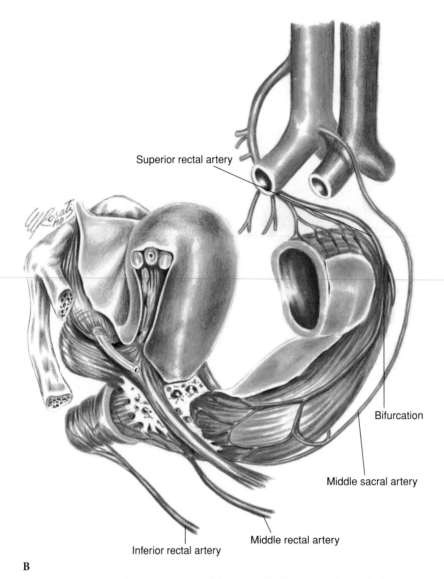

Superior rectal artery

Bifurcation

Middle sacral artery

Middle rectal artery

Inferior rectal artery

B

Figure 10.3.2. (*Continued*) (**B**) The ureters are at risk because of infiltrating endometriosis.

Hydrodissection is useful to identify and develop the dissection plane, which is ablated or excised, using a laser or dissecting scissors or any other cutting instrument.

Peritoneal Implants

In treating peritoneal endometriosis, the implants should be destroyed in the most effective and least traumatic manner to minimize postoperative adhesions. Although different modalities have been used, hydrodissection and a high-power superpulse or ultrapulse CO_2 laser are the best choices for treatment.[89] This laser does not penetrate water, and a fluid backstop (hydrodissection) allows the surgeon to work on selected tissue with a greater safety margin than would otherwise be available (Figure 10.3.3). A small opening is made in the retroperitoneum with the laser or scissors, and lactated Ringer's solution is injected beneath the lesion to provide a protective cushion of fluid between the lesion to be excised and the underlying ureter or blood vessels. The fluid under the implant absorbs the CO_2 laser energy, buffering the underlying tissue. For retroperitoneal disease, the lesion is picked up with grasping forceps, pulled medially, and removed, using sharp or blunt dissection.

Superficial peritoneal endometriosis is vaporized with the laser, coagulated with monopolar or bipolar current, or excised. Implants less than 2 mm are coagulated, vaporized, or excised. When lesions exceed 3 mm, vaporization or excision is needed. For lesions greater than 5 mm, deep vaporization or excisional techniques are used. Superficial implants on the pelvic side wall are ablated with the CO_2 laser (3500 to 5500 W/cm^2). Low-power densities cause greater damage and more charring. High-power densities penetrate too deeply and injure underlying normal structures or cause unnecessary bleeding. Firing in a continuous mode will ablate the lesion from the surface to its base, where the peritoneal fat should appear as unpigmented and soft rather than fibrotic, like endometriosis or scars. To suction the laser plume and irrigate the lesion base, the suction–irrigator is placed next to or behind the lesion, removing char and identifying any vascular structure within the operative field. If carbon is allowed to accumulate, the field is obscured. In either situation, carbon may be mistaken for endometriosis. Therefore, if vaporization is chosen, it is important to copiously irrigate and remove the charred areas to confirm complete removal of the lesion and avoid confusing endometriosis with a carbon deposit.

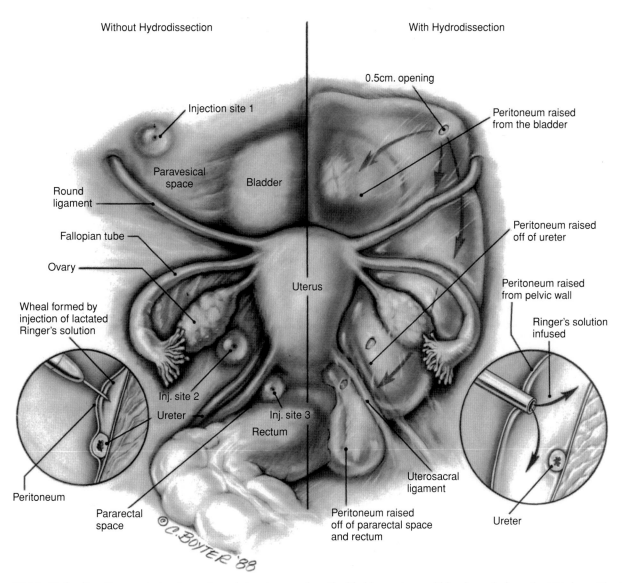

Figure 10.3.3. Hydrodissection protects retroperitoneal structures such as the bladder, ureter, and blood vessels from the CO_2 laser. The *insets* show the creation of retroperitoneal space.

When used in the superpulse/ultrapulse mode, this laser achieves more rapid vaporization and decreased carbonization.

Resection of Ovarian Endometriosis

The ovaries are a common site for endometriosis. Ovarian endometriosis causes adhesions between the ovarian surface and the broad ligament. In 1921, Sampson [90] noted that the histologic findings varied in different portions of the same cyst. Some implants also developed from spilling of the contents of endometriomas after rupture, resulting in the invasion of functional cysts by these surface implants. Large endometriomas could develop because of secondary involvement of follicular or luteal cysts by surface implants. Ovarian implants are similar to endometriosis in extra-ovarian sites and are limited in size by fibrosis and scarring. Endometriomas might originate from metaplasia of the celomic epithelium that lines the cystic epithelial inclusions that frequently are found in the ovaries.[91,92] Sampson [90] believed that there was local spread of endometriosis by salpingeal reflux.

The accepted histologic criterion for the diagnosis of endometriosis is the presence of endometrial glands and stroma.[93] Chernobilsky and Morris [94] described a variety of epithelial characteristics found in ovarian endometriosis. Nissole-Pochet and associates [95] studied 113 instances of ovarian endometriosis before and after hormone therapy. Those authors could identify typical endometrial glandular epithelium and stroma. In 18%, only the endometrial epithelium lined the cyst. Areas with ciliated cells representing oviduct-like epithelium were observed in 47%. In the others, flattened endometrial epithelium and typical glandular and stromal structures were seen. Martin and Berry [96] examined 41 "chocolate" cysts and found that 61% were endometriomas, 27% were corpora lutea, and in 12%, no lining was found. Vercellini and coworkers [84] confirmed 97.7% of visually diagnosed endometriomas by using at least two of the following microscopic patterns to diagnose them: (1) the presence of endometrial epithelium, (2) endometrial glands or glandlike structures, or (3) endometrial stroma and hemosiderin-laden macrophages.

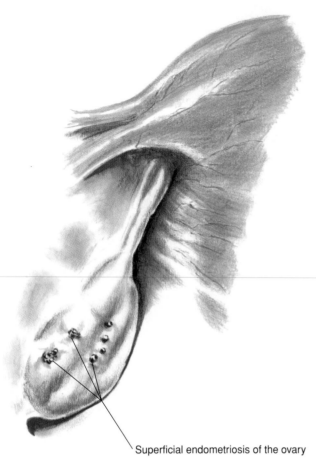

Superficial endometriosis of the ovary

Figure 10.3.4. Superficial implants are seen on this ovary.

Endometriotic implants or endometriomas less than 2 cm in diameter are coagulated, laser ablated, or excised, using scissors, biopsy forceps, lasers, or electrodes (Figure 10.3.4). For successful eradication, all visible lesions and scars must be removed from the ovarian surface. Entrapment of oocytes within the luteinized ovarian follicle, as reported in experimental animal models, must be avoided.[97] Draining the endometrioma or partially resecting its wall is inadequate because the endometrial tissue lining the cyst can remain functional and may cause the symptoms to recur.[98] However, photocoagulation of the cyst wall has been equally therapeutic and occasionally less difficult.[41,99,100] Brosens and Puttemansi [99] recommended cytology and biopsy of the cyst wall before ablating the cyst. When a double optic laparoscope, which involves the passage of a smaller operative endoscope through the channel of the main laparoscope, is used, the ovarian cyst is punctured and drained, the fluid is sent for cytology, and the lining is inspected visually. Any suspicious area is biopsied, and the specimen is sent for frozen section. Once it has been ascertained that the cyst is not malignant, its wall is ablated to a depth of 3 to 4 mm using a laser or an electrocoagulator introduced through the operative channel of the second laparoscope. This procedure is analogous to endometrial ablation and seems to be successful, with no recurrence on follow-up ultrasound or second-look laparoscopy.

Endometriomas can be classified as types I to IV. Type I endometriomas are 1 to 2 cm in size and contain dark fluid (Figure 10.3.5). They develop from surface endometriotic implants

and are difficult to excise. Microscopically, endometrial tissue is seen in all of them. Although small, these endometriomas are difficult to remove intact because of associated fibrosis and adhesions. They can be biopsied, drained, and vaporized by using a laser or electrosurgery or removed in pieces.

Type IIA endometriomas are hemorrhagic cysts and grossly look like endometriomas. The cyst wall is separated easily from the ovarian tissue. Endometriotic implants are superficial and adjacent to a hemorrhagic cyst, which is either follicular or luteal in origin; microscopically, no endometrial lining is seen.

In type IIA lesions, the peri-ovarian adhesions are lysed, the ovarian cortex is evaluated, and the cyst is aspirated. Superficial ovarian implants adjacent to the cyst are vaporized or excised. The cyst is opened, its wall is examined, and a biopsy specimen is taken for frozen section. If it has a yellowish appearance, removal is easy (Figure 10.3.6). Postoperatively, either danazol 800 mg/day or a gonadotropin-releasing hormone (GnRH) analogue may be used for 6 to 8 weeks.

In type IIB lesions, the cyst lining is separated easily from the ovarian capsule and stroma, except near the endometrial implant. In type IIC lesions, surface endometrial implants penetrate deeply into the cyst wall, making excision difficult. Histologic findings of endometriosis are seen in the cyst wall in these two subtypes. The basis for differentiating between these two subtypes is the progressive difficulty in removing the cyst wall.

Type IIB and type IIC endometriomas are large and are associated with peri-ovarian adhesions that attach them to the pelvic side wall and the back of the uterus. When suction and irrigation are alternated, the contents are removed. The inside of the cyst is examined, and the portion of ovarian cortex involved with endometriosis is removed. Using the grasping forceps and the suction–irrigator probe, the cyst wall is grasped and separated from the ovarian stroma by traction and countertraction.[101] Small blood vessels from the ovarian bed and bleeding from the ovarian hilum are controlled with bipolar electrocoagulation.

In type IIC lesions, it is difficult to develop a cleavage plane between the cyst wall and the ovarian stroma. The portion of the ovary attached to the cyst wall is removed until a clear boundary is found so that the entire cyst can be extirpated. The remainder of the procedure is similar to that which was described earlier. The edges of the ovarian defect are brought together with a low-power laser or electrosurgery. Low-power, continuous laser or bipolar coagulation applied to the inside wall of the redundant ovarian capsule causes it to invert. Excessive coagulation of the adjacent ovarian stroma must be avoided. If sutures are needed, they are placed inside the capsule, and 4-0 polyglycolic material is used. Fewer sutures result in fewer adhesions.[102]

The least invasive and technically simplest approach to endometriomas involves laparoscopic fenestration and removal of "chocolate" fluid without cystectomy or ablation of the cyst wall. However, fenestration and irrigation are ineffective, as evidenced by a 50% recurrence rate. Fayez and Vogel [103] made a wide opening in the cyst wall to drain its contents. They claimed that their technique created fewer periadnexal adhesions (27%). Vercellini and associates [99] showed that aspiration of the cyst and irrigation of the endometriomas were ineffective. In 33 women, most endometriomas recurred, although many patients took GnRH analogues postoperatively. Hasson [98] noted recurrences in eight of nine endometriomas treated by fenestration alone.

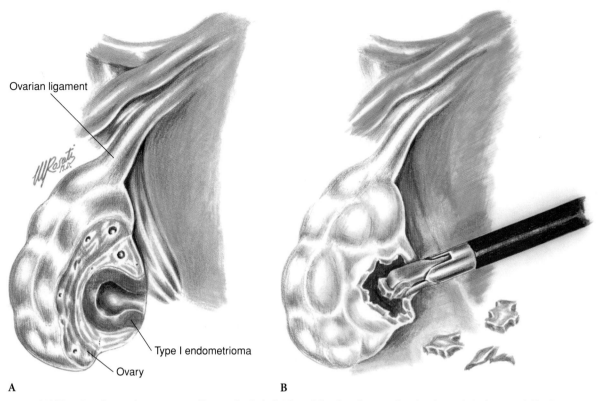

Figure 10.3.5. (**A**) Type I endometriomas are small, contain dark fluid, and develop from surface implants. (**B**) They are difficult to remove intact because of associated adhesions and fibrosis.

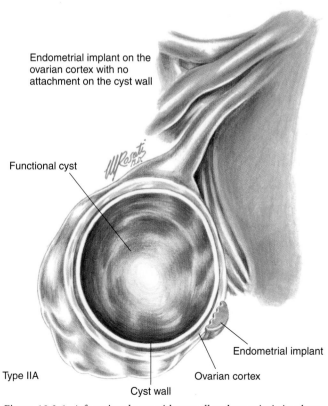

Figure 10.3.6. A functional cyst with a small endometriotic implant.

For endometriomas over 2 cm in diameter, the cyst is punctured with the 5-mm trocar and aspirated with the suction–irrigator probe. Using high-pressure irrigation at 500 to 800 mm Hg, the cyst is irrigated, causing it to expand, and is aspirated several times.[104] This procedure allows examination of the cyst wall. After the repeated expansion and shrinkage with irrigation and suction, the cyst wall should separate from the surrounding ovarian stroma (Figure 10.3.7). If it does not, 5 to 20 mL of lactated Ringer's solution is injected between the stroma and the cyst wall. The cyst wall is removed by grasping its base with laparoscopic forceps and peeling it from the ovarian stroma (Figure 10.3.8). If this is not successful, the wall is separated from the ovarian cortex with forceps at the puncture site. A cleavage plane is created by pulling the two forceps apart and cutting between the structures. Use of the laser or electrosurgery minimizes bleeding because the blood vessels supplying the endometrioma are usually small enough to be cut and coagulated simultaneously. Another method involves hydrodissection of the plane between the cyst wall and the ovarian stroma.[23,43] These techniques may be applied successfully to completely remove the cyst wall, which should be sent for histologic evaluation to rule out malignancy. If the entire cyst cannot be separated from the ovary, the adherent sections are ablated or coagulated.[98–100,104] When the entire cyst wall is ablated, representative biopsy specimens are taken for histologic diagnosis. These endometriomas tend to rupture during separation because of their adherence to other pelvic structures. Because it is difficult to develop a plane between the cyst wall and the ovarian stroma, the portion of the ovary attached to the

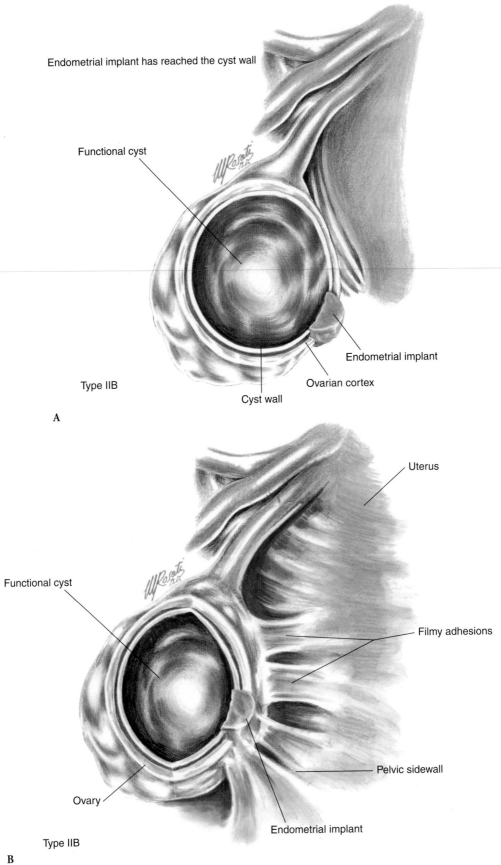

Endometrial implant has reached the cyst wall

Functional cyst

Endometrial implant

Ovarian cortex

Cyst wall

Type IIB

A

Uterus

Functional cyst

Filmy adhesions

Pelvic sidewall

Ovary

Endometrial implant

Type IIB

B

Figure 10.3.7. (**A**) A type IIB endometrioma with features of a functional cyst involved deeply with histologic findings of endometriosis in the cyst wall. The cyst wall is separated easily from the ovarian capsule and stroma except where adjacent to the areas of endometriosis. (**B**) In this type IIB lesion, the endometriotic implant has reached the cyst wall. (*Continued*)

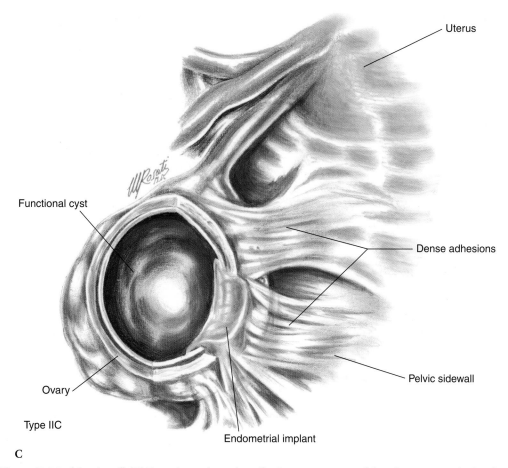

Uterus

Functional cyst

Dense adhesions

Ovary

Pelvic sidewall

Type IIC

Endometrial implant

C

Figure 10.3.7. (*Continued*) (**C**) Extensive peri-ovarian adhesions are present, and there is more extensive involvement of the cyst wall with endometriotic implants. When suction and irrigation are alternated, the inside of the cyst can be explored.

cyst wall is removed until an area is located to produce a line of cleavage.

Cyst wall closure is not necessary, according to animal experiments [105] and clinical experience.[106] For large defects that result from resecting endometriomas larger than 5 cm, the edges of the ovarian cortex are approximated with a single suture placed within the ovarian stroma. The knot is tied inside the ovary so that no part of the suture penetrates the ovarian cortex or is exposed to the ovarian surface to minimize adhesion formation. Fibrin sealant has been described to atraumatically approximate the edges of large ovarian defects (Figure 10.3.9).[107]

Rare patients present with localized symptoms and severe involvement of the ovary with disease and adhesions while the opposite ovary is normal, requiring unilateral salpingo-oophorectomy. When the diseased ovary is removed, the risk of disease recurrence is minimized, and the fertility potential is improved by limiting ovulation to the healthy side. In a prospective trial, Beretta and coauthors [108] randomly allocated 64 patients with advanced stages of endometriosis to undergo either cystectomy of the endometrioma or drainage of the endometrioma and bipolar coagulation of the inner lining. The 24-month cumulative recurrence rates of dysmenorrhea, deep dyspareunia, and nonmenstrual pelvic pain were lower in the patients who underwent cystectomy than in those who did not (dysmenorrhea, 15.8% vs. 52.9%; deep dyspareunia, 20% vs. 75%; nonmenstrual pelvic pain, 10% vs. 52.9%). The median interval between the operation and the recurrence of moderate to severe pelvic

pain was longer after cystectomy: 19 months compared with 5 months. The 24-month cumulative pregnancy rate was higher after cystectomy: 66.7% compared with 23.5%. For the treatment of ovarian endometriomas, a better outcome with a similar rate of complications is achieved with laparoscopic cystectomy than with drainage and coagulation.

The efficacy of laparoscopy done by applying the stripping technique was compared retrospectively with that of microsurgery by laparotomy in 132 women under 40 years of age with ovarian endometriotic cysts at least 3 cm in diameter, stages III and IV endometriosis, rAFS classification.[109] The recurrence rate of ovarian cysts, symptomatic improvement, and the reproductive outcome were found to be comparable for the two groups. However, as was expected, laparoscopy resulted in less postoperative febrile morbidity and a significantly shorter duration of hospitalization. The long-term results of laparoscopic fenestration and coagulation of ovarian endometriomas were investigated in a case-control study and compared with the results of ovarian cystectomy done by either laparotomy or laparoscopy.[110] The study enrolled 156 premenopausal women with ovarian endometriomas at least 3 cm in diameter, stages III and IV endometriosis, rAFS classification. The mean time to first pregnancy was shorter in the 80 patients who underwent laparoscopic ovarian fenestration and coagulation (1.4 years) than it was in the 23 patients who underwent laparoscopic ovarian cystectomy (2.2 years) or the 53 patients who underwent ovarian cystectomy by laparotomy and a microsurgical technique (2.4 years).

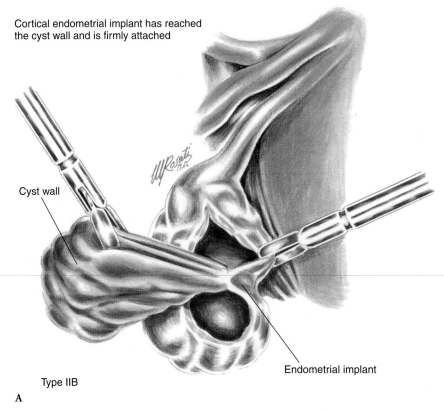

Cortical endometrial implant has reached the cyst wall and is firmly attached

Cyst wall

Endometrial implant

Type IIB

A

Figure 10.3.8. (**A**) The lining is separated easily from the ovarian capsule and stroma except where adjacent to the areas of endometriosis.

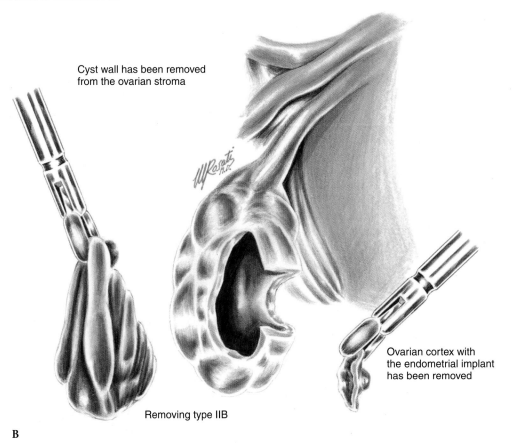

Cyst wall has been removed from the ovarian stroma

Ovarian cortex with the endometrial implant has been removed

Removing type IIB

B

Figure 10.3.8. (**B**) The cyst wall has been removed, and a piece of the ovarian cortex with the endometrial implant has been excised. Using the grasping forceps and the suction–irrigator probe, the cyst wall is separated from the ovarian cortex by traction and countertraction.

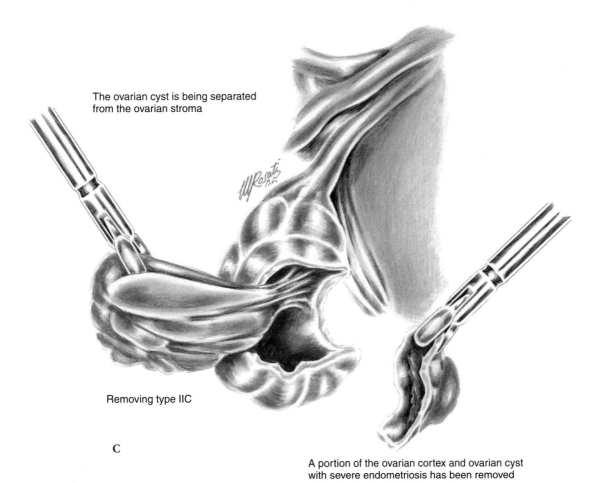

The ovarian cyst is being separated from the ovarian stroma

Removing type IIC

C

A portion of the ovarian cortex and ovarian cyst with severe endometriosis has been removed

Figure 10.3.8. (*Continued*) (**C**) Surface implants penetrate the cyst wall deeply, making excision difficult. The degree of invasion of the cyst wall forms the basis for differentiating these subgroups.

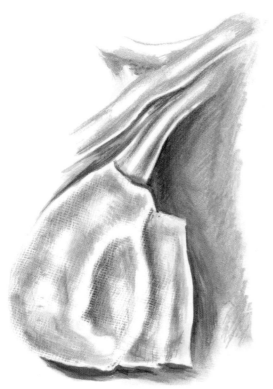

Figure 10.3.9. The resected ovary and adjacent side wall of the pelvis are wrapped with Interceed (Gynecare).

The difference in the recurrence rate and between the cumulative clinical pregnancy rates in the three groups was not statistically significant after 36 months of follow-up. The investigators concluded that laparoscopic ovarian fenestration and coagulation of endometriomas led to faster conception than did ovarian cystectomy by laparotomy. Furthermore, laparoscopic ovarian fenestration and coagulation of endometriomas were associated with cumulative clinical pregnancy rates and recurrence rates over 36 months that were similar to those associated with ovarian cystectomy.

Genitourinary Endometriosis

Endometriosis may spread to the urinary system in 1% to 2% of women with symptomatic endometriosis. Endometriosis of the urinary tract tends to be superficial but may be invasive and cause complete ureteral obstruction.[111] Decreased bladder capacity and stability unresponsive to conventional therapy may result. Goldstein and Brodman [112] reported one case of bladder endometriosis that they monitored cystometrically for 4 years. They found that decreased bladder capacity and bladder instability that were not responsive to conventional parasympatholytic therapy were corrected after surgical destruction of superficial bladder endometriosis. When bladder symptoms recurred 2 years later, a course of danazol again reversed bladder instability. Clinicians should consider endometriosis in cases of refractory and unexplained urinary complaints. If urinary tract endometriosis is suspected, an intravenous pyelogram (IVP), ultrasound of the kidneys, and a routine blood and urine work-up are indicated. In selected cases of recurrent hematuria, cystoscopy is suggested.

Superficial implants over the ureter are treated with a variation of hydrodissection. Approximately 20 to 30 mL of lactated Ringer's solution is injected subperitoneally on the lateral pelvic wall; this elevates the peritoneum and backs it with a bed of fluid. The CO_2 laser may be used to create a 0.5-cm opening on this elevation. The opening in the peritoneum is made anteriorly and laterally, close to the corresponding round ligament. The hydrodissection probe is inserted into the opening, and approximately 100 mL of lactated Ringer's solution is injected under 300 mm Hg pressure into the retroperitoneal space along the course of the ureter. The fluid surrounds the ureter, moves it posteriorly, and allows superficial laser dissection or vaporization of the area.

After a water bed is created, a superpulse or ultrapulse CO_2 laser or any other cutting device (20 to 80 W) may be used to vaporize or excise the lesion with a circumference of 1 to 2 cm. When the lesions are large or excision is preferred, a circular line with a 1- to 2-cm margin is made around the lesion. The peritoneum is held with an atraumatic grasping forceps and peeled away with the help of a cutting instrument and the suction–irrigator probe. If the endometrial implant is embedded and has formed scarring down to the subperitoneal connective tissue, hydrodissection allows water to tunnel beneath the lesion, often separating scar tissue. Then the lesion can be treated safely. After vaporization or excision of these lesions, the area is irrigated and washed to remove all charcoal and verify that the nonpenetrating endometriosis (to the lumen of ureter bladder) has been treated properly. In more than 500 consecutive procedures (275 bladder and 250 ureter), there were no major complications involving vesical or ureteral injury.[15] Two patients were unable to void immediately postoperatively. An indwelling catheter was placed and removed the day after surgery, and then those women were able to void. Four patients with bladder endometriosis experienced minimal hematuria that resolved several hours postoperatively. After hydrodissection of the broad ligaments and the pelvic side wall, about 5% of the patients developed swelling of the external genitalia, most likely from the penetration of water through the inguinal canal to the labia majora. This swelling resolved in most patients within 1 to 2 hours without sequelae.

The surgical management of 28 women who had deeply infiltrating urinary tract endometriosis has been described.[113] All procedures were accomplished laparoscopically: seven involved the bladder, and 21 the ureter. Patients who had vesical endometriosis underwent partial cystectomy and primary repair. Partial ureteral obstruction was found in 17 women; 10 underwent ureterolysis and excision of endometriosis, and seven had partial wall resection. Four patients with ureteral involvement had complete obstruction. Three underwent partial resection and ureteroureterostomy, and one had ureteroneocystostomy. Severe infiltrative endometriosis of the bladder and the ureter may present without specific symptoms and may cause silent compromise of renal function.

Laparoscopic closure of intentional or unintentional bladder lacerations during operative laparoscopy was done in 19 women with one layer using interrupted absorbable polyglycolic suture or polydioxanone suture (PDS) followed by 7 to 14 days of transurethral drainage.[114] Complications were limited to

one vesicovaginal fistula that required reoperation. After 6 to 48 months of follow-up, all these patients had a good outcome. A new laparoscopic technique for the treatment of infiltrative ureteral endometriosis, a laparoscopic vesicopsoas hitch, was described. In a 36-year-old woman with infiltrative endometriosis of the ureter after partial ureteral resection, it was noted that a tension-free anastomosis to the bladder was not possible. Thus, a laparoscopic vesicopsoas hitch was done.[115]

As a result, depending on the extent of ureteral involvement, ureterolysis with or without ureteral resection can be performed safely and effectively with the laparoscopic approach. The ultimate goal is to avoid ureteral obstruction and loss of renal function. Success is dependent on careful preoperative evaluation, surgical planning, and careful postoperative follow-up. Radiologic imaging, laparoscopy, and ureteroscopy are useful techniques for disease staging that the laparoscopic surgeon should be familiar with. Complete resection remains the mainstay of therapy in cases refractory to conservative medical management. Urinary symptoms generally resolve, and recurrence generally does not occur provided that the lesion is completely resected. In experienced hands, laparoscopy is not only feasible but also has become the standard of care in many centers.

Ureteral Involvement

Ureteral involvement by endometriosis is rare and occurs in 0.1% to 0.4% of cases. It most commonly affects the distal ureter, less commonly the mid-ureter, and rarely the proximal ureter.[116–118] Lesions are typically extrinsic, with a smaller fraction of cases involving the lumen of the ureter (i.e., intrinsic). The extrinsic-to-intrinsic ratio has been reported at 3:1 to 4:1, and the left ureter appears to be more frequently involved.[116,117,119] In cases of ureteral involvement, the patient typically has concomitant pelvic endometriosis that causes external compression, inflammation, and fibrosis of the involved ureter. The patient may present with symptoms of renal colic, hematuria, or silent urinary obstruction with loss of renal function. The latter presentation is worrisome, and early recognition is of key importance in preventing irreversible damage to the kidneys.[118,120–122] Thus, ureteral endometriosis must be on the differential diagnosis in a premenopausal woman with unilateral or bilateral ureteral obstruction of uncertain etiology.

DIAGNOSIS

Silent obstruction with loss of renal function occurs in 5% to 30% of women with endometriosis; thus, early disease recognition is critical.[123,124] Diagnosis is most easily made by laparoscopy with tissue biopsy, and in cases of primary intrinsic ureteral endometriosis, retrograde pyelogram and ureteroscopy are useful.[117,124] Radiologic imaging of the ureter, including IVP, retrograde pyelograms, and computed tomographic IVP, is useful in defining the extent of ureteral involvement and for preoperative planning.

SURGICAL TECHNIQUE

Preoperative assessment of the location and extent of ureteral involvement is key to successful surgical management. Intraoperatively, ureterolysis is performed, and the goal is to treat all pelvic endometriosis with excision or ablation. The surgical techniques of laparoscopic ureterolysis for endometriosis are similar to that first described for the treatment of retroperitoneal fibrosis when the technique was first described.[125,126] During ureterolysis, care is taken to preserve the periureteral vascular supply if the ureter is not directly affected by endometriosis, fibrosis, or inflammation. The blood supply to the distal ureter typically comes laterally from the iliac artery, whereas the mid- and proximal ureters' blood supply comes medially from the aorta. There is also a fine network of vessels that travel along the length of the ureter. Thus, ureterolysis must preserve the periureteral tissue and adventitia of the ureter. In cases in which extrinsic ureteral involvement is minimal, ureterolysis alone may be all that is needed.[127] The principles of success include atraumatic handling of the ureter and when feasible, interposition of normal tissue, such as omentum.

In cases in which the ureter is strictured and directly affected, the goal is to resect all of the diseased ureter and then reconstitute urinary continuity. Surgical principles of ureteral surgery are the same in laparoscopy. The ureter should be spatulated, and fine interrupted absorbable sutures such as 5-0 or 4-0 are used. In the majority of cases, only the distal third of the ureter is involved, and when the length of the involved ureter is short (≤ 2 cm), resection followed by an end-to-end ureteroureterostomy may be performed.[128] However, when involvement of the distal ureter is more extensive, ureteral reimplantation to the dome of the bladder in a refluxing, tension-free manner may be needed. To identify the most appropriate location for the reimplant, the bladder may be filled with saline, and the cystoscope may be used to "light" a location on the dome of the bladder that can be reached easily by the spatulated ureter. A simple 5-0 holding stitch is placed laparoscopically onto the bladder detrusor at the cystoscope light. A transmural cystotomy can then be created precisely around this stitch for the reimplant.

If additional ureter length is needed, a vesicopsoas hitch with or without a vesical flap may be performed.[116] The detrusor fiber of the bladder is tacked down to the psoas with either absorbable or nonabsorbable suture to minimize tension on the reimplanted ureter. The laparoscopic surgeon should be aware of the location of the genital–femoral nerve as it crosses the surface of the psoas. The stitch is usually placed parallel to the nerve either lateral or medial to it to avoid nerve entrapment. Should additional length be required, the contralateral superior vesical pedicles can be divided to give upward mobility to the bladder. Rarely, a vesical flap or an ileal ureter may also be used for replacement of the entire ureter.[116,129] However, the laparoscopic approach for complete ureteral substitution is technically demanding and beyond the scope of our discussion. Nevertheless, it is important to note that in selecting a vesical flap, a bladder of sufficient capacity is required.

Except for simple cases of ureterolysis in which ureter manipulation is minimal, a double-J ureteral stent is placed and left indwelling for 3 to 6 weeks. In clinic follow-up, the stent is removed and an IVP is typically obtained in 3 to 4 weeks to assess ureter anatomy and to rule out strictures. A renal bladder ultrasound may also be useful in assessment of hydronephrosis.

Ureteral Obstruction

The incidence of ureteral obstruction by endometriosis is low, and conventional therapy previously consisted of laparotomy and resection of the obstructed segment of the ureter. Laparoscopic ureteroureterostomy was accomplished in 1990 by Nezhat and

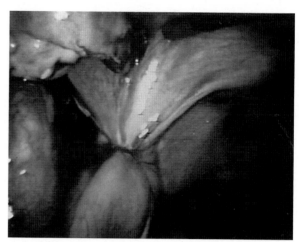

Figure 10.3.10. At laparoscopy, a 3- to 4-cm nodule was found over the left ureter about 4 cm above the bladder, distorting the course of the ureter.

colleagues [130] on a 36-year-old woman with long-term ureteral obstruction caused by endometriosis. The condition had been diagnosed previously at laparoscopy. The patient refused conventional laparotomy and had a nephrostomy tube for 4 years. At laparoscopy, a 3- to 4-cm fibrotic nodule over the left ureter was seen, approximately 4 cm above the bladder, distorting the course of the ureter (Figure 10.3.10). This corresponded to the level of obstruction seen on radioimaging techniques. Under direct laparoscopic observation, an attempt to place a retrograde catheter was unsuccessful, and so the nodule was excised. The left retroperitoneal space was entered at the pelvic brim. After all associated endometriosis, fibrosis, or adhesions were treated, the ureter was dissected (Figure 10.3.11). The nodule involved the entire thickness of the ureter; a partial resection was done (Figure 10.3.12).

Under cystoscopic guidance, a 7F ureteral catheter was passed through the ureterovesical junction, at which level the ureter was excised. Indigo carmine was injected into the patient's intravenous line to ensure patency of the proximal ureter. The distal ureter was transected over the stent, and the obstructed portion was removed. The ureteral stent was introduced into the

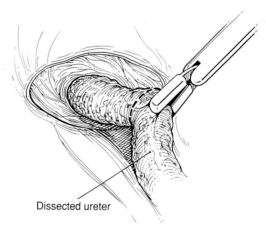

Dissected ureter

Figure 10.3.11. After all associated endometriosis, fibrosis, and adhesions were treated, the ureter was dissected with the CO_2 laser.

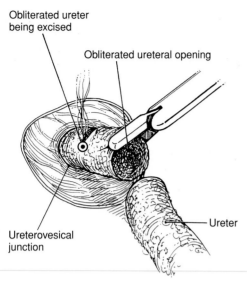

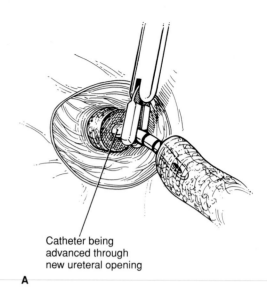

A

Figure 10.3.12. During dissection, it was discovered that the nodule involved the entire thickness of the ureter; a partial resection was done.

proximal ureter and advanced into the renal pelvis (Figure 10.3.13). Finally, the edges of the ureter were reapproximated with sutures. To accomplish anastomosis, four interrupted 4-0 PDS were placed at 6, 12, 9, and 3 o'clock to approximate the proximal and distal ureteral ostia (Figure 10.3.14). The patient went home the next day. The postoperative course was uncomplicated. An IVP confirmed ureteral patency and renal function (Figure 10.3.15). Estimated blood loss was less than 100 mL, and the procedure lasted 117 minutes. The pathology report confirmed severe endometriosis and fibrosis of the resected ureter.

Since that time, 12 more patients with severe ureteral endometriosis in whom endometriosis and fibrosis caused partial or complete ureteral obstruction have been treated. All these patients had a known history of endometriosis and underwent different surgical and medical treatments. In four women, the ureteral endometriosis was removed completely without entering the ureteral lumen. In three women, the obstructed ureter required a complete segmental resection. One right and one left ureteroureterostomy and one anastomosis of the left ureter to the bladder (ureteroneocystostomy) were achieved, using four through-and-through interrupted 4-0 PDS to approximate the edges over the ureteral catheter. In five women, the ureter was involved partially. The severe retroperitoneal and ureteral endometriosis was excised or vaporized cautiously with the CO_2 laser until ureterotomy occurred. In three women, the ureterotomy was very small and was detected by intravenous injection of indigo carmine. A ureteral stent was left in place, and no suture was required. In two patients, the ureterotomy was repaired using 4-0 PDS to overlap the laceration after stent placement. Histologic examination of the resected specimen revealed fibrosis, endometriosis, or both in all the women. A rare case of endometriosis with focal severely atypical hyperplasia was found in the specimen of a 46-year-old woman. She had undergone total abdominal hysterectomy and BSO followed by HRT at another institution. All the patients had an uneventful intra- and postoperative course and reported symptomatic relief of their symptoms. Imaging techniques revealed patent ureters with a functioning kidney in all these patients except one, a 24-year-old woman

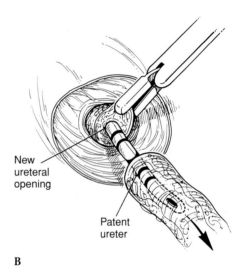

B

Figure 10.3.13. The ureteral stent was introduced into the proximal ureter and advanced into the renal pelvis.

who had been diagnosed several months earlier with pelvic endometriosis that was treated partially at initial laparoscopy, followed by GnRH analogue therapy postoperatively. During a

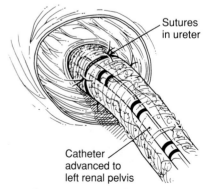

Figure 10.3.14. To do an anastomosis, four interrupted 4-0 polydioxanone sutures were placed at 6, 12, 9, and 3 o'clock to approximate the proximal and distal ureteral edges.

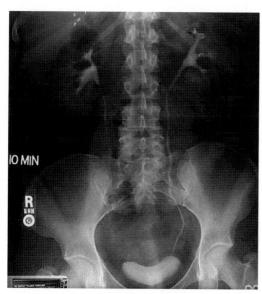

Figure 10.3.15. An IVP confirmed bilateral patency and renal function.

second laparoscopy, she was found to have severe endometriosis involving left uterosacral ligament, left pelvic sidewall, and ureter causing complete ureteral obstruction. Segmental resection and ureteroureterostomy were accomplished. Intraoperative intravenous injection of indigo carmine did not reveal any leakage from the ureter and raised the question of a nonfunctioning kidney. Postoperative follow-up and imaging revealed a 10% to 20% functioning kidney. However, the ureter was noted to be patent. The authors suggested that in such cases, a ureteral stent is left in the ureter. This stent remains in place for approximately 2 months postoperatively. The patient's follow-up should include IVP, ultrasound, or excretion scans.

Recently, clinical results of six patients who underwent successful laparoscopic ureteroneocystostomy and vesicopsoas hitch were published.[131] Five of the six patients had a history of endometriosis, and their obstructions were diagnosed during prior surgeries. The other patient was diagnosed with severe endometriosis of the rectum, bladder, and ureter at the time of the procedure. All patients had a normal cystogram performed 10 to 14 days postoperatively prior to Foley catheter removal. Stents were kept in place for 6 to 8 weeks, and an IVP was done 2 weeks after removal. All patients had a normal renal ultrasound, computer tomography, or IVP at least 1 year postoperatively. As a conclusion, laparoscopic vesicopsoas hitch can be a safe and effective alternative to laparotomy with the known benefits of laparoscopy.

Vesical Endometriosis

Although the bladder wall is one of the sites least frequently involved with endometriosis, the bladder is the most commonly affected site in the urinary system, followed by the ureter and the kidney in a ratio of 40:5:1.[123–133] Patient presentation is quite variable, and symptoms may consist of suprapubic discomfort, pelvic pain, dysmenorrhea, dysuria, urinary frequency, urgency, microscopic hematuria, and even cyclical gross hematuria. Endometriomas are typically solitary and most frequently involve the dome and posterior wall of the bladder because of the

relative location of the uterus to the bladder. However, involvement of other locations of the bladder may occur. The lesions tend to invade the detrusor musculature in an extrinsic fashion and often remain submucosal.[112]

DIAGNOSIS

Prompt diagnosis requires clinical acumen and vigilance. Often, patients will give a history of pelvic endometriosis, cesarean delivery, or other gynecologic surgery.[134] Direct visualization of the endometrioma via cystoscopy and laparoscopy is important. Cystoscopically, lesions appear as solitary submucosal lesions that are slightly raised, with little surrounding mucosal edema in the absence of concomitant cystitis or infection. Transurethral biopsy or resection may be inadequate for histologic diagnosis because of the submucosal nature of the lesion. Extravesically, the lesions can be identified by laparoscopy, and direct biopsy remains the gold standard of disease diagnosis and staging. However, the actual extent of bladder involvement may be difficult to completely visualize in laparoscopy. Thus, a combined cystoscopic and laparoscopic approach is needed during definitive surgical resection.

SURGICAL MANAGEMENT

Although medical management can be transiently effective in some patients, surgical resection of the endometrioma in toto remains the most definitive therapy. Minimally invasive approaches using combined cystoscopy and laparoscopy techniques are becoming the standard of care for solitary lesions. If the lesions are superficial, hydrodissection and vaporization or excision may be adequate for removal (Figure 10.3.16). Using hydrodissection, the areolar tissue between the serosa and muscularis beneath the implants is dissected. The lesion is circumcised, and fluid is injected into the resulting defect. The lesion is grasped with forceps and dissected. Frequent irrigation is necessary to remove char, ascertain the depth of vaporization or excision, and ensure that the lesion does not involve the muscularis and the mucosa.

Endometriosis extending to the muscularis but without mucosal involvement can be treated laparoscopically, and any residual or deeper lesions may be treated successfully with postoperative hormone therapy. In selected cases in which the endometrioma is small and clearly submucosal, a mucosal-sparing approach may be used. In this approach, the light of the cystoscope is simply directed close to the endometrioma to provide "backlighting" for laparoscopic dissection. If successful, postoperative irritative voiding symptoms as well as hematuria may be avoided in the patients.

When endometriosis involves full bladder wall thickness, the lesion is excised and the bladder is reconstructed.[135] Four cases of full-thickness bladder endometriosis were treated by excision and a one-layer reconstruction. The exposure seemed to be better than that at laparotomy. Simultaneous cystoscopy is performed, and bilateral ureteral catheters are inserted. The bladder dome is held near the midline with the grasping forceps, and the endometriotic nodule is excised 5 mm beyond the lesion (Figure 10.3.17).

In intravesical endometriosis cases in which the lesion is located in the dome, lateral walls, or posterior wall, partial cystectomy with primary repair of cystotomy is the treatment of choice if adequate postresection capacity can be maintained.[135,136]

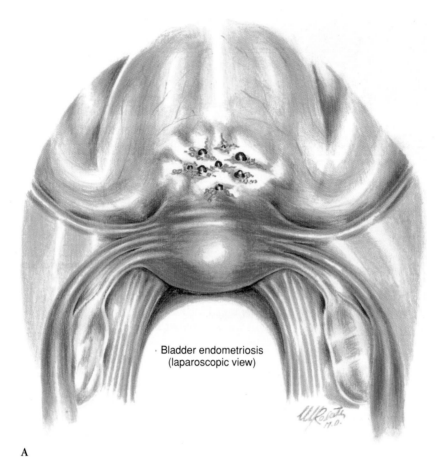

A

Figure 10.3.16. (**A**) Endometriosis involves the anterior lower uterine segment and the bladder. The extent of vesical involvement cannot be ascertained from this view.

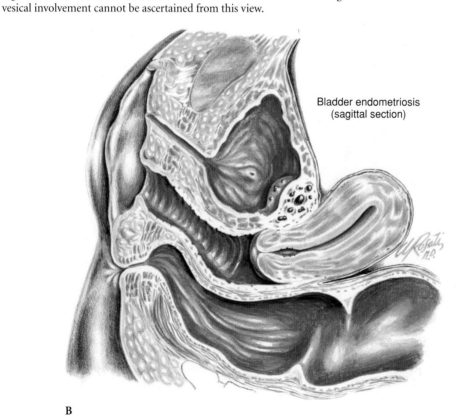

B

Figure 10.3.16. (**B**) The sagittal sections show that the muscularis and mucosal surface of the bladder are involved.

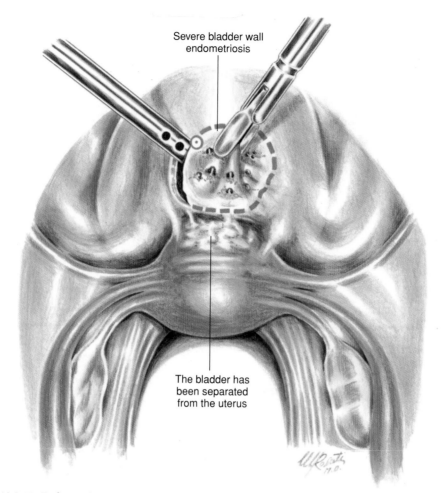

Figure 10.3.17. Endometriosis involving the bladder is being excised with the CO_2 laser after the bladder has been separated from the uterus. The lesion involves the full thickness of the bladder. Bilateral ureteral catheters were inserted during simultaneous cystoscopy. The endometrial implants were excised 5 mm beyond the lesion.

In rare cases in which the lesions involve areas of the trigone or near either ureteral orifice, partial cystectomy with ureteral reimplantation may be necessary. With either approach, cystoscopy is first used to characterize the full extent of the lesion. Then, using an electrocautery cutting device through the cystoscope, the lesion is marked circumferentially. The light intensity of the laparoscope is turned down to a minimum so that the light of the cystoscope can be visualized transvesically. The cystoscopically guided dissection is carried deep into the detrusor musculature but without bladder perforation. The bladder should be moderately distended during this dissection to avoid inadvertently taking too much normal tissue around the endometrioma. Of note, overdistention must also be avoided because of the increased risk of bladder perforation. Once the lesion is marked intravesically, the surgeon turns to extravesical dissection with laparoscopic guidance. Cutting "toward the light" of the cystoscope will provide accuracy. Often, the peritoneal covering over the dome of the bladder must first be incised to gain access to lesions located near the trigone of deep in the posterior wall of the bladder.

The specimen is removed from the abdominal cavity with a long grasping forceps through the operative channel of the laparoscope. Alternatively, once resected, the lesion is placed into a laparoscopic retrieval device for later removal. CO_2 gas distends the bladder cavity, allowing excellent observation of its interior (Figure 10.3.18). After the ureters have been identified and the bladder mucosa has been examined again, the bladder is closed with several interrupted or continuous 4-0 through-and-through PDS using extracorporeal or intracorporeal knotting (Figure 10.3.19). The bladder can be closed with resorbable sutures in one or two layers. In one-layer closures, it is important to take transmural stitches with more detrusor than mucosa for inversion of the suture line. Once the cystotomy is closed, the bladder is tested for leaks with retrograde filling using methylene blue mixed in saline. Leaks are readily visualized and repaired with simple interrupted sutures. A closed-suction drain is often placed in the pelvis and kept for the first 24 to 48 hours but is not absolutely necessary given the transperitoneal nature of surgery. The duration of laparoscopic segmental cystectomy is approximately 35 minutes. Patients are discharged the following day and instructed to take trimethoprim-sulfamethoxazole for 2 weeks. A urinary catheter is left indwelling for 10 to 14 days and removed when the postoperative voiding cystourethrogram or retrograde cystogram demonstrates no leakage at follow-up. Anticholinergics such as oxybutynin or tolterodine may be useful during early recovery to minimize bladder spasms. Blood loss is minimal. In these reports on excisional treatment for full-thickness bladder endometriosis, the pathology report confirmed severe endometriosis and fibrosis of the resected bladder wall. No

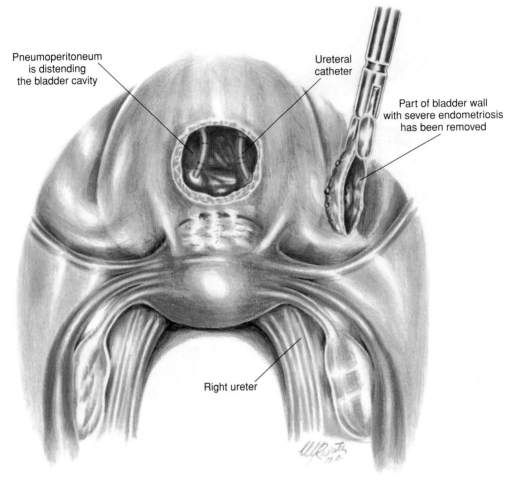

Figure 10.3.18. The lesion is removed with a grasping forceps through a 10-mm trocar sleeve.

intraoperative or postoperative complications were noted. Ten to 13 months postoperatively, the women were doing well.

Gastrointestinal Involvement

Gastrointestinal endometriosis was described in 1909 by Sampson [137] during the histologic examination of resected sigmoid colon that had been diagnosed intraoperatively as a carcinoma. The gastrointestinal tract is believed to be involved in 3% to 37% of women with endometriosis.[138–139] However, in a specialized practice, the number of patients with bowel involvement may be as high as 50% if patients with serosal and subserosal lesions are included. Endometriotic implants may be found between the small intestine and the anal canal. The clinical presentation varies from an incidental finding at celiotomy to bowel obstruction.[140]

Severe endometriosis commonly involves the uterosacral ligaments, rectovaginal septum, and rectosigmoid colon with partial or complete posterior cul-de-sac obliteration. Patients may present with lower abdominal pain, back pain, dysmenorrhea, dyspareunia, diarrhea, constipation, tenesmus, and occasionally rectal bleeding.[138] Symptoms usually occur cyclically at or about the time of menstruation.

Intestinal endometriosis should be suspected in women of childbearing age who present with gastrointestinal symptoms and a history of endometriosis. Proctoscopy and colonoscopy are suggestive, but the lesions usually are not identified before laparoscopy. Although microscopic examination of the bowel mucosa may reveal endometrial glands, colonoscopic biopsy is usually not diagnostic.[141] In patients with severe symptoms, medical therapy rarely yields satisfactory long-term results. Surgical intervention is necessary to dissect and resect infiltrating bowel endometriosis. These patients generally undergo videolaparoscopy after previous surgical or hormonal management fails to relieve their discomfort. Large bowel resection for obstructing endometriosis of the sigmoid colon was reported in 1909 by Mackenrodt.[142] Colonic resection has been shown to be safe, with low morbidity, and to provide satisfactory pain relief and favorable pregnancy rates.[143]

Intestinal endometriosis involves the rectum and sigmoid colon in 76% of cases, the appendix in 18%, and the cecum in 5%. Operative laparoscopy is done to treat endometriotic implants on the intestinal wall, appendix, and rectovaginal space.

APPENDICEAL ENDOMETRIOSIS

Reports evaluating gastrointestinal endometriosis suggest that the appendix is the second most common site of involvement, with only the rectosigmoid colon being more commonly affected.[144,145] During laparoscopic surgery of patients with chronic pelvic pain and endometriosis, surgeons should be alert to the possible contribution of appendiceal pathology to the pelvic

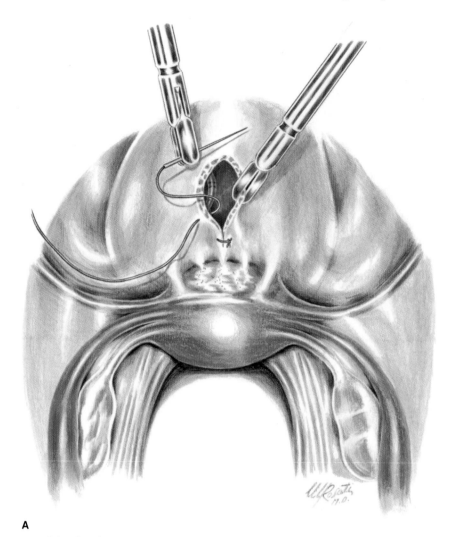

A

Figure 10.3.19. (**A**) After the ureteral orifices and the ureteral catheters have been identified, the bladder is closed with several interrupted through-and-through PDS, using extracorporeal and intracorporeal knot tying. Cystoscopy is done to identify any leaks. (*Continued*)

discomfort of patients with endometriosis. Recently, we have reported the frequency and spectrum of histologically proven diseases of the appendix in patients undergoing laparoscopic surgery for chronic pelvic pain in conjunction with endometriosis.[146] Of the 231 patients with pelvic endometriosis, concomitant appendiceal pathology was present in 115. Notably, of the 231 patients with pelvic endometriosis, 51 (22.1%) had histologic evidence of appendiceal endometriosis. Pathology other than endometriosis was found in 64 (27.7%) of the 231 patients. In another study of 65 women with symptomatic endometriosis and preoperative right lower quadrant pain, 52 underwent appendectomy as part of the endoscopic surgery when Gastrografin enema screening or the visual appearance of appendix was abnormal.[147] Thirty-nine (75%) had histologically confirmed pathology. The current approach for surgical treatment of endometriosis is to excise or fulgurate all suspected areas. The appendix also should be carefully evaluated among all patients undergoing laparoscopy for the evaluation and treatment of endometriosis. However, more prospective, randomized studies may be required before "routine" appendectomy can be recommended in women with chronic pelvic pain and endometriosis.

BOWEL RESECTION

In patients who have severe disease of the bowel wall, resection may be necessary. Laparoscopically assisted anterior rectal wall resection and anastomosis were described in 1991 to treat symptomatic, infiltrative rectosigmoid endometriosis.[148,149] Preoperative mechanical and antibiotic bowel preparation is necessary. Three 5-mm suprapubic trocars are placed, one each in the midline, right, and left lower quadrants for the insertion of grasping forceps, Endoloop suture applicators, a suction–irrigator probe, and a bipolar electrocoagulator.

The technique includes laparoscopic mobilization of the lower colon, transanal or transvaginal prolapse, resection, and anastomosis.[150–153] When the lesion involves only the anterior rectal wall near the anal verge, the rectovaginal septum is delineated by simultaneous vaginal and rectal examinations effected by an assistant. The rectum is mobilized along the rectovaginal septum anteriorly to within 2 cm of the anus. Mobilization continues along the left and right pararectal spaces by electrodesiccating and dividing branches of the hemorrhoidal artery and partially posteriorly. When the rectum is mobilized sufficiently, the lesion is prolapsed vaginally or anally and the

Interceed

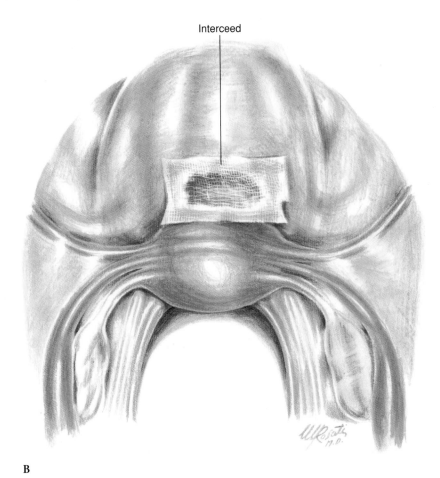

B

Figure 10.3.19. (*Continued*) (**B**) The suture line is covered with Interceed.

nodule is excised. Two staple applications may be required to traverse the width of the involved mucosa. The rectum is returned to the pelvis under direct observation, and closure is confirmed by insufflating the rectum while the cul-de-sac is filled with lactated Ringer's solution.

In patients with circumferential lesions, the entire rectum is mobilized, the lateral rectal pedicles are electrocoagulated, and the presacral space is entered to the level of the levator ani muscles to allow mobilization of the bowel. The branches of the inferior mesenteric vessels of the bowel segment to be resected are coagulated and cut. The rectum is transected proximal to the lesion, and the proximal limb is either prolapsed vaginally or into the distal limb, using Babcock clamps (Figure 10.3.20). A 2-0 purse-string suture is inserted to the end of the proximal bowel to secure the opposing anvil of a number 29 or 33 ILS stapler (Ethicon; Figure 10.3.21). The anvil is replaced transanally or transvaginally into the pelvis along with the proximal bowel.

The rectal stump, containing the endometrial lesion, is prolapsed through the anal canal or vagina and transected proximal to the lesion using an RL60 linear stapler (Ethicon; Figure 10.3.22). The resected segment is sent for pathologic diagnosis. The rectal stump is replaced through the anal canal or vagina into the pelvis. The ILS stapler is placed into the rectum, and the anvil in the proximal limb of the bowel is inserted into the stapling device by using the laparoscope. The device is fired, creating an end-to-end anastomosis. A proctoscope is used to examine

the anastomosis for structural integrity and bleeding. The pelvis is filled with lactated Ringer's solution and observed with the laparoscope as the rectum is insufflated with air to check for leakage. Air leaks can be corrected with 2-0 polyglactin sutures placed transanally. This technique is identical to resection at laparotomy.[154]

Another method uses a 60-mm Endostapler (Ethicon) to resect the bowel intra-abdominally. The Endostapler is fired distal to the lesion. The proximal limb of the colon is delivered from the abdomen and exteriorized through a small (2- to 4-cm) incision. The lesion is amputated, and the anvil of the stapler is inserted in the lumen after the placement of a purse-string suture. At this stage, anastomosis is completed with the stapler gun.

Another method to treat severe disease of the anterior wall of the colon eliminates stapling devices.[155] The extent of the lesion is evaluated visually and by palpation, using the tip of the suction–irrigator probe. If the lesion is low enough, an assistant can identify it by doing a rectal examination. A sigmoidoscope is used to further delineate the lesion and guide the surgeon. After the ureters are identified to avoid inadvertent injury, the lower colon is mobilized in all aspects except posteriorly. Depending on the location of the lesion, the right or left pararectal area is entered, and the colon is separated from the adjacent organs. Full-thickness shaving excision, if necessary, is carried out, beginning above the area of visible disease. After the normal tissue is identified, the lesion is held at its proximal end with grasping forceps.

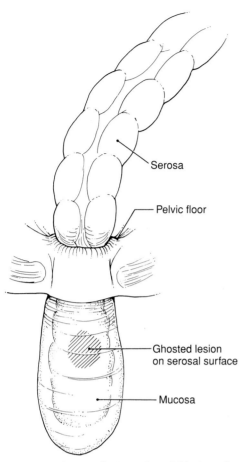

Figure 10.3.20. In patients with circumferential lesions, the rectum is transected distal to the lesion and the proximal limb is prolapsed into the distal bulb.

An incision is made through the bowel serosa and muscularis, and the lumen is entered. The lesion is excised entirely from the anterior rectal wall. After complete excision of the lesion, the pelvic cavity is irrigated and suctioned. Debris is extracted through the operative channel of the laparoscope by using a long grasping forceps, or from the anus by using polyp forceps, and submitted for pathology. The bowel is repaired transversely in one layer. Two traction sutures are applied to each side of the defect, transforming it to a transverse opening (Figure 10.3.23). The stay sutures are brought out through the right and left lower quadrant trocar sleeves. The sleeves are removed and then replaced in the peritoneal cavity next to the stay sutures, and the sutures are secured outside the abdomen. The bowel is repaired by placing several interrupted through-and-through sutures in 0.4- to 0.6-cm increments until it is completely anastomosed (Figure 10.3.24). Polyglactin or polydioxanone sutures with a straight needle (Ethicon) and extracorporeal knot tying are used. At the end of the procedure, sigmoidoscopy is done to ensure that the closure is watertight and that there is no bowel stricture. Results from our center's experience with its use during laparoscopic treatment of adhesions, endometriosis, and associated disease of the bowel also are provided. Intraoperative sigmoidoscopy is a safe and efficacious procedure that can aid in the evaluation and treatment of pelvic pathology and facilitate identification and management of bowel injuries. It should be considered a valu-

able adjunct when such cases are encountered by gynecologic and pelvic surgeons.[156,157] As an alternative, at times it is possible to excise the nodule and staple it; the defect closes simultaneously by articulated vascular staplers.

CUL-DE-SAC RESTORATION

Cul-de-sac obliteration, which is common among patients with severe endometriosis and pain, suggests rectovaginal involvement with deep endometriosis and dense adhesions and significant distortion of the regional anatomy involving the bowel, vaginal apex, posterior cervix, ureter, and major blood vessels (Figure 10.3.25). Transrectal ultrasonography is sensitive and specific for diagnosing the presence of rectovaginal endometriosis.[158] In one study, infiltration of the rectal and vaginal walls was identified correctly in all the patients in whom it was present, but rectal infiltration in three women was not confirmed by the surgeon and the pathologic specimen. Rectal endoscopic ultrasonography was shown by other researchers to provide a reliable indication of the presence of deep bowel infiltration in patients with retroperitoneal endometriotic lesions.[159] The preoperative use of endoscopic ultrasonography as a diagnostic instrument may facilitate preparing a patient for laparoscopic surgery.

Cul-de-sac restoration should not be attempted by an inexperienced laparoscopist or a gynecologist unfamiliar with bowel and urinary tract operations. Most of these situations involve the rectum and the rectovaginal space and do not require bowel resection. To aid in identifying anatomic landmarks and tissue planes, an assistant stands between the patient's legs and does a rectovaginal examination with one hand while holding the uterus up with a rigid uterine elevator. An uninvolved area of peritoneum is identified and injected with 5 to 8 mL of diluted vasopressin (10 U in 100 mL of lactated Ringer's solution) with an 18-gauge laparoscopic needle. Using the CO_2 laser, scissors, electrosurgical knife, needle, or harmonic scalpel, the peritoneal adhesions are cut. With the high-power CO_2 laser and hydrodissection, the rectum attached to the uterosacral ligaments and the back of the cervix is separated. If rectal involvement is more extensive, a sigmoidoscope can be used to guide the surgeon and rule out bowel perforation. After complete separation of the rectum, lesions on the rectum or rectovaginal septum are removed or vaporized (Figure 10.3.26). The cul-de-sac is filled with irrigation fluid and is observed through the laparoscope while air is introduced into the rectum through the sigmoidoscope. Air bubbles observed in the cul-de-sac fluid indicate perforation. As the assistant guides the gynecologist by doing a rectovaginal examination, the rectum is freed from the back of the cervix. Generalized oozing or bleeding is controlled with an injection of 3 to 5 mL of vasopressin solution (one ampule in 100 mL of lactated Ringer's solution), laser, or bipolar electrocoagulator. Bleeding from the stalk vessels caused by dissection or vaporization of the fibrotic uterosacral ligaments and pararectal area is controlled with a bipolar electrocoagulator, clips, or sutures.

The ureters are usually lateral to the uterosacral ligaments. If the dissection is extended lateral to the uterosacral ligaments, the ipsilateral ureter should be identified by opening the overlying peritoneum and tracing it to the area of the lesion. The ureter, uterine arteries, and uterine veins are exposed. Bipolar forceps or hemoclips must be available and fully functional to control unexpected bleeding.

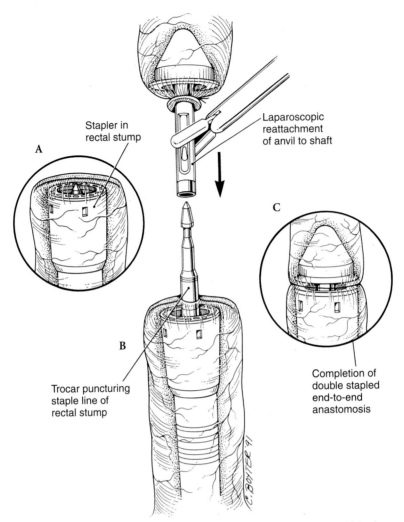

Figure 10.3.21. (**A**) The ILS stapler is placed into the rectum. (**B**) The anvil trocar within the proximal bowel is inserted into the stapling device using the laparoscope. (**C**) The device is fired, creating an end-to-end anastomosis.

For patients who have posterior cul-de-sac nodularity and infiltration of endometriosis toward the vagina, dissection and resection of the nodularity continue as an assistant palpates the nodule to ensure its removal.[160–162] Endometriosis rarely penetrates the mucosa of the colon but commonly involves the serosa, subserosa, and muscularis. When significant portions of both muscularis layers have been excised or vaporized and the mucosa is reached, the bowel wall is reinforced by interrupted 4-0 PDS. The procedure requires maximal coordination between the assistant and the surgeon.

When the rectovaginal space is dissected and hemostasis is accomplished, the pelvis is filled with lactated Ringer's solution to observe the cul-de-sac and the area of dissection under water. This magnifies and clarifies the dissected tissue to help identify residual disease, verify the intact anatomy of the ureters and bowel, and coagulate small bleeders. The raw surfaces of the rectum or cul-de-sac are not reperitonealized because several studies have demonstrated that reperitonealization is not necessary and promotes adhesion formation.[95,96,138,139]

This procedure was accomplished in 185 women age 25 to 41 years. Eighty patients had complete posterior cul-de-sac obliteration. All were managed successfully by laparoscopy and dis-charged within 24 hours, except for nine patients with bowel perforation and one with a partial bowel resection, who were discharged after 2 to 4 days. The procedures lasted from 55 to 245 minutes. Among 185 patients, 174 were available for follow-up after 1 to 5 years. Moderate to complete pain relief was observed in 162 of 174 patients (93%). Thirteen (8%) required two procedures, and four required three procedures. Twelve (7%) had persistent or worse pain postoperatively.[163]

In an unpublished study by one of the authors (B.B.), a series of 356 women who underwent laparoscopic treatment of bowel endometriosis with different techniques, two patients required intraoperative laparotomy early in the authors' experience. The first patient underwent laparotomy for repair of enterotomy after treatment of infiltrative rectal endometriosis. The other patient required laparotomy for anastomosis after an unsuccessful attempt to place a purse-string suture around the patulous rectal ampulla. Significant postoperative complications occurred in 1.7% of these patients. Two women developed leaks and pelvic infections. One required a temporary laparoscopic colostomy with subsequent takedown and repair, and one was managed with prolonged drainage. One woman had a bowel stricture requiring resection and anastomosis by laparotomy.

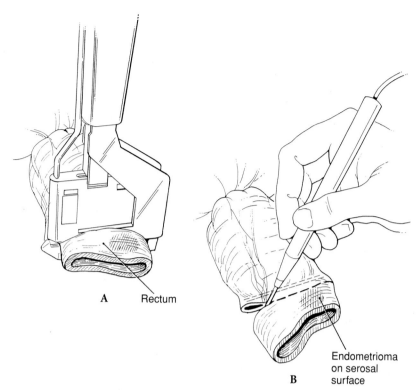

A Rectum

B Endometrioma on serosal surface

Figure 10.3.22. The rectal stump, containing the endometrial lesion, is prolapsed through the anal canal. (**A**) The RL60 linear stapler is applied. (**B**) Using a sharper electrosurgical knife (Ethicon), the rectal stump is transected proximal to the lesion.

One developed a pelvic abscess and subsequently underwent laparoscopic right salpingo-oophorectomy. One patient had an immediate rectal prolapse that was reduced without surgical management. Her original bowel symptoms persisted, and she finally had a colectomy.

Minor complications included skin ecchymosis, temporary urinary retention, temporary diarrhea or constipation, and dyschezia. Donnez and coworkers [160] described a series of 500 women who underwent a laparoscopic procedure with excision of deep fibrotic endometriotic nodules of the rectovaginal septum for pelvic pain or infertility. Excision of the endometriotic nodules resulted in considerable pain relief. Histologically, the rectovaginal nodule was similar to an adenomyoma, as it was a circumscribed nodular aggregate of smooth muscle and endometrial glands and stroma. The variations in estrogen receptor and progesterone receptor content suggested a regulatory mechanism different from that of eutopic endometrium. On the basis of these observations, the authors suggested that nodules of the rectovaginal septum should be considered an entity distinct from peritoneal and ovarian endometriosis and originating from the mullerian rests present in the rectovaginal septum.[164]

Hepatic Endometriosis

Hepatic endometriosis is rare and was first described in 1986.[165] So far, 15 cases of hepatic endometriosis have been reported in the literature. This rare condition raises several diagnostic and therapeutic challenges. When symptomatic, endometriosis of the liver is difficult to diagnose. It is often confused with other pathologies of the liver. Recently, we described two patients with hepatic endometriosis managed laparoscopically.[166] The diagnosis of extrapelvic endometriosis is difficult, and it is often made many years after the onset of symptoms. On the other hand, hepatic endometriosis is so uncommon that such a diagnosis before surgical exploration demands a high degree of suspicion. Women should be evaluated for upper abdominal pain associated with the onset of the menstrual cycle. However, this is not the most common manifestation of the hepatic endometriosis encountered in the cases reported in the literature. Excluding one, all patients described in the literature had epigastric or right upper quadrant pain; including one of our patients, only two patients complained of characteristic cyclic pain related with menses. These findings demonstrate that medical history regarding pain may not be that helpful in diagnosing hepatic endometriosis. One of the significant advantages of laparoscopy is the ability to explore the upper abdominal region, which may be a difficult task when performing a laparotomy for the treatment of pelvic endometriosis. This benefit of laparoscopy always should be exploited. Regardless of the indication for surgery, complete visual inspection of the entire abdominal cavity, including the upper abdominal region, should be performed routinely. The laparoscopic approach may be recommended as an option for the treatment of hepatic endometriosis in proper settings.

Diaphragmatic Endometriosis

The diaphragm rarely is a reported site of endometriosis.[169] Women should be asked about pleuritic, shoulder, or upper abdominal pain occurring with menses because they do not make the connection between these distant anatomic landmarks. The laparoscope is excellent for diagnosing and possibly treating

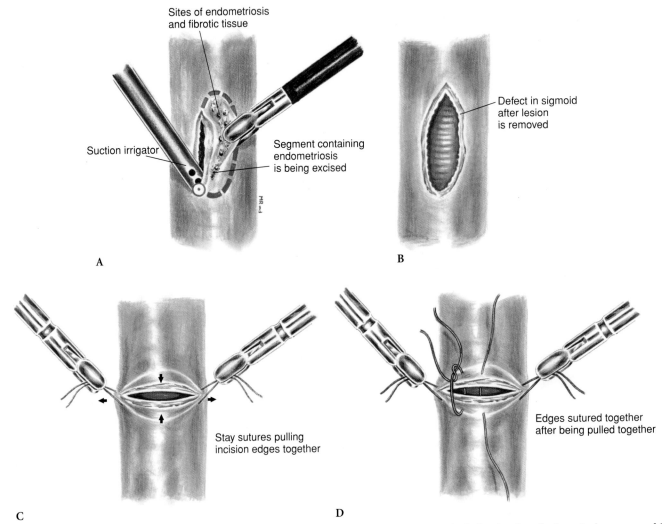

Figure 10.3.23. (**A**) Schematic representation of a bowel segment shows endometrial implants. The lesion involves the intestinal mucosa and is excised. (**B**) The pelvic cavity has been irrigated and suctioned. The longitudinal defect is seen. (**C**) The bowel is repaired transversely in one layer. Two traction sutures are applied to each side, transforming it into a transverse opening. The right and left stay sutures, held with grasping forceps, are secured outside the abdominal cavity and are used to pull the incisional edges together. (**D**) The bowel is repaired by using several interrupted through-and-through 0 polyglactin or polydioxanone sutures on a straight needle. Extracorporeal knot tying is used.

endometriosis on the diaphragm, which is difficult to reach by laparotomy.[168]

Before diaphragmatic endometriosis is treated by laparotomy or laparoscopy, other options are discussed with the patient because an operation at this location may injure the diaphragm, phrenic nerve, lungs, or heart.

For women interested in preserving their reproductive organs, medical treatment should be administered. If the patient does not want to preserve her reproductive organs, bilateral oophorectomy may relieve her symptoms, and further intervention may not be necessary. However, if she does want to preserve her fertility potential and symptoms are not responsive to medical therapy, surgical intervention may be attempted after all possible complications have been discussed.

Most implants are superficial and cause no discomfort. Symptomatic diaphragmatic lesions were found in eight of 4875 patients at our center. Most women prefer BSO, and so it rarely is necessary to treat these implants surgically. Others benefit from medical therapy, and the chance of recurrence on the diaphragm is low.

Endoscopic treatment begins by introducing a 10-mm laparoscope at the umbilical port and placing three additional trocars in the upper quadrant (right or left, according to implant location), similar to the arrangement for laparoscopic cholecystectomy. Two grasping forceps are used to push the liver from the operative field and allow better exposure of the diaphragm. Lesions are removed with hydrodissection and vaporization or excision. If a diaphragmatic defect is formed, it is repaired with 4-0 PDS or staples.

After the procedure, the patient should be evaluated by a cardiopulmonary consultant. The pharynx, larynx, and trachea are examined with a rigid bronchoscope. A flexible scope is introduced to examine the distal trachea and proximal main bronchi. Symptomatic diaphragmatic endometriosis implants were treated in eight women at our center. In three patients, the lesions were directly over the phrenic nerve or the diaphragmatic vasculature. The lesions were excised in three, and vaporization was accomplished in three others. In one patient, the lesion was treated by combined laser and ultrasound (Cavitational Ultrasonographic Surgical Aspirator [CUSA], Valleylab, Boulder, CO). In the remaining patient, only a BSO was done. No intraoperative

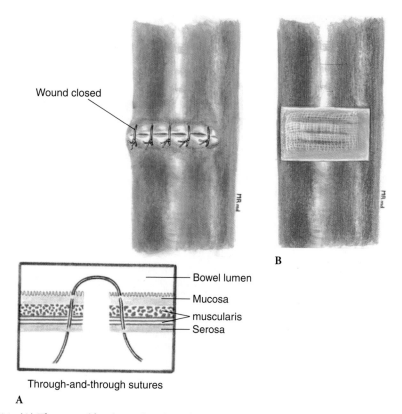

Figure 10.3.24. (**A**) The wound has been closed. At the end of the operation, sigmoidoscopy is done to ensure that the closure is watertight and that there is no bowel stricture. The *inset* shows the through-and-through suture technique to close the defect. (**B**) Interceed has been applied to cover the suture line.

or postoperative complications were noted. Six patients were without pain 6 to 36 months later. In one woman, the pain returned after 1 year, and another experienced no significant pain relief. Both responded to hormone suppressive therapy.

Experience with 24 women with endometriosis of the diaphragm was summarized.[169] Operative findings in 17 patients included two to five spots of endometriosis on the diaphragm measuring 1 cm or less. Some women had numerous lesions scattered across the diaphragm. Lesions were bilateral in eight patients, limited to the right hemidiaphragm in 14 patients, and limited to the left hemidiaphragm in two patients. In seven patients, six endometriosis lesions were directly in the line of the left ventricle and three lesions were adjacent to the phrenic nerve. Endometriosis was infiltrating into the muscular layer of the diaphragm in seven patients. The symptoms in all seven symptomatic patients decreased significantly after treatment, with a minimal follow-up period of 12 months. No postoperative complications occurred.

Restoration of Tubo-Ovarian Anatomy

Once all lesions are resected or ablated and the adnexa are freed of adhesions, the anatomic relation between the ovary and ipsilateral tube is evaluated and any distortion caused by adhesions is corrected. The mesosalpinx often adheres to the ovarian cortex along the ampullary segment of the tube. These adhesions cover a significant part of the surface of the ovarian cortex and may interfere with the ovulatory process at oocyte release. Moreover, the fimbriae frequently are agglutinated, inhibiting their ability

to capture the oocyte. Adhesiolysis along the ovarian surface and mesosalpinx can be accomplished, the ovary and tube are grasped with atraumatic forceps and pulled apart, and the plane between them is dissected with a laser, electrode, or scissors. However, fimbrial adhesions should be resected with laparoscopic microscissors only under water or with an ultrapulse CO_2 laser with high millijoules. Adhesiolysis effected under water offers a clearer view of the anatomy than is provided with the pneumoperitoneum alone. The pelvis is filled with lactated Ringer's solution to allow the fimbriae to float freely in the clear fluid away from each other and from the filmy adhesions. The lighter fimbriae float higher and separate from the normal tissue. As they float away from the fimbrial folds, adhesions are grasped with a fine forceps and atraumatically divided with microscissors without bleeding or injury to the normal tissues.

RELIEF OF PAIN

Besides infertility, the most common complaint of patients with endometriosis is pain, usually in the pelvis, frequently worse at menses and occasionally during coital activity. The classic symptom triad of infertility, dysmenorrhea, and dyspareunia, although not diagnostic of endometriosis, strongly suggests the disease. The existence of a relationship between chronic pelvic pain (CPP) symptoms and endometriosis is widely accepted by gynecologists. The nature of this relationship remains poorly understood, however. No correlation is found between the stage of endometriosis according to the rAFS classification and the severity of CPP.

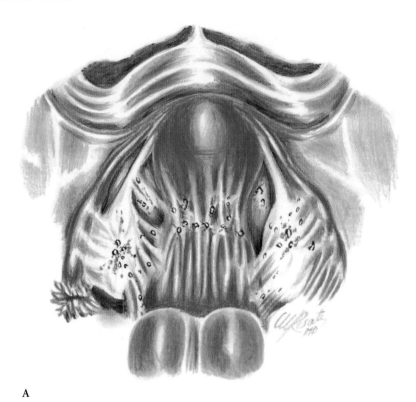

A

Figure 10.3.25. (**A**) Diffuse endometriosis involves the posterior cul-de-sac and both ovaries associated with dense periadnexal adhesions.

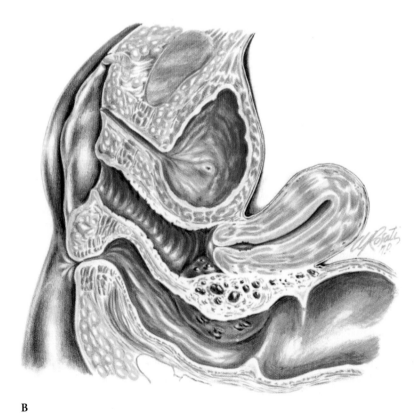

B

Figure 10.3.25. (*Continued*) (**B**) Sagittal view reveals obliteration of the posterior fornix with cul-de-sac nodularity and dense adhesions between the rectum and uterus.

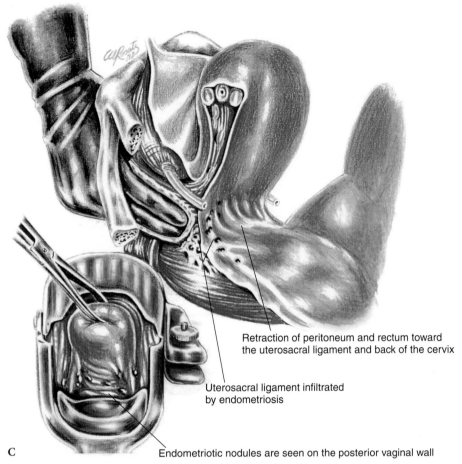

Retraction of peritoneum and rectum toward
the uterosacral ligament and back of the cervix

Uterosacral ligament infiltrated
by endometriosis

C · · · · · · · Endometriotic nodules are seen on the posterior vaginal wall

Figure 10.3.25. (*Continued*) (**C**) Dissection and resection of these nodularities require an assistant to palpate
them to assure their removal. The *inset* shows endometrial implants on the posterior vaginal wall.

Focal or localized pain associated with endometriosis usually responds to removal or destruction of endometriosis and associated adhesions. However, in some women, the pain is disproportionate to the extent of the disease or does not improve after resection of endometriosis and adhesions. For intractable or diffuse pain, interruption of pelvic nerves by uterosacral resection or presacral neurectomy is advised.[170–172] Definitive surgery consisting of hysterectomy and salpingo-oophorectomy is very effective for relieving endometriosis-associated pain. This therapeutic approach would be indicated in women who do not respond satisfactorily to medical and/or conservative surgical treatment and can accept loss of fertility. Women who have completed childbearing and desire a more definitive approach to their symptoms may elect to proceed with this treatment as the primary option. In some cases, symptoms may persist because of adhesions or other peritoneal lesions that remain in situ.[173]

Sutton and coworkers [176] were able to assess in a prospective, randomized, double-blind controlled clinical study the efficacy of laser laparoscopic operations in the treatment of pain associated with minimal, mild, and moderate endometriosis. At the time of laparoscopy, they randomized 63 patients with pain (dysmenorrhea, pelvic pain, or dyspareunia) and minimal to moderate endometriosis to laser ablation of endometriotic deposits and laparoscopic uterine nerve ablation or expectant management.

The study was unique in that both the women and the nurse who assessed them postoperatively were unaware of the treatment. The study showed that laser laparoscopy results in significant pain relief compared with expectant management 6 months postoperatively. Among the patients treated by laser laparoscopy, 62.5% reported improvement or resolution of symptoms, compared with 22.6% in the expectant group. Results were poorest for those with minimal disease, and if only patients with mild and moderate disease are included, 73.7% of the patients achieved pain relief. There were no operative or laser complications in this series. Long-term follow-up of this study revealed that symptom relief continued at 1 year in 90% of those who initially responded.[175] All symptomatic controls had a second-look procedure, which showed disease progression in seven (29%), disease regression in seven (29%), and static disease in 10 (42%). The benefits of laser laparoscopy for painful pelvic endometriosis continue in the majority of patients at 1 year. In most untreated patients, painful endometriosis progresses or remains static, but it may spontaneously improve in others.

Recently, a randomized, blinded, crossover study was done to examine the effect on pain and quality of life for women with all stages of endometriosis undergoing laparoscopic surgery compared with placebo surgery.[176] Thirty-nine women were randomized to receive initially either a diagnostic procedure or full

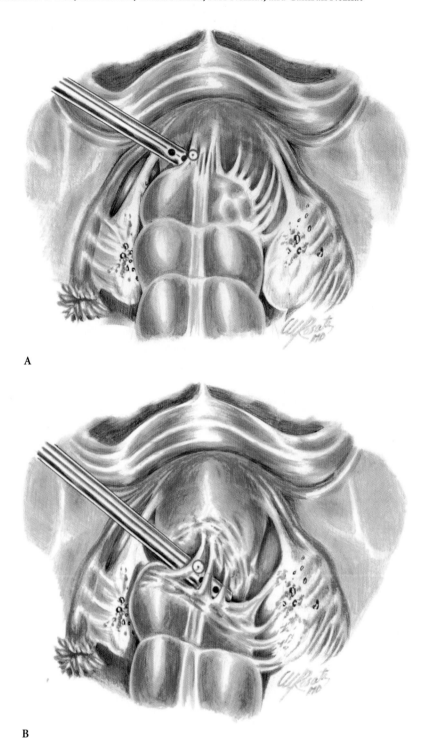

A

B

Figure 10.3.26. (**A**) Adherent sigmoid is removed from the posterior aspect of the uterus. The probe serves as a backstop for the laser, for irrigation, and to put the adhesions on stretch. (**B**) The dissection continues. (*Continued*)

excisional surgery. After 6 months, repeat laparoscopy was performed, with removal of any pathology present. More women in the group who were operated on according to protocol reported symptomatic improvement after excisional surgery than in the placebo group: 16 of 20 (80%) versus six of 19 (32%). Other aspects of quality of life were also significantly improved 6 months after excisional surgery but not after placebo. Progression of disease at second surgery was demonstrated for women having only an initial diagnostic procedure in 45% of cases, with disease

remaining static in 33% and improving in 22% of cases. Nonresponsiveness to surgery was reported in 20% of cases. As a conclusion, laparoscopic excision of endometriosis was more effective than placebo at reducing pain and improving quality of life.

Both presacral neurectomy and uterosacral neurectomy (uterine nerve resection or transection of the uterosacral ligament) have been recommended for relief of chronic pelvic pain associated with endometriosis, based mostly on data from observational studies. Presacral neurectomy has been evaluated, however,

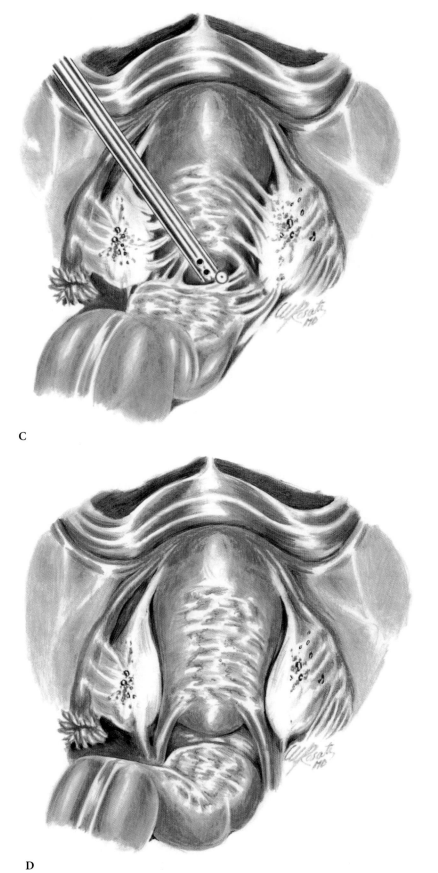

C

D

Figure 10.3.26. (*Continued*) (**C**) Adhesiolysis proceeds until the back of the cervix and the uterosacral ligaments come into view. (**D**) The rectosigmoid colon is mobilized, and most of the adhesions have been removed. (*Continued*)

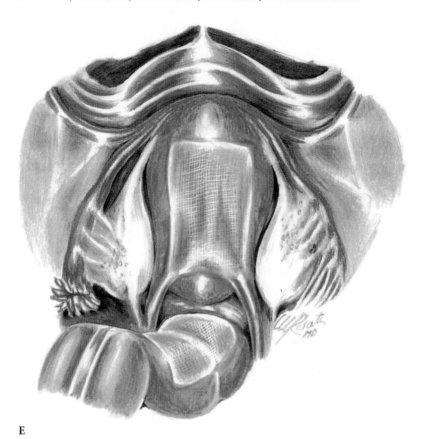

E

Figure 10.3.26. (*Continued*) (**E**) Interceed has been placed over the raw surfaces.

in at least two randomized clinical trials.[177,178] Taken together, these two trials suggest that presacral neurectomy has a role in conservative surgery for endometriosis, but is most effective for the treatment specifically of midline dysmenorrhea. There appears to be a small effect, if any, on nonmenstrual pelvic pain or dyspareunia. Uterosacral neurectomy, also called laparoscopic uterosacral nerve ablation or laparoscopic uterosacral nerve ablation, in a randomized clinical trial has been shown to offer no additional benefit to laparoscopic surgery for treatment of endometriosis-associated pelvic pain.[179]

FERTILITY OUTCOMES AFTER ENDOSCOPIC SURGERY OF ENDOMETRIOSIS

In 1986, we reported our results for the treatment of endometriosis-associated infertility patients with videolaseroscopy.[180] The CO_2 laser has been used laparoscopically for the removal of endometriotic implants, excision of endometrioma capsules, and lysis of adnexal adhesions in 102 patients. Of 102 patients presenting with infertility attributed to endometriosis, 60.7% conceived within 24 months after laser laparoscopy. The rates of conception after surgery were as follows: 75% for patients with mild endometriosis, 62% for patients with moderate endometriosis, 42.1% for patients with severe endometriosis, and 50% for patients with extensive endometriosis. Controversy remains regarding the benefit of surgical treatment of endometriosis with respect to improvement in fecundity at the time of laparoscopy.[58,181] However, because of the progressive nature of the disease in many patients, combined with the largest prospective, randomized trial demonstrating improved fecundity with therapy at the time of surgery, it appears prudent to ablate endometriotic lesions at the time of endoscopic surgery in patients with minimal and mild endometriosis.[57,182,183] Because there are no prospective, randomized studies yet, we are unable to draw any conclusions as to whether endoscopic treatment of advanced endometriosis will improve reproductive outcome; however, there is no reason to be pessimistic. Hence, if the multiple aspects of the reproductive cycle are found to be impaired in women with endometriosis or endometriomas as some investigators claim, it can be normalized by surgery. Supporting this, a 50% pregnancy rate was obtained after laparoscopic management in a series of 814 women with endometriomas.[184] It could be that the removal or destruction of endometriomas provides further benefit than simply restoring the normal anatomy and ovarian structure.

However, it has been suggested that ovarian surgery in cases of ovarian endometriomas could be deleterious for the residual normal ovarian tissue either by removing ovarian stroma with oocytes together with the capsule or by thermal damage provoked by coagulation. In a case controlled study, Aboulghar et al. [185] reported that the outcome of in vitro fertilization (IVF) in stage IV endometriosis with previous surgery was significantly lower compared with an age-matched group of patients with tubal factor infertility. Some investigators reported a marked reduction in the number of both dominant follicles and retrieved oocytes in the operated ovary.[186–188] In contrast, others failed to observe this difference.[189,190] The results from these studies are

Table 10.3.1: Studies Comparing the Number of Follicles in the Operated and in the Contralateral Nonoperated Ovary during IVF Techniques in Endometrioma Cases

Reference	Surgical Technique	Cycles, no.	Follicles, no.		P
			Control Ovary	Operated Ovary	
Nargund et al., 1996 [186]	Not reported	90	8.9 ± 5.1	6.3 ± 5.2	≤0.001
Loh et al., 1999 [190]	Cyst enucleation	12	3.6	4.6	NS
Donnez et al., 2001 [189]	Cyst wall vaporization	87	6.6 ± 3.5	5.2 ± 3.0	NS
Ho et al., 2002 [187]	Cyst enucleation	38	3.3 ± 2.1	1.9 ± 1.5	≤0.001
Somigliana et al., 2003 [188]	Cyst enucleation	46	4.2 ± 2.5	2.0 ± 1.5	≤0.001

NS, not significant.

summarized in Table 10.3.1. The results from randomized trials comparing laser vaporization and stripping enucleation for the treatment of endometrioma are warranted to draw definitive conclusions on this topic. The decreased ovarian response may not be related to the surgical procedure. In this regard, based on histologic analysis, it has been reported recently that the ovarian tissue surrounding the cyst wall in endometriomas is morphologically altered and possibly not functional, thus suggesting that a functional disruption may already be present before surgery.[191] Therefore, the decreased ovarian response, which may be observed in patients previously treated for a large ovarian endometrioma, may also be a consequence of the disease. This needs to be taken into account when proposing nonsurgical management of these patients.

EFFECT OF ENDOMETRIOSIS ON IVF CYCLES: VALUE OF ENDOSCOPIC SURGERY

With the advances obtained in IVF, a large number of patients, especially when age is a factor, opt to proceed with IVF without undergoing adequate surgical evaluation and treatment of endometriosis. Although IVF is one of the options that may be offered to an infertile couple with endometriosis, its success rate is lower compared with that of women undergoing IVF for other indications. Numerous studies have compared IVF outcome in terms of fertilization rate, embryo development, and implantation and pregnancy rates in women with endometriosis with other diagnostic entities. The question of whether the presence of endometriosis affects the outcome of women undergoing IVF has not been resolved, with some authors noting negative associations and others noting no association. In a meta-analysis, Barnhart et al. [192] investigated the IVF outcome for patients with endometriosis. It was demonstrated that patients with endometriosis have a more than 50% reduction in pregnancy rate after IVF compared with women with tubal factor infertility.

Multivariate analysis also demonstrated a decrease in fertilization and implantation rates, and a significant decrease in the number of oocytes retrieved for endometriosis patients. These data therefore suggest that the presence of endometriosis affects multiple aspects of the reproductive cycle, including oocyte quality, embryogenesis, and/or the receptivity of the endometrium. Thus, it is unlikely that the effect of endometriosis is solely the result of alterations of normal pelvic anatomy, and an effect on the developing follicle, oocyte, and embryo is suggested. Further evidence of poor oocyte quality, and thus reduced implanting ability of embryos, is strengthened by studies showing no adverse effect on implantation rates in women with endometriosis using donated oocytes, and the receipt of oocytes from donors with endometriosis may result in lower implantation rates.[101,182,183] Currently, in advanced endometriosis cases, there are no randomized, controlled trials comparing the outcome of endoscopic infertility surgery and IVF to definitively lead us to a conclusion. On the bases of the accumulated data, we believe that laparoscopic diagnosis and treatment of endometriosis will be useful in increasing the probability of conception either spontaneously or with IVF treatment. This should also be valid for patients with multiple IVF failures. In May 2004, The Practice Committee of the ASRM developed a report.[193] According to its recommendations, when laparoscopy is performed, the surgeon should consider safely ablating or excising visible lesions of endometriosis. In women with stage I/II endometriosis-associated infertility, expectant management or superovulation/intrauterine insemination (IUI) after laparoscopy may be considered for younger patients. Women 35 years of age or older should be treated with superovulation/IUI or IVF embryo transfer. In women with stage III/IV endometriosis-associated infertility, conservative surgical therapy with laparoscopy and possible laparotomy is indicated.

In conclusion, because it is a well-known fact that endometriosis is more prevalent in the setting of infertility, with proper patient selection, a meticulously performed laparoscopic surgery is an excellent option that provides these patients with the potential to achieve repeated future pregnancies. The inability to thoroughly treat the endometriosis might have also been a contributing factor to the contradictory results of the studies. Patients with endometriomas also have an increased rate of accompanying peritoneal endometriosis, which should be thoroughly treated in patients who desire to get pregnant. Another possible factor is the declining number of endoscopic surgeries being performed in response to the increasing numbers of patients opting for IVF. This phenomenon results in fewer physicians who develop adequate proficiency in performing these technically advanced procedures.

MINIMIZING RECURRENCES

Recurrence or persistence of endometriosis after treatment is one of the most vexing problems of gynecology and is based on the known unpredictability of the disease. Endometriosis recurrence rates vary from 2% to 47%. The highest recurrence rate is documented for retrocervical (or deep infiltrative) endometriosis, based on difficulties in estimating the real borders of the infiltrate, as well as the conscious rejection of more aggressive approaches to removal of the lesions, which are located near vital organs. The surgical treatment of endometriosis involves destroying endometrial implants (coagulation, vaporization, resection) and associated adhesions and restoring normal anatomy. The anatomic, physiologic, and genetic factors that predispose each patient to developing endometriosis are not altered by the treatment. Therefore, recurrence is unavoidable unless endometrial proliferation, menstruation, or the predominantly estrogenic environment of the patient is altered. For those who desire pregnancy, an early success will be therapeutic because the 9-month gestational period, besides precluding menstrual flow, results in a predominantly progestational medium that reduces endometrial proliferation and the extent of disease. Patients who do not desire pregnancy have an increased risk of earlier recurrence and may benefit from preventive measures targeted at decreasing known risk factors, such as short length of menstrual cycles, lack of exercise, menorrhagia, and outflow obstruction. Mullerian anomalies that predispose a patient to outflow obstruction should be corrected.[194] Postoperatively, exercise and hormone therapy (progestational agents or low-dose oral contraceptives) are suggested. For the first 9 months postoperatively, medroxyprogesterone (Provera, Pfizer) 30 mg daily is given to induce amenorrhea in more than 75% of patients and regression of residual disease.[195] In using the Provera regimen, a change to low-dose oral contraceptives may cause hypomenorrhea and may be therapeutic. If symptoms recur, medroxyprogesterone acetate therapy or a GnRH analogue can control pain.

Continuous oral contraceptive pills may be prescribed for certain patients. Recently, in a prospective study, continuously administered monophasic oral contraceptive treatment was found not only to significantly reduce pain scores, but also the required radical operative solution (hysterectomy plus bilateral adnexectomy) for CPP by oral contraceptive users.[196] A recent, small pilot study of 10 reproductive-aged women with treatment-resistant endometriosis investigated the effects of the aromatase inhibitor letrozole (2.5 mg/day), administered with the progestin norethindrone acetate (2.5 mg/day), calcium, and vitamin D for 6 months. This treatment significantly reduced pelvic pain scores in nine of 10 patients and achieved marked reduction of laparosc-

ically visible lesions in all 10 women, with no significant change in bone marrow density.[197] Although promising, these results require confirmation in randomized clinical trials. Second-look laparoscopy may be necessary to treat recurrent or persistent endometriosis. Supracervical hysterectomy is not advisable for patients with severe endometriosis because persistent pelvic pain subsequently requires the removal of the cervical stump.

FUTURE DEVELOPMENT

New developments in fiberoptic endoscopes with diameters less than 1 mm have enabled a gynecologist to diagnose and stage the disease in an office setting under local anesthesia, possibly at earlier stages. Further development of laser surgery and photodynamic therapy may make therapeutic microendoscopy possible in an office setting.[198] Manyak and colleagues [199] conducted experiments evaluating photodynamic therapy for endometriosis using rabbit endometriotic implants. After the intravenous injection of dihydroporphyrin ether (DHE), the rabbits were treated with a low-energy argon laser, which is absorbed mainly by the endometriotic implants but not the surrounding normal tissues. The selective absorption of the laser energy by the DHE enables the low-power laser energy to destroy only the endometriotic lesions containing DHE, sparing the normal tissue. Because DHE is absorbed by both gross and microscopic disease, a more thorough resection of endometriosis is possible with photodynamic therapy, which is less invasive and safer. The ability to diagnose and treat disease at earlier stages and in an office setting may prevent the progression and invasion of endometriosis, reducing its adverse impact on health, quality of life, and fertility potential. Operative microlaparoscopy can be safe in the office under local anesthesia with conscious sedation for the diagnosis and treatment of CPP.[200] The diagnostic accuracy achieved for endometriosis with 2-mm microlaparoscopy is comparable to that achieved with standard 10-mm laparoscopy.[201] However, one study found discordant findings for mild or minimal endometriosis.[202]

Microlaparoscopy allows conscious pain mapping, fulguration of endometriotic lesions, adhesiolysis, and laparoscopic uterosacral nerve ablation.[203]

Pelvic pain mapping during laparoscopy under conscious sedation can provide useful information about visceral and somatic sources of CPP. A diagnostic superior hypogastric plexus block under direct laparoscopic observation is possible. The pelvis is mapped to ascertain whether painful areas are supplied by hypogastric plexuses. The results of mapping allow a more informed selection of patients for presacral neurectomy.[204]

REFERENCES

1. Hasson HM. Incidence of endometriosis in diagnostic laparoscopy. *J Reprod Med*. 1976;16:135.
2. Schmidt LC. Endometriosis: a reappraisal of pathogenesis and treatment. *Fertil Steril*. 1985;44:157.
3. Giudice LC, Kao LC. Endometriosis. *Lancet*. 2004;364(9447): 1789–1799.
4. Williams TJ, Pratt JHL. Endometriosis in 1000 consecutive celiotomies: incidence and management. *Am J Obstet Gynecol*. 1977;129:245.

5. American Society for Reproductive Medicine. Revised American Society for Reproductive Medicine classification of endometriosis: 1996. *Fertil Steril.* 1997;67:817–821.

6. Rokitansky C. Ueber Uterusdrusen-Neubildung in uterus and ovarial sarcomen. *Z Gesellschaft Aertz Wein.* 1860;16:755.

7. Williams TJ. Endometriosis. In: Thompson JD, Rock JA, eds. *Te Linde's Gynecology.* 7th ed. Philadelphia: Lippincott; 1992.

8. Gomel V, McComb P. Microsurgery in gynecology. In: Silver JS, ed. *Microsurgery.* Baltimore: Williams & Wilkins; 1979.

9. Cook AS, Rock JA. The role of laparoscopy in the treatment of endometriosis. *Fertil Steril.* 1991;4:663.

10. Nezhat C, Winer WK, Cooper JD, Nezhat F, Nezhat C. Endoscopic infertility surgery. *J Reprod Med.* 1989;34(2):127–134.

11. Nezhat C, Hood J, Winer W, Nezhat F, Crowgey SR, Garrison CP. Videolaseroscopy and laser laparoscopy in gynaecology. *Br J Hosp Med.* 1987;38(3):219–224.

12. Nezhat C, Nezhat F, Nezhat CH, Admon D. Videolaseroscopy and videolaparoscopy. *Baillieres Clin Obstet Gynaecol.* 1994;8(4):851–864.

13. Nezhat C, Nezhat FR. Safe laser endoscopic excision or vaporization of peritoneal endometriosis. *Fertil Steril.* 1989;52:149.

14. Martin DC. CO_2 laser laparoscopy for the treatment of endometriosis associated with infertility. *J Reprod Med.* 1985;30:409.

15. Nezhat C, Crowgey S, Nezhat F. Surgical treatment of endometriosis via laser laparoscopy. *Fertil Steril.* 1986;45:778.

16. Nezhat C, Crowgey S, Nezhat F. Videolaseroscopy for the treatment of endometriosis associated with infertility. *Fertil Steril.* 1989;51:123.

17. Adamson DG, Subak LL, Pasta DJ, et al. Comparison of CO_2 laser laparoscopy with laparotomy for the treatment of endometriomata. *Fertil Steril.* 1992;57:965.

18. Adamson DG, Hurd SJ, Pasta DJ, et al. Laparoscopic endometriosis treatment: is it better? *Fertil Steril.* 1993;59:35.

19. Ranney BR. Endometriosis III: complete operations. *Am J Obstet Gynecol.* 1971;109:1137.

20. Wilson EA. Surgical therapy for endometriosis. *Clin Obstet Gynecol.* 1988;31:857.

21. Ray G. The effectiveness of laparoscopic excision of endometriosis. *Curr Opin Obstet Gynecol.* 2004;16(4):299–303.

22. The American Fertility Society. Revised American Fertility Society classification of endometriosis: 1985. *Fertil Steril.* 1985;43:351–352.

23. Nezhat C, Nezhat F, Nezhat CH. Operative laparoscopy (minimally invasive surgery): state of the art. *J Gynecol Surg.* 1992;8:111.

24. Luciano AA, Lowney J, Jacobs SL. Endoscopic treatment of endometriosis-associated infertility: therapeutic, economic and social benefits. *J Reprod Med.* 1992;37:573.

25. Davis CJ, McMillan L. Pain in endometriosis: effectiveness of medical and surgical management. *Curr Opin Obstet Gynecol.* 2003;15(6):507–512.

26. Moen MH, Schei B. Epidemiology of endometriosis in a Norwegian county. *Acta Obstet Gynecol Scand.* 1997;76:559–562.

27. Eskenazi B, Warner M, Bonsignore L, et al. Validation study of non-surgical diagnosis of endometriosis. *Fertil Steril.* 2001;76: 929–935.

28. Husby GK, Haugen RS, Moen MH. Diagnostic delay in women with pain and endometriosis. *Acta Obstet Gynecol Scand.* 2003;82:649–653.

29. Olive DL, Martin DC. Treatment of endometriosis associated infertility with CO_2 laser laparoscopy: the use of 1- and 2-parameter exponential models. *Fertil Steril.* 1987;48:18.

30. Filmar S, Gomel V, McComb P. Operative laparoscopy versus open abdominal surgery: a comparative study on postoperative adhesion formation in the rat model. *Fertil Steril.* 1987;48:486.

31. Luciano AA, Maier DB, Nulsen ZC, et al. A comparative study of postoperative adhesion formation following laser surgery by laparoscopy versus laparotomy in the rabbit model. *Obstet Gynecol.* 1989;74:220.

32. Maier DB, Klock A, Nulsen J, et al. Laser laparoscopy vs laparotomy in lysis of dense and incidental pelvic adhesions. *J Reprod Med.* 1992;37:965.

33. Diamond MP, Daniell SF, Feste J, et al. Adhesion reformation and de novo formation after reproductive pelvic surgery. *Fertil Steril.* 1987;47:864.

34. Luciano AA, Moufauino-Oliva M. Comparison of postoperative adhesion formation – laparoscopy versus laparotomy. *Infert Reprod Med Clin North Am.* 1994;5:437.

35. Marana R, Luciano AA, Morendino VE, et al. Reproductive outcome after ovarian surgery: microsurgery versus CO_2 laser. *J Gynecol Surg.* 1991;7:159.

36. Lundorff P, Hahlin M, Kallfelt B, et al. Adhesion formation after laparoscopic surgery in ectopic pregnancy: a randomized trial versus laparotomy. *Fertil Steril.* 1991;55:91.

37. Trimbos-Kemper TCM, Trimbos JB, van Hall EV. Adhesion formation after tubal surgery: results of the 8 day laparoscopy in 188 patients. *Fertil Steril.* 1985;43:395.

38. Nezhat C, Nezhat F, Metzger DA, et al. Adhesion reformation after reproductive surgery by videolaseroscopy. *Fertil Steril.* 1990;53:1008.

39. Operative Laparoscopy Study Group. Postoperative adhesion development after operative laparoscopy evaluation at early second look procedures. *Fertil Steril.* 1991;55:700.

40. Donnez J. Carbon dioxide laser laparoscopy in infertile women with endometriosis and women with adnexal adhesions. *Fertil Steril.* 1987;48:190.

41. Fayez JA, Collazo LM. Comparison between laparotomy and operative laparoscopy in the treatment of moderate and severe endometriosis. *Int J Fertil.* 1990;35:272.

42. Nezhat C, Silfen SL, Nezhat F, et al. Surgery for endometriosis. *Curr Opin Obstet Gynecol.* 1991;3:385.

43. Gomel V. Laparoscopic tubal surgery in infertility. *Obstet Gynecol.* 1975;46:4752.

44. Gomel V. Salpingo-ovariolysis by laparoscopy in infertility. *Fertil Steril.* 1983;40:607.

45. Chong AP, Luciano AA, O'Shaughnessy AM. Laser laparoscopy versus laparotomy in the treatment of infertility patients with severe endometriosis. *J Gynecol Surg.* 1990;6:179.

46. Crosignani PG, Vercellini P, Biffignandi F, et al. Laparoscopy versus laparotomy in conservative surgical treatment for severe endometriosis. *Fertil Steril.* 1996;66:706.

47. Soong YK, Chang FH, Chou HH, et al. Life table analysis of pregnancy rates in women with moderate or severe endometriosis comparing danazol therapy after carbon dioxide laser laparoscopy plus electrocoagulation or laparotomy plus electrocoagulation versus danazol therapy only. *J Am Assoc Gynecol Laparosc.* 1997;4:225.

48. Busacca M, Fedele L, Bianchi S, et al. Surgical treatment of recurrent endometriosis: laparotomy versus laparoscopy. *Hum Reprod.* 1998;13(8):2271–2274.

49. Revelli A, Modotti M, Ansaldi C, Massobrio M. Recurrent endometriosis: a review of biological and clinical aspects. *Obstet Gynecol Surv.* 1995;50:747–754.

50. Schenken SR, Malinak RL. Reoperation after initial treatment of endometriosis with conservative surgery. *Am J Obstet Gynecol.* 1978;131:416.

51. Wheeler JH, Malinak LR. Recurrent endometriosis: incidence, management, and prognosis. *Am J Obstet Gynecol.* 1983;146: 247.

52. Murphy AA, Green WR, Bobbie D, et al. Unsuspected

endometriosis documented by scanning electron microscopy in visually normal peritoneum. *Fertil Steril.* 1986;46:522.

53. Nezhat F, Allan JC, Nezhat C, et al. Nonvisualized endometriosis at laparoscopy. *Int J Fertil.* 1991;36:340.

54. Vasquez G, Cornille F, Brosens IA. Peritoneal endometriosis: scanning electron microscopy and histology of minimal pelvic endometriotic lesions. *Fertil Steril.* 1984;42:696.

55. Adamson GD, Pasta DJ. Surgical treatment of endometriosis-associated infertility: meta-analysis compared with survival analysis. *Am J Obstet Gynecol.* 1994;171:1488.

56. Marcoux S, Maheux R, Berube S. Canadian Collaborative Group on Endometriosis: laparoscopic surgery in infertile women with minimal or mild endometriosis. *N Engl J Med.* 1997;337:217.

57. Parazzini F. Ablation of lesions or no treatment in minimal-mild endometriosis in infertile women: a randomized trial. Gruppo Italiano per lo Studio dell'Endometriosi. *Hum Reprod.* 1999;14:1332–1334.

58. Chang FH, Chou HH, Soong YK, et al. Efficacy of isotopic $13CO_2$ laser laparoscopic evaporation in the treatment of infertile patients with minimal and mild endometriosis: a life table cumulative pregnancy rates study. *J Am Assoc Gynecol Laparosc.* 1997;4:219.

59. Tulandi T, al-Took S. Reproductive outcome after treatment of mild endometriosis with laparoscopic excision and electrocoagulation. *Fertil Steril.* 1998;69:229.

60. Chapron C, Fritel X, Dubuisson JB. Fertility after laparoscopic management of deep endometriosis infiltrating the uterosacral ligaments. *Hum Reprod.* 1999;14:329–332.

61. Magos A. Endometriosis: radical surgery. *Baillieres Clin Obstet Gynaecol.* 1993;7(4):849–864.

62. Nezhat C, Nezhat F. Operative laparoscopy for the management of ovarian remnant syndrome. *Fertil Steril.* 1992;57:1003.

63. Nezhat F, Nezhat C, Silfen SL. Videolaseroscopy for oophorectomy. *Am J Obstet Gynecol.* 1991;165:1323.

64. Betts WJ, Buttram CVJ. A plan for managing endometriosis. *Contemp Ob Gyn.* 1980;15:121.

65. Ranney BR. Endometriosis: conservative operations. *Am J Obstet Gynecol.* 1970;107:743.

66. Barbieri RL. Hormonal therapy of endometriosis. *Infertil Reprod Med North Am.* 1992;3:187.

67. Dover RW, Chen J, Torode H. Oophorectomy at the time of surgery for moderate endometriosis: a survey of Australian gynaecologists. *Aust N Z J Obstet Gynaecol.* 2000;40(4):455–458.

68. Namnoum AB, Hickman TN, Goodman SB, Gehlbach DL, Rock JA. Incidence of symptom recurrence after hysterectomy for endometriosis. *Fertil Steril.* 1995;64:898–902.

69. Fedele L, Bianchi S, Raffaelli R, Zanconato G. Comparison of transdermal estradiol and tibolone for the treatment of oophorectomized women with deep residual endometriosis. *Maturitas.* 1999;32(3):189–193.

70. Goumenou AG, Chow C, Taylor A, Magos A. Endometriosis arising during estrogen and testosterone treatment 17 years after abdominal hysterectomy: a case report. *Maturitas.* 2003;46(3):239–241.

71. Cohn MN, Altaras S, Lew R, Tepper Y. Ovarian endometrioid carcinoma and endometriosis developing in a postmenopausal breast cancer patient during tamoxifen therapy: a case report and review of the literature. *Gynecol Oncol.* 1994;55:443–447.

72. Lam AM, French M, Charnock FM. Bilateral ureteric obstruction due to recurrent endometriosis associated with hormone replacement therapy. *Aust New Zealand J Obstet Gynaecol.* 1992;32:83–84.

73. Matorras R, Elorriaga MA, Pijoan JI, Ramon O, Rodriguez-Escudero FJ. Recurrence of endometriosis in women with bilateral adnexectomy (with or without total hysterectomy) who received hormone replacement therapy. *Fertil Steril.* 2002;77(2):303–308.

74. Brunson GL, Barclay DL, Sanders M, Araoz CA. Malignant extraovarian endometriosis: two case reports and review of the literature. *Gynecol Oncol.* 1988;30:123–130.

75. Spaczynski RZ, Duleba AJ. Diagnosis of endometriosis. *Semin Reprod Med.* 2003;21(2):193–208.

76. Martin DC, Hubert GD, Vander-Zwaag R, et al. Laparoscopic appearances of pelvic endometriosis. *Fertil Steril.* 1989;51:63.

77. Redwine DB. Age-related evolution in color appearance of endometriosis. *Fertil Steril.* 1987;48:1062.

78. Vernon MW, Beard JS, Graves K, et al. Classification of endometriotic implants by morphologic appearance and capacity to synthesize prostaglandin. *Fertil Steril.* 1990;53:984.

79. Nisolle M, Donnez J. Peritoneal endometriosis, ovarian endometriosis, and adenomyotic nodules of the rectovaginal septum are three different entities. *Fertil Steril.* 1997;68:585–596.

80. Cornillie FJ, Ooosterlynck D, Lauweryns JM, et al. Deeply infiltrating pelvic endometriosis: histology and clinical significance. *Fertil Steril.* 1990;53:978.

81. Crain LJ, Luciano AA. Peritoneal fluid evaluation in infertility. *Obstet Gynecol.* 1983;61:1591.

82. Nisolle M, Paindavene B, Boudon A, et al. Histologic study of peritoneal endometriosis in infertile women. *Fertil Steril.* 1990;53:984.

83. Redwine DB. Peritoneal blood painting: an aid in the diagnosis of endometriosis. *Am J Obstet Gynecol.* 1989;161:865.

84. Vercellini P, Vendola N, Bocciolone L, et al. Reliability of the visual diagnosis of ovarian endometriosis. *Fertil Steril.* 1991;56:1198–1200.

85. Candiani GB, Vercelli P, Fedele L. Laparoscopic ovarian puncture to correct staging of endometriosis. *Fertil Steril.* 1990;53:984.

86. Demco L. Mapping the source and character of pain due to endometriosis by patient-assisted laparoscopy. *J Am Assoc Gynecol Laparosc.* 1998;5:241.

87. Goldman EL. ACOG advises against videotaping of deliveries. *Ob.Gyn. News.* 1999.

88. Prystowsky JB, Stryker SJ. Ujiki GT, et al. Gastrointestinal endometriosis: incidence and indications for resection. *Arch Surg.* 1988;7:855.

89. Nezhat CH, Nezhat F, Roemisch M, et al. Laparoscopic trachelectomy for persistent pelvic pain and endometriosis after supracervical hysterectomy. *Fertil Steril.* 1996;66:925.

90. Sampson JA. Perforating hemorrhagic (chocolate) cysts of the ovary. *Arch Surg.* 1921;3:245.

91. Blaustein A, Kantius M, Kaganowicz A, et al. Inclusions in ovaries of females aged 1–30 years. *Int J Gynecol Pathol.* 1982;1:145.

92. Kerner H, Gaton E, Czernobilsky B. Unusual ovarian, tubal and pelvic mesothelial inclusions in patients with endometriosis. *Histopathology.* 1981;5:277.

93. Sternberg SS, ed. *Histology for Pathologists.* Philadelphia: Lippincott Williams & Wilkins; 1992.

94. Chernobilsky B, Morris WJ. A histologic study of ovarian endometriosis with emphasis on hyperplastic and atypical changes. *Obstet Gynecol.* 1979;53:318.

95. Nissole-Pochet M, Casanas-Roux F, Donnez J. Histologic study of ovarian endometriosis after hormonal therapy. *Fertil Steril.* 1988;49:423.

96. Martin DC, Berry JD. Histology of chocolate cysts. *J Gynecol Surg.* 1990;6:43.

97. Luciano AA, Marana R, Krakta S, et al. Ovarian function after incision of the ovary by scalpel, CO_2 laser and microelectrode. *Fertil Steril.* 1991;56:349.

98. Hasson HM. Laparoscopic management of ovarian cysts. *J Reprod Med.* 1990;25:863.

99. Brosens I, Puttemansi P. Double optic laparoscopy. *Ballieres Clin Obstet Gynaecol.* 1989;3:595.

100. Keye WR, Hansen LW, Astin M, et al. Argon laser therapy of endometriosis: a review of 92 consecutive patients. *Fertil Steril.* 1987;47:208.

101. Nezhat F, Nezhat C, Allan CJ, et al. A clinical and histologic classification of endometriomas: implications for a mechanism of pathogenesis. *J Reprod Med.* 1992;37:771.

102. Nezhat C, Nezhat F. Postoperative adhesion formation after ovarian cystectomy with and without ovarian reconstruction. Presented at: 75th Annual Meeting of the American Fertility Society; October 19–24, 1991; Orlando, FL.

103. Fayez JA, Vogel MF. Comparison of different treatment methods of endometriomas by laparoscopy. *Obstet Gynecol.* 1991;78:660.

104. Nezhat F, Nezhat C, Allan CJ, et al. A clinical and histologic classification of endometriomas: implications for a mechanism of pathogenesis. *J Reprod Med.* 1992;37:771.

105. Marana R, Luciano AA, Muzii L, et al. Reproductive outcome after ovarian surgery. Suturing versus nonsuturing of the ovarian cortex. *J Gynecol Surg.* 1991;7:155.

106. Nezhat C, Nezhat F. Postoperative adhesion formation after ovarian cystectomy with and without ovarian reconstruction. Abstract O-012 presented at: 47th Annual Meeting of the American Fertility Association; October 21–24, 1991; Orlando, FL.

107. Donnez J, Nisolle M. Laparoscopic management of large ovarian endometrial cyst: use of fibrin sealant. *Surgery.* 1991;7:163.

108. Beretta P, Franchi M, Ghezzi F, et al. Randomized clinical trial of two laparoscopic treatments of endometriomas: cystectomy versus drainage and coagulation. *Fertil Steril.* 1998;70:1176.

109. Catalano GF, Marana R, Caruana P, et al. Laparoscopy versus microsurgery by laparotomy for excision of ovarian cysts in patients with moderate or severe endometriosis. *J Am Assoc Gynecol Laparosc.* 1996;3:267.

110. Hemmings R, Bissonnette F, Bouzayen R. Results of laparoscopic treatments of ovarian endometriomas: laparoscopic ovarian fenestration and coagulation. *Fertil Steril.* 1998;70:527.

111. Stanley EK, Utz DC, Dockerty MB. Clinically significant endometriosis of the urinary tract. *Surg Gynecol Obstet.* 1965;120:491.

112. Goldstein MS, Brodman ML. Cystometric evaluation of vesical endometriosis before and after hormonal or surgical treatment. *Mt Sinai J Med.* 1990;57:109.

113. Nezhat C, Nezhat F, Nezhat CH, et al. Urinary tract endometriosis treated by laparoscopy. *Fertil Steril.* 1996;66:920.

114. Nezhat CH, Seidman DS, Nezhat F, et al. Laparoscopic management of intentional and unintentional cystotomy. *J Urol.* 1996;156:1400.

115. Nezhat CH, Nezhat FR, Freiha F, Nezhat CR. Laparoscopic vesicopsoas hitch for infiltrative ureteral endometriosis. *Fertil Steril.* 1999;71:376.

116. Antonelli A, Simeone C, Frego E, Minini G, Bianchi U, Cunico SC. Surgical treatment of ureteral obstruction from endometriosis: our experience with thirteen cases. *Int Urogynecol J Pelvic Floor Dysfunct.* 2004;15:407–412.

117. Zanetta G, Webb MJ, Segura JW. Ureteral endometriosis diagnosed at ureteroscopy. *Obstet Gynecol.* 1998;91:857–859.

118. Gagnon RF, Arsenault D, Pichette V, Tanguay S. Acute renal failure in a young woman with endometriosis. *Nephrol Dial Transplant.* 2001;16:1499–1502.

119. Vercellini P, Pisacreta A, Pesole A, Vicentini S, Stellato G, Crosignani PG. Is ureteral endometriosis an asymmetric disease? *BJOG.* 2000;107:559–561.

120. Klein RS, Cattolica EV. Ureteral endometriosis. *Urology.* 1979; 13:477–482.

121. Kerr WS Jr. Endometriosis involving the urinary tract. *Clin Obstet Gynecol.* 1966;9:331–357.

122. Yohannes P. Ureteral endometriosis. *J Urol.* 2003;170:20–25.

123. Abeshouse BS, Abeshouse G. Endometriosis of the urinary tract: a review of the literature and a report of four cases of vesical endometriosis. *J Int Coll Surg.* 1960;34:43–63.

124. Horn LC, Minh MD, Stolzenburg JU. Intrinsic form of ureteral endometriosis causing ureteral obstruction and partial loss of kidney function. *Urol Int.* 2002;73:181–184.

125. Kavoussi LR, Clayman RV, Brunt LM, Soper NJ. Laparoscopic ureterolysis. *J Urol.* 1992;147:426–429.

126. Loison G, Almeras C, Chartier-Kastler E. Ureterolysis: technique, indications. *Ann Urol (Paris).* 2005;39:1–9.

127. Watanabe Y, Ozawa H, Uematsu K, Kawasaki K, Nishi H, Kobashi Y. Hydronephrosis due to ureteral endometriosis treated by transperitoneal laparoscopic ureterolysis. *Int J Urol.* 2004;11:560–562.

128. Nezhat C, Nezhat F. Laparoscopic repair of ureter resected during operative laparoscopy. *Obstet Gynecol.* 1992;80:543–544.

129. Castillo OA, Litvak JP, Kerkebe M, Olivares R, Urena RD. Early experience with the laparoscopic boari flap at a single institution. *J Urol.* 2005;173:862–865.

130. Nezhat C, Nezhat F, Green B. Laparoscopic treatment of obstructed ureter due to endometriosis by resection and ureteroureterostomy: a case report. *J Urol.* 1992;148:659.

131. Nezhat CH, Malik S, Nezhat F, Nezhat C. Laparoscopic ureteroneocystostomy and vesicopsoas hitch for infiltrative endometriosis. *JSLS.* 2004;8(1):3–7.

132. Stillwell TJ, Kramer SA, Lee RA. Endometriosis of ureter. *Urology.* 1986;28:81–85.

133. Stanley KE Jr, Utz DC, Dockerty MB. Clinically significant endometriosis of the urinary tract. *Surg Gynecol Obstet.* 1965;120:491–498.

134. Comiter CV. Endometriosis of the urinary tract. *Urol Clin North Am.* 2002;29:625–635.

135. Nezhat C, Nezhat F. Laparoscopic segmental bladder resection for endometriosis: a report of two cases. *Obstet Gynecol.* 1993;81:882.

136. Ferzli G, Wenof M, Giannakakos A, Raboy A, Albert P. Laparoscopic partial cystectomy for vesical endometrioma. *J Laparoendosc Surg.* 1993;3:161–165.

137. Sampson JA. Intestinal adenomas of endometrial type. *Arch Surg.* 1922;5:217.

138. Jenkinson EL, Brown WH. Endometriosis: a study of 117 cases with special reference to constricting lesions of the rectum and sigmoid colon. *JAMA.* 1943;122:349.

139. Samper ER, Sagle GW, Hand AM. Colonic endometriosis, its clinical spectrum. *South Med J.* 1984;77:912.

140. Ponka JL, Brush BE, Hodgkinson CP. Colorectal endometriosis. *Dis Colon Rectum.* 1973;16:490.

141. Meyers WC, Kelvin FM, Jones RS. Diagnosis and surgical treatment of colonic endometriosis. *Arch Surg.* 1979;114:169.

142. Mackenrodt R. Uber entzundliche heterage Epithelwucherungen in weiblichen Genital-gebiete und uber cine bir in die Wurzel des Mescolon ausgedehnte benigne Wucherung des Darmepithels. *Virchows Arch Pathol Anat.* 1909;195:487.

143. Coronado C, Franklin RR, Lotze EC, et al. Surgical treatment of symptomatic colorectal endometriosis. *Fertil Steril.* 1990;3:411.

144. Cameron IC, Rogers S, Collins MC, et al. Intestinal endometriosis: presentation, investigation, and surgical management. *Int J Colorectal Dis.* 1995;10:83–86.

145. Redwine DB. Ovarian endometriosis: a marker for more extensive pelvic and intestinal disease. *Fertil Steril.* 1999;72:310–315.

146. Berker B, Lashay N, Davarpanah R, Marziali M, Nezhat CH, Nezhat C. Laparoscopic appendectomy in patients with endometriosis. *J Minim Invasive Gynecol.* 2005;12(3):206–209.

147. Harris RS, Foster WG, Surrey MW, et al. Appendiceal disease in women with endometriosis and right lower quadrant pain. *J Am Assoc Gynecol Laparosc*. 2001;8:536–541.

148. Nezhat C, Pennington E, Nezhat F, Silfen SL. Laparoscopically assisted anterior rectal wall resection and reanastomosis for deeply infiltrating endometriosis. *Surg Laparosc Endosc*. 1991;1:106.

149. Nezhat C, Nezhat F, Pennington E. Laparoscopic proctectomy for infiltrating endometriosis of the rectum. *Fertil Steril*. 1992;57:1129.

150. Nezhat F, Nezhat C, Pennington E, Ambroze W. Laparoscopic segmental resection for infiltrating endometriosis of the rectosigmoid colon: a preliminary report. *Surg Laparosc Endosc*. 1992;2:212.

151. Sharpe DR, Redwine DB. Laparoscopic segmented resection of the sigmoid and the recto sigmoid colon for endometriosis. *Surg Laparosc Endosc*. 1992;2:120.

152. Redwine DB, Koning M, Sharpe DR. Laparoscopically assisted transvaginal segmental resection of the rectosigmoid colon for endometriosis. *Fertil Steril*. 1996;65:193.

153. Jerby BL, Kessler H, Falcon S, Milsom JW. Laparoscopic management of colorectal endometriosis. *Surg Endosc*. 1999;13:1125.

154. Nezhat C, Nezhat F, Pennington E, et al. Laparoscopic disk excision and primary repair of the anterior rectal wall for the treatment of full-thickness bowel endometriosis. *Surg Endosc*. 1994;8:682.

155. Nezhat C, Nezhat F, Ambroze W, Pennington E. Laparoscopic repair of small bowel, colon, and rectal endometriosis: a report of twenty-six cases. *Surg Endosc*. 1993;7:88.

156. Nezhat C, de Fazio A, Nicholson T, Nezhat C. Intraoperative sigmoidoscopy in gynecologic surgery. *J Minim Invasive Gynecol*. 2005;12(5):391–395.

157. Nezhat C, Seidman D, Nezhat F, Nezhat C. The role of intraoperative proctosigmoidoscopy in laparoscopic pelvic surgery. *J Am Assoc Gynecol Laparosc*. 2004;11(1):47–49.

158. Fedele L, Bianchi S, Portuese A, et al. Transrectal ultrasonography in the assessment of rectovaginal endometriosis. *Obstet Gynecol*. 1998;91:444.

159. Chapron C, Dumontier I, Dousset B, et al. Results and role of rectal endoscopic ultrasonography for patients with deep pelvic endometriosis. *Hum Reprod*. 1998;13:2266.

160. Donnez J, Nisolle M, Gillerot S, et al. Rectovaginal septum adenomyotic nodules: a series of 500 cases. *Br J Obstet Gynaecol*. 1997;104:1014.

161. Martin DC. Laparoscopic and vaginal colpotomy for the excision of infiltrating cul-de-sac endometriosis. *J Reprod Med*. 1988;33:806.

162. Redwine DB. Laparoscopic en bloc resection for treatment of the obliterated cul-de-sac in endometriosis. *J Reprod Med*. 1992;37:695.

163. Nezhat C, Nezhat F, Pennington E. Laparoscopic treatment of lower colorectal and infiltrative rectovaginal septum endometriosis by the technique of video-laseroscopy. *Br J Obstet Gynaecol*. 1992;99:664.

164. Donnez J, Nisolle M, Smoes P, et al. Peritoneal endometriosis and "endometriotic" nodules of the rectovaginal septum are two different entities. *Fertil Steril*. 1996;66:362.

165. Finkel L, Marchevsky A, Cohen B. Endometrial cyst of the liver. *Am J Gastroenterol*. 1986;81:576–578.

166. Nezhat C, Kazerooni T, Berker B, Lashay N, Fernandez S, Marziali M. Laparoscopic management of hepatic endometriosis: report of two cases and review of the literature. *J Minim Invasive Gynecol*. 2005;12(3):196–200.

167. Shiraishi T. Catamenial pneumothorax: report of a case and review of the Japanese and non-Japanese literature. *Thorac Cardiovasc Surg*. 1991;39:304.

168. Nezhat F, Nezhat C, Levy JS. Laparoscopic treatment of symptomatic diaphragmatic endometriosis: a case report. *Fertil Steril*. 1992;58:614.

169. Nezhat C, Seidman DS, Nezhat F, Nezhat C. Laparoscopic surgical management of diaphragmatic endometriosis. *Fertil Steril*. 1998;69:1048.

170. Black WT. Use of presacral sympathectomy in the treatment of dysmenorrhea: a second look after twenty-five years. *Am J Obstet Gynecol*. 1964;89:16.

171. Lee RB, Stone K, Magelssen D, et al. Presacral neurectomy for chronic pelvic pain. *Obstet Gynecol*. 1986;68:517.

172. Tjaden B, Schlaff WD, Kimball A, et al. The efficacy of presacral neurectomy for the relief of midline dysmenorrhea. *Obstet Gynecol*. 1990;76:89.

173. Adamson D. Surgical management of endometriosis. *Semin Reprod Med*. 2003;21(2):223–234.

174. Sutton CJ, Ewen SP, Whitelaw N, Haines P. Prospective, randomized, double-blind, controlled trial of laser laparoscopy in the treatment of pelvic pain associated with minimal, mild, and moderate endometriosis. *Fertil Steril*. 1994;62:696.

175. Sutton CJ, Pooley AS, Ewen SP, Haines P. Follow-up report on a randomized controlled trial of laser laparoscopy in the treatment of pelvic pain associated with minimal to moderate endometriosis. *Fertil Steril*. 1997;68:1070.

176. Abbott J, Hawe J, Hunter D, Holmes M, Finn P, Garry R. Laparoscopic excision of endometriosis: a randomized, placebo-controlled trial. *Fertil Steril*. 2004;82(4):878–884.

177. Tjaden B, Schlaff WD, Kimball A, Rock JA. The efficacy of presacral neurectomy for the relief of midline dysmenorrhea. *Obstet Gynecol*. 1990;76:89.

178. Candiani GB, Fedele L, Vercellini P, Bianchi S, Di-Nola G. Presacral neurectomy for the treatment of pelvic pain associated with endometriosis: a controlled study. *Am J Obstet Gynecol*. 1992;167:100–103.

179. Sutton C, Pooley AS, Jones KD, Dover RW, Haines P. A prospective, randomized, double-blind controlled trial of laparoscopic uterine nerve ablation in the treatment of pelvic pain associated with endometriosis. *Gynaecol Endosc*. 2001;10:217–222.

180. Nezhat C, Crowgey SR, Garrison CP. Surgical treatment of endometriosis via laser laparoscopy. *Fertil Steril*. 1986;45(6):778–783.

181. Hughes EG, Fedorkow DM, Collins JA. A quantitative overview of controlled trials in endometriosis-associated infertility. *Fertil Steril*. 1993;59:963–970.

182. Buyalos RP, Agarwal SK. Endometriosis-associated infertility. *Curr Opin Obstet Gynecol*. 2000;12(5):377–381.

183. Winkel CA. Evaluation and management of women with endometriosis. *Obstet Gynecol*. 2003;102:397–408.

184. Donnez J, Nisolle M, Gillet N, Smets M, Bassil S, Casanas-Roux F. Large ovarian endometriomas. *Hum Reprod*. 1996;11:641–646.

185. Aboulghar MA, Mansour RT, Serour GI, Al-Inany HG, Aboulghar MM. The outcome of in vitro fertilization in advanced endometriosis with previous surgery: a case-controlled study. *Am J Obstet Gynecol*. 2003;188:371–375.

186. Nargund G, Cheng WC, Parsons J. The impact of ovarian cystectomy on ovarian response to stimulation during in-vitro fertilization cycles. *Hum Reprod*. 1996;11:81–83.

187. Ho HY, Lee RK, Hwu YM, Lin MH, Su JT, Tsai YC. Poor response of ovaries with endometrioma previously treated with cystectomy

to controlled ovarian hyperstimulation. *J Assist Reprod Genet.* 2002;19:507–511.

188. Somigliana E, Ragni G, Benedetti F, Borroni R, Vegetti W, Crosignani PG. Does laparoscopic excision of endometriotic ovarian cysts significantly affect ovarian reserve? Insights from IVF cycles. *Hum Reprod.* 2003;18(11):2450–2453.

189. Donnez J, Wyns C, Nisolle M. Does ovarian surgery for endometriomas impair the ovarian response to gonadotropin? *Fertil Steril.* 2001;76(4):662–665.

190. Loh FH, Tan AT, Kumar J, Ng SC. Ovarian response after laparoscopic ovarian cystectomy for endometriotic cysts in 132 monitored cycles. *Fertil Steril.* 1999;72:316–321.

191. Muzii L, Bianchi A, Croce C, Manci N, Panici PB. Laparoscopic excision of ovarian cysts: is the stripping technique a tissue-sparing procedure? *Fertil Steril.* 2002;77:609–614.

192. Barnhart K, Dunsmoor-Su R, Coutifaris C. Effect of endometriosis on in vitro fertilization. *Fertil Steril.* 2002;77(6):1148–1155.

193. The Practice Committee of the American Society for Reproductive Medicine. Endometriosis and infertility. *Fertil Steril.* 2004;81(5):1441–1446.

194. Olive DL, Henderson DY. Endometriosis and müllerian anomalies. *Obstet Gynecol.* 1987;69:412.

195. Moghissi KS, Boyce CR. Management of endometriosis with oral medroxyprogesterone acetate. *Obstet Gynecol.* 1976;47:265.

196. Szendei G, Hernadi Z, Devenyi N, Csapo Z. Is there any correlation between stages of endometriosis and severity of chronic pelvic pain? Possibilities of treatment. *Gynecol Endocrinol.* 2005;21(2):93–100.

197. Ailawadi RK, Jobanputra S, Kataria M, Gurates B, Bulun SE. Treatment of endometriosis and chronic pelvic pain with letrozole and norethindrone acetate: a pilot study. *Fertil Steril.* 2004;81:290–296.

198. Henzi MR, Corson SL, Moghissi K, et al. Photodynamic therapy of rabbit endometrial implants: a model treatment of endometriosis. *Fertil Steril.* 1989;52:140.

199. Manyak MJ, Nelson LM, Solomon D, et al. Photodynamic therapy of rabbit endometrial implants: a model treatment of endometriosis. *Fertil Steril.* 1989;52:140.

200. Almeida OD Jr, Val-Gallas JM. Office microlaparoscopy under local anesthesia in the diagnosis and treatment of chronic pelvic pain. *J Am Assoc Gynecol Laparosc.* 1998;5:407.

201. Faber BM, Coddington CC 3d. Microlaparoscopy: a comparative study of diagnostic accuracy. *Fertil Steril.* 1997;67:952.

202. Evans SF, Petrucco OM. Microlaparoscopy for suspected pelvic pathology – a comparison of 2mm versus 10mm laparoscope. *Aust N Z J Obstet Gynaecol.* 1998;38:215.

203. Steege JF. Superior hypogastric block during microlaparoscopic pain mapping. *J Am Assoc Gynecol Laparosc.* 1998;5:265.

204. Yang JZ, Van Dijk-Smith JP, Van Vugt DA, et al. Fluorescence and photosensitization of experimental endometriosis in the rat after systemic 5-aminolevulinic acid administration: a potential new approach to the diagnosis and treatment of endometriosis. *Am J Obstet Gynecol.* 1996;174:154.

11 | LAPAROSCOPIC ADHESIOLYSIS AND ADHESION PREVENTION

Bulent Berker, Senzan Hsu, Ceana Nezhat, Farr Nezhat, and Camran Nezhat

Adhesions are defined as connections between opposing serosal and/or nonserosal surfaces of the internal organs and the abdominal wall, at sites where there should be no connection. This connection can be a band, which is vascular or avascular, and filmy/transparent or dense/opaque, or it could be a cohesive connection of surfaces without an intervening adhesion band.[1] Adhesion formation is an almost unavoidable consequence of abdominal surgery. Although not all patients with intra-abdominal adhesions develop symptoms, the clinical implications, such as early and late bowel obstruction, infertility, and chronic abdominal pain, remain a common problem in general surgical and gynecologic practice.[2] In addition, adhesion formation is associated with increased socioeconomic costs.

THE RISK FACTORS AND CLINICAL SIGNIFICANCE OF ADHESIONS

The risk factors for pelvic adhesions include a history of pelvic inflammatory disease (PID), prior surgery, perforated appendix, endometriosis, and inflammatory bowel diseases.[3] Other recognized causes of adhesions include bacterial peritonitis, radiotherapy, chemical peritonitis, foreign body reaction, long-term continuous ambulatory peritoneal dialysis, endometriosis, and pelvic inflammatory disease.[4] However, the greatest contribution of these risk factors is a previous history of an intra-abdominal operative procedure.

Adhesion formation after abdominal and pelvic operations remains extremely common and is a source of considerable morbidity. Menzies and Ellis [5] confirmed that after an intra-abdominal operation, most patients developed adhesions. They found that after merely one previous abdominal operation, 93% of patients had adhesions. In contrast, the prevalence rate of intra-abdominal adhesions among patients who had never experienced a laparotomy was 10.4%. More importantly, within 1 year of laparotomy, 1% of patients developed adhesion-related intestinal obstruction.[5] The recurrence rate of adhesion-related intestinal obstruction after surgery is 11% to 12%.[6] Gynecologists manage more than 20% of all female patients with intestinal obstruction. It has been reported that abdominal hysterectomy is among the most commonly performed operations contributing to intestinal obstruction associated with postoperative adhesions.[7] Myomectomy is associated with a high degree of adnexal adhesions, especially after incision performed on the posterior uterine wall.[8]

Patients undergoing laparoscopy after a previous laparotomy should be considered at risk for the presence of adhesions between the old scar and the bowel and omentum. Patients with midline abdominal incisions had more adhesions than did those with Pfannenstiel incisions. Patients with midline incisions done for gynecologic indications had more adhesions than did patients with any abdominal incision made for obstetric indications. The presence of adhesions in patients with previous obstetric operations was not affected by the type of incision. Adhesions to the bowel were more common after midline incisions above the umbilicus. Twenty-one women had direct injury to adherent omentum and bowel during the laparoscopic procedure.[9]

Pelvic adhesions may cause infertility and pain. Adhesions may result in infertility by causing mechanical blockage to the fallopian tubes, thus preventing oocyte retrieval. Fifteen percent to 20% of female infertility is caused by adhesions.[10] Caspi and associates [11] reported an inverse relation between the severity of pelvic adhesions and pregnancy rates. After adhesiolysis, pregnancy rates vary according to the extent of adnexal damage and, to a lesser degree, the severity of the adhesions.[11–14] Pregnancy rates are increased by 38% to 52% among previously infertile patients following adhesiolysis.[15] Para-ovarian peritubal adhesions inhibit follicular growth by possible ovarian entrapment from adhesions around the ovaries.[16] Peritubal as well as intratubal adhesions may affect tubal motility and ovum transport. The slowing or prevention of the embryo's arrival in the uterus may lead to either infertility or an ectopic pregnancy. Ectopic pregnancies have been implicated as possible sequelae of peritubal or intratubal adhesions. Infertility may be caused not only by tubal dysfunction but also by adhesion formation following treatment of an ectopic gestation either by laparotomy or laparoscopy.[17]

Chronic pelvic pain (CPP) is one of the sequelae of intraperitoneal adhesions. Pelvic adhesive diseases, either postoperative or from pelvic inflammatory reactions, and endometrioses are the most common morphologic changes seen in women with pelvic pain.[18] Unilateral pelvic pain is usually associated with adhesions on the same side as the symptom. A number of studies have shown that division of adhesions at surgery is useful in the treatment of CPP.[19,20] Nezhat and colleagues [21] evaluated the short- and long-term results of laparoscopic enterolysis in patients with CPP following hysterectomy. In their study, 48 patients were evaluated at time intervals from 2 weeks to 5 years after laparoscopic enterolysis. Patients were asked to rate postoperative relief of their pelvic pain as complete/near-complete relief (80% to 100% pain relief), significant relief (50% to 80% pain relief), or less than 50% or no pain relief. They found that after 2 to 8 weeks, 39% of patients reported complete/near-complete pain relief, 33% reported significant pain relief, and 28% reported less than 50% or no pain relief. Six months to 1 year post laparoscopy, 49% of patients reported complete/near-complete pain relief, 15% reported significant pain relief, and 36% reported less than 50% or no pain relief. Two to 5 years after laparoscopic enterolysis, 37% of patients reported complete/near-complete pain relief, 30% reported significant pain relief, and 33% reported less than 50% or no pain relief. Some patients required between one and three subsequent laparoscopic adhesiolysis procedures. The authors concluded that laparoscopic enterolysis may offer significant long-term relief of CPP in some patients. A detailed discussion of CPP management may be found in Chapter 15.

Intra-abdominal adhesions lead to significant morbidity and severely affect the quality of life of millions of people worldwide. In the United States, 303,836 hospitalizations resulted from surgeries that were performed primarily for adhesiolysis of adhesions of the digestive and female reproductive systems in 1994. These procedures resulted in 846,415 days of inpatient care at a cost of $1.3 billion.[22] A study from Sweden revealed direct costs of $5695 per patient for the nonoperative and operative treatment of adhesion-related bowel obstruction.[23] Moreover, it was estimated that obstructive bowel disease may cause 2330 hospital admissions annually, which are associated with direct costs of about $13 million.

Because the development of postoperative adhesions is a major factor in deciding the outcome of fertility-promoting operative procedures, gynecologists should understand the mechanism of their formation, use optimal techniques for adhesiolysis, and apply agents or devices to reduce their development.

FORMATION OF ADHESIONS AND THE VALUE OF MINIMALLY INVASIVE SURGERY

Before the action of various adhesio-preventive strategies can be assessed, the key components and interactions involved in the process of peritoneal healing itself must be thoroughly understood. At the time of surgery, the initial mesothelial injury exposes a denuded and acellular surface that serves as the nidus for wound healing and/or tissue–tissue adhesion. This submesothelial damage and unveiling of the submesothelial matrix occurs with simultaneous activation of the coagulation cascade and deposition of fibrin at the site of injury. Under normal conditions, this fibrinous exudate serves as a platform for appropriate healing to progress, but under certain pathologic circumstances, the deposited fibrin may instead serve as a bridge between unrelated, neighboring tissues. Within a very short period of time, the wound and its surrounding area are invaded by inflammatory cells that migrate from the peritoneal vasculature or from the peritoneal fluid itself.[24] Normal fibrinolytic activity usually prevents fibrinous attachments (fibrinous exudate) for 72 to 96 hours after injury. Mesothelial repair occurs within 5 days of trauma. A single cell layer of mesothelium covers the injured raw area, replacing the fibrinous exudate. Next, the injured wound surface is evenly reperitonealized by the combined effort of multiple foci of proliferating mesothelial cells. Reperitonealization continues for 7 to 10 days, during which the entire surface becomes covered by a contiguous sheet of mesothelium.

The fibrinolytic system clearly plays a significant role in adhesion formation/re-formation. There are also interactions between the fibrinolytic system and other proteinases, particularly the metalloproteinases and tissue inhibitors of metallo-

Table 11.1: Predisposing Factors for Adhesions

Ischemia

Drying of serosal surfaces

Excessive suturing

Omental patches

Traction of peritoneum

Blood clots retained in peritoneal cavity

Prolonged operations

Adnexal trauma

Infection

proteinases. However, if the fibrinolytic activity of the peritoneum is suppressed, fibroblasts will migrate, proliferate, and form fibrous adhesions with collagen deposition and vascular proliferation.[25] The factors that suppress fibrinolytic activity and promote the formation of postoperative adhesions are listed in Table 11.1.

Peritoneal healing differs from that of skin. Skin reepithelialization takes place through proliferation of epithelial cells from the periphery toward the center of the skin wound. By contrast, regardless of the size of the injury, the peritoneum becomes mesothelialized simultaneously, with new mesothelium developing from islands of mesothelial cells that later proliferate into sheets of cells. Consequently, large skin injuries take longer to reepithelialize than do small skin injuries. Larger peritoneal wounds remesothelialize about as quickly as small peritoneal wounds, within 5 to 6 days for the parietal peritoneum and within 5 to 8 days for both the visceral mesothelium.[26]

Meticulous surgical technique with careful tissue handling and application of the rules of microsurgery may prevent the adhesion formation. Microsurgery includes the use of magnification, gentle handling of tissues, constant irrigation, meticulous hemostasis, the use of microsurgical instruments, the use of fine nonreactive sutures, and precise approximation of tissue. Fertility-promoting operations done by laparotomy often are followed by re-formation of adhesions and the development of new adhesions even when proper microsurgical techniques are applied. Re-formation of adhesions is found at 37% to 72% of operative sites [27,28], and 51% of patients develop new adhesions after reproductive procedures by laparotomy.[28]

The introduction of laparoscopic surgery into the armament of general surgery and gynecology was associated with the expectation of markedly reduced adhesion formation. Several animal and clinical studies compared the formation of postoperative adhesions after fertility-promoting operations by laparoscopy and laparotomy. With few exceptions, operative laparoscopy resulted in the development of fewer re-formed and new adhesions.[13,29–32] These results are consistent with the observations made a century ago by Von Dembrowski [33] and later confirmed by Ellis.[34] They reported that uncomplicated peritoneal injuries, such as those likely to occur at operative laparoscopy, heal without the development of adhesions (Table 11.2).

Table 11.2: Historical Perspective

Author	Year	Contribution
Von Dembrowski [33]	1898	Peritoneal defects in dogs heal mostly without adhesions.
DeRenzi and Boeri [100]	1903	Ischemia is a major factor in the formation of adhesions.
Thomas [101]	1950	Oversewing serosal defects increases rather than decreases adhesions.
Ellis [34]	1971	Excision of parietal peritoneum from rats healed without adhesions in 52 of 58 experiments. "Meticulous" repair of peritoneal defects in 16 of 19 experiments resulted in fibrous adhesions.
Ryan et al. [102]	1971	The combination of tissue drying and bleeding is a major promoter of adhesions.

Even if adhesiolysis can be completely conducted initially, there is a high failure rate after follow-up because of adhesion re-formation and de novo adhesion formation. Adhesion formation and re-formation after either diagnostic or operative laparoscopy or after a laparotomy have been studied, but there is no unified classification. The most comprehensive classification of adhesion re-formation was the one introduced by Diamond and Nezhat in 1993 [35]:

Type 1. De novo adhesions: adhesions occurring at sites with no previous adhesion.

Type 1a. Adhesions at sites where no surgical procedure was performed, such as adhesions caused by indirect trauma.

Type 1b. Adhesions at sites of a surgical procedure other than adhesiolysis, such as adhesions caused by direct trauma.

Type 2. Re-formed adhesions: adhesions re-forming at sites of previous adhesiolysis.

Type 2a. Adhesions occurring at sites of adhesiolysis only.

Type 2b. Adhesions occurring at sites of adhesiolysis, plus sites of another procedure, such as treatment of endometriosis.

Wiseman et al. [36] conducted a review of the topic based on the stratification system of Diamond and Nezhat.[35] They compared laparoscopy versus laparotomy and found that the adhesion-free outcome was actually greater after laparotomy (54.2% de novo type 1b; 26.6% re-formed) than after laparoscopy (37.2% de novo type 1b; 14.3% re-formed).

Decreased adhesion formation after laparoscopic procedures has been attributed to the reduced presence of foreign bodies within the peritoneum that tend to stimulate more numerous and dense adhesions.[37] Laparoscopic operations may lead to fewer adhesions because tissue trauma distant from the site of adhesions increases their formation. The type of injury to the peritoneum can control the formation of intra-abdominal adhesions. The potential to form adhesions is significantly higher in visceral than in parietal peritoneal lesions.[38] Transperitoneal laparoscopy did not increase adhesions compared with extraperitoneal laparotomy in an animal model.[39] The transperitoneal laparoscopy approach also induced fewer adhesions than did transperitoneal laparotomy. A presumed advantage of the extraperitoneal approach is the avoidance of adhesions because the peritoneum is not entered and direct contact with intra-abdominal structures is avoided.

When the peritoneum is dissected from the abdominal wall, it is partially devascularized, leading to scars and potential adhesions. Dissection of the peritoneum from the overlying abdominal wall in a murine model may cause intra-abdominal adhesions. The totally extraperitoneal approach may not avoid the risk of intra-abdominal adhesions.[40]

A laparoscopic approach to surgery is more convenient for the patient, is considered to be less traumatic to tissue, and is associated with reduced inflammatory response, which is presumed to lower the risk of postsurgical adhesion formation.[41] Summarizing the results, laparoscopy indeed reduces postoperative adhesion formation experimentally and in humans. Table 11.3 shows the advantages of laparoscopic procedures for preventing adhesion formation. Although laparoscopic procedures result in fewer adhesions than do laparotomy procedures, adhesions may develop even after laparoscopy. To minimize the formation of adhesions, good surgical technique involves the basic principles of microsurgery, liberal irrigation of the abdominal cavity, and instillation of a large amount of lactated Ringer's solution at the completion of the procedure.[42] Alternatively, an early second-look laparoscopy after laparoscopy may be useful for assessing the degree of postoperative adhesions, allow technically easy adhesiolysis, and result in lower adhesion scores, as shown by third-look procedures.[43]

THE VALUE OF ADJUVANTS

Despite much interest in prevention, the formation of peritoneal adhesions continues to be a significant and common side effect of intra-abdominal surgery. Although microsurgical techniques and operative laparoscopy may reduce the formation of adhesions, the benefit derived from various adjuvants remains controversial despite their widespread use. An optimal adhesive barrier should be easy to apply in the operating room (e.g., sprayable), have the appropriate chemical and physical properties and kinetics (e.g., dissolve after 1 to 2 weeks), and be nontoxic and biocompatible.[24] Moreover, the ideal barrier,

Table 11.3: Advantages of Laparoscopic Procedures for Preventing Adhesion Formation

Decreased peritoneal injury

Minimized tissue handling

Decreased immune and stress response

Prevention of air pollution in the abdominal cavity

Reduced drying of the peritoneal surface

Intact peritoneal phospholipid layer

Reduced impairment of gut motility

Table 11.4: Pharmacological Interventions to Prevent Adhesions

Nonsteroidal anti-inflammatory drugs

Corticosteroids

Antihistamines

Progesterone/estrogen

Anticoagulants

Fibrinolytics

Antibiotics

besides being safe and effective, should be noninflammatory and nonimmunogenic, persist during the critical remesothelialization phase, stay in place without sutures or staples, remain active in the presence of blood, and be completely biodegradable. In addition, it should not interfere with healing, promote infection, or cause adhesions.[26] We still do not have an ideal adhesion-preventing substance. Following is a summary of the most commonly used adhesion-reducing substances.

Pharmacologic Interventions

A classical approach to adhesion prevention has been the use of drugs to inhibit or retard adhesion formation without providing a physical barrier to tissue contact (Table 11.4). These pharmacologic interventions include the use of anticoagulants and fibrinolytics (e.g., tissue plasminogen activator, heparin, and low molecular weight heparins), anti-inflammatory agents (e.g., nonsteroidal anti-inflammatory drugs and steroids), growth factor inhibitors and modulators, and various other medications to attenuate the formation of postsurgical adhesions. Steroids and antihistamines are used infrequently because of their questionable efficacy and potential adverse effects, such as delayed wound healing and the risk of wound dehiscence.[44] Unfortunately, a global examination of the literature suggests there are very little clinical data supporting the use of any one of these interventions as the standard of care.[24] Other most commonly known adhesion barriers are listed in Table 11.5 and evaluated in the following paragraphs.

Peritoneal Instillates

Crystalloids

Absorption of water and electrolytes from the peritoneal cavity is rapid, with up to 500 mL of iso-osmolar sodium chloride absorbed in less than 24 hours.[45] Because it takes 5 to 8 days for peritoneal surfaces to remesothelialize, a crystalloid solution should be absorbed well before the processes of fibrin deposition and adhesion formation are complete. From a theoretical point of view, intraperitoneal crystalloid instillates are not expected to prevent adhesion formation.[26] A substantial body of clinical data is available to assess the benefit of crystalloid instillates, such as saline and lactated Ringer's solution, in adhesion prevention. During the early 1980s, many clinical studies were pub-

lished that compared dextran with crystalloid used as instillates. A combination of these studies showed an adhesion re-formation rate of approximately 80% in patients who received crystalloid instillates.[46] To significantly reduce adhesion formation and re-formation, the device must effectively separate damaged surfaces during the crucial phases of postsurgical repair. The rapid rate of absorption of crystalloid solution from the peritoneal cavity (35 to 60 mL/hour) may preclude its residence during the crucial time of adhesion formation. Meta-analysis of clinical studies using crystalloid solution conclusively showed no reduction in adhesion with instillation of lactated Ringer's solution or saline.[36]

32% Dextran 70 (Hyskon)

Hyskon (Medisan Pharmaceuticals Inc., Parsippany, NJ), a high molecular weight form of dextran, is absorbed from the peritoneal cavity over 7 to 10 days. Its osmotic effect draws fluid into the peritoneal cavity to float mobile peritoneal organs, reducing adherence between intraperitoneal structures. Through dilution,

Table 11.5: Barriers to Prevent Adhesions

Peritoneal Instillates

Crystalloids

32% Dextran 70 (Hyskon)

Hyaluronic acid

    Hyaluronic acid with ferric ion (Intergel)

    Combined hyaluronic acid and carboxymethylcellulose (Sepracoat)

Hydrogel (SprayGel)

Viscous gel

    Carboxymethylcellulose and polyethylene glycol (viscoelastic gel)

    Auto–cross-linked hyaluronan gel (Hyalobarrier)

Solid Adhesion Barriers

Oxidized regenerated cellulose (Interceed)

Expanded polytetrafluoroethylene (Gore-Tex)

Combined hyaluronic acid and carboxymethylcellulose (Seprafilm)

dextran also diminishes local fibrin concentration, preserves local plasminogen activators, and interferes with polymorphonuclear neutrophil expression of adhesion molecules.[47,48] Some studies in animals [49] and humans [49,50] have shown reduced postoperative adhesions, but inconsistent results suggest limited efficacy. In addition, there have been reports of allergic reactions [51,52], infections, and complications of fluid overload.

Hyaluronic Acid

Hyaluronic acid (HA) is a naturally occurring glycosaminoglycan and a major component of the extracellular matrix, including connective tissue, skin, cartilage, and vitreous and synovial fluids. HA is biocompatible, nonimmunogenic, nontoxic, and naturally bioabsorbable. Like carboxymethylcellulose, it is negatively charged at physiologic pH and freely soluble.[26] HA coats serosal surfaces and provides a certain degree of protection from serosal desiccation and other types of injury. However, its use after tissue injury is ineffective.

HYALURONIC ACID WITH FERRIC ION (INTERGEL)

Cross-linking HA with ferric ion (FeHA) increases its viscosity and half-life. The first marketed derivative of FeHA is Intergel (Lifecore, Johnson and Johnson Gynecare Unit, New Brunswick, NJ). Intergel Adhesion Prevention Solution is a single-use, sterile, nonpyrogenic 0.5% ferric hyaluronate gel. This amber-colored aqueous gel of sodium hyaluronate has been ionically cross-linked with ferric ions and adjusted to isotonicity with sodium chloride. It is packaged in a bellows-type container designed to deliver 300 mL of Intergel solution. Intergel solution functions by providing a viscous, lubricated coating on the peritoneal surfaces, minimizing tissue apposition during the critical period of fibrin formation and mesothelial regeneration. Lymphatic drainage appears to be the major elimination pathway for intraperitoneally administered Intergel solution. The elimination half-life ($t_{1/2}$) of Intergel solution in humans has been estimated from animal studies to be approximately 51 hours. The 300-mL Intergel solution instillation is expected to clear from the peritoneal cavity in 5 to 7 days.

Intergel solution has been shown to be easy to use in a multicenter randomized study and to reduce the number, severity, and extent of postoperative adhesions after gynecologic surgery.[53] The product was withdrawn from the market because of several reports of late-onset postoperative pain requiring repeated surgery. Other reported side effects are foreign body reactions and tissue adherence.[54]

COMBINED HYALURONIC ACID AND CARBOXYMETHYLCELLULOSE (SEPRACOAT)

Sepracoat (Genzyme Corp., Cambridge, MA) is composed of chemically derived sodium hyaluronate and carboxymethylcellulose (HAL-C). Sepracoat is bioresorbable, with an intraabdominal residence time of 24 hours or less and complete clearance in 5 days or less. It acts by decreasing tissue desiccation. This solution coats tissues with a temporary, protective, viscous barrier.[55] Preclinical studies have shown Sepracoat to be safe and effective in reducing and preventing de novo adhesion formation in animal models.[56] In animal studies, tissue precoating with Sepracoat significantly reduced de novo adhesion formation compared with nontreated control animals.[56,57] Consistent with those observations, in a multi-center randomized clinical trial, Sepracoat significantly increased the percentage of patients who were free of de novo adhesion formation to 13.1%, compared with 4.6% of the control group.[58] The use of Sepracoat also was associated with significant reductions in the proportion of available sites with de novo adhesion formation, as well as the severity and extent of de novo adhesion formation.

Hydrogel (SprayGel)

SprayGel Adhesion Barrier (Confluent Surgical, Waltham, MA) is a synthetic hydrogel that forms when two polyethylene glycol (PEG)-based liquids are sprayed onto target tissue, where the precursor liquids cross-link within seconds to form an absorbable, flexible, adherent gel barrier in situ. The delivery system is a 5-mm–diameter, air-assisted sprayer that can be used in either laparoscopic or open procedures. The gel barrier remains intact at the site of application for approximately 5 to 7 days, protecting the target tissue during the normal wound-healing period, and then gradually breaks down through hydrolysis into PEG constituent molecules that are resorbed and rapidly cleared by the kidneys. The material has been shown to be highly biocompatible.[59,60]

Mettler et al. [61] evaluated 66 women who underwent myomectomy with or without SprayGel application. A second-look laparoscopy was performed in 40 women. The investigators reported that seven of 22 patients (31.8%) in the SprayGel group and two of 18 patients (11.1%) in the control group were free of adhesions. This product might be well suited for infertility surgery, endometriosis, pelvic floor repair, and any surgeries carried out for adhesiolysis, but this needs to be further investigated.

Viscous Gel

The carboxymethylcellulose and PEG formulation is a transparent, viscoelastic gel that is readily administered to the specific anatomic sites where adhesion formation is a concern. This ease of use includes single-unit packaging stored at room temperature, which, when opened, delivers the sterile gel and applicator directly to the operating field. The gel viscosity allows the surgeon to control directly the rate of gel delivery to the surgical site. When the surgeon stops depressing the syringe, gel stops flowing. Gel residing within the applicator tube does not harden, allowing for continued application at the convenience of the surgeon. In a small randomized series, 15 mL of viscoelastic gel was instilled to the adnexal area in 25 patients. The results were compared with those of 24 patients who underwent surgery without the use of the gel.[62] The authors reported that the use of viscoelastic gel showed a significant reduction in the number of adnexa that developed adhesions following surgery. In the viscoelastic gel–treated group, 93% of the adnexa did not have a worse adhesion category in contrast to 56% of the control adnexa at the time of second look. These differences were highly significant and demonstrated the overall benefit of viscoelastic gel when used with good surgical technique to enhance the likelihood of a good response to surgical therapy. The gel was safe and no complications or adverse events were observed in the treatment group.

A highly viscous gel of HA derivatives obtained through an auto–cross-linking process that does not introduce foreign bridge molecules, namely auto–cross-linked hyaluronan gel (Hyalobarrier, FAB-Fidia), has recently been developed. The auto–cross-linked polymer is an inter- and intramolecular ester of HA in which a proportion of the carboxyl groups is esterified with hydroxyl groups belonging to the same and/or different molecules of the polysaccharide, thus forming a mixture of lactones and intermolecular ester bonds. The level of cross-linking can be varied by modulating the reaction conditions. The absence of foreign bridge molecules ensures the release of native HA only during degradation, whereas the auto–cross-linking process improves the viscoelastic properties of the gel compared with unmodified HA solutions of the same molecular weight.[63]

Preclinical trials in animal models have shown that auto–cross-linked hyaluronan gel reduces the incidence and severity of postoperative adhesions.[64,65] Moreover, preliminary clinical studies in hysteroscopic surgery as well as laparotomic and laparoscopic myomectomy have suggested that auto–cross-linked hyaluronan gel may reduce the incidence and severity of postoperative adhesions in pelvic surgery [66,67], with improvement in the pregnancy rate in infertile patients who were submitted to laparoscopic myomectomy.[68]

Recently, Mais and et al. [69] investigated the applicability, safety, and efficacy of an auto–cross-linked hyaluronan gel in preventing adhesion formation after laparoscopic myomectomy. Fifty-two patients were randomly allocated to receive either the gel or no adhesion prevention. At second look, the incidence and severity of postoperative adhesions were assessed laparoscopically after 12 to 14 weeks. A nonsignificantly higher proportion of patients receiving the gel were free from adhesions (13 of 21; 62%) compared with control patients (nine of 22; 41%), with a statistically significant difference between the severity of uterine adhesions at baseline and at second look. The authors suggested that the auto–cross-linked hyaluronan gel might have a favorable safety profile and efficacious antiadhesive action following laparoscopic myomectomy.

Solid Adhesion Barriers

Oxidized Regenerated Cellulose (Interceed)

Interceed (Gynecare, Johnson & Johnson Medical, Somerville, NJ) is an absorbable adhesion barrier made of oxidized regenerated cellulose (ORC). Evidence has shown that Interceed is safe and effective in reducing the incidence of postoperative adhesions in patients undergoing various laparoscopic operations.[70] ORC is the first commercially marketed adhesion barrier. ORC prevents adhesion formation by its transformation into a gelatinous mass covering the damaged peritoneum. When applied to a raw peritoneal surface, it becomes gel within 8 hours. ORC can be applied easily by laparoscopy, follows the contour of the organ, and does not need suturing.

It has been postulated that ORC may compete for the macrophage scavenger receptor because of its polyanionic nature. Results from in vitro studies suggest that the interaction of Interceed with macrophages with scavenger receptors results in decreased secretion of matrix components, inflammatory mediators, and cellular growth factors. Thus, Interceed cellulose may function as a biologic barrier in preventing adhesions.[71] In two multicenter clinical studies [72,73], Interceed was placed on only one pelvic side wall at the conclusion of the operation, although both areas had been treated for comparable disease. At a second-look laparoscopy, fewer adhesions re-formed on the side treated with Interceed, although postoperative adhesions were not elim-

inated completely. Haney and Doty [74] applied Interceed in the abdominal cavity of normal mice. They found peritoneal injury and new adhesions between the abdominal peritoneum and the intra-abdominal viscera. Pagidas and Tulandi [75] found that Interceed was not effective in decreasing postoperative adhesions in rats. Fewer adhesions were found in animals treated with Gore-Tex (W. L. Gore & Associates, Inc., Flagstaff, AZ) and lactated Ringer's solution than in control and Interceed-treated animals.[75] On the other hand, in the rabbit model, Interceed reduced the incidence and score of postoperative ovarian adhesions and improved the reproductive outcome.[76] Azziz [77] observed in a prospective, randomized trial involving 134 patients undergoing adhesiolysis by standard microsurgical techniques at laparotomy that 90% benefited from the use of Interceed.

Randomized prospective studies showed a significant reduction in the formation of postoperative adhesions after laparoscopic ovarian operations [78,79], myomectomy [80], and surgical treatment of endometriosis.[81] Interceed is supplied as a sterile unit of 7.6 cm × 10.2 cm and is cut to the appropriate size to be applied on the desired organ. It is essential that complete hemostasis be achieved before ORC is placed on the peritoneal surface, as the presence of intraperitoneal blood negates any beneficial effect. Because hemostasis at the myomectomy incision is rarely absolute, its use could be precluded.[82] Fixation of Interceed by placing 6-0 Vicryl sutures [83] and the addition of heparin [84] did not enhance the adhesion-reducing capacity. Rather than support bacterial growth, ORC exhibits antibacterial properties in vivo. Interceed appears to play an important role and may provide beneficial effects in preventing and reducing postoperative adhesion development. The efficacy of this absorbable barrier is limited to situations in which the traumatized area can be covered completely. Effective application is limited by technical difficulties, including the need for hemostasis and removal of excess peritoneal fluid.[70]

Expanded Polytetrafluoroethylene (Gore-Tex)

Another barrier material is an expanded polytetrafluoroethylene (PTFE) Gore-Tex surgical membrane. This material is a nonabsorbable, nonreactive surgical membrane that has been used to repair and reconstruct the pericardium and peritoneum.[85] Expanded PTFE is an antithrombogenic, nontoxic synthetic fabric with small pores that inhibit cellular transmigration and tissue adherence. The use of PTFE is strictly reserved for noncontamination operations. This barrier should be sutured to the tissue, overlapping the incision by more than 1 cm. It prevents adhesion formation and re-formation regardless of the type of injury or whether hemostasis is achieved.[82]

Animal studies by Boyers and associates [86] revealed that the Gore-Tex surgical membrane was effective in reducing primary adhesions after pelvic operations. Gore-Tex membrane was applied over the raw surface of the peritoneal wall or uterus after adhesiolysis or myomectomy by laparotomy. At second-look laparoscopy, when the surgical membrane was removed, the mean postoperative adhesion score had been reduced from 10.13 ± 0.35 to 0.75 ± 2.12 ($P \leq 0.001$).[86] The Gore-Tex surgical membrane may reduce postmyomectomy adhesions.[87] At laparoscopy, 15 of 27 incisions covered with PTFE (55.6%) and only two of 27 uncovered sites (7.4%) were completely free of adhesions. A randomized, prospective crossover study in nonhuman primates found that the Gore-Tex surgical membrane was

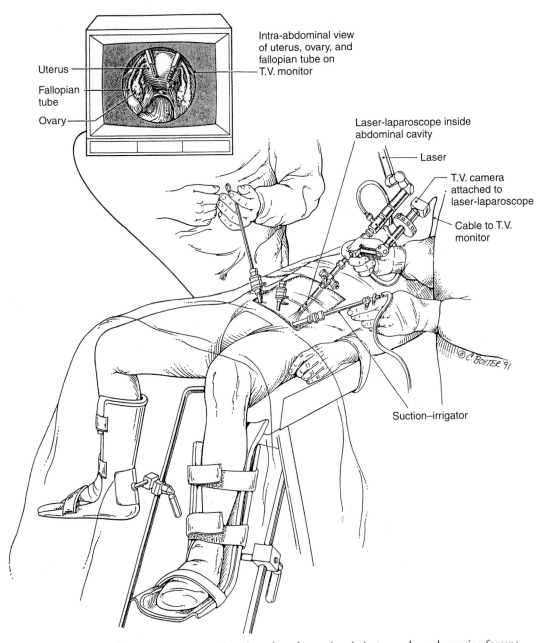

Figure 11.1. Suprapubic punctures are made to introduce the suction–irrigator probe and grasping forceps.

better than Interceed with respect to the size of the adhesion area, tenacity, and vascularity, with a significant improvement in the total adhesion score.[88] These results were confirmed in a multicenter, nonblinded randomized clinical trial that enrolled 32 women with bilateral pelvic side wall adhesions undergoing reconstructive pelvic operations and second-look laparoscopy. Expanded PTFE was associated with fewer postsurgical adhesions to the pelvic side wall compared with Interceed.[89]

The Gore-Tex surgical membrane may be used laparoscopically.[89] It is easy to introduce and position over a peritoneal defect because its handling properties do not diminish with wetting. Fixation is secured with laparoscopic staples.[90] Removal of the PTFE barrier at early second-look laparoscopy 11 days after myomectomy was not associated with adhesions.[91] Various studies compared the efficacy of the two adhesion barriers

in women undergoing reconstructive pelvic surgery and found that PTFE was associated with fewer postsurgical adhesions to the pelvic sidewall than was ORC.[92,93] However, as a result of its nonabsorbable nature, most gynecologists are reluctant to use PTFE.

Combined Hyaluronic Acid and Carboxymethylcellulose (Seprafilm)

Seprafilm (Genzyme Corp., Cambridge, MA), which is composed of modified HA and carboxymethylcellulose (HA-CMC), is effective as a surgical adjuvant for the reduction of adhesions. HA is a normal constituent of the extracellular matrix, connective tissue, synovial fluid, umbilical cord, and vitreous humor. Carboxymethylcellulose is a commonly used filler found in food, cosmetics, and pharmaceuticals; it has no known toxic effects and has been shown in animal studies to be effective in reducing postoperative adhesions. The Seprafilm barrier has significantly reduced the incidence, extent, and severity of postoperative adhesions in a variety of animal models [94,95] and also in two large prospective randomized, controlled multicenter clinical studies. One of these studies involved gynecologic surgery using myomectomy in which patients randomly received Seprafilm wrapped over the entire uterus or no treatment.[96] The other study involved general surgery in which patients undergoing colectomy and ileal pouch–anal anastomosis with diverting loop ileostomy randomly did or did not receive Seprafilm placed under the midline incision before closure of the abdomen.[97] In both trials, Seprafilm significantly reduced postoperative adhesion development.

Seprafilm is a useful adjuvant in reducing the incidence, extent, and severity of abdominal and pelvic postoperative adhesions. In the field of gynecology, it is also effective in reducing the area of postoperative uterine adhesions after myomectomy. Seprafilm is placed by the surgeon on the traumatized surfaces of the operated tissues in the abdomen by the end of surgery, before surgical closure. It is biocompatible, safe, nontoxic, and nonimmunogenic, and it acts as a temporary adhesion barrier that keeps tissue surfaces separated during the early days of wound healing, when adhesions form. Seprafilm hydrates to a gel within 24 to 48 hours following placement and then slowly resorbs from the abdominal cavity in about 5 to 7 days. It is excreted from the body within 28 days. Although Seprafilm barrier was shown to be safe and effective in all human clinical trials, its use did not eliminate adhesions in all patients. Efficacy of this barrier is limited to surgical situations in which the area in question can be completely covered. Physician acceptance is constrained by technical difficulties as well as limitations in application and handling properties within the surgical field.[98]

LAPAROSCOPIC ADHESIOLYSIS

Before adhesiolysis is attempted, the surgeon should consider whether (1) lysis of the adhesion would benefit the patient, (2) whether a sharp or blunt technique should be used, and (3) which side of the adhesion should be excised to reduce the risk of injury to vital organs. To do laparoscopic adhesiolysis adequately, three or four abdominal punctures are required: the infraumbilical incision for the operative laparoscope and two to three lower, lateral suprapubic punctures about 4 cm below the level of the iliac crests (Figure 11.1). Through the lateral trocar, on the side of the assistant, an atraumatic grasping forceps is inserted to hold the adhesion or involved organ, stretch it, and identify its boundaries and avascular planes. The opposite trocar, on the side of the primary surgeon, is used for microscissors or the suction–irrigator probe. That probe can serve as a manipulator or backstop when the CO$_2$ laser is used (Figure 11.2).

Adhesions are cut close to the affected organ at both ends and, if possible, removed from the abdomen. Vascular adhesions are coagulated with lasers or microelectrodes. When scissors are used, filmy and avascular adhesions are stretched and then cut (Figures 11.3, 11.4).[103] Thick, vascular adhesions must be coagulated before being cut (Figures 11.5, 11.6).

Intestinal adhesions are severed first, followed by peri-ovarian adhesions and peritubal adhesions. This approach allows pro-

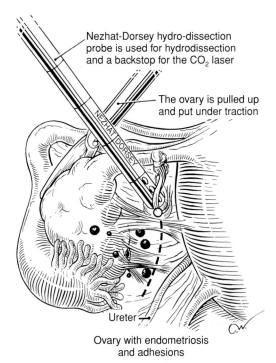

Nezhat-Dorsey hydro-dissection probe is used for hydrodissection and a backstop for the CO$_2$ laser

The ovary is pulled up and put under traction

Ureter

Ovary with endometriosis and adhesions

Figure 11.2. The left ovary is grasped and put under traction. The suction–irrigator is used for a backstop, and the adhesions are cut using the CO$_2$ laser.

gressive exposure of the pelvic structures. Once the intestines are freed from adjacent structures, they are pushed gently cephalad. Adherent ovaries are freed from the pelvic side wall, broad ligament, tubes, and uterus. Grasping forceps are essential for applying traction to the ovary, tube, intestines, or abdominal wall so that a plane of dissection can be identified.

Bleeding areas are coagulated with the laser or a bipolar electrocoagulator. Whenever possible, either the adhesions or the ovarian ligaments are grasped instead of the ovarian cortex to reduce trauma. Once the ovaries are lifted from the cul-de-sac and mobilized, the peritubal adhesions are removed.

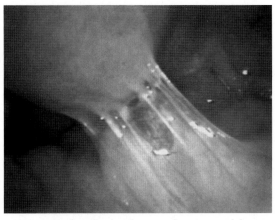

Figure 11.3. Avascular adhesions between the uterus and the omentum are put under stretch before dissection with scissors.

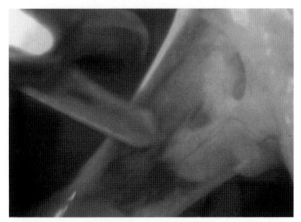

Figure 11.4. Avascular adhesions are dissected with scissors.

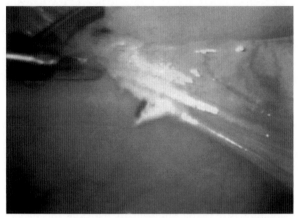

Figure 11.6. A coagulated vascular adhesion is cut with scissors.

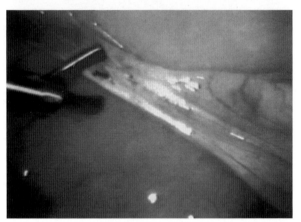

Figure 11.5. Thick vascular adhesions are coagulated before dissection.

and anterior abdominal wall), hydrodissection with the suction–irrigator probe is useful to create tissue planes before dissection.

Because an intestinal injury may occur during enterolysis, patients with a history of previous laparotomies or severe endometriosis should undergo a preoperative bowel preparation. Inadvertent enterorrhaphy can be repaired with the use of a one-layer closure of 0 polyglactin (Vicryl, Ethicon) or an Endoloop (Ethicon).

Once the pelvic structures are freed and hemostasis is achieved, the cul-de-sac is filled with lactated Ringer's solution and the adnexa are allowed to float in the clear fluid (Figure 11.7).[99] Filmy adhesions that are difficult to identify on the surface of the ovary become visible as they float from the ovarian cortex. These adhesions are grasped with the forceps, cut, and removed from their attachments, using laparoscopic microscissors. They are filmy and avascular, and so coagulation is not required.

Agglutinated fimbrial folds are caused by fine avascular adhesions. As the fimbrial folds float and disperse in the fluid, the adhesions become visible; they are grasped, stretched, and sharply cut

Adhesions can be coagulated effectively and incised with a CO_2 laser, superpulse (40 W) laser, ultrapulse (20 to 80 W and 25 to 200 millijoules), fiber laser (15 to 25 W), or microelectrode (15 to 20 W, cutting mode). When there are dense adhesions among different organs (bowel, uterus, ovaries, pelvic side wall,

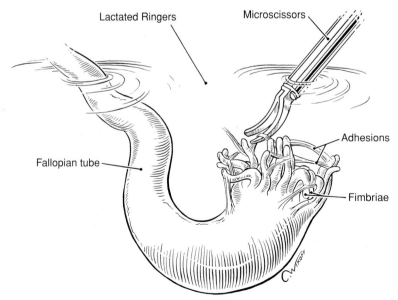

Figure 11.7. Hydroflotation of the tube and fimbria is used to detect and remove filmy adhesions.

with fine scissors or an ultrapulse laser. The laser beam (other than ultrapulse) delivered through the laparoscope is at least 1 mm in diameter and is too wide for these narrow bands of adhesions. Thermal damage may occur with electrosurgery and the fiber laser (neodymium: yttrium–aluminum–garnet, potassium titanyl phosphate, or argon). For delicate microscopic procedures of fimbriolysis and salpingo-ovariolysis, the microscissors or ultrapulse laser is preferable.

CONCLUSION

Although significant progress has been made toward understanding the development of postoperative adhesions and their prevention, the use of adjuvants and microsurgery have not eliminated them. Operative laparoscopy may be more effective than laparotomy in reducing their formation and should be the first procedure in their management.

REFERENCES

1. Hammoud A, Gago LA, Diamon MP. Adhesions in patients with chronic pelvic pain: a role for adhesiolysis? *Fertil Steril.* 2004;82(6):1483–1491.
2. Scott-Coombes DM, Vipond MN, Thompson JN. General surgeons' attitudes to the treatment and prevention of abdominal adhesions. *Ann R Coll Surg Engl.* 1993;75:123–128.
3. Monk BJ, Berman ML, Montz FJ. Adhesions after extensive gynecologic surgery: clinical significance, etiology, and prevention. *Am J Obstet Gynecol.* 1994;170:1396–1403.
4. Cheong YC, Laird SM, Li TC, Shelton JB, Ledger WL, Cooke ID. Peritoneal healing and adhesion formation/reformation. *Hum Reprod Update.* 2001;7(6):556–566.
5. Menzies D, Ellis H. Intestinal obstruction from adhesion: how big is the problem? *Ann R Coll Surg Engl.* 1990;72:60–63.
6. Ellis H. The clinical significance of adhesions: focus on intestinal obstruction. *Eur J Surg Suppl.* 1997;577:5–9.
7. Stricker B, Blanco J, Fox HE. The gynecologic contribution to intestinal obstruction in females. *J Am Coll Surg.* 1994;178:617–620.
8. Tulandi T, Murray C, Guralnick M. Adhesion formation and reproductive outcome after myomectomy and second-look laparoscopy. *Obstet Gynecol.* 1993;82:213–215.
9. Brill AI, Nezhat F, Nezhat CH, Nezhat C. The incidence of adhesions after prior laparotomy: a laparoscopic appraisal. *Obstet Gynecol.* 1995;85:269.
10. Luijendijk RW, de Lange DCD, Wauters CCAP, et al. Foreign material in postoperative adhesions. *Ann Surg.* 1996;223:242–248.
11. Caspi E, Halperin Y, Bukovski I. The importance of periadnexal adhesions in tubal reconstruction surgery for infertility. *Fertil Steril.* 1979;31:296.
12. Hulka JF. Adnexal adhesions: a prognostic staging and classification system based on a five year survey of fertility surgery results at Chapel Hill, North Carolina. *Am J Obstet Gynecol.* 1982;144:141.
13. Nezhat C, Metzger MD, Nezhat F, et al. Adhesion formation following reproductive surgery by videolaseroscopy. *Fertil Steril.* 1990;53:1008.
14. Donnez J, Casanas-Roux F. Prognostic factors of fimbrial surgery. *Fertil Steril.* 1986;45:778.
15. di Zerega GS. Biochemical events in peritoneal tissue repair. *Eur J Surg Suppl.* 1997;577:10–16.
16. Mahadevan MM, Wiseman D, Leader A, et al. The effects of ovarian adhesive disease upon follicular development in cycles of controlled stimulation for in vitro fertilization. *Fertil Steril.* 1985;44:489–492.
17. Mecke H, Semm K, Freys I, et al. Incidence of adhesions in the pelvis after pelviscopic operative treatment of tubal pregnancy. *Gynecol Obstet Invest.* 1985;28:202–204.
18. Duffy DM, di Zerega GS. Adhesion controversies: pelvic pain as a cause of adhesions, crystalloids in preventing them. *J Reprod Med.* 1996;41:19–26.
19. Mueller MD, Tschudi J, Herrmann U, Klaiber C. An evaluation of laparoscopic adhesiolysis in patients with chronic abdominal pain. *Surg Endosc.* 1995;9(7):802–804.
20. Saravelos HG, Li TC, Cooke ID. An analysis of the outcome of microsurgical and laparoscopic adhesiolysis for chronic pelvic pain. *Hum Reprod.* 1995;10(11):2895–2901.
21. Nezhat FR, Crystal RA, Nezhat CH, Nezhat CR. Laparoscopic adhesiolysis and relief of chronic pelvic pain. *JSLS.* 2000;4(4):281–285.
22. Ray NF, Denton WG, Thamer M, Henderson SC, Perry S. Abdominal adhesiolysis inpatient care and expenditures in the United States in 1994. *J Am Coll Surg.* 1998;186:1–9.
23. Ivarsson ML, Homdahl L, Franzen G, Risberg B. Costs of bowel obstruction from adhesions. *Eur J Surg.* 1997;163:679–684.
24. Boland GM, Weigel RJ. Formation and prevention of postoperative abdominal adhesions. *J Surg Res.* 2006;132(1):3–12.
25. DiZerega GSD, Holtz G. Cause and prevention of postsurgical pelvic adhesions. In: Osofsky H, ed. *Advances in Clinical Obstetrics and Gynecology.* Baltimore: Williams & Wilkins; 1982.
26. Liakakos T, Thomakos N, Fine PM, Dervenis C, Young RL. Peritoneal adhesions: etiology, pathophysiology, and clinical significance. Recent advances in prevention and management. *Dig Surg.* 2001;18(4):260–273.
27. Trimbos-Kemper TCM, Trimbos JB, van Hall EV. Adhesion formation after tubal surgery: results of the 8 day laparoscopy in 188 patients. *Fertil Steril.* 1985;43:395.
28. Gomel V, McComb P. Microsurgery in gynecology. In: Silver JS, ed. *Microsurgery.* Baltimore: Williams & Wilkins; 1979.
29. Luciano AA, Maier DB, Koch E, et al. A comparative study of postoperative adhesions following laser surgery by laparoscopy versus laparotomy in the rabbit model. *Obstet Gynecol.* 1989;4:220.
30. Operative Laparoscopy Study Group. Postoperative adhesion development after operative laparoscopy: evaluation at early second-look procedures. *Fertil Steril.* 1991;55:700.
31. Lundorff P, Hahlin M, Kallfelt B, et al. Adhesion formation after laparoscopic surgery in tubal pregnancy: a randomized trial versus laparotomy. *Fertil Steril.* 1991;55:911–915.
32. Schippers E, Tittel A, Ottinger A, Schumpelick V. Laparoscopy versus laparotomy: comparison of adhesion-formation after bowel resection in a canine model. *Dig Surg.* 1998;15:145.
33. Von Dembrowski T. Ueber die ursachen der peritoneum ashasionennach cirugischen: eiugriffen mit rucksieht auf die frage des ileus nach laparotomien. *Arch Klin Chir.* 1898;37:745.
34. Ellis H. The cause and prevention of postoperative intraperitoneal adhesions. *Surg Gynecol Obstet.* 1971;133:497.
35. Diamond MP, Nezhat F. Letter to the editor: adhesions after resection of ovarian endometriomas. *Fertil Steril.* 1993;59:934–935.
36. Wiseman DM, Trout R, Diamond MP. The rates of adhesion development and the effects of crystalloid solutions on adhesion development in pelvic surgery. *Fertil Steril.* 1998;70:702–711.
37. Garrard CL, Clements RH, Nanney L, et al. Adhesion formation is reduced after laparoscopic surgery. *Surg Endosc.* 1999;13:10.
38. Wallwiener D, Meyer A, Bastert G. Adhesion formation of the parietal and visceral peritoneum: an explanation for the

controversy on the use of autologous and alloplastic barriers? *Fertil Steril*. 1998;69:132.

39. Chen MD, Teigen GA, Reynolds HT, et al. Laparoscopy versus laparotomy: an evaluation of adhesion formation after pelvic and paraaortic lymphadenectomy in a porcine model. *Am J Obstet Gynecol*. 1998;178:499.

40. Halverson AL, Barrett WL, Bhanot P, et al. Intraabdominal adhesion formation after preperitoneal dissection in the murine model. *Surg Endosc*. 1999;13:14.

41. Parker JD, Sinaii N, Segars JH, Godoy H, Winkel C, Stratton P. Adhesion formation after laparoscopic excision of endometriosis and lysis of adhesions. *Fertil Steril*. 2005;84(5):1457–1461.

42. Tulandi T. How can we avoid adhesions after laparoscopic surgery? *Curr Opin Obstet Gynecol*. 1997;9:239.

43. Ugur M, Turan C, Mungan T, et al. Laparoscopy for adhesion prevention following myomectomy. *Int J Gynaecol Obstet*. 1996;53:145.

44. Jansen BPS. Failure of intraperitoneal adjuncts to improve the outcome of pelvic operations in young women. *Am J Obstet Gynecol*. 1983;153:363.

45. Shear L, Swartz C, Shinaberger J, et al. Kinetics of peritoneal fluid absorption in adult man. *N Engl J Med*. 1965;272:123–127.

46. diZerega GS, Campeau JD. Use of instillates to prevent intraperitoneal adhesions: crystalloid and dextran. *Infert Reprod Med Clinics North Am*. 1994;5:463–478.

47. Menzies D. Peritoneal adhesions: incidence, cause, and prevention. *Surg Annu Surg*. 1992;24:27–45.

48. Wiseman D. Polymers for the prevention of surgical adhesions. In: Domb AJ, ed. *Polymeric Site-Specific Pharmacotherapy*. New York: Wiley; 1994:370–421.

49. Luciano AA, Hauser KS, Benda J. Evaluation of commonly used adjuvants in the prevention of postoperative adhesions. *Am J Obstet Gynecol*. 1983;146:88.

50. Rosenberg SM, Board JA. High-molecular-weight dextran in human fertility surgery. *Am J Obstet Gynecol*. 1984;148:380.

51. DiZerega GS. Reduction of postoperative pelvic adhesions with intraperitoneal 32% dextran 70: a prospective randomized clinical trial. *Fertil Steril*. 1983;40:612.

52. Borten M, Seibert CP, Taymor ML. Recurrent anaphylactic reaction to intraperitoneal dextran 75 used for prevention of postsurgical adhesions. *Obstet Gynecol*. 1983;61:755.

53. Johns DB, Keyport GM, Hoehler F, diZerega GS; Intergel Adhesion Prevention Study Group. Reduction of postsurgical adhesions with Intergel adhesion prevention solution: a multicenter study of safety and efficacy after conservative gynecologic surgery. *Fertil Steril*. 2001;76:595–604.

54. Tulandi T, Al-Shahrani A. Adhesion prevention in gynecologic surgery. *Curr Opin Obstet Gynecol*. 2005;17(4):395–398.

55. Kelekci S, Yilmaz B, Oguz S, et al. The efficacy of a hyaluronate/carboxymethylcellulose membrane in prevention of postoperative adhesion in a rat uterine horn model. *Tohoku J Exp Med*. 2004;204:189–194.

56. Burns JW, Skinner K, Colt J, et al. Prevention of tissue injury and postsurgical adhesions by precoating tissues with hyaluronic acid solutions. *J Surg Res*. 1995;59:644–652.

57. Urman B, Gomel V. Effect of hyaluronic acid on postoperative intraperitoneal adhesion formation in the rat model. *Fertil Steril*. 1991;56:563–567.

58. Diamond MP; Sepracoat Adhesion Study Group. Reduction of de novo postsurgical adhesions by intraoperative precoating with Sepracoat (HAL-C) solution: a prospective, randomized, blinded, placebo-controlled multicenter study. *Fertil Steril*. 1998;69:1067–1074.

59. Dunn R, Lyman MD, Edelman PG, Campbell PK. Evaluation of the SprayGel adhesion barrier in the rat cecum abrasion and rabbit uterine horn adhesion models. *Fertil Steril*. 2001;75:411–416.

60. Ferland R, Mulani D, Campbell PK. Evaluation of a sprayable polyethylene glycol adhesion barrier in a porcine efficacy model. *Hum Reprod*. 2001;16:2718–2723.

61. Mettler L, Audebert A, Lehmann-Willenbrock E, et al. A randomized, prospective, controlled, multicenter clinical trial of a sprayable, site-specific adhesion barrier system in patients undergoing myomectomy. *Fertil Steril*. 2004;82:398–404.

62. Lundorff P, Donnez J, Korell M, Audebert AJM, Block K, diZerega GS. Clinical evaluation of a viscoelastic gel for reduction of adhesions following gynaecological surgery by laparoscopy in Europe. *Hum Reprod*. 2005;20:514–520.

63. Renier D, Bellato P, Bellini D, Pavesio A, Pressato D, Borrione A. Pharmacokinetic behaviour of ACP gel, an autocrosslinked hyaluronan derivative, after intraperitoneal administration. *Biomaterials*. 2005;26:5368–5374.

64. Belluco C, Meggiolaro F, Pressato D, et al. Prevention of postsurgical adhesions with an autocrosslinked hyaluronan derivative gel. *J Surg Res*. 2001;100:217–221.

65. Pucciarelli S, Codello L, Rosato A, Del Bianco P, Vecchiato G, Lise M. Effect of antiadhesive agents on peritoneal carcinomatosis in an experimental model. *Br J Surg*. 2003;90:66–71.

66. Acunzo G, Guida M, Pellicano M, et al. Effectiveness of auto–cross-linked hyaluronic acid gel in the prevention of intrauterine adhesions after hysteroscopic adhesiolysis: a prospective, randomized, controlled study. *Hum Reprod*. 2003;18:1918–1921.

67. Guida M, Acunzo G, Di Spiezio Sardo A, et al. Effectiveness of auto–crosslinked hyaluronic acid gel in the prevention of intrauterine adhesions after hysteroscopic surgery: a prospective, randomized, controlled study. *Hum Reprod*. 2004;19:1461–1464.

68. Pellicano M, Guida M, Bramante S, et al. Reproductive outcome after autocrosslinked hyaluronic acid gel application in infertile patients who underwent laparoscopic myomectomy. *Fertil Steril*. 2005;83:498–500.

69. Mais V, Bracco GL, Litta P, Gargiulo T, Melis GB. Reduction of postoperative adhesions with an auto-crosslinked hyaluronan gel in gynaecological laparoscopic surgery: a blinded, controlled, randomized, multicentre study. *Hum Reprod*. 2006;21(5):1248–1254.

70. Larsson B. Efficacy of Interceed in adhesion prevention in gynecologic surgery: a review of 13 clinical studies. *J Reprod Med*. 1996;41:27.

71. Reddy S, Santanam N, Reddy PP, et al. Interaction of Interceed oxidized regenerated cellulose with macrophages: a potential mechanism by which Interceed may prevent adhesions. *Am J Obstet Gynecol*. 1997;177:1315.

72. Interceed (TC7) Barrier Adhesion Study Group. Prevention of postsurgical adhesions by Interceed (TC7), an absorbable adhesion barrier: a prospective randomized multicenter clinical study. *Fertil Steril*. 1989;51:933.

73. The Obstetrics and Gynecology Adhesion Prevention Committee. Use of Interceed (TC7) absorbable adhesion barrier to reduce postoperative adhesion reformation in infertility and endometriosis surgery. *Obstet Gynecol*. 1992;79:518.

74. Haney AF, Doty E. Murine peritoneal injury and de novo adhesion formation caused by oxidized-regenerated cellulose (Interceed [TC7]) but not expanded polytetrafluoroethylene (Gore-Tex surgical membrane). *Fertil Steril*. 1992;57:202.

75. Pagidas K, Tulandi T. Effects of Ringer's lactate, Interceed (TC7) and Gore-Tex surgical membrane on PST surgical adhesion formation. *Fertil Steril*. 1992;57:199.

76. Marana R, Catalano GF, Caruana P, et al. Postoperative adhesion formation and reproductive outcome using Interceed after

ovarian surgery: a randomized trial in the rabbit model. *Hum Reprod.* 1997;12:1935.

77. Azziz R. Microsurgery alone or with Interceed Absorbable Adhesion Barrier for pelvic sidewall adhesion re-formation: the Interceed (TC7) Adhesion Barrier Study Group II. *Surg Gynecol Obstet.* 1993;177:135.

78. Franklin RR. Reduction of ovarian adhesions by the use of Interceed: Ovarian Adhesion Study Group. *Obstet Gynecol.* 1995;86:335.

79. Keckstein J, Ulrich U, Sasse V, et al. Reduction of postoperative adhesion formation after laparoscopic ovarian cystectomy. *Hum Reprod.* 1996;11:579.

80. Mais V, Ajossa S, Piras B, et al. Prevention of de-novo adhesion formation after laparoscopic myomectomy: a randomized trial to evaluate the effectiveness of an oxidized regenerated cellulose absorbable barrier. *Hum Reprod.* 1995;10:3133.

81. Mais V, Ajossa S, Marongiu D, et al. Reduction of adhesion reformation after laparoscopic endometriosis surgery: a randomized trial with an oxidized regenerated cellulose absorbable barrier. *Obstet Gynecol.* 1995;86:512.

82. Al-Jaroudi D, Tulandi T. Adhesion prevention in gynecologic surgery. *Obstet Gynecol Surv.* 2004;59(5):360–367.

83. Ramsewak S, Narayansingh G, Bassaw K, et al. Fixation of Interceed does not improve its efficacy against adhesion formation in rats. *Clin Exp Obstet Gynecol.* 1996;23:147.

84. Bulletti C, Polli V, Negrini V, et al. Adhesion formation after laparoscopic myomectomy. *J Am Assoc Gynecol Laparosc.* 1996;3:533.

85. Minale C, Nikol S, Hollweg G, et al. Clinical experience with expanded polytetrafluoroethylene Gore-Tex surgical membrane for pericardial closure: a study of 110 cases. *J Cardiac Surg.* 1988;3:193.

86. Boyers SP, Diamond MP, DeCherney AH. Reduction of postoperative pelvis adhesions in the rabbit with Gore-Tex surgical membrane. *Fertil Steril.* 1988;49:1066.

87. The Myomectomy Adhesion Multicenter Study Group. An expanded polytetrafluoroethylene barrier (Gore-Tex Surgical Membrane) reduces post-myomectomy adhesion formation. *Fertil Steril.* 1995;63:491.

88. Haney AF. Removal of surgical barriers of expanded polytetrafluoroethylene at second-look laparoscopy was not associated with adhesion formation. *Fertil Steril.* 1997;68:721.

89. Crain J, Curole D, Hill G, et al. Laparoscopic implant of Gore-Tex surgical membrane. *J Am Assoc Gynecol Laparosc.* 1995;2:417.

90. The Surgical Membrane Study Group. Prophylaxis of pelvic sidewall adhesions with Gore-Tex surgical membrane: a multicenter clinical investigation. *Fertil Steril.* 1992;57:921.

91. Haney AF. Removal of surgical barriers of expanded polytetrafluoroethylene at second-look laparoscopy was not associated with adhesion formation. *Fertil Steril.* 1997;68:721.

92. Haney A, Hesla J, Hurst B, et al. Expanded polytetrafluoroethylene (Gore-Tex Surgical Membrane) is superior to oxidized regenerated cellulose (Interceed TC7) in preventing adhesions. *Fertil Steril.* 1995;63:1021–1026.

93. Grow DR, Seltman HJ, Coddington CC, et al. The reduction of postoperative adhesions by two different barrier methods versus control in cynomolgus monkeys: a prospective randomized cross over study. *Fertil Steril.* 1994;61:1141–1146.

94. Alponat A, Lakshminarasappa SR, Yavuz N, Goh PM. Prevention of adhesions by Seprafilm, an absorbable barrier: an incisional hernia model in rats. *Am Surg.* 1997;63:818–819.

95. Burns JW, Colt MJ, Burgess LS, Skinner KC. Preclinical evaluation of Seprafilm bioresorbable membrane. *Eur J Surg Suppl.* 1997;577:40–48.

96. Diamond MP; Seprafilm Adhesion Study Group. Seprafilm (HAL-F) reduces postoperative adhesions: initial results of a multicenter gynecologic clinical study. Abstract 053 presented at: Fourth Congress of the European Society for Gynaecological Endoscopy; December 6–9, 1995; Brussels, Belgium.

97. Becker JM, Dayton MT, Fazio W, et al. Prevention of postoperative abdominal adhesions by a sodium hyaluronate–based bioresorbable membrane: a prospective, randomized, double-blind multicenter study. *J Am Coll Surg.* 1996;183:297–306.

98. Gago LA, Saed GM, Chauhan S, Elhammady EF, Diamond MP. Seprafilm (modified hyaluronic acid and carboxymethylcellulose) acts as a physical barrier. *Fertil Steril.* 2003;80(3): 612–616.

99. Nezhat F, Winer WK, Nezhat C. Fimbrioscopy and salpingoscopy in patients with minimal to moderate pelvic endometriosis. *Obstet Gynecol.* 1990;75:15.

100. DeRenzi E, Boeri G, Das Hetz als Schutzorgen. *Bed Klin Wochenschr.* 1903;40:773.

101. Thomas JW, Continued hyaluronidase on the formation of intraperitoneal adhesions in rats. *Prosc Soc Exp Biol Med.* 1950; 74:497.

102. Ryan GB, Groberty J, Majino G. Postoperative peritoneal adhesions: a study of the mechanisms. *Am J Pathol.* 1971;675: 117.

12 | LEIOMYOMAS

Section 12.1. Minimally Invasive Approaches to Myomectomy

Mark H. Glasser

As more articles debating the prevalence of hysterectomies appear in the lay press and on the Internet, increasing numbers of women are demanding alternative procedures. A recent *New York Times* article decrying the prevalence of hysterectomies stated that by the age of 60, one in three women in the United States will have had her uterus removed.[1] By comparison, in Italy the figure is one in six, whereas in France, it is one in 18 women. Of the 600,000 hysterectomies performed annually in the United States, one third are done for leiomyomas.[2] This number rises dramatically for women over the age of 40 and for those in certain ethnic groups. For African American women, 61.3% of hysterectomies are done for leiomyomas, and for women in the 45-to-54–year age group, 53% of all hysterectomies, regardless of race, are done for this indication. It is estimated that more than 25% of women over the age of 36 have one or more leiomyomas, with 50% of these being symptomatic.[3]

Uterine leiomyomas (myomas) are benign smooth muscle tumors arising from the myometrium. Despite the fact that myomas are quite common, very little is known about their etiology. They are monoclonal – arising from a single myometrial cell. Different karyotypes of multiple myomas have been found in the same patient. What causes abnormal myometrial cells to transform into clinically detectable myomas is also unknown. There are, however, more estrogen receptors in myomas than in the surrounding myometrium and less estradiol conversion, so hormonal factors certainly play a role. There has also been speculation that chromosome rearrangement may contribute to tumor initiation and growth as well as stimulation by growth hormone and other insulin-like growth factors. Myomas are heterogeneous; some women have solitary myomas, whereas others have multiple myomas. Myomas may be subserous, intramural, pedunculated, or submucous. There are even different classifications of submucous myomas according to the percentage of the myoma that is within the endometrial cavity versus the percentage within the myometrium. Treatment options depend greatly on careful classification of the myoma or myomas present in an individual patient and on what symptoms are most bothersome to her and require treatment.

Most myomas do not cause any symptoms, and the first lesson physicians must learn is that if the patient is asymptomatic, no treatment is necessary. The presence of an abdominal mass is not an indication for a hysterectomy or myomectomy unless it is of significant concern to the patient. Also, the old teaching that a hysterectomy is necessary in uteri larger than 12 gestational weeks because the adnexa cannot be adequately examined is no longer true in the age of modern imaging technology such as ultrasound, computed tomography (CT), and magnetic

resonance imaging (MRI). Patients with myomas may present with a wide variety of symptoms, including menometrorrhagia, dyspareunia, pelvic pressure or discomfort, urinary frequency, bowel or back discomfort, infertility or repeated pregnancy loss, and the presence of a large pelvic mass.[4] Symptoms very often are related to the size, type, and location of the myoma as well as the lifestyle of the individual patient. The criteria for intervention as outlined by the American College of Obstetrics and Gynecology in their published Quality Assurance criteria sets are:

- Clinically apparent myomas that are a significant concern to the patient, even if otherwise asymptomatic
- Myomas causing excessive bleeding and/or anemia
- Myomas causing acute or chronic pain
- Myomas causing significant urinary problems not due to other abnormalities

Various modalities besides the bimanual pelvic and rectal examination have been used to diagnose and classify myomas, the mainstay being transabdominal and transvaginal ultrasound. MRI has been used for more accurate myoma "mapping" as well as differentiation of pedunculated myomas from adnexal masses. To evaluate whether or not an intracavitary component is present, saline infusion sonography as well as hysteroscopy are valuable tools. Hysterosalpingography is useful in the evaluation of infertile patients with myomas because tubal patency, as well as the size and shape of the uterine cavity, can be assessed.

The treatment of symptomatic leiomyomas for women who have completed childbearing has been, in the vast majority of cases, hysterectomy. Perimenopausal women are often given no choice other than hysterectomy, with myomectomy offered in only a small number of cases. Recent advances in the nonsurgical management of leiomyomas, including medical management with gonadotropin-releasing hormone (GnRH) analogues or antagonists, mifepristone, raloxifene, and progesterone receptor modifiers as well as uterine artery embolization, have been promising for these patients but may be inappropriate for those who want to preserve childbearing, because none has been shown to enhance fertility.[5] Certainly, for women in the reproductive-age group wanting to maintain fertility, a myomectomy remains the "gold standard." Abdominal myomectomy, however, is associated with significant morbidity, including excessive blood loss, a high rate of blood transfusion, infection, and postoperative adhesions.[6] Recurrence rates have been reported to be between 5% and 30%, with 20% to 25% of patients requiring a subsequent hysterectomy.[7]

LAPAROSCOPIC MYOMECTOMY

Laparoscopic myomectomy is an alternative to the abdominal approach, with fewer complications, shortened hospital stay, and less disability [8,9], but it is a difficult and tedious operation. Widespread acceptance of this procedure has been limited because of the advanced skills required, but the advent of better insufflators, light sources, and cameras as well as the electronic morcellator has increased the use of this procedure. It is felt by some authors that women with large intramural myomas who want to bear children should not be managed laparoscopically because meticulous repair of the uterus is difficult. Parker [10] has established selection criteria for patients with symptomatic myomas for laparoscopic myomectomy, which include uterine size equal to or less than 14 weeks after a 3-month course of GnRH agonist therapy, no individual myoma larger than 7 cm, no myoma near the uterine artery or near the tubal ostia if fertility is desired, and at least 50% of the myoma subserosal, to be accessible and to allow adequate repair through the laparoscope.[11] Certainly there are several highly skilled laparoscopists in the world who are comfortable managing larger myomas, but the vast majority of practicing gynecologists would resort to standard laparotomy in these cases. Sinha et al. [11], in a study published in 2003, removed 78 myomas in 51 patients. Three patients had two myomas between 5 cm and 9 cm (in addition to one ≥ 9 cm), and one had three myomas between 5 cm and 9 cm (in addition to one ≥ 9 cm). Mean number of myomas removed per patient was 1.53 ± 1.17 (range, 1 to 6); 12 women (23.5%) had multiple myomectomy. The largest myoma removed was 21 cm. Mean myoma weight was 698.47 ± 569.13 g (range, 210 to 3400 g). Mean operating time was 136.67 ± 38.28 minutes (range, 80 to 270 minutes). Mean blood loss was 322.16 ± 328.2 mL (range, 100 to 2000 mL). One patient developed a broad ligament hematoma, two developed postoperative fever, and one underwent open subtotal hysterectomy 9 hours after surgery for dilutional coagulopathy. Twenty women (39.2%) were given blood transfusions postoperatively; 10 received a single unit, six were given 2 U, three were given 3 U, and one was given 4 U.[12] This study has a far higher incidence of blood transfusion than any study in the literature and may be explained by different criteria for transfusion in India. Nezhat and associates [9] reported on myomectomy in 137 women, from whom 196 leiomyomas were removed. The fibroids ranged in size from 2 to 14 cm. The operations lasted from 50 to 160 minutes (mean, 116 minutes). Estimated blood loss was between 10 mL and 600 mL, and two women received transfusions because of intraoperative blood loss. The hospital stay ranged from 7 to 48 hours, with a mean of 19.6 hours. In a retrospective multicenter study comparing myomectomy by laparoscopy and laparotomy, Marret et al. [12] found that compared with women undergoing laparoscopic myomectomy, women undergoing open myomectomy had more myomas that were larger and that were generally interstitial and anterior. More of them received GnRH analogues. Excised myomas weighed four times more, the decrease in hemoglobin was greater (1 g/dL), fever was more frequent, and nine patients needed transfusions (compared to none for laparoscopic myomectomy). There were 37 conversions to laparotomy (29%) after laparoscopic myomectomy. The conversion rate was high for inexperienced surgeons. Length of hospital stay was reduced by half for laparoscopic myomectomy (without conversion). Recurrence rate at 2 years was 2.5% for laparoscopic myomectomy versus 3.6% for open myomectomy ($P = 0.506$). The authors concluded that preoperative evaluation by ultrasound was essential to establish myoma number, size, type, and location to choose the most appropriate surgical procedure. The ideal candidate for laparoscopic myomectomy is a patient with fewer than three myomas, none larger than 8 to 9 cm. Those with pedunculated myomas are ideal for a minimally invasive approach regardless of the size. Patients with multiple myomas whose imaging studies report "fibroids too numerous to count" are not candidates for myomectomy because the myometrial damage created by excising them would be like doing a virtual hysterectomy. Certainly these patients should be counseled to accept hysterectomy if future childbearing is not desired. If the patient strongly desires keeping her uterus, she should be referred for uterine fibroid embolization.

Surgical Technique

The patient is placed in the low lithotomy position using Allen stirrups (Allen Medical Systems, Cleveland, OH). Ten milliliters of a dilute vasopressin solution (2 U in 60 mL NaCl) is then injected intracervically about 1 to 2 cm deep at both the 8 and 4 o'clock positions. Laparoscopic myomectomy is facilitated by the use of a uterine manipulator. Although manipulators that use a balloon for stabilization of the device within the uterus work well for most laparoscopic procedures, these may be counterproductive in myomectomy. If the uterine cavity is entered, as occasionally occurs inadvertently or intentionally during the course of myoma enucleation, the balloon may be ruptured, causing the manipulator to fall out. We prefer the MHI uterine manipulator (Medical Horizons, Fair Oaks, CA; Figure 12.1.1) or the Pelosi manipulator (Apple Medical, Marlborough MA; Figure 12.1.2). The procedure is facilitated by the use of four ports, the sizes of which are dependent on which suturing technique is employed or whether an electronic morcellator is used. Generally, one can perform most laparoscopic myomectomies with an 11-mm umbilical port, a high lateral port on each side placed 3 cm below the umbilicus and 6 to 8 cm lateral to the midline. The lateral ports may be placed above the umbilicus for larger uteri. Finally, a suprapubic 11- to 12-mm port is placed, through which the morcellator can be inserted after dilating the port site to 15 mm. Alternatively, this port may be placed in the left lower quadrant. Before proceeding with the insertion of multiple accessory ports, the size and position of the myomas are carefully assessed. If there is any doubt about the safe performance of the myomectomy via laparoscopy, such as the presence of large inaccessible posterior or broad ligament myomas, a conventional laparotomy should be performed.

A dilute vasopressin solution (2 U in 60 mL of normal saline) is then injected into the serosa and myometrium overlying the myoma until the tissue blanches. This is easily accomplished using a control-top syringe and a 4-inch 22-gauge spinal needle, which is inserted percutaneously over the uterus. The tip of the needle is then guided into the proper sites along the myoma with a 5-mm grasper from a lateral port. The use of vasopressin for gynecologic surgery has been controversial but is widely accepted in the United States. In two prospective randomized studies, dilute vasopressin

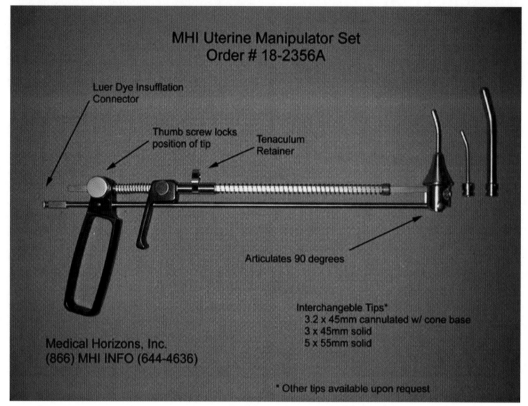

Figure 12.1.1. The MHI uterine manipulator.

solution was found to decrease blood loss at time of myomectomy by laparotomy compared with placebo or a tourniquet.[13] An alternative to the use of vasopressin is to inject 0.25% bupivacaine with epinephrine into the serosa and myometrium in the same fashion. This also has a vasoconstrictive effect and has been found in one randomized study to decrease the need for postoperative pain medication in women undergoing laparoscopic myomectomy as well as to decrease blood loss.[14]

Pedunculated myomas are the least difficult to manage laparoscopically. After the dilute vasopressin solution is injected into the stalk, the myoma is removed by cutting and coagulating the stalk. Care must be taken to stay close to the myoma and avoid thermal damage to the normal myometrium from which the stalk arises. An alternative technique is to place one or two ties around the pedicle (Endoloops [Ethicon] may be used) and to excise the myoma by electrosurgically cutting through the serosa around its base about 1 to 2 cm above the insertion of the pedicle. The pedicle can then be oversewn to assure hemostasis. This technique minimizes the risk of later uterine rupture, which has been reported during pregnancy following laparoscopic removal of a pedunculated myoma.[15]

The removal of subserous myomas is less challenging than the removal of deep intramural myomas. Dilute vasopressin is injected in multiple sites between the myometrium and the fibroid capsule. An incision is made on the serosa overlying the leiomyoma, using the CO_2 laser (superpulse or ultrapulse mode), a monopolar electrode, a fiber laser, or harmonic scalpel. The incision is extended until it reaches the capsule. The myometrium retracts as the incision is made and the myoma bulges outward.

Two grasping, toothed forceps hold the edges of the myometrium, and the suction–irrigator can be used as a blunt probe to shell the leiomyoma from its capsule. A myoma screw is inserted into the tumor to apply traction while the suction–irrigator is used as a blunt dissector. An alternative is to insert a finger through the 12-mm suprapubic port site incision and manually dissect the myoma free from the myometrium. Once this is accomplished, the cannula is reinserted. Vessels are electrocoagulated before being cut. After complete removal of the myoma, the uterine defect is irrigated. Bleeding points are identified and controlled with bipolar or monopolar electrocoagulation. Point coagulation of identifiable vessels can be accomplished by using short bursts of cutting current while the vessel is grasped with a Maryland dissecting forceps, much as one would do in an open case with a hemostat. The edges of the uterine defect are approximated by superficial suturing.

Deep intramural or broad ligament intramural myomas are the most difficult to properly manage laparoscopically and should be done only by surgeons skilled in laparoscopic suturing. This is especially true if the patient plans future childbearing. The gold standard of myometrial closure after open myomectomy is a three-layered closure beginning at the base of the defect to obliterate the dead space with figure-of-eight or horizontal mattress sutures. A second layer of continuous suture is then placed to further approximate the myometrium and finally ending with a continuous imbricating "baseball" stitch on the serosa. Synthetic absorbable polyglactin sutures (Vicryl, Ethicon, Somerville, NJ; Polysorb, USSC, Norwalk, CT) are recommended because they produce less inflammatory reaction than catgut.

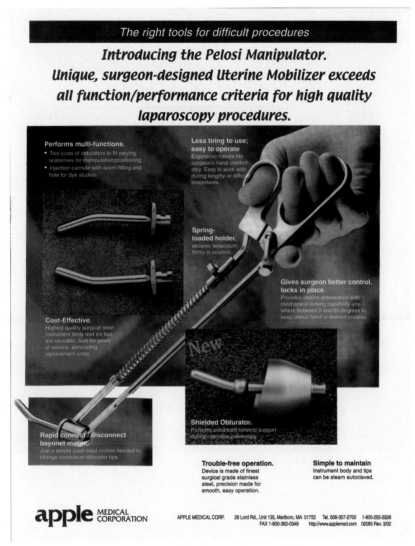

Figure 12.1.2. The Pelosi uterine manipulator.

Intraligamentous and broad ligament myomas require careful observation of the course of the ureters and large blood vessels. Depending on the location of the myoma, an incision is made on the anterior or posterior leaf of the broad ligament. The myoma is removed with the techniques described above for subserosal and intramural tumors. Throughout the procedure, the location of the ureters is noted. Hemostasis is obtained with the sutures, clips, or bipolar forceps. None of the available lasers, despite the power setting or focus of the beam, can adequately coagulate bleeding myometrial vessels. A bipolar forceps, monopolar fine dissecting forceps (Maryland), or argon beam coagulator is excellent for this purpose. The broad ligament and peritoneum are not closed but allowed to heal spontaneously. Drains are used infrequently.

Stringer and associates [16] described a simplified way of closing deep myometrial defects using the Endo Stitch automatic suturing device (United States Surgical, Norwalk CT).[16] Multiple layers of continuous interlocking sutures are placed using this device, which captures the 9-mm needle in the opposite jaw when the handles are squeezed (Figure 12.1.3). The suture is held taut by the assistant, and finally an intracorporeal knot is tied with the device (Figure 12.1.4). The Endo Stitch must be used through a 10-mm port. Its limitations are a semi-straight needle that is relatively short. Once adept at using the device, one can often stitch faster than by using conventional open suturing techniques.

Recently, the da Vinci surgical robot (Intuitive Surgical) has been advocated as a suturing aid in performing laparoscopic myomectomy. The initial published report done in a university hospital setting showed a conversion rate of 8.6% to laparotomy and an average operating time of 230.8 ± 83 minutes. The average length of stay was 1 day.[17] Although this technology is certainly "space age," it is very expensive in capital outlay, per case cost, and annual service contract cost. This device performs suturing precisely and because of its high cost, will be available only in a very few centers. The average operating time of close to 4 hours as reported above is unacceptable and far longer than the average operating time for laparoscopic myomectomy in the published literature. The degree of precision the system affords is hardly necessary or appropriate for myomectomy, which can be accomplished safely by many of the techniques discussed in this chapter. Until good data are presented clearly demonstrating the superiority of this instrument, gynecologists should approach it with a critical eye.

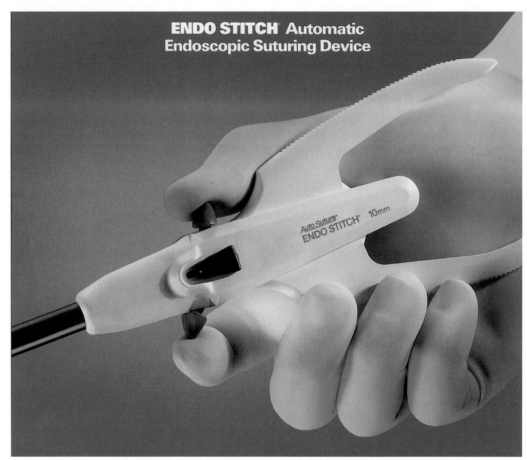

Figure 12.1.3. The Endo Stitch automatic suturing device.

Specimen Removal Techniques

Other than laparoscopic suturing, the greatest challenge and often the most frustrating step in laparoscopic myomectomy is specimen removal. For multiple small myomas, the enucleated specimens can be placed in a specimen retrieval bag, brought up to the largest port site, and morcellated in the bag at the skin line using a #11 scalpel blade. Another technique for intra-abdominal morcellation of larger myomas is to grasp opposite sides of the myoma with strong toothed graspers from each lateral port and to suspend it in the lower abdominal airspace near the anterior peritoneum. A narrow scalpel with a #11 blade is then passed

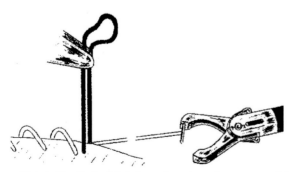

Figure 12.1.4. The Endo Stitch is used to tie an intracorporeal knot after a line of continuous suture.

through the suprapubic 12-mm port, and the myoma is cut into small segments, placed in a specimen retrieval bag, and removed through the umbilical or suprapubic port site after the cannula is removed. The port site incision can be made larger to facilitate this. If the cannula needs to be reinserted, a disposable cone-shaped adaptor or a Hasson cannula can be used.

The laparoscopic morcellator has been a significant advance for specimen removal during laparoscopic myomectomy and has saved many patients from major laparotomies. The most widely used device in the United States is made by Gynecare (Johnson & Johnson, Somerville, NJ). Other excellent electronic morcellators are made by Karl Storz, WISAP, and Richard Wolf. Because the morcellator blade is very sharp and turns at a high rate of speed, it is most important that the cutting edge of the blade be kept in view at all times. The morcellator is best inserted through the lateral or suprapubic port and held parallel to the abdominal wall. A full pneumoperitoneum must be maintained to maximize the airspace and minimize the risk of a loop of bowel or other structure being injured by coming into contact with the active blade. The myoma should be grasped with a heavy claw forceps or laparoscopic tenaculum and drawn into the morcellator blade without changing position of the morcellator. Slow, gentle pressure will withdraw the morcellated myoma in a single strip from the end of the morcellator. Excess traction should be avoided because it will sever the strip and necessitate regrasping. The surgeon should work from the periphery of the myoma and around it, almost like peeling a fruit. It is not advisable to drill through the center of the myoma because this technique takes much longer and increases the risk of injury to organs hidden from view by the myoma. It is also important to not lose sight of any fragments of myoma that have been morcellated and dropped into the abdomen or any small myomas that have been enucleated. Transfixing these small myomas with a single suture and suspending them from the anterior abdominal wall is a good way to prevent their loss in the abdomen. One study reported the loss of a 6-cm myoma during a laparoscopic supracervical hysterectomy. The specimen became entangled and fixed to the mesentery of the small bowel in the upper abdomen and caused a bowel obstruction, resulting in the need for an exploratory laparotomy.[18] Seeding of port sites with malignant cells or endometriosis is a well-known sequela of laparoscopic procedures. This may also occur with morcellated myoma tissue, as was shown in a case report by Ostrzenski.[19]

In a randomized trial, Sinha and associates [20] evaluated two groups of patients undergoing laparoscopic myomectomy with at least one myoma 7 cm in diameter to assess the feasibility of enucleation of myomas by morcellation while the myoma is still attached to the uterus compared with standard enucleation and morcellation as described above. The mean weight of the myomas removed in each group was about 600 g. Blood loss, length of stay, and complication rates were similar in both groups, but operating time was significantly decreased in the group employing the technique of morcellation of the myomas while still attached to the uterus. The authors speculate that this technique may allow larger myomas to be managed laparoscopically. In situ morcellation of large myomas is the technique employed in minilap myomectomy, which is discussed at length later in this chapter.

Another variation of laparoscopic myomectomy used as an alternative to the morcellator is specimen removal through a colpotomy incision. The colpotomy incision can be done vaginally below the cervix between the uterosacral ligaments. This is facilitated by transfixing the myoma with a tumor screw and pushing it into the cul-de-sac laparoscopically. This allows the vaginal surgeon to make the colpotomy incision directly over the myoma without fear of injury to intra-abdominal structures. Once the peritoneum is opened, the myoma is grasped vaginally with a tenaculum or Leahy clamp and removed intact or progressively morcellated using a coring technique. Alternatively, the vagina can be identified laparoscopically by the uterine manipulator, vaginal probe, or a sponge stick placed in the posterior fornix vaginally. An incision is then made laparoscopically using an electrosurgical needle or scissors, harmonic scalpel, or CO_2 laser. The disadvantage of this approach is the pneumoperitoneum is rapidly lost, making it difficult to bring the myoma into the cul-de-sac. A wet lap pad may be placed in the vagina to facilitate restoring the pneumoperitoneum to view the pelvis. Multiple small myomas can be removed with a specimen retrieval bag placed through the colpotomy incision. The colpotomy incision can be sutured laparoscopically, but it is far quicker and easier to close the colpotomy vaginally.

In a retrospective cohort study, Ou and associates [21] compared two groups of patients undergoing laparoscopic myomectomy with specimen removal by colpotomy versus morcellation. They found that multiple myomas can be removed more quickly via posterior colpotomy than by morcellation. The incisions were closed vaginally and then inspected laparoscopically to ensure hemostasis. Certainly, avoiding the use of electronic morcellators and the high cost of disposable morcellator blades is an economical way of performing laparoscopic myomectomy.

VAGINAL MYOMECTOMY AND LAPAROSCOPICALLY ASSISTED VAGINAL MYOMECTOMY

Several authors have reported on vaginal myomectomy and laparoscopically assisted vaginal myomectomy (LAVM), a version of laparoscopic myomectomy in which the dominant myoma is incised and partially enucleated by the techniques described above and the enucleation is completed through a transverse colpotomy incision. Smaller myomas are then incised and enucleated vaginally. The fundus is then delivered through the colpotomy and the defects repaired.[22,23] This technique is possible only if there is adequate room vaginally and the cul-de-sac can be reached easily. For large dominant posterior myomas, the use of the laparoscope may not be necessary. In a small pilot study, Birsan and associates [24] compared two similar groups of women undergoing laparoscopic myomectomy versus vaginal myomectomy for large posterior myomas. There was no difference in parity or myoma size between the two groups. Vaginal myomectomy was found to be feasible and safe and was associated with a shorter operating time and lower morphine consumption than laparoscopic myomectomy.[24] LAVM through an anterior approach was reported by Chin and associates.[25] Seven women with symptomatic fundal and anterior wall myomas were treated by laparoscopically placing a suture through the myoma and bringing it down through the anterior cul-de-sac into the vagina via an anterior colpotomy. Resection and suturing were performed transvaginally. There were no complications, although four patients developed transient hematuria.

LAPAROSCOPICALLY ASSISTED MYOMECTOMY/MINILAP MYONECTOMY

First reported by Nezhat et al. [26] in 1994, laparoscopically assisted myomectomy (LAM) is a safe alternative to laparoscopic myomectomy. It is less difficult and requires less time to complete than other modes of myomectomy. These considerations are summarized in Table 12.1.1. The decision to do LAM usually is made in the operating room after the diagnostic laparoscopy and treatment of other pelvic abnormalities are completed. The criteria for LAM are a myoma greater than 8 cm, many myomas requiring extensive morcellation, and a deep, large, intramural myoma that requires uterine repair in multiple layers.

A combination of laparoscopy with a 2- to 4-cm abdominal incision may enable more gynecologists to apply this technique. The conventional uterine suturing in two or three layers reduces the potential for uterine dehiscence, fistulas, and adhesions. Better pelvic exposure during the laparoscopy allows the gynecologist to diagnose and treat associated endometriosis or adhesions.

Three major objectives of LAM are reduction of blood loss, prevention of postoperative adhesions, and maintenance of myometrial integrity. LAM with morcellation and conventional suturing reduces the duration of the operation and the need for more extensive laparoscopic experience.

Table 12.1.1: Results of Types of Myomectomy

Studied Parameter	LAM (57 patients), mean ± SEM	LM (64), mean ± SEM	Lap (22), mean ± SEM	P(LM)* P(Lap)†
Leiomyoma weight, g	247 ± 30.1	58 ± 7.16	337 ± 77.4	P(LM) ≤ 0.00001
				P(Lap) = 0.27
Uterine size, weeks	12 ± 26	8 ± 14	10 ± 24	
Operative time, minutes	127 ± 7.62	136 ± 9.6	134 ± 9.95	P(LM) = 0.36
				P(Lap) = 0.59
Blood loss, mL	267 ± 54.4	143 ± 35.6	245 ± 56.1	P(LM) = 0.0068
				P(Lap) = 0.78
Postoperative hospital stay, days	1.28	0.91	3.3 ± 0.39	P(LM) = .0141
				P(Lap) = .00004
Days to resume normal activity	12.2	11.2	39.2	P(LM) = 0.43
				P(Lap) ≤ 0.0001
Days for complete "100%" recovery	23.1	20.9	70.0	P(LM) = 0.41
				P(Lap) = 0.0002

LAM, laparoscopically assisted myomectomy; Lap, laparotomy; LM, laparoscopic myectomy; SEM, standard error of the mean.
*P(LM) compares LAM and LM.
†P(Lap) compares LAM and myomectomy by laparotomy.
Source: Nezhat [9] p206, 715-2.

The use of minilaparotomy in surgery for benign gynecologic disease has been well established.[27] In a randomized controlled trial, Benassi and associates [28] evaluated the efficacy and applicability of the minilaparotomy technique in abdominal myomectomies and compared it with traditional laparotomy. They found duration of surgery and days of postoperative hospital stay were significantly lower in the minilaparotomy group, as well as higher treatment satisfaction reported by the patients ($P \leq 0.05$). Moreover, each minilaparotomy operation ended up saving 620 euros.

Based on a review of 139 cases, Glasser [29] found that myomectomy performed through a 3- to 6-cm minilaparotomy incision affords the advantage of same-day discharge as well as the ability to palpate the uterus and close the defect using a standard three-layered suturing technique. Of the original 139 patients, 66 had LAM, during which the laparoscope was used to identify and mark the incision site or to perform adhesiolysis. The vast majority of those procedures were done during our early experience. For the last 4 years, virtually all myomectomies were done without the use of the laparoscope. All patients with leiomyomas complaining of "bulk" symptoms and desiring intervention were offered minilap myomectomy as one of their treatment options. Those who had completed childbearing were also offered vaginal or minilap supracervical hysterectomy, uterine artery embolization, or medical therapy if they were perimenopausal.

Laparoscopic myolysis was also offered as a treatment option. Laparoscopic myolysis was our first choice for the management of large symptomatic myomas in the mid-1990s. We did perform 102 myolysis procedures from 1994 to 2001 but have not done any in the past 4 years. The procedure is technically much easier to perform than myomectomy, blood loss is less, and operating time is shorter. Over time, however, both patients and physicians found this procedure to be distasteful. Patients, in particular, were unhappy with leaving "dead fibroids" in their uterus. We did see some regrowth, and subsequent hysterectomies done on myolysis patients were difficult secondary to adhesions. As our skill level with minilap myomectomy improved, more of our physicians encouraged this procedure as a first option – even when fertility was not an issue. Certainly, myomectomy is always the first option in patients desiring future childbearing.

All patients underwent pelvic ultrasonography to assess uterine size, individual myoma size, and number and location of myomas. Those with equivocal sonography and those with multiple myomas desiring future fertility underwent MRI studies to "map" the uterus more accurately. Those with abnormal uterine bleeding underwent diagnostic office hysteroscopy and hysteroscopic resection at the time of myomectomy if submucous myomas were present. Myomas larger than 2 cm were removed transmyometrially. Patients with more than five measurable myomas on imaging studies and not desiring future fertility were strongly urged to undergo hysterectomy or uterine artery embolization. The "ideal" patient for this procedure is thin, with a single large anterior fundal myoma. We have, however, performed this procedure on patients weighing as much as 280 lb and on those with multiple or posterior myomas.

Pretreatment with GnRH analogues was used in all patients in the early part of the study, but this practice has largely been abandoned. GnRH analogues are given only to reduce massive bulk in uteri greater than 20 weeks' gestational size or to patients who are anemic (Hgb <10 GMS.) to create amenorrhea and increase hemoglobin levels. An 8-week course is generally sufficient to achieve these results. The results of this series are summarized in Table 12.1.2. The average age of the patients was 38.9

Table 12.1.2: Minilap Myomectomy in 139 Patients*

Patient Characteristic	Median	Range	Interquartile Range
Age, years	30	23–56	8
Myoma weight, g	275	30–975	270
Estimate blood loss, mL	300	50–2000	200
Operating room time, minutes	110	44–260	61
Length of stay, hours	6	2–48	9
Additional procedures	Three hysterectomies: one due to emergency hemorrhage and two due to recurrent fibroids		

*Performed at Kaiser San Rafael January 1, 1995, [29], to December 31, 2003.

years, with a range of 23 to 56 years. There were also a few perimenopausal patients who were poor candidates for either vaginal hysterectomy (nulliparous, no uterine decensus and huge fibroids) or laparoscopic supracervical hysterectomy (LSH) and wanted a minimally invasive approach rather than a conventional abdominal hysterectomy. Those patients are now offered minilap supracervical hysterectomy as an alternative.

The average weight of the myomas removed was 285.6 g, with a range of 30 to 925 g. The patient with a 30-g myoma was an infertility patient with a 5-cm type 2 myoma penetrating the entire myometrium. Two patients had 15 separate myomas removed that were not evident on preoperative imaging studies. Seventy of 139 patients had pretreatment with GnRH analogues.

The average length of stay was 13.6 hours, with a range of 4 to 48 hours. One of the two patients who spent 48 hours in the hospital developed a fever, probably secondary to atelectasis, and was kept for observation. The other patient had nausea and vomiting, which resolved with antiemetics. Twenty-four of 139 patients were discharged within 4 hours of surgery and 61 within 8 hours. Of the 51 patients discharged between 8 and 23 hours post surgery, 27 lived more than 50 miles from the hospital and chose to spend the night rather than drive home.

Average operating time for this procedure was 110 minutes, with a range of 55 to 260 minutes. The operating time was, to some degree, related to the skill and experience of the surgeon. There was a direct relationship between operating time and number of myomas, rather than size, although individual myomas larger than 10 cm took longer to morcellate.

The average blood loss was 330 mL, with a range of 50 to 2000 mL. The patient with the 2000-mL blood loss had a large broad ligament myoma that was avulsed by too vigorous upward traction before being completely morcellated. She had uncontrolled bleeding at the myoma bed and underwent emergency hysterectomy after efforts at uterine artery ligation failed. She was the only patient to undergo a blood transfusion in our series. This complication occurred early in our series in a procedure performed by a relatively inexperienced surgeon.

The two other hysterectomies performed in this group were for recurrent myomas. Both these patients had multiple myomas at the time of initial myomectomy. One had a hematometra

following surgery and gradual uterine growth over a 6-month period. Her bulk symptoms recurred, and she elected to have an abdominal hysterectomy at that time. The second patient had multiple myomas removed at age 38 and had recurrence of symptoms 5 years later. She underwent a supracervical hysterectomy for a uterus that weighed 900 g and contained multiple myomas.

Surgical Technique

If LAM is being performed, the following technique is used. In patients with multiple myomas, the most prominent myoma is injected at its base with 3 to 7 mL of diluted vasopressin. A vertical incision is made over the uterine serosa onto the surface of the tumor and extended until the capsule of the leiomyoma is reached. A corkscrew manipulator is inserted into the leiomyoma and used to elevate the uterus toward the midline suprapubic puncture. With the trocar and manipulator attached to the myoma, this midline 5-mm puncture is enlarged to a 4-cm transverse skin incision. After the incision of the fascia transversely, the rectus muscle is divided using a monopolar electrode. If the inferior epigastric vessels are found, they are coagulated. This approach provides excellent access to the abdominal cavity.

The peritoneum is entered transversely, and the leiomyoma is observed. It is brought to the laparotomy incision by using the corkscrew manipulator to raise the uterus. A corkscrew manipulator is replaced with two Lahey tenacula. The tumor is shelled and morcellated sequentially, and after its complete removal, the uterine wall defect shows through the incision. If uterine size allows, the uterus is exteriorized to complete the repair. When multiple leiomyomas are found, as many as possible are removed through one uterine incision if it can be accomplished without excessive tunneling. When other myomas are located that cannot be removed through the initial uterine incision, the 4-cm abdominal opening is approximated temporarily with two or three Allis clamps or an inflated latex glove. The laparoscope is reintroduced, and the remaining myomas are identified and brought to the level of the abdominal incision. They are removed under laparoscopic control. The uterus is exteriorized through the 4-cm abdominal incision. The myometrium is closed in layers with 2-0 and 0 polydioxanone sutures. The serosa is closed microsurgically with 5-0 sutures. The uterus is palpated to ensure that no small intramural leiomyomas remain. It is returned to the peritoneal cavity. The fascia is closed with a 1-0 polyglactin suture, and the skin is closed in a subcuticular manner. The laparoscope is used to evaluate hemostasis. The pelvis is observed to detect and treat endometriosis and adhesions that may have been obscured previously by myomas. Copious irrigation is used, blood clots are removed, and Interceed (Gynecare, Somerville, NJ) is applied over the uterus to help prevent adhesions.

Intraoperatively, injections of dilute vasopressin into the myoma help reduce blood loss. Vertical uterine incisions bleed less than do transverse incisions [4], and pneumoperitoneum seems to decrease intraoperative bleeding.

A recent innovation in LAM is the use of the LAP DISK abdominal wall sealing device (Ethicon Endosurgery, Somerville, NJ), which allows the surgeon to place a hand in the abdomen during laparoscopic surgery, facilitating exposure and dissection. In a retrospective study of 43 patients who underwent LAM using the LAP DISK, Tanaguchi and associates [30] in Japan removed myomas that ranged in weight from 40 to 700 g (mean, 208 g) and diameter from 2 to 10 cm (mean, 5.4 cm). Mean blood loss was 42.3 mL. Half of the 18 patients who had been diagnosed with primary infertility for 2 years or longer became pregnant without postoperative assisted reproductive techniques. The authors concluded that the LAP DISK abdominal wall sealing device was useful for LAM, allowing surgeons to remove myomas safely and repair uterine defects effectively while minimizing blood loss and trauma.

In minilap myomectomy without the use of laparoscopy, the patient is placed in the low lithotomy position using Allen stirrups (Allen Medical Systems, Cleveland, OH). Ten milliliters of a dilute vasopressin solution (6 U in 60 mL NaCl) is then injected intracervically about 1 to 2 cm deep at both the 8 and 4 o'clock positions according to the technique described by Phillips et al. [31], and we have noticed a marked blanching of the entire uterus when this is done before making the abdominal incision. A firm uterine manipulator with a 5-mm obturator (Medical Horizons, Fair Oaks, CA) is then placed in the cervix (Figure 12.1.1). A Pelosi (Figure 12.1.2) or Valtchev manipulator also works well. It is important not to use a uterine manipulator with an inflatable balloon because it may be mistaken for a myoma on palpation. The midline is identified on the abdomen and a 3- to 5-cm horizontal line is drawn on the skin about two to three finger breaths above the top of the symphysis. The incision should be made slightly higher if the myoma is posterior. Also, the incision should be made slightly longer for patients with central obesity. For patients who are massively obese with a large pannus, this can be raised and taped to the top of the table with 6-inch cloth tape secured with tincture of benzoin. The incision then is made at the skin fold above the pubic bone, which is often the thinnest part of the abdomen.

The operation is performed using a cruciate incision. The cruciate incision, as described by Pelosi [32] for minilaparotomy, affords excellent exposure. By dissecting the fascia vertically rather than horizontally, the abdominal opening is round rather than ovoid, giving an increased working area. Before making the skin incision, 10 mL of 0.25% bupivacaine (Marcaine, AstraZeneca) with epinephrine solution is injected superficially, extending laterally beyond the limits of the incision. The skin and subcutaneous tissue are opened horizontally to the level of the fascia, and a finger is used to bluntly tunnel under the subcutaneous fat close to the fascia in the midline both cephalad toward the umbilicus and caudad to the pubic bone. The fascia is then opened in the midline for a total length of about 6 cm. The rectus muscle is then separated in the midline and the peritoneum grasped, nicked, and entered longitudinally. Care must be taken not to injure the bladder when extending the peritoneal incision downward. Once the peritoneum is opened, the surgeon's finger is swept circumferentially, to make sure there are no adhesions to the anterior abdominal wall. A Mobius elastic retractor (Apple Medical, Marlborough, MA) is then inserted (Figure 12.1.5). The bottom blue ring of the retractor is first inserted under the peritoneum, and the polyethylene membrane is then rolled up on the top yellow ring. This is facilitated by the surgeon grasping the top ring at the 10 and 2 o'clock positions and twisting it down toward the abdominal wall. The assistant then completes the twist while the surgeon holds the top ring firmly. Usually two or three twists are sufficient to create a nice round opening in the abdominal wall with a diameter equal to the length of the skin incision. The Mobius elastic self-retaining retractor [33] enhances this expo-

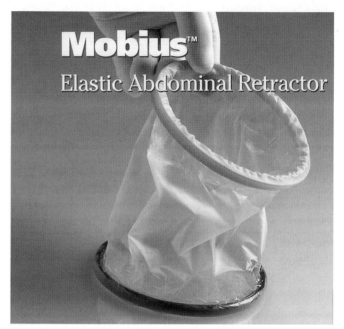

Figure 12.1.5. The Mobius retractor.

sure, and the incision can be moved to the areas of dissection using small Deaver or Lorenz vein retractors. A 4-cm incision results in a working area of 12.5 cm^2, whereas a 6-cm incision will increase this working area to 28 cm^2. The retractor gently compresses the layers of the abdominal wall and allows the specimen to be elevated to the skin line. Also, the retractor allows the skin to stretch so that much larger specimens can be removed. This is not possible using a fixed metal self-retaining retractor. There is also minimal trauma to the rectus muscles. The vast majority of our patients require only oral analgesics in the immediate postoperative period and manage well on nonsteroidal anti-inflammatory drugs or acetaminophen at home. The retractor is soft and very atraumatic to the tissues of the abdominal wall while it keeps subcutaneous fat, muscle, and peritoneum out of the operative field. We have found that a 4- to 5-cm incision gives us adequate room to remove myomas by morcellation and repair the uterine defect by conventional suturing techniques.

Before proceeding with the myomectomy, the size and position of the myomas are carefully assessed. If there is any doubt about the safe performance of the procedure via minilap, such as the presence of large inaccessible posterior or broad ligament myomas, a conventional laparotomy should be performed. This can easily be accomplished by removing the Mobius retractor, extending the skin and fascial incisions, and reinserting the Mobius to its full 6-inch diameter. Conversion to laparotomy when the myoma is partially dissected results in increased blood loss secondary to the delay, so this decision should be made early. Assessment as to where the uterine incision should be placed is the next step. We prefer anterior midline fundal incisions for large solitary intramural myomas. If multiple myomas are present, a strategic incision site through which most of the myomas can be removed is attempted, but it is sometimes preferable to make separate incisions for each myoma. Posterior myomas can usually be approached through a transverse incision well below the tubal insertions. For large subserosal myomas, it is important to make the initial incision high on the myoma, usually 2 to 3 cm distal to the junction between the myoma and the uterus. This allows for easier closure of the defect. Also, pedunculated myomas should be incised above where the pedicle inserts on the myoma to avoid cautery damage to the fundal myometrium. Attempts should be made to avoid the cornual region, thus minimizing trauma to the tubal ostia.

Using the uterine manipulator, the uterus is elevated to the abdominal incision. The serosa and myometrium along the course of the proposed incision is then injected with the same dilute vasopressin solution used intracervically to a depth of 1 to 2 cm. This is easily accomplished with the use of a standard 22-gauge 1.5-inch needle. Additional vasopressin is injected deeply into the myoma. Subserous myomas should be injected at the base, directing the needle both into the myoma and into the uterus. A distinct blanching of the myoma becomes readily apparent. Usually, 10 to 15 mL of vasopressin is sufficient to achieve hemostasis. A 4- to 6-cm incision is then made through the serosa and myometrium and carried down through the pseudocapsule of the myoma. The myoma usually bulges out at this point. Small "army–navy," Jarit "S," or Lorenz vein retractors are then inserted between the myoma and the myometrium inside the pseudocapsule (Figure 12.1.6). The myoma is grasped with Lahey thyroid clamps and strong upward traction applied. This tamponades the uterine incision against the upper abdominal wall and markedly reduces blood loss. The myoma is then progressively morcellated, much as one would do in a vaginal hysterectomy using a #10 scalpel blade on a long handle (Figure 12.1.7). This is more ergonomic and thus less tiring than using a short-handled scalpel. It is most important to regrasp a remaining edge of the myoma before the morcellated core of tissue is removed so that upward traction and tamponade are maintained (Figure 12.1.8). Attempts to enucleate the large myoma should be avoided because this tears blood vessels both in the periphery and at the base of the myoma. Careful dissection around the capsule of the myoma with coagulation of blood vessels as they are encountered significantly reduces blood loss. The large blood vessels at the base are easily identified and desiccated when the remains of the myoma are brought through the incision (Figure

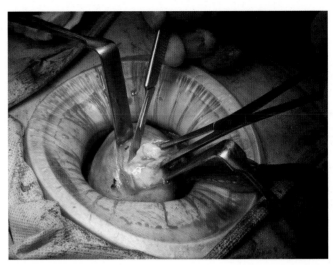

Figure 12.1.7. Morcellation of the myoma using a #10 scalpel.

12.1.9). Careful palpation at this point allows additional myomas to be identified and, if possible, removed through this incision by a combination of morcellation and enucleation. Also, palpation of the obturator of the manipulator identifies the uterine cavity. If additional myomas are identified in other areas, it is more prudent to first close the original uterine incision and approach the others through separate incisions using the same technique described above.

The uterine elevator is helpful in bringing the uterus up to the anterior abdominal wall, where the edges of the uterine incision are then grasped with Pennington clamps. The Pennington clamps are placed as deep as possible into the myometrial defect and an attempt is made to evert the edges. The entire uterine defect can often be exteriorized completely for easy repair on the abdomen (Figure 12.1.10). This allows placement of deep figure-of-eight or horizontal mattress sutures. We use #1 Polysorb on an HGS 21 needle (USSC, Norwalk, CT) and take deep myometrial bites to close off the base of the incision and approximate the

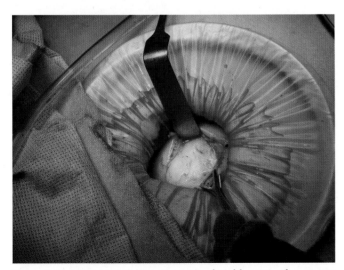

Figure 12.1.6. Lorenz vein retractors are placed between the myoma and the myometrium before morcellation.

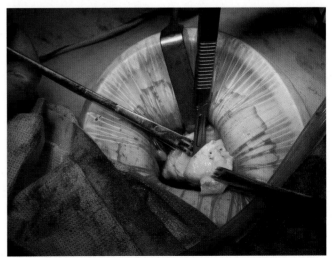

Figure 12.1.8. Upward traction on the myoma is maintained with an additional Leahy clamp before the morcellated core is removed.

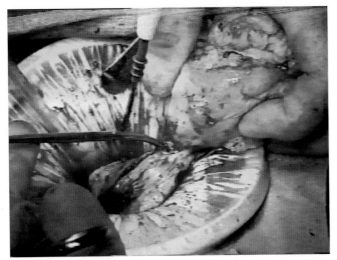

Figure 12.1.9. The dominant vessels are clamped and coagulated after the morcellated myoma is delivered through the minilap incision.

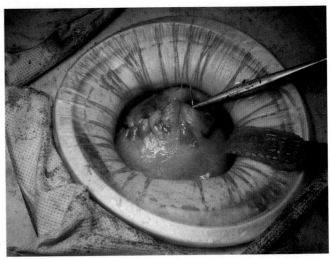

Figure 12.1.11. The serosa is closed with an imbricating baseball closure using fine suture on a vascular needle.

myometrium. A second layer of continuous 0 Polysorb or interrupted horizontal mattress sutures are placed to further approximate the myometrium. The serosa is then closed with a continuous "baseball" imbricating layer using 3-0 Polysorb on a V20 (vascular) needle for minimal trauma and adhesion prevention (Figure 12.1.11). All anterior and pedunculated myomas should be removed first so that the uterus can be sharply anteflexed by the uterine manipulator to approach posterior lower-segment myomas. We have been surprised that even posterior cervical myomas can be removed by this technique.

Large pedunculated fundal myomas are most easily managed by minilap because extensive deep suturing usually is not necessary. Usually, a 3-cm incision suffices. Once the myoma pedicle is identified, it is injected with the dilute vasopressin solution as described above. A large, blunt right-angled vascular clamp (Grover or Satinsky) is placed under the myoma pedicle and a

0.5-inch Penrose drain is drawn under and tightly tied around the myoma pedicle (Figure 12.1.12). Using the electrosurgical pencil, a circumferential mark is made at the myoma base about 1 to 2 cm above the tourniquet. The top of the myoma is then brought to the incision (Figure 12.1.13) and progressively morcellated with a scalpel until the mark at the base is reached (Figure 12.1.14). It is then carefully dissected free from the pedicle (Figure 12.1.15). A horizontal mattress suture is then placed in the fundus of the uterus incorporating the base of the pedicle and

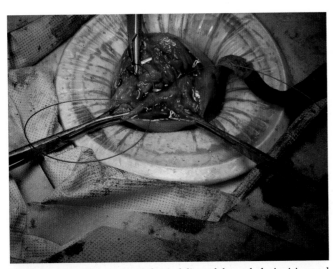

Figure 12.1.10. The uterine defect is delivered through the incision and the edges grasped with Pennington clamps. The defect is closed with multiple layers to eliminate any myometrial "dead space."

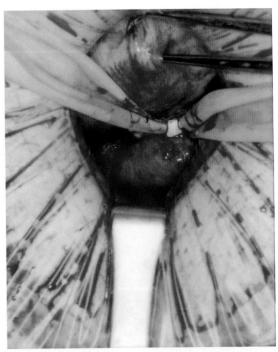

Figure 12.1.12. A 0.5-inch Penrose drain is placed under the pedicle of a 7-cm pedunculated myoma, which has been grasped by a tenaculum. The drain is tied tightly to form a tourniquet. The uterus is visible below the Penrose drain.

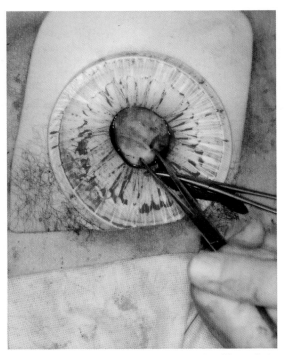

Figure 12.1.13. The top of the myoma is grasped and brought into the skin incision, where it will be progressively morcellated.

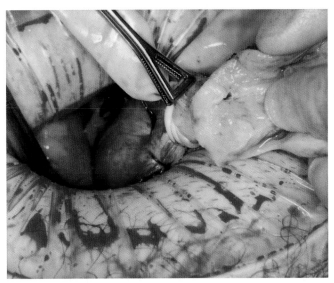

Figure 12.1.15. The edge of the pedicle is grasped with a Pennington clamp 1–2 cm above the Penrose drain around the pedicle and the myoma dissected free.

tied tightly (Figure 12.1.16). The tourniquet is then removed and the edges of the pedicle sutured and imbricated (Figure 12.1.17). This technique assures that the myometrium at the fundus of the uterus is not subject to electrosurgical or thermal injury.

After hemostasis is assured in the uterine incision, the uterus is dropped back into the pelvis and the pelvis is irrigated with copious amounts of lactated Ringer's solution or normal saline. Interceed adhesion prevention barrier is placed over the uterine incisions. The minilaparotomy incision is repaired in layers, with

an attempt to eliminate the dead space in the subcutaneous tissue to prevent seroma formation. A subcuticular closure for the skin is used after Marcaine 0.25% with epinephrine is injected in the fascia and the skin edges. Steri-Strips (3M) and a large Band-Aid are placed on the incision, and a vertical pressure dressing is applied until the patient is discharged.

Most patients receive ketorolac 60 mg intramuscularly (Toradol, Roche Pharmaceuticals, Nutley, NJ) and dexamethasone 8 mg intravenously (IV) (Decadron, Merck & Co., West Point, PA) intraoperatively and are discharged after approximately 4 hours in our ambulatory surgery recovery area. Patients who have late-afternoon surgery or are insufficiently recovered are discharged the following morning. All patients

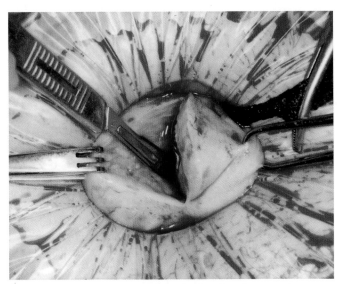

Figure 12.1.14. The myoma is grasped with Lahey clamps and progressively morcellated with a #10 scalpel.

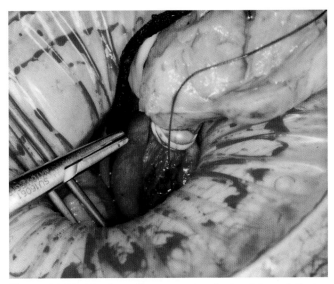

Figure 12.1.16. A horizontal mattress suture is placed through the top of the fundus of the uterus around the pedicle.

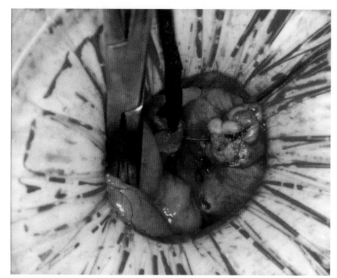

Figure 12.1.17. After the myoma is removed, the edges of the pedicle are imbricated with fine suture.

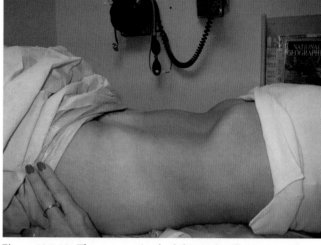

Figure 12.1.19. The same patient's abdominal wall contour at her 4-week postoperative checkup. She left the hospital 4 hours after surgery.

without cephalosporin allergies are given cefazolin 1 g IV preoperatively. Figures 12.1.18 through 12.1.20 show the pre- and postoperative abdominal wall contours of a 49-year-old patient who had an 848-g myoma excised through a 5-cm minilap incision. The patient left the hospital 4 hours postoperatively and went shopping for shoes 4 days postoperatively.

Use of GnRH Agonists

Pretreatment with GnRH agonists before myomectomy remains controversial. In a systematic review of randomized controlled trials of the use of GnRH analogues before hysterectomy and myomectomy, it was found that pre- and postoperative blood counts were improved, uterine and myoma volume decreased, and operative time and blood loss reduced by GnRH agonist therapy.[34] Reduction in leiomyoma size makes the procedure

less time consuming because a smaller uterine incision can be made and less morcellation is required. The individual myomas, however, are softer, which often results in the Lahey clamps tearing through the tissue, resulting in the loss of upward traction, which is counterproductive and may result in increased

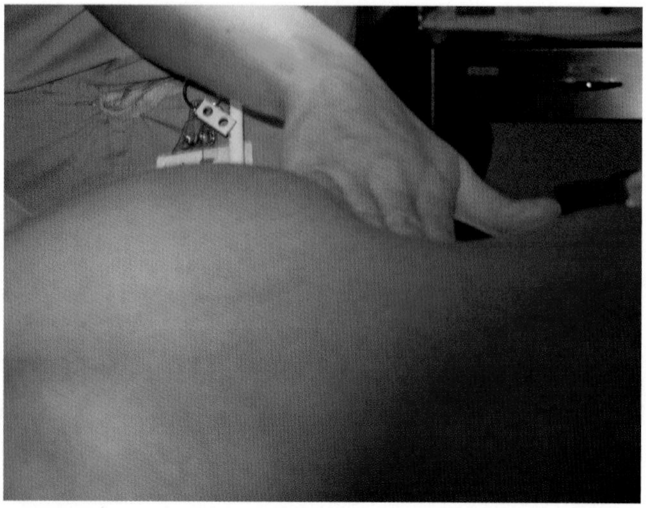

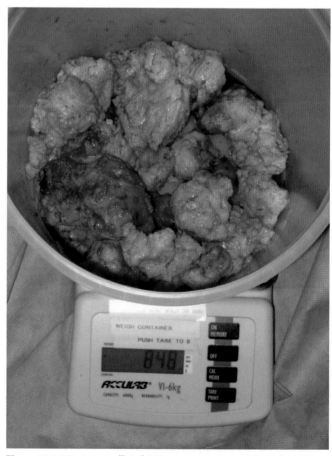

Figure 12.1.20. A morcellated 848-g myoma removed from the patient.

Figure 12.1.18. Preoperative abdominal contour of a 49-year-old woman with a 17-cm dominant intramural fundal myoma.

bleeding. For anemic patients, preoperative GnRH treatment may enable restoration of a normal hematocrit, decrease the size of the myoma, and reduce the need for transfusion.[35] Although GnRH agonist use may soften the myoma (facilitating morcellation) and shorten operative times, it also may increase the duration of laparoscopic or minilap myomectomy.[36] However, not all studies have shown the benefits described above. Increased difficulty in identifying and dissecting the cleavage planes and shrinking small myomas to the point at which they cannot be seen or palpated may increase recurrence.[37] We do not use preoperative GnRH agonists unless the patient is anemic or the myoma is above the umbilicus.

Adhesion Prevention

Although myomectomy is done to preserve fertility, postoperative adhesions may jeopardize this goal. Single, vertical, anterior, and midline uterine incisions cause fewer adhesions.[4] Although sutures predispose patients to adhesions [38], they are always necessary to close the uterine defect. Although several adhesion barriers are either available or under development, none is completely effective.[39] A prospective, randomized, blinded multicenter study evaluated 127 women undergoing uterine myomectomy with at least one posterior uterine incision 1 cm or greater in length.[40] Patients were randomized to Seprafilm (HAL-F) bioresorbable membrane (Genzyme Corporation, Cambridge, MA) or to no treatment. At second-look laparoscopy, the incidence, measured as the mean number of sites adherent to the uterine surface, was significantly lower in the treated group as were the mean uterine adhesion severity scores and mean area of adhesions. In another study, 50 premenopausal, nonpregnant women who underwent laparoscopic myomectomy were randomized to the control group (25 patients) with surgery alone or to the treatment group (25 patients) using Interceed, an oxidized regenerated cellulose.[41] At second-look laparoscopy 12 to 14 weeks later, 12% (three) of the women in the control group were adhesion-free, compared with 60% (15) of those treated with Interceed ($P \leq 0.05$).

In a randomized, prospective, controlled, multicenter clinical trial of a sprayable, site-specific adhesion barrier system (SprayGel, Confluent Surgical, Waltham, MA) in 66 women with a mean age at surgery of 34.9 years (range, 23 to 52 years) undergoing laparoscopic or open uterine myomectomy, Mettler and associates [42] found when compared with initial surgery, the mean adhesion tenacity score of adhesions seen at second-look laparoscopy was significantly reduced in treatment patients compared with control patients (0.6 vs. 1.7, a 64.7% reduction). Mean adhesion extent score at second-look laparoscopy compared with initial surgery was 4.5 cm^2 versus 7.2 cm^2, and the mean adhesion incidence score was 0.64 versus 1.22. Of 64 patients, 40 (62.5%) returned for second-look laparoscopy. The Mettler group's conclusions were that this adhesion barrier was safe and well tolerated and demonstrated efficacy in a population of patients known to be at risk for adhesion formation. There were no adverse effects attributable to the product and no patients in whom it could not be applied.

Regardless of the adhesion prevention material used, most are ineffective in the absence of hemostasis. This was shown very early in a study on animal models by Linsky and associates.[43] Using an imbricating baseball-type closure on the uterine serosa is both hemostatic and minimizes the presence of raw edges, which also predispose to adhesion formation.

LAPAROSCOPIC MYOMECTOMY AND LAPAROSCOPICALLY ASSISTED (MINILAP) MYOMECTOMY: COMPARISON OF RESULTS

Nezhat and associates [9] evaluated 143 charts from their practice, including those of patients who had myomectomy by laparotomy (15.3%), laparoscopic myomectomy (44.7%), or LAM (39.8%) (Table 12.1.1). The 22 myomectomies by laparotomy were done before the development of LAM. Because LAM replaced myomectomy by laparotomy and patient selection criteria were comparable, the myoma weights of the two groups were similar.

Mean operating times were the same for laparoscopic myomectomy and LAM despite larger myomas, difficult locations of intramural myomas, and adjunctive laparoscopy in the latter group. The leiomyoma weights were greater in the LAM group than in the laparoscopic myomectomy group ($P \leq 0.05$).

The mean estimated blood loss of the LAM and laparotomy groups was not different. In contrast, blood loss among the laparoscopic myomectomy patients was significantly lower, and this may be attributed to the smaller leiomyomas. In comparing the hospitalization time of the LAM and laparoscopic myomectomy patients, that of the LAM group appeared to be longer ($P(LM) = 0.014$). This may be explained by the initial reluctance of some physicians to discharge LAM patients on the day of the operation or on postoperative day 1. After the initial 10 to 15 operations, all the women underwent LAM on an outpatient basis. In fact, when the initial 15 cases are removed from the LAM group, the mean hospital stay drops to 1.06 days. This period is not statistically different from that for the laparoscopic myomectomy group.

The comparison of postoperative recovery times shows important distinctions between the LAM and laparoscopic myomectomy groups. Here, despite the differences in size and location of myomas, the recovery time can be compared because of the diverse incisions. The time elapsed before patients resumed work or regular activity was similar ($P \leq 0.05$). Introducing a 4-cm incision in the LAM group did appear to prolong ($P \leq 0.05$) the subjectively perceived time for the women to achieve 100% recovery.

Previous studies [44,45] underscored the need to decrease the operative time of laparoscopic myomectomy. Whereas myomas less than 8 cm are managed laparoscopically, larger tumors and intramural lesions require prolonged morcellation and laparoscopic suturing of the uterine defect. The largest reported myomas removed by laparoscopy were 15 to 16 cm [9,44], and one group wrote that 10 cm was its limit.[46] Both laparoscopic morcellation and myometrial suturing are difficult and prolong operations. Hospitalization was much longer for the patients who underwent myomectomy by laparotomy ($P \geq 0.05$) compared with both the LAM and the laparoscopic myomectomy groups.

Second-look laparoscopies done on postmyomectomy patients who had pedunculated and superficial subserosal myomas without sutures showed complete uterine healing. In contrast, intramural myomas were associated with granulation tissue and indentation of the uterus proportional to the size of the

Table 12.1.3: Incidence of Adhesions after Laparoscopic Myomectomy with or without the Use of Sutures

Leiomyoma Size, cm	No Suture Used				Suture Used			
	0*	1	2	3	0	1	2	3
≤3	18/21	3/21	0/21	0/21	NA	NA	NA	NA
>3	10/16	5/16	1/16	0/16	0/19	4/19	12/19	5/19

NA, not applicable: suture was not used for myomas ≤3 cm in size.
*Adhesion score: 0 = no adhesions; 1 = filmy and nonvascular; 2 = thick and nonvascular; 3 = thick, vascular, and bowel.
Source: Nezhat [9], p 267

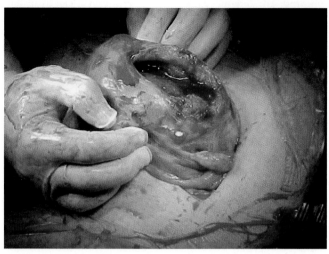

Figure 12.1.21. A posterior uterine rupture at 27 weeks' gestation in a patient who had undergone a previous laparoscopic myomectomy (courtesy of Riccardo Marana, M.D.).

leiomyoma excised unless sutures were used. The use of sutures is associated with more adhesions (Table 12.1.3).[9]

Most patients are observed in an outpatient unit and discharged the morning after the operation, although some can leave the hospital on the afternoon or evening of the procedure.

UTERINE RUPTURE FOLLOWING MYOMECTOMY

Women of childbearing age who plan a future pregnancy and require a myomectomy for an intramural tumor should probably undergo a minilaparotomy or standard laparotomy to ensure proper closure of the myometrial incision unless the surgeon is very skilled in laparoscopic suturing. A cesarean delivery is safest for such patients. The laparoscopic approach is appropriate for pedunculated or subserosal tumors because smaller intramural tumors may be missed by the laparoscopic approach. Also, the necessity for complete closure of the defect cannot be emphasized enough. It is inadequate to place two or three large through-and-through interrupted sutures in a deep myometrial defect if the patient plans future childbearing. Recent reports of uterine rupture following laparoscopic myomectomy [47–49] emphasize the importance of adequate closure of the myometrial defect. A dramatic photograph of a uterine rupture at 27 weeks' gestation submitted by Riccardo Marana's group in Rome appeared on the cover of the July/August issue of the *Journal of Minimally Invasive Gynecology* (Figure 12.1.21).[50] A recent study reported the appearance of myomectomy scars in 15 women undergoing elective cesarean section because of previous myomectomy.[51] The scars in the five women who had the myomectomies performed laparoscopically were all described as "strained with thinned tissue and ill-defined edges" despite being sutured. In the 10 women who had their myomectomy performed by laparotomy, the majority of scars were symmetric, with the tissue being of uniform thickness compared with the surrounding myometrium. Certainly the liberal use of electrocautery for hemostasis might be the etiologic factor in uterine rupture.

Spontaneous rupture of the uterine scar after laparoscopically assisted minilaparotomy has also been reported.[52] Chromic catgut was used to close the uterine defect in that case, but whether or not this played a role is a matter of conjecture. In summary, patients must be thoroughly counseled about the possibility of uterine rupture at any time during the pregnancy and be made aware of the possibility of losing the baby and also losing the uterus if hemorrhage cannot be controlled. They must be followed very carefully and all complaints of abdominal pain taken seriously.

PREGNANCY FOLLOWING MYOMECTOMY

Pregnancy rates after myomectomy, both open and laparoscopic, have been variable. One study comparing reproductive outcomes after laparoscopic or abdominal myomectomy showed no significant difference between the two approaches.[53] There are many factors that determine the reproductive outcome following myomectomy, including the age of the patient and the number, size, and location of the myomas. In a retrospective study of 67 women who had undergone myomectomy, the majority of which were done by laparotomy, Sudik and associates [54] reported higher pregnancy rates in women with fewer than six myomas removed. Although myoma location did not influence the results in this study, women with a larger volume (≥100 mL) of myomas removed had higher pregnancy rates. Age of the patient was not a factor in this study because there was no significant difference in the age of women who did not become pregnant (33.8 ± 5.1 years) and those who did (31.4 ± 4.5 years). In a retrospective review of 103 women who had undergone laparoscopic myomectomy in France, Desolle and associates [55] found a significantly higher pregnancy rate in women with unexplained infertility, those less than 35 years of age, and those with less than 3 years of infertility. Neither the number of myomas removed nor their location or size had any significant influence on pregnancy rates. The authors concluded other factors involved in the patients' infertility were probably more important than the characteristics of the myomas. In a 5-year review of the anticipated benefits of myomectomy, Olufowobi and associates [56] in the United Kingdom found that the symptomatic benefit was less (36%) in the "infertility group." Following an observation period of 12 to 36 months, 17 patients in the infertility group were lost to follow-up. Two of the 14 patients (14%) who attempted in vitro fertilization (IVF) were successful. In the non-IVF group, 13 of the 28 (46%)

achieved natural conception. These results suggested that symptomatic improvement and fertility enhancement may be possible in some patients with fibroids. It was also the feeling of the authors that in view of the risks and potential failure of treatment associated with myomectomy, their results, yet again, support the fact that patients should be properly counseled before embarking on myomectomy. They strongly advocate local data to form the basis of the advice given during the consultation rather than what is published in the literature.

In a retrospective analysis of 72 women with intramural and subserosal myomas, Marchionni and associates [57] in Italy found the conception rate was 28% before myomectomy and 70% after surgery. The corresponding figures were 69% and 25% for pregnancy loss and 30% and 75% for live birth rate, respectively. Age 30 years or younger and number of fibroids removed were the only significant and independent predictors of obstetric outcome by multivariate analysis. Their results suggested that abdominal myomectomy might improve reproductive outcome in patients with intramural and subserosal fibroids. The reproductive performance was particularly good when the patients were younger than 30 years and had a single myoma to remove. In a prospective randomized study of 131 women comparing myomectomy by laparoscopy versus laparotomy, Seracchioli and associates [58] found pregnancy rates were no different (55.9% in the laparotomy group compared with 53.6% in the laparoscopy group).

In a retrospective study comparing reproductive outcomes after uterine artery embolization for fibroids versus laparoscopic myomectomy, Goldberg and associates [59] found that pregnancies after uterine artery embolization had higher rates of preterm delivery (odds ratio, 6.2; 95% CI, 1.4–27.7) and malpresentation (odds ratio, 4.3; 95% CI, 1.0–20.5) than did pregnancies after laparoscopic myomectomy. The risks of postpartum hemorrhage (odds ratio, 6.3; 95% CI, 0.6–71.8) and spontaneous abortion (odds ratio, 1.7; 95% CI, 0.8–3.9) after uterine artery embolization were similarly higher than the risks after laparoscopic myomectomy; however, these differences were not statistically significant. They concluded that pregnancies in women with fibroids who were treated by uterine artery embolization, compared with pregnancies after laparoscopic myomectomy, were at increased risk for preterm delivery and malpresentation.

Surrey and associates [60] evaluated the impact of myomectomy on in vitro fertilization–embryo transfer (IVF-ET) and oocyte donation cycle outcome. The study was carried out within one center and involved treatment of myomas that distorted the uterine cavity only, whether submucosal or intramural. A total of 101 patients underwent surgical treatment for leiomyomas: 46 submucosal with hysteroscopic resection and 55 intramural treated with open laparotomy. Patients who underwent surgical myomectomy for what was felt to be clinically significant leiomyomas had assisted reproductive technology cycle outcomes similar to those of a control population with regard to implantation, ongoing pregnancy, and early pregnancy loss. Neither the size nor the surgical approach altered the outcome. Pregnancy rates in the donor oocyte group were higher in patients who underwent surgical myomectomy as opposed to the control group, with no increase in biochemical pregnancies. Size was not the criterion for a surgical approach in this study; uterine cavity distortion was the criterion used. The study also mandated a diagnostic hysteroscopy in all patients to rule out any cavity distortions or endometrial lesions, including postoperatively. The authors stress the lack of strong correlation between either hysterosalpingography or traditional standard transvaginal sonography and hysteroscopic findings. As would be expected, the mean number and size of leiomyomas were significantly larger in patients who underwent abdominal myomectomy. However, neither ongoing pregnancy nor implantation rates were significantly different in comparison with controls among either oocyte donor recipients (group A – hysteroscopic resection: 86.7%, 57.8%; group B – myomectomy: 84.6%, 55.2%; group C – no surgery: 77%, 49.1%). The findings were similar for those undergoing IVF-ET in comparison with controls (group 1: 61%, 24%; group 2: 52%, 26%; group 3: 53%, 23%).

Oliveira and associates [61] in Brazil did a study to further evaluate the effects of intramural and subserosal uterine fibroids on the outcome of IVF-ET when there is no compression of the endometrial cavity. In a retrospective, matched-control study from January 2000 to October 2001 done in a private IVF center, 245 women with subserosal and/or intramural fibroids that did not compress the uterine cavity (fibroid group) and 245 women with no evidence of fibroids anywhere in the uterus (control group) were studied. The type of fibroid (intramural, subserosal) and the number, size (centimeters), and location of intramural leiomyomas (fundal, corpus) were recorded and outcomes of IVF–intracytoplasmic sperm injection (ICSI) cycles were compared between the two groups. There was no correlation between location and number of uterine fibroids and the outcomes of IVF-ICSI. Patients with subserosal or intramural fibroids 4 cm or smaller had IVF-ICSI outcomes (pregnancy, implantation, and abortion rates) similar to those of controls. Patients with intramural fibroids 4 cm or greater had lower pregnancy rates than did patients with intramural fibroids 4 cm or less. There were no statistical differences related to delivery rates (31.5% vs. 32%, respectively) between all patients with fibroids and controls. The authors concluded that patients having subserosal or intramural leiomyomas 4 cm or smaller not encroaching on the uterine cavity have IVF-ICSI outcomes comparable to those of patients without such leiomyomas. Therefore, these patients might not require myomectomy before being scheduled for assisted reproduction cycles. However, the investigators recommend caution for patients with fibroids 4 cm or larger and that such patients be submitted to treatment before they are enrolled in IVF-ICSI cycles.

In summary, there is no consensus as to superior pregnancy rates associated with a laparoscopic route versus myomectomy by laparotomy versus no intervention at all. Preemptive myomectomy in the asymptomatic patient who wants fertility remains one of the most controversial subjects in gynecology. One must remember that myomectomy carries the risk of emergency hysterectomy in about 1% of cases.[4] Also, the chance of infection and adhesion formation might in itself cause infertility. In a review of fibroids in pregnancy, Cooper and Okolo stated that "the true incidence of fibroids during pregnancy is, however, unknown, but reported rates vary from as low as 0.1% of all pregnancies to higher rates of 12.5%. It seems that pregnancy has little or no effect on the overall size of fibroids despite the occurrence of red degeneration in early pregnancy. Fibroids, however, affect pregnancy and delivery in several ways, with abdominal pain, miscarriage, malpresentation, and difficult delivery being the most frequent complications. The size, location, and number of fibroids and their relation to the placenta are critical factors."[62]

It stands to reason that a 4-cm intracavitary myoma will certainly interfere with the ability to get pregnant or maintain a pregnancy. It is our practice to perform preemptive myomectomies on all intramural myomas 6 cm or greater in diameter in asymptomatic patients desiring pregnancy. If patients are symptomatic from their myomas, then they should be treated for the symptoms that bother them. It is most important that gynecologists employ only the minimally invasive techniques they are skilled in performing and not be afraid to convert to standard laparotomy if they encounter difficulty.

REFERENCES

1. Angler NA. Different battle over a woman's womb. *New York Times.* February 17, 1997.

2. Farquahar CM, Steiner CA. Hysterectomy rates in the United States 1990–1997. *Obstet Gynecol.* 2002;99:229–234.

3. Pokras R. *Hysterectomy: Past, Present and Future. Statistical Bulletin of Metropolitan Life Insurance Company.* New York: Metropolitan Life Insurance Company; 1989.

4. Buttram VC, Reiter RC. Uterine leiomyomata: etiology, symptomatology and management. *Fertil Steril.* 1981;36:433–445.

5. Olive DL, Lindheim SR, Pritts EA. Non-surgical management of leiomyomata: impact on fertility. *Curr Opin Obstet Gynecol.* 2004;16(3):239–243.

6. Berkeley AS, DeCherney AH, Polon ML. Abdominal myomectomy and subsequent infertility. *Surg Gynecol Obstet.* 1983;156:319–322.

7. Candiani GB, Fedele L, Parazzini F, Villa L. Risk of reoccurrence after myomectomy. *Br J Obstet Gynaecol.* 1991;98:385–389.

8. Daniell JF, Gurley LD. Laparoscopic treatment of clinically significant symptomatic uterine fibroids. *J Gynecol Surg.* 1991;7:37.

9. Nezhat C, Nezhat F, Silfen SL, et al. Laparoscopic myomectomy. *Int J Fertil.* 1991;36:275–280.

10. Parker WH, Rodie IA. Patient selection for laparoscopic myomectomy. *J Am Assoc Gynecol Laparosc.* 1994;2:23–26.

11. Sinha R, Hegde A, Warty N, Patil N. Laparoscopic excision of very large myomas. *J Am Assoc Gynecol Laparosc.* 2003;10(4):461–468.

12. Marret H, Chevillot M, Giraudeau B. A retrospective multicentre study comparing myomectomy by laparoscopy and laparotomy in current surgical practice. What are the best patient selection criteria? *Eur J Obstet Gynecol Reprod Biol.* 2004;117:82–86.

13. Fletcher H, Frederick J, Hardie M, et al. A randomized comparison of vasopressin and tourniquet as hemostatic agents during myomectomy. *Obstet Gynecol.* 1996;87:1014–1018.

14. Zullo F, Palomba S, Corea D, et al. Bupivacaine plus epinephrine for laparoscopic myomectomy (a randomized placebo-controlled trial). *Obstet Gynecol.* 2004;104:243–249.

15. Lieng M, Istre O. Uterine rupture after laparoscopic myomectomy. *J Am Assoc Gynecol Laparosc.* 2004;11(1):92–93.

16. Stringer NH, McMillan NA, Jones RI, Nezhat A, Park E. Uterine closure with the endo stitch 10-mm laparoscopic suturing device – a review of 50 laparoscopic myomectomies. *Int J Fertil Womens Med.* 1997;42(5):288–296.

17. Advincula AP, Song A, Burke W. Preliminary experience with robot assisted laparoscopic myomectomy. *J Am Assoc Gynecol Laparosc.* 2004;11(4):511–518.

18. Hutchins FL, Reinoehl EM. Retained myoma after laparoscopic supracervical hysterectomy with morcellation. *J Am Assoc Gynecol Laparosc.* 1998;5:293–295.

19. Ostrzenski A. Uterine leiomyoma particle growing in an abdominal-wall incision after laparoscopic retrieval. *Obstet Gynecol.* 1997;89:853–854.

20. Sinha R, Hegde A, Warty N. Laparoscopic myomectomy: enucleation of the myoma by morcellation while it is still attached to the uterus. *J Minim Invasive Gynecol.* 2005;12(3):284–289.

21. Ou CS, Harper A, Liu YH, et al. Laparoscopic myomectomy technique (use of colpotomy and the harmonic scalpel). *J Reprod Med.* 2002;47:849–853.

22. Pelosi MA 3d, Pelosi MA. Laparoscopic-assisted transvaginal myomectomy. *J Am Assoc Gynecol Laparosc.* 1997;4:241–246.

23. Goldfarb HA, Fanarjian MA. Laparoscopc-assisted transvaginal myomectomy: a case report and literature review. *J Soc Laparosc Surg.* 2001;5:81–85.

24. Birsan A, Deval B, Detchev R. Vaginal and laparoscopic myomectomy for large posterior myomas: results of a pilot study. *Eur J Obstet Gynecol Reprod Biol.* 2003;10(1):89–93.

25. Chin HY, Lee CL, Yen CF, et al. Laparoscopic-assisted vaginal myomectomy through an anterior approach. *J Laparoendosc Adv Surg Tech A.* 2004;14(3):135–138.

26. Nezhat C, Nezhat F, Bess O. Laparoscopically assisted myomectomy: a report of a new technique in 57 cases. *Int J Fertil Menopausal Stud.* 1994;39:39–44.

27. Benedetti-Panici P, Maneschi F, Cutillo G. Surgery by minilaparotomy in benign gynecologic disease. *Obstet Gynecol.* 1996;87:456–459.

28. Benassi L, Marconi L, Benassi G, et al. Minilaparotomy vs laparotomy for uterine myomectomies: a randomized controlled trial. *Minerva Ginecol.* 2005;57(2):159–163.

29. Glasser MH. Minilaparotomy myomectomy: a minimally invasive alternative for the large fibroid uterus. *J Minim Invasive Gynecol.* 2005;12(3):275–283.

30. Tanaguchi F, Harada T, Iwabe T, et al. Use of the LAP DISK (abdominal wall sealing device) in laparoscopically assisted myomectomy. *Fertil Steril.* 2004;81(4):1120–1124.

31. Phillips DR, Nathanson HG, Millim SJ. The effect of dilute vasopressin on blood loss during hysteroscopy: a randomized controlled trial. *Obstet Gynecol.* 1996;88:761–766.

32. Pelosi MA 3d, Pelosi MA. The suprapubic cruciate incision for laparoscopic-assisted microceliotomy. *JSLS.* 1997;1(3):269–272.

33. Pelosi MA 2d, Pelosi MA 3d. Self-retaining abdominal retractor for minilaparotomy. *Obstet Gynecol.* 2000;96:775–778.

34. Lethaby A, Vollenhoven B, Sowter M. Efficacy of pre-operative gonadotrophin releasing hormone analogues for women with uterine fibroids undergoing hysterectomy or myomectomy: a systematic review. *Br J Obstet Gynaecol.* 2002;109(10):1097–1108.

35. Freidman AJ, Rein NS, Harrison-Atlas D, et al. A randomized, placebo-controlled, double blind study evaluating leuprolide acetate depot treatment before myomectomy. *Fertil Steril.* 1989;52:728.

36. Campo S, Garcea N. Laparoscopic myomectomy in premenopausal women with and without preoperative treatment using gonadotrophin-releasing hormone analogues. *Human Reprod.* 1999;14:44–48.

37. Vercellini P, Trespidi L, Zaina B, Vicentini S, Stellato G, Crosignani PG. Gonadotropin-releasing hormone agonist treatment before abdominal myomectomy: a controlled trial. *Fertil Steril.* 2003;79(6):1390–1395.

38. Operative Laparoscopy Study Group. Postoperative adhesion development after operative laparoscopy: evaluation at early second-look procedures. *Fertil Steril.* 1991;55:700.

39. Bayers SP, Jansen D. Gore-Tex surgical membrane. In: DeCherney A, Diamond MP, eds. *Treatment of Post-Surgical Adhesions.* New York: Wiley-Liss; 1990.

40. Diamond MP. Reduction of adhesions after uterine myomectomy by Seprafilm membrane (HAL-F): a blinded, prospective, randomized, multicenter clinical study. Seprafilm Adhesion Study Group. *Fertl Steril.* 1996;66:904.

41. Melis GB, Ajossa S, Piras B, et al. A randomized trial to evaluate the prevention of de novo adhesion formation after laparoscopic myomectomy using oxidized regenerated cellulose (Interceed) barrier. *J Am Assoc Gynecol Laparosc.* 1995;2:S31.

42. Mettler L, Audebert A, Lehmann-Willenbrock E, et al. A randomized, prospective, controlled, multicenter clinical trial of a sprayable, site-specific adhesion barrier system in patients undergoing myomectomy. *Fertil Steril.* 2004;82(2):398–404.

43. Linsky CB, Diamond MP, DiZerega GS. Effect of blood on the efficacy of barrier adhesion reduction in the rabbit uterine horn model. *Infertility.* 1988;11:273.

44. Fedele L, Vercellmi P, Bianchi S, et al. Treatment with GnRH agonists before myomectomy and the risk of short-term myoma recurrence. *Br J Obstet Gynaecol.* 1990;97:393.

45. Hasson HM, Rotman C, Rana N, et al. Laparoscopic myomectomy. *Obstet Gynecol.* 1992;80:884.

46. Dubuisson JB, Lecuru F, Herve F, et al. Myomectomy by laparoscopy. *Fertil Steril.* 1991;56:827.

47. Dubuisson JB, Chavet X, Chapron C, et al. Uterine rupture during pregnancy after laparoscopic myomectomy. *Hum Reprod.* 1995;10(6)1475–1477.

48. Friedman W, Maier RE, Luttkus A, et al. Uterine rupture after laparoscopic myomectomy. *Acta Obstet Gynecol Scand.* 1996; 75(7):683–684.

49. Malberti S, Ferrari L, Milani R. Spontaneous uterine rupture in the third trimester of gestation after laparoscopic myomectomy. A case report. *Minerva Ginecol.* 2004;56(5):479–480.

50. Grande N, Catalano GF, Ferrari S, Marana R. Spontaneous uterine rupture at 27 weeks of pregnancy after laparoscopic myomectomy. *J Minim Invasive Gynecol.* 2005;12(4):301.

51. Cobellis L, Pecori E, Cobellis G, et al. Comparison of intramural myomectomy scar after laparotomy or laparoscopy. *Int J Gynaecol Obstet.* 2004;84:87–88.

52. Hockstein S. Spontaneous uterine rupture in the early third trimester after laparoscopically assisted myomectomy (a case report). *J Reprod Med.* 2000;45:139–141.

53. Campo S, Campo V, Gambadauro P. Reproductive outcome before and after laparoscopic or abdominal myomectomy for subserous or intramural myomas. *Eur J Obstet Gynecol Reprod Biol.* 2003;110(2):215–219.

54. Sudik R, Husch K, Steller J, et al. Fertility and pregnancy outcome after myomectomy in sterility patients. *Eur J Obstet Gynaecol Reprod Biol.* 1996;65:209–214.

55. Dessolle L, Soriano D, Poncelet C, et al. Determinants of pregnancy rate and obstetric outcome after laparoscopic myomectomy for infertility. *Fertil Steril.* 2001;76:370–374.

56. Olufowobi O, Sharif K, Papainnou S, et al. Are the anticipated benefits of myomectomy achieved in women of reproductive age? A 5-year review of the results at a UK tertiary hospital. *J Obstet Gynecol.* 2004;24(4):434–440.

57. Marchionni M, Fambrini M, Zambelli V, et al. Reproductive performance before and after abdominal myomectomy (a retrospective analysis). *Fertil Steril.* 2004;82:154–159.

58. Seracchioli R, Rossi S, Govoni F, et al. Fertility and obstetric outcome after laparoscopic myomectomy of large myomata (a randomized comparison with abdominal myomectomy). *Hum Reprod.* 2000;15:2663–2668.

59. Goldberg J, Pereira L, Berghella V, et al. Pregnancy outcomes after treatment for fibromyomata: uterine artery embolization versus laparoscopic myomectomy. *Am J Obstet Gynecol.* 2004;191(1):18–21.

60. Surrey ES, Minjarez DA, Stevens JM, Schoolcraft WB. Effect of myomectomy on the outcome of assisted reproductive technologies. *Fertil Steril.* 2005;83(5):1473–1479.

61. Oliveira FG, Abdelmassih VG, Diamond MP, et al. Impact of subserosal and intramural uterine fibroids that do not distort the endometrial cavity on the outcome of in vitro fertilization–intracytoplasmic sperm injection. *Fertil Steril.* 2004;81(3):582–587.

62. Cooper NP, Okolo S. Fibroids in pregnancy–common but poorly understood. *Obstet Gynecol Surv* 2005;60(2):132–138.

Section 12.2. Uterine Fibroid Embolization

Mahmood K. Razavi

Uterine leiomyomas are the most common solid tumors in the female reproductive tract, occurring in 20% to 40% of women in the reproductive age. They are highly vascular estrogen-responsive benign tumors and frequently increase in size during pregnancy. Conditions that cause elevated estrogen levels, such as anovulatory states or granulosa–theca cell tumors, increase the incidence and size of fibroids. After menopause, tumor regression occurs, often leading to calcification.

The majority of fibroids are asymptomatic and in the absence of substantial growth, should be treated conservatively. Symptoms may include abnormal uterine bleeding, dysmenorrhea, dyspareunia, abdominal distention, and impaired fertility. In addition, compression of adjacent organs may cause symptoms such as urinary frequency, urgency, constipation, back pain, and radiculopathy. Both patients and physicians frequently overlook the correlation between fibroids and the latter two symptoms.

Current therapies offered to patients with symptomatic fibroids include medical and surgical treatments. Medical management consists of GnRH agonists. This treatment reduces estrogen levels, thereby leading to a reduction in fibroid number and size. However, because of the risk of osteoporosis and development of symptoms of menopause, treatment is recommended only for a short time, and following discontinuation, the symptoms may recur. Surgical therapy has mainly consisted of hysterectomy. Of the more than 600,000 hysterectomies performed in the United States annually, leiomyomas are the most common indication, accounting for approximately one third of the cases. Hysterectomies, however, occur at the expense of fertility and have a long recovery period. Despite the reported low mortality of hysterectomy (0.1%), complications such as hemorrhage, peritonitis, sepsis, pulmonary embolism, and injury to bowel, bladder, ureter, or adjacent vessels may occur. Furthermore, removal of the uterus in itself may be emotionally distressful for the patient.

Less invasive uterine-sparing procedures, such as myomectomy, are hence attractive alternatives, particularly for women of childbearing age who desire future pregnancy. Potential disadvantages of myomectomy include the relatively high risk of recurrence of fibroids and uterine wall weakening, which may interfere with future delivery. In addition, surgical complications such as infection, adhesions, bowel obstruction, infertility, and ectopic pregnancies may result.

Because of the limitations of these surgical approaches, uterine fibroid embolization (UFE) has emerged as an effective, less invasive alternative therapy. The purpose of this section is to provide an overview of UFE, including preprocedural evaluation, technical principles, postprocedural monitoring, and clinical results.

EMBOLIZATION

The procedure of therapeutic embolization is not new. It has been used to treat various conditions, such as traumatic bleeds, gastrointestinal bleeds, tumors, vascular malformations, and aneurysms, for the past three to four decades. More recently, the application of embolization as an adjunct to transvascular targeted drug delivery for treatment of cancer is gaining wide acceptance in the field of oncology.

There are various embolic agents commercially available to achieve the desired clinical effect in the wide variety of pathologies to which embolization is applied. These range from large coils and flow occluders for larger vessels to liquid agents and particles microns in diameter for the treatment of vascular malformations and tumors.

The first reported application of embolization in the obstetric field was in 1979.[1] In this case, embolization was employed to control postpartum hemorrhage in a patient in whom surgical ligation of the internal iliac arteries was unsuccessful. Since then, embolization has been widely used for various conditions, including postpartum, post-cesarean, or postabortion hemorrhage, as well as pre- and postoperative gynecologic hemorrhage.[2]

UTERINE FIBROID EMBOLIZATION

The features of uterine fibroids that make them suitable targets for embolization therapy are their vascularity and hormone responsiveness. The arteries feeding the fibroids are typically larger in diameter, are more numerous, and have a lower resistance as compared with the normal arteries of the muscle of the uterus (spiral arteries). Embolization takes advantage of this pathologic preferential flow to the fibroids. During the procedure, embolic particles of a particular size are selected to preferentially target the tumor vascularity and its blood supply. This has two advantages. First, the resultant ischemia causes coagulative necrosis of the fibroid, leading to a decrease in the size of the tumors. Second, absence of circulation to the fibroids prevents tumor exposure to the systemic hormones and growth stimuli, such as estrogen. Furthermore, lack of flow results in cessation of fibroid-related bleeding.

In 1995, the first report on the results of the clinical application of uterine artery embolization for fibroids was published in the literature.[3] Several other groups reported their results soon after, confirming the technical and clinical merits of this approach.[4–8] Since these original publications, there has been a substantial growth in both the clinical volume and scientific evaluation of UFE worldwide.

PATIENT EVALUATION FOR UFE

As with any other medical procedure, the treating physician must perform a complete history and physical examination. Coexistence of other conditions that may cause patients' symptoms should be investigated. Additionally, comprehensive preprocedural counseling and assessment by the treating physician are essential. Technical details, risks, complications, and postprocedural expectations should be reviewed with patients. Careful assessment of patients' expectations is essential to establish whether UFE is the appropriate next step.

Medical history, physical examination, imaging, and/or laboratory evaluation are directed toward confirming that symptoms are related to fibroids and ensuring that there are no contraindications to UFE. In addition, a focused vascular examination is also performed. Routine pre-angiography laboratory tests, such as serum electrolytes, renal panel, and complete blood count, also are obtained.

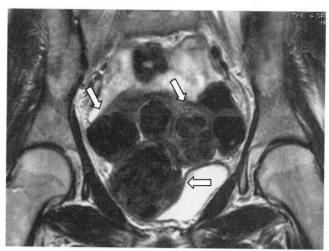

Figure 12.2.1. T2-weighted non-enhanced MRI of the pelvis demonstrating multiple myometrial fibroids (arrows).

Contraindications

Pregnancy is an absolute contraindication to UFE. Embolization for the treatment of fibroids should also be avoided in the setting of known or suspected pelvic malignancy. Although frequently used for palliation, embolization is not a replacement for surgery in such cases. Active infection is also a contraindication to UFE because of the increased risk of abscess formation. With the exception of adenomyosis, UFE may not be of much benefit if the symptoms are the result of etiologies other than fibroids. Patients must also be evaluated for any contraindications to angiography.

Relative contraindications include presence of large submucosal or pedunculated large subserosal fibroids, desire for cosmetic relief, and unrealistic patient expectations.

Imaging

Because of its superior soft tissue resolution, MRI is the imaging modality of choice for women undergoing evaluation for UFE. Office ultrasound is an insufficient imaging tool for this purpose. MRI confirms the presence of fibroids and provides information on other anatomic and physiologic features that are important correlates of UFE outcome, such as the precise location of the fibroids, degree of vascularity and extrauterine blood supply, and presence of spontaneous infarction (Figure 12.2.1). Additionally, other causes of pelvic pain, menorrhagia, uterine/abdominal enlargement, and compression syndrome are excluded. Similarly, uterine volume and other uterine pathologies, such as adenomyosis and malignancy, are better evaluated. Limitations of MRI include increased cost and longer scan duration. Additionally, claustrophobic patients may have difficulty completing the examination.

TECHNIQUE OF UFE

Performing UFE requires complete familiarity with angiographic principles and techniques, vascular anatomy of the pelvis and uterus, and the procedure of embolization. Hence, physicians experienced with UFE obtain the best outcome.

The procedure is most commonly performed by placing a standard 5F introducer sheath in one of the common femoral arteries. A nonselective pelvic arteriogram should first be obtained to evaluate the number and size of the arterial feeders to the uterus and fibroids. This is usually accomplished by placing a pigtail catheter at the level of the renal arteries and performing digital subtraction angiography (Figure 12.2.2). An initial nonselective injection of contrast typically identifies any potential ovarian or other extrauterine blood supply to the fibroids.

Uterine arteries are then selected individually using one of many selective catheters (Figure 12.2.2). In cases of uterine arteries with a small caliber or very tortuous proximal course, microcatheters are used in a coaxial fashion. The catheter tip is usually placed in a position distal to the cervicovaginal branch of the uterine artery, and embolic particles are injected.

The choice of embolic particle size depends on the type of particle chosen. A variety of embolic particles and sizes are available for this purpose. The most common embolic agents used are either polyvinyl alcohol (PVA) or trisacryl gelatin microsphere (Embosphere, BioSphere Medical). These are considered to be permanent embolic particles, which preferentially reside in the microvasculature of the tumor and occlude the flow.

The commonly accepted end point of embolization is stasis of flow in the main uterine arteries (Figure 12.2.2).

Following adequate embolization, the catheter and introducer sheath are removed and hemostasis obtained at the puncture site.

EFFICACY OF UFE

A high technical success rate has been reported for UFE, exceeding 98%. Technical success rate is defined as the ability to catheterize and embolize the fibroid blood supply. Clinical efficacy of UFE in the early studies was reported to be between 80% and 95% and depended on the nature of the symptoms.[4–9] Relief from menorrhagia has the highest consistent success rate of 90% to 95% with UFE and is immediate. This is hardly surprising because fibroids become devoid of vasculature after UFE. Recurrence of pelvic bleeding may be the result of incomplete embolization of

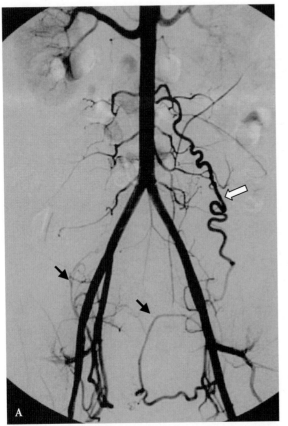

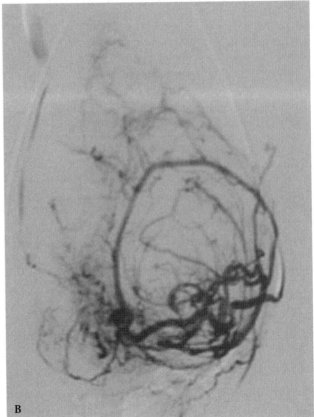

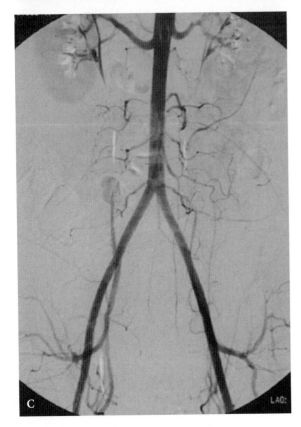

Figure 12.2.2. **A.** Non-selective abdominal and pelvic angiography showing uterine arteries feeding an enlarged uterus (arrows). Note the presence of hypertrophied left ovarian artery that provides extra-uterine supply to the fibroids (open arrows). **B.** Selective left uterine arteriogram showing a hypervascular fibroid. **C.** Post embolization arteriogram showing devascularization of the fibroids.

the existing fibroid, presence of extrauterine blood supply, growth of new fibroids, or etiologies other than myomas.

Resolution of dysmenorrhea and bulk-related symptoms has been reported to be in the 80% to 90% range. The potential reasons for lack of complete response in these patients are discussed below.

In a recent study of 2112 eligible patients, a change in symptom severity and health-related quality of life among patients treated with UFE was reported.[10] At 12 months, symptom improvement was observed in 94.53% of patients, with the mean symptom score improving from 58.61 to 19.23 ($P \leq 0.001$). The mean health-related quality-of-life score improved from 46.95 to 86.68 ($P \leq 0.001$). Hysterectomy was required in only 2.9% of patients in the first 12 months.

Reduction in the volume of the fibroids depends on the tumors' initial size, vascularity, and presence or absence of previous spontaneous infarcts. It averages around 50% to 60% decrease in volume and is continuous over time, with the maximum rate of shrinkage occurring in the first 6 to 12 months post embolization.[8] The degree of reduction in the volume of leiomyomas after UFE is unpredictable and cannot be guaranteed in any one patient. For this reason, we recommend surgery to women who seek cosmetic relief from fibroids. Despite the emphasis of many physicians and patients on the size of fibroids, there appears to be no correlation between reduction in fibroid volume and degree of relief from symptoms after UFE.

Studies addressing the long-term efficacy of UFE have confirmed the durability of this procedure in patients with symptomatic fibroids. Spies et al. [11] followed 200 consecutive patients who had undergone UFE. Of the 182 patients with complete follow-up data, 73% remained symptom-free at 5 years.

Although UFE results in a decrease in fibroid size and stops the pathologic preferential flow away from the muscle of the uterus, its role in the treatment of fibroid-related infertility has not been comprehensively studied to date. For this reason, UFE is not recommended for treatment of infertility until more data become available.

CAUSES OF UFE FAILURE

Clinical failure of UFE occurs in a relatively small number of patients. There are several causes for failure, including coexistence of other pelvic pathologies not responding to UFE, unrealistic patient expectations, and inadequate embolization leading to suboptimal fibroid infarction, which may be the result of extrauterine arterial flow to the fibroids. Ovarian arteries are the most important source of such collateral flow.

The majority of vascular communications between the uterus and ovary are too small to be visualized at angiography and do not affect the outcome of UFE. However, three main types of ovarian-to-uterine artery anastomosis that are of prognostic significance have been described at angiography.[12]

The most common anastomosis is type I, which occurs in approximately 28% of women with symptomatic fibroids. The ovarian artery connects to the intramural uterine artery via the tubal segment, with flows toward the uterus. Type I anastomosis is a substantial source of collateral flow to the uterus and fibroids. In this type, ovarian artery supply is not a likely source of UFE failure because the embolization typically occurs distal to

the point anastomosis. Fibroid devascularization is hence unaffected. Disruption of flow at any point proximal to these anastomoses, which may occur with uterine artery ligation, will not cause fibroid infarction and lasting symptom relief in women with this type of anastomosis.

In type II anastomosis, direct parasitization of the flow from the ovarian arteries to the fibroids occurs. Although connections to the intramural uterine artery may exist, flow to the fibroid is anatomically independent of uterine artery. This occurs in approximately 8% of women and may be an important cause of procedural failure after UFE.[12]

Conversely, in type III anastomosis, the ovarian supply is mainly from the uterine artery through the tubal arteries. Independent ovarian arteries are not seen. At angiography, the observed flow is therefore toward the ovary. This pattern of flow has been observed in approximately 6% of arteries. This pattern of flow will not change the efficacy of fibroid devascularization but may be a cause of ovarian failure.

UFE VERSUS SURGERY

Several studies have compared UFE with surgery, either abdominal myomectomy or hysterectomy. In the first such study, the outcomes of two uterine-sparing procedures (UFE and abdominal myomectomy) were retrospectively compared in 111 patients.[9] Efficacy, complication, and recovery periods were the main study outcome measures of this analysis. Results are summarized in Tables 12.2.1 and 12.2.2.

Statistical analysis of these results revealed that UFE is significantly better than myomectomy in relieving menorrhagia, with both procedures being equally effective in controlling pelvic pain. There was a trend toward better improvement in symptoms of mass effect, such as urinary frequency and constipation, after myomectomy.

Comparison of other outcome measures, such as postprocedural pain, recovery period, and complications, all favored UFE

Table 12.2.1: Percent Response after Abdominal Myomectomy (AM) and UFE

Response Category	Menorrhagia, %		Pain Number,%		Mass Effect Number,%	
	AM	UFE	AM	UFE	AM	UFE
6 (resolved)	27	60	38.5	29.5	65	19
5 (significantly improved)	36	32	15.5	44	26	57
4 (moderately improved)	23	6	38	23.5	9	19
3 (no change)	9	2	4	3	0	5
2 (moderately worse)	4.5	0	4	0	0	0
1 (significantly worse)	0	0	0	0	0	0
% Improvement	**86.5**	**98**	**92**	**97**	**100**	**95**

Adapted from Razavi MK, et al. [9].

Table 12.2.2: Comparison of Other Outcome Measures

	AM, mean (range)	UFE, mean (range)	P value
Inpatient hospital days	2.9 (2–7)	0	≤ 0.05
Days on pain medications	8.7 (2–47)	5.1 (1–21)	≤ 0.05
Days to normal activity	36 (7–120)	8 (1–49)	≤ 0.05
Secondary interventions,%	10	8	NS
Estimated blood loss, mL	376 (50–2000)	Minimal	
Complications,%	25	10	≤ 0.5

NS, not significant.
Adapted from Razavi MK, et al. [9]

(Table 12.2.2). The need for secondary interventions during the study period was similar in both groups.

The complications included nonautologous blood transfusion (n = 3), wound infection (n = 2), adhesion (n = 2), readmission for ileus (n = 1), and chronic pelvic pain (n = 2) among the myomectomy patients. Complications in the fibroid embolization group included endometritis requiring readmission for intravenous antibiotics (n = 1), readmission for pelvic pain (n = 1), and menopause (n = 4). All those who experienced menopause after fibroid embolization were older than 46 years.

In a prospective randomized study of 63 women with intramural fibroids larger than 4 cm who desired future fertility, Mara et al. [13] compared UFE to myomectomy. Similar to the study by Razavi et al. [9], UFE was associated with fewer hospital days, procedure time, blood loss, and disability period. Complication rate and follicle-stimulating hormone (FSH) levels were similar at 6 months, although the UFE group reported a lower rate of symptom relief.

UFE has also been compared with hysterectomy. Pinto et al. [14] conducted a prospective analysis of hysterectomy versus UFE in 60 patients. UFE was associated with fewer complications and a shorter hospital stay. Spies et al. [15], in a prospective multicenter trial of UFE versus hysterectomy, reported similar results. In this study, pain relief was more common among those with hysterectomy, with both groups experiencing marked improvement in other symptoms and quality-of life-scores, with no difference between them. Complications were more frequent in the hysterectomy group (50% vs. 27.5%).

In a cost-effectiveness analysis, Beinfeld et al. [16] developed a decision model to compare the costs and effectiveness of UFE and hysterectomy. They concluded that UFE is less expensive and more effective than hysterectomy. In their model, however, when the quality-of-life adjustment was eliminated, the two procedures were equally effective.

UFE AND PREGNANCY

The issue of pregnancy after UFE has been addressed in only a small number of studies. Kim et al. [17] reviewed their experience in 94 patients and concluded that UFE with PVA particles does not seem to affect fertility among women who do not use contraception.

Based on their study of 671 women who underwent UFE, Carpenter et al. [18] observed no increased obstetric-associated risk, with the exception of the number of patients who underwent cesarean section. In a similar large multicenter clinical registry of 555 patients with a mean age of 43 years, the enrolled women were followed prospectively.[19] Thirty-one percent of the patients were younger than 40 years. Although it is unclear as to what fraction of women who were trying to get pregnant actually did, 24 pregnancies were reported in women who were an average age of 34 years. There were four spontaneous abortions and four preterm deliveries. Abnormal placentation was seen in three women. The authors concluded "women are able to achieve pregnancies after uterine artery embolization, and most resulted in term deliveries and appropriately grown newborns." Close monitoring of placental status, however, was recommended in this study.

In comparison with myomectomy, McLucas et al. [20] and Goldberg et al. [21] reached opposite conclusions. The McLucas group observed no difference in pregnancy outcome between those who underwent UFE versus those who had myomectomy, whereas the Goldberg group reported a higher incidence of complications in UFE patients. It should be noted that both these studies suffer from major methodologic flaws, and their results should be interpreted with caution.

COMPLICATIONS OF UFE

Serious complications after UFE are rare. In a large prospective multicenter study of 3160 patients enrolled in 72 sites, major in-hospital complications occurred in 0.66% of patients.[22] The 30-day complication rate was 4.8%, with no reported deaths. The most common complication was inadequate pain control requiring a hospital visit by 2.4% of patients. One percent required additional surgical procedures within the first 30 days, with 0.1% undergoing hysterectomy. Multivariate analysis showed modest increased odds for an adverse event for African Americans, smokers, and those with prior leiomyoma procedures.[22]

Endometritis has been reported to occur in 1% to 4% of patients after UFE. The most common risk factors for infection are the presence of large submucosal fibroids or preexistence of an undetected or incompletely treated pelvis infection. In these patients, aggressive therapy with antibiotics is warranted to prevent further progression, which may lead to sepsis and/or hysterectomy.

A long-term complication of UFE is ovarian failure and early menopause. The risk of ovarian failure is age dependent and highest in women over the age of 45. Review of the literature reveals that less than 1% of women under the age of 40 develop menopause after UFE. This risk increases to 15% for those older than 45 years.[12,23]

Other, less common complications occurring in less than 1% of patients include vessel injury, deep vein thrombosis, and pulmonary embolism.

POSTPROCEDURAL CARE AND FOLLOW-UP

As mentioned above, the most common reason for postprocedural physician visits after UFE is inadequate pain control. Because of the less invasive nature of UFE, occasionally the treating physicians have a tendency to underprescribe pain medications. According to the published studies, women will experience pelvic discomfort for an average of 3 to 4 days after the procedure and may require oral analgesics. The degree of pain is highly variable, with no reliable preprocedural indicator. Rarely, pain may last longer, but persistent pelvic discomfort for a period longer than 3 weeks or recurrence of pain after an initial abatement requires evaluation.

Postembolization syndrome is a constellation of symptoms including nausea, low-grade fever, and malaise and is common after UFE. This syndrome may last for 4 to 7 days post procedure, and the treatment is supportive, including the use of antiemetic and anti-inflammatory medications.

A self-limiting vaginal spotting with a brownish discharge is also a common finding and may occur for several weeks after embolization. In fewer than 10% of women, the discharge may be associated with passing of tissue and clot, which have been shown histologically to be fibroid fragments. Transcervical expulsion of leiomyomas may occur in 1% to 2% of patients and is associated with pain and bleeding. These are typically submucosal fibroids, which detach into the uterine cavity about 4 to 12 weeks after embolization. Incomplete passage is associated with a high risk of infection and may require hospitalization and intravenous antibiotics. Delayed passage of leiomyomas for up to a year after UFE has also been reported.[24]

After the initial postprocedural follow-up, patients are seen in follow-up approximately 3 months later. Follow-up MRI is obtained 6 to 12 months later.

Temporary amenorrhea occurs in approximately 5% to 8% of women during the first 3 months following the procedure. Menses resumes in the majority of these women, with no permanent sequela. No specific therapy is prescribed in these patients. If amenorrhea persists, a serum FSH may be obtained to evaluate for menopause.

SUMMARY

UFE is a uterine-sparing alternative to hysterectomy that has been shown to be an effective therapy for women with fibroids. By permanently eliminating the blood flow to the fibroids, UFE alleviates symptoms and reduces fibroid volume and uterine size. Advantages include the elimination of surgical risks, treatment of the entire fibroid burden with one therapy, preservation of fertility, and reduction of hospitalization and recovery times. Although the role of UFE in the treatment algorithm for leiomyomas remains controversial, it should be offered to women who do not desire surgery or those who have failed medical or less invasive surgical therapies before hysterectomy is advised.

REFERENCES

1. Brown BJ, Heaston DK, Poulson AM, Gabert HA, Mineau DE, Miller FJ Jr. Uncontrollable postpartum bleeding: a new approach to hemostasis through angiographic arterial embolization. *Obstet Gynecol*. 1979;54(3):361–365.
2. Vedantham S, Goodwin SC, McLucas B, Mohr G. Uterine artery embolization: an underused method of controlling pelvic hemorrhage. *Am J Obstet Gynecol*. 1997;176(4):938–948.
3. Ravina JH, Herbreteau D, Ciraru-Vigneron N, et al. Arterial embolisation to treat myomata. *Lancet*. 1995;346:671–672.
4. Spies JB, Ascher SA, Roth AR, Kim J, Levy EB, Gomez-Jorge J. Uterine artery embolization for uterine leiomyomata. *Obstet Gynecol*. 2001;98:29–34.
5. Goodwin SC, McLucas B, Lee M, et al. Uterine artery embolization for the treatment of uterine leiomyomata: midterm results. *J Vasc Interv Radiol*. 1999;10:1159–1165.
6. Worthington-Kirsch RL, Popky GL, Hutchins FL Jr. Uterine arterial embolization for the management of leiomyomas: quality-of-life assessment and clinical response. *Radiology*. 1998;208:625–629.
7. Hutchins FL Jr, Worthington-Kirsch R. Embolotherapy for myoma-induced menorrhagia. *Obstet Gynecol Clin North Am*. 2000;27:397–405.
8. Spies JB, Roth AR, Jha RC, et al. Leiomyomata treated with uterine artery embolization: factors associated with successful symptom and imaging outcome. *Radiology*. 2002;222:45–52.
9. Razavi MK, Hwang G, Jahed A, Modanloo S, Chen B. Abdominal myomectomy versus uterine fibroid embolization in the treatment of symptomatic uterine leiomyomas. *AJR Am J Roentgenol*. 2003;180(6):1571–1575.
10. Spies JB, Myers ER, Worthington-Kirsch R, Mulgund J, Goodwin S, Mauro M; the FIBROID Registry Investigators. The FIBROID Registry: symptom and quality-of-life status 1 year after therapy. *Obstet Gynecol*. 2005;106(6):1309–1318.
11. Spies JB, Bruno J, Czeyda-Pommersheim F, Magee ST, Ascher SA, Jha RC. Long-term outcome of uterine artery embolization of leiomyomata. *Obstet Gynecol*. 2005;106(5):933–939.
12. Razavi MK, Wolanske K, Hwang G, Sze D, Kee S, Dake M. Angiographic classification of ovarian to uterine artery anastomoses: incidence and significance in UFE. *Radiology*. 2002;294:707–712.
13. Mara M, Fucikova Z, Maskova J, Kuzel D, Haakova L. Uterine fibroid embolization versus myomectomy in women wishing to preserve fertility: preliminary results of a randomized controlled trial. *Eur J Obstet Gynecol Reprod Biol*. 2006;126(2):226–233.
14. Pinto I, Chimeno P, Romo A, et al. Uterine fibroids: uterine artery embolization versus abdominal hysterectomy for treatment – a prospective, randomized, and controlled clinical trial. *Radiology*. 2003;226(2):425–431.
15. Spies JB, Cooper JM, Worthington-Kirsch R, Lipman JC, Mills BB, Benenati JF. Outcome of uterine embolization and hysterectomy for leiomyomas: results of a multicenter study. *Am J Obstet Gynecol*. 2004;191(1):22–31.
16. Beinfeld MT, Bosch JL, Isaacson KB, Gazelle GS. Cost-effectiveness of uterine artery embolization and hysterectomy for uterine fibroids. *Radiology*. 2004;230(1):207–213.
17. Kim MD, Kim NK, Kim HJ, Lee MH. Pregnancy following uterine artery embolization with polyvinyl alcohol particles for patients with uterine fibroid or adenomyosis. *Cardiovasc Intervent Radiol*. 2005;28(5):611–615.
18. Carpenter TT, Walker WJ. Pregnancy following uterine artery embolisation for symptomatic fibroids: a series of 26 completed pregnancies. *Br J Obstet Gynaecol*. 2005;112(3):321–325.
19. Pron G, Mocarski E, Bennett J, Vilos G, Common A, Vanderburgh L; Ontario UFE Collaborative Group. Pregnancy after uterine artery embolization for leiomyomata: the Ontario multicenter trial. *Obstet Gynecol*. 2005;105(1):67–76.
20. McLucas B, Goodwin S, Adler L, Rappaport A, Reed R, Perrella R. Pregnancy following uterine fibroid embolization. *Int J Gynaecol Obstet*. 2001;74(1):1–7.

21. Goldberg J, Pereira L, Berghella V, et al. Pregnancy outcomes after treatment for fibromyomata: uterine artery embolization versus laparoscopic myomectomy. *Am J Obstet Gynecol.* 2004;191(1): 18–21.

22. Worthington-Kirsch R, Spies JB, Myers ER, et al.; FIBROID Investigators. The Fibroid Registry for outcomes data (FIBROID) for uterine embolization: short-term outcomes. *Obstet Gynecol.* 2005;106(1):52–59.

23. Chrisman HB, Sakter MB, Ryu RK, et al. The impact of uterine fibroid embolization on resumption of menses and ovarian function. *J Vasc Interv Radiol.* 2000;11:699–703.

24. Spies JB, Spector A, Roth AR, Baker CM, Mauro L, Murphy-Skrynarz K. Complications after uterine artery embolization for leiomyomas. *Obstet Gynecol.* 2002;100(5 pt 1):873–880.

13 | HYSTERECTOMY
Section 13.1. Laparoscopy and Hysterectomy

Farr Nezhat and Jyoti Yadav

The number of hysterectomies, a frequently practiced major surgical procedure, varies between different regions and cultures of the world. It reflects differences in health care systems, education, and psychosocial attitudes. The highest rates of hysterectomy are found in the United States and Australia (36% and 40%, respectively) and the lowest in Italy (15.5%) and France (8.5%).[1–3]

INDICATIONS

Most hysterectomies are performed for leiomyomas, uterine prolapse, endometriosis, and gynecologic cancer.[4] The number of hysterectomies for endometriosis doubled between 1965 and 1984, exceeding the increase observed for any other indication and probably reflecting an increased recognition of endometriosis. Other indications are abnormal uterine bleeding, pelvic infection and its sequelae, ovarian tumors, and complications of pregnancy. These indications account for 15% to 21% of all hysterectomies.

About 75% of all hysterectomies are done abdominally and 25% vaginally.[4,5] The vaginal approach is primarily used for uterine prolapse. Abdominal hysterectomy is usually done for women with significant pelvic disease, such as endometriosis or pelvic adhesions, which can make a vaginal removal more difficult (Table 13.1.1).[6] Compared to those having a vaginal hysterectomy, women having an abdominal operation have more febrile morbidity, receive more blood transfusions [5,7], and have a longer postoperative hospitalization and convalescence. If more women had a vaginal rather than an abdominal approach for their hysterectomy, therapeutic, economic, and social benefits would result.[8]

The route selected depends on the clinical assessment of the pelvic disorder, which is based on the medical history, pelvic examination, ultrasound studies, review of prior operative notes, and the surgeon's experience in vaginal surgery.[8]

The role of the laparoscope in assisting vaginal hysterectomy has been described by Semm since 1984.[9,10] Laparoscopic hysterectomy using bipolar electrocautery and the endoscopic stapler was first described in 1989 [11] and 1990 [12], respectively. Kovac and coworkers [13] performed diagnostic laparoscopy in 46 patients scheduled for abdominal hysterectomy who, on the basis of clinical indicators, were thought to have a serious pelvic abnormality that contraindicated vaginal hysterectomy. Based on the laparoscopic findings, 42 of the 46 women (91%) were candidates for vaginal hysterectomy, which was done under the same anesthesia. Because clinical assessment of pelvic disease may not be accurate, laparoscopy can reveal whether a vaginal approach is appropriate. For these women,

diagnostic or operative laparoscopy provided the benefits of both vaginal and abdominal approaches without their disadvantages (Table 13.1.2). A comparison of the results of abdominal hysterectomy versus laparoscopic hysterectomy in 20 cases was reported by Nezhat et al. in 1992.[14] That report established the validity of laparoscopically assisted vaginal hysterectomy (LAVH) and suggested that it could replace most abdominal hysterectomies for benign lesions. The indications for laparoscopically assisted hysterectomy in this series were similar to those listed for abdominal rather than vaginal hysterectomy. All hysterectomies were completed successfully endoscopically without significant complications. Patients had reduced morbidity, blood loss, postoperative discomfort, hospitalization, and recovery time.

A review of the literature reveals many definitions of a laparoscopically assisted hysterectomy. A suggested classification follows:

1. *Total laparoscopic hysterectomy (TLH)*. The hysterectomy is done laparoscopically; the vaginal cuff may be closed laparoscopically or vaginally.
2. *Subtotal laparoscopic hysterectomy (SLH)*. A supracervical hysterectomy is done laparoscopically.
3. *LAVH*. The hysterectomy starts laparoscopically, but most steps, especially the uterosacral and cardinal ligaments, are done vaginally.

A laparoscopic approach allows the treatment of intra-abdominal and pelvic disease and the dissection or removal of adnexa. Patients who have suspected pelvic endometriosis undergo a diagnostic laparoscopy to inspect the pelvis. Significant pelvic disease is treated endoscopically, and if necessary, adnexectomy is performed. The hysterectomy is completed vaginally.[13] Usually, a combined laparoscopic and vaginal approach is used to dissect and remove uterine attachments.[15–19] The extent of laparoscopic and vaginal dissection depends on the gynecologist's preference and experience with laparoscopic and vaginal operations. A more experienced endoscopist can do the entire hysterectomy laparoscopically.[20] However, TLH may be time consuming, especially if the uterus is more than 16 to 18 weeks' gestational size. Laparoscopic hysterectomy is useful if the vagina is small and narrow and significant infiltrative pelvic endometriosis is present, which would make a vaginal operation difficult. Almost all abdominal hysterectomies for endometriosis can be converted to LAVH.[21] Patients who have the indications for traditional vaginal hysterectomy should not undergo LAVH, vaginally assisted laparoscopic hysterectomy, or laparoscopic hysterectomy.[22]

Table 13.1.1: Indications for Hysterectomy

	Abdominal Hysterectomy, %	Vaginal Hysterectomy, %
Leiomyomas	38	1
Uterine prolapse	1	76
Endometriosis	3	0
Abnormal bleeding	13	9
Adenomyosis	9	8
Pelvic pain/adhesions	5	0
Ovarian tumors	10	0
Uterine neoplasia	15	3

Source: Dicker et al.[5]

Table 13.1.2: Advantages and Disadvantages of Abdominal, Vaginal, and Laparoscopically Assisted Vaginal Hysterectomy (LAVH)

	Abdominal	Vaginal	LAVH
Exposure	Excellent	Limited	Excellent
Associated pelvic disease	Easily treated	Reduced access	Easily treated
Incision	Abdominal	Vaginal	Abdominal/vaginal
Hospitalization, days	3	2–3	1–2
Cost	Average	Average	More expensive
Morbidity, %	30	10	10
Surgical expertise	Average gynecologist	Average gynecologist	Experienced endoscopist
Oophorectomy	Easy	≤25%	Easy

PREOPERATIVE EVALUATION

Routine preoperative tests include a complete blood count with differential, serum electrolytes, bleeding time, and urinalysis. More comprehensive blood studies, thrombin time, partial thrombin time, electrocardiography (ECG), chest radiography, and endometrial biopsy are done as indicated. A mechanical and, at times, an antibiotic bowel preparation is advised. Consultations with a urologist, colorectal surgeon, and oncologist are sought as necessary. Appropriate informed consent is obtained from the patient after a thorough explanation of the planned operation, its potential risks and benefits, the possibility of laparotomy, and therapeutic alternatives. After an overnight fast, the patient is admitted to the ambulatory surgical unit the morning of her operation.

TECHNIQUE

Laparoscopically Assisted Vaginal Hysterectomy

The patient's initial position is the same as that for standard laparoscopy. The 10-mm trocar is inserted transumbilically for placement of the operative laparoscope, and two to four accessory trocars are positioned suprapubically. For the vaginal portion, the patient's legs are readjusted to allow vaginal access (Allen Universal stirrups, Allen Medical Systems). With an adjustment under the drapes, the legs are flexed and abducted without redraping. Some gynecologists prefer to place the patient's legs in candy-cane stirrups for the vaginal portion. Various types of uterine manipulators can be placed inside the uterus of facilitate manipulation intraoperatively.

Every operative laparoscopy begins with exploration of the abdominal and pelvic cavity to assess the extent of disease. Anatomic landmarks, anomalies, distortions, and alterations are identified. The locations of the bladder, ureters, colon, rectum, and major blood vessels are noted. The omentum and small bowel are evaluated for disease and checked for Veress needle or trocar injury.

After the diagnostic portion, the operator uses the CO_2 laser or other cutting instrument and hydrodissection to resect, ablate, or coagulate implants of endometriosis. An electrocoagulator,

clips, staplers, or Endoloops (Ethicon) are used to coagulate or ligate large vessels. Monopolar electrodes, fiber lasers, or the harmonic scalpel may be used for smaller bleeders.[23] Other instruments include bipolar forceps (middle port), suction–irrigator probe (left), and grasping forceps (right).

The bowel is freed from the pelvic organs to expose the pelvis. Ovaries and tubes are dissected from the cul-de-sac or pelvic side wall, and endometriosis or other abnormalities are treated.

Ureteral Evaluation and Dissection

The direction and location of both ureters are identified from the pelvic brim to the cardinal ligaments, where they are no longer visible. This is undertaken early in the operation, before pelvic side wall peritoneum becomes edematous or opaque and ureteral peristalsis is inhibited due to irritation by the CO_2 pneumoperitoneum or hydrodissection. The course of the ureters is marked superiorly with the laser or electrocoagulation so that they can be identified while the broad ligament and adnexa are dissected (Figure 13.1.1). For extensive endometriosis, very wide dissection, as is done during radical hysterectomy, is sometimes necessary.[16,17] To identify the ureters at the level of the cardinal ligaments, the peritoneum is opened above or below the ureter and hydrodissection is carried out. A peritoneal incision is made, and the ureter is identified toward its course to the bladder. Small bleeding vessels are coagulated by laser or electrosurgery. If the uterosacral ligaments are dissected, the ureter is retracted laterally and the uterosacral ligaments are dissected at their origin from the cervix. The uterine vessels run superiorly. They are isolated and safely coagulated. When the pelvic anatomy is distorted, it may be safer to do a cystoscopy and place catheters in both ureters for better identification.

Upper Broad Ligament and Adnexa

If adnexectomy is indicated, after electrocoagulation and transection of the round ligaments 2 to 3 cm from the uterus, the infundibulopelvic ligament is coagulated and cut. If the endoscopic linear stapler is used, the appendage is grasped with

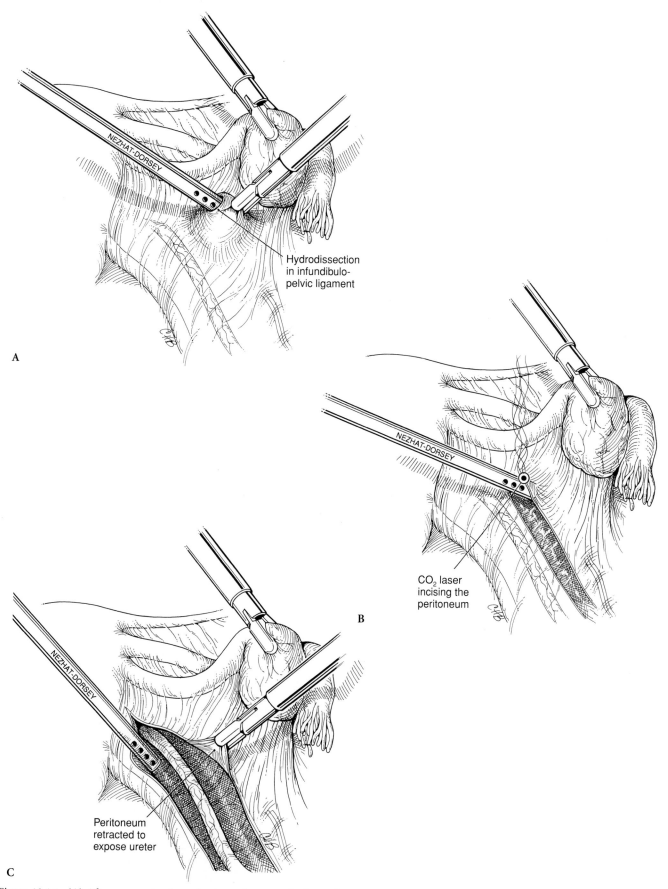

Figure 13.1.1. (**A**) After an opening is made above the ureter in the peritoneum, retroperitoneal hydrodissection is carried out. (**B**) Using the suction–irrigator probe as a backstop, an opening is made above the ureter with the CO_2 laser. (**C**) The ureter is dissected from the pelvic brim to the back of the bladder by using blunt hydrodissection.

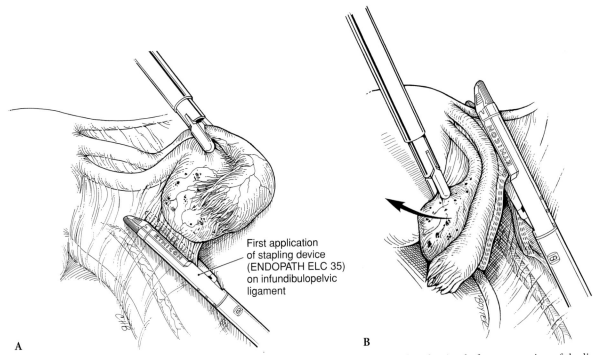

A   **B**

Figure 13.1.2. (**A**) The linear stapler is applied across the infundibulopelvic ligament. Ureteral evaluation before transection of the ligament is very important. (**B**) Second application of the stapler across the infundibulopelvic ligament. The round ligament may be included.

forceps. It is retracted medially and caudally to stretch and outline the infundibulopelvic ligament, which is grasped and secured with the stapler. A uterine manipulator (HUMI [Cooper Surgical] or other uterine manipulator) placed inside the uterus vaginally is helpful in retracting the uterus in the opposite direction, facilitating the stretch on the infundibulopelvic ligament. The stapler is not fired until the contained tissue is identified and the ureteral position is confirmed. Once it is transected, the staple line is examined for placement and hemostasis. After infundibulopelvic ligament transection, the adnexa and uterine fundus are retracted in the opposite direction. Tissue of the upper broad ligament, including the round ligament, is grasped, secured, and cut after safe margins have been established (Figure 13.1.2A). The infundibulopelvic ligament and the round ligament occasionally are cut with a single staple application (Figure 13.1.2B). Any other hemostatic cutting device (LigaSure, Valleylab; Harmonic ACE, Ethicon Endo-Surgery) may be used in a similar fashion on all vascular pedicles.

Development of the Bladder Flap

If the adnexa are preserved, the round ligament is coagulated and cut approximately 3 cm from the uterus (Figure 13.1.3). Using hydrodissection, the anterior leaf of the broad ligament is opened toward the vesicouterine fold and the bladder flap is developed (Figure 13.1.4). The anterior leaf of the broad ligament is grasped with forceps, elevated, and dissected from the anterior lower uterine segment with hydrodissection and the CO_2 laser, monopolar scissors, or any harmonic device (Figure 13.1.5). The utero-ovarian ligament, proximal tube, and mesosalpinx are electrodesiccated and cut, and the posterior leaf of the broad ligament is opened (Figure 13.1.6). Similarly, the round ligament, fallop-

ian tube, and utero-ovarian ligament can be grasped close to their insertion into the uterus with the endoscopic linear stapler and then secured, stapled, and severed (Figure 13.1.7). The distal end of the stapler or bipolar forceps must be kept free of the bladder and ureter.

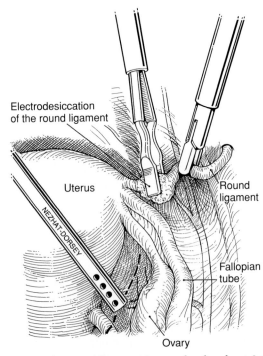

Figure 13.1.3. The round ligament is coagulated and cut 2 to 3 cm lateral to the uterus.

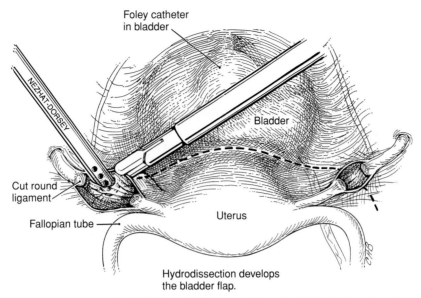

Figure 13.1.4. While the anterior leaf of the broad ligament is elevated with hydrodissection, the anterior leaf of the broad ligament is opened toward the vesicouterine fold.

The uterovesical peritoneum is identified, grasped, and elevated with forceps while scissors, laser, or a harmonic device is used to dissect the bladder off the cervix. The bladder pillars are identified, coagulated, and cut. The bladder is dissected from the uterus by pushing downward with the tip of a blunt probe along the vesicocervical plane until the anterior cul-de-sac is exposed completely (Figure 13.1.8).

In patients who have severe anterior cul-de-sac endometriosis or adhesions or a history of previous cesarean deliveries, sharp dissection of the vesicouterine fold often is necessary. Injecting 5 to 10 mL of indigo carmine in the patient's intravenous line and looking for its presence in the peritoneal cavity is one way to detect bladder trauma. However, the best method to identify bladder injury is either by cystoscopy or by distending the bladder with 300 to 400 mL of sterile milk and performing a careful laparoscopic inspection for any leaks.

Uterine Vessels

After the bladder is dissected from the anterior cervix, the uterine vessels are identified, desiccated, and cut to free the lateral borders of the uterus (Figure 13.1.9). If single clips or linear staplers are used, the vessels are skeletonized to prevent slippage of the clips. As the uterine vessels are grasped and cut, the safety and position of the ureters should be checked. This can be done more easily if they are marked, exposed, or catheterized at the beginning of the procedure. The hysterectomy is completed vaginally or continued laparoscopically.

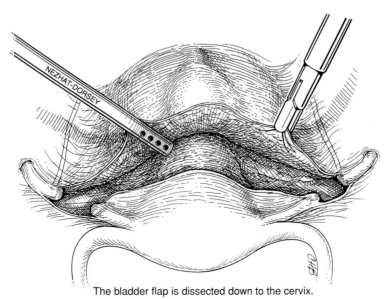

The bladder flap is dissected down to the cervix.

Figure 13.1.5. The bladder is elevated and further separated from the cervix. It is pushed downward using sharp and blunt dissection and hydrodissection.

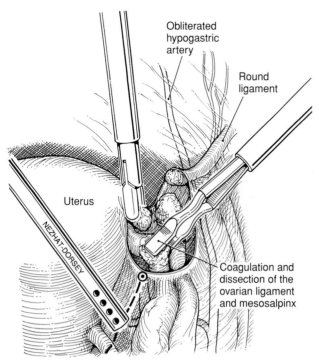

Figure 13.1.6. The proximal tube, mesosalpinx, and utero-ovarian ligament are coagulated and cut.

Cardinal Ligament

At the level of the cardinal ligaments, the ureter and the descending branches of the uterine artery are close to one another and the cervix. Therefore, cardinal ligament dissection must be precise to prevent bleeding and ureteral injury. The linear stapler is used only if the parametrium is dissected with ample margins

as the width of the linear stapler is 12 mm. Because of the short distance between the cervix and the ureter, the risk of ureteral injury by the stapler increases. Using contralateral retraction of the uterus, the cardinal ligament is dissected to identify tissue planes, vessels, and the ureter. Once the ureter is displaced laterally, the cardinal ligament tissue closest to the cervix is coagulated and transected (Figure 13.1.10). Alternatively, the linear stapler is applied on both the uterine vessels and the cardinal ligament (Figure 13.1.11). The harmonic scalpel or LigaSure may be used as an alternative.

Anterior and Posterior Culdotomy

A folded wet gauze in a sponge forceps or on the tip of a right-angle Heaney retractor marks the anterior or posterior vaginal fornix. The vaginal wall is tented and transected horizontally (Figures 13.1.12, 13.1.13). Newer uterine manipulators on the market are fitted with cups of varying sizes (KOH Colpotomizer, Cooper Surgical) that fit onto the cervix and delineate the vaginal fornices, enabling easy transaction of the vaginal cuff. Additionally, they are fitted with a balloon that maintains the pneumoperitoneum once the vagina is opened.

Vaginal Portion of Hysterectomy

The laparoscopic portion temporarily ends before or after the anterior or posterior culdotomy. Dissecting and resecting the uterus are done vaginally using standard techniques. Once the uterus is removed, the vaginal cuff is closed. To ensure support of the vaginal vault, the vaginal angles are attached to the uterosacral and cardinal ligaments with absorbable sutures. The vaginal cuff is closed transversely or vertically, and any coexisting cystocele or rectocele is repaired. Once the vaginal part is completed and the cuff is closed, the laparoscopic procedure resumes.

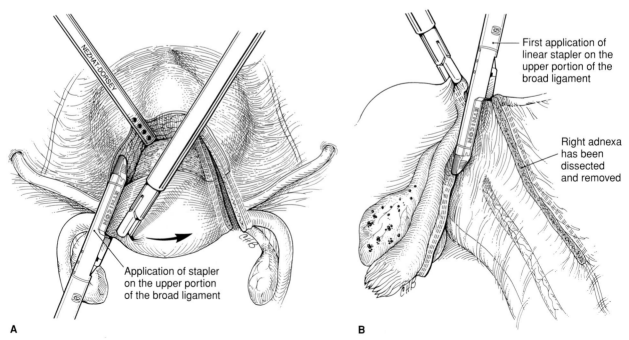

A **B**

Figure 13.1.7. (**A**) The linear stapler is applied on the upper portion of the broad ligament while preserving the adnexa. (**B**) The linear stapler is applied on the upper broad ligament while removing the adnexa.

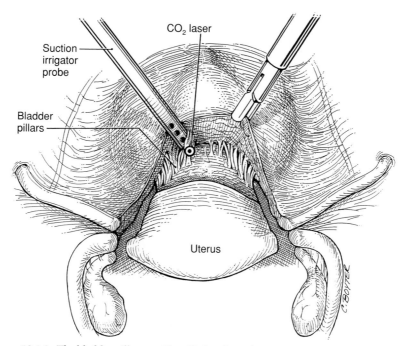

Figure 13.1.8. The bladder pillars are identified and cut close to the cervix with the CO_2 laser.

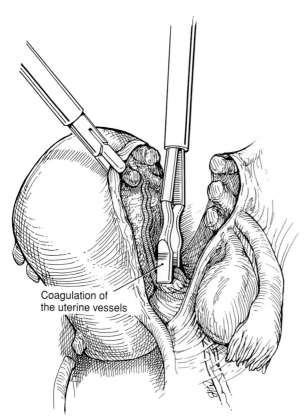

Figure 13.1.9. While the ureter is observed, the uterine vessels are skeletonized, coagulated, and cut.

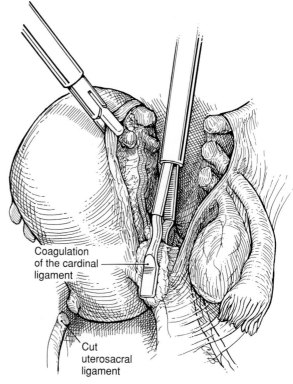

Figure 13.1.10. The uterus is pulled to the opposite side with a grasping forceps. The ureter must be observed to ensure that it is not damaged by the bipolar forceps during coagulation and cutting of the cardinal ligament.

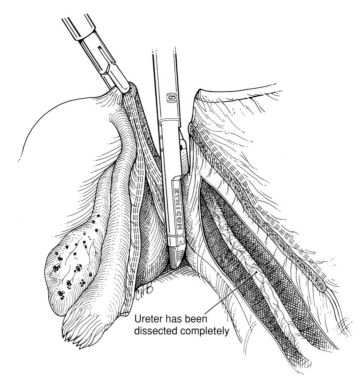

Figure 13.1.11. The linear stapler is applied across the uterine vessels and cardinal ligament. The ureter is dissected and held away from the stapler jaws.

Prevention of Enterocoele (Moschcowitz Procedure)

By obliterating the posterior cul-de-sac, this procedure helps prevent enterocele and should be considered, especially in patients with a deep pelvis. A continuous nonabsorbable or delayed absorbable suture is placed through the various structures of the posterior cul-de-sac, preventing herniation into the rectovaginal space. The suture is started laterally over the periureteral area after the ureter is located. It is passed through the serosa of the

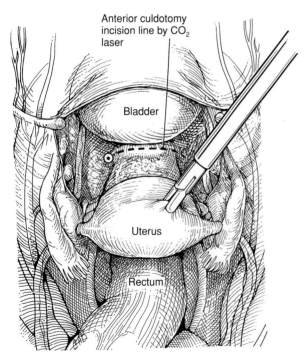

Figure 13.1.12. The uterus is elevated, and as the assistant identifies the posterior fornix, a laparoscopic posterior culdotomy is done. The gynecologist must select the correct location so that the rectum is not involved.

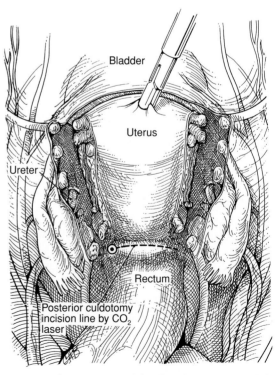

Figure 13.1.13. The uterus is mobilized, and as it is pushed down, a laparoscopic anterior culdotomy is created by using the CO_2 laser.

rectosigmoid colon posteriorly, the contralateral side to include the opposite periureteral area, and the anterior vaginal wall. When it is tied, the posterior cul-de-sac is obliterated. Injury to the ureter, rectum, and bladder is avoided by meticulous suturing. Several variations to the Moschcowitz procedure (e.g., Halban's technique) that may be used alternatively have been described in the literature.

Final Laparoscopic Evaluation

The pelvic and abdominal cavities are evaluated laparoscopically, irrigated, and cleared of blood clots and debris. The pelvis is filled with 300 to 500 mL of lactated Ringer's solution, and the pedicles and vaginal cuff are inspected for any bleeding with the patient in reverse Trendelenburg position.[18] Intra-abdominal pressure is reduced and the pedicles are reinspected to confirm hemostasis. The vaginal cuff is examined to ensure that no small bowel or omental tissue is included in its closure. At this point, the fluid in the pelvis should be clear and a look at the ureters should confirm normal peristalsis and anatomic integrity. To avoid incisional omental or bowel strangulation after the removal of any trocars more than 5 mm in size, the fascia is repaired with delayed absorbable sutures.[24]

HYSTERECTOMY FOR EXTENSIVE PELVIC ENDOMETRIOSIS AND ADHESIONS

In women who have extensive endometriosis, the rectosigmoid colon often is densely adherent to the posterior aspect of the uterus (Figure 13.1.14). Similarly, if the ovaries are affected by endometriosis and endometriomas, they may become attached to the pelvic side wall. To coagulate the uterine artery, it may be necessary to dissect the pelvic side wall and identify the uterine vessel at its origin from the hypogastric artery. Bipolar forceps, harmonic scalpel, clips, or sutures are used. The rectosigmoid colon is separated from the posterior uterus incrementally, and the bowel endometriosis is resected or vaporized (Figures

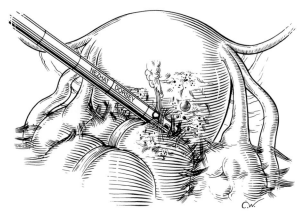

Figure 13.1.15. The dissection of the rectosigmoid colon is continued.

13.1.15, 13.1.16). The high-power ultrapulse CO_2 laser is very precise, and with a penetration of only 100 μm, the possibility of delayed bowel necrosis is very low. The CO_2 laser is an excellent instrument for the treatment of endometriosis. Hemostasis not obtained with the CO_2 laser is controlled with cautious application of the bipolar electrocoagulator. Endometriosis of the rectum, rectovaginal septum, and uterosacral ligament is treated by vaporization, excision, or a combination of the two, and the posterior cul-de-sac is freed (Figures 13.1.17, 13.1.18). Bipolar forceps are used to achieve hemostasis. If the endometriosis has penetrated deeply to the bowel muscularis or mucosa and has caused a stricture requiring anterior or complete resection and repair, this procedure is done after the hysterectomy.

The hysterectomy starts with coagulation and transection of the round ligament close to the pelvic side wall (Figure 13.1.19). The peritoneum is opened, and the pelvic side wall is dissected and developed. This technique allows excellent visualization of retroperitoneal major vessels and ureter (Figure 13.1.20).

The bladder serosa is injected with lactated Ringer's solution. The bladder flap is developed with the CO_2 laser or any cutting device. After division of scar tissue in the vesicouterine fold, the suction–irrigator probe is used for blunt dissection and

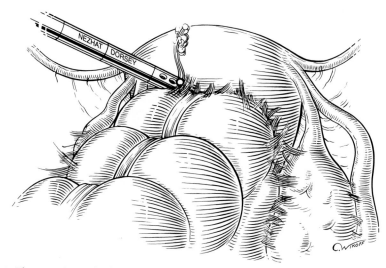

Figure 13.1.14. The rectosigmoid colon is attached to the posterior aspect of the uterus with dense adhesions and endometriosis. Using the hydrodissection probe and CO_2 laser, the adhesions are lysed and the rectosigmoid colon is separated from the uterus.

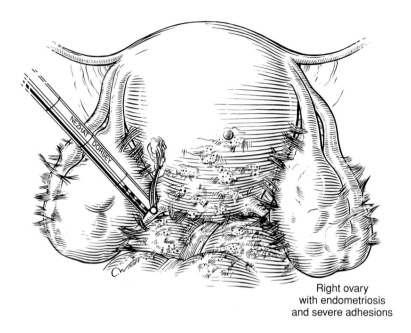

Right ovary
with endometriosis
and severe adhesions

Figure 13.1.16. The rectum, the back of the cervix, and the uterosacral ligaments are dissected.

mobilization of the bladder. The infundibulopelvic ligaments are desiccated and transected (Figure 13.1.21).

The uterine vessels are coagulated close to the hypogastric artery (Figures 13.1.22, 13.1.23) and retracted medially and removed from the ureter. The anterior parametrium is transected. The ureters are freed from the peritoneum and skeletonized down to the bladder with the suction–irrigator probe and the laser, harmonic scalpel, scissors, or electric knife.

At the level of the cardinal ligaments, the ureter and the descending branches of the uterine artery are close to one another and to the cervix. Therefore, cardinal ligament dissection must be precise to prevent bleeding and ureteral injury. The Liga-Sure device is 10 mm and the linear stapler is 12 mm wide, which considering the short distance between the cervix and the ureter, increases the risk of ureteral injury with these instruments. Using contralateral retraction of the uterus, the cardinal ligament is dissected to identify tissue planes, vessels, and the ureter (Figure 13.1.24). Once the ureter is displaced laterally, the cardinal ligament tissue closest to the cervix is coagulated and transected. The bladder pillars are transected close to the cervix (Figure 13.1.25).

After the uterosacral ligaments are dissected, folded wet gauze in a sponge forceps or the tip of a right-angle Heaney retractor is used to mark the anterior or posterior vaginal fornix. The vaginal wall is tented and transected horizontally with a laser or electrode (Figures 13.1.26, 13.1.27). Bipolar electrocoagulation may be used to control bleeding. The remainder of the procedure is done vaginally.

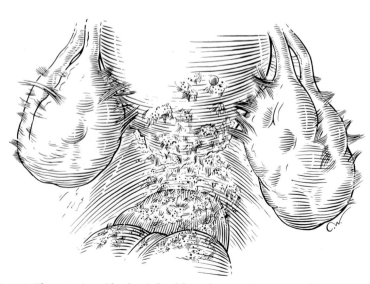

Figure 13.1.17. The rectosigmoid colon is freed from the posterior aspect of the uterus and cervix.

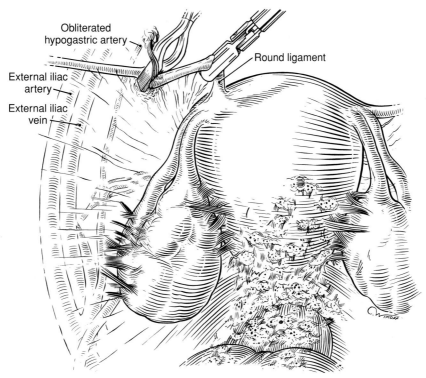

Figure 13.1.18. While the uterus is pulled to the right, the left round ligament is coagulated close to the pelvic side wall.

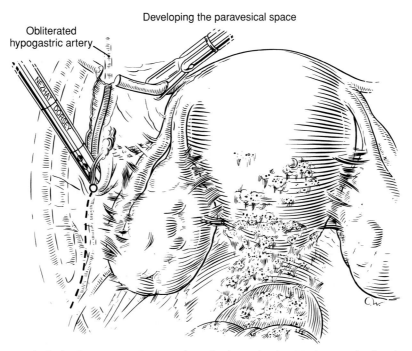

Figure 13.1.19. The hydrodissection probe is used as a backstop for the CO_2 laser to develop the paravesical space. The gynecologist must be careful to avoid injury to the major pelvic side wall vessels and the ureter.

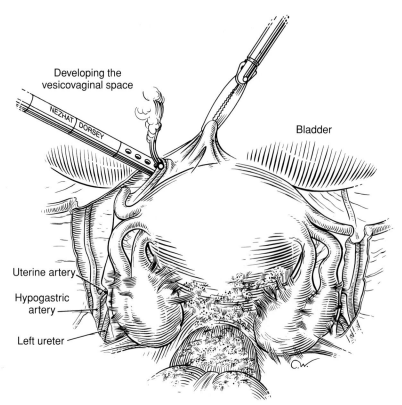

Figure 13.1.20. The anterior leaf of the left broad ligament is dissected with hydrodissection and the CO_2 laser to develop the vesicovaginal space.

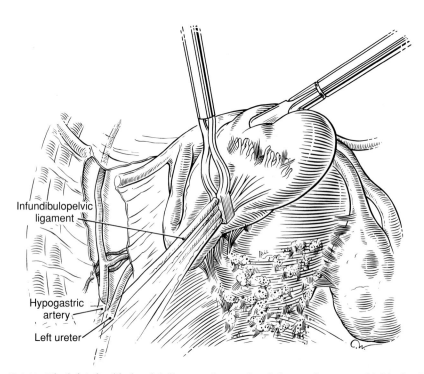

Figure 13.1.21. The left infundibulopelvic ligament is coagulated close to the ovary with bipolar forceps.

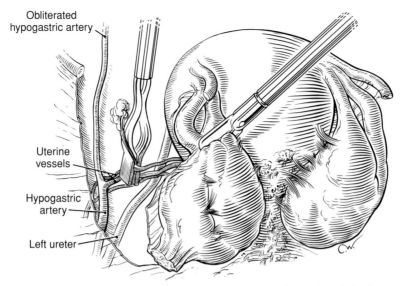

Figure 13.1.22. The paravesical space is developed, and the uterine vessels are identified. The uterine artery at its origin from the hypogastric artery is coagulated with bipolar forceps. The ureter is observed, and excessive heat is avoided to prevent ureteral injury.

HYSTERECTOMY FOR LARGE MYOMAS

The safety of the laparoscopic approach to hysterectomy for large myomatous uteri has been demonstrated in numerous studies. Both Wattiez et al. [25] and Seracchioli [26] et al. reported on laparoscopic hysterectomies for uteri weighing more than 500 g, with comparable complication rates and operating times and shorter convalescence versus the abdominal approach.

The following factors must be considered in selecting patients for this procedure:

1. The patient must have adequate hemoglobin and hematocrit to decrease the possibility of transfusion.

2. Gonadotropin-releasing hormone (GnRH) analogues are advisable if the uterus is more than 18 weeks' gestational size.

3. The primary trocar should be inserted between the umbilicus and the xiphoid if the uterus is more than 18 weeks' gestational size. The secondary trocars should be placed nearer to the umbilicus than usual.

A uterus more than 16 weeks' gestational size with multiple large leiomyomas is more difficult to manipulate laparoscopically. Three and, at times, four secondary trocars are introduced to provide adequate traction to the uterus if the anatomy is distorted, and ureteral dissection may be recommended in this situation. Although it is possible to completely dissect the uterus

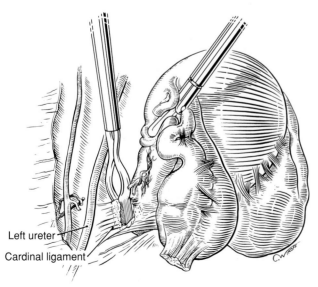

Figure 13.1.23. While the uterus is pulled to the right, bipolar forceps are used to coagulate the cardinal ligaments close to the cervix. The ureter is distanced from the bipolar forceps.

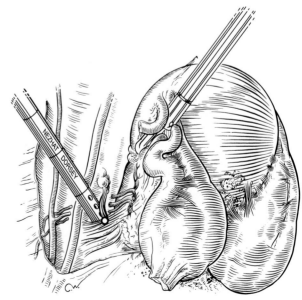

Figure 13.1.24. The cardinal ligament is dissected with the CO_2 laser.

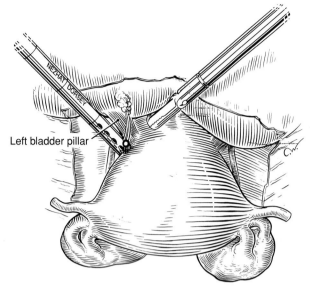

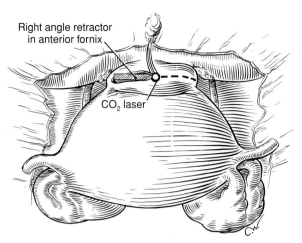

Figure 13.1.26. An assistant places a right-angle Heaney retractor in the anterior fornix, and the CO_2 laser is used to create an anterior culdotomy.

Figure 13.1.25. The vesicocervical fascia (bladder pillars) is dissected close to the cervix with the CO_2 laser.

laparoscopically, it takes longer and a combination of laparoscopic and vaginal approaches is preferred. If there is a large pedunculated leiomyoma interfering with the exposure and laparoscopic manipulation, myomectomy is done first. The laparoscopic approach is continued until the cardinal ligaments are reached, and the remaining portion of the procedure is completed vaginally. After the uterosacral and cardinal ligaments are ligated and cut vaginally, the uterus is morcellated and removed vaginally.

TOTAL LAPAROSCOPIC HYSTERECTOMY

TLH is a technically challenging procedure. Proficiency and comfort with this procedure require years of experience. In the largest

series of total laparoscopic hysterectomies by Wattiez et al. [27], comprising 1647 cases over 10 years, the average operating time was 102.5 minutes, with an average uterine weight of 235 g and a 3.4% major complication rate.

If TLH is planned, two 4×4 wet sponges are placed in a surgical latex glove and inserted into the vagina to prevent loss of pneumoperitoneum. When contralateral traction is applied to the uterus, the vaginal wall surrounding the cervix is outlined, coagulated with the unipolar scissors or bipolar forceps, and cut circumferentially until the cervix is separated (Figure 13.1.28). The specimen is pulled to mid-vagina but not removed, to preserve pneumoperitoneum. Alternatively, a colpotomizer, several of which are available on the market, may be used to delineate the vaginal cuff. This allows the cervix to be circumscribed at a higher level while preserving the uterosacral–cardinal ligament complex and has been referred to in the literature as total laparoscopic intrafascial hysterectomy (TLIH).[28] The vaginal cuff is

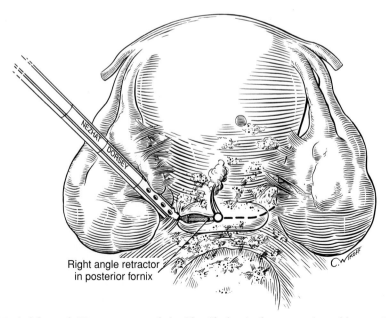

Figure 13.1.27. A right-angle Heaney retractor helps identify the site for a posterior culdotomy. The CO_2 laser cuts the remainder of the uterosacral and cardinal ligaments.

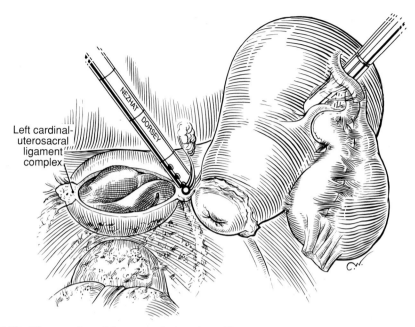

Figure 13.1.28. After anterior culdotomy and posterior culdotomy are achieved, the remainder of the cardinal and uterosacral ligaments on each side is dissected. The cervix is amputated from the vagina. The uterus is removed.

irrigated and inspected for active bleeding. Once hemostasis is achieved, vaginal angles are sutured to the adjacent cardinal and uterosacral ligaments; care is taken to avoid the ureters. The rest of the vaginal cuff is closed with polydioxanone (PDS) or polyglactin (Vicryl) suture on a straight or curved needle using the extracorporeal or intracorporeal knot-tying technique (Figures 13.1.29, 13.1.30). Endoscopic suturing is difficult and time consuming for an unskilled surgeon, and the cuff closure should be done vaginally in such cases. Thermal electrocoagulation or a harmonic device should be used cautiously at the vaginal cuff to prevent tissue necrosis and subsequent breakdown if sutures are placed in nonviable tissue.

Because of the close proximity of the bladder, ureters, rectum, and uterine arteries to one another, the most difficult aspect of TLH involves ligation and transection of the uterosacral–cardinal ligament. An expert laparoscopist will be able to place adequate traction on the uterus to avoid injury to these pelvic structures; however, concomitant pelvic disease may distort the anatomy. A rectum that is adherent to the posterior cul-de-sac may be thought to be a thickened uterosacral ligament. A ureter may be mistaken for pelvic vasculature in the case of extensive pelvic adhesions or an anomalous renal system. In contrast, employing a vaginal approach when ligating the uterosacral–cardinal ligament complex affords the laparoscopist the benefit of tactile

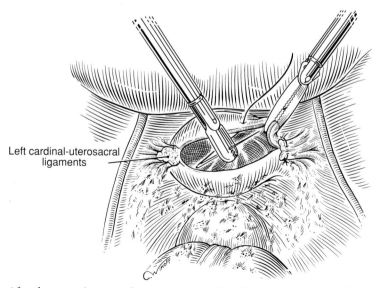

Figure 13.1.29. After the uterus is removed, two sponges are placed in a surgical glove and left inside the vagina to prevent the loss of pneumoperitoneum. The vaginal angles are sutured to the uterosacral–cardinal ligament complex, and the cuff is closed with 0 Vicryl laparoscopic sutures and intracorporeal or extracorporeal knot tying.

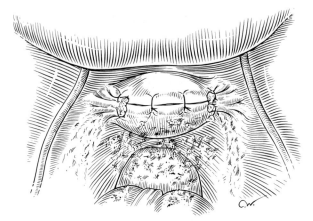

Figure 13.1.30. The vaginal cuff is repaired laparoscopically. The round ligaments and upper portion of the broad ligaments have been cut and suture ligated.

inspection of the cervix and vagina, using hands instead of endoscopic instruments. In doing so, the bladder, ureters, and other pelvic structures can be felt more confidently to avoid injury.

SUPRACERVICAL (SUBTOTAL) LAPAROSCOPIC HYSTERECTOMY

Supracervical hysterectomy is requested by patients and preferred by some gynecologists who believe that the cervix affects sexuality and orgasm and helps provide better vaginal support. A comparison [29] of the risks and benefits of subtotal hysterectomy with those of total hysterectomy in women at low risk for cervical cancer revealed the following operative complication rates and ranges for total abdominal hysterectomy and subtotal hysterectomy, respectively: infection 3% (3% to 20%) and 1.4% (1% to 5%), hemorrhage 2% (2% to 15.4%) and 2% (0.7% to 4%), adjacent organ injury 1% (0.7% to 2%) and 0.7% (0.6% to 1%). The study design was a decision analysis and concluded that proposed benefits from subtotal hysterectomy had not been proven. More recent reports by Munro [30] and Learmen et al. [31] were also unable to demonstrate any significant difference in short- and long-term outcomes between supracervical hysterectomy and total abdominal hysterectomy. The procedure may be performed laparoscopically, and the specimen is morcellated before removal from the peritoneal cavity through a small abdominal incision. An electric morcellator is recommended for this purpose (e.g., 15-, 20-, and 25-mm morcellators by Gynecare [Johnson & Johnson] and Semm [WISAP]). A comparison among laparoscopic supracervical hysterectomy (LSH), LAVH, and TLH failed to demonstrate any clear benefit with LSH.[32–34]

The uterine vessels are coagulated and cut at the level of the cardinal ligaments above the uterosacral ligaments. The uterus is retracted, and its lower segment is amputated with scissors, a unipolar endoscopic electrode, or laser. After the uterus is transected from the cervix, the uterine manipulator is removed vaginally, the cervical stump is irrigated, and hemostasis is achieved. The endocervical epithelium lining the cervical canal is vaporized or coagulated with the laser or electrosurgery. The rest of the endocervical canal is ablated vaginally or laparoscopically to reduce the risk of intraepithelial cervical neoplasia

(0.4% to 1.4%), menstrual bleeding (25%), and vaginal discharge (10%).[35] Approximately 22% of patients require a second procedure for persistent symptoms following supracervical hysterectomy.[36] The uterus is morcellated and removed through a 10- to 20-mm trocar with an electric morcellator. The cervical stump is closed with interrupted absorbable sutures and covered with peritoneum sewn transversely with either continuous or interrupted sutures. Peritoneal washing and inspection of the pelvis and abdomen are done at the end of the procedure.

If the vagina was not entered, there are fewer sexual restrictions. These patients are advised of the continued risk of cervical neoplasia and the need for annual examinations and Papanicolaou smears.

CLASSIC INTRAFASCIAL SUPRACERVICAL HYSTERECTOMY

Semm [37] described coring the cervix intrafascially without colpotomy by using a calibrated resection tool (CURT) that removes the transformation zone to prevent the subsequent potential development of cervical carcinoma (Figures 13.1.31–13.1.34). The pelvic floor support is maintained, the ureters are not jeopardized, and sexual function is not compromised. Semm suggested that the classic intrafascial supracervical hysterectomy (CISH) technique should replace total hysterectomy in 80% of patients.[38] It preserves the blood supply to the lower pelvis and prevents subsequent uterine prolapse. Mettler and coworkers [39] described an approach for doing endoscopic intrafascial supracervical hysterectomy using a serrated-edged macromorcellator. When the endoscopic approach for dissection and uterine extraction was used with the morcellator, a colpotomy was avoided. Another modification involved nearly complete excision (95%) of the endocervical mucosa with the calibrated resection instrument. Maintaining the cardinal ligaments provides support to the cervical stump, and the risks of hemorrhage and genitourinary complications are reduced by avoiding dissection of the parametrium at the level of the endocervix.

An evaluation of the efficacy of CISH was ascertained in 90 patients.[40] No major complications occurred, even in women who had large myomas. The average operating time was 170 minutes, blood loss was lower than that from conventional hysterectomy, and no procedure was converted to a laparotomy. Kim and coauthors [41] compared CISH with TLH and LAVH. They found among three groups that CISH resulted in lowest blood loss and the fewest complications and suggested that CISH was preferable for patients with myomas.

COMPARISON OF OUTCOMES FOR VAGINAL, ABDOMINAL, AND LAPAROSCOPIC HYSTERECTOMIES

There is ample evidence in the literature that laparoscopic hysterectomy compares favorably with abdominal hysterectomy, offering reduced morbidity, expense, and discomfort.[42–44] In a multicenter randomized comparison of 34 women undergoing LAVH and 31 women undergoing abdominal hysterectomy [45], although the mean operating time was significantly longer for LAVH (179.8 vs. 146 minutes), LAVH required a considerably

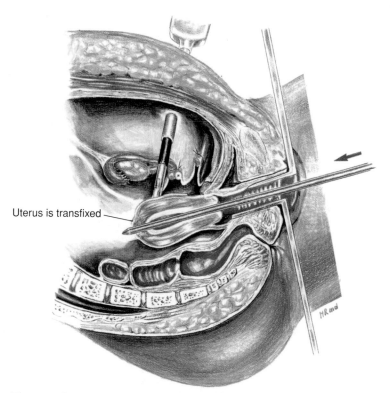

Uterus is transfixed

Figure 13.1.31. The uterus has been transfixed with the CURT instrument. With the classic intrafascial supracervical hysterectomy procedure, the inner part of the cervix is excised by clockwise rotation of the cutting cylinder of the CURT instrument. The instrument has perforated the fundus.

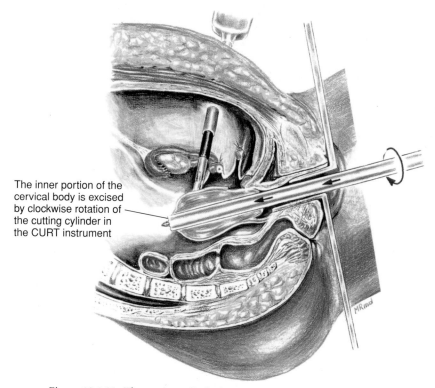

The inner portion of the cervical body is excised by clockwise rotation of the cutting cylinder in the CURT instrument

Figure 13.1.32. The cutting cylinder has removed a portion of the cervix.

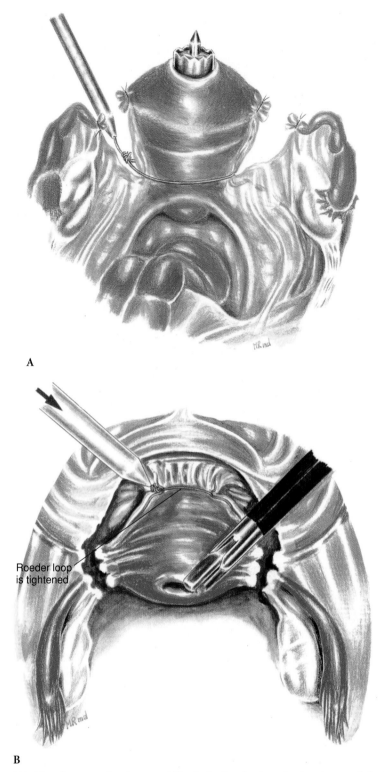

A

B

Figure 13.1.33. (**A**) After the uterus has been mobilized, the Roeder loop is placed around the lower uterine segment. (**B**) The loop is tightened around the cervix as the metal cylinder is removed.

shorter mean hospital stay (2.1 days) and convalescence (28 days) than abdominal hysterectomy (4.1 days and 38.0 days, respectively). There were no important differences in mean hospital charges, blood loss, or intraoperative complication rates between the study groups. A higher incidence of wound complications in the abdominal hysterectomy group was noted. Slightly less optimistic experience with laparoscopic hysterectomy was reported by Bruhat and coauthors [22] in a series of 36 patients. Twenty-seven (75%) were treated successfully by laparoscopy, whereas nine (25%) were converted to laparotomy. Gynecologists had difficulty achieving hemostasis (six patients) and locating anatomic landmarks (three patients) because of large uteri, myomas, or a long cervix. Nevertheless, the authors concluded that LAVH is an alternative to abdominal hysterectomy in properly selected patients. Recent studies have reported a conversion rate of 10%.[46]

The opposite is true when LAVH is compared with standard vaginal hysterectomy, as reported by Summit and colleagues.[19] Among 56 women scheduled to undergo vaginal hysterectomy in an outpatient setting, 29 were randomized to LAVH and 27 to standard vaginal hysterectomy. In the latter group, all surgical procedures were completed and the patients were discharged within 12 hours of admission. In the LAVH group, one patient had a bladder laceration repaired, and the hysterectomy was completed endoscopically. A second patient experienced bleeding from the inferior epigastric vessels. It was not controlled endoscopically, and she underwent exploratory laparotomy with abdominal hysterectomy. When the two groups were compared, the LAVH group required more pain medication, experienced greater blood loss and more intraoperative complications, and incurred higher surgical expenses – a mean of $7905 compared with $4891 for the standard vaginal group. Similar outcomes have been demonstrated in several randomized

Table 13.1.3: Type of Laparoscopic Hysterectomy

Types of Hysterectomy	Procedures, no.			
		BSO	RSO	LSO
Laparoscopically assisted vaginal hysterectomy	24	14	2	3
Vaginally assisted laparoscopic hysterectomy	148	94	12	13
Total laparoscopic hysterectomy	176	114	15	29
Subtotal laparoscopic hysterectomy	13	6	0	1
Total	361	228	29	46

BSO, bilateral salpingo-oophorectomy; LSO, left salpingooophorectomy; RSO, right salpingo-oophorectomy.
Source: Nezhat et al. [51]

comparisons.[47–49] A large retrospective review of 10,110 hysterectomies from Europe reported a higher complication rate, specifically infectious morbidity and bowel injury, blood loss, hospital stay, and recovery, following vaginal hysterectomy versus laparoscopic hysterectomy.[50] Notably, the number of hysterectomies performed vaginally ($n = 1801$) was the least of all the approaches (abdominal hysterectomy, $n = 5875$; laparoscopic hysterectomy, $n = 2434$), indicating a relative lack of experience with vaginal surgery, which may account for the findings of the study. Overall, there are strong data to support the recommendation that LAVH should replace abdominal, not vaginal, hysterectomy.

Nezhat et al. [51] reported on 361 women who fulfilled the criteria for abdominal hysterectomy but underwent LAVH

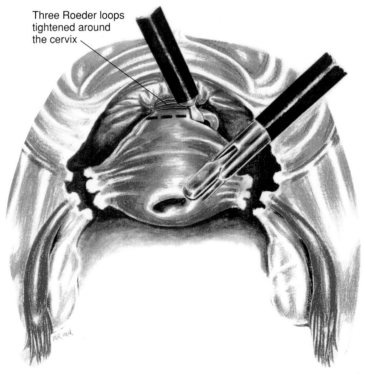

Three Roeder loops tightened around the cervix

Figure 13.1.34. The corpus is amputated above the suture using an electrosurgical knife.

Table 13.1.4: Summary of Women Who Underwent LAVH, TLH, or SLH

Mean age, years (range)	42.5 (25–72)
Gravidity, no. of pregnancies (range)	1.6 (0–7)
Parity, no. of live births (range)	1.3 (0–5)
Mean duration of procedure (range)	2.3 hours (55 minutes–6.5 hours)
Uterine size, weeks' gestation	4–26
Mean uterine weight, g (range)	178.38 (36–1530)
Average blood loss, mL (range)	73 (50–800)
Average hospitalization duration (range)*	21 hours (20 hours–5 days)
Time to full recovery post operation (range)†	3.3 weeks (3 days–13 weeks)
Length of time postoperative pain medication was needed, days (range)‡	3.3 days (0–21 days)

*From termination of procedure until discharge from hospital.
†This information was obtained from office visits, written questionnaires, and telephone interviews.
‡After the patient was discharged from the hospital.

Table 13.1.5: Inoperative and Pathologic Findings in 361 Women

Finding	Patients, no.
Mild to extensive endometriosis	212
Mild to extensive adhesions	189
Uterine fibroids (uterine size 8–26 weeks' size)	116
Uterine adenomyosis	119
Endometriomas (5–15 cm in diameter)	22
Endometrial polyp	13
Endometrial hyperplasia	2
Cervical dysplasia	4
Large cornual pregnancy	1
Hydrosalpinx	7
Pelvic abscess	1
Asherman's syndrome	2
Benign cystic teratoma	3
Serous cyst	2
Mucinous cyst	2
Para-ovarian cyst	2

Source: Nezhat et al.[51]

Table 13.1.6: Additional Procedures Carried Out with Hysterectomy

Procedure	Patients, no.
Treatment of mild to extensive endometriosis	212
Lysis of mild to extensive abdominal and/or pelvic adhesions	189
Ureterolysis	129
Appendectomy	47
Marshall–Marchetti–Krantz or Burch procedure	43
Moschcowitz procedure	88
Bowel resection	11
Cystocele repair	13
Rectocele repair	24
Enterocele repair	6
Vaginal sacral colposuspension	2
Cholecystectomy	2
Removal of ovarian remnant	4
Removal of pelvic abscess	1

Source: Nezhat et al.[51]

Table 13.1.7: Complications after Hysterectomy in 361 Women

Complication, Type	Complications, no.	Incidence per 100 Women
Mortality	0	0.00
Intraoperative		
Vascular		
Inferior epigastric vessel injury	3	0.83
Hemorrhage requiring transfusion	2	0.55
Major blood vessel injury	0	0.00
Gastrointestinal		
Small bowel injury	1	0.27

Source: Nezhat et al.[15]

(172), TLH (176), or SLH (13) from July 1987 through July 1993 (Table 13.1.3). Bipolar forceps and the CO_2 laser were used for hemostasis and cutting, respectively. Patients who required suturing, staples, or clips for hemostasis or had malignancy were excluded from the study. Preoperative indications for hysterectomy included chronic pelvic pain (116 women), chronic pelvic pain with abnormal uterine bleeding (148 women), abnormal uterine bleeding (40 women), and enlarging leiomyoma (28 women). Other indications were endometrial hyperplasia, cervical dysplasia, pelvic abscess, ectopic pregnancy, and pelvic relaxation. The demographic, surgical, and postoperative characteristics of women who underwent hysterectomy are listed in Table 13.1.4. There were no conversions to laparotomy, although one patient with bowel endometriosis and stricture underwent laparotomy for bowel resection and anastomosis. Intraoperative and pathologic findings are summarized in Table 13.1.5. Most patients underwent one or more additional procedures (Table 13.1.6), and the complication rate was 10% (Table 13.1.7).

CONCLUSION

Currently, 25% of hysterectomies are done vaginally, the least traumatic, safest, and most cost-effective way to remove the uterus. Seventy-five percent of hysterectomies are conducted abdominally. Laparoscopically assisted hysterectomy is an excellent alternative when the standard vaginal approach seems difficult. Laparoscopically assisted hysterectomy offers many advantages and will become an integral part of gynecologic surgery, replacing the abdominal hysterectomy. Therefore, efforts no longer should be directed toward validating such surgery but toward providing gynecologists with more opportunities for training. In five reports [51–55], the complication rate was less than 10% (Table 13.1.8) and was lower than those from abdominal and vaginal hysterectomy. Most of these complications involve ureteral and bladder injuries.[50,56] Therefore, particular attention should be paid to identifying and localizing the ureters and dissecting the bladder during an LAVH or laparoscopic hysterectomy. The rate of complications is directly related to the level of expertise and experience of the surgeon. Wattiez et al. [27] reported a decline in major complications from 5.6% to 1.3% with increasing operator experience. Though hard to determine, several studies have attempted to define the number of cases needed to attain proficiency and a low complication rate with LAVH and

laparoscopic hysterectomy. A large Finnish study with more than 2400 laparoscopic hysterectomies demonstrated a statistically significant drop in all complications after 30 procedures.[50] Similar experiences have been reported by others.[57]

Although laparoscopically assisted hysterectomy takes longer, this approach tends to result in less postoperative pain, requires shorter hospitalization, and allows a more rapid recovery. Specific indications and contraindications for LAVH and laparoscopic hysterectomy must be established on the basis of outcome data. Such information is essential for the gynecologist to ascertain the best method for removal of the uterus in each instance. The authors recommend that the use of laparoscopic assistance during hysterectomy be considered in cases in which intra-abdominal pathology or adnexal pathology is suspected, as in cases of endometriosis, adhesions, or an adnexal mass. The extent of laparoscopic dissection should be determined based on the surgeon's experience and comfort with laparoscopic and vaginal procedures.

REFERENCES

1. Selwood T, Wood C. Incidence of hysterectomy in Australia. *Med J Aust.* 1978;2:201.
2. Van Keep PA, Wildemeersch D, Lehert P. Hysterectomy in six European countries. *Maturitas.* 1983;5:69.
3. Porkas R, Hufnagel VG. Hysterectomy in the United States, 1964–84. *Am J Public Health.* 1988;78:852.
4. Bachmann GA. Hysterectomy: a critical review. *J Reprod Med.* 1990;35:839.
5. Dicker RC, Scally MJ, Greenspan JR, et al. Hysterectomy among women of reproductive age. *JAMA.* 1982;248:323.
6. White SC, Wartel LJ, Wade ME. Comparison of abdominal and vaginal hysterectomy: a review of 600 operations. *Obstet Gynecol.* 1971;37:530.
7. Wingo PA, Huezo CM, Rubin GL, et al. The mortality risk associated with hysterectomy. *Am J Obstet Gynecol.* 1985;152:803.
8. Lee NC, Dicker RC, Rubin GL, et al. Confirmation of the preoperative diagnoses for hysterectomy. *Am J Obstet Gynecol.* 1984;150:283.
9. Semm K. *Operationslehre für endoskopische Abdominalchirugie–operative Pelviskopie.* Stuttgart, Germany: Schattauer; 1984.
10. Semm K. *Operative Manual for Endoscopic Abdominal Surgery.* Friedrich ER, trans. Chicago: Year Book Medical Publishers; 1987.
11. Reich H, DeCaprio J, McGlynn F. Laparoscopic hysterectomy. *J Gynecol Surg.* 1989;5:213.
12. Nezhat C, Nezhat F, Silfen SL. Laparoscopic hysterectomy and bilateral salpingo-oophorectomy using multifire GIA surgical stapler. *J Gynecol Surg.* 1990;6:185.
13. Kovac RS, Cruishank SH, Retto HF. Laparoscopy-assisted vaginal hysterectomy. *J Gynecol Surg.* 1990;6:185.
14. Nezhat C, Nezhat F, Gordon S, et al. Laparoscopic versus abdominal hysterectomy. *J Reprod Med.* 1992;37:247.
15. Nezhat C, Nezhat F, Silfen SL. Laparoscopic hysterectomy and bilateral salpingo-oophorectomy using multifire GIA with standard vaginal hysterectomy in an outpatient setting. *Obstet Gynecol.* 1992;80:895.
16. Nezhat C, Burrell MO, Nezhat FR, et al. Laparoscopic radical hysterectomy with para-aortic and pelvic node dissection. *Am J Obstet Gynecol.* 1992;166:864.
17. Nezhat CR, Nezhat FR, Ramirez CE, et al. Laparoscopic radical hysterectomy and laparoscopic assisted vaginal radical hysterectomy with pelvic and paraaortic node dissection. *J Gynecol Surg.* 1993;9:105.

Table 13.1.8: Complications of Laparoscopic Hysterectomy

Author(s)	Cases, no.	Complications, no. (%)
Nezhat et al. [51]	361	40 (11.0)
Hill et al. [52]	220	35 (15.9)
Liu [53]	518	30 (5.8)
Jones [54]	252	18 (7.1)
Chapron et al. [55]	210	21 (10.0)
Total	1561	144 (9.2)

18. Nezhat C, Nezhat F, Burrell M. Laparoscopically assisted hysterectomy for the management of a borderline ovarian tumor: a case report. *J Laparoendosc Surg.* 1992;2:167.

19. Summit RL, Stovall TG, Lipscomb GH, et al. Randomized comparison of laparoscopy-assisted vaginal hysterectomy with standard vaginal hysterectomy in an outpatient setting. *Obstet Gynecol.* 1992;80:895.

20. Nezhat C, Nezhat F, Nezhat C. Operative laparoscopy (minimally invasive surgery): state of the art. *J Gynecol Surg.* 1992;8:111.

21. Nezhat F, Nezhat C, Levy JS. A report of laparoscopic injuries and complications over a 10-year period. Presented at: 41st Annual Clinical Meeting of the American College of Obstetricians and Gynecologists; May 3–6, 1993; Washington, DC.

22. Bruhat MA, Mage G, Pouly JL, et al. *Laparoscopic Hysterectomy in Operative Laparoscopy.* New York: McGraw-Hill; 1992.

23. Nezhat C, Nezhat F, Winer W. Salpingectomy via laparoscopy: a new surgical approach. *J Laparosc Surg.* 1991;1:91.

24. Nezhat C, Nezhat F, Bess O, et al. Injuries associated with the use of a linear stapler during operative laparoscopy: review, diagnosis, management, and prevention. *J Gynecol Surg.* 1993;3:145.

25. Wattiez A, Soriano D, Fiaccavento A, et al. Total laparoscopic hysterectomy for very enlarged uteri. *J Am Assoc Gynecol Laparosc.* 2002;9(2):125–130.

26. Seracchioli R, Venturoli S, Vianello F, et al. Total laparoscopic hysterectomy compared with abdominal hysterectomy in the presence of a large uterus. *J Am Assoc Gynecol Laparosc.* 2002;9(3):333–338.

27. Wattiez A, Soriano D, Cohen SB, et al. The learning curve of total laparoscopic hysterectomy: comparative analysis of 1647 cases. *J Am Assoc Gynecol Laparosc.* 2002;9(3):339–345.

28. Lee PI. Total laparoscopic intrafascial hysterectomy. *J Am Assoc Gynecol Laparosc.* 1996;3(suppl 4):S25.

29. Scott JR, Sharp HT, Dodson MK, et al. Subtotal hysterectomy in modern gynecology: a decision analysis. *Am J Obstet Gynecol.* 1997;176:1186.

30. Munro MG. Supracervical hysterectomy: a time for reappraisal. *Obstet Gynecol.* 1997;89:133–139.

31. Learmen LA, Summitt RL, Varner RE, et al.; Total or Supracervical Hysterectomy (TOSH) Reasearch Group. A randomized comparison of total or supracervical hysterectomy: surgical complications and clinical outcomes. *Obstet Gynecol.* 2003;102(3):453–462.

32. Richards SR, Simpkins S. Laparoscopic supracervical hysterectomy versus laparoscopic assisted vaginal hysterectomy. *J Am Assoc Gynecol Laparosc.* 1995;2(4):431–435.

33. Lalonde CJ, Daniell JF. Early outcomes of laparoscopic-assisted vaginal hysterectomy versus laparoscopic supracervical hysterectomy. *J Am Assoc Gynecol Laparosc.* 1996;3(2):251–256.

34. Milad MP, Morrison K, Sokol A, Miller D, Kirkpatrick L. A comparison of laparoscopic supracervical hysterectomy vs laparoscopically assisted vaginal hysterectomy. *Surg Endosc.* 2001;15:286–288.

35. van der Stege JG, van Beek JJ. Problems related to the cervical stump at follow-up in laparoscopic supracervical hysterectomy. *JSLS.* 1999;3(1):5–7.

36. Okaro EO, Jones KD, Sutton C. Long term outcome following laparoscopic supracervical hysterectomy. *BJOG.* 2001;108(10):1017–1020.

37. Semm K. Hysterectomy via laparotomy or pelviscopy: a new CISH method without colpotomy. *Geburtshilfe Frauenheilkd.* 1991;51:996.

38. Semm K. Endoscopic subtotal hysterectomy without colpotomy: classic intrafascial SEMM hysterectomy: a new method of hysterectomy by pelviscopy, laparotomy, per vagina or functionally by total uterine mucosal ablation. *Int Surg.* 1996;81:362.

39. Mettler L, Semm K, Lehmann-Willenbrock L, et al. Comparative evaluation of classical intrafascial–supracervical hysterectomy (CISH) with transuterine mucosal resection as performed by pelviscopy and laparotomy – our first 200 cases. *Surg Endosc.* 1995;9:418.

40. Kim DH, Lee JC, Bae DH. Clinical analysis of pelviscopic classic intrafascial SEMM hysterectomy. *J Am Assoc Gynecol Laparosc.* 1995;2:289.

41. Kim DH, Bae DH, Hur M, et al. Comparison of classic intrafascial supracervical hysterectomy with total laparoscopic and laparoscopic-assisted vaginal hysterectomy. *J Am Assoc Gynecol Laparosc.* 1998;5:253.

42. Marana R, Busacca M, Zupi E, Garcea N, Paparella P, Catalano GF. Laparoscopically assisted vaginal hysterectomy versus total abdominal hysterectomy: a prospective, randomized, multicenter study. *Am J Obstet Gynecol.* 1999;180(2 pt 1):270–275.

43. Falcone T, Paraiso MF, Mascha E. Prospective randomized clinical trial of laparoscopically assisted vaginal hysterectomy versus total abdominal hysterectomy. *Am J Obstet Gynecol.* 1999;180(4):955–962.

44. Olsson J, Ellstrom M, Hahlin M. A randomized prospective trial comparing laparoscopic and abdominal hysterectomy. *Br J Obstet Gynaecol.* 1999;180:270–275.

45. Summitt RL Jr, Stovall TG, Steege JF, Lipscomb GH. A multicenter randomized comparison of laparoscopically assisted vaginal hysterectomy and abdominal hysterectomy in abdominal hysterectomy candidates. *Obstet Gynecol.* 1998;92:321.

46. Cristofororni PM, Palmieri A, Gerbaldo D, Montz FJ. Frequency and cause of aborted laparoscopic-assisted vaginal hysterectomy. *J Am Assoc Gynecol Laparosc.* 1995;3(1):33–37.

47. Ottosen C, Lingman G, Ottosen L. Three methods for hysterectomy: a randomised, prospective study of short term outcome. *BJOG.* 2000;107(11):1380–1385.

48. Kovac SR. Hysterectomy outcomes in patients with similar indications. *Obstet Gynecol.* 2000;95(6 pt 1):787–793.

49. Soriano D, Goldstein A, Lecuru F, Darai E. Recovery from vaginal hysterectomy compared with laparoscopy-assisted vaginal hysterectomy: a prospective, randomized, multicenter study. *Acta Obstet Gynecol Scand.* 2001;80(4):337–341.

50. Makinen J, Johansson J, Tomas C, et al. Morbidity of 10,110 hysterectomies by type of approach. *Hum Reprod.* 2001;13:431–436.

51. Nezhat F, Nezhat CH, Admon D, et al. Complications and results of 361 hysterectomies performed at laparoscopy. *J Am Coll Surg.* 1995;180:307.

52. Hill D, Maher PJ, Wood CE, et al. Complications of laparoscopic hysterectomy. *J Am Assoc Gynecol Laparosc.* 1994;1:159.

53. Liu CY. Complications of total laparoscopic hysterectomy in 518 cases. *Gynecol Endosc.* 1994;3:203.

54. Jones RA. Complications of laparoscopic hysterectomy: 250 cases. *Gynecol Endosc* 1995;4:95.

55. Chapron CM, Dubuisson JB, Ansquer Y. Is total laparoscopic hysterectomy a safe procedure? *Hum Reprod.* 1996;11:2422.

56. Meikle SF, Nugent EW, Orleans M. Complications and recovery from laparoscopy-assisted vaginal hysterectomy compared with abdominal and vaginal hysterectomy. *Obstet Gynecol.* 1997;89(2):304–311.

57. Altgassen C, Michels W, Schneider A. Learning laparoscopic-assisted hysterectomy. *Obstet Gynecol* 2004;104(2):308–313.

Section 13.2. Laparoscopic Excision of a Rudimentary Uterine Horn

Togas Tulandi

During embryogenesis, complete atresia of one of the two mullerian ducts results in the development of one of the uterine horns only (unicornuate uterus), whereas partial development of the mullerian duct results in a rudimentary horn.

The American Society for Reproductive Medicine classified unicornuate uterus as type II.[1] It is further divided into four subcategories. Types IIa and IIb are unicornuate uteri with and without a communicating rudimentary horn, respectively; type IIc is a unicornuate uterus with a noncavitated uterine horn; and type IId is a unicornuate uterus without a rudimentary horn (Figure 13.2.1).

In most cases, there is no communication between the uterine cavity proper and the cavity of the rudimentary horn (Figure 13.2.2, type IIb). As a result, menstrual blood will accumulate in the rudimentary horn (hematometra), causing cyclic abdominal pain. It also predisposes to the development of endometriosis. Approximately 25% of unicornuate uteri are associated with a cavitated noncommunicating rudimentary uterine horn.[2] The rudimentary horn may be separated from the unicornuate uterus by fibrous tissue (Figure 13.2.2), or the horn may be adherent to the uterus.

As with the normal uterus, polyps, fibroids, or adenomyosis may be found in the rudimentary uterine horn (Figure 13.2.3).

Pregnancy may be located in the rudimentary uterine horn. Its incidence is estimated to be between one in 100,000 and one in 140,000 pregnancies.[3] It occurs as the result of transperitoneal migration of a fertilized ovum or spermatozoa. Although most reported cases of pregnancy have been in the noncommunicating rudimentary horn, pregnancy in the communicating horn has also been reported.[4] In any event, pregnancy in the rudimentary horn, whether communicating or noncommunicating, carries the risk of uterine rupture.[5–9]

DIAGNOSIS

The most common symptom of a cavitated rudimentary uterine horn is primary dysmenorrhea, sometimes associated with dyspareunia. The diagnosis is best established by magnetic resonance imaging (MRI). However, a noncavitated rudimentary horn may be misinterpreted as a pedunculated uterine fibroid. Another important imaging technique is ultrasound. The best time to perform ultrasound is in the second half of the cycle, when the endometrium is thick and echogenic. A cavitated uterine horn can be easily identified.

Concomitant findings of a blind vagina and a rudimentary uterine horn are found in Mayer–Rokitansky–Küster–Hauser (MRKH) syndrome. Other associated findings of MRKH syndrome are urinary tract abnormalities and endometriosis.

TREATMENT

The noncavitated rudimentary uterine horn is asymptomatic and does not require treatment. In contrast, excision of a cavitated uterine horn is recommended because of the symptoms of cyclic abdominal pain, the need to reduce possible endometriosis, and more importantly, the possibility of pregnancy in the horn with functional endometrium. Because of the high risk of uterine rupture, early discovery of a pregnancy in the uterine horn is best terminated with methotrexate and local injection of potassium chloride. Laparoscopic removal of the rudimentary horn may be performed several months later.

Fedele et al. [2] reported a series of 10 women with unicornuate uterus associated with a cavitated uterine horn. They and others [10–16] demonstrated that excision of a uterine horn by laparoscopy is effective.

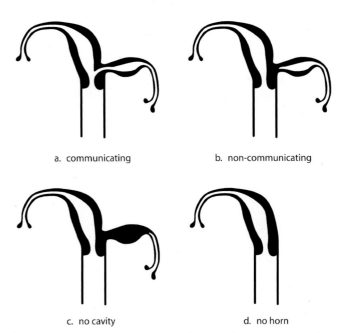

a. communicating　　　b. non-communicating

c. no cavity　　　d. no horn

Figure 13.2.1. The American Society for Reproductive Medicine classifications of unicornuate uterus.

363

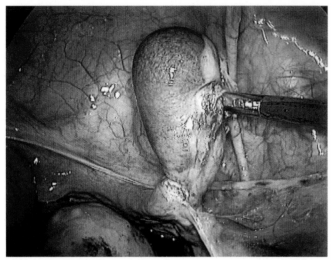

Figure 13.2.2. The most common type of rudimentary uterine horn (cavitated and noncommunicating). The horn is separated from the unicornuate uterus by a fibrous band. This case is unusual. The two horns are seperated by a long fibrous band.

SURGICAL TECHNIQUE

Standard laparoscopy is performed with one primary trocar for the laparoscope and two secondary trocars. A thorough examination of the abdominal cavity should be performed. The presence of endometriosis might distort the anatomy, including the course of the ureter. In any event, the ureter ipsilateral to the rudimentary horn is often located higher than the opposite side.

The horn may be separated from the uterus or closely attached to it with a poorly defined cleavage plane. To prevent the occurrence of tubal ectopic pregnancy, the fallopian tube attached to the rudimentary horn should be removed. Excision of the rudimentary horn is similar to that of hysterectomy. The round ligament, proximal part of the fallopian tube, and ovarian ligament are electrocoagulated and divided, allowing access to the retroperitoneal space and visualization of the uterine vessels. The bladder

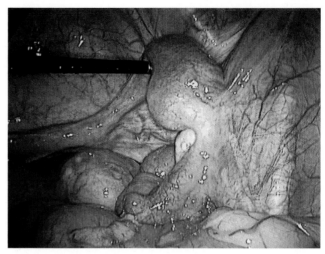

Figure 13.2.4. Right rudimentary uterine horn in the same patient.

peritoneum anterior to the uterine horn is hydrodissected and divided, and the bladder is dissected off the lower part of the uterine horn.

Figures 13.2.4 through 13.2.6 show rudimentary uterine horns in a patient with MRKH syndrome. The two horns are completely separated with a long fibrous band. In this case, mobilization of the bladder was not required.

Separation of the horn from the uterus is easy when there is merely a band of fibrous tissue between them. The fibrous band can be simply coagulated and divided. The procedure is more complex when the horn is closely attached to the uterus. Separation of the horn can be accomplished with sharp dissection at the point where they join. Identification of the surgical plane can be further enhanced by hysteroscopic illumination. Hemostasis is achieved using bipolar coagulation, and the uterine defect is closed with a few sutures.

The excised rudimentary horn is extracted intact either through a colpotomy incision or an extended lateral port. This will allow confirmation as to whether the horn is cavitated.

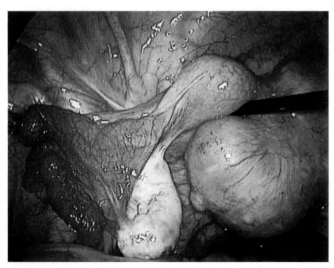

Figure 13.2.3. Left rudimentary uterine horn with a subserous fibroid in a patient with Mayer–Rokitansky–Küster–Hauser syndrome.

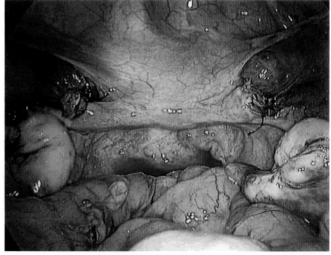

Figure 13.2.5. Because of the wide separation of the two horns, in this case the bladder does not need to be mobilized.

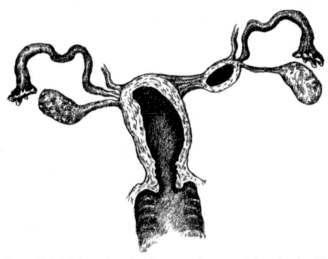

Figure 13.2.6. The cavitated rudimentary horns and the tube should be excised, leaving the fibrous bands that connected the two uterine horns.

SUMMARY

The most common type of rudimentary uterine horn is communicating and cavitated uterine horn (type IIb of the American Society for Reproductive Medicine classification). Pregnancy in the rudimentary uterine horn, whether communicating or non-communicating, carries the risk of uterine rupture. Because of this risk and the symptoms of cyclic abdominal pain, excision of a cavitated uterine horn is recommended. This can be achieved effectively by laparoscopy.

REFERENCES

1. American Fertility Society. The American Fertility Society classifications of the adnexal adhesions, distal tubal occlusion, tubal occlusion secondary to tubal ligation, tubal pregnancy, mullerian anomalies and intrauterine adhesions. *Fertil Steril.* 1998;49:944–955.
2. Fedele L, Bianchi S, Zanconato G, Berlanda N, Bergamini V. Laparoscopic removal of the cavitated noncommunicating rudimentary uterine horn: surgical aspects in 10 cases. *Fertil Steril.* 2005;83:432–436.
3. Johansen K. Pregnancy in a rudimentary uterine horn. *Obstet Gynecol.* 1983;61:565–567.
4. Elsayegh A, Nwosu EC. Rupture of pregnancy in the communicating rudimentary uterine horn at 34 weeks. *Human Reprod.* 1998;13:3566–3568.
5. Heinonen PK. Unicornuate uterus and rudimentary horn. *Fertil Steril.* 1997;68:224–230.
6. Daskalakis G, Pilalis A, Lykeridou K, Antsaklis A. Rupture of noncommunicating rudimentary uterine horn pregnancy. *Obstet Gynecol.* 2002;100:1108–1110.
7. Oral B, Guney M, Ozsoy M, Sonal S. Placenta accreta associated with a ruptured pregnant rudimentary uterine horn. Case report and review of the literature. *Arch Gynecol Obstet.* 2001;265:100–102.
8. Panayotidis C, Abdel-Fattah M, Leggott M. Rupture of rudimentary uterine horn of a unicornuate uterus at 15 weeks' gestation. *J Obstet Gynaecol.* 2004;24:323–324.
9. Shinohara A, Yamada A, Imai A. Rupture of noncommunicating rudimentary uterine horn at 27 weeks' gestation with neonatal and maternal survival. *Int J Gynaecol Obstet.* 2005;88:316–317.
10. Amara DP, Nezhat F, Giudice L, Nezhat C. Laparoscopic management of a noncommunicating uterine horn in a patient with an acute abdomen. *Surg Laparosc Endosc.* 1997;7:56–59.
11. Cutner A, Saridogan E, Hart R, Pandya P, Creighton S. Laparoscopic management of pregnancies occurring in non-communicating accessory uterine horns. *Eur J Obstet Gynecol Reprod Biol.* 2004;113:106–109.
12. Giatras K, Licciardi FL, Grifo JA. Laparoscopic resection of a non-communicating rudimentary uterine horn. *J Am Assoc Gynecol Laparosc.* 1997;4:491–493.
13. Kadir RA, Hart J, Nagele F, O'Connor H, Magos AL. Laparoscopic excision of a noncommunicating rudimentary uterine horn. *Br J Obstet Gynaecol.* 1996;103:371–372.
14. Panayotidis C, Abdel-Fattah M, Leggott M. Rupture of rudimentary uterine horn of a unicornuate uterus at 15 weeks' gestation. *J Obstet Gynaecol.* 2004;24:323–324.
15. Perrotin F, Bertrand J, Body G. Laparoscopic surgery of unicornuate uterus with rudimentary uterine horn. *Hum Reprod.* 1999;14:931–933.
16. Silva PD, Welch HD. Laparoscopic removal of a symptomatic rudimentary uterine horn in a perimenarchal adolescent. *J Soc Laparoendosc Surg.* 2002;6:377–379.

14 | PELVIC FLOOR

Section 14.1. Laparoscopic Burch Colposuspension

Jim W. Ross and Mark R. Preston

Retropubic Burch colposuspension has been considered by many to be the "gold standard" procedure for the treatment of female stress urinary incontinence for almost 40 years. Vancaillie and Schuessler [1] introduced the laparoscopic approach to retropubic colposuspension in 1991. Numerous reports followed in subsequent years describing laparoscopic colposuspensions and their efficacy. Analysis of the outcomes of these various laparoscopic "Burch" colposuspensions is difficult because many of the techniques are not true Burch procedures but rather other modified retropubic colposuspensions. In this section, we describe the laparoscopic Burch colposuspension, including patient selection, preoperative evaluation, operative technique, possible complications, and efficacy. We review the efficacy of the laparoscopic Burch colposuspension studies that use the Burch–Tanagho procedure and compare these techniques to other popular anti-incontinence procedures. The many modified laparoscopic retropubic procedures are not addressed.

BURCH COLPOSUSPENSION: THE EVOLUTION OF A PROCEDURE

In 1961, Burch [2] published the description of a new female anti-incontinence procedure, based on a technique started in 1958. The technique involved entering the space of Retzius via a paramedian incision. After clearing the periurethral tissue of its overlying fat and areolar tissue, three 2-0 chromic sutures were placed at the mid-urethra and the bladder neck and then fixed to Cooper's ligament. Burch [3] reported a subjective cure rate of 92% in 143 patients with 10 to 60 months of follow-up.

Tanagho [4] suggested several refinements to increase the cure rate and decrease complications for the Burch colposuspension (Table 14.1.1). He stressed the importance of the surgical repair "is to preserve the initially intact sphincteric mechanism, to restore its proper position and to provide it with adequate support." He stressed staying at least 2 cm lateral to the urethra and urethrovesical junction when removing overlying fat. After placing absorbable sutures at the mid-urethra and lateral to the urethra–vesical junction, the anterior vaginal wall is elevated by the surgeon. Each suture is placed through Cooper's ligament and brought 2 cm below the ligament to be tied. Tanagho stressed the formation of a "hammock" of support without compressing the urethra against the pubic bone. We feel the laparoscopic colposuspension must include the Burch–Tanagho gold standard technique to be called a laparoscopic Burch colposuspension.

LAPAROSCOPIC COLPOSUSPENSIONS

The first reported retropubic surgery performed via the laparoscopic approach was described by Vancaillie and Schuessler in 1991.[1] Their techniques resembled a Marshall–Marchetti–Krantz (MMK) rather than a Burch colposuspension. Albala et al. [5] reported on a series of laparoscopic MMK and Burch colposuspensions. In subsequent years, larger case series were reported by numerous authors.[6–8] One goal of this section is to show that the laparoscopic Burch colposuspension, when performed in a fashion identical to the open Burch with good laparoscopic technique, is comparable to laparotomy and provides several advantages for patient care.

SELECTION, EVALUATION, AND ANATOMY

Patient Selection

Any patient with genuine stress incontinence (GSI) is a candidate for laparoscopic colposuspension. Once the diagnosis is made, the decision for surgery is made by the physician and patient jointly, usually after a trial of more conservative treatment. Possible contraindications to the laparoscopic approach are history of severe abdominal or pelvic adhesions, prior incontinence procedures, intrinsic sphincter deficiency, or the necessity of other abdominal procedures requiring laparotomy. Many physicians advocate treating only primary GSI with a retropubic Burch, but we [9,10] and others [11] have successfully treated recurrent GSI laparoscopically. Prior procedures, such as anterior vaginal repair, needle suspensions, MMK, Burch, and bone anchor procedures, are not absolute contraindications. Laparoscopic Burch has been used successfully in patients with low urethral closure pressure and/or low Valsalva leak point pressure (VLPP) in conjunction with urethral hypermobility. Laparoscopic Burch is not the surgery of choice for intrinsic sphincter deficiency (ISD) with a fixed, frozen urethra.

Evaluation

The basic evaluation consists of a history and physical exam, cough stress test (CST), urine culture and sensitivity, assessment of postvoid residual volume, and 24-hour voiding diary. A basic filling cystometrogram with VLPP is essential if multichannel urodynamic testing is not available. Multichannel urodynamic testing is considered necessary in patients with prior incontinence procedures and in the elderly. Quality-of-life (QOL) questionnaires, cystoscopy, and bladder neck ultrasound can also be used. In the history, a detailed inquiry concerning urinary complaints

Table 14.1.1: The Tanagho Principles for Burch Colposuspension

Remove paraurethral fat out to lateral sidewalls

Keep dissection 2 cm from urethra and bladder neck

Elevate paraurethral tissue with vaginal hand during dissection and suture placement

Clean off Cooper's ligament

Place a right and left suture through the paraurethral tissue 2 cm lateral to the mid-urethra and up through Cooper's ligament

Keep paraurethral tissue elevated with vaginal hand while tying

Repeat bilateral suture placement 2 cm lateral to the bladder neck and through Cooper's ligament

Do not overcorrect when tying the sutures, leaving 2 cm between the pubic ramus and the urethra

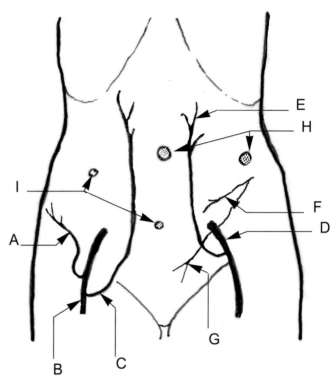

Figure 14.1.1. Abdominal wall vessels and nerves at risk during laparoscopy and trocar sites for laparoscopic Burch. *A*, superficial circumflex artery; *B*, femoral artery; *C*, superficial inferior epigastric artery; *D*, external iliac artery; *E*, inferior epigastric artery; *F*, iliohypogastric nerve; *G*, ilioinguinal nerve; *H*, 10-mm trocar sites; *I*, 5-mm trocar sites.

and pelvic support problems is essential. In addition, patients are questioned about obstructive defecation and fecal incontinence. In our clinic, 23% of the patients with severe GSI or pelvic organ prolapse have fecal incontinence, which is in agreement with findings of others.[12–15] Obstructive defecation is often associated with rectal prolapse, rectocele, and intussusception.[16,17] When either condition is present, anal manometry, anal ultrasound, and pudendal nerve terminal motor latency studies should be included in the evaluation.

Surgical Anatomy

There are several vessels and nerves that come into play with laparoscopic pelvic procedures. The first vessels at possible risk from trocar placement are the great vessels under the infraumbilical site. The umbilicus is at the L3-4 level, and in women with thin to normal body habitus the aortic bifurcation is at L4-5. In obese women, the umbilicus is lower. In thin to normal-size women, the infraumbilical trocar is placed at a 45° angle toward the pelvis, whereas in an obese female, the trocar can be placed close to a 90° angle. The left common iliac vein crosses over the lateral half of the lower lumbar vertebrae and may be inferior to the umbilicus, making it susceptible to injury at trocar insertion or when exposing the sacral promontory. The common iliac arteries course 5 to 6 cm lateral from the midline before bifurcating into the internal and external common iliac vessels.

The inferior epigastric, coming off the distal portion of the external iliac artery, crosses the medial border of the inguinal ligament and runs below and lateral to the rectus sheath to anastomose with the superior epigastric vessels coming from the internal mammary arteries in the upper abdominal wall (Figure 14.1.1). Two inferior epigastric veins accompany the artery. The superficial epigastric artery arises from the femoral artery 1 cm below the inguinal ligament and passes through the femoral sheath to supply the superficial area of the abdominal wall up to the umbilicus. If the patient is thin, this vessel can be transilluminated when placing trocars through the abdominal wall.

The obturator artery is one of the terminal branches of the internal iliac artery and is found on the lateral pelvic sidewall, leaving the pelvis via the obturator canal along with the obtura-

tor nerve (Figure 14.1.2A). It gives off a pubic branch that anastomoses with the pubic branch of the inferior epigastric artery to supply the posterior surface of the symphysis. An accessory obturator artery is present 25% of the time, arising from the inferior epigastric (Figure 14.1.2B). In approximately 5% of patients, both obturator and accessory obturator branches are present. Care must be taken with these vessels because they complete an anastomotic circle of vessels between the internal and external iliac arteries, referred to as the circle of death in surgical texts. Damage to any vessel in this circle may result in significant hemorrhage.

Neuropathies may occur from nerve damage or entrapment in laparoscopic surgery. Lateral trocar placement can damage the iliohypogastric and ilioinguinal nerve, leading to sharp pain in the suprapubic or groin area (Figure 14.1.1).[18] Obturator nerve damage may occur during dissection of the space of Retzius or with paravaginal repairs, causing sensory loss to the medial thigh and difficulty ambulating.

SURGICAL PROCEDURE

The patient's legs are placed in low Allen stirrups, and the three-way Foley catheter is placed in the bladder. The patient should be flat and not in Trendelenburg, as Trendelenburg positioning can bring the pelvic vessels closer to the anterior abdominal wall. The infraumbilical area is infiltrated with Marcaine (Hospira) 0.25% (as are all of the trocar sites), and an infraumbilical stab

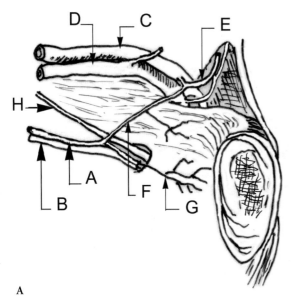

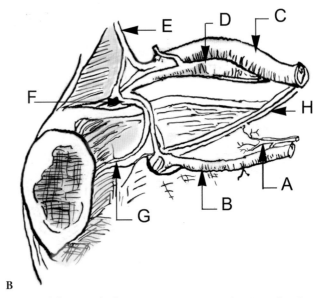

A   **B**

Figure 14.1.2. Normal obturator artery and accessory obturator artery anatomy. (**A**) Normal obturator artery, present in 70% of patients. *A*, obturator artery; *B*, obturator vein; *C*, external iliac artery; *D*, external iliac vein; *E*, inferior epigastric artery; *F*, obturator branch anastomosing with pubic branch of the inferior epigastric artery; *G*, pubic artery branch; *H*, obturator nerve. (**B**) Accessory obturator, present in 25% of patients. Five percent of patients have a combination of a normal obturator artery and an accessory obturator. *A*, obturator artery; *B*, obturator vein; *C*, external iliac artery; *D*, external iliac vein; *E*, inferior epigastric artery; *F*, pubic branch of the inferior epigastric artery; *G*, pubic artery branch supplying pubic ramus; *H*, obturator nerve.

incision is made. Preemptive anesthesia significantly decreases postoperative pain. The abdominal wall is elevated manually and the Veress needle is passed into the abdominal cavity; if the initial abdominal pressure is 8 mm Hg or less, the gas is turned on. Many surgeons feel the open technique is safer if the patient has had multiple surgical procedures. The literature shows that the open procedure prevents great vessel injury, but there is no difference in bowel injury.[19]

Once the abdominal pressure reaches 15 mm Hg, the infraumbilical trocar is passed into the abdomen through the umbilical aponeurosis. The laparoscope, with video camera, is put in place. A left lateral 10-mm and right lateral and suprapubic 5-mm trocars are then introduced under direct visualization. Now the patient can be placed in Trendelenburg to visualize the pelvis. After an initial inspection of the abdomen and pelvis is completed, approximately 150 mL of sterile saline or water stained with indigo carmine (or methylene blue) is instilled through the Foley to delineate the borders of the bladder. A transverse incision is made approximately 2 cm above the bladder reflection. It is important to remember that the patient is in Trendelenburg position and to dissect in an upward fashion, or the bladder may be entered. This will help prevent inadvertent cystotomy. Identification of loose areolar tissue confirms dissection in the correct plane (Figure 14.1.3A). The loose areolar tissue and fat in this space are swept away with the spatula until the pubic bone is reached. As small vessels are encountered, they are coagulated. Once the pubic bone is reached, the overlying loose tissue is bluntly dissected away to expose the bone and Cooper's ligament (Figure 14.1.3B). This dissection is carried out inferiorly to the lateral attachments of the anterior vaginal wall and laterally to the obturator notch.

The surgeon places his or her left hand in the vagina. The Foley balloon and urethra are identified, and the paraurethral

tissue is cleared of its overlying adipose tissue, which is elevated with the vaginal hand (Figure 14.1.3C). To minimize bleeding and avoid damaging the nerve supply to the urethra, care is taken to stay at least 2 cm lateral to the urethra, and the adipose tissue overlying the urethra is not removed. The rich venous plexus adherent to pubocervical fascia can be coagulated as necessary.

The first suture is placed 2 cm lateral to the mid-urethra as this tissue is elevated with the vaginal hand. A large bite of tissue is taken. A figure-of-eight suture is not necessary, as demonstrated by Burch and Tanagho.[2,4] The needle is passed up through Cooper's ligament, and while the vaginal tissue is elevated, the suture is tied with an extracorporeal knot. The vaginal tissue is not pulled all the way up to Cooper's ligament as this will result in overcorrection of the urethrovesical angle and possibly kink the ureter. A suture bridge of approximately 2 cm and a similar space between the urethra and pubic arch are the desired end point. The second suture is placed 2 cm lateral to the bladder neck and tied using the same technique. The contralateral sutures are then placed in a similar fashion. At completion, the four sutures elevate the pubocervical fascia to form "dog ears," creating a hammock of vaginal wall under the mid-urethra and bladder neck (Figures 14.1.3D, 14.1.4).

As the last two sutures are being placed, the anesthetist is instructed to give intravenous indigo carmine. Once all sutures have been tied down, cystoscopy is performed. It is essential that dye is seen coming from both ureteral orifices and that no sutures have penetrated the bladder wall. If no dye is seen, the sutures must be removed from that side and replaced. Most ureteral obstruction is the result of excessive elevation of the trigone, which crimps the ureter, preventing flow.[20] After cystoscopy, the space of Retzius is closed with a continuous delayed absorbable suture.

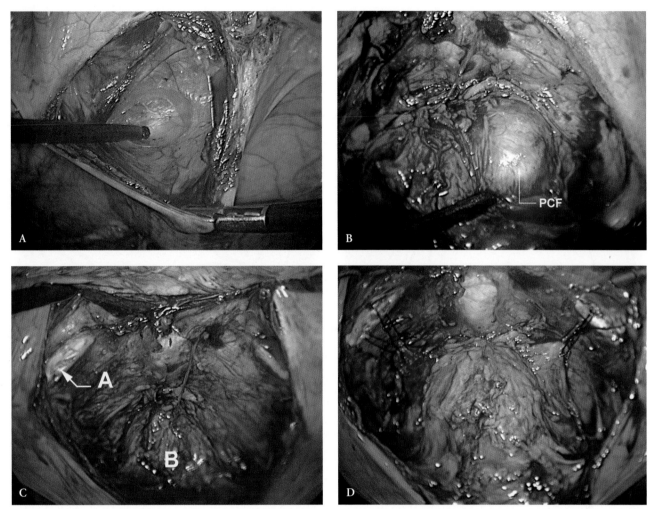

Figure 14.1.3. (**A**) Opening of the space of Retzius. Notice the fine areolar tissue. This is an avascular plane. We use the adage "Fat is your friend." (**B**) The pubocervical fascia (PCF) has been elevated with the vaginal hand and the adipose tissue has been removed, staying 2 cm lateral to the urethra and bladder neck. Elevation aids in the placement of the Burch sutures. (**C**) Cooper's ligament is cleaned off before suture placement. The Foley bulb is seen elevating the bladder proximal to the bladder neck. *A*, Cooper's ligament; *B*, bulge of the Foley bulb at the bladder neck. (**D**) The completed Burch colposuspension with the typical "dog ears" created by elevation of the pubocervical fascia.

Most surgeons believe that the Burch procedure should be the last repair if it is being done with concomitant procedures. Other repairs done after the Burch may affect the urethrovesical angle, secondary to changes in the pelvic axis. In any patient demonstrating vaginal support weakness, we usually perform some type of colpopexy before the Burch to prevent prolapse at the vault or in the posterior pelvic compartment. Laparoscopic Burch has been combined with anterior and posterior support procedures, paravaginal repair, sacrocolpopexy [9], laparoscopic hysterectomy, external anal sphincteroplasty [12], and rectopexy.

ENTRY INTO THE SPACE OF RETZIUS

Both intraperitoneal (or transperitoneal) and extraperitoneal approaches to the space of Retzius have been described and may be used for performing the laparoscopic Burch procedure. The choice of approach depends on the surgeon's preference and on whether concomitant procedures will be performed requiring intraperitoneal access.

Suggested advantages of the extraperitoneal approach include the avoidance of entering the intraperitoneal cavity, better visualization [21], decreased risk of vascular and bowel injury, the bypassing of intra-abdominal adhesions, and the ability to use regional anesthesia.[21–23] Additionally, decreased blood loss has been reported by some and is thought to be the result of instillation of CO_2 gas at 20 mm Hg into the extraperitoneal space, causing compression of capillaries.[23] The extraperitoneal approach also allows lower placement of trocars, making it easier to reach the operative field. At one center, extraperitoneal Burch was cheaper than open Burch ($3100 vs. $6000).[21] In several reports, this technique is considered faster and cheaper, with cure rates comparable to those of open or laparoscopic transperitoneal Burch and high patient satisfaction.[22,24–26]

Potential drawbacks and complications of the extraperitoneal approach include higher rates of cystotomy, subcutaneous emphysema, inadvertent entry into the peritoneal cavity, conversion to open or intraperitoneal Burch, and exclusion of patients with prior retropubic surgery.[21,22,25] Prior surgery is not a contraindication in some centers.[26,27] Additionally,

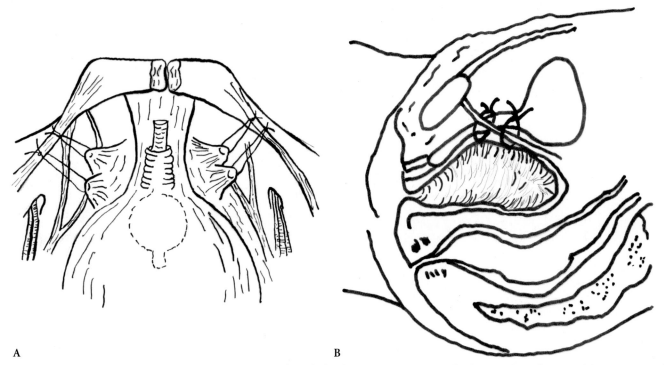

A   B

Figure 14.1.4. (**A**) The laparoscopic view of a completed Burch, with the classic two sutures per side elevating the pubocervical fascia up toward Cooper's ligament. (**B**) A parasagittal view of a Burch colposuspension.

extraperitoneal laparoscopy may result in greater degrees of carbon dioxide absorption than with transperitoneal surgery, increasing the chance of pneumomediastinum and pneumothorax.[25,28]

Extraperitoneal access can be via balloon dissector (Origin Medsystems, Menlo Park, CA), operative laparoscope, direct-vision trocar (Visaport, U.S. Surgical Corp., Norwalk, CT), regular trocar or the surgeon's finger (Origin Medsystems, Menlo Park, CA; Spacemaker, General Surgical Innovations, Cupertino, CA; Visaport, U.S. Surgical Corp, Norwalk, CT). The technique involves making a small incision in the abdominal midline that is opened down to the preperitoneal space. Then, a balloon or trocar is placed in this potential space and carbon dioxide is instilled, opening the space of Retzius. Two 5-mm ports are placed 3 cm above the suprapubic bone and 2 cm lateral to midline, avoiding the inferior epigastric vessels. The remainder of the procedure is carried out in the same fashion as if by the intraperitoneal approach.

As it is uncommon to see a patient who requires only a Burch colposuspension and no other procedure, the intraperitoneal approach is more common in most centers.[10,29–31] Most patients requiring pelvic reconstructive surgery need additional procedures, such as a vault suspension, paravaginal repair, anterior and/or posterior vaginal repair, or other intra-abdominal procedure.[32]

OUTCOMES AND COMPLICATIONS

Outcomes

When assessing colposuspension outcomes, it is important that one differentiate between procedures done with the true Burch–Tanagho technique and those done using surgical modifications called "Burch" procedures. The lack of differentiation accounts for the varied outcomes reported for the laparoscopic "Burch." The following studies represent the Burch–Tanagho procedure done laparoscopically. The importance of this distinction is made clear by a randomized, controlled study of 161 patients by Persson and Wolner-Hanssen [33] that demonstrated the importance of placing two sutures per side, as opposed to only one, in the laparoscopic Burch colposuspension. In their randomized, controlled trial, one group of 78 had a single suture placed on each side and the other group of 83 had two sutures on each side. At 1 year, the objective cure rate was 58% and 83%, respectively ($P = 0.001$). These findings support the necessity of two sutures per side for optimum results and give a possible reason for the high failure rate reported by many with a single suture per side. Persson stopped this study early because of the poor outcome with one suture per side.

Laparoscopic Burch success rates of 89% to 100% with 1- to 2-year follow-up have been reported in several series. [6–8,31,34–38] Liu [6] reported on 107 cases with a 97% subjective cure rate over a follow-up of 3 to 27 months. He had a 10% complication rate, including four cystotomies and one kinked ureter. Patient satisfaction was high.

Extracting data from six different studies [8–10,12,39,40], we had an objective cure rate of 91% at 1 year in 178 patients (Table 14.1.2). The majority of these patients were assessed postoperatively by multichannel urodynamic testing. In most of these studies, patients with detrusor instability and ISD were excluded. The de novo detrusor instability rate was less than 9% at 1- to 2-year follow-up, which is lower than that reported in most open Burch colposuspension studies.[41–44] Urodynamic testing demonstrated a significant increase in pressure transmission ratio, functional urethral length, and maximum bladder capacity. There was no significant change in maximal flow rate. Multiple

Table 14.1.2: Laparoscopic Burch Colposuspensions with Sutures

Study	Study Type*	Patients, No.	F/U, Months	Suture Type†	Suture No.	Cure Type of F/U‡	%	Major Comps, %
Abala et al. [5]	R	10	7	P	2	S	100	0
Liu [6]	R	107	3–27	P	4	O	97	7.4
Nezhat et al. [7]	R	62	8–30	P	4	O	100	10
Radomski & Herschorn [36]	P	34	17	P	4	S	85	11.8
Papasakelariou & Papasakelarious [31]	P	32	24	P	4	S	91	6.3
Saidi et al. [22]	P	70	12.9	P	4	S	91	NR
Ross [8]	P	32	12	DA	4	O	94	6.3
Ross [39]	P	35	12	DA	4	O	91	
Ross [9]	P	19	12	DA	4	O	93	
Ross [10]	P	48	24	DA	4	O	89	
Ross [12]	P	40	12	DA	4	O	89	
Ross [40]	P	87	>60	DA	4	O	84	

Comps, complications; F/U, follow-up; NR, not reported.
*Study type: R, retrospective; P, prospective.
†Suture type: P, permanent; DA, delayed absorbable.
‡Type of follow-up: S, subjective; O, objective.

concomitant laparoscopic procedures for total vaginal vault prolapse and GSI were performed in these patients [9], including the first reported laparoscopic paravaginal repair. With Burch alone, 97% of patients were discharged home in less than 24 hours and 93% voided spontaneously before discharge. When combined with multiple repairs, including laparoscopic hysterectomy, posterior vaginal repair, apical vault repair, and sacrocolpopexy, 91% of patients were discharged in less than 48 hours. There were two common factors in the few patients who experienced delayed voiding: substantial posterior repairs or a preoperative maximum flow rate of 15 mL per second or less.

In their retrospective study of 113 women, Cooper et al. [38] reported an 87% subjective cure rate with transperitoneal (93 patients) or extraperitoneal colposuspension (20 patients) after a mean follow-up of 8 months. Fourteen percent of these patients had mixed incontinence preoperatively. Complications included 10 cystotomies, one inferior epigastric vessel injury, one vaginal tear, one suture in the bladder, and one possible enterotomy. A subjective cure rate of 91% at 2 years has been reported by Papasakelariou.[31] Using a gasless extraperitoneal approach, Flax [45] obtained a 90% cure rate (defined as no pad usage) in 47 patients, with a mean follow-up of 8.2 months. We have a 83% objective cure rate at 5 years in 163 patients (Ross JW, unpublished data).

Complications

Most studies do not differentiate between major and minor complications. Overall complication rates range from 0% to greater than 20%.[5,34,38,46] Major complications include bladder injury, ureteral damage or kinking, abscess formation in the space of Retzius, failed procedure requiring additional surgery, de novo detrusor instability, new-onset ISD, urinary retention, voiding dysfunction, and a possible increase in posterior compartment prolapse.

In a study of 171 patients who underwent laparoscopic colposuspension, Speights et al. [47] found a 2.3% rate of lower urinary tract (LUT) injury. All four injuries noted were inadvertent cystotomies, two following prior MMK and staple–mesh procedures. All were in the dome of the bladder, and all were repaired laparoscopically at the time of surgery. No ureteral injuries were seen. These authors point out that this injury rate is lower than the 10% injury rate observed in a series of open colposuspensions.[48] A French center [49] reported a 3% injury rate in 104 laparoscopic Burch procedures: two cystotomies and one partial ureteral transection. Ferland and Rosenblatt [20] reported ureteral obstruction in two patients. Cystoscopy revealed a transmural passage of suture anterior and lateral to the urethral orifice in one patient and puckering and lateral displacement of the right trigone causing ureteral obstruction in the other. Both these injuries were on the patient's right side, similar to other reports.[50,51] Ferland suggests that when the surgeon stands on the patient's left side, suture placement tends to be lateral to medial with the right sutures, increasing the risk of entrapment of the right bladder wall and intramural ureter (Figure 14.1.5A). He recommends passing the right sutures medial to lateral to prevent this complication (Figure 14.1.5B), not seen on the left side because the natural suture placement is medial to lateral, away from the bladder for a right-handed surgeon.

Dwyer et al. [52] reported three bladder sutures and three ureteral obstructions by suture in 178 patients, giving an overall LUT injury rate of 3.4%. Cooper et al. [38] reported

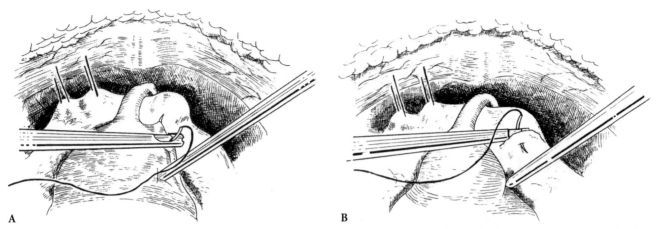

A   **B**

Figure 14.1.5. (**A**) The incorrect lateral-to-medial placement of a Burch suture, increasing the likelihood of ureteral compression.[19] (**B**) The correct medial-to-lateral placement of a Burch suture, decreasing the chance of ureteral or trigone injury.

10 cystotomies and one bladder suture in 113 patients, resulting in a 9.7% LUT injury rate. The overall laparoscopic injury rate for the LUT in all gynecologic cases ranges from 0.02% to 1.70%, which is not different from that seen in open gynecologic procedures. The inadvertent cystotomies reported were more common in patients with prior surgery in the space of Retzius and were bladder dome injuries easily recognized and repaired at the time of surgery. Several of these reports were made in the early development of these surgeons' laparoscopic skills. It is essential that intraoperative cystoscopy be performed to identify occult bladder and ureteral injuries.

Data on de novo detrusor instability are scant and not well reported in most studies. The range appears to be approximately 3% to 13%.[30,38,53–55] Cardozo et al. [44] reported a rate of 18.5% de novo detrusor instability in open Burch, supported by others.[42,56,57] Jarvis [58] reported a 9.6% mean incidence of laparoscopic de novo detrusor instability in a meta-analysis, with a range of 4% to 18%, and suggests this is less than that seen in open procedures. One possible explanation is less scarring in the laparoscopic procedure, although this has not been clearly demonstrated. In more than 300 cases, our de novo detrusor instability rate following laparoscopic Burch has been 8% (Ross JW, unpublished data, 2004).

Several published series report no significant voiding dysfunction with laparoscopic Burch.[6,10,37] Lavin et al. [55] found significantly less subjective voiding dysfunction after 2 years in laparoscopic versus open Burch: 16% and 52%, respectively. Su et al. [59] reported 4.3% voiding dysfunction in both laparoscopic and open Burch. No good long-term follow-up studies are available. As many as 20% of our patients report positional changes to empty their bladders in the first 6 months following laparoscopic Burch, usually with resolution by the end of the first year. Many studies have found less blood loss with laparoscopic Burch [22,55,59,60], early spontaneous voiding [22,59,61], and decreased length of stay in the hospital with laparoscopic Burch.[60]

Abdominal wall vascular injury is usually secondary to lateral trocar placement, resulting in inferior epigastric vessel damage [8], with a reported incidence of 0.5% and less frequent with cone-shaped or blunt trocars (0%) as compared with sharp-cutting

ones (0.83%).[62] Major bleeding requiring transfusion has been reported after injury to these vessels.[63]

A major advantage of laparoscopic surgery is the significantly lower ventral hernia formation.[62] Most hernias that develop at trocar sites are the result of lack of closure and are entirely preventable. The majority of these hernias are extraumbilical, the contents are usually small bowel (84.2%) and less often colon and omentum, and they often involve less than full herniation (Richter's hernia).[64] Margossian et al. [65] reported a preperitoneal herniation of the terminal ileum through the right lateral 10-mm port in which the fascia had been closed (Figure 14.1.6). We had a similar experience with a left 10-mm trocar site. To prevent this complication, it is necessary to close the peritoneum, muscle, and fascia at large trocar sites. Several companies have simple devices to use for this purpose (Inlet Closure Carter-Thomason Closure, Inlet Medical, Inc., Trumbull, CT; Endoclose, U.S. Surgical Corp., Norwalk, CT; Storz reusable fascial closure, Karl Storz, Culver City, CA), and the closure adds very little time to the operative procedure (Figure 14.1.7).

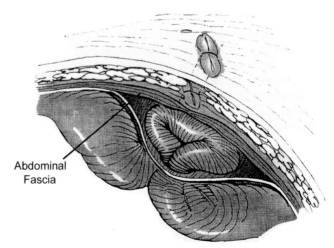

Abdominal
Fascia

Figure 14.1.6. An example of a Richter's hernia with small bowel entrapped between the abdominal muscles and fascia after improper closure of the trocar site.

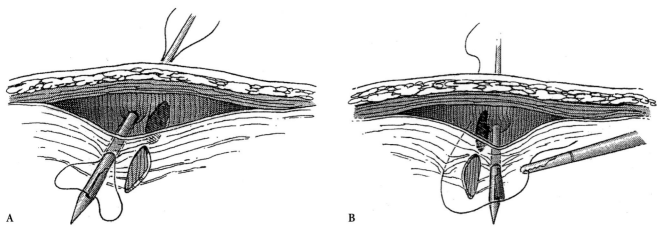

Figure 14.1.7. A trocar closure device needle passes a suture through the abdominal wall into the peritoneal cavity on one side of the trocar site. The needle is removed and passed through the opposite site, and the suture is grasped and pulled out to be tied extracorporeally.

COMPARATIVE RESULTS

Ideally, comparisons among surgical procedures should be based on the long-term results of direct, head-to-head studies in which cohorts of similar patients are prospectively randomized to undergo one of the different procedures to be studied, and follow-up evaluation is conducted by practitioners blinded as to which procedure the patients have undergone. Unfortunately, it is often hard to get patients to agree to randomization, making randomized, controlled studies difficult. The following studies compare the clinical outcomes of the laparoscopic Burch colposuspension to (1) open Burch colposuspension, (2) laparoscopic colposuspension with mesh and staples, (3) tension-free vaginal tape (TVT) suburethral sling, and (4) bone anchor suburethral slings.

Laparoscopic versus Open Burch Colposuspension

Six prospective randomized, controlled studies comparing open and laparoscopic colposuspension have been reported. Four of these studies used the classic Burch–Tanagho technique, and two modified the technique by using one suture per side in most cases.

In 2003, Cheon et al. [66] published results of a prospective randomized trial comparing laparoscopic and open Burch colposuspension. Forty-three patients were included in the open arm and 47 in the laparoscopic arm. In both arms, suture number and placement technique were identical. The authors found no difference in subjective or objective outcomes at 1-year follow-up, with subjective success of 86% versus 81% and objective success of 86% versus 85% in the open and laparoscopic arms, respectively.

The three other studies using the Burch–Tanagho technique were reported in abstract form only. Burton [67,68] published a randomized, controlled trial comparing open and laparoscopic Burch using absorbable suture (Table 14.1.3). In each arm of the study, 30 patients with moderate to severe GSI were followed for 3 years postoperatively. Superior results, in terms of both subjective and objective cure, were noted in the open arm during follow-up at both 1 and 3 years. At 1 year, objective cure, defined as no GSI on video cystourethrography, was observed in 97% of the open cases and 73% of the laparoscopic cases. The open procedure

maintained a 93% objective cure rate at 3 years, whereas the laparoscopic cure rate dropped to 60%. One criticism of this study is that Burton reported doing fewer than 20 laparoscopic procedures before the onset of the study – a rather small number given the steep and long learning curve of this relatively advanced procedure.

Two multicenter studies subsequently demonstrated no significant difference in outcomes between the two procedures. Carey et al. [69] randomized 200 patients with proven GSI to open or laparoscopic Burch colposuspension. He reported 6-month objective urodynamic cure rates of 80% and 69% and subjective success rates of 95% and 100% for the two procedures, respectively. Neither difference was statistically significant. In another multicenter trial involving 28 laparoscopic procedures and 34 open procedures, Summitt et al. [70] observed objective 1-year success rates of 92.9% for the laparoscopic Burch and 88.2% for the open Burch.[70] Saidi et al. [22] compared 70 patients with extraperitoneal laparoscopic Burch to 87 patients with open Burch and reported 91% and 92% objective cure rates, respectively, at 12 months.

Prospective randomized studies in which one stitch per side was used in the laparoscopic colposuspensions have shown mixed results. Su et al. [59] used two to three stitches per side for open colposuspensions but only one stitch per side in most of their laparoscopic colposuspensions. They reported objective cure rates – defined as dry on urodynamic testing – of 80.4% and 95.6% for laparoscopic and open colposuspensions, respectively, with a minimum 1-year follow-up. Interestingly, on a 1-hour extended pad test, the laparoscopic group showed a slightly greater improvement than the open group, though there was no statistically significant difference between the groups pre- or postoperatively. As discussed earlier in this section, the difference between one stitch and two per side likely accounts for the differences in outcomes. The Su group stated the reason for only one suture in the laparoscopic group was lack of room for suture placement through the laparoscope.

In 2001, Fatthy et al. [54] published a study in which one stitch per side was used for both the open and laparoscopic colposuspensions. There was no statistically significant difference in objective cure by urodynamic testing at 18-month follow-up,

Table 14.1.3: Comparison of Laparoscopic versus Open Burch Colposuspension

Author (Reference no.)	Study Type	N		Months Follow-up Mean (range)		Objective Cure (%)			Subjective Cure (%)		
		LSC	Open	LSC	Open	LSC	Open	p value	LSC	Open	p value
Burton (67, 68)	P	30	30	12/36	12/36	73/60	97/93	<0.05/<0.05	NR	NR	
Ross (8)	R	32	30	12	12	94	93	NS	NR	NR	
Polascik (60)	R	12	10	20.8 (8–29)	35.6 (11–50)	83	70	NS	NR	NR	
Su (59)	P	46	46	>12	>12	80*	96	0.04	NR	NR	
Lavin (55)	R	116	52	6	6	73	77		81	73	
Miannay (72)	R	36	36	12/24	12/24	NR	NR		79/68*	69/64	NS/NS
Saidi (22)	R	70	87	12.9 (2–24)	16.3 (6–30)	NR	NR		91.4	91.9	NS
Summitt (70)	P	28	34	12	12	93	88	NS	NR	NR	
Carey (69)	P	96	104	6	6	69	80	0.1	100	95	0.12
Fatthy (54)	P	34	40	18	18	88*	85*	NS	NR	NR	
Huang (71)	R	82	75	12	12	NR	NR		84	89	0.49

*Modified Burch with one suture per side
Study Type: P = Prospective, R = Retrospective
NR, Not reported

with no leakage reported in 87.9% of the laparoscopic cases and 85% of open cases.

Three published retrospective cohort studies compared open with laparoscopic Burch, and one used a one-suture-per-side technique for the laparoscopic colposuspensions. In a cohort study involving 30 patients followed prospectively in the laparoscopic arm and 32 patients reviewed retrospectively in the open arm, we reported objective cure rates at 1-year follow-up of 94% and 93%, respectively (Table 14.1.2).[8] That same year, Polascik et al. [60] published the results of a retrospective cohort study showing a subjective cure rate of 83% using the laparoscopic approach, with a mean follow-up of 20.8 months, versus 70% via the abdominal route, with a mean follow-up of 35.6 months. More recently, a retrospective cohort study by Huang and Yang [71] found subjective cure rates of 84% and 89% at 1 year for laparoscopic and open Burch colposuspensions, respectively. There were no statistically significant differences in cure rates between the two approaches in any of these three studies. Miannay et al. [72] also found no difference in subjective cure rates at 1- and 2-year follow-up between open and laparoscopic colposuspension, even though only one stitch per side was used in the laparoscopic cases.

Where reported, data seem to support the general perceived benefits to the patient of laparoscopy versus laparotomy. A shorter length of stay with the laparoscopic approach was noted in all but one study in which this parameter was investigated.[8,54,60,66,70–73] Likewise, less postoperative pain [54,60,66,72,73] and a quicker return to normal activity have

been noted in most laparoscopic groups.[8,54,72,73] Complications do not differ statistically where reported.

Laparoscopic Burch versus Tension-free Vaginal Tape Suburethral Sling

Ten years have passed since Ulmsten et al. [74] described their tension-free vaginal tape (TVT) mid-urethral sling procedure and reported on its early successes. The rapid rise in popularity of the TVT procedure coincided with, and has now mostly surpassed, the rise in popularity of the laparoscopic Burch colposuspension. Both procedures have their proponents. Advocates of the laparoscopic Burch colposuspension cite the longer track record of the Burch procedure, the ability to visualize the surgical field, and the lack of concern over erosion, whereas TVT advocates point to shorter duration of surgery, slightly shorter recovery, relative ease of the procedure, and perceived lower cost. To date, three prospective randomized, controlled trials have been published comparing the two procedures. Additionally, one large prospective randomized, controlled trial comparing TVT with the open Burch procedure has been published.

Persson et al. [75] in a prospective randomized trial comparing laparoscopic Burch with TVT, with 31 patients in the laparoscopic arm and 37 patients in the TVT arm, found no significant difference in efficacy between the two procedures (Table 14.1.4). Objective cure rates (defined as a negative short pad test) were 87% for the laparoscopic Burch and 89% for the TVT. Interestingly, subjective cure rates based on a

Table 14.1.4: Comparison of Laparoscopic Burch versus TVT

Author (year)	No. of Patients			Months Follow-up Mean (range)		Objective Cure (%)			Subjective Cure (%)		
	LSC	TVT	Type	LSC	TVT	LSC	TVT	p value	LSC	TVT	p value
Persson (76)	31	37	P	12	12	87	89	NS	52	57	NS
Usten (77)	23	23	P	13.5	11.3	82.6	82.6	NS	NR	NR	
Ward (78)	108*	137	P	24*	24	80*	81	NS	62*	60	NS

questionnaire were markedly lower in both groups — 52% and 57%, respectively.

Ustun et al. [76] reported results of a study of 46 patients with GSI randomized to undergo laparoscopic Burch ($n = 23$) or TVT ($n = 23$) who were followed for up to 24 months postoperatively. An objective cure rate of 82.6% was seen in both the laparoscopic Burch group, with a mean follow-up of 13.5 months, and the TVT group, with a mean follow-up of 11.3 months. Patients were considered "cured" if they were subjectively dry, had a negative stress test, and had had no leakage on urodynamic testing performed at 3 months. TVT patients did have a significant decrease in maximum urinary flow, suggesting more obstruction.

Most recently, Paraiso et al. [77] published the results of a randomized prospective trial comparing laparoscopic Burch colposuspension with TVT. Thirty-five patients were enrolled in the colposuspension arm and 36 in the TVT arm. At 1 year, 33 and 30 patients were available for follow-up in the colposuspension and TVT arms, respectively; at 2 years, 17 and 16 patients were evaluated in the respective arms. Objectively, urodynamic testing at 1 year demonstrated a higher rate of stress urinary incontinence (SUI) in the colposuspension group (18.8% vs. 3.2%) and a higher rate of detrusor overactivity in the TVT group (19.3% vs. 6.2%); however, neither result achieved statistical significance. Subjectively, although Kaplan–Meier survival curve analysis showed statistically significant earlier development of both stress and urge incontinence symptoms in the colposuspension group, there were no differences noted with regard to patient satisfaction, pad usage, Urinary Distress Inventory/Incontinence Impact Questionnaire (UDI/IIQ) scores, or incontinence episodes per week at either 1 or 2 years. The actual percentages of patients experiencing recurrent SUI symptoms at 1 and 2 years were not reported.

There are few studies reporting direct comparisons of complication rates, costs, length of stay, and perioperative convalescence between laparoscopic Burch colposuspension and TVT. In all three prospective comparison trials, a statistically shorter operative time was noted in the TVT group. For the most part, these data are consistent with noncomparative data on TVT, which typically show operating time shorter than that reported in most studies for laparoscopic Burch. In general, the more experienced the laparoscopist, the smaller the difference in time between the two procedures. Despite the shorter operating room (OR) time, Persson et al. [75] found the total cost of TVT to be higher than that of the laparoscopic Burch because of the high cost of the TVT set. Cost comparisons are notoriously difficult, not only because of differences in surgery times among different surgeons but also because OR costs per minute differ among different locations.

In the Paraiso study [77], overall complication rates were not significantly different between the two procedures, but it was noted that the TVT complications were of a more serious nature. Estimated blood loss, change in hematocrit, and days to catheter removal were similar between the TVT and colposuspension groups. There was a strong trend toward increased detrusor overactivity in the TVT group, but it did not reach statistical significance. There were no differences in voiding dysfunction. Persson et al. [75] did not address complications in their study. Numerous internal discrepancies in the Ustun group's paper [76] preclude making any conclusions regarding complication rates between the two procedures, although complications appeared to be few in both.

In a prospective randomized study comparing immediate outcomes of laparoscopic mesh colposuspension and TVT, Valpas et al. [78] noted no major differences in intraoperative or postoperative complications. They did find that return to normal voiding was quicker and pain medication use lower in the TVT group. Similarly, in a retrospective review of all 800 female anti-incontinence procedures performed at their hospital over 13 years, Debodinance et al. [79] found no major differences in intraoperative or immediate postoperative complications between TVT and laparoscopic Burch colposuspension; they did note, however, higher de novo voiding difficulties (18.5% vs. 0%) and de novo urgency (11.0% vs 4.8%) in TVT when compared with laparoscopic Burch colposuspension.

In summary, laparoscopic Burch colposuspension and the TVT sling appear to have similar efficacy, at least over the short to medium term. There are no published long-term data beyond 2 years. Operative time and time to resumption of normal voiding appear to be slightly shorter with TVT versus laparoscopic Burch colposuspension. Complication rates appear to be low with both procedures, though good comparative data are lacking.

Although TVT – and more recently, tension-free obturator tape (TOT) – have become the procedures of choice for many physicians because of the ease of performing the procedure, short operative time, excellent efficacy, and low complication rate, we feel laparoscopic Burch still has a role in the treatment of female stress incontinence. In particular, laparoscopic Burch colposuspension may be the procedure of choice in patients who are allergic to or do not desire polypropylene mesh, those in whom suprapubic bowel adhesions are suspected, those who have femoral–femoral bypass grafts, or those who are undergoing other laparoscopic procedures, especially paravaginal defect repair, in which placement of the colposuspension sutures would add relatively little time to the procedure.

REFERENCES

1. Vancaillie T, Schuessler W. Laparoscopic bladder neck suspension. *J Laparoendosc Surg.* 1991;13:169–173.

2. Burch JC. Urethrovaginal fixation to Cooper's ligament for correction of stress incontinence, cystocele, and prolapse. *Am J Obstet Gynecol.* 1961;81:281–290.

3. Burch JC. Cooper's ligament urethovesical suspension for stress incontinence. Nine years' experience – results, complications, technique. *Am J Obstet Gynecol.* 1968;100(6):764–774.

4. Tanagho E. Colpocystourethropexy: the way we do it. *J Urol.* 1976;116:751–753.

5. Abala D, Schuessler WE, Vancaillie TG. Laparoscopic bladder suspension for the treatment of stress incontinence. *Semin Urol.* 1992;10:222.

6. Liu C. Laparoscopic retropubic colposuspension (Burch procedure). A review of 58 cases. *J Reprod Med.* 1993;38:526–530.

7. Nezhat CH, Nezhat F, Nezhat CR, Rottenberg H. Laparoscopic retropubic cystourethropexy. *J Am Assoc Gynecol Laparosc.* 1994;1(4):339–349.

8. Ross J. Laparoscopic Burch repair compared to laparotomy Burch for cure of urinary stress incontinence. *Int Urogynecol J.* 1995;6:323–328.

9. Ross J. Techniques of laparoscopic repair of total vault eversion after hysterectomy. *J Am Assoc Gynecol Laparosc.* 1997;4:173–183.

10. Ross J. Multichannel urodynamic evaluation of laparoscopic Burch colposuspension for genuine stress incontinence. *Obstet Gynecol.* 1998;91:55–59.

11. Moore RD, Speights SE, Miklos JR. Laparoscopic Burch colposuspension for recurrent stress urinary incontinence. *J Am Assoc Gynecol Laparosc.* 2001;8(3):389–392.

12. Ross JW. 2001. Laparoscopic Burch colposuspension and overlapping sphincteroplasty for double incontinence. *JSLS.* 2001;5(3):203–209.

13. Jackson SL, Weber AM, Hull TL, Mitchinson AR, Walters MD. Fecal incontinence in women with urinary incontinence and pelvic organ prolapse. *Obstet Gynecol.* 1997;89(3):423–427.

14. Sultan AH, Kamm MA, Hudson CN, Thomas JM, Bartram CI. 1993. Anal-sphincter disruption during vaginal delivery. *N Engl J Med.* 1993;329:1905–1911.

15. Sultan A, Kamm MA, Hudson CN, Bartram CI. Third degree obstetric anal sphincter tears: risk factors and outcome of primary repair. *Br Med J.* 1994;308:887–891.

16. Goei R, Baeten C. Rectal intussusception and rectal prolapse: detection and postoperative evaluation with defecography. *Radiology.* 1990;174:124–126.

17. Healy JC, Halligan S, Reznek RH, Watson S, Phillips RK, Armstrong P. Patterns of prolapse in women with symptoms of pelvic floor weakness: assessment with MR imaging. *Radiology.* 1997;203(1):77–81.

18. El-Minawi AM, Howard FM. Iliohypogastric nerve entrapment following gynecologic operative laparoscopy. *Obstet Gynecol.* 1998;91(5):871.

19. Magrina JF. Complications of laparoscopic surgery. *Clin Obstet Gynecol.* 2002;45(2):469–480.

20. Ferland RD, Rosenblatt P. Ureteral compromise after laparoscopic Burch colpopexy. *J Am Assoc Gynecol Laparosc.* 1999;6(2):217–219.

21. Hannah SL, Roland B, Gengenbacher PM. Extraperitoneal retropubic laparoscopic urethropexy. *J Am Assoc Gynecol Laparosc.* 2001;8(1):107–110.

22. Saidi MH, Gallagher MS, Skop IP, Saidi JA, Sadler RK, Diaz KC. Extraperitoneal laparoscopic colposuspension: short-term cure rate, complications, and duration of hospital stay in comparison with Burch colposuspension. *Obstet Gynecol.* 1998;92(4 pt 1):619–621.

23. Lee CL, Yen CF, Wang CJ, Jain S, Soong YK. Extraperitoneal approach to laparoscopic Burch colposuspension. *J Am Assoc Gynecol Laparosc.* 2001;8(3):374–377.

24. Batislam E, Germiyanoglu C, Erol D. Simplification of laparoscopic extraperitoneal colposuspension: results of two-port technique. *Int Urol Nephrol.* 2000;32(1):47–51.

25. Meltomaa S, Haarala M, Makinen J, Kiilholma P. Endoscopic colposuspension with simplified extraperitoneal approach. *Tech Urol.* 1997;3(4):216–221.

26. Froeling FM, Deprest JA, Ankum WM, Mendels EL, Meijer DW, Bannenberg J. Controlled balloon dilatation for laparoscopic extraperitoneal bladder neck suspension in patients with previous abdominal surgery. *J Laparoendosc Adv Surg Tech A.* 2000;10(1):27–30.

27. Smith ML, Perry C. Simplified visual preperitoneal access to the space of Retzius for laparoscopic urethrocolpopexy. *J Am Assoc Gynecol Laparosc.* 1996;3(2):295–298.

28. Wolf J, Monk TG, McDougall EM, McClennan BL, Clayman RV. The extraperitoneal approach and subcutaneous emphysema are associated with greater absorption of carbon dioxide during laparoscopic renal surgery. *J Urol* 1995;154:959–963.

29. Liu CY, Paek W. Laparoscopic retropubic colposuspension (Burch procedure). *J Am Assoc Gynecol Laparosc.* 1993;1(1):31–35.

30. Liu CY. Laparoscopic treatment for genuine urinary stress incontinence. *Baillieres Clin Obstet Gynaecol.* 1994;8(4):789–798.

31. Papasakelariou C, Papasakelariou B. Laparoscopic bladder neck suspension. *J Am Assoc Gynecol Laparosc.* 1997;4(2):185–189.

32. Ross J. Apical vault repair, the cornerstone of pelvic vault reconstruction. *Int Urogynecol J.* 1997;8:146–152.

33. Persson J, Wolner-Hanssen P. Laparoscopic Burch colposuspension for stress urinary incontinence: a randomized comparison of one or two sutures on each side of the urethra. *Obstet Gynecol.* 2000;95:151–155.

34. Langebrekke A, Dahlstrom B, Eraker R, Urnes A. The laparoscopic Burch procedure. A preliminary report. *Acta Obstet Gynecol Scand.* 1995;74(2):153–155.

35. Carter JE. Laparoscopic bladder neck suspension. *Endosc Surg Allied Technol.* 1995;3(2):81–87.

36. Radomski SB, Herschorn S. Laparoscopic Burch bladder neck suspension: early results. *J Urol.* 1996;155(2):515–518.

37. Lam AM, Jenkins GJ, Hyslop RS. Laparoscopic Burch colposuspension for stress incontinence: preliminary results. *Med J Aust.* 1995;162(1):18–21.

38. Cooper MJ, Cario G, Lam A, Carlton M. A review of results in a series of 113 laparoscopic colposuspensions. *Aust N Z J Obstet Gynaecol.* 1996;36(1):44–48.

39. Ross JW. Two techniques of laparoscopic Burch repair for stress incontinence: a prospective, randomized study. *J Am Assoc Gynecol Laparosc.* 1996;3:351–357.

40. Ross J. 5-Year outcome of laparoscopic Burch for stress incontinence. *J Am Assoc Gynecol Laparosc.* 1999;6(3):48S.

41. Eriksen B, Hagen B, Eik-Nes SH, Molne K, Mjolnerod OK, Romslo I. Long-term effectiveness of the burch colposuspension in female urinary stress incontinence. *Acta Obstet Gynecol Scand.* 1990;69:45–50.

42. Feyereisl J, Dreher E. Long-term results after Burch colposuspension. *Am J Obstet Gynecol.* 1994;171:647–652.

43. Alcalay M, Monga A, Stanton SL. Burch colposuspension: a 10–20 year follow up. *Br J Obstet Gynaecol.* 1995;102(9):740–745.

44. Cardozo LD, Stanton SL, Williams JE. Detrusor instability following surgery for genuine stress incontinence. *Br J Urol.* 1979;51(3):204–207.

45. Flax S. The gasless laparoscopic Burch bladder neck suspension: early experience. *J Urol.* 1996;156(3):1105–1107.

46. Lobel R, Davis G. Long-term results of laparoscopic Burch urethropexy. *J Am Assoc Gynecol Laparosc.* 1997;4:341–345.

47. Speights SE, Moore RD, Miklos JR. Frequency of lower urinary tract injury at laparoscopic Burch and paravaginal repair. *J Am Assoc Gynecol Laparosc.* 2000;7(4):515–518.

48. Harris R, Cundiff GW, Theofrastous JP, Yoon H, Bump RC, Addison WA. The value of intraoperative cystoscopy in urogynecologic and reconstructive pelvic surgery. *Am J Obstet Gynecol.* 1997;177:1367–1371.

49. Soulie M, Salomon L, Seguin P, et al. Multi-institutional study of complications in 1085 laparoscopic urologic procedures. *Urology.* 2001;58(6):899–903.

50. Aslan P, Woo H. Ureteric injury following laparoscopic colposuspension. *Br J Obstet Gynaecol.* 1997;104:266–268.

51. Dietz HP, Wilson PD, Samalia KP, Walton J, Fentiman G. Ureteric injury following laparoscopic colposuspension. *Br J Obstet Gynaecol.* 1997;104(10):1217.

52. Dwyer PL, Carey MP, Rosamilia A. Suture injury to the urinary tract in urethral suspension procedures for stress incontinence. *Int Urogynecol J Pelvic Floor Dysfunct.* 1999;10(1):15–21.

53. Lawton V, Smith AR. Laparoscopic colposuspension. *Semin Laparosc Surg.* 1999;6(2):90–99.

54. Fatthy H, El Hao M, Samaha I, Abdallah K. Modified Burch colposuspension: laparoscopy versus laparotomy. *J Am Assoc Gynecol Laparosc.* 2001;8(1):99–106.

55. Lavin JM, Foote AJ, Hosker GI, Smith AR. Laparoscopic Burch colposuspension: a minimum of 2 year's follow up and comparison with open colposuspension. *Gynaecol Endosc.* 1998;7:251–258.

56. Bergman A, Ballard CA, Koonings PP. Comparison of three different surgical procedures for genuine stress incontinence: prospective randomized study. *Obstet Gynecol.* 1989;160:1102–1106.

57. Wang AC. Burch colposuspension vs. Stamey bladder neck suspension. A comparison of complications with special emphasis on detrusor instability and voiding dysfunction. *J Reprod Med.* 1996;41(7):529–533.

58. Jarvis GJ. Surgery for genuine stress incontinence. *Br J Obstet Gynaecol.* 1994;101(5):371–374.

59. Su T, Wang KG, Hsu CY, Wei HJ, Hong BK. 1997. Pospective comparison of laparoscopic and traditional colposuspensions in the treatment of genuine stress incontinence. *Acta Obstet Gynecol Scand.* 1997;76:576–582.

60. Polascik TJ, Moore RG, Rosenberg MT, Kavoussi LR. Comparison of laparoscopic and open retropubic urethropexy for treatment of stress urinary incontinence. *Urology.* 1995;45(4):647–652.

61. Kohli N, Jacobs PA, Sze EH, Roat TW, Karram MM. Open compared with laparoscopic approach to Burch colposuspension: a cost analysis. *Obstet Gynecol.* 1997;90(3):411–415.

62. Hashizume M, Sugimachi K. Needle and trocar injury during laparoscopic surgery in Japan. *Surg Endosc.* 1997;11:1198–1201.

63. Hurd W, Pearl ML, DeLancey JO, Quint EH, Garnett B, Bude RO. Laparoscopic injury of abdominal wall blood vessels: a report of three cases. *Obstet Gynecol.* 1993;82S:673–676.

64. Boike G, Miller CF, Spirtos NM. Incisional bowel herniations after operative laparoscopy: a series of nineteen cases and review of the literature. *Am J Obstet Gynecol.* 1995;172:1726.

65. Margossian H, Pollard RR, Walters MD. Small bowel obstruction in a peritoneal defect after laparoscopic Burch procedure. *J Am Assoc Gynecol Laparosc.* 1999;6(3):343–345.

66. Cheon W, Mak JH, Liu JY. Prospective randomised controlled trial comparing laparoscopic and open colposuspension. *Hong Kong Med J.* 2003;9(1):10–14.

67. Burton G. A randomized comparison of laparoscopic and open colposuspension. *Neurourol Urodyn.* 1993;13:497–498.

68. Burton G. A three year prospective randomized urodynamic study comparing open and laparoscopic colposuspension. *Neurourol Urodyn.* 1997;16:353–354.

69. Carey MR, Maher C, Cronish A, et al. Laparoscopic versus open colposuspension: a prospective multicentre randomised single-blind comparison. *Neurourol Urodyn.* 2000;19:389–390.

70. Summitt RL, Lucente V, Karram MM, Shull BL, Bent AE. Randomized comparison of laparoscopic and transabdominal Burch urethropexy for the treatment of genuine stress incontinence. *Obstet Gynecol.* 2000;95(4):S2.

71. Huang WC, Yang JM. Anatomic comparison between laparoscopic and open Burch colposuspension for primary stress urinary incontinence. *Urology.* 2004;63(4):676–681.

72. Miannay E, Cosson M, Lanvin D, Querleu D, Crepin G. Comparison of open retropubic and laparoscopic colposuspension for treatment of stress urinary incontinence. *Eur J Obstet Gynecol Reprod Biol.* 1998;79:159–166.

73. Kung RC, Lie K, Lee P, Drutz HP. The cost-effectiveness of laparoscopic versus abdominal Burch procedures in women with urinary stress incontinence. *J Am Assoc Gynecol Laparosc.* 1996;3(4):537–544.

74. Ulmsten U, Henriksson L, Johnson P, Varhos G. An ambulatory surgical procedure under local anesthesia for treatment of female urinary incontinence. *Int Urogynecol J.* 1996;7:81–86.

75. Persson J, Teleman P, Eten-Bergquist C, Wolner-Hanssen P. Cost-analyzes based on a prospective, randomized study comparing laparoscopic colposuspension with a tension-free vaginal tape procedure. *Acta Obstet Gynecol Scand.* 2002;81(11):1066–1973.

76. Ustun Y, Engin-Ustun Y, Gungor M, Tezcan S. Tension-free vaginal tape compared with laparoscopic Burch urethropexy. *J Am Assoc Gynecol Laparosc.* 2003;10(3):386–389.

77. Paraiso M, Walters MD, Karram MM, Barber MD. Laparoscopic Burch colposuspension versus tension-free vaginal tape: a randomized trial. *Obstet Gynecol.* 2004;104(6):1249–1258.

78. Valpas A, Kivela A, Penttinen J, et al. Tension-free vaginal tape and laparoscopic mesh colposuspension in the treatment of stress urinary incontinence: immediate outcome and complications – a randomized clinical trial. *Acta Obstet Gynecol Scand* 2003;82(7):665–671.

79. Debodinance P, Cosson M. Prolapse in the young woman: study of risk factors. *Gynecol Obstet Fertil.* 2002;31(3):320–321.

Section 14.2. Minimally Invasive Slings

Alan D. Garely and Cedric K. Olivera

More than 10 million women in the United States suffer from stress urinary incontinence.[1] Leakage of urine during coughing, laughing, or sneezing is the most common complaint. It is estimated that stress incontinence and other types of urinary incontinence cost over $9 billion per year in health care spending.[2–4] These costs include medical and surgical therapy but also paper products for adult diapers and nursing home care.

Stress incontinence is a disease that affects quality of life. This means that activities of daily living (shopping, working, and socializing) may be curtailed, which ultimately can affect the patient's psychological well-being. Depression is common, and afflicted individuals often isolate themselves to avoid embarrassing situations.[5–7] Nobody likes to smell like urine or to be around others who smell bad. Coupling this with injuries that occur from falls while trying to rush to the bathroom, especially at night, many of these people end up in nursing homes.

Significant improvement has been made in treating overactive bladder conditions with new anticholinergic medications. Stress incontinence has also seen tremendous improvements in treatment since the advent of the tension-free vaginal tape (TVT). Although the TVT was the first sling of its type, other approaches and methods have continued this momentum, making stress incontinence treatment a safe, quick, and outpatient procedure.

This section discusses the pathophysiology, work-up, and treatment of stress incontinence. Unless specified, the term *minimally invasive sling (MIS)* is used to discuss all the minimally invasive slings, regardless of brand or approach.

ANATOMY OF STRESS INCONTINENCE

The vagina receives its support in three dimensions (Figures 14.2.1, 14.2.2). The roof of the vagina (anterior wall) supports the bladder and the urethra. Distally, the connective tissue anterior to the vaginal epithelium attaches to the pubic bone. Laterally, the tissue (commonly called the pubocervical fascia) is attached to the arcus tendineus fascia via the fascia endopelvina. This arcus tendineus runs from the pubic symphysis to the ischial spine bilaterally. The obturator internus muscle and the iliococcygeus muscle (part of the levator ani) are separated by the arcus tendineus (Figures 14.2.3, 14.2.4). Anterior wall defects are called cystoceles and may be further divided into central and lateral defects.

If the anterior vaginal wall connective tissue separates from the arcus tendineus fascia on either one or both sides, this is considered a lateral or paravaginal defect. If the lateral attachments are well supported but a "drop" in the anterior wall is seen, this is a central or midline defect (Figure 14.2.5).

The apex of the vagina is supported by the cardinal ligament and the uterosacral ligaments. The cardinal ligament runs across the pelvis from ischial spine to ischial spine, and lends support by encircling the cervix. This forms a critical component of the pericervical ring at the level of the ischial spines, along with the pubocervical fascia, the pubourethral ligaments, the uterosacral ligaments, and the rectovaginal septum. The cardinal ligament bridges the pubocervical fascia to the posterior rectovaginal fascia (which serves a similar purpose on the posterior vaginal wall). The uterosacral ligaments join posteriorly to the cervix and attach to the sacrum.[8–10]

When the supportive tissue of the vaginal apex becomes injured or attenuated, apical support decreases and the vagina starts to invert like an inside-out pocket. This is called an enterocele. As the apex further descends toward the introitus, the anterior vaginal wall usually separates from the lateral arcus tendineus fascia, exacerbating the anterior wall cystocele.

Posteriorly, the vaginal connective tissue separates the rectal wall from the vaginal epithelium. Like the anterior vaginal wall, the posterior connective tissue is also attached laterally, but to the arcus tendinous via the fascia endopelvina. Breaks or attenuation of this tissue create a rectocele.

PHYSIOLOGY OF STRESS INCONTINENCE

In a normal anatomic pelvis at rest, the closure pressure of the urethra (Pu) exceeds the intravesical pressure (Pves). This means that the pressure inside the bladder is lower than the pressure inside the urethra. As long as Pu is greater than or equal to Pves, no leakage of urine should occur. It is very important for Pu to be less than Pves when needed, or otherwise normal micturition cannot occur. Our problem begins when Pves is greater than Pu at times in between voluntary voiding. This indicates incontinence.

Assuming the patient is not voiding intentionally, to maintain an intact continence mechanism, the Pu must always be greater than Pves, even under events of stress (i.e., coughing, laughing, and sneezing). In the perfectly intact pelvis, this means that the intra-abdominal pressures are equally transmitted to both the bladder and the urethra, thereby canceling out the momentary rise in pressure. This can work only if the urethra is well supported. This is easy to picture by thinking about a garden hose on a driveway. If water is running through the hose and you step on it, the water will stop. If the same hose is placed on a trampoline, which lacks support, it is unlikely that stepping on the hose will stop the flow of water. Applying this principle to the urethra and

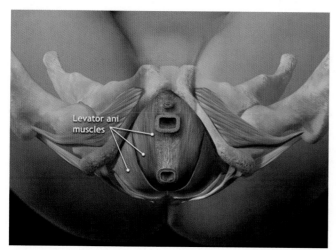

Figure 14.2.1. Frontal view showing vaginal support and surrounding structures. (Permission granted by Gynecare.)

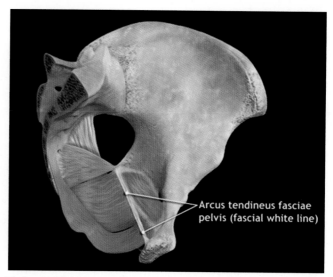

Figure 14.2.3. Arcus tendineus fascia pelvis (the white line). (Permission granted by Gynecare.)

bladder neck, it becomes clear how a cystocele can increase the risk of incontinence.[11–13]

Not all stress incontinence will occur in the presence of a cystocele, and not all cystoceles are accompanied with stress incontinence. The urethra itself has an intrinsic resting tone, which is often high enough to compensate for lack of anterior wall support. The converse of this occurs in patients with stress incontinence in whom the anterior vaginal wall support is excellent. In these cases, the intrinsic resting tone of the urethra is poor, despite a solid "backboard" (Figure 14.2.6).

The three factors known to increase the risk of developing stress incontinence are age, genetic predisposition to weak connective tissue (hernia formation), and a history of vaginal childbirth. Looking at each of these individually, we can see how they influence the continence mechanism.

As the pelvic floor ages, even intact support may begin to weaken. This is probably why stress incontinence increases with age. Factors such as decreased estrogen may contribute, but the studies are not conclusive and are often contradictory.

For reasons not completely understood, certain ethnicities appear to be at a higher risk of incontinence secondary to connective tissue strength. Although studies are ongoing, this increased risk is most likely related to collagen composition and deposition. Populations from northern Europe seem predisposed, whereas prevalence in African-based populations is lower.

Vaginal deliveries cause both stretching and crushing of the pelvic floor tissues, muscles, and nerves. Some women recover without any sequelae. Like a rubber band stretched to its limits, the pelvic floor does not always "snap" back to its original position. If the injury involves nerves, the intrinsic resting tone of the urethra may decrease. If it involves the muscles, a cystocele may develop, decreasing anterior wall support.

EVOLUTION OF SURGICAL REPAIR

Before 1996, the approach to stress incontinence surgery was determined more by specialty than by technique and outcome. The gynecologists favored anterior repairs and retropubic urethropexies (MMK and Burch), whereas urologists chose needle suspensions (Stamey, Raz, and Pereyra) and open slings.

Anterior Repair

Anterior repairs (Kelly plication) are done transvaginally at the time of other vaginal surgery and are often combined with vaginal hysterectomy and posterior repairs. These procedures rarely are performed with cystoscopy, as most gynecologists do not have privileges to use the cystoscope. The anatomic basis of the anterior repair is to plicate the connective tissue under the bladder and urethra (just anterior to the vaginal epithelium). The vaginal epithelium lying lateral to the plication is trimmed and closed with a running or interrupted absorbable suture (Figure 14.2.7). This pulls the tissue together under the midline of the anterior vaginal wall. This increased tension under the bladder neck and

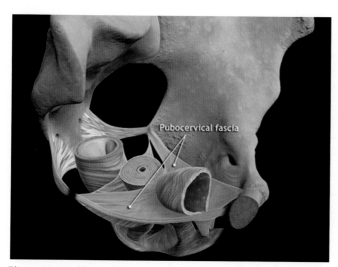

Figure 14.2.2. 3D model showing pubocervical fascia and anterior vaginal wall support. (Permission granted by Gynecare.)

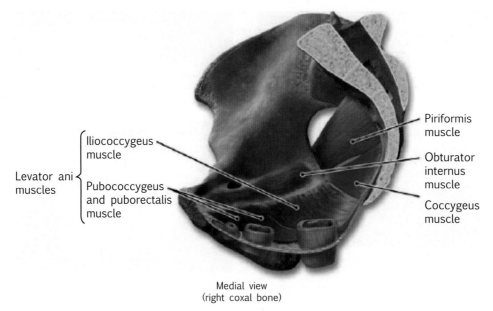

Figure 14.2.4. Iliococcygeus and obturator internus muscle forming arcus tendineus fascia pelvis. (Permission granted by Gynecare.)

urethra was thought to increase the urethral closure pressure, decreasing stress incontinence.

Two problems with this approach were long-term success rates and anatomic distortion of the vagina. Objective cure rates with more than 2 years of follow-up ranged from 54% to 79% [14–16], with some studies showing failure as high as 80%. Because the anterior vaginal wall is "pulled" together in the midline, the pubocervical fascia is also pulled off of its lateral attachment from the arcus tendineus fascia. Detaching tissue from the arcus tendineus causes the most common anterior wall defect, called a lateral cystocele. It is probably not a coincidence that cystoceles are associated with stress incontinence, as the bladder neck and urethra lose support. The anterior repair has a place in repairing central cystoceles, but its use in stress incontinence is not supported by the data.

Retropubic Urethropexies

Retropubic urethropexies are based on the concept of urethral stabilization. Suture is placed next to the urethra starting at the bladder neck and is often followed by additional sutures lateral to the urethra. These sutures are then placed through the periosteum of the symphysis (MMK) or through Cooper's ligament (Burch). The suture tension is tied so that the bladder neck rests with little elevation. This is done by creating a "suture bridge" effect with the suture. The physiologic goal is to "fool" the urethra into behaving as if it were at rest during stress events (Figure 14.2.8).

In properly selected cases, success rates should be greater than 80% at 5 years. Although success rates are similar for the MMK and Burch, the MMK is rarely associated with osteitis pubis, an often debilitating and chronic disorder. Retropubic urethropexies require dissection of the space of Retzius (retropubic space). This

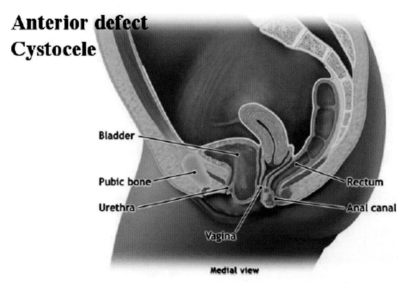

Figure 14.2.5. Central anterior wall defect known as a cystocele. (Permission granted by Gynecare.)

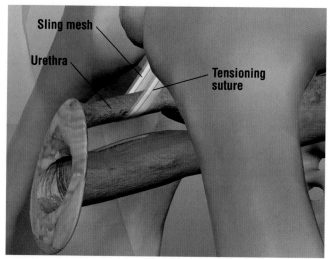

Figure 14.2.6. Sling providing "backboard" support under urethra. (Permission granted by AMS.)

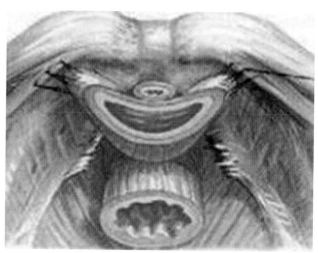

Figure 14.2.8. Retropubic urethropexy (Burch). (Permission granted by AMS.)

area frequently has a vast plexus of superficial veins that may cause a rapid and profound blood loss. Unless this area is approached laparoscopically, an abdominal incision is required.

Stress incontinence can be objectively graded on a continuum ranging from mild to severe by looking at urethral closure pressures or leak point pressures. The lower the pressure, the lower the intrinsic resting tone of the urethra. We know that stress incontinence with an objective assessment of good intrinsic urethral resting tone (higher pressure) will respond well to a retropubic urethropexy. Cases with poor urethral tone are associated with higher failure rates and should probably be treated with a sling.

Failures in this group occur because there is a lack of support directly under the urethra. Lateral support is just not enough to coapt the urethra during stress events.

Although cystoscopy has not been the standard of care with retropubic urethropexies, recent studies have shown urinary tract injury rates as high as 4.9%.[17–19] These injuries include placement of sutures into the bladder and urethra and kinking of the ureters. Permanent suture in the bladder acts as a nidus for stone formation. Given these injuries, cystoscopy should be required to assure decreased morbidity.

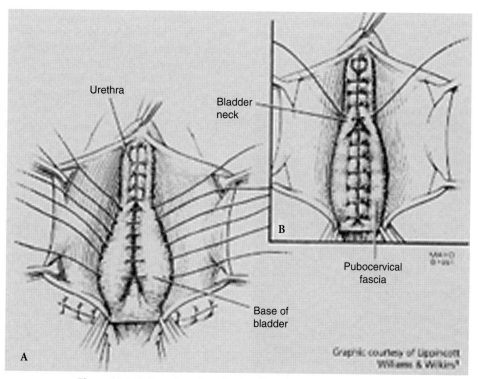

Figure 14.2.7. Anterior colporrhaphy. (Permission granted by AMS.)

Needle Suspensions

In the past, urologists have favored needle suspensions. Sutures are placed next to the bladder neck and urethra (like a retropubic urethropexy) and then anchored to the rectus fascia instead of the pubic symphysis. Depending on the way the suture is secured next to the bladder neck (whether with a pledget or just suture) determines the name of the approach (Raz, Stamey, or Pereyra). The sutures are pulled up to the rectus fascia with a "needle." The needle is a long, thin metal rod that is sharp enough to puncture through the intervening layers between vagina and rectus. This approach also requires an abdominal skin incision.

Overall success rates for needle suspensions are 81%.[20–22] This rate is lower than that of retropubic suspensions at 85%.[20–22] The limitations for needle suspensions are similar to those for the retropubic urethropexies, including the lack of direct suburethral support. Although the MMK and Burch are "fixed" to immobile tissue, the needle suspensions are totally dependent on mobile, distensible tissue. This contributes to failure on two fronts. First, it gives two separate places for suture to pull or rip out. Second, it gives two places for the soft tissue to stretch, decreasing the ability to support the urethra.

Placement of the sutures with the needle is done blindly and with a tactile feel for anatomic landmarks. Cystoscopy must be performed after each pass of the needle to ensure urinary tract integrity.

Open Slings

Before the advent of the MIS, the traditional sling was considered the domain of the urologist or specially trained urogynecologist. This "open" sling required opening the vaginal epithelium under the bladder neck, cutting the abdomen, and placing a sling or hammock under the bladder neck and urethra (Figure 14.2.9). Although many materials were used for the sling, the most common material was autologous fascia or muscle. Fascia was usually taken from the upper thigh (fascia lata) or the abdomen (rectus

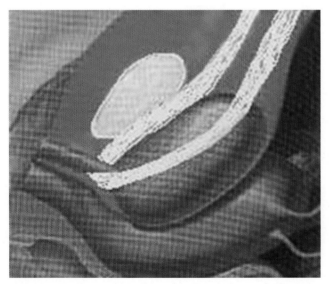

Figure 14.2.9. Sling under bladder neck. (Permission granted by AMS.)

fascia). The rectus muscle was used because of its proximity to the vagina. The sling was then brought above the rectus fascia and then tied either to the fascia or across the midline to the other end of the sling.

Because the sling was tied down, the risk of urinary retention was high. Traditional slings were also associated with infections and blood loss because of the dissection needed to properly place the sling. When certain nonabsorbable materials were used as the sling substrate (mesh made of Prolene, Marlex, Gore-Tex, etc.), erosion into the urethra and vagina was common. Muscle herniation was also noted in the upper thigh and abdomen, depending on the site of fascial harvest.

Traditional slings may be used for treatment of the entire range of stress incontinence, and success rates can exceed 85%. This "take-all-comers" flexibility, along with a high success rate, served as the impetus for developing a safer, easier, and faster sling. This would also include making the sling "minimally invasive."

MINIMALLY INVASIVE SLINGS

The advent of the MIS was initially met with a high degree of skepticism. Long-term success was unknown. Placing the sling at the mid-urethra instead of the bladder neck was a new idea. The choice of material was also controversial given the history of urethral erosions with Prolene mesh. Medical "politics" also contributed to doubts about the MIS. Urologists had been the surgeons doing slings, but the MIS was developed by a gynecologist and was being taught to gynecologists. The rate-limiting step of the procedure that kept it from most gynecologists was the absolute need to do a cystoscopy during the case.

Westby and other authors [23–25] postulated that when looking at a urethral pressure profile, the mid-portion of the urethra has the highest resting closure pressure. It is easier to augment coaptation at the area that already has the highest intrinsic pressure. Anatomically, support of the mid-urethra causes less distortion and less "kinking" than does support at the distal meatus or at the bladder neck.

By applying the principles of tension-free surgery, the sling is placed under the urethra, with a spacer temporarily interposed between sling and urethra. The sling is then pulled through the intervening tissue and not tied or secured to any tissue. This is the crucial step in the "tension-free" description.

Since the first TVT was introduced by Ulmsten, several similar devices have come to market. The first generation of MIS was based on retropubic placement. The main differences between each proprietary sling are in the weave of the mesh, the type of material used, and whether the sling is placed by pushing the mesh from the vagina through the abdominal incisions or the mesh is pulled up from the abdominal side.

The second-generation MIS used a transobturator approach instead of passing through the retropubic space.[26–28] Again, different proprietary products strive to achieve the same result with variations on material and on direction of placement.

The third generation of MIS is readjustable. This allows the sling to be tightened or loosened either during the surgery or at any time after. All three types of sling are described in detail in the following paragraphs.

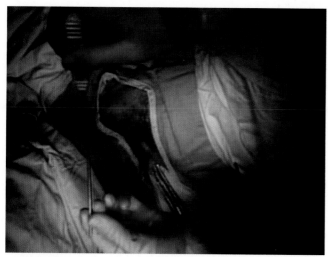

Figure 14.2.10. First-generation TVT device. (Permission granted by Gynecare.)

TENSION-FREE VAGINAL TAPE

In 1998, Ulmsten et al. presented "A Multicenter Study of Tension-Free Vaginal Tape (TVT) for Surgical Treatment of Stress Urinary Incontinence."[29] It was noted by Ulmsten that "a long series of experiments proceeding the current TVT operation have shown that placing a sling under the midurethra without tension is the best way to provide a dynamic kinking of the organ, and hence to close the urethra in stress situations."[30–32] This led to a patent by Dr. Ulmsten and subsequent sale of the device to Johnson & Johnson. The device is marketed under the name TVT (Figure 14.2.10).

Preoperative Evaluation

No patient should ever have a stress incontinence procedure unless stress incontinence is visually witnessed. Without actually seeing the leakage, you run the risk of operating on a patient who really has urge incontinence. If the patient does not have stress incontinence, her urge incontinence symptoms may worsen because of the obstruction placed on the urethra. Although bedside urodynamic evaluation done with a simple catheter and syringe are usually reliable, complex testing should be done to help aid in determining the final tensioning of the sling. Patients with very low leak point pressures will probably need the sling to abut the suburethral tissue, whereas patients with higher leak point pressures can have the sling placed looser.

Slings work best when placed under the urethra in the presence of a well-supported anterior vaginal wall. Although it is difficult to quantitate when a cystocele is too big, the surgeon must be mindful that the anterior vaginal wall will not rotate around the sling (which stabilizes the urethra) like a fulcrum, contributing to urethral kinking and urinary retention. Proper surgical planning may mean that the patient is not a candidate for an isolated sling but may require a larger pelvic reconstructive surgery.

Although slings may be considered minor outpatient procedures, they are still surgical procedures done with anesthesia and associated risks. These operations should be taken seriously, with great attention paid to the patient's medical history and medications. Proper planning will help ensure a safe and effective operation.

Technique

When doing these cases for the first time, general anesthesia is essential. This will keep the patient absolutely still, allowing the surgeon to concentrate on the dissection and placement of the sling. Even in the hands of an experienced surgeon, a moving patient makes it hard to achieve an optimal outcome. After the surgeon is comfortable with the procedure, a combination of local anesthesia with sedation may be attempted if necessary. The entire procedure should take less than an hour, and patients recover rapidly with few side affects from general anesthesia. If the sling is to be done with other gynecologic procedures, local anesthesia with sedation may not be possible.

Local anesthesia with epinephrine is given to all patients regardless of whether the procedure is done under general anesthesia or sedation. The epinephrine will greatly reduce blood loss by causing vasoconstriction. The local component will decrease pain sensation by numbing the pain receptors prior to incision. Vasopressin may also be substituted for the epinephrine component to achieve hemostasis.

The patient is brought to the operating room and placed in the dorsal lithotomy position. Positioning the patient's buttock a little lower than usual will aid in visualization of the field and placement of the sling. The patient is prepped and draped for combined abdominal/vaginal approach surgery. The drape should also have a cysto bag to help prevent a flood during the cystoscopy portion of the procedure.

A preoperative dose of antibiotic should be given intravenously. A weighted speculum is placed in the vagina to expose the anterior vaginal wall. A marking pen is used to make two 0.5-cm marks 5 cm apart, symmetric to the midline, at the level of the pubic symphysis. Lidocaine with epinephrine or Marcaine with epinephrine should be injected at the marked spots and into the retropubic space along the pubic symphysis. The same anesthetic should be injected under the urethra and lateral to the urethra aiming at the ipsilateral shoulder. An 18F Foley catheter should then be placed into the bladder and allowed to drain the urine. Placing the catheter before injecting can inadvertently cause the catheter balloon to pop, requiring a new Foley.

A #14 surgical knife should be used to make small puncture incisions at the marked spots on the abdomen. The knife should then be used to cut a 3-cm vertical incision under the urethra starting just distal to the urethra vesical junction. Using a very sharp plastic surgical Metzenbaum or tenotomy scissors, flaps should be gently developed on the left and right sides of the midline incision. Injuries that occur with sharp dissection are almost always easier to repair than those created with blunt dissection or spreading. Care should be taken not to go too deep, as this may cause immediate entry into the urethra or bladder, or may contribute to delayed erosion in these structures. Superficial dissection may lead to cutting through the vaginal epithelium. This is called a "button hole." A button hole makes it easy to place the sling through the inside of the flap, out into the vagina, and then back into the flap. This will leave the patient with a small piece of exposed mesh in the vagina. Dissection should stop short of perforating into the retropubic space (Figure 14.2.11).

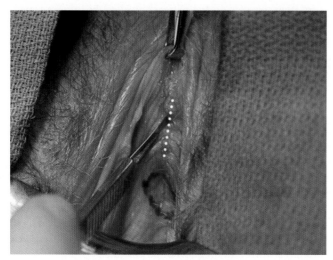

Figure 14.2.11. Initial dissection of vagina for placement of a midurethral sling. (Permission granted by AMS.)

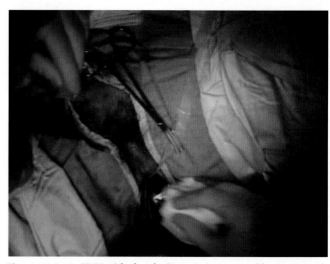

Figure 14.2.13. TVT with sheath. (Permission granted by Gynecare.)

The rigid catheter guide is placed into the Foley, and the catheter is deflected to the same side that the first needle will be passed. Assuming the first pass is on the left side, the Foley is deflected to the left. Because of limited space, the catheter and guide may be clamped onto the drape at an angle slightly above the horizontal plain of the urethra. The rigid catheter guide deflects the uterovesical junction away from the TVT needle when it is passed. This decreases the risk of injury to the urethra and bladder (Figure 14.2.12).

The TVT device consists of two separate needles swedged onto either end of a strip of Prolene mesh. This is covered by two overlapping pieces of a plastic sheath. The overlapping area of the two sheaths can be clamped with one click from a hemostat to prevent early separation of the sheaths. This decreases the possibility that the mesh will twist or stretch. Other than aiding in sling placement, the sheath protects the sling from exposure to vaginal flora, thereby decreasing the risk of surgical infection in the surrounding tissue (Figure 14.2.13).

The TVT needle on one side is screwed tightly into the reusable TVT handle. Using a toothed forceps, the cut vaginal edge on the left side is lifted. Working in the left flap, the surgeon should use his or her left hand to hold the TVT handle and position the tip of the needle into the flap. With the surgeon's right hand, two fingers should be placed into the vagina, outside the flap. The right hand should then cradle the curve of the TVT needle, aiming it at a 45° angle toward the left shoulder. The tip should be adjacent to the pubic symphysis. The surgeon's left hand should be exerting gentle pressure while the right hand guides the needle into the retropubic space (Figure 14.2.14).

Once the pubocervical fascia is perforated, a "give" should be palpated and the pushing halted. This indicates that the TVT needle tip is safely anterior and lateral to the urethra and bladder. The angle of the TVT handle should then be corrected to aim toward the patient's head and not the shoulder. The tip can be gently "walked" off the symphysis with a touch-and-push technique (Figure 14.2.15).

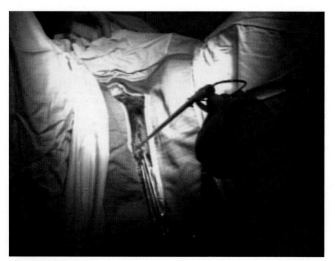

Figure 14.2.12. TVT Foley catheter guide. (Permission granted by Gynecare.)

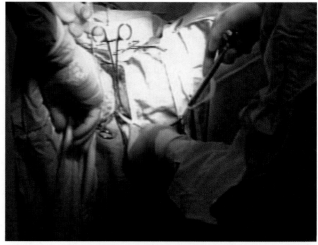

Figure 14.2.14. Placement of the TVT needle. (Permission granted by Gynecare.)

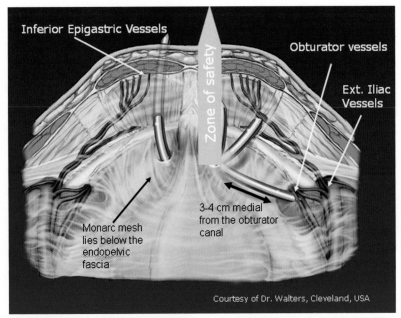

Figure 14.2.15. TVT needle next to pubic bone. (Permission granted by AMS.)

The surgeon should identify his or her incision on the left side of the patient's abdomen and aim for that spot. With a little effort, the TVT needle should be easily pushed through the incision and the procedure halted. The rigid catheter guide should be removed and the Foley opened to drainage. Evaluation of urine color may sometimes signal a bladder perforation. Even in the presence of a perforation, the urine is often clear because the injuries are small and do not always bleed. The bladder should be filled with a least 300 mL of water, but more fluid is preferable as it is easy to miss "in–out" injuries in the bladder that catch a small area of tissue. A 70° cystoscope should be used to visualize the bladder and urethra. Most bladder injuries occur at the 10 and 2 o'clock positions.[33–35] If an injury is detected, the needle should be removed, the bladder emptied, and the entire procedure for that side restarted. Gentle movement of the TVT handle should show the TVT needle gliding in the tissue lateral to the bladder. If the tissue moves with the needle, the placement is probably too close to the bladder, and the needle should be removed and replaced.

If the needle was well placed, the bladder is emptied with the Foley, and the TVT handle is unscrewed from the TVT needle. The needle is pushed up, pulled through the abdominal incision, and left to rest on the abdomen.

The rigid catheter guide is reinserted into the Foley, and the same procedure is done on the right side, but with reversal of the surgeon's hands and displacement of the catheter guide to the right side.

Once both needles are safely resting on the abdomen, the surgeon or assistant can slowly pull up equally on both needles until the sheath is about 2 cm from the urethra. The hemostat may be removed, and a spacing device should be placed between the sheath and urethra. The wide part of a closed Metzenbaum or a #8 Hegar dilator may be used. The needles should be cut free from the sheaths and mesh. The sheath on each side should be grasped with a Kelly clamp. To avoid injury to the mesh, one arm of the clamp is placed on the outside and one arm on the inside of the sheath (Figure 14.2.16).

While the surgeon holds countertraction between the sheath and the urethra, the Kelly clamps are pulled upward, causing the sheaths to separate in the midline, leaving the mesh sitting under the urethra with no "tension" (Figure 14.2.17).

The mesh is cut at the abdominal incisions, pulling up gently on the mesh and pushing down with the suture scissors on the skin. This ensures that the mesh does not irritate the incision site. The mesh is inspected and palpated through the vaginal incision to ensure that it is not too tight. The vaginal incision is then closed with a 2-0 absorbable running, nonlocking suture. The skin incisions can be closed with Dermabond (Ethicon, Inc.; Figure 14.2.18).

Personal preference will determine how and when the Foley catheter is removed. Some surgeons will leave the operating room with the Foley out and then wait up to 4 hours or until the patient

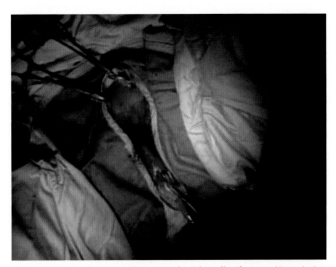

Figure 14.2.16. TVT sheaths grasped with Kelly clamps. (Permission granted by Gynecare.)

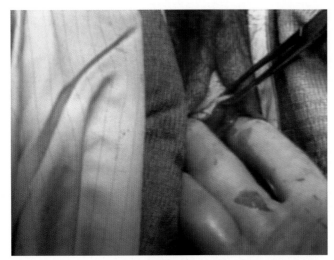

Figure 14.2.17. Midurethral placement of tension-free mesh. (Permission granted by Gynecare.)

feels the need to void (whichever comes first) to do a passive voiding trial. If the patient is able to void, the bladder is catheterized within 15 minutes to check for the postoperative residual. A residual less than 75 mL is usually considered acceptable.

Others will leave the Foley in place at the completion of the case and then wait about 1 to 2 hours before doing an active voiding trial. This involves filling the bladder with water through the Foley until the patient feels full, or until at least 200 mL is instilled. The catheter is removed, and the patient voids within 15 minutes into a graduated hat or cup. The voided amount is subtracted from the instilled amount for the postvoid residual. Experience has shown that the surgical assistants and recovery room nurses who manage these patients prefer the active voiding trial as it creates less work for them.

Variations

The SPARC device (American Medical Systems) is also a retropubic MIS but uses the "top-down" approach. Instead of pushing

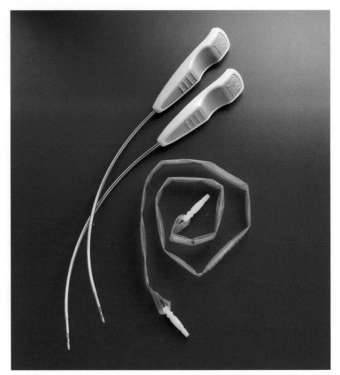

Figure 14.2.19. SPARC system. (Permission granted by AMS.)

the mesh up through the abdominal incisions, the SPARC needles are pushed down into the anterior vaginal wall incision and the mesh is pulled up. Urologists who have experience with needle suspensions often feel more comfortable with this approach than through the vagina (Figure 14.2.19).

Numerous studies have shown that the SPARC has success and complication rates similar to those for the TVT.[36,37] One study showed a lower success rate, but this has not been duplicated in other studies.[38] Because of the learning curve needed for all these procedures, it is difficult to judge outcome unless the surgeon has extensive experience with a specific technique before initiation of a study.

TRANSOBTURATOR TAPE

In 2001, an article was published by Delorme [26] that described the next generation of suburethral slings. Because of the anatomic position, this was called the transobturator urethral suspension or transobturator tape (TOT) procedure. The original abstract states: "This tape has two original features: its non-woven polypropylene structure is coated with silicone on the urethral surface in order to limit retraction of polypropylene and to establish a barrier to extension of periurethral fibrosis. Transmuscular insertion, through the obturator and puborectalis muscles, reproduces the natural suspension fascia of the urethra while preserving the retropubic space"(Figures 14.2.20, 14.2.21).

The concept of avoiding the retropubic space was very appealing for many reasons. Most complications associated with the TVT procedure (see below) would be decreased, if not eliminated. Going through the obturator fossa would be associated with a new set of problems, but anatomically, none seemed as

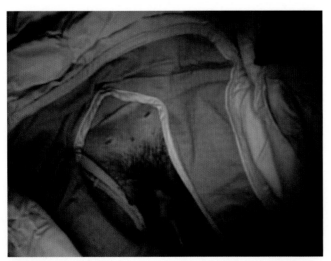

Figure 14.2.18. Sutureless closure of incision with glue. (Permission granted by Gynecare.)

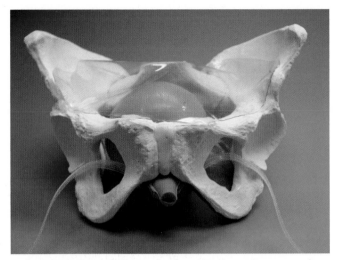

Figure 14.2.20. Transobturator passage of TOT avoiding space of Retzius. (Permission granted by Caldera.)

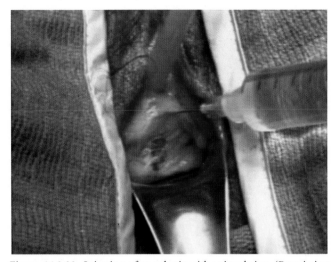

Figure 14.2.22. Injection of anesthetic with epinephrine. (Permission granted by Gynecare.)

severe as those with the TVT. Similar to the TVT, the TOT was embraced rapidly by the medical community, with little or no long-term data with regard to safety or success. Despite these limitations, the technique appears to be as good as the original TVT, with fewer injuries.

Technique

Preoperative preparation and anesthesia are the same as those for the TVT. The patient is positioned at the end of the table in the dorsal lithotomy position. A weighted speculum is placed on the posterior vaginal wall. A marking pen is used to make a transverse line at the level of the urethra onto the vulva. "X" marks are made 2 cm superior to this line on both sides of the midline just at the medial aspect of the obturator foramen. This spot is usually easily palpable, even in obese patients. Anesthetic with epinephrine is injected at these two spots. Using a small-blade scalpel, stab incisions are made at the injection spots.

The same anesthetic is injected under the urethra and lateral toward the obturator foramen (aiming at a 45° angle). A #14 blade scalpel is used to make a 3-cm vertical incision under the urethra. The incision is safely made without entering the urethra if the vaginal epithelium blanches white from the injection. This will also decrease significant blood loss (Figure 14.2.22).

Using either the tenotomy or plastic surgical Metzenbaum scissors, flaps are developed toward the obturator foramen on both sides. Once the flap is started, the space should accommodate the diameter of an index finger. Gentle digital dissection to the obturator foramen will make the operation safer because this will limit the distance that the TOT needle will be out of sight or palpation (Figure 14.2.23).

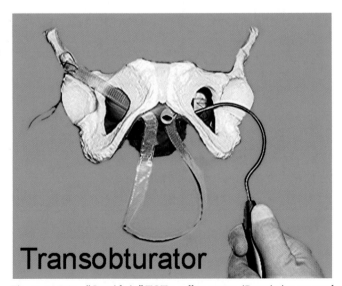

Figure 14.2.21. "Outside in" TOT needle passage. (Permission granted by Caldera.)

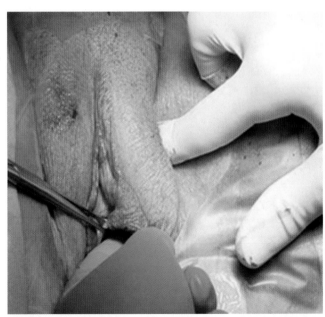

Figure 14.2.23. Palpation of landmarks during TOT procedure. (Permission granted by Caldera.)

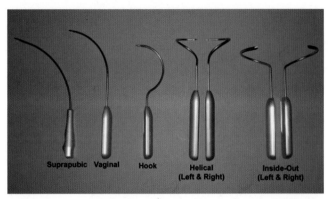

Figure 14.2.24. Minimally invasive sling needles. (Permission granted by Caldera.)

The TOT needle is introduced into the vulvar incision on either side and gently rotated or pushed into the flap on that side. The needle will traverse the obturator foramen and then puncture through the pubocervical fascia into the flap under the guidance of the surgeon's contralateral index finger. There are differently shaped TOT needles made by different companies, but they all accomplish the same goal (Figure 14.2.24).

Once the needle is in the flap, the preferred mesh/sheath system is fastened onto the needle, which is then backed out, pulling the mesh/sheath with it. The sheath can be clamped onto the drape to keep it out of the way while the same technique is done on the other side, with the other end of the sheath.

Once both sides have been done, the Foley is removed and cystourethroscopy is performed. If there are no injuries, the bladder is emptied and the sling is adjusted using the same tensioning technique as for the retropubic TVT (Figure 14.2.25).

Variations

The tension-free vaginal tape-obturator (TVT-O) is an "inside-out" TOT that pushes the mesh from inside the vagina and then out through the vulvar incisions. The TVT-O uses a winged guide that acts like a shoe horn for the TVT-O needle. The guide is pierced into the obturator foramen through the vaginal flaps.

The needle glides over the guide, through the obturator foramen, and then out through the vulvar incisions.

There are two basic designs for the transobturator needles. One has a corkscrew appearance, and the other looks like a hook. One company (Caldera) offers both types of needles as reusable, and they can be used with different types of sling material (permanent or delayed absorbable mesh). Other systems are designed to clamp onto a proprietary coupling device.

READJUSTABLE SLINGS

The first Food and Drug Administration (FDA)-approved readjustable sling was developed in Spain and approved for use in the United States in 2004.[39–41] This sling uses minimally invasive techniques with the advantage of allowing the surgeon to adjust the tension at the time of placement, and at any time in the future. Because of the permanent presence of the tensioning device above the fascia, this sling is best reserved for patients with previous incontinence surgery failures. Before the adjustable sling, bulking agents such as Contigen (C. R. Bard, Inc.) were used to increase coaptation of the urethral walls. If the bulking did not help, the only other option was to redo the entire sling.

The kit consists of a small piece of polypropylene mesh, two tensioning sutures (Prolene), a tensioning device, and a screwdriver set (Figure 14.2.26).

As with a TVT-type MIS, the mesh is placed under the bladder neck or mid-urethra through a vaginal incision. The lateral sides of the mesh are stitched with the Prolene tensioning sutures. These sutures are pulled up through the retropubic space as with the SPARC approach. A small suprapubic incision allows the tensioning device to be fastened to the two proline sutures. Cystoscopy must be performed to confirm urinary tract integrity. The device is tightened with the screwdriver until it rests directly on top of the rectus fascia. The screwdriver is left exposed through the skin incision. After leaving the operating room, the patient's bladder is filled with water, and in the standing position, the patient performs cough and Valsalva maneuvers. The screwdriver is used to make incremental changes in the suture tension. When the patient achieves continence, she is asked to void, and a postvoid residual is obtained. Assuming the patient can empty well and is

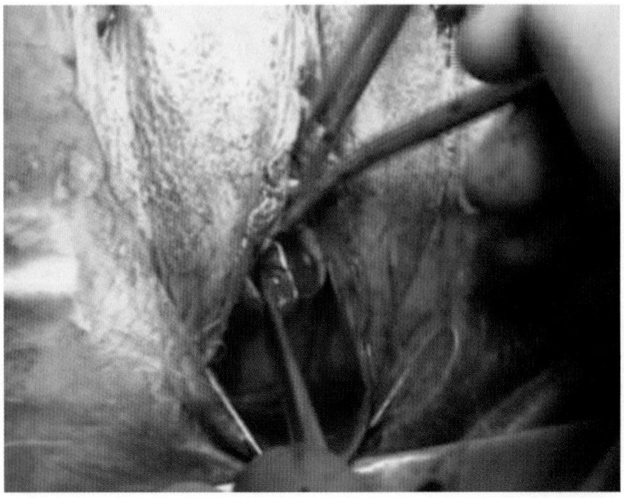

Figure 14.2.25. TOT sling tensioning. (Permission granted by AMS.)

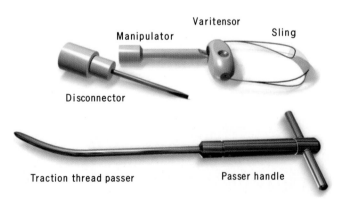

Figure 14.2.26. Remeex kit. (Permission granted by Neomedic/Tri-Anim.)

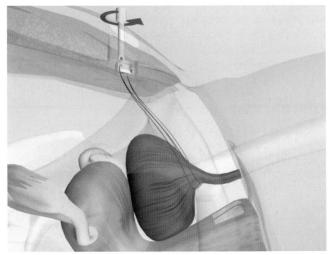

Figure 14.2.27. Tensioning of the Remeex device. (Permission granted by Neomedic/Tri-Anim.)

dry, the screwdriver is detached from the tensioning device and the incision is closed (Figures 14.2.27, 14.2.28).

Because of the presence of a prosthesis, antibiotic coverage for 7 to 10 days is recommended to avoid infection, although at least one study suggests that routine antibiotic use in an uncomplicated patient may not be of significant value.[42–44] If the patient develops recurrent incontinence, readjustment of the sling is possible by opening the incision just enough to allow entry of the screwdriver. The same test protocol is used again. Because there is adequate support under the urethra secondary to the Prolene mesh, leak point pressure can be increased by tightening the lateral sutures.

Although long-term data on the adjustable sling are lacking, preliminary studies indicate cure rates in the range of 95.5%.[38–40] For patients with continued leakage, improvement is also significant. Given the unique nature of the readjustable sling, it warrants further investigation.

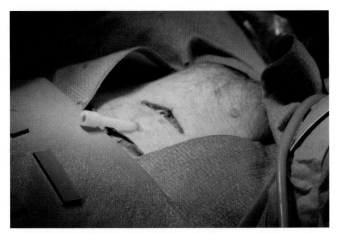

Figure 14.2.28. Closure of the skin with Remeex screwdriver in place. (Permission granted by Neomedic/Tri-Anim.)

COMPLICATIONS

Among all types of MIS, complications are common. Early studies show that the retropubic approach probably has more overall injuries than do the transobturator slings. Most retropubic sling injuries are minor and resolve spontaneously. This is probably related more to the anatomic placement of the sling than to the absolute skill of the surgeon. There have been severe injuries reported, some resulting in death. Attention to detail is imperative to ensure a positive outcome. Skill alone will help, but complications will never be eliminated.

Bladder Perforations

In retropubic MIS, bladder perforations occur in up to 5% of cases [17–19], although the frequency decreases precipitously with surgical experience. As long as the perforation site is not bleeding, nothing more needs to be done. If bleeding is seen, the bladder may be filled with sterile water for a few minutes. This is usually enough to stop the bleeding by tamponade. When active bleeding is seen, it is best to leave a Foley in place until the urine is clear for at least 24 hours. This is typically enough time for the cystotomy to heal itself. If multiple cystotomies are seen, or if the hole is larger than the diameter of the needle, longer bladder drainage may be indicated.

The TOT slings are inserted lateral to the urethra and are a few centimeters away from the bladder. Although bladder perforations do occur with TOT slings, the rate of these injuries is significantly lower ($\leq$2%) than those of TVTs.[45–47] It has been suggested by some of the companies producing TOT slings that cystoscopy is not indicated. Some surgeons consider this to be a marketing gimmick to sell more slings to physicians who do not have cystoscopy privileges. Although bladder and urethral injuries are uncommon, they do occur. Most experienced surgeons would consider cystoscopy an essential part of any incontinence procedure.

Patients receiving the readjustable sling have had numerous anti-incontinence procedures in the past. Complication rates will probably be increased in this population. Cystoscopy with the use of indigo carmine dye to visualize ureteral patency is advised during the case.

Vascular Injury

Retropubic slings such as the TVT are associated with a very low incidence of vascular injury. Because the needles are placed blindly, relying on anatomic landmarks, the needles may sometimes wander. A small change in the angle of placement can mean the difference between being safely lateral to the bladder and perforating the external iliac or obturator vessels. These vessels are only 4 to 6 cm away from where the needle should be passed.[47,48]

If a major blood vessel is injured, the patient typically will show symptoms. She may experience a drop in blood pressure, swelling or ecchymosis in the lower abdomen or vulva. She may also have visible blood pouring out of the vaginal or abdominal incisions. If there is bleeding only at the suburethral incision, the blood most likely is from the superficial plexus of veins. Firm pressure held in the vagina for 5 or 10 minutes can stop or slow blood loss, allowing the procedure to be completed. Packing can be left in the vagina and removed in the recovery room a few hours later.

Bleeding that does not slow down or that starts coming through the abdominal incision is more worrisome. This may indicate a major vessel injury and requires immediate decision making. If the blood is oozing out of the incisions only, firm pressure held over the lower abdomen and from the vagina for 5 or 10 minutes should be attempted first. Extra tamponade can be provided by retrograde filling of the bladder with water through the Foley catheter.

If the bleeding does not significantly slow down after 10 minutes, an abdominal incision may be warranted. Superficial vessels can be ligated or coagulated. Larger vessels may need repair, and a vascular surgery consult may be indicated. Overall transfusion rates are much less than 1% in experienced hands.[18, 50, 57]

Postoperative hematomas are common and usually asymptomatic. If the size of the hematoma appears stable and the patient is without complaint, observation only is indicated. If the hematoma appears to be enlarging or if the patient is becoming symptomatic, sonographic imaging is helpful to determine its size. In some cases, the hematoma can be drained under sonographic guidance. Infected hematomas are rare, but antibiotic augmentation may be considered.

Bowel Injury

Bowel injuries are always considered life threatening and require immediate intervention once they are recognized. Unfortunately, most bowel injuries go unnoticed until the patient has signs of an acute abdomen or sepsis. It seems difficult to picture how the bowel could be perforated with an MIS needle until one does cadaveric dissections and sees how close the intraperitoneal contents are to the retropubic space. Bowel injuries have been reported in the literature during suprapubic catheter placement.[52–54] Patients who have had previous surgery in the retropubic space are at an increased risk of injury, as the bowel may have slid into the space. This is why the peritoneum must be closed during any concurrent abdominal procedure (open or laparoscopic) to prevent herniation of the small bowel into the space anterior to the bladder.

Patients undergoing the readjustable sling need to be treated a little differently. Many candidates for this procedure have had multiple prior surgeries. Patients with a history of prior abdominal approach pelvic surgery are at increased risk of bowel injury. Overnight observation may be warranted. Any clinical signs of peritonitis require an extensive and immediate work-up.

Patients with a bowel injury may present with an acute abdomen, nausea, vomiting, and diarrhea. Fever and elevated white blood count are frequently seen. These patients look sick. When a patient complains of any lower abdominal pain postoperatively, she must be taken seriously.

Evaluation for bowel injury may include a flat plate and upright radiograph to look for free air, bowel obstruction, or ileus. A computed tomography (CT) scan can show changes consistent with bowel injury, including free air. A sonogram may also be helpful. Bowel injuries require aggressive management with resection, drainage, and possible colostomy if indicated.

Wound Infections

Surgical site infections are very rare secondary to prophylactic antibiotics. It is has been suggested that the outer sheath reduces the bacteria load after they are removed. Some surgeons soak the MIS in an antibiotic solution before starting the case. One animal study using a polymer mesh soaked for 15 minutes in rifampicin, vancomycin, and gentamicin showed decreased infection rates when the mesh was reimplanted into rabbit tissue.[33,55–57]

POSTOPERATIVE MANAGEMENT

Incomplete Bladder Emptying

If the patient has failed the voiding trial, either an indwelling Foley catheter is left in place or the patient begins intermittent self-catheterization. Most commonly, the patient is sent home with the catheter, a leg bag, and a night bag. The Foley will stay in place for 2 to 4 days, after which another voiding trial will be attempted. Repeated failure of the voiding trial results in approximately 3% to 5% of patients with less than 1% needing a sling revision.[58–60] Early intervention in the first 2 weeks will allow the sling to be loosened by opening up the vaginal incision and gently pulling down on the lateral sides of the exposed sling. This allows the sling to remain flat under the urethra, without disrupting its integrity. After 2 weeks, the sling will have started to have tissue ingrowth, and it is best to wait for 4 to 6 weeks after surgery to cut the sling in the midline. In cases in which the patient has no urine output, resection of the mid-portion of the sling may be indicated if the sling cannot be loosened. Continued continence with good bladder emptying occurs in over 85% of patients undergoing revision. Patients with borderline high residuals will often require occasional self-catheterization. In this small subgroup of patients, many will prefer to continue self-catheterizing rather than risk becoming incontinent again.

As a rule, tight slings can be loosened by cutting them under the urethra. Loose slings need to be redone or improved with bulking agents. Experienced surgeons will often make the sling "tighter" rather than "looser."

Antibiotic therapy with nitrofurantoin 50 mg/day is helpful in preventing urinary tract infections in patients with an indwelling catheter. Antibiotics are not indicated in patients who use the intermittent self-catheterization technique.

Vaginal and Urethral Erosions

It is difficult to determine whether a sling has eroded into the vagina or was inadvertently placed there at the time of surgery. This difficulty applies to slings found in the urethra as well. The time from surgery that the erosion is found probably gives the best indication of the cause. If the sling is found within the first month, it is probably the result of surgical error. This is not always the case, however, as suture lines can break down and some patients have decreased tissue vascularity secondary to prior medical conditions.

Mesh in the vagina often presents with persistent vaginal discharge or odor, or the patient's partner may complain of pain during sexual relations, which may be accompanied by the finding of small lacerations on the partner's penis (which does not require examination). This problem is best dealt with in the operating room, with the patient under anesthesia. The visible mesh should either be resected or be completely covered over with healthy vaginal epithelium. In most cases, resection will be the easiest approach, and the entry and exit sites should be closed with absorbable suture. Cases in which only a small amount of mesh is palpable but not seen, may respond to 8 to 12 weeks of topical estrogen cream.

Urethral erosions require removal of the material. This can be attempted transurethrally but usually requires a vaginal approach. Developing a few layers of inverted u-flaps under the urethra helps to identify the sling and also preserves the urethral sphincter. By taking down the tissue in thin layers, minimal damage is done to the urethra itself, allowing a repair that decreases the risk of urethra–vaginal fistula. If the erosion into the urethra requires extensive repair, it is best to leave a transurethral catheter in place for 5 days to prevent stricture of the healing urethra. In these cases, a suprapubic catheter is also placed for up to 10 days to divert urine flow and allow adequate healing.

Pain

Pain control is rarely a problem. A few days of nonsteroidal anti-inflammatory drug (NSAID) therapy is usually enough. Patients who demand or require stronger medication warrant immediate evaluation because of the unusual nature of the complaint. Continued pain may be caused by a range of conditions, with most being self-limited. A urinary tract infection should always be looked for first. A digital exam of the vagina will rapidly rule out the presence of mesh in the vagina. Rarely, patients are sent home without removal of the vaginal packing. Retained packing presents as "pressure" that quickly resolves once it is taken out.

Complaints of protracted pain may occur along the path of the sling placement. This is not dependent on improper technique, as the patient may be completely continent, with good bladder emptying. There is no "one cause" for this occurrence, but most symptoms abate after 4 to 8 weeks of NSAIDs. If pain is present after 12 weeks, excision or release of the sling is advised. It is not easy to excise the sling in its entirety because of tissue ingrowth.[61–65] It is usually possible to remove most of the sling to the obturator foramen bilaterally or near the pubocervical fascia.

Failures

Patients with continued incontinence require reassessment. In most cases, the anterior vaginal wall is still well supported but the sling is just too loose. Retesting with urodynamics is the best place to start. Confirmation that the patient has stress incontinence and not de novo urge incontinence is helpful from a practical and legal perspective. Some patients may think they have stress incontinence, but the leakage is really caused by a contraction of the detrusor muscle of the bladder. Reoperating on patients without true stress incontinence will only make their symptoms worse. These patients will respond to anticholinergic medical therapy. Patients who continue to have stress incontinence have a few treatment options.

When the incontinence is severe, repeating the initial MIS is probably the best place to start. Patients who have already had more than one anti-incontinence procedure will probably benefit from the readjustable sling. For patients who have improved with the MIS, urethral bulking should be considered. Different bulking agents are available, and improvement in the condition can be expected, but this may require more than one session of injections. Long-term cure has not been seen with these products, and they may require yearly repeat injections. These injections can be easily applied and performed in the office if necessary.

New in-office modalities using radiofrequency therapy are now FDA approved but still lack long-term data. Clinical trials are under way and show improvement in up to 80% of patients treated. It is unclear how this therapy will affect the urethra in cases in which a sling will be placed at a later time. If this therapy demonstrates encouraging results, it may be considered a first-line treatment in patients who either do not want surgery or are poor surgical risks.

Patients who develop hypermobility of the anterior vaginal wall after a sling has been placed are at increased risk not only of recurrent stress incontinence but also of urinary retention.[66–69] Retention occurs when the sling, acting as a fulcrum, causes kinking of the urethra and bladder neck as the anterior vaginal wall descends. These patients will have stress incontinence secondary to overflow from incomplete bladder empting. Re-support of vaginal mobility will usually correct the problem without having to redo the sling. Placing a pessary into the vagina will sometimes cure the problem by relieving the kink. Although not always an accurate predictor of success, the pessary can give a good indication of how corrective surgery will work.

SLINGS WITH CONCOMITANT SURGERY

The sling should be the last procedure performed when combined with other surgery. This is because it is important to have the anterior vaginal wall and urethra resting at the point where the sling is placed. If the vaginal wall and urethra are moved in any direction (i.e., posterior repair or apical suspension), this may increase or decrease the tension placed on the sling. This can increase the risk of retention or continued incontinence.

For surgeons who are doing laparoscopy, the Burch or MMK procedure may be their primary incontinence procedure. By avoiding the retropubic space, decreased morbidity and increased success rates may be achieved by switching to a MIS. Overall, the MIS is applicable to a wider range of patients than is any retropubic bladder neck suspension. It may also decrease operative time.

CONCLUSION

The MIS is now considered the "gold standard" for stress incontinence therapy. Long-term safety data confirm low morbidity and mortality rates.[70–73] Cases can be done in the ambulatory setting and do not require extensive recovery periods. Familiarity of pelvic anatomy and a thorough understanding of the pathophysiology of bladder dysfunction are essential. This will ensure the proper choice of both the procedure and the technique. Despite any marketing ploy to the contrary, cystourethroscopy should still be considered essential during these procedures.

REFERENCES

1. Fantl JA, Newman DK, Colling J, et al. *Urinary Incontinence in Adults: Acute and Chronic Management*. Rockville, MD: US Dept of Health and Human Services, Agency for Health Care Policy and Research; 1996.

2. Hu TW, Wagner TH. Health-related consequences of overactive bladder: an economic perspective. *BJU Int*. 2005;96(suppl 1):43–45.

3. Hughes DA, Dubois D. Cost-effectiveness analysis of extended-release formulations of oxybutynin and tolterodine for the management of urge incontinence. *Pharmacoeconomics*. 2004;22:1047–1059.

4. Hu TW, Wagner TH, Bentkover JD, et al. Estimated economic costs of overactive bladder in the United States. *Urology*. 2003;61:1123–1128.

5. Irwin DE, Milsom I, Kopp Z, Abrams P, Cardozo L. Impact of overactive bladder symptoms on employment, social interactions and emotional well-being in six European countries. *BJU Int*. 2006;97:96–100.

6. Davis K, Kumar D. Pelvic floor dysfunction: a conceptual framework for collaborative patient-centred care. *J Adv Nurs*. 2003;43:555–568.

7. Black NA, Bowling A, Griffiths JM, Pope C, Abel PD. Impact of surgery for stress incontinence on the social lives of women. *Br J Obstet Gynaecol*. 1998;105:605–612.

8. Delancey JO. Anatomic aspects of vaginal eversion after hysterectomy. *Am J Obstet Gynecol*. 1992;166(6 pt 1):1717–1724.

9. Ross JW. Apical vault repair, the cornerstone or pelvic vault reconstruction. *Int Urogynecol J Pelvic Floor Dysfunct*. 1997;8:146–152.

10. Gabriel B, Denschlag D, Gobel H, et al. Uterosacral ligament in postmenopausal women with or without pelvic organ prolapse. *Int Urogynecol J Pelvic Floor Dysfunct*. 2005;16:475–479.

11. DeLancey JO. Structural support of the urethra as it relates to stress urinary incontinence: the hammock hypothesis. *Am J Obstet Gynecol*. 1994;170:1713–1723.

12. Delancey JO, Ashton-Miller JA. Pathophysiology of adult urinary incontinence. *Gastroenterology*. 2004;126(suppl 1):S23–S32.

13. Yamada T, Hayashi T, Kamata S, Ohno R, Horiuchi S. New hammock hypothesis-based method for the treatment of stress urinary incontinence: the first 29 urethral supports with a small fascial patch. *Int J Urol*. 2005;12:806–809.

14. Thaweekul Y, Bunyavejchevin S, Wisawasukmongchol W, Santingamkun A. Long term results of anterior colporrhaphy with Kelly plication for the treatment of stress urinary incontinence. *J Med Assoc Thai*. 2004;87:357–360.

15. Park GS, Miller EJ Jr. Surgical treatment of stress urinary incontinence: a comparison of the Kelly plication, Marshall–Marchetti–Krantz, and Pereyra procedures. *Obstet Gynecol*. 1988;71:575–579.

16. Guner H, Ahmed S, Nas T, Yildirim M. Surgical treatment alternatives in stress incontinence. *Int J Gynaecol Obstet*. 1996;52:255–258.

17. Karram MM, Segal JL, Vassallo BJ, Kleeman SD. Complications and untoward effects of the tension-free vaginal tape procedure. *Obstet Gynecol*. 2003;101(5 pt 1):929–932.

18. Kolle D, Tamussino K, Hanzal E, et al.; Austrian Urogynecology Working Group. Bleeding complications with the tension-free vaginal tape operation. *Am J Obstet Gynecol*. 2005;193:2045–2049.

19. Quicios Dorado C, Fernandez Fernandez E, Gomez Garcia I, Perales Cabanas L, Arias Funez F, Escudero Barrilero A. Treatment of female stress urinary incontinence with TVT system (tension-free vaginal tape): complications in our first 100 cases [in Spanish]. *Actas Urol Esp*. 2005;29:750–756.

20. Serels S, Stein M. Meta-analysis for four different surgical treatments for stress urinary incontinence. *Can J Urol*. 1997;4:300–304.

21. El-Barky E, El-Shazly A, El-Wahab OA, Kehinde EO, Al-Hunayan A, Al-Awadi KA. Tension free vaginal tape versus Burch colposuspension for treatment of female urinary incontinence. *Int Urol Nephrol*. 2005;37:277–281.

22. Akpinar H, Cetinel B, Demirkesen O, Tufek I, Yaycioglu O, Solok V. Long-term results of Burch colposuspension. *Int J Urol*. 2000;7:119–125.

23. Westby M, Asmussen M, Ulmsten U. Location of maximum intraurethral pressure related to urogenital diaphragm in the female studied by simultaneous urethrocystometry and voiding urethrocystography. *Am J Obstet Gynecol*. 1982;144:408–412.

24. Lose G. Urethral pressure and power generation during coughing and voluntary contraction of the pelvic floor in females with genuine stress incontinence. *Br J Urol*. 1991;67:580–585.

25. Thind P, Lose G, Colstrup H. Initial urethral pressure increase during stress episodes in genuine stress incontinent women. *Br J Urol*. 1992;69:137–140.

26. Delorme E. Transobturator urethral suspension: mini-invasive procedure in the treatment of stress urinary incontinence in women. *Prog Urol*. 2001;11:1306–1313.

27. Roumeguere T, Quackels T, Bollens R, et al. Trans-obturator vaginal tape (TOT) for female stress incontinence: one year follow-up in 120 patients. *Eur Urol*. 2005;48:805–809.

28. Mellier G, Benayed B, Bretones S, Pasquier JC. Suburethral tape via the obturator route: is the TOT a simplification of the TVT? *Int Urogynecol J Pelvic Floor Dysfunct*. 2004;15:227–232.

29. Ulmsten U, Falconer C, Johnson P, Jomaa M, Lanner L, Nilsson CG, Olsson I. A multicenter study of tension-free vaginal tape (TVT) for surgical treatment of stress urinary incontinence. *Int Urogynecol J Pelvic Floor Dysfunct*. 1998;9(4):210–213.

30. Letter to the Editor. *Int Urogynecol J*. 2000;11:130–132.

31. Ulmsten U. An introduction to tension-free vaginal tape (TVT) – a new surgical procedure for treatment of female urinary incontinence. *Int Urogynecol J Pelvic Floor Dysfunct*. 2001;12(suppl 2):S3–S4.

32. Petros PP, Ulmsten U. An anatomical classification – a new paradigm for management of female lower urinary tract dysfunction. *Eur J Obstet Gynecol Reprod Biol*. 1998;80:87–94.

33. Kuuva N, Nilsson CG. A nationwide analysis of complications associated with the tension-free vaginal tape (TVT) procedure. *Acta Obstet Gynecol Scand*. 2002;81:72–77.

34. Tsivian A, Mogutin B, Kessler O, Korczak D, Levin S, Sidi AA. Tension-free vaginal tape procedure for the treatment of female stress urinary incontinence: long-term results. *J Urol*. 2004;172:998–1000.

35. Canis Sanchez D, Bielsa Gali O, Cortadellas Angel R, Arango Toro O, Placer Santos J, Gelabert i Mas A. Results and complications of TVT procedure in the surgical treatment of female stress incontinence [in Spanish]. *Actas Urol Esp*. 2005;29:287–291.

36. Andonian S, Chen T, St-Denis B, Corcos J. Randomized clinical trial comparing suprapubic arch sling (SPARC) and tension-free vaginal tape (TVT): one year results. *Eur Urol*. 2005;47:537–541.

37. Tseng LH, Wang AC, Lin YH, Li SJ, Ko YJ. Randomized comparison of the suprapubic arc sling procedure vs tension-free vaginal taping for stress incontinent women. *Int Urogynecol J Pelvic Floor Dysfunct*. 2005;16:230–235.

38. Gandhi S, Abramov Y, Kwon C, et al. TVT versus SPARC: comparison of outcomes for two midurethral tape procedures. *Int Urogynecol J Pelvic Floor Dysfunct*. 2005;17:125–130.

39. Sousa-Escandon A, Lema Grille J, Rodriguez Gomez JI, Rios Tallon L, Uribarri Gonzalez C, Marques-Queimadelos A. Externally readjustable device to regulate sling tension in stress urinary incontinence: preliminary results. *J Endourol*. 2003;17:515–521.

40. Sousa-Escandon A, Rodriguez Gomez JI, Uribarri Gonzalez C, Marques-Queimadelos A. Externally readjustable sling for treatment of male stress urinary incontinence: points of technique and preliminary results. *J Endourol*. 2004;18:113–118.

41. Palma PC, Dambros M, Thiel M, et al. Readjustable transobturator sling: a novel sling procedure for male urinary incontinence. *Urol Int.* 2004;73:354–356.

42. Gomelsky A, Dmochowski RR. Antibiotic prophylaxis in urologic prosthetic surgery. *Curr Pharm Des.* 2003;9:989–996.

43. Abouassaly R, Steinberg JR, Lemieux M, et al. Complications of tension-free vaginal tape surgery: a multi-institutional review. *BJU Int.* 2004;94:110–113.

44. Garcia Florez D, Perez Sanz P, Briones Mardones G, et al. Surgical management and complications of urinary stress incontinence: our experience in 385 patients operated on during the last 25 years [in Spanish]. *Actas Urol Esp.* 2003;27:92–96.

45. Roumeguere T, Quackels T, Bollens R, et al. Trans-obturator vaginal tape (TOT) for female stress incontinence: one year follow-up in 120 patients. *Eur Urol.* 2005;48:805–809.

46. Smith PP, Appell RA. Transobturator tape, bladder perforation, and paravaginal defect: a case report. *Int Urogynecol J Pelvic Floor Dysfunct.* 2007;18:99–101.

47. Mellier G, Benayed B, Bretones S, Pasquier JC. Suburethral tape via the obturator route: is the TOT a simplification of the TVT? *Int Urogynecol J Pelvic Floor Dysfunct.* 2004;15:227–232.

48. Abbas Shobeiri S, Gasser RF, Chesson RR, Echols KT. The anatomy of midurethral slings and dynamics of neurovascular injury. *Int Urogynecol J Pelvic Floor Dysfunct.* 2003;14:185–190.

49. Agostini A, Bretelle F, Franchi F, Roger V, Cravello L, Blanc B. Immediate complications of tension-free vaginal tape (TVT): results of a French survey. *Eur J Obstet Gynecol Reprod Biol.* 2006; 124:237–239.

50. Bourrat M, Armand C, Seffert P, Tostain J. Complications and medium-term functional results of TVT in stress urinary incontinence [in French]. *Prog Urol.* 2003;13:1358–1364.

51. Kobashi KC, Govier FE. Perioperative complications: the first 140 polypropylene pubovaginal slings. *J Urol.* 2003;170:1918–1921.

52. Noller KL, Pratt JH, Symmonds RE. Bowel perforation with suprapubic cystostomy: report of two cases. *Obstet Gynecol.* 1976; 48(suppl 1):67S–69S.

53. Farina LA, Palou J. Re: suprapubic catheterisation and bowel injury. *Br J Urol.* 1993;72:394.

54. Parikh A, Chapple CR, Hampson SJ. Suprapubic catheterisation and bowel injury. *Br J Urol.* 1992;70:212–213.

55. Goeau-Brissonniere O, Leflon V, Letort M, Nicolas MH. Resistance of antibiotic-bonded gelatin-coated polymer meshes to *Staphylococcus aureus* in a rabbit subcutaneous pouch model. *Biomaterials.* 1999;20:229–232.

56. Debodinance P, Delporte P, Engrand JB, Boulogne M. Complications of urinary incontinence surgery: 800 procedures [in French]. *J Gynecol Obstet Biol Reprod (Paris).* 2002;31:649–662.

57. Kochakarn W. Tension-free vaginal tape procedure for the treatment of stress urinary incontinence: the first experience in Thailand. *J Med Assoc Thai.* 2002;85:87–91.

58. Meschia M, Pifarotti P, Bernasconi F, et al. Tension-free vaginal tape: analysis of outcomes and complications in 404 stress incontinent women. *Int Urogynecol J Pelvic Floor Dysfunct.* 2001;12(suppl 2):24–27.

59. Marteinsson VT. Reoperations on lower urinary tract due to foreign body after urinary incontinence surgery [in Icelandic]. *Laeknabladid.* 2005;91:237–241.

60. Kato K, Hirata T, Suzuki K, Yoshida K, Murase T. Sling removal after the Vesica sling and tension-free vaginal tape (TVT) procedures [in Japanese]. *Nippon Hinyokika Gakkai Zasshi.* 2004;95:17–24.

61. Hermieu JF, Milcent S. Synthetic suburethral sling in the treatment of stress urinary incontinence in women [in French]. *Prog Urol.* 2003;13:636–647.

62. Gonzalez R, Fugate K, McClusky D 3rd, et al. Relationship between tissue ingrowth and mesh contraction. *World J Surg.* 2005;29:1038–1043.

63. Matthews BD, Pratt BL, Pollinger HS, et al. Assessment of adhesion formation to intra-abdominal polypropylene mesh and polytetrafluoroethylene mesh. *J Surg Res.* 2003;114:126–132.

64. Slack M, Sandhu JS, Staskin DR, Grant RC. In vivo comparison of suburethral sling materials. *Int Urogynecol J Pelvic Floor Dysfunct.* 2006;17:106–110.

65. Junge K, Klinge U, Rosch R, Klosterhalfen B, Schumpelick V. Functional and morphologic properties of a modified mesh for inguinal hernia repair. *World J Surg.* 2002;26:1472–1480.

66. Hammad FT, Kennedy-Smith A, Robinson RG. Erosions and urinary retention following polypropylene synthetic sling: Australasian survey. *Eur Urol.* 2005;47:641–646.

67. Thiel DD, Pettit PD, McClellan WT, Petrou SP. Long-term urinary continence rates after simple sling incision for relief of urinary retention following fascia lata pubovaginal slings. *J Urol.* 2005;174:1878–1881.

68. Sweeney DD, Leng WW. Treatment of postoperative voiding dysfunction following incontinence surgery. *Curr Urol Rep.* 2005;6:365–370.

69. Palma PC, Dambros M, Riccetto CL, Thiel M, Netto NR Jr. Transvaginal urethrolysis for urethral obstruction after anti-incontinence surgery [in Spanish]. *Actas Urol Esp.* 2005;29:207–211.

70. Rackley RR, Abdelmalak JB, Tchetgen MB, Madjar S, Jones S, Noble M. Tension-free vaginal tape and percutaneous vaginal tape sling procedures. *Tech Urol.* 2001;7:90–100.

71. Rutman M, Itano N, Deng D, Raz S, Rodriguez LV. Long-term durability of the distal urethral polypropylene sling procedure for stress urinary incontinence: minimum 5-year followup of surgical outcome and satisfaction determined by patient reported questionnaires. *J Urol.* 2006;175:610–613.

72. Flynn BJ, Yap WT. Pubovaginal sling using allograft fascia lata versus autograft fascia for all types of stress urinary incontinence: 2-year minimum followup. *J Urol.* 2002;167(2 pt 1):608–612.

73. Morgan TO Jr, Westney OL, McGuire EJ. Pubovaginal sling: 4-year outcome analysis and quality of life assessment. *J Urol.* 2000;163:1845–1848.

Section 14.3. Laparoscopic Uterine Suspension, Sacrocolpopexy, Vault Suspension

James E. Carter and Senzan Hsu

LAPAROSCOPIC UTERINE SUSPENSION FOR PAIN AND UTERINE RETROVERSION

Uterine retroversion is a backward displacement of the uterus into the pouch of Douglas from its normal anteverted position.[1] Uterine retroversion may be congenital or may result from adhesions and fibrosis. The condition occurs in 20% to 30% of women. Commonly reported symptoms include dysmenorrhea, dyspareunia, and backache. Laparoscopic ventral suspension has been performed to successfully treat symptomatic retroversion and significantly reduce symptoms.[1–17] Long-term follow-up of 5 to 20 years has demonstrated continued relief of chronic pelvic pain and deep dyspareunia by uterine suspension.[14] Several techniques have been described to treat uterine retroversion. These include suspension of round ligament at midpoint, modified Olshausen uterine suspension, and the Uterine Positioning by Ligament Investment, Fixation, and Truncation (UPLIFT) technique.

Ventral Suspension of the Round Ligaments at the Midpoint

This procedure involves the placement of two 5-mm suprapubic trocars and the introduction of grasping forceps into the pelvis through them. Alternatively, long Kelly clamps are inserted through suprapubic stab incisions. Both round ligaments are grasped near their midpoints, and partial escape of pneumoperitoneum is allowed. The knuckle of the round ligament is pulled gently and firmly through the fascial incision (Figure 14.3.1.1). The round ligaments are sutured to the rectus fascia with 2-0 Ethibond nonabsorbable sutures (Ethicon, Somerville, NJ). Uterine position is confirmed with the laparoscope, and one must avoid kinking the fallopian tubes.[18,19]

Potential complications with this procedure include avulsion of the round ligaments secondary to inadequate fascial incision and undue tension or positioning of the round ligaments with full pneumoperitoneum. The inferior epigastric arteries may be lacerated during placement of the suprapubic trocars. Although transilluminating the abdomen often helps prevent this complication, it is difficult in obese patients. For most patients, incisional pain and discomfort are managed with mild analgesics and a heating pad. Occasionally, patients who experience more significant postoperative pain from secondary spasms of the recti muscles are relieved with heat, muscle relaxants, and analgesics. Patients are advised to avoid strenuous exercise for 4 to 6 weeks postoperatively.

Modified Olshausen Uterine Suspension

A delayed absorbable or permanent suture is passed transabdominally at the suprapubic trocar site, using a swaged-on needle. While the round ligament is placed on stretch, several areas are taken where the round ligament enters the inguinal canal moving toward the uterus. Approximately 2 cm from the uterus, the direction of the needle is reversed and a similar maneuver is performed along the length of the round ligament to the inguinal canal. The needle is passed transabdominally. After both sides have been completed, pneumoperitoneum is decreased, and the suture is tied above the fascia (Figure 14.3.1.2). The result is a plication of the round ligaments.

The UPLIFT Procedure

The UPLIFT laparoscopic uterine suspension is performed with a Carter-Thomason 2-mm needlepoint suture passer. A tiny skin incision is made near the exit point of the round ligament into the inguinal canal (Figure 14.3.1.3). Size 0 (3.5 metric) monofilament polybutester suture is used to make two passes subcutaneously and transfascially into the extraperitoneal space and within and along the round ligament (Figure 14.3.1.4A–F). The first pass's exit point of the suture is 0.5 to 1.0 cm from the uterus in the fibrous portion of the ligament. The second pass starts 1 to 2 cm cephalad or caudad from the previous puncture site. The exit point of the suture from the ligament is approximately 1 to 2 cm proximal to the exit point of the previously placed suture. The suture is retrieved and withdrawn to outside of the skin and tied. This technique creates a pledget of round ligament and a bridge of fascial tissue. The ligament imbricates within itself as it is pulled up by the suture. This moderately anteverts the uterine position by ligament investment, fixation, and truncation (Figure 14.3.1.5).

Use of this technique has resulted in an average operating time of less than 15 minutes for this portion of the patient's surgery. In one series of 75 patients [20], the average time to discharge was 4 hours. Mild incisional and abdominal wall discomfort, which occurred in most patients for the first 24 hours, was readily relieved with mild oral analgesics. There were no intraoperative complications. After the UPLIFT and associated laparoscopic procedures, immediate and sustained relief of pelvic pain has been reported in majority of patients.[20,21]

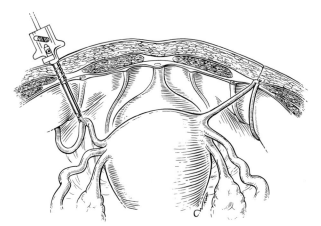

Figure 14.3.1.1. The round ligaments at midpoint are pulled through the suprapubic incision and tied to the rectus fascia.

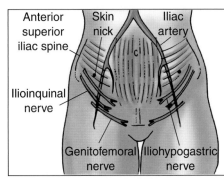

Figure 14.3.1.3. Position of the skin nicks relative to the exiting point of the round ligament through the inguinal canal. The retroverted uterus is pictured before uterine suspension. (Courtesy of Inlet Medical, Inc.)

Multiple procedures for uterine suspension have been described in the literature that involve folding, plicating, bending, and fixing the round ligament to the anterior abdominal wall, and these procedures have been reported as being successful. The UPLIFT procedure avoids potential problems with bowel herniation into the anterior cul-de-sac, which may occur with some of the other procedures. It also results in an anatomically correct anteversion, with the suspension at the lateral extension of the round ligaments.

LAPAROSCOPIC UTERINE SUSPENSION FOR DESCENSUS

Maher and colleagues [22] described laparoscopic suture hysteropexy for uterine prolapse in women wishing uterine preservation. As Maher pointed out, "Vaginal hysterectomy remains the accepted surgical treatment for women with uterine prolapse. The Manchester repair is favored in women wishing uterine preservation. Vaginal hysterectomy alone fails to address the pathological cause of the uterine prolapse. The Manchester repair has a high failure rate and may cause difficulty sampling the cervix and uterus in the future. The laparoscopic suture hysteropexy offers physiologic repair of uterine prolapse."

Maher performed surgery as follows: Surgery was performed in a low lithotomy position. The bladder was drained with a Foley catheter, and a Pelosi uterine manipulator (Apple Medical, Bolton, MN) was used to obtain exaggerated anteversion of the uterus. A steep Trendelenburg position facilitated mobilization of the bowel from the pouch of Douglas. Following placement of two 5-mm ports for performance of the surgery, the bowel was removed from the pouch of Douglas, and the course of the ureters was followed from the pelvic rim along the lateral sidewall. As the cul-de-sac at this stage is an expansive hernia-like area between the bowel posteriorly and the cervix and posterior vaginal wall anteriorly, the uterosacral ligaments are frequently deficient. A Moschcowitz culdoplasty was performed using a size 0 polydioxanone purse-string suture. The uterosacral ligaments were independently plicated using two size 1 Gore-Tex sutures (CV-2, Gore, Flagstaff, AZ). The uterosacral ligament plication started midway along the uterosacral ligament between the sacrum and the cervix. The ligaments were reattached to their point of physiologic insertion on the posterior aspect of the cervix. At the completion of surgery, a 3- to 4-cm gap was left between the sacrum and the plicated uterosacral ligaments to ensure normal large bowel function. The course of the ureters was checked. If kinking was present, a peritoneal releasing incision was performed between the ureter and uterosacral ligaments

In the 43 women who underwent this procedure for symptomatic uterine prolapse to or beyond the introitus with straining, Maher reported that the mean operating time for the laparoscopic suture hysteropexy was 42 ± 15 minutes and the mean blood loss was 50 mL or less. Intraoperatively, one woman had broad ligament hematoma resulting from laceration of the left uterine artery. Peritoneal releasing incisions were performed in two women in whom the ureter was kinked medially, close to the plicated uterosacral ligament. No postoperative complications were reported. With a mean length of follow-up of 12 months (range 5–19 months), majority of women had no symptoms of or no objective evidence of prolapse (81% and 79%, respectively). Seven women (16%) underwent additional surgeries for symptomatic uterine prolapse such as abdominal and sacral colpopexy, vaginal hysterectomy, and sacrospinous vault suspension and sacrospinous hysteropexy. Two women subsequently

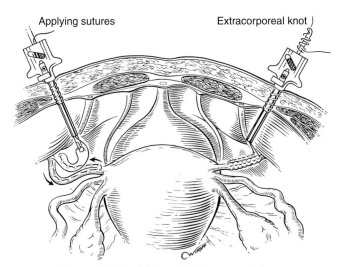

Figure 14.3.1.2. Modified Olshausen technique.

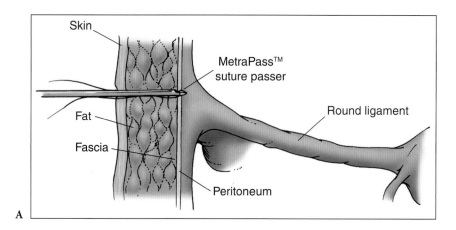

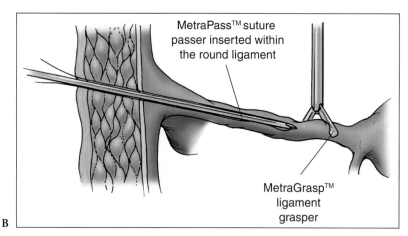

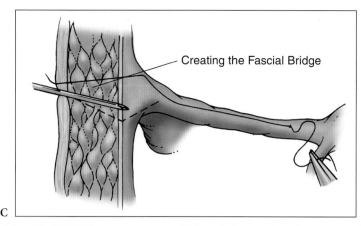

Figure 14.3.1.4. The UPLIFT procedure creates thickened, shortened, and strengthened round ligaments. (**A**) The polybutester suture is grasped and passed subcutaneously. (**B**) The suture exits the round ligament 0.5 to 1.0 cm from the uterus in the fibrous portion of the ligament. (**C**) The empty suture passer is passed 1 to 2 cm cephalad to caudad from the first pass. (*continued*)

completed term pregnancies, delivered by cesarean section, and were without prolapse at follow-up.

Yen et al.[23], believing that uterine retrodisplacement itself was associated with dyspareunia, chronic pelvic pain and uterine prolapse in the absence of organic disease, described the efficacy of a modified technique to treat a symptomatic retrodisplaced uterus with a combination of laparoscopic shortening and plication of the uterosacral ligaments and modified Gilliam round ligament suspension.

The surgery began by noting the anatomic relationship of rectum, ureters, and uterosacral ligaments to avoid injury. Four size 0 propylene sutures were placed (two on the left uterosacral ligament and two on the right) to make a circle. Beginning with the left uterosacral ligament, the first suture was placed at the lower level near the pelvic wall beside the junction with the rectal margin. A deep bite of the ligament was included while care was taken to avoid the rectum and ureter. The second suture was placed at the upper part of the left uterosacral ligament at the

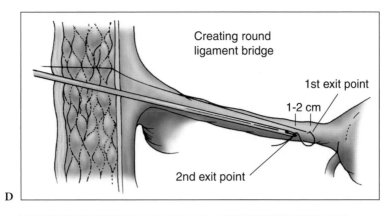

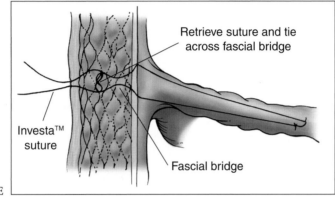

Figure 14.3.1.4. (*continued*) (**D**) The second pass exits 1 to 2 cm from the first exit point near the uterus. (**E**) The suture ends are retrieved and tied to create a fascial bridge. (**F**) The round ligament is shortened and strengthened, repositioning the uterus. (**A–F** courtesy of Inlet Medical, Inc.)

junction of the ligament and the uterus. Care was taken to avoid adjacent vessels, especially engorged varicose veins, which may lie close to the ligaments and may result in hemorrhage. To complete a full circle, a third suture was placed on the upper part of the right uterosacral ligament and a fourth suture was placed on the lower part of the ligament opposite the previous sutures. Finally, the suture was carried out of the body and used to perform extracorporeal knot tying. When the knot was tied down, the upper and lower sites were brought closer and the ligaments were plicated together bilaterally, yielding an effective shortening and tightening of the ligaments. Therefore, the upper and lower sutures should be separated as far apart as possible to achieve better ligament shortening.

The modified Gilliam suspension of the round ligaments was then performed. The accessory cannula in the lower abdomen was removed, the skin incision was extended to 1 to 2 cm, and the underlying rectus fascia was exposed. A grasping forceps was pushed into the pelvic cavity to grasp the round ligament at a point about 2 to 3 cm lateral to its insertion on the uterus. This point could be adjusted and changed slightly to ensure proper tension and ideal degree of uterine suspension. Improper traction on the fallopian tubes was avoided. The round ligament was withdrawn

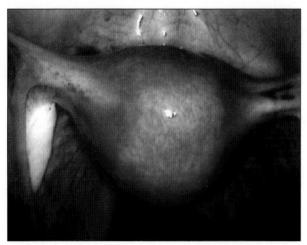

Figure 14.3.1.5. Anteverted uterus has a normal, uniform color following the UPLIFT procedure. (Courtesy of Dr. James E. Carter.)

shortened a little in some women, but only around 1.0 cm and without symptoms.

This procedure restores the normal relationship between the uterus and intra-abdominal pressure. As the uterus is completely fixed into an anteverted and anteflexed position, intra-abdominal pressure falls on the posterior surface of the uterus and to some degree prevents conversion of the uterine position.

Margossian et al.[24] reported on a technique of laparoscopic uterosacral ligament plication and shortening for pelvic organ prolapse. The authors pointed out pelvic organ prolapse can occur when pelvic support structures are subjected to increased intra-abdominal pressure. Commonly, there is an intrinsic defect of the pelvic floor. The clinical manifestation of pelvic organ prolapse reflects this specific fascial defect.

The procedure these authors described is as follows:

After inserting the laparoscope, we carefully identify the ureters. An incision is made in the peritoneum medial to the ureters. In this way, when the uterosacral ligaments are plicated, there is no kinking of the ureters. We used permanent sutures to plicate and shorten the uterosacral ligaments. The plication sutures are placed in the uterosacral ligament at its insertion into the cervix and through the posterior wall of the vagina and then tied with an extracorporeal knot-tying technique. Additional sutures are placed between the uterosacral ligaments to close the cul-de-sac. To shorten the uterosacral ligament, a suture is placed near its insertion in the sacrum and then through its insertion on the uterus. This is repeated on the opposite side. Only after both sutures are placed are they tied. The uterosacral ligament in between the sutures is allowed to fold medially.

into the incision and sutured to and through the anterior rectus fascia in a figure-of-eight manner with size 0 Vicryl (Ethicon Inc., Somerville, NJ). The same procedures were repeated on the opposite side.

Operating time was 24.1 ± 4.7 minutes, with blood loss of 30 mL or less in all cases. No intraoperative or postoperative complications occurred. At the first clinic visit 1 week later, all patients felt only slight lower abdominal traction and could walk freely without discomfort.

All the patients had an anteverted, anteflexed uterus without failure, and all declared they experienced marked improvement of deep dyspareunia, with a mean follow-up of 3.3 ± 1.0 years. The technique lengthened the vagina a little in most patients. Average vaginal lengths before and after surgery were 5.9 ± 0.7 cm and 7.0 ± 0.3 cm, respectively. In 2 years of follow-up, vaginal length

Results obtained with the procedure were not reported.

More recently, a technique using the ELEVEST device has been describe[25–27] (Figure 14.3.1.6A-F). It involves uterine

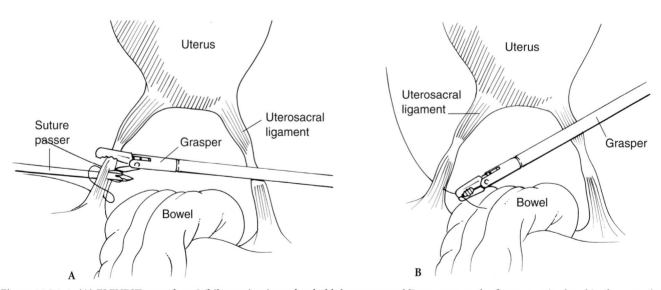

Figure 14.3.1.6. (**A**) ELEVEST procedure. While traction is used to hold the uterosacral ligament taut, the first suture is placed in the posterior one third of the ligament. (Courtesy of Inlet Medical, Inc.) (**B**) The suture is released, and the suture passer is removed from the uterosacral ligament. The suture is passed through the uterosacral ligament at the uterosacral ligament cervical junction. (Courtesy of Inlet Medical, Inc.) (*Continued*)

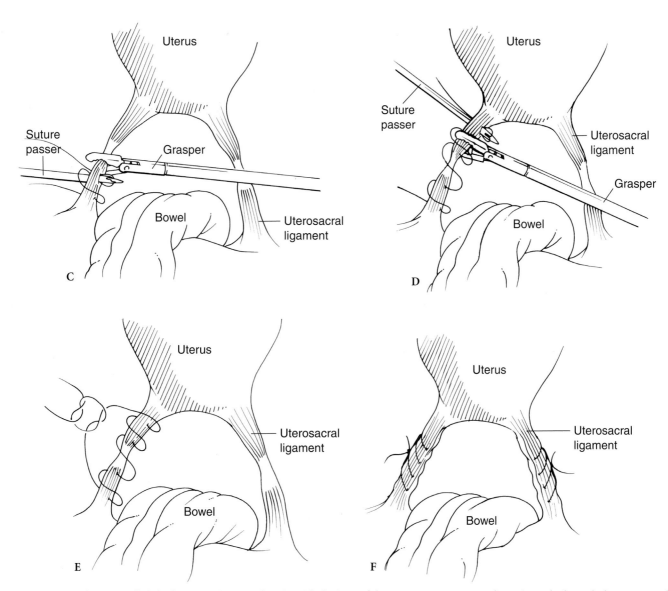

Figure 14.3.1.6. (*Continued*) (**C**) The suture is grasped again with the jaws of the suture passer. A second pass is made through the uterosacral ligament. (**D**) Three or four passes are made with the suture, with the last pass placed near the cervix. A second suture may be passed to reinforce the repair. (**E**) An extracorporeal knot is tied and tightened down to the level of the uterosacral ligament, thereby shortening and strengthening the ligament. (**F**) The procedure is completed with suture placement. (Figures courtesy of Inlet Medical, Inc.)

hysteropexy with round ligament suspension using specialized needlepoint suture passer that does not require a laparoscopic needle driver suturing technique. There were no major complications in these small series. Although 1 patient required a second operation to remove one of the round ligament sutures due to pain and 1 patient had recurrent prolapse [26], follow-up at 37 weeks for 21 patients [26] and at 18 months for 1 patient [27] revealed satisfactory results.

CONCLUSION

Treatment of uterine descensus by uterine suspension by a combination of round ligament and uterosacral ligament plication and shortening has been demonstrated in a number of series, some with long-term follow-up of up to 3.3 ± 1.0 years, and is a valid option for women who desire uterine preservation.

REFERENCES

1. Rasian F, Lynch CB, Rix J. Symptoms relieved by endoscopic ventral suspension. *Gynecol Endosc*. 1995;4:101–104.
2. Massouda D, Ling FW, Muram D, et al. Laparoscopic uterine suspension with Falope rings. *J Reprod Med*. 1987;32:859–861.
3. Candy JW. Modified Gilliam uterine suspension using laparoscopic visualization. *Obstet Gynecol*. 1976;47:242–243.
4. Mann WJ, Stenger VG. Uterine suspension through the laparoscope. *Obstet Gynecol*. 1978;51:563–566.
5. Yoong FE. Laparoscopic ventrosuspension: a review of 72 cases. *Am J Obstet Gynecol*. 1990;163:1151–1153.

6. Perry CP, Sarria C. Minimal incision Pereyra needle uterine suspension. *J Laparosc Surg*. 1991;1:151–155.

7. Ivey JL. Laparoscopic uterine suspension as an adjunctive procedure at the time of laser laparoscopy for the treatment of endometriosis. *J Reprod Med*. 1992;37:757–765.

8. Gordon SF. Laparoscopic uterine suspension. *J Reprod Med*. 1992;37:615–616.

9. Koh L, Tang F, Huang M. Preliminary experience in pelviscopic uterine suspension using Webster–Baldy and Franke's method. *Acta Obstet Gynecol Scand*. 1996;75:575–578.

10. Nezhat CR, Nezhat FR, Luciano AA, et al. *Uterine Surgery in Operative Gynecologic Laparoscopy Principles and Techniques*. New York: McGraw-Hill; 1995.

11. Daniell JF, Lalonde CJ. Advanced laparoscopic procedures for pelvic pain and dysmenorrhea. *Baillieres Clin Obstet Gynaecol*. 1995;9:795–808.

12. Metzger DA. Uterine suspension. In: Steege JF, Metzger DA, Levy BS, eds. *Chronic Pelvic Pain: An Integrated Approach*. Philadelphia: Saunders; 1998.

13. Ortega I. Uterine suspension for deep dyspareunia using Carter-Thomason needle point suture passer. Presented at: The International Society of Gynecologic Endoscopists World Conference; March 15–18, 1998; Sun City, South Africa.

14. Halperin R, Padoa A, Schneider D, Bukovsky I, Pansky M. Long-term followup (5–20 years) after uterine ventrosuspension for chronic pelvic pain and deep dyspareunia. *Gynecol Obstet Invest*. 2003;55:216–219.

15. Ou CS, Liu YH, Joki JA, Rowbotham R. Laparoscopic uterine suspension by round ligament plication. *J Reprod Med*. 2002;47:211–216.

16. Batioglu S, Zeyneloglu HB. Laparoscopic plication and suspension of the round ligament for chronic pelvic pain and dyspareunia. *J Am Assoc Gynecol Laparosc*. 2000;7:547–551.

17. Gargiulo T, Leo L, Gomel V. Laparoscopic uterine suspension using 3-stitch technique. *J Am Assoc Gynecol Laparosc*. 2000;7:233–236.

18. Smith DB, Kelsey JF, Sherman RL, et al. Laparoscopic uterine suspension. *J Reprod Med*. 1977;18:98.

19. Steptoe PC. *Laparoscopy and Gynecology*. London: Livingstone; 1967.

20. Carter JE. Carter-Thomason uterine suspension and positioning by ligament investment, fixation, and truncation (UPLIFT). *J Reprod Med*. 1999;44:417–422.

21. Perry CP, Presthus J, Nieves A. Laparoscopic uterine suspension for pain relief: a multicenter study. *J Repro Med*. 2005;50:567–570.

22. Maher CF, Carey MP, Murray CJ. Laparoscopic suture hysteropexy for uterine prolapse. *Obstet Gynecol*. 2001;97:1010–1014.

23. Yen CF, Wang CJ, Lin SL, Lee CL, Soong YK. Combined laparoscopic uterosacral and round ligament procedures for treatment of symptomatic uterine retroversion and mild uterine descensus. *J Am Assoc Gynecol Laparosc*. 2002;9:359–366.

24. Margossian H, Walters MD, Falcone T. Laparoscopic management of pelvic organ prolapse. *Eur J Obstet Gynecol Reprod Biol*. 1999;85:57–62.

25. Presthus J. Uterine prolapse: a new technique for uterine preservation. Video presented at: Annual Meeting of the Society of Laparoendoscopic Surgeons; May 16, 2003; New York, NY.

26. Sobolewski C, Glazerman L, Abbott K, Presthus J, Schwartz M. ELEVEST: a new technique for laparoscopic treatment of uterine prolapse without hysterectomy. Poster presented at: Annual Meeting of the American Association of Gynecologic Laparoscopists; November 16–22, 2003; Las Vegas, NV.

27. Abbott KR. A new technique for laparoscopic uterine prolapse repair: 18-month followup. Internet communication, Athena Gynecology Medical Group, San Carlos, CA, 2003.

PART 2: LAPAROSCOPIC VAGINAL VAULT SUSPENSION

Laparoscopic vaginal vault suspension is performed to treat apical enteroceles and vault descensus and to reposition the vaginal vault after hysterectomy.[1]

To properly perform pelvic vault reconstruction, specifically apical enterocele repair and vaginal vault suspension, a paradigm shift in the understanding of the anatomy of the pelvis is required. Defects in pelvic support are now viewed as defects in the actual fascia, which can be understood to constitute a "hernia." Richardson [2] described the anatomic defects in the apical enterocele. Ross [3] elegantly reviewed apical vault repair, which is the cornerstone of pelvic vault reconstruction.

Vaginal prolapse occurs when the upper one third of the vagina that is suspended by the cardinal–uterosacral ligament complex breaks free of its attachments to the sacrum via the uterosacral ligament. Additionally, the middle one third of the vagina, which is maintained by lateral attachments, is frequently broken free. Lateral defects are often found in the anterior quadrant of these patients and can be unilateral or bilateral. These are paravaginal defects or detachments of the pubocervical fascia from its lateral attachment to the fascia of the obturator internus muscle at the level of the arcus tendineus fascia of the pelvis. The arcus tendineus pelvic fascia is the tendinous aponeurosis of the obturator internus muscle anteriorly and the levator ani complex posteriorly.[4–7] All pelvic support defects must be addressed to ensure the integrity of the vagina and to correct associated stress incontinence if it exists. This section focuses on laparoscopic techniques for reconstruction of the vaginal apex with correction of vaginal vault prolapse.

ANATOMY

The apex of the vagina after hysterectomy is formed by the connection of the pubocervical fascia to the rectovaginal (Denonvilliers') septum (rectovaginal fascia). The rectovaginal fascia is a distinct fibrous tissue layer between the vagina and rectum in a diaphragm-like configuration. The principle attachments are located peripherally; cranially to the cul-de-sac peritoneum, the uterosacral ligaments, and the base of the cardinal ligaments; caudally to the perineal body; and laterally to the fascial covering of the levator ani muscles. The rectovaginal fascia merges in the cul-de-sac with the fibers of the uterosacral ligaments. It merges into the more lateral fibers of the cardinal–uterosacral complex in the area lateral to the upper vagina. An enterocele may occur if the pubocervical fascia separates from the rectovaginal fascia in the midline (Figure 14.3.2.1). [2–8]

Pelvic support defects are similar to hernias. They are not associated with protrusions of peritoneal sacs containing intraabdominal contents with the exception of enteroceles such as those described here. However, pelvic support defects do exhibit disruptions in the continuity of their supporting connective tissues as is the case with midline cystoceles and in rectocele defects.[9] These disruptions in supporting connective tissues are also seen in paravaginal defects. These defects can be made visible in preoperative and intraoperative inspection. They behave

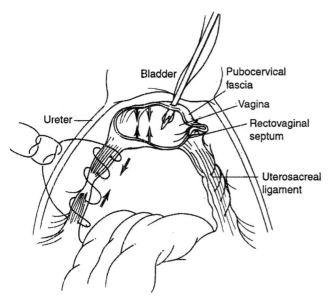

Figure 14.3.2.1. Vaginal vault suspension and enterocele repair. A beginning enterocele. Notice the separation of the pubocervical fascia at the anterior wall from the rectovaginal fascia of the posterior vaginal wall. From Carter JE.[9] Reprinted with permission of A. Cullen Richardson, MD.

just as other hernias and either remain stable or increase in size. Failure to accurately identify and properly repair each of these defects may result in failure of the operation. Therefore, operative repair of pelvic floor support defects must address each anatomic defect posteriorly, laterally, and anteriorly as described by Richardson [2,6–8] and Shull.[10]

Clinical evaluation of women with pelvic floor defects is performed using the techniques described by Shull.[11] The effectiveness of addressing fascial defects for rectocele has been demonstrated.[8,12,13] The effectiveness of a defect-specific approach to the paravaginal area involving reattachment of the pubocervical fascia laterally to the fascia of the obturator internus muscle at the level of the arcus tendineus fascia of the pelvis

has been demonstrated by Shull [10], Richardson et al. [6,7] and Liu.[14] Therefore, transverse, midline, and lateral ligament defects in the anterior vaginal wall must be addressed when performing laparoscopic vaginal vault suspension and enterocele repair as described by Richardson.[6,7]

Ross [3] described apical vault repair as the cornerstone of pelvic floor reconstruction. The techniques available for apical vault repair, including laparoscopic vaginal vault suspension using the uterosacral ligaments, have been described by several authors.[9,15–17] Laparoscopic vaginal vault support may also be provided by laparoscopic sacrocolpopexy with or without the use of mesh.[18,19]

TECHNIQUE AND RESULTS

Uterosacral Ligament Suspension

There are two laparoscopic techniques to treat vaginal vault prolapse: uterosacral ligament suspension and sacrocolpopexy. This section concentrates on laparoscopic uterosacral ligament suspension.

After general endotracheal anesthesia has been induced, careful pelvic exam is performed. The abdomen is insufflated with CO_2, and trocars are selected and placed depending on the surgeon's preferences regarding suturing techniques and instrumentation.[1,9,17] The patient is placed in Trendelenburg position, and the bowel is swept out of the pelvis. Using a rectal sizer placed in the vaginal vault, the vault is inverted so that the peritoneal lining overlying the separated rectovaginal and pubocervical fascia is visible in the pelvic cavity (Figure 14.3.2.2). The uterosacral ligaments are identified bilaterally, with care also taken to identify the course of the ureters anterolateral to the uterosacral ligaments. The uterosacral ligaments are examined as they enter the sacrum. The unbroken portion of the uterosacral ligament is tagged with suture bilaterally and used for reattachment of the vaginal apex (Figure 14.3.2.3). The peritoneum overlying the break between the pubocervical and rectovaginal fasciae is opened. The pubocervical fascia is identified ventrally between the vagina and the bladder by sharp dissection. The rectovaginal fascia is identified posteriorly (Figure 14.3.2.4). Redundant

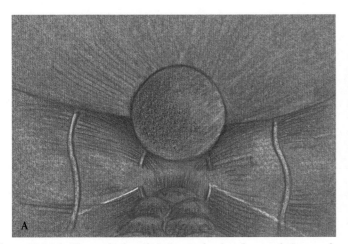

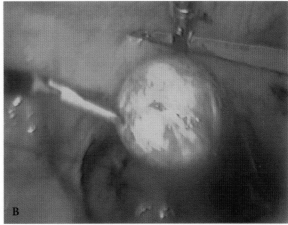

Figure 14.3.2.2. The vaginal vault is inverted using the rectal sizer so that it can be visualized within the pelvic cavity. The peritoneal lining overlying the rectovaginal and pubocervical fascia can be clearly seen. From Carter JE.[9]

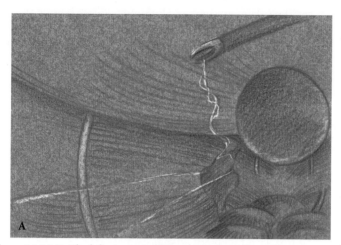
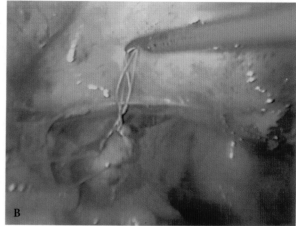

Figure 14.3.2.3. The left uterosacral ligament is shown here. The uterosacral ligaments are visualized as they enter the sacrum and are tagged by suture for later identification. From Carter JE.[9]

peritoneum and excess vagina are excised. Corner stitches are then placed on each side that approximate the edges of the pubocervical to the rectovaginal fascia overlying the vaginal mucosa. Permanent suture can be used for all aspects of the repair. The corner stitch is then incorporated into the ipsilateral uterosacral ligament, which had been previously tagged (Figure 14.3.2.5). The corner of the now reapproximated pubocervical and rectovaginal fascia along the edges and corner of the vaginal apex is then incorporated into the ipsilateral uterosacral ligament as it courses to the sacrum. In this way, the rectovaginal–pubocervical complex is sutured to the unbroken portion of the uterosacral ligament, forming a very secure attachment of the vaginal apical corner (Figure 14.3.2.6). This procedure is performed on both sides of the apical vault, providing a very secure support for the lateral and upper corner of the vaginal vault.

The rectovaginal fascia is then approximated to the pubocervical fascia across the center of the vaginal vault with interrupted sutures (Figure 14.3.2.7). Reinforcing sutures from the uterosacral ligaments to the posterior rectovaginal fascia are then placed bilaterally. These sutures do not cross the midline but rather reinforce the attachment of the corner of the vaginal

vault to the ipsilateral uterosacral complex. Thus, they provide an appropriate anatomic connection to the rectovaginal septum and maintain the maximum possible transverse dimension of the upper portion of the vagina (Figure 14.3.2.8). Cystoscopy is performed to visualize the ureteral orifice and assure the ureters were not kinked during suspension of the uterosacral ligaments to the vaginal vault.

Lin et al. [17] reviewed 133 cases of laparoscopic vaginal vault suspension using uterosacral ligaments. Efficacy and anatomic outcome were assessed by the Baden–Walker halfway scoring system before and after the surgical procedure. Preoperatively, all patients showed evidence of grade 2 or greater prolapse (descent to the level of the hymen). Fifty-one patients (38.4%) had uterovaginal prolapse, and 82 patients (61.6%) had vaginal vault prolapse. The patients were reevaluated at 1, 6, and 12 months postoperatively and yearly thereafter. In postoperative follow-up ranging from 2.0 to 7.3 years, 112 patients (87.2%) had no recurrence of prolapse and 17 patients (12.8%) had recurrence of prolapse. The major complication rate was 2.25% and involved only three patients. One patient developed a deep vein thrombosis and pulmonary embolus on day 5. A second patient developed

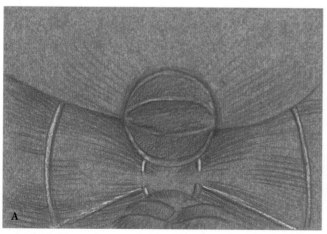
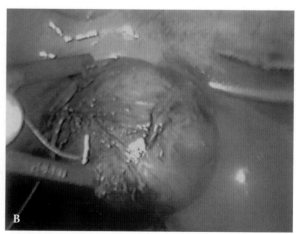

Figure 14.3.2.4. The peritoneum has been divided, and with sharp dissection, the pubocervical and rectovaginal fascia has been identified. The break between them is clearly visible. From Carter JE.[9]

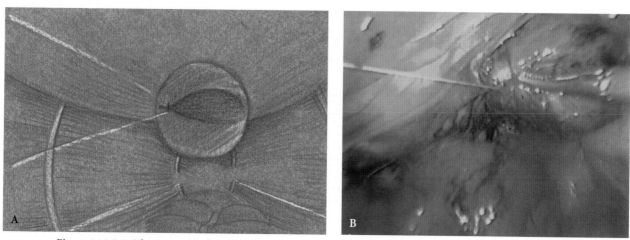

Figure 14.3.2.5. The corner stitch is placed through the pubocervical and rectovaginal fascia. From Carter JE.[9]

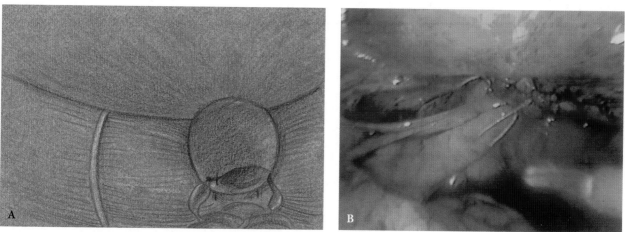

Figure 14.3.2.6. The lateral edges and apical corner of the vaginal vault are secured to the unbroken portion of the uterosacral ligament as it courses to the sacrum. The left apical corner is shown here. From Carter JE.[9]

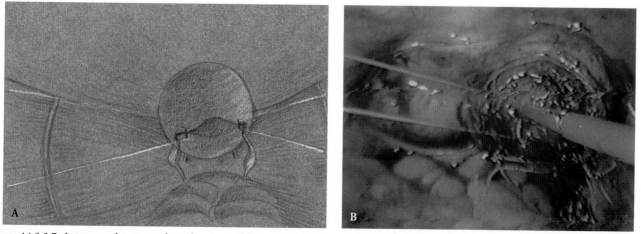

Figure 14.3.2.7. Interrupted sutures close the apex of the vaginal vault, restoring the integrity of the attachment of the pubocervical to the rectovaginal fascia. From Carter JE.[9]

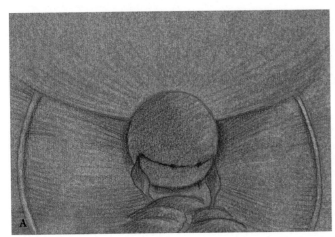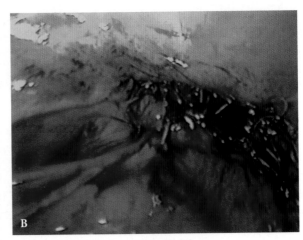

Figure 14.3.2.8. Completed vaginal vault apical support is visualized. From Carter JE.[9]

persistent pelvic pain, and a third patient developed an erosion of a suburethral sling graft through the vaginal mucosa; the graft had been placed as part of a concomitant procedure. There were no ureteral injuries or blood transfusions. The authors concluded that laparoscopic vaginal vault suspension is a safe, efficacious, and durable alternative for the management of vaginal vault prolapse.

Margossian [20] described laparoscopic uterosacral ligament plication and shortening techniques for supporting both the uterus in place and the vaginal apex but did not report results. Seman [21] reported an objective success rate of 100% in 10 selected patients with defects in the apical compartment, with up to 12 months of follow-up The overall success rate in the series of 73 patients was 90% over a 2-year duration.

Another technique using the AVESTA kit (Inlet Medical, Eden Prairie, MN) involves the use of specialized instrumentation for the investment and placation of the uterosacral ligaments at the vaginal vault after closure of the apex. It has been reported to have satisfactory result in a series of 24 patients with a mean follow-up of 6 months.[1]

Wattiez et al. [22] commented that regardless of the reconstruction method used, all authors agree that the anatomic defect leading to vaginal vault prolapse is detachment of the pubocervical and rectovaginal fasciae from each other and from their apical supports – the sacrouterine and cardinal ligaments. Hence, the principles of reconstruction should include a global reattachment of all of the cervical ring fascial components.

Laparoscopic Sacrocolpopexy

Laparoscopic sacrocolpopexy represents the adaptation of abdominal sacrocolpopexy to different instrumentation. Nezhat et al. [18], Lyons and Winer [19], Wattiez et al. [22], and Ross [23,24] have all described laparoscopic techniques to perform sacrocolpopexy.

As described by Ross [23], the surgical repair was performed in the following order depending on the pelvic defects present: anal sphincteroplasty, posterior colporrhaphy, anterior colporrhaphy, laparoscopic sacrocolpopexy, laparoscopic paravaginal repair, and laparoscopic Burch colposuspension. This surgical order was used to ensure appropriate urethrovesical elevation for the Burch colposuspension or other anterior compartment repairs. Anterior midline and posterior vaginal vault repairs were performed with site-specific vaginal repairs as described in detail by Ross.[24]

In Ross's technique for laparoscopic sacrocolpopexy, the laparoscope is placed through an infraumbilical trocar site after establishing a pneumoperitoneum. One midline suprapubic and two lateral ports are placed for instrumentation under direct vision. A vaginal probe is placed at the apex of the vagina for dissection support. The peritoneum at the vaginal apex is mobilized until the pubocervical fascia and rectovaginal septum are found anteriorly and posteriorly. Thinned out vaginal wall, primarily mucosa, is treated as a hernia sac and amputated to the level of the ischial spine. A piece of polypropylene mesh (Ethicon, Inc., Somerville, NJ) is precut so that it extends posteriorly from the vaginal apex to the sacral promontory lengthwise, loosely following the curve of the sacral hollow. A second piece of mesh is placed anteriorly and sutured with polypropylene suture 3 to 4 cm from the distal end of the posterior piece of mesh, making a Y. In cases of descending perineum, the posterior strip of mesh extends down to the perineal body. The added length necessary is measured by approximation with a grasper. The posterior rim of the mesh is secured distally to the perineal body and the posterior vaginal wall with three to five polypropylene sutures (Ethicon, Inc., Somerville, NJ). The anterior rim of the mesh is fixed to the pubocervical fascia with two to three sutures per side. This technique reestablishes the paracervical ring almost completely with sutures through mesh into the rectovaginal fascia posteriorly and pubocervical fascia anteriorly.

After vaginal attachment, the sacral promontory is identified and the loose peritoneum covering is elevated and incised. Using blunt dissection, the sacral anterolateral ligaments are exposed. The iliac vessels and ureter are visualized on the right. The left common iliac vein often crosses over the midline sacral promontory and must be identified. The peritoneal incision is continued down to the sacral hollow, just right of midline, to the apical vaginal vault. Laterally, the peritoneal dissection is opened to the edge of the colon on the left and to the uterosacral ligament on the right. The proximal end of the mesh is fixed to the anterior longitudinal sacral ligaments with three to four interrupted polypropylene sutures or hernia staples at the promontory. The mesh should create a tension-free suspension. The peritoneum is closed to completely cover the polypropylene mesh. Finally, the anterior pelvic compartment procedure and cystoscopy are performed.[23]

There were no intraoperative complications in Ross' report.[23] Postoperatively, one patient developed a perineal hematoma after surgery, which was treated conservatively. Two patients (4%) experienced small bowel obstructions on days 10 and 14 postoperatively resulting in bowel resection. Four patients (8%) had mesh erosion into the vagina.

In long-term follow-up, there were only three patients with recurrent apical vault prolapse. The failures were at 6, 14, and 15 months, resulting in 98% (and 93%) 1- and 5-year objective cure rates. Forty-one patients (80%) had reported impaired coitus before surgery. At 5-year followup, only 17 patients (43%) continued to report impaired coitus.

Wattiez et al. [22] described a technique for laparoscopic sacrocolpopexy using the following steps:

1. Dissection and identification of the pubocervical fascia
2. Dissection and identification of the cardinal–uterosacral complex (uterosacral ligaments are dissected up to their origin, the most solid part)
3. Dissection of the rectovaginal space down to the puborectalis muscle, lateral to the anorectal junction
4. Subtotal hysterectomy (optional)
5. Dissection and identification of the prevertebral ligament and peritoneal incision laterally to the direction of the cul-de-sac of Douglas
6. Fixation of the posterior part of the synthetic mesh to the puborectal muscle, the cardinal–uterosacral complex
7. Fixation of the anterior part of the above-mentioned mesh to the pubocervical fascia
8. Attachment of both parts of the mesh together lateral to the cervix and reconstruction of the fascial pericervical ring
9. Fixation of the uterosacral ligaments to the mesh complex and re-creation of a double vaginal axis
10. Fixation of the mesh to the promontorium
11. Peritonization
12. Dissection of the space of Retzius and identification of the paravaginal defects
13. Paravaginal defect repair, as required
14. Burch colposuspension, if needed

In Wattiez et al.'s study [22], 125 patients underwent laparoscopic sacrocolpopexy as described with a mean follow-up of 32 months. The objective overall success rate was 93.4%, and the subjective overall success rate was 100%.

It was concluded that the benefits of a global laparoscopic reconstructive repair using mesh include better assessment, a more precise and correct anatomic repair, the use of strong and acceptable materials instead of the weak native tissue, faster recovery, and excellent anatomic and functional results. The authors' later results improved on the results originally obtained using the technique they described in 2001.[25]

Nezhat et al. [18] demonstrated early that laparoscopic sacrocolpopexy is an effective technique for treatment of vaginal vault prolapse. The authors reported 100% success for a series of 15 patients with apical vault prolapse, with a follow-up of 3 to 40 months. Lyons and Winer [19] reported a series of 20 patients with a cure rate of 80% in 1-year follow-up.

CONCLUSION

As pointed out by Nezhat [26], the introduction of videolaparoscopy and videolaseroscopy has revolutionized chest, abdominal, and pelvic surgery. Abdominal colpopexy performed by suspending a mesh hammock between the prolapsed vaginal vault and sacrum provides good results in carefully selected patients. By following the surgical principles in restoring correct anatomical position of the vault, the use of laparoscopic route is an alternative to abdominal sacrocolpopexy for patients who are not candidates for a vaginal approach.

REFERENCES

1. Glazerman L, Abbott K, Schwartz M, Presthus J. Interim results of a multicenter study of a minimally interventional technique for treating vaginal vault prolapse [abstract]. *JSLS.* 2005;9:S50.
2. Richardson AC. The anatomic defects in rectocele and enterocele. *J Pelv Surg.* 1995;1:214–221.
3. Ross JW. Apical vault repair, the cornerstone of pelvic vault reconstruction. *Int Urogynecol J.* 1997;8:146–152.
4. DeLancey JOL. Anatomy and biomechanics of genital prolapse. *Clin Obstet Gynecol.* 1993;36:897–909.
5. DeLancey JOL. Pelvic organ prolapse. In: Scott JR, DiSaia PJ, Hammond CP, Spellacy WN, eds. *Danforth's Obstetrics and Gynecology.* 7th ed. Philadelphia: JB Lippincott Co.; 1994:803–825.
6. Richardson AC, Lyon JB, Williams NL. New look at pelvic relaxation. *Am J Obstet Gynecol.* 1976;126:568–573.
7. Richardson AC. Hernias of the pelvic wall, perineum and pelvic floor. In: Skandalakis LJ, ed. *Modern Hernia Repair: The Embryological and Anatomical Basis of Surgery.* New York: Parthenon Publishing Group; 1996:271–378.
8. Richardson AC. The rectovaginal septum revisited: its relationship to rectocele and its importance to rectocele repair. *Clin Obstet Gynecol.* 1993;36:976–983.
9. Carter JE, Winter M, Mendelsohn S, Saye W, Richardson AC. Vaginal vault suspension and enterocele repair by Richardson–Saye laparoscopic technique: description of training technique and results. *JSLS.* 2001;5:29–36.
10. Shull BL, Benn SJ, Kuehl TJ. Surgical management of prolapse of the anterior vaginal segment: an analysis of support defects, operative morbidity and anatomic outcome. *Am J Obstet Gynecol.* 1994;171:1429–1439.
11. Shull BL. Clinical evaluation of women with pelvic support defects. *Clin Obstet Gynecol.* 1993;36:939–951.
12. Porter W, Steele A, Kohli N, et al. The anatomic and functional outcomes of defect-specific rectocele repair. *Am J Obstet Gynecol.* 1999;181:1353.
13. Kenton K, Shott S, Brubaker L. Outcome after rectovaginal fascia attachment for rectocele repair. *Am J Obstet Gynecol.* 1999;181:1360–1364.
14. Liu CY. Laparoscopic cystocele repair: paravaginal suspension. In: Liu CY, ed. *Laparoscopic Hysterectomy and Pelvic Floor Reconstruction.* Cambridge, MA: Blackwell Science; 1996:330–344.
15. Saye W. Laparoscopic enterocele repair and vaginal vault suspension. Presented at: Society of Laparoscopic Surgeons Postgraduate Course on Laparoscopic Pelvic Floor Reconstruction and

Treatment of Stress Urinary Incontinence; December 9, 1998; San Diego, CA.

16. Miklos JR, Kohli N, Lucente V, et al. Site-specific fascial defects in the diagnosis and surgical management of enterocele. *Am J Obstet Gynecol*. 1998;179:1418–1423.

17. Lin LL, Phelps J, Liu CY. Laparoscopic vaginal vault suspension using uterosacral ligaments: review of 133 cases. *J Minim Invasive Gynecol*. 2005;12:216–220.

18. Nezhat CH, Nezhat F, Nezhat C. Laparoscopic sacrocolpopexy for vaginal vault prolapse. *Obstet Gynecol*. 1994;84:885–888.

19. Lyons TL, Winer WK. Vaginal vault suspension. *Endosc Surg*. 1995;3:88–92.

20. Margossian H, Walters MD, Falcone T. Laparoscopic management of pelvic organ prolapse. *Eur J Obstet Gynecol Reprod Biol*. 1999;85:57–62.

21. Seman EI, Cook JR, O'Shea RT. Two-year experience with laparoscopic pelvic floor repair. *J Am Assoc Gynecol Laparosc*. 2003;10:38–45.

22. Wattiez A, Mashiach R, Donoso M. Laparoscopic repair of vaginal vault prolapse. *Curr Opin Obstet Gynecol*. 2003;15:315–319.

23. Ross JW, Preston M. Laparoscopic sacrocolpopexy for severe vaginal vault prolapse: five-year outcome. *J Minim Invasive Gynecol*. 2005;12:221–226.

24. Ross JW. Techniques of laparoscopic repair of total vault eversion after hysterectomy. *J Am Assoc Gynecol Laparosc*. 1997;4:173–183.

25. Wattiez A, Canis M, Mage G, et al. Promontofixation for the treatment of prolapse. *Urol Clin North Am*. 2001;28:151–157.

26. Nezhat C. Videolaseroscopy: a new modality for treatment of diseases of the reproductive organs. *Colposc Gynecol Laser Surg*. 1986;2:221–224.

Section 14.4. Laparoscopic Repair of Cystourethrocele, Vesicovaginal Fistula, and Vaginal Vault Prolapse

Bulent Berker, Babac Shahmohamady, Naghmeh Saberi, and Camran Nezhat

Pelvic organ prolapse may occur when pelvic support structures are subjected to increased intra-abdominal pressure. Commonly, there is an intrinsic defect of the pelvic floor. There are several theories regarding the etiology of pelvic organ prolapse; none fully explains the origin and natural history of the process. Proposed causes include denervation of the pelvic floor musculature, direct injury to the pelvic floor musculature, abnormal synthesis or degradation of collagen, and defects in endopelvic fascia.[1] Although support for the pelvic viscera, the vagina, and neighboring structures involves a complex interplay among muscles, fascia, nerve supply, and appropriate anatomic orientation, the endopelvic fascia and pelvic floor muscles provide most of the support function in the female pelvis.[2]

Loss of support of the pelvic organs may involve any or all of the three following areas: anterior, posterior, and apical compartments. Defects in the anterior vaginal compartment result in cystourethrocele formation and sometimes stress urinary incontinence. Posterior compartment defects result in rectocele and enterocele. Apical defects result in uterovaginal prolapse and vaginal vault prolapse.[3] Usually, pelvic floor defects occur in several places, requiring multiple procedures in the same patient. The existence of numerous surgical techniques for treating genitourinary prolapse and incontinence demonstrates that no single method is completely satisfactory.

The anatomy, pathophysiology, and treatment of pelvic organ prolapse have significantly evolved over the last decade, with increasing understanding of anatomy and development of minimally invasive surgical procedures.[2] The introduction of videolaparoscopy by Nezhat has revolutionized modern-day gynecologic and general surgery.[4–6] Although operative laparoscopy has been used for decades, only recently has it gained widespread popularity for major operative procedures. The increasing application of operative laparoscopy is the result of advances in laparoscopic techniques and equipment.[6,7] Laparoscopic reconstructive pelvic surgery requires a thorough knowledge of pelvic floor anatomy and its supportive components before repair of defective anatomy is attempted.

REPAIR OF CYSTOURETHROCELE

Prolonged, bothersome vaginal protrusions and pelvic pressure that worsens with ambulation and daily activity are common symptoms in women who have vaginal prolapse. Other symptoms include difficulty walking, voiding, or defecating; urinary incontinence; recurrent mucosal irritation; ulceration; and coital difficulty. Improvement of the quality of life is achievable in certain patients with behavioral modification and nonsurgical vaginal devices.

The arcus tendinous fascia pelvis is a band of dense regular connective tissue stretched between the pubic bone and the ischial spine. The pubocervical fascia forms a trapezoidal layer spanning the area between the two arcus tendineae.[1] Paravaginal repair is required when cystourethrocele results from a separation of the pubocervical fascia from its lateral attachment to the pelvic side wall. If this defect is accompanied by GUSI, the paravaginal repair almost always will correct the problem.[8]

Dissection during anterior colporrhaphy splits the vaginal muscularis, and vaginal repair involves plication of the muscularis and adventitia in the midline and can pull the lateral attachments farther from the pelvic side wall. Paravaginal repair restores the lateral attachments to the pelvic side wall at the linea alba. Reported failure rates range from 0% to 20% for anterior colporrhaphy and from 3% to 14% for paravaginal repair.[9]

In determining the correct surgical approach, preoperative clinical assessment of the patient is very important. Successful surgical correction of the cystocele depends on the type of defect found in the pubocervical fascia. On examination of the anterior vagina, anterolateral support should be confirmed. If one or both anterolateral sulci are absent and vaginal rugation is present, then a detachment of the pubocervical fascia from the fascial white line – a paravaginal defect – should be suspected.[2] Four different pubocervical fascial defects can cause cystocele. Distinguishing these defects is important, as each type requires a different operative procedure.

1. The paravaginal defect results from detachment of the pubocervical fascia from its lateral attachment to the fascia of the obturator internal muscle at the level of the arcus tendineus fascia of the pelvis.[10–12] This is the most common cause of cystourethrocele. The repair consists of reestablishing the lateral pelvic side wall attachments of the pubocervical fascia and restoring the stability of this "hammock" by correcting the fundamental anatomic defect.
2. The transverse defect is caused by transverse separation of the pubocervical fascia from the pericervical ring into which the cardinal and uterosacral ligaments insert. The base of the bladder herniates into the anterior vaginal fornix and forms a cystocele without displacing the urethra or urethrovesical junction.
3. The midline or central defect results from a break in the central portion of the hammock between its lateral, dorsal, or ventral attachments.

4. With the distal defect, the distal urethra becomes avulsed or separated from its attachment to the urogenital diaphragm as it passes under the pubic symphysis.

Technique

Many operations have been described to correct loss of pelvic support. The abnormalities are identified, and the operation is planned with the intention of correcting each defect to achieve the optimal outcome.[13] The patient should be able to tolerate general anesthesia, increased intra-abdominal pressure, and the Trendelenburg position.

The principles of the transabdominal approach used at laparotomy are employed during laparoscopy. This technique has evolved as an alternative in reconstructive pelvic operations.[14,15] Laparoscopy involves a smaller incision, eliminates the need for abdominal packing, causes less manipulation of the viscera, affords a better view of the pelvis, and allows precise hemostasis.

The patient is given intravenous antibiotics prophylactically. After induction of general endotracheal anesthesia and placement, a 10- to 11-mm umbilical trocar is inserted. Three lower abdominal 5-mm ancillary trocars also are placed; two are lateral to the epigastric vessels at the level of the iliac crest, and one is in the midline 5 cm above the pubic symphysis. The patient is put in the Trendelenburg position and tilted to the left to shift the bowel away from the operating field. After evaluation of the peritoneal cavity and completion of other indicated procedures, the pelvic reconstruction can proceed. The retropubic space is entered and dissected. The pubic symphysis, obturator foramen, and obturator neurovascular bundle are identified. The paravaginal defect (the lateral vaginal sulci) can be seen detached from the arcus tendineus fascia (Figures 14.4.1, 14.4.2).

The bladder is mobilized medially, and the pubocervical fascia is exposed. The ischial spine can be located digitally by placing the operator's fingers inside the vagina while viewing through the laparoscope. During mobilization of the bladder, the lateral

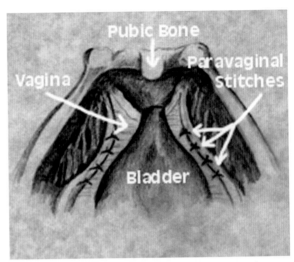

Figure 14.4.2. Laparoscopic surgical approach to repair of paravaginal defect.

superior sulcus of the vagina is lifted by the assistant's fingers in the vagina to facilitate dissection.

Separation of the lateral sulcus from the pelvic side wall can be seen laparoscopically. Permanent sutures (2-0 Prolene) are used to attach the superior lateral sulcus of the vagina to the arcus tendineus fascia (white line). The superior lateral sulcus of the vagina is elevated with the assistant's fingers in the vagina. Beneath the prominent paraurethral vascular plexus, the vagina is sutured to the linea alba of the pelvic side wall.

The paraurethral vascular plexus runs longitudinally along the axis of the vagina and is electrodesiccated before the placement of sutures. Otherwise, bleeding may occur if the plexus is penetrated by the needle. Such bleeding invariably stops when the suspension sutures are tied. To avoid bleeding, the first paravaginal suspension stitch should be placed close to the ischial spine. Figure-of-eight sutures are used for the suspension stitches to obtain good hemostasis and suspension. After placement of the first stitch, additional sutures are placed through the vaginal sulcus with its overlying fascia and the arcus tendineus fascia ventrally toward the pubic symphysis. The last stitch should be as close as possible to the pubic ramus.

Before this first suture is placed, the gynecologist should identify the ischial spine by vaginal palpation and by viewing through the laparoscope to avoid injuring the pudendal vessels and nerve. The initial stitch is placed through the linea alba approximately 1.0 to 1.5 cm ventral to the ischial spine.[16] Frequent vaginal examinations are done while suturing to assist the proper placement of the stitches, assess the adequacy of suspension, and establish anterior support. The procedure is completed by bladder neck suspension.

VESICOVAGINAL FISTULA REPAIR

The primary etiology of vesicovaginal fistula in developed countries is surgical trauma associated with gynecologic procedures. Most fistulas occur after hysterectomy for benign conditions because these procedures are far more common than surgery

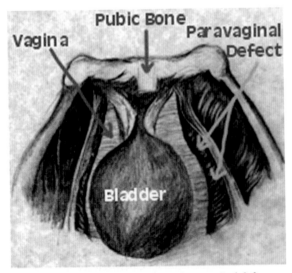

Figure 14.4.1. A representation of paravaginal defect.

for cancer. However, the risk of fistula formation is higher after radical surgery because of the scope of surgery, the presence of tumor, and, in some cases, radiation-induced changes. In contrast, urogenital fistulas in developing countries are usually associated with childbirth. Despite the best efforts of the surgeon, injuries to the urinary tract may still occur as part of the healing process in pelvic surgery. Tissue necrosis follows tissue ischemia, attributable to external pressure (crush or clamp injury), kinking of urinary tract tissue (proximity to a ligated pedicle), or marked inflammation with tissue fibrosis. Direct injury to the urinary tract by laceration or puncture usually results in immediate urine leakage, whereas delayed injury from retroperitoneal fibrosis, tissue pressure, or partial obstruction may not result in fistula formation and urine leakage for days or weeks.

Postoperative patients with a vesicovaginal fistula usually are easily diagnosed with urine leaking through the vagina. Classically, fistulas occur between the seventh and the 12th day after obstetric or gynecologic surgery. The diagnosis can be confirmed by filling the bladder with a dilute solution of methylene blue. The vaginal vault is then directly inspected to visualize the fistula. If no defect is clearly seen, then cystoscopy can be a valuable diagnostic help. In a patient who is experiencing urinary incontinence, the tampon test, in which a tampon is inserted into the vagina after filling the bladder with a dilute solution of methylene blue and have the patient ambulate, can help confirm the diagnosis. In addition to the cystoscopy and the cystourography, an intravenous pyeloureterogram is recommended to rule out concomitant ureteral fistulas before proceeding with the surgical repair.[17]

There is debate in the literature regarding the most appropriate period of time to wait before proceeding to surgery should the defect not heal, with the number of surgeons advocating early intervention (1 to 3 months) approximately equal to the number advocating later intervention (more than 3 months). The purpose of waiting is to allow recovery from inflammation, infection, and tissue necrosis. Although this might be true for complicated fistula and postpartum fistula, extensive infection and tissue necrosis are uncommon with gynecologic surgery–related fistula. Thus, waiting is less relevant for fistula following hysterectomy.

Vesicovaginal fistulas are treated with different surgical techniques, depending on their cause and location.[18] Small vesicovaginal fistulas that are not responsive to nonsurgical management usually are repaired easily.[19] The edges of the fistula are removed, and the defect is closed. Latzko's technique [20] is used commonly for fistulas that are surrounded by severe fibrosis and close to the bladder neck or urethral meatus. Lee and coworkers [21] recommended an abdominal approach for fistulas in the upper part of a narrow vagina, multiple fistulas, and those associated with other pelvic abnormalities or close to the ureter. A combined abdominal and vaginal approach is used in some instances.[22] Nezhat et al. [23] first reported the laparoscopic approach in 1994. Laparoscopic repair of vesicovaginal fistula may offer the patient less morbidity and a quicker recovery. The laparoscopic approach significantly reduces the access trauma of traditional laparotomy, with additional advantages of magnified vision of pelvic organs and less traumatic tissue handling.

Technique

The basic principles for repair include adequate exposure, excision of fibrous tissue from the edges of the fistula, approximation of the edges without tension, the use of suitable suture material, and efficient postoperative bladder drainage.[21]

A 10-mm infraumbilical incision is made for the insertion of the operative laparoscope. Three 5-mm trocars are inserted in the lower abdomen for the suction–irrigator probe, grasping forceps, and bipolar forceps. A simultaneous cystoscopy is done, and both ureters are catheterized to aid in their identification and protection during excision and closure of the fistula. A ureteral catheter is pulled through the fistula into the vagina to facilitate identification during excision.

A digital rectovaginal examination is carried out to exclude rectal involvement. An opening is made in the vagina, avoiding the bladder and rectum, and an inflated glove in the vagina helps maintain pneumoperitoneum. The anterior vaginal wall is elevated with a grasping forceps, and the fistula is identified with the previously inserted catheter, which also delineates the posterior bladder wall. The bladder is filled with water, and a cystotomy is made above the fistula. The water is evacuated as the bladder is distended by the pneumoperitoneum from the cystotomy. The fistula tract, vesicovaginal space, and ureters are observed laparoscopically (Figures 14.4.3, 14.4.4, and 14.4.5). The vesicovaginal space is developed laparoscopically with the CO_2 laser and hydrodissection or any other cutting modality. The bladder is freed posteriorly from the vaginal wall. The fistula is identified, held with a grasping forceps, and excised. Adequate bladder dissection and mobilization are essential to eliminate tension upon suturing.

Initially, the vaginal wall opening of approximately 1.5 cm is closed with one layer of interrupted polyglactin suture (Figure 14.4.6). Then the vesical defect is repaired in one layer with interrupted 1-0 Endoknot polyglactin sutures (Ethicon), using extracorporeal knotting. Defects in the vagina and bladder are closed separately. Hemostasis in the vesicovaginal space and fistula area is essential. A peritoneal flap is obtained superior and lateral to the bladder dome, close to the round ligament and diverted toward the bladder base. The flap is used to separate the vesicovaginal space. It is secured with two interrupted polyglactin sutures. The dissected peritoneal area heals secondarily. No intraperitoneal drainage is used. After the procedure, a suprapubic or transurethral catheter is inserted and the ureteral catheters are removed.

VAGINAL VAULT PROLAPSE

Vaginal vault prolapse is seen whenever the apex of the vagina descends below the introitus, turning the vagina inside out. It is uncommon in the United States, affecting between 900 and 1200 women annually.[24] Vaginal vault prolapse occurs as a result of damage to the supporting structures of the vaginal apex, the cardinal or the uterosacral ligaments. The most common cause of this condition is hysterectomy with failure to adequately reattach the cardinal–uterosacral complex to the pubocervical fascia and rectovaginal fascia at the vaginal cuff. Other predisposing factors include enterocele, damage to the endopelvic fascia or pelvic floor ligaments during labor and delivery, and postmenopausal

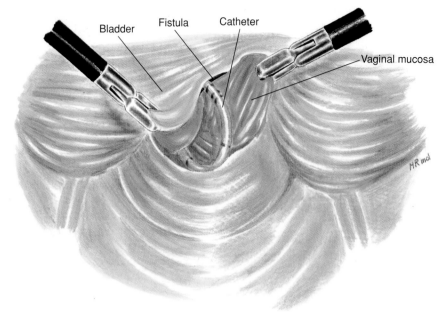

Figure 14.4.3. The fistula tract, vesicovaginal space, and ureters are observed laparoscopically.

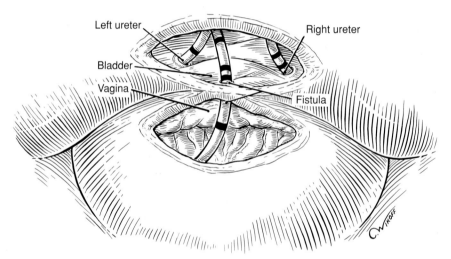

Figure 14.4.4. The bladder has been freed posteriorly from the vaginal wall.

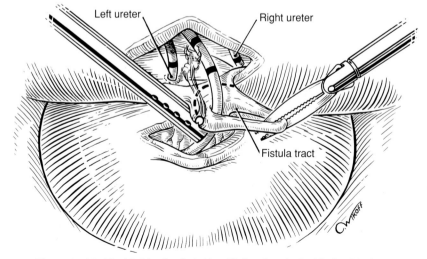

Figure 14.4.5. The bladder fistula is identified and excised with the CO_2 laser.

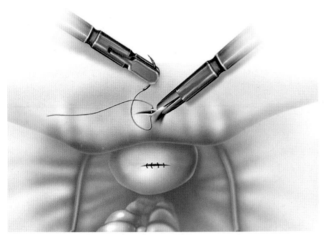

Figure 14.4.6. The vaginal wall repair is complete, and the bladder opening repair is in progress.

atrophy. Vaginal vault prolapse is usually associated with cystocele, rectocele, enterocele, or a combination of these defects.[1,6,25]

The approaches to the treatment of vaginal vault prolapse include the use of a pessary, vaginal reconstruction, and vaginal closure. For the obliterative approach, patient selection criteria should include the patient's physiologic age, sexual desires, general health status, and symptoms. Total colpocleisis is not an option for sexually active women.

The goal of vaginal vault suspension is to correct all anatomic defects, maintain or restore normal bowel and bladder function, and restore a functioning vagina. Transvaginal sacrospinous vault suspension and needle urethropexy may result in a satisfactory outcome in most operations.[26] The vaginal route may be used in women whose preference or medical disorders contraindicate the abdominal approach. However, studies have shown a 33% rate of recurrent prolapse associated with sacrospinous fixation and transvaginal needle suspension. The probability of an optimal surgical outcome is twice as great with a transabdominal operation.

Among the proposed surgical techniques to prevent and correct this condition is abdominal sacral colpopexy using the interposition of a synthetic suspensory hammock between the prolapsed vaginal vault and the anterior surface of the sacrum. [13,14,26] However, this technique usually requires a midline abdominal incision, abdominal packing, and extensive bowel manipulation. It has a potential for infection, wound separation or dehiscence, and ileus or bowel obstruction. To minimize these drawbacks, sacral colpopexy can be carried out laparoscopically. Laparoscopic sacrocolpopexy was first described by Nezhat et al. in 1994.[27] This procedure is discussed in more detail in Chapter 14.3.

CONCLUSION

Laparoscopic pelvic reconstructive surgeries may be complex and require advanced laparoscopic skills. However, when performed by experienced surgeons, the success rates of these procedures are comparable to traditional routes of repair.[12,16,23,27,28].

REFERENCES

1. Deval B, Haab F. What's new in prolapse surgery? *Curr Opin Urol.* 2003;13(4):315–323.
2. Miklos JR, Moore RD, Kohli N. Laparoscopic surgery for pelvic support defects. *Curr Opin Obstet Gynecol.* 2002;14(4):387–395.
3. Birnbaum SJ. Rational therapy for the prolapsed vagina. *Am J Obstet Gynecol.* 1973;115(3):411–419.
4. Nezhat C. Videolaparoscopy and videolaseroscopy: a new modality for the treatment of endometriosis and other diseases of reproductive organs. *Colposc Gynecol Laser Surg.* 1986;2:221–224.
5. Nezhat C, Siegler A, Nezhat F, et al. Appendectomy. In: *Operative Gynecologic Laparoscopy, Principles and Techniques.* 2nd ed. New York: McGraw-Hill;2000:339–353.
6. Tadir Y, Fisch B. Operative laparoscopy: a challenge for general gynecology. *Am J Obstet Gynecol.* 1993;169:7–12.
7. Margossian H, Walters MD, Falcone T. Laparoscopic management of pelvic organ prolapse. *Eur J Obstet Gynecol Reprod Biol.* 1999; 85(1):57–62.
8. Richardson AC. How to correct prolapse paravaginally. *Contemp Obstet Gynecol.* 1990;35:100.
9. Weber AM, Walters MD. Anterior vaginal prolapse: review of anatomy and techniques of surgical repair. *Obstet Gynecol.* 1997; 89:311.
10. Richardson AC, Lyon JB, Williams NL. A new look at pelvic relaxation. *Am J Obstet Gynecol.* 1976;126:568.
11. Baden WF, Walker TA. Urinary stress incontinence: evolution of paravaginal repair. *Female Patient.* 1987;12:89.
12. Liu CY. Laparoscopic cystocele repair: paravaginal suspension. In: Liu CY, ed. *Laparoscopic Hysterectomy and Pelvic Floor Reconstruction.* Cambridge, MA: Blackwell; 1996.
13. Arthur HG, Savage D. Uterine prolapse and prolapse of vaginal vault treated by sacral hysteropexy. *J Obstet Gynaecol Br Emp.* 1957;64:355.
14. Randall CL, Nichols DH. Surgical treatment of vaginal inversion. *Obstet Gynecol.* 1971;38:327.
15. Symmonds RE, Williams TJ, Lee RA, Webb MJ. Posthysterectomy enterocele and vaginal vault prolapse. *Am J Obstet Gynecol.* 1981;140:852.
16. Nezhat C, Nezhat F, Gordon S, Wilkins E. Laparoscopic versus abdominal hysterectomy. *J Reprod Med.* 1992;37:247.
17. Angioli R, Penalver M, Muzii L, et al. Guidelines of how to manage vesicovaginal fistula. *Crit Rev Oncol Hematol.* 2003;48(3):295–304.
18. Drutz HP. Urinary fistulas. *Obstet Gynecol Clin North Am.* 1989;16:11.
19. Falk HC, Orkin LA. Nonsurgical closure of vesicovaginal fistulas. *Obstet Gynecol.* 1957;9:538.
20. Latzko W. Behandlund hochsitzender blasen und mastdarmscheidenfisteln nach uteruseztipation mit hohom schedienverschluss. *Zentralbl Gynakol.* 1914;38:904.
21. Lee RA, Symmonds RE, William TJ. Current status of genitourinary fistula. *Obstet Gynecol.* 1988;72:313.
22. Taylor JS, Hewson AD, Rachow P. Synchronous combined transvaginal repair of vesicovaginal fistulas. *Aust N Z J Surg.* 1980;50:23.
23. Nezhat CH, Nezhat F, Nezhat LC, Rottenberg II. Laparoscopic repair of a vesicovaginal fistula: a case report. *Obstet Gynecol.* 1994;83:899.
24. Dunton JD, Mikuta J. Post-hysterectomy vaginal vault prolapse. *Postgrad Obstet Gynecol.* 1988;8:1.

25. Drutz HP, Alnaif B. Surgical management of pelvic organ prolapse and stress urinary incontinence. *Clin Obstet Gynecol.* 1998;41(3):786–793.

26. Sze EH, Miklos JR, Partoll L, et al. Sacrospinous ligament fixation with transvaginal needle suspension for advanced pelvic organ prolapse and stress incontinence. *Obstet Gynecol.* 1997;89:129.

27. Nezhat CH, Nezhat F, Nezhat C. Laparoscopic sacral colpopexy for vaginal vault prolapse. *Obstet Gynecol.* 1994;84(5):885–888.

28. Sotelo R, Mariano MB, García-Segui A, Dubois R, Spaliviero M, Keklikian W, Novoa J, Yaime H, Finelli A. Laparoscopic repair of vesicovaginal fistula. *J Urol.* 2005;173(5):1615–1618.

Section 14.5. Laparoscopic Rectovaginal Fistula Repair

Ceana Nezhat, Patrick Yeung, and Deidre T. Fisher

The discovery of a rectovaginal fistula is distressing to both the patient and her surgeon. This socially crippling condition likely includes the uncontrolled passage of flatus or stool from the anorectal canal through the fistulous tract into the vagina. Fortunately, fistulas between the anorectal canal and vagina are relatively uncommon, accounting for less than 5% of all anorectal fistulas.[1]

ANATOMY

Fistulas occurring caudad or adjacent to the external anal sphincter are termed anovaginal fistulas and are managed differently from rectovaginal fistulas. Fistulas occurring more than 3 cm above the anal canal are true rectovaginal fistulas. There are several classification systems for rectovaginal fistulas.[2–6] Although some surgeons have classified fistulas as "high" or "low," we favor classification with respect to condition of the perineal body and rectovaginal septum. The first three types are classified as (i) loss of perineal body *without* evidence of a fistulous tract, (ii) loss of perineal body *with* a fistulous tract in the lower third of the vagina, and (iii) an *intact* perineal body *with* a fistulous tract in the lowest third of the vagina. A vaginal approach is commonly used to repair these three types of rectovaginal fistulas, whereas types IV and V fistulas, which involve the middle and upper thirds of the vagina, respectively, require either a transabdominal or laparoscopic approach.

ETIOLOGY

The etiology of rectovaginal fistulas includes obstetric trauma, congenital anomalies, endometriosis, carcinoma, irradiation damage, inflammatory bowel disease, and complications of gynecologic and colorectal surgery.[7] Obstetric injuries are, by far, the most common etiology and usually arise as a complication of a repaired fourth-degree perineal tear.[5] Obstetric risk factors include prolonged labor, difficult forceps delivery, shoulder dystocia, and midline episiotomy. Reassuringly, only 0.1% of vaginal deliveries result in fistula formation.[5] Rectovaginal fistulas may result from direct surgical injury to the rectum or vagina or indirectly, as a result of tissue necrosis or postoperative infection. Fistulas may be secondary to surgical trauma, malignancy, or an inflammatory process and may occur anywhere along the vaginal wall, including the apex. In fact, the most common cause of high fistulas is repeated episodes of diverticulitis with abscess formation. Rectovaginal fistulas are associated with inflammatory bowel disease in 10% of patients.[5] Crohn's disease may result in complex fistulas, especially because the lesions may be transmural.[8,9] These fistulas have little chance of healing in the presence of severe proctitis; therefore, intensive medical treatment of inflammatory disease is indicated before surgical methods are employed.

DIAGNOSIS

Symptoms include vaginal passage of flatus, foul discharge, diarrhea, or frank stool. Also, patients may complain of abdominal or pelvic pain, rectal bleeding, or a mucus-like discharge, depending on the size and complexity of the fistula. Usually, symptoms occur between 7 and 10 days postoperatively and coincide with tissue breakdown and/or infection.

The first step in making the diagnosis is to consider rectovaginal fistula as a possible diagnosis. Therefore, a detailed clinical evaluation including a detailed history and physical examination is warranted. This includes a thorough examination of the vagina; the integrity of the rectum, external and internal anal sphincters, and puborectalis; and perineum, including the perineal body. Type IV and V fistulas may not readily be apparent on physical examination or vaginal inspection and may even be missed by endoscopy.[3] If no fistula is seen but one seems likely because of history and symptoms, there are a number of maneuvers that can be performed in the office or under anesthesia in the operating room to help identify the fistula. With the patient in pelvic tilt or Trendelenburg position, air can be injected via a Foley catheter or a bulb syringe into the rectum while observing for bubble formation in a saline-filled vagina. We have used sigmoidoscopy or vaginoscopy, with either the submersion of a hysteroscope or cystoscope in the saline-filled vagina, to visualize the bubbles from air simultaneously injected into the rectum to identify the precise location of the fistula. Similarly, an indigo carmine dye enema may be given, and a tampon inserted into the vagina may indicate the presence of a fistula. However, the most useful studies include direct visualization with proctosigmoidoscopy with gentle passage of a probe through the fistulous tract into the rectal canal. This also allows for assessment of intestinal mucosa and identification of additional defects or fistulas. In addition, rectogram and barium enema studies are helpful to confirm the presence of a type IV or V fistula, whereas occasionally CT and magnetic resonance imaging (MRI) with oral contrast may also uncover the underlying etiology. Lastly, if there is any concern of malignancy, biopsy should be considered.

SURGICAL MANAGEMENT

General Principles

The repair of the rectovaginal fistula can be surgically managed using a vaginal, anal, abdominal, or laparoscopic route. In addition to the surgeon's expertise, one must consider the location, size, and complexity of the fistula; accessibility; status of anal sphincter; and the original etiology for the defect. Basic principles used for successful repair include adequate exposure to allow for complete excision of the fistulous tract and fibrosis to ensure healthy, well-vascularized tissue for reapproximation.[10–13] In addition, the fistula site must be free of infection, induration, and fecal contamination. In fact, preoperatively, several days of a liquid diet with a full mechanical and chemical bowel preparation will decrease chances of contamination of the repair site. If the patient has Crohn's disease, she may require high-dose systemic steroids and/or chemotherapeutic agents to bring her disease into remission before repair. If significant fecal contamination, prior surgery, or persistent abscess is present, a diverting colostomy or ileostomy may be considered. Lastly, suitable suture material and a tension-free closure will help minimize chances of a failed repair.

Technique

Although the usual surgical repair of high rectovaginal fistulas is traditionally via a laparotomy approach, there have been several reports of the procedure performed laparoscopically. Schwenk et al. [14] reported a laparoscopic resection of the sigmoid colon with the fistulous tract and intracorporeal colorectal anastomosis in 1997. Pelosi et al. [15] performed laparoscopic upper rectovaginal mobilization to facilitate the transvaginal repair of a recurrent rectovaginal fistula. Total laparoscopic repair is still rare because of the complexity of the procedure and the need for keen suturing technique. However, Nezhat et al. [4] reported two cases of total laparoscopic rectovaginal fistula repair. Most recently, Kumaran et al. [3] reported a laparoscopic rectovaginal fistula repair following a laparoscopic-assisted vaginal hysterectomy. Our laparoscopic surgical treatment for type IV and V rectovaginal fistulas is similar to that used for laparoscopic treatment of infiltrative endometriosis involving the rectovaginal septum.[4,11–13] After general anesthesia, a multiple-puncture operative laparoscopy technique is used and the patient is placed in modified dorsolithotomy position with a slight Trendelenburg position. A detailed inspection of the abdomen and pelvis is performed. At times, extensive adhesiolysis and mobilization of the bladder from the vagina are necessary, and sometimes bilateral ureterolysis is necessary to restore normal anatomy (Figure 14.5.1).

Rectovaginal examination along with concomitant rigid sigmoidoscopy by the assistant are then used to identify correct planes, and the bowel is suctioned of its contents. Dissection to the pararectal areas down to the level of levator ani muscles may be necessary for optimal exposure and adequate mobilization. At this point, various maneuvers may be used to identify the course of the fistulous tract. For example, indigo carmine dye may be injected into the peritoneal end of the fistula while the surgeon observes leakage of dye using the proctosigmoidoscope. The fistulous opening may be seen as a small dimple or pit and

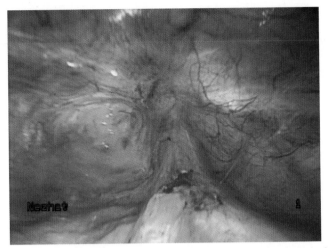

Figure 14.5.1. Survey of the pelvis revealed adhesions between vaginal apex and rectosigmoid colon.

occasionally can be gently probed for confirmation. The simultaneous use of both laparoscopy and proctosigmoidoscopy should reveal the presence of the fistulous tract. The vaginal wall should be elevated with grasping forceps (Figures 14.5.2, 14.5.3) and the rectovaginal space developed with CO_2 laser and hydrodissection or sharply until the fistula is apparent.

The fistula is then excised with CO_2 laser or scissors to healthy and vascularized margins (Figure 14.5.4). Adequate rectum dissection and mobilization are essential to eliminate tension upon suturing. Rectal and vaginal defects are then closed separately with several interrupted 1.0 polyglactin sutures (Figure 14.5.5).

With the pelvis filled with fluid, air is injected transanally to allow visualization of the repair site under water. This will help ensure that the repair is airtight. A piece of omentum is then interposed between vaginal and rectal repairs. Meticulous hemostasis in the rectovaginal space is imperative; therefore, a drain is not usually necessary. If a temporary colostomy is required, the hollow of the sacrum is entered and the rectosigmoid colon is mobilized. At this stage, the rectosigmoid colon is transected approximately 25 cm from the anal verge with a 60-mm

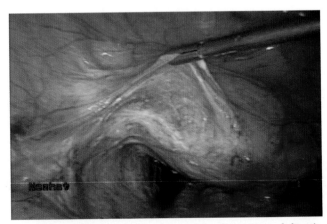

Figure 14.5.2. Fistulous tract can be seen after dissection and elevation of the vagina.

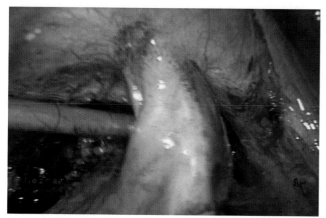

Figure 14.5.3. Development of rectovaginal space with CO_2 laser.

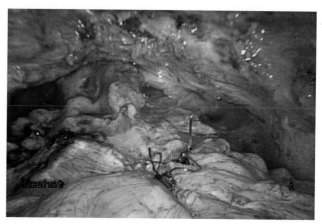

Figure 14.5.5. Rectal and vaginal defects are closed separately with sutures.

stapling device (Endopath; Endosurgery Inc., Cincinnati, OH) and the proximal end of the colon is transfixed to the skin of the 30-mm cannula site, thus performing a diverting colostomy.

POSTOPERATIVE CARE

Attention to the details of postoperative care is vital to prevent complications after a rectovaginal fistula repair. A low-residue diet, adequate hydration, abstaining from laxatives, and no rectal instrumentation (including digital examination, enemas, and suppositories) will prevent both direct mechanical trauma and hyperstimulation of the bowel when infection is present. In addition, a 2-week course of broad-spectrum antibiotics providing coverage of bowel and vaginal flora will prevent subsequent infection of the repair.[5,10] Sigmoidoscopic evaluation of the repair site 6 weeks later will ensure successful closure of the fistula. If a temporary colostomy was performed, before consideration of colostomy reversal either by minilaparotomy or laparoscopy, examination under anesthesia is performed. A careful vaginal examination and rigid proctosigmoidoscopy will ensure a healed fistula and normal rectal mucosa.

CONCLUSION

Although the discovery of a rectovaginal fistula is often disruptive both psychosocially and sexually, it can be successfully managed and depends on the location and etiology of the defect. Operative laparoscopy has revolutionized abdominal surgery and is a reasonable alternative to laparotomy for increasing numbers of indications. These advances extend to treatment of rectosigmoid colon and rectovaginal septum pathology. Advantages of the laparoscopic approach to rectovaginal septum are better visualization in this deep and small space, with Trendelenburg position, magnification, and lighting. With the patient in lithotomy position, one can use the sigmoidoscope simultaneously. This allows the surgeon to view the rectum from its mucosal as well as peritoneal surface for identification, precise dissection, and resection of the fistula. Lastly, as with all minimally invasive procedures, its advantages include less postoperative pain, minimal wound complications, and a quicker recovery.

REFERENCES

1. Fry RD, Kodner IJ. Rectovaginal fistula. *Surg Ann*. 1995;27:113–131.
2. Rosenshein NB, Genadry RR, Woodruff JF. An anatomic classification of rectovaginal septal defects. *Am J Obstet Gynecol*. 1980;137:439–443.
3. Kumaran SS, Palanivelu C, Kavalakat SJ, Parthasarathi R, Neelayathatchi M. Laparoscopic repair of high rectovaginal fistula: is it technically feasible? *BMC Surg*. 2005;5:20.
4. Nezhat CH, Bastidas JA, Pennington E, Nezhat FR, Raga F, Nezhat CR. Laparoscopic treatment of type IV rectovaginal fistula. *Am Assoc Gynecol Laparosc*. 1998;5:297–299.
5. Aronson MP, Lee RA. Fecal incontinence and rectovaginal fistulas. In: Rock J, Jones HW, eds. *TeLinde's Operative Gynecology*. Philadelphia: Lippincott Williams & Wilkins; 2003;1121–1160.
6. Ettayebi E, Behamou M. Anorectal malformation: treatment by laparoscopy. *Pediatr Endosurg Innov Technol*. 2001;5:209–213.
7. Pickhardt PJ, Bhalla S, Balfe DM. Acquired gastrointestinal fistulas: classification, etiologies, and imaging evaluation. *Radiology*. 2002;224:9–23.
8. Radcliffe AG, Ritchie JK, Hawley RP. Anovaginal and rectovaginal fistulas in Crohn's disease. *Dis Colon Rectum*. 1988;31:94–97.

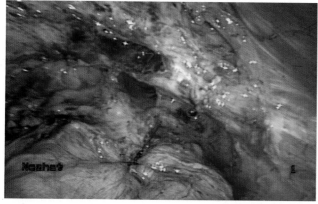

Figure 14.5.4. Fistulous tract is excised with adequate margin with CO_2.

9. Ludwig KA, Milson JW, Church JM, et al. Preliminary experience with laparoscopic intestinal surgery for Crohn's disease. *Am J Surg.* 1996;67:817–821.

10. Stenchever MA, Fenner DE. Anatomic defects of the abdominal wall and pelvic floor. In: Stenchever M, Droegemueller W, Herbst A, et al., eds. *Comprehensive Gynecology.* St. Louis: Mosby; 2001:565–606.

11. Nezhat C, Gary SB, Nezhat FR, et al. *Endometriosis: Advanced Management and Surgical Techniques.* New York: Springer-Verlag; 1995.

12. Nezhat C, Nezhat FR, Pennington E. Laparoscopic treatment of infiltrative rectosigmoid colon and rectovaginal septum endometriosis by the technique of videolaparoscopy and the CO_2 laser. *Br J Obstet Gynaecol.* 1992;99:664–667.

13. Nezhat C, Nezhat FR, Luciano AA, et al., eds. *Operative Gynecologic Laparoscopy: Principles and Techniques.* 2nd ed. New York: McGraw-Hill; 2000.

14. Schwenk, Bohm B, Muller J. Laparoscopic resection of high rectovaginal fistula with intracorporeal colorectal anatomosis and omentoplasty. *Surg Endosc.* 1997;11:147–149.

15. Pelosi MA, Pelosi MA. Transvaginal repair of recurrent rectovaginal fistula with laparoscopic-assisted rectovaginal mobilization. *J Laparoendosc Adv Surg Tech A.* 1997;7:379–383.

Section 14.6. Laparoscopically Assisted Neovaginoplasty

Luigi Fedele, Stefano Bianchi, Nicola Berlanda, Eleonora Fontana, and Alessandro Bulfoni

Surgical creation of the neovagina has been performed for more than a century according to various techniques and for a multitude of congenital and acquired causes of partial or total absence of the vaginal canal. The most frequent indication for neovaginoplasty is the Mayer–Rokitansky–Küster–Hauser syndrome, or simply Rokitansky syndrome. New surgical techniques in which laparoscopy has replaced traditional surgery have been recently proposed to treat rare congenital anomalies.

THE ROKITANSKY SYNDROME

The Rokitansky syndrome is a complex malformation comprising an absent vagina and uterus, grouped as class IE of the Buttram and Gibbons classification of genital tract abnormalities. The occurrence of a nonfunctioning vagina has been reported since ancient times. Hippocrates described a membranous obstruction of the vagina in the book *On the Nature of Women*. A few centuries later, Celsius presented a complete description of vaginal atresia.[1] Mayer in 1829 [2] and Rokitansky in 1838 [3] described a syndrome that included agenesis of the uterus and vagina due to an anomalous development of the mullerian ducts. Subsequently, Küster [4] recognized urologic associations whereas Hauser [5] distinguished Rokitansky syndrome from testicular feminization. The exact incidence of Rokitansky syndrome is unknown, although a recent epidemiologic study [6] estimated it to be one in 1500 to one in 4000 people born female. Following gonadal dysgenesis, Rokitansky syndrome is the major cause of primary amenorrhea.

The etiology of Rokitansky syndrome is not yet understood. It occurs sporadically but has been described in sisters with a normal karyotype and in a pair of monozygotic twins. The majority of patients have a normal female karyotype, although some show a mosaicism of the sex chromosomes (45X/46XX; 46XX/47XXX). It has been hypothesized that exposure to a teratogenic agent during the fourth gestational week may be responsible for Rokitansky syndrome as well as for the frequently associated anomalies of the skeletal and urinary systems. Indeed, in this intrauterine stage, the pronephric duct and the cervicothoracic somite blastema are closely linked.

The genital anatomy of Rokitansky syndrome is distinguished by normal external genitalia and the absence of the upper two thirds of the vagina (Figure 14.6.1). Another common finding is a blind retrohymenal pouch that may be as deep as 2 cm. The uterus is absent; whereas in most cases, two fibromuscular cords are found originating from the medial aspect of the tubal extremities and fused along the median line, resembling a double rudimentary uterus (Figure 14.6.2). Asymmetric and distinct rudimentary horns are seldom found and are usually of a greater size (Figure 14.6.3). Sometimes these horns may appear hollow and lined with endometrial tissue that is generally hyporesponsive to cyclic hormonal modifications. The horns may be also rarely a site of menstruation as seen in reports of subjects with Rokitansky syndrome developing hematometra in one or both rudimentary horns.[7] The salpinges and ovaries are usually normal, although rarely there may be ovarian anomalies, such as occurrences of unilateral agenesis.

Rokitansky syndrome is also distinguished by a frequent association with malformations of the urinary and skeletal systems. There may also be congenital cardiac anomalies. Urinary tract malformations are present in about 40% of cases, especially unilateral renal agenesis or ectopy, which is demonstrated in around 15% of patients.[8] Skeletal malformations affect the spine, limbs, and ribs. Recently, Pittock et al. [9] found vertebral anomalies in 44% of patients, whereas Strubbe et al. [10] showed that over 50% have some abnormalities on hand radiography. The most frequently described combination in Rokitansky syndrome has been uterovaginal agenesis, renal agenesis/ectopy, and cervical somite dysplasia. Such association is also known as MURCS, and is found in just over 10% of cases.[11]

Symptoms

If functioning endometrial tissue is present inside the rudimentary uterine bodies, cyclic pelvic pain will consequently develop as soon as secondary sexual characteristics appear. Symptoms are generally primary amenorrhea and sexual dysfunction. Amenorrhea is present and is associated with a normal endocrine work-up and normal development of secondary sexual features. Sexual intercourse is almost always problematic – in fact, not infrequently, the presence of just a brief portion of vagina above the vestibular area may still imply initial difficulties, but after a certain period, sexual activity may become satisfactory due to stretching of the ectodermal vaginal residue.

Diagnosis

Diagnosis of Rokitansky syndrome is usually apparent on a clinical examination, which demonstrates normal external genitalia and the absence of a vagina. Rectal examination often confirms the absence of the uterus or the presence of a small fibrous nodule. The presence of normal pubic and axillary hair growth permits exclusion of Androgen Insensitivity syndrome. A transabdominal ultrasound scan usually confirms absence of the uterus and,

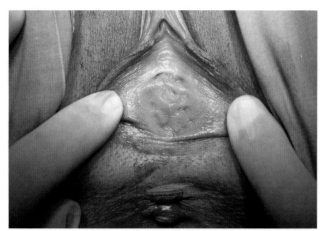

Figure 14.6.1. Normal external genitalia and absence of vagina in a patient with Rokitansky syndrome.

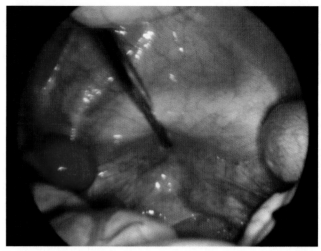

Figure 14.6.3. Laparoscopic view in a patient with Rokitansky syndrome. Note the absence of the uterus and the presence of two rudimentary horns.

where present, shows a median rudimentary uterus or two laterally displaced rudimentary horns. MRI is the imaging method that best defines the anatomic features of Rokitansky syndrome, especially the subperitoneal structures and possible endometrial cavitations. Presence of endometrium within a rudimentary horn may then be confirmed during laparoscopy by an endoscopic ultrasound probe (Figure 14.6.4). Such demonstration permits removal of the rudimentary horn or, if the horn is of adequate size, surgery could be attempted to join the horn to the neovagina to allow outflow of menstrual blood and possibly restore gestational capability.[12]

Treatment

In spite of numerous surgical and nonsurgical techniques proposed in the past (Table 14.6.1), a standardized and internationally acknowledged treatment for correction of Rokitansky syndrome still does not exist. All experimental methods aim at creating a neovagina by means of separating the rectal–urethrovesical space as well as maintaining an open cavity, thus ensuring its reepithelization. Excellent results have been described when the nonsurgical method proposed by Frank in 1938 [13] has

been applied in subjects with a relatively deep (2 to 3 cm) retrohymenal pouch. The author observed that some patients with Rokitansky syndrome were able to achieve a vagina of adequate depth and caliber solely with sexual activity. Among the most widely known surgical approaches is probably the operation proposed by McIndoe in 1938 [14], which requires surgical creation of a tunnel in the rectal–urethrovesical space, which is then coated with a strip of skin taken from the buttocks or from the medial aspect of the thigh. Among the surgical operations requiring dissection of the rectal–urethrovesical space for the creation of a neovagina, the best results can be achieved by the method proposed by Davydov [15] and Rothman [16], in which the tunnel formed by surgical dissection is coated by pelvic peritoneum that is mobilized and pulled downward toward the hymen. In Europe during the past 30 years, the most frequently used method for creation of a neovagina has been that proposed by Vecchietti in 1965.[17]

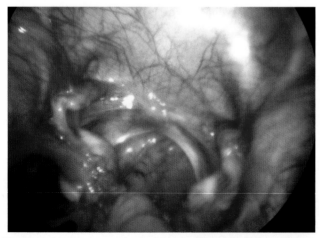

Figure 14.6.2. Laparoscopic view in a patient with Rokitansky syndrome. Note the absence of the uterus and the presence of two fibromuscular cords originating from the medial aspect of the tubes.

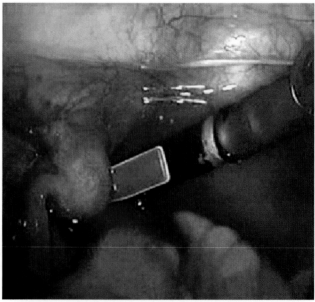

Figure 14.6.4. Laparoscopic ultrasound of a rudimentary horn to assess the presence of endometrial tissue.

Table 14.6.1: Methods for the Creation of a Neovagina

Author	Method
Frank (1938) [13]	Intermittent use of vaginal dilators
D'alberton (1972) [27]	Sexual activity ("functional" method)
Ingram (1981) [28]	Intermittent pressure with bicycle seat
Baldwin (1904) [29]	Double ileal segment transplantation
Popoff (1910) [30]	Rectal segment transplantation
Schubert (1911) [31]	Sigmoid segment transplantation
Graves (1921) [32]	Pedunculated skin flaps from vulva and thigh
Frank and Geist (1927) [33]	Cylindric dermo-epidermal flaps from thigh
Brindeau (1934) [34]	Perineal dissection and transplantation of amniotic membrane and insertion of vaginal stent for continuous dilatation
Wharton (1938) [35]	Perineal dissection and insertion of a balsa wood vaginal stent for continuous dilatation
McIndoe (1938) [14]	Perineal dissection and transplantation of skin flaps and insertion of vaginal stent for continuous dilatation
Williams (1964) [36]	Creation of a vulvovaginal pouch
Vecchietti (1965) [17]	Traction from above on the hymenal pseudomembrane
Davydov (1969) [37]	Perineal dissection and transplantation of peritoneum and insertion of vaginal stent for continuous dilatation

This technique is essentially a surgical variant of the traditional method by Frank. Instead of applying pressure from below on the retrohymenal tissue, constant traction is maintained from above.

LAPAROSCOPIC SURGERY FOR CREATION OF A NEOVAGINA

The first approach for creation of a neovagina via laparoscopy was introduced by Semm in 1983.[18] In this case, the sole purpose of laparoscopy was to supervise the creation of a neovagina in the vesicorectal space starting from the perineum. In 1992, two laparoscopic versions of Vecchietti's laparotomy procedure were proposed. Gauwerky et al. [19] and Popp and Ghirardini [20] described two relatively similar approaches, which made use of Vecchietti's original idea – that is, a proper device producing upward traction from the retrohymenal pouch on an acrylic olive, which acts as a wedge through the rectovesical space, thus creating between the two viscera an adequate space that can be maintained by dilators and sexual activity. These authors' suggestions have not achieved popularity, probably because of their excessive complexity.

There are only two laparoscopic procedures that have been used experimentally on a sufficient number of subjects and can therefore be adequately evaluated: the laparoscopic modification of the original operation of Rothman [16] and Davydov [15]

proposed by Soong et al. [21] and the laparoscopic modification of the original laparoscopic operation of Vecchietti [17] proposed by Fedele et al.[22]

Laparoscopically Assisted Neovaginoplasty through the Pelvic Peritoneum

In 1994, Soong et al. [21] first published a description of laparoscopically assisted neovaginoplasty through the pelvic peritoneum as well as this technique's results in four patients; in 1996, they reported a technical variation and its results in another 14 subjects.[23] The procedure is a laparoscopic adaptation of the creation of a neovagina through the peritoneal pull-down technique according to Adamyan [24], and in its latest version, it consists of the following steps. First, the round ligament is cut. Loosening peritoneal incisions are then made lateral to the infundibulopelvic ligament on each side and above the bladder to facilitate the pulling down of the loosest, most dependent deep cul-de-sac peritoneum to the vaginal introitus. Dissection of the pelvic peritoneum above the pouch of Douglas is gently performed to obtain a continuation of the bilateral pelvic incisions. Complete excision of the uterine remnant is performed after the peritoneum is loosened. A vaginal vault is then created through blunt dissection of the new vaginal canal, in the plane between the bladder and rectum, by means of the surgeon's index finger in the vagina, and is dissected with scissors via laparoscopy. A Kelly clamp is then inserted transvaginally to grasp and pull down the peritoneum, relaxed previously, and the tip of the peritoneum is fixed with a 0 Vicryl suture to the upper edge of the neovaginal orifice on each side. A temporary vaginal stent is inserted into the previously prepared vaginal space. The top of the reconstructed vagina is formed by approximating the peritoneum with 2-0 Vicryl suture.

The main complication occurring in this series was a rectovaginal fistula that appeared 18 months after surgery and was repaired via laparotomy. Vaginal bleeding occurred rather frequently, especially in the first 2 months. The authors reported good results from both an anatomic and a functional point of view. Mean length of the neovagina was greater than 8 cm, with a diameter of 3 cm; among the 16 patients experiencing sexual activity after the procedure, 14 (84%) reported satisfactory sexual intercourse. According to the authors, obtaining adequate vaginal length was not problematic, and there was no tendency toward contraction, narrowing, or stenosis, provided that the pelvic peritoneum was loosened extensively and that anastomosis to the hymen region was generous. No cases of enterocele or prolapse of the neovaginal vault were reported during follow-up. The new vaginal epithelium was squamous and had the normal appearance of a vagina, with minimal granulation in the vaginal cuff in 16 cases and moderate granulation in two. These observations account for the functional success of the procedure but also explain the postcoital spotting that may persist in some patients long after surgery.

Laparoscopic Modification of the Vecchietti Operation

Instrumentation required to perform laparoscopic modification of the Vecchietti operation includes a thread-bearing cutting needle (Figure 14.6.5), a traction device, and a mobile intruder. The traction device and the acrylic olive originally developed

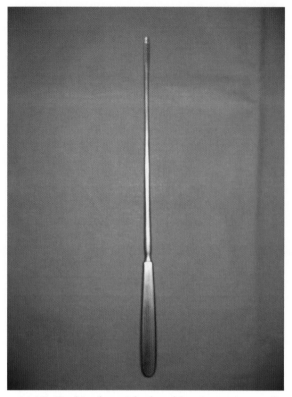

Figure 14.6.5. Vecchietti's straight thread-bearing cutting needle.

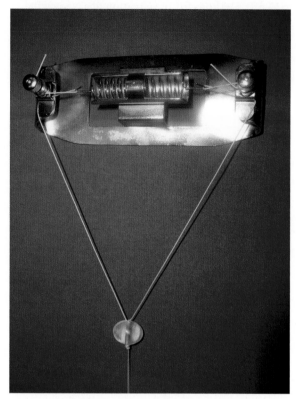

Figure 14.6.6. Vecchietti's original instrument set for creation of a neo-vagina.

by Vecchietti are shown in Figure 14.6.6. The traction device and the pluggable segmented dummy recently developed by Storz (Karl Storz Endoscopy, Tuttlingen, Germany) are shown in Figure 14.6.7.

After the bladder is emptied by catheterization, adequate pneumoperitoneum is obtained and a laparoscope is introduced into the umbilicus. The traction device along with the threads is temporarily placed on the suprapubic region, and the points at which the threads pass are marked on the skin. Adjacent to the markings, two ancillary trocars are introduced to allow accurate exploration of the abdominal and pelvic organs. The trocars are then removed, and one is replaced by Vecchietti's straight thread-bearing cutting needle, which is passed through the loose subperitoneal connective tissue downward and medially until it has reached the fold between the bladder and uterine rudiment. Because it is difficult to separate the peritoneum from the rudiment, the thread-bearing needle is brought out of the peritoneal cavity and reinserted in the subperitoneum immediately below the uterine rudiment. At this point, the direction is changed from lateromedial to craniocaudal so that the cutting needle crosses the space between the bladder and rectum and reaches the pseudo-hymen. Before perforating the pseudo-hymen, the laparoscopist should guide the tip of the instrument, aided by the insertion of middle finger inserted in the rectum (Figure 14.6.8A). At the same time, the integrity of the bladder is checked by cystoscopy. The pseudo-hymen is perforated centrally, and the threads attached to the mobile intruder are hooked (Figure 14.6.8B). When the needle is withdrawn, the threads are brought back into the peritoneal cavity and are then both brought outward

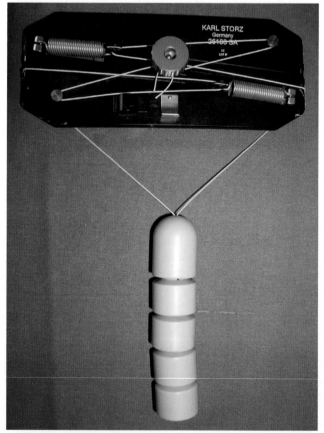

Figure 14.6.7. Instrument set recently developed by Storz for creation of a neovagina.

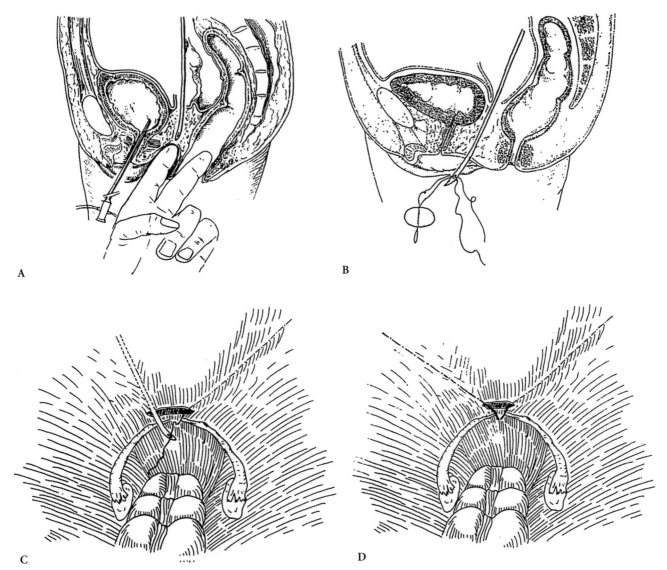

Figure 14.6.8. Surgical steps of the laparoscopic Vecchietti operation. The thread-bearing cutting needle crosses the recto-vesical space guided by the operator's finger. At the same time, the integrity of both the rectum and the bladder is checked (**A**). The pseudo-hymen is perforated and the threads hooked (**B**). The needle is withdrawn and the threades are brought inside the pelvis (**C**) and then passed subperitoneally through the abdominal wall (**D**).

and passed subperitoneally through the abdominal wall (Figure 14.6.8C,D).

In the last stage of the procedure, the threads are attached to the traction device and its tension is graduated. When the traction device is first positioned, traction on the mobile intruder must be applied to allow downward movement of the olive by approximately 1 cm if countertraction is applied. Subsequent traction must be gradual and progressive, as excessive traction could cause necrosis of the foveal epithelium, whereas limited traction would not allow lengthening of the vagina. Graduation of traction is therefore empiric, but it can be evaluated adequately using the degree of distention of the two springs on the traction device as a reference. Correct traction is achieved if the tension of the two springs is constantly intermediate between maximum and minimum tension and identical on both sides.

The traction device and mobile intruder are removed after the neovagina has progressed to at least 7 to 8 cm in depth, which may be obtained between the sixth and ninth day after surgery. Patients can be discharged from hospital 48 to 72 hours after surgery and then may be seen every 48 hours to adjust the thread tension. Adequate analgesic therapy is usually necessary on the day the traction is readjusted.

After this initial period, all women are instructed to use dilators, starting with the smallest and keeping it inserted in the neovagina for approximately 8 to 10 hours per day during the first month. Although there are various types of dilators, we recommend those that are soft and blunt (Figure 14.6.9). The decision to progress to a larger dilator is made by the physician at follow-up examination. After the first month and the start of sexual activity, the use of dilators is recommended for shorter periods of time, taking into consideration the frequency of intercourse as well as the width, length, and epithelialization of the neovagina.

The dilators are made of soft latex, measure 10 cm long, and come in three diameters: 1.5, 2, and 2.5 cm. After use, they are washed and sterilized with antiseptic solution or otherwise simply washed and covered with a condom. Intercourse is generally allowed 20 days after removal of the acrylic olive.

Results

From June 1993 to November 2004, we performed the laparoscopic creation of a neovagina in 106 patients with Rokitansky syndrome. Anatomic success was defined as a neovagina 6 cm or longer allowing easy introduction of two fingers within 6 months after corrective surgery. The report of satisfactory sexual intercourse was considered a functional success. The anatomic and functional results of the laparoscopic creation of a neovagina are shown in Table 14.6.2. Anatomic success was obtained in 104 (98%) of the 106 operated patients. In two subjects, the operation did not succeed. One patient refused to use vaginal dilators after the operation. In the other patient, a small rectal perforation was observed 2 days after the operation. Consequently, the Vecchietti device was removed, and the lesion healed spontaneously without need for surgical repair; the patient was scheduled for a repeat procedure after a few months.

All patients started experiencing sexual intercourse within 30 days after removal of the device. One hundred and three patients (97%) reported satisfactory sexual intercourse starting from 6 months after surgery. Only three patients (2.8%) did not obtain functional success. Two of these patients failed to achieve a satisfactory sexual life because of inadequate length of the neovagina. A third patient complained of unsatisfactory intercourse 1 year or more after surgery despite having an anatomically adequate vagina. She had been diagnosed with Rokitansky syndrome dur-

Table 14.6.2: Results of Laparoscopic Treatment for Creation of a Neovagina in 106 Patients

	Number of patients	Percent
Anatomic success*		
≤6 months	97	(91.5%)
6–12 months	2	(1.9%)
No success	2	(1.9%)
Functional success†		
≤6 months	40	(37.7%)
6–12 months	53	(50.0%)
≥12 months	10	(9.5%)
No success	3	(2.8%)

*Presence of a neovagina at least 6 cm long allowing easy introduction of two fingers.
†Report of satisfactory sexual intercourse.
Source: Fedele L., unpublished data

ing adolescence but had waited until she was 34 to request the creation of a neovagina.

Vaginoscopy, Schiller's test, and vaginal biopsies were also performed in some patients to compare the epithelium of the neovagina with that of a normal vagina. Vaginoscopy showed a vaginal-type epithelium with passive reaction to the Schiller test, coating 90% of the neovagina 6 months after surgery. All biopsies of the neovagina showed a normal squamous stratified epithelium

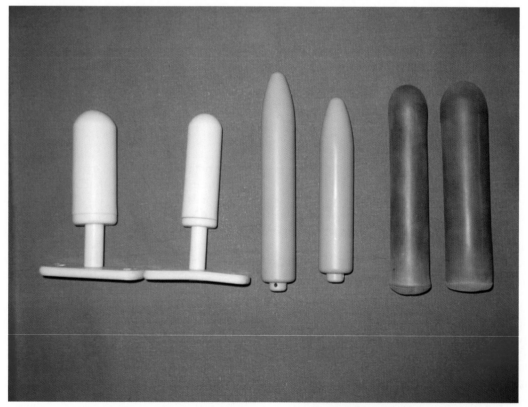

Figure 14.6.9. Different sets of vaginal dilators. The original Vecchietti dilators (*left*), Storz dilators (*center*), and blunt and soft dilators (*right*).

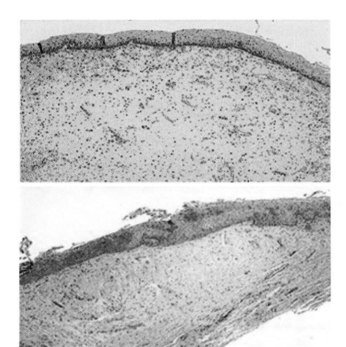

Figure 14.6.10. Histologic characteristics of a neovagina (*lower image*) and a normal vagina (*upper image*). The two epithelial layers are very similar. (Hematoxylin & eosin, original magnification ×100.)

of adequate thickness, rich in glycogen and very similar to that of the normal vagina (Figure 14.6.10).

Compared with the other laparoscopic modifications of Vecchietti's procedure, we believe the approach proposed by our group to be the most advantageous. In fact, our approach does not require dissection of the urethral–vesicorectal space, provides an almost entirely subperitoneal route for the traction threads, and is performed in a single laparoscopic stage without the need for a perineal stage.

Finally, this procedure holds two other important advantages. In case of failure, a new surgical operation can be undertaken by any other technique. In addition, if uterine transplantation [26] becomes available in the future, Vecchietti's approach seems the best approach to permit adequate grafting of the transplanted organ in the pelvis.

REFERENCES

1. Robert M, Goldwyn MD. History of attempts to form a vagina. *Plast Reconstr Surg.* 1977;59:319–329.
2. Mayer CA. Uber Verdoppelungen des Uterus und ihre Arten, nebst Bemerkungen uber Hasenscharte und Wolfsrachen. *J Chir Augenheilkd.* 1829;13:525–564.
3. Rokitansky C. Uber die sogenennten Verdoppelungen des Uterus. *Med Jb Osterreich Staates.* 1938;26:39–77.
4. Küster H. Uterus bipartitus solidus rudimentarius cum vagina solida. *Z Geburtshilfe Gynakol.* 1910;67:692–718.
5. Hauser GA, Schreiner WE. Das Mayer–Rokitansky–Kuster–Syndrom. Uterus bipartitus solidus rudimentarius cum vagina solida. *Schweiz Med Wochschr.* 1961;91:381–384.
6. Aittomaki C, Eroila H, Kajanoja P. A population-based study of the incidence of mullerian aplasia in Finland. *Fertil Steril.* 2001;76:624–625.
7. Deligeoroglou E, Christopoulous P, Creatsas G. A unique case of descending salpingitis and functioning endometrium in a mullerian remnant in a woman with Mayer–Rokitansky–Küster–Hauser syndrome. *Fertil Steril.* 2005;83:1545–1547.
8. Willemsen WNP. Renal-skeletal-ear and facial anomalies in combination with the Mayer–Rokitansky–Küster syndrome. *Eur J Obstet Gynecol Reprod Biol.* 1982;14:121–130.
9. Pittock ST, Babovic-Vuksanovic D, Lteif A. Mayer–Rokitansky–Küster–Hauser anomaly and its associated malformations. *Am J Med Genet A.* 2005;135:314–316.
10. Strubbe EH, Thijn CJ, Willemsen WN, Lappohn R. Evaluation of radiographic abnormalities of the hand in patients with the Mayer–Rokitansky–Küster–Hauser syndrome. *Skeletal Radiol.* 1987;16:227–231.
11. Strubbe EH, Cremers CW, Willemsen WN, et al. The Mayer–Rokitansky–Küster–Hauser syndrome without and with associated features: two separate entities? *Clin Dysmorphol.* 1994;3:192–199.
12. Fedele L, Bianchi S, Berlanda N, Bulfoni A, Fontana E. Laparoscopic creation of a neovagina and recovery of menstrual function in a patient with Rokitansky syndrome: a case report. *Hum Reprod.* 2006;21(12):3287–3289. Epub 2006 Aug 17
13. Frank RT. The formation of an artificial vagina without operation. *Am J. Obstet Gynecol.* 1938;135:1053–1055.
14. McIndoe AH, Bannister JB. An operation for the cure of congenital absence of the vagina. *J Obstet Gynaecol Br Emp.* 1938;45:490–494.
15. Davydov SN. 12-year experience with colpopoiesis using the peritoneum. *Gynakologe.* 1980;13:120–121.
16. Rothman D. The use of peritoneum in the construction of a vagina. *Obstet Gynecol.* 1972;40:835–838.
17. Vecchietti G. Creation of an artificial vagina in Rokitansky–Küster–Hauser syndrome. *Attual Obstet Gynecol.* 1965;11:131–147.
18. Semm K. Pelviskopische Kontrolle der neovaginalen Operatiostechnik uber eine Gliederoptik. *Alete Wissenschaftlicher Dienst.* 1983;93:24–27.
19. Gauwerky JFH, Wallwiener D, Bastert G. An endoscopically assisted technique for reconstruction of a neovagina. *Arch Gynecol Obstet.* 1992;252:59–63.
20. Popp LW, Ghirardini G. Creation of a neovagina by pelviscopy. *J Laparoendosc Surg.* 1992;2:165–173.
21. Soong YK, Chang FH, Lee CL, Lai YM. Vaginal agenesis treated by laparoscopically assisted neovaginoplasty. *Gynecol Endosc.* 1994;3:217–220.
22. Fedele L, Busacca M, Candiani M, Vignali M. Laparoscopic creation of a neovagina in Mayer Rokitansky Kuster Hauser syndrome by modification of Vecchietti operation. *Am J Obstet Gynecol.* 1994;171:268–297.
23. Soong YK, Chang FH, Lai YM, et al. Results of modified laparoscopically assisted neovaginoplasty in 18 patients with congenital absence of vagina. *Hum Reprod.* 1996;11:200–203.
24. Adamyan LV. Therapeutic and endoscopic perspectives. In: Nichols DH, Clarke-Pearson DL, eds. *Gynecologic, Obstetric, and Related Surgery.* 2nd ed. St. Louis: Mosby; 2000:1209–1217.
25. Fedele L, Bianchi S, Berlanda N, Fontana E, Raffaelli R, Bulfoni A, Braidotti P. Neovaginal mucosa after Vecchietti's laparoscopic operation for Rokitansky syndrome: structural and ultrastructural study. *Am J Obstet Gynecol.* 2006;195(1):56–61.
26. Altchek A. Uterus transplantation. *Mt Sinai J Med.* 2003;50:154–162.
27. D'Alberton A, Santi F. Formation of a neovagina by coitus. *Obstet Gynecol.* 1972;40:763–764.
28. Ingram J.M. The bicycle seat stool in the treatment of vaginal agenesis and stenosis: a preliminary report. *Am J Obstet Gynecol.* 1981;140:867–873.

29. Baldwin J.F. The formation of an artificial vagina by intestinal transplantation. *Ann Surg.* 40:398–403, 1904.

30. Popoff DD. Russk. Vrach. St Petersburg 1910;60:1512–1514.

31. Schubert G. Uber Schidenbildung bei Angeborene Vaginal Defekt. *Zentralbl Gynacol.* 1911;35:1017.

32. Graves WP. Surg Clin N Amer. Chapter I, 1921;611–612.

33. Frank RT, Geist SH. The formation of an artificial vagina by a new plastic technique. *Am J Obstet Gynecol.* 1927;14:721–728.

34. Brindeau A. Kunstliche Scheide mit Hilfe einer reifen Eihaut. *Zentralbl Gynak.* 1934;59:1196–1197.

35. Wharton LR. A simple method of constructing a vagina. *Ann Surg.* 1938;107:842–849.

36. Williams EA. Congenital absence of the vagina. A simple operation for its relief. *J Obstet & Gynecol Br Commonw.* 1964;71:511–512.

37. Davydov SN. Colpopoiesis from the peritoneum of the uterorectal space. *Akush Ginekol (Mosk).* 1969;45:55–57.

15 | LAPAROSCOPIC TREATMENT OF CHRONIC PELVIC PAIN

Section 15.1. Presacral Neurectomy

James E. Carter

Presacral neurectomy is useful in the treatment of severe, disabling dysmenorrhea secondary to endometriosis and pelvic pain associated with pelvic inflammatory disease.[1] The efficacy of presacral neurectomy for the relief of midline dysmenorrhea was confirmed by a randomized study performed at the Johns Hopkins University School of Medicine.[2] Tjaden used the surgical technique first described in 1899 by Jaboulay [3] and Ruggi.[4] Black [5] estimated a 75% to 80% success in 9937 cases of presacral neurectomy. Laparoscopic techniques for presacral neurectomy have been described by Perez [6], Biggerstaff [7], Carter [8], Chen [9], and Nezhat.[10] Kwok [11] reviewed laparoscopic presacral neurectomy and concluded that patients for whom this operation is recommended should be carefully selected. They should have midline dysmenorrhea as the main symptom and should have failed or not tolerated medical therapy. Presacral neurectomy has been shown to have long-run effectiveness for the treatment of severe dysmenorrhea due to endometriosis.[12] As has been pointed out by Stones and Jacobson [13,14], a percentage of women with chronic pelvic pain and/or dysmenorrhea do not respond or respond poorly to medical treatment. Surgery may represent the final therapeutic option for these patients. In a prospective double-blind randomized, controlled study, Zullo et al. [15] demonstrated the effectiveness of presacral neurectomy for women with severe dysmenorrhea due to endometriosis who had been treated with conservative laparoscopic surgical intervention. The authors continued to follow their patients for an additional year and published on the 2-year success of this procedure. They found a significant reduction in the frequency and severity of dysmenorrhea, dyspareunia, and chronic pelvic pain observed 24 months after surgery. The addition of presacral neurectomy was also associated with significant improvement in quality of life. In the conclusion to the study, Zullo et al. [12] stated, "We demonstrate that presacral neurectomy is a safe and useful surgical procedure to improve the cure rate and the quality of life in patients with severe dysmenorrhea treated with laparoscopic conservative surgery based on a long-term followup of two years, but chronic constipation and/or urinary urgency may be consequences of this therapy."

ANATOMY

Pain impulses from the cervix, the body of the uterus, and the proximal fallopian tube are transmitted through afferent fibers that accompany sympathetic nerves into the spinal cord at the thoracic and lumbar levels. The sympathetic nerves that emerge from the uterus pass through the uterosacral ligament along the cardinal ligament and join the pelvic plexus. Parasympathetic fibers from S1 through S4 travel with the phrenic nerve through the pelvic plexuses (Frankenhäuser ganglia) lateral to the cervix to reach the bladder, rectum, and uterus.

The presacral nerve is a plexus of nerves known as the superior hypogastric plexus. Kwok [11] elegantly summarized the anatomy of the pelvic autonomic nerves as originally described by Curtis [16]:

> The lumbar and lower thoracic sympathetic ganglia, and the superior, middle, and inferior hypogastric plexus provide the afferent pathways for the pelvic viscera. However, an exception to this is the pain afferent fibers from the ovaries and distal fallopian tubes, which travel to the ovarian plexus, and then via the infundibulopelvic ligaments to the aortic and renal plexuses. The sigmoid colon sends visceral afferents to the inferior mesenteric plexus. Interruption of the presacral plexus will affect a decrease in central pain perception and perhaps also a change in the function of the sigmoid colon. Pain afferents from the uterus and cervix and proximal part of the fallopian tubes travel with the sympathetic nerves and travel via the uterosacral and cardinal ligaments to join with the pelvic plexus. (Frankenhauser's ganglion, uterovaginal ganglion)
>
> The fibers from the pelvic plexus course proximally to become the inferior, the middle hypogastric plexus over the sacral promontory, and then the superior hypogastric plexus. The 'presacral nerve', the common name for the superior hypogastric plexus, is a misnomer because it is actually pre-lumbar in position and lies in front of the fifth lumbar vertebrae. In addition, it is usually not a nerve but rather a nerve plexus. It is a single trunk in only approximately 20% of the anatomical sections.[11]
>
> The presacral nerve is a direct extension of the aortic plexus below the aortic bifurcation. This plexus spreads out behind the peritoneum in the loose areolar tissue lying over the fourth and fifth lumbar vertebrae. Between the vertebrae and the presacral nerve lies the middle sacral artery, which may be traumatized during surgical dissection. In a series of 30 cadaveric dissections, Curtis et al. [16] reported 75% of the time the superior and middle hypogastric plexus lie on the left, 25% in the midline, and none on the right. On the right of the presacral nerve, lie the right ureter and common iliac vein and artery. On the left lie the sigmoid colon, inferior mesenteric vessels, and the left ureter. The left ureter is seen less commonly in surgical dissections because it is obscured by the sigmoid colon.[11]

425

When performing presacral neurectomy, the surgeon will encounter variable anatomic findings. For this reason, the nerve-bearing tissue, especially on the left, should be thoroughly exposed when performing the procedure.[17] In 8% to 15% of dissections, the mesocolon was over the area of the presacral nerve, making neurectomy difficult or impossible.[17] Labate [18] found a single nerve in 8% to 13% of dissections. In 75 dissections, he found a plexus in 84% of the cases, parallel nerve trunks in 8%, and single nerves in 8%.

Within the interiliac trigone, the common iliac artery and ureter are on the right and the common iliac vein is on the left. The inferior mesenteric, superior hemorrhoidal, and midsacral arteries are in the center of the prelumbar space. This trigone is defined caudally by the sacral promontory and laterally by the common iliac arteries. The superior edge of the triangle is delineated by the aortic bifurcation. Centrally and to the left, multiple nerve fibers, sometimes in bundles, run caudally from the aortic plexus above and through the interiliac trigone to form the superior hypogastric plexus. These fibers, representing the presacral nerve, are buried in loose areolar tissue. They display no particular patterns and vary among individuals. Both ureters, which lie to the right and left of the trigone, are identified before transection of the nerve bundle continues. The left ureter is more difficult to see because it lies underneath the rectosigmoid and mesocolon.

INDICATIONS

The presacral neurectomy is indicated for patients who have disabling midline dysmenorrhea and pelvic pain and have not responded to appropriate and adequate medication. The operation is likely to relieve pain in 50% to 75% of patients. When associated with complete resection of endometriosis, cure rates are improved.

Presacral neurectomy does not alleviate adnexal pain because ovarian innervation originates from the ovarian plexus, a meshwork of nerve fibers that arise from the aortic and renal plexuses and accompany the ovarian artery throughout its course.

TECHNIQUE

After associated pelvic abnormalities have been treated, the steep Trendelenburg position is used and the patient is tilted slightly to the left. The aortic bifurcation, common iliac arteries and veins, ureters, and sacral promontory are identified. The peritoneum overlying the promontory is elevated with grasping forceps, and a small opening is made with the CO_2 laser, scissors, or other cutting modality (Figure 15.1.1).

The suction–irrigator is inserted through this opening, and the peritoneum is elevated by hydrodissection. The peritoneum is incised horizontally and vertically, and the opening is extended cephalad to the aortic bifurcation (Figure 15.1.2). Bleeding from the peritoneal vessels is controlled with the bipolar electrocoagulator. Retroperitoneal fatty tissue is removed before the hypogastric plexus is reached. The mesocolon does not cover the sacral promontory in most patients. If the mesocolon covers the sacral promontory, the procedure is more difficult, and the surgeon must avoid injuring the inferior mesenteric artery and

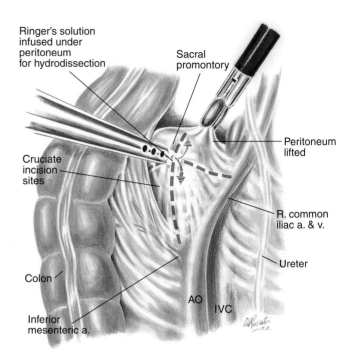

Figure 15.1.1. The peritoneum over the promontory is elevated with grasping forceps, and a small opening is made with the CO_2 laser or scissors or any other cutting modality. The suction–irrigator is inserted, and the peritoneum is elevated by hydrodissection. The peritoneum is excised horizontally and vertically, and the opening is extended cephalad until the bifurcation of the aorta is seen. From Nezhat et al.[28]

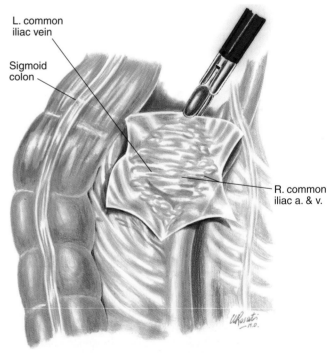

Figure 15.1.2. Retroperitoneal fatty tissue is removed before the hypogastric plexus is reached. Hemostasis is achieved with bipolar electrocoagulation. From Nezhat et al.[28]

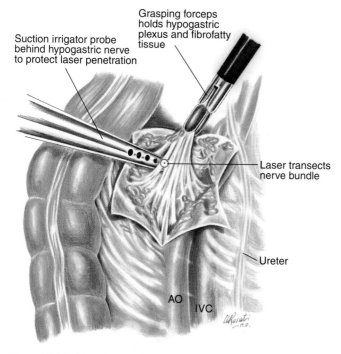

Figure 15.1.3. The plexus of nerves is grasped with atraumatic forceps. The nerves are skeletonized, coagulated, and excised. Nerves that lie within the boundaries of the interiliac triangle are removed along with the fibers entering the area from underneath the common aortic arteries. From Nezhat et al.[28]

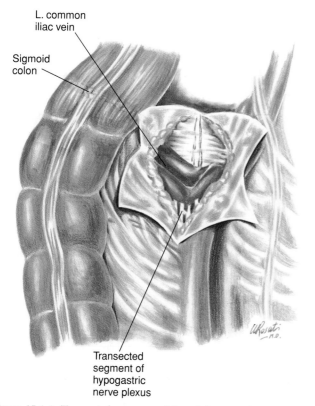

Figure 15.1.4. Transected segments of the pelvic nerve. Sutures are not required to close the defect. The excised tissue is sent for histologic examination. From Nezhat et al.[28]

its branches. Hemostasis is obtained with bipolar electrocoagulation.

The nerve plexus is grasped with an atraumatic forceps. Using blunt and sharp dissection, the nerve fibers are skeletonized, coagulated, and excised (Figure 15.1.3). All the nerves that lie within the boundaries of the interiliac triangle are removed, including any fibers entering the area from under the common iliac arteries (Figure 15.1.4). The retroperitoneal space is irrigated, and bleeding points are coagulated. Sutures are not required. The excised tissue is sent for histologic confirmation of nerve removal. At second-look laparoscopy, the presacral area should appear healed. Usually, no small bowel is attached to this area. If a mesocolon detachment is required at the initial procedure, the mesocolon usually reattaches itself to the presacral area.

RESULTS

Cotte [19] reported favorable results with presacral neurectomy in 1500 selected patients with only a 2% failure rate. Meigs [20] reported an 85% relief rate. In a review of 2516 patients, Black [5] noted 70% of the patients experienced relief, 19% were improved, and 11% were unimproved. Polan and DeCherney [1] reported in 1980 that 14 of 20 patients (70%) were relieved of pain after presacral neurectomy. In the control group, 14 of 54 (26%) showed significant pain relief. Lee and colleagues [21] reported a 74% success rate, with 14% experiencing a partial cure. There was a 12% failure rate. Perez [6] studied 25 patients and concluded that 96% experienced pain relief. The mean preoperative score for patients in the study was 8.5 (on a scale of 0 to 10, with 0 being no pain and 10 being the worst pain), whereas the postoperative mean score was 2.2. In a randomized prospective study on the efficacy of presacral neurectomy initiated by Tjaden and colleagues [2], 17 of the 26 patients had a presacral neurectomy. Fifteen of the 17 (88%) noted relief, whereas two (12%) had no improvement. Pain persisted in all nine of the patients who did not undergo presacral neurectomy. In 1992, Nezhat and Nezhat [22] described a simplified method of presacral neurectomy in one of the earliest reports on the laparoscopic approach. The authors performed laparoscopic presacral neurectomy in 52 patients with dysmenorrhea unresponsive to medical treatment. The severity of endometriosis varied among the patients (31 had minimal, 13 had mild, five had moderate, and three had severe endometriosis). Forty-eight of the 52 patients (92.3%) reported relief of dysmenorrhea, including 27 (51.2%) who reported complete pain relief. Of the 27 patients reporting complete pain relief, 16 (59%) had minimal, six (22%) had mild, three (11%) had moderate, and two (8%) had severe endometriosis. Carter [8] reported on presacral neurectomy in 20 patients with follow-up of up to 18 months. The pain level in these women decreased from an average of 9.4 to 2.0 (on a scale of 0 to 10, with 0 being no pain and 10 the worst).

Chen and coworkers [23] reported on presacral neurectomy in 67 patients with primary dysmenorrhea who had a poor response to medical treatment. The patients were divided into two groups, with 33 undergoing laparoscopic presacral neurectomy and 34 undergoing LUNA. The efficacy of the two procedures was identical after 3 months, but after 12 months, laparoscopic presacral neurectomy was significantly more effective than LUNA. The authors concluded that presacral neurectomy was

Table 15.1.1: Pain Reduction after Laparoscopic Presacral Neurectomy by Stage of Endometriosis. The Long-Term Outcome of Laparoscopic Presacral Neurectomy Is Satisfactory in Most Patients

	Degree of Improvement				
	>80%	50–80%	<50%	None	No Response
Pelvic pain					
Stage I (n = 53)	18 (34.0)	19 (35.8)	10 (18.9)	5 (9.4)	1 (1.9)
Stage II (n = 22)	13 (59.1)	4 (18.2)	3 (13.6)	2 (9.1)	0
Stage III (n = 7)	2 (28.6)	3 (42.9)	1 (14.3)	1 (14.3)	0
Stage IV (n = 13)	8 (61.5)	3 (23.1)	2 (15.4)	0	0
Total (n = 95)	41 (43.2)	29 (30.5)	16 (16.8)	8 (8.4)	1 (1.1)
Dysmenorrhea					
Stage I (n = 53)	12 (22.6)	16 (30.2)	14 (26.4)	5 (9.4)	6 (11.3)
Stage II (n = 22)	10 (45.5)	5 (22.7)	3 (13.6)	2 (9.1)	2 (9.1)
Stage III (n = 7)	2 (28.6)	3 (42.7)	0	2 (28.6)	0
Stage IV (n = 13)	7 (53.8)	2 (15.4)	1 (7.7)	1 (7.7)	2 (15.4)
Total (n = 95)	31 (32.6)	26 (27.4)	18 (18.9)	10 (10.5)	10 (10.5)

preferable to uterine nerve ablation for long-term relief of primary dysmenorrhea. In a retrospective review of 655 patients who had laparoscopic conservative surgery and laparoscopic presacral neurectomy, Chen and Soong [9] found that 527 (80%) reported significant alleviation of pain. Cure was achieved in 22 (52%) of the 42 patients with adenomyosis, 75 (73%) of the 103 patients with moderate to severe endometriosis with dysmenorrhea, 123 (75%) of the 164 patients with minimal to mild endometriosis with dysmenorrhea, 64 (77%) of the 83 patients with primary dysmenorrhea, and 84 (62%) of the 135 patients with chronic pelvic pain. Nezhat et al. [10] evaluated long-term outcomes of laparoscopic presacral neurectomy in 176 women who underwent presacral neurectomy and treatment of endometriosis. More than 50% alleviation of pain was reported in 69.8% of the women with stage I endometriosis (using the revised classification of the American Fertility Society), 77.3% of those with stage II, 71.4% with stage III, and 84.6% with stage IV (Table 15.1.1). The authors concluded that long-term outcome of laparoscopic presacral neurectomy is satisfactory in most patients, and the stage of endometriosis is not related directly to the degree of pain improvement achieved.

Zullo [12] reported on a 2-year study of presacral neurectomy for the treatment of severe dysmenorrhea due to endometriosis. The frequency and severity of dysmenorrhea, dyspareunia, and chronic pelvic pain, and quality of life were evaluated at entry and 24 months postoperatively. At follow-up visit, the 83.3% cure rate ($P \leq 0.05$) was significantly higher in the group with laparoscopic surgery and presacral neurectomy than the 53.3% cure rate in the group with only conservative laparoscopic surgical intervention. The frequency and severity of dysmenorrhea, dyspareunia, and chronic pelvic pain were significantly lower in both groups compared with baseline values ($P \leq 0.05$), and only severity was significantly lower in the group with presacral neurectomy and endometriosis surgery ($P \leq 0.05$). A significant improvement in quality of life was observed after surgery in both groups ($P \leq 0.05$) and was significantly better in the presacral neurectomy group ($P \leq 0.05$) compared with the conservative surgery–only group. Zullo concluded that presacral neurectomy improves long-term cure rates and quality of life in women treated with conservative laparoscopic surgery for severe dysmenorrhea due to endometriosis.

COMPLICATIONS

Bleeding is the most important intraoperative complication of presacral neurectomy. The middle sacral vessels are in the midline between the presacral nerve and the periosteum of the sacral promontory. Usually, the nerve is dissected anterior to the vessels and ligation is not necessary. Hemostasis is obtained by ligation or coagulation. However, an injury to the common iliac vein or vena cava may require an immediate laparotomy.

Ureteral injury, urinary urgency, and poor bladder emptying are potential complications. Meigs [20] noted urinary urgency in some patients that persisted for 7 years postoperatively and persistent constipation in 32% of the patients. Black [5] reported the need for catheterization in 13 of 26 patients postoperatively (four for 1 day, six for 2 days, and one each for 3, 5, and 6 days). Lee et al. [21] noted bladder problems and urgency and constipation problems in 4% of 50 patients. Eight (18%) of 45 patients who benefited from presacral neurectomy initially had a return of bladder pain within 19 months. Jones and Rock [24] cited vaginal dryness that usually resolved within 6 months as a complication in 10% to 15% of patients. Lee et al. [21] noted one operative complication involving an estimated 1500-mL blood loss from a damaged presacral vein. Davis [25] recognized a vascular injury to the left common iliac vein that was repaired. Cotte [19] reported one incidence of damage to the left ureter among 1500 operations and noted postoperative bleeding in four other patients. Two required a second operation and repair of the posterior peritoneum. The other two cases, which involved sub-peritoneal blood infiltrating the posterior rectal areas, resolved spontaneously. Chen and coworkers [26] reported four cases of chylous ascites after laparoscopic presacral neurectomy. This rare complication is caused by intraoperative injury to the retroperitoneal lymphatic plexus. Of the four injuries, two were treated successfully with bipolar cauterization. One was managed by compression with Gelfoam (Pharmacia & Upjohn Inc., Peapack, NJ), and closure of the peritoneum was achieved by laparoscopic suturing. The fourth patient had persistent chylous leakage from the drainage tube. This complication was resolved by conservative management, removal of the drainage tube, and a low-fat diet. Yen [27] reported postlaparoscopic vulvar edema in two cases after laparoscopic presacral neurectomy. This was associated with chyloperitoneum. Both cases were managed expectantly. Yen now closes the presacral neurectomy wound with bipolar coagulation to seal the cutting edge and the cannula wound with precise and layer-by-layer repair, and no further cases of chyloperitoneum and vulvar edema have occurred in 2 years since that modification was introduced.

Zullo [15] reported constipation and urinary urgency as a complication of presacral neurectomy performed concomitantly with laparoscopic surgery for endometriosis. Constipation was reported in 21 (3.3%) and nine patients (14.3%) at 6- and 12-month follow-up, respectively. In 15 of 21 cases (71.4%), constipation was treated successfully with medical therapies. At the 6- and 12-month follow-up visits, urinary urgency was observed in three patients (4.8%).

CONCLUSION

Laparoscopic presacral neurectomy is an effective, safe operation for patients who have incapacitating central dysmenorrhea that is not relieved by medication. The procedure is empiric because success rates are not predictable. Complications and mortality rates have been minimal. Poor patient selection and incomplete neurectomy due to neurologic variability or failure to remove all nerve tissue within the interiliac trigone are the most common reasons for poor results.

REFERENCES

1. Polan M, DeCherney A. Presacral neurectomy for pelvic pain in infertility. *Fertil Steril.* 1980;34:557–560.
2. Tjaden B, Schlaff WD, Kimball A, Rock JA. The efficacy of presacral neurectomy for the relief of midline dysmenorrhea. *Obstet Gynecol.* 1990;76:89–91.
3. Jaboulay M. Le traitment de la neuralgie pelvienne par la paralysie du sympathetique sacre. *Lyon Med.* 1899;90:102.
4. Ruggi T. Della sympathectamia al collo ed ale avome. *Policlinico.* 1899;1:193.
5. Black WT. Use of presacral sympathectomy in the treatment of dysmenorrhea. *Am J Obstet Gynecol.* 1964;89:16–22.
6. Perez JJ. Laparoscopic presacral neurectomy. Results of the first 25 cases. *J Reprod Med.* 1990;35:625–630.
7. Biggerstaff ED 3rd, Foster SN. Laparoscopic presacral neurectomy for treatment of midline pelvic pain. *J Am Assoc Gynecol Laparosc.* 1994;2:31–35.
8. Carter JE. Laparoscopic presacral neurectomy utilizing contact-tip Nd: YAG laser. *Keio J Med.* 1996;45:332–335.
9. Chen FP, Soong YK. The efficacy and complications of laparoscopic presacral neurectomy in pelvic pain. *Obstet Gynecol.* 1998; 91:701–704.
10. Nezhat CR, Nezhat FR, Luciano AA, et al. *Uterine Surgery in Operative Gynecologic Laparoscopy: Principles and Techniques.* New York: McGraw-Hill; 1995.
11. Kwok A, Lam A, Ford R. Laparoscopic presacral neurectomy: a review. *Obstet Gynecol Surv.* 2001;56:99–104.
12. Zullo F, Palomba S, Zupi E, et al. Long-term effectiveness of presacral neurectomy for the treatment of severe dysmenorrhea due to endometriosis. *J Am Assoc Gynecol Laparosc.* 2004, 11:23–28.
13. Stones RW, Mountfield J. Interventions for treating chronic pelvic pain in women. *Cochrane Database Syst Rev.* 2000:CD000387.
14. Jacobson TZ, Barlow DH, Garry R, et al. Laparoscopic surgery for pelvic pain associated with endometriosis. *Cochrane Database Syst Rev.* 2001:CD001300.
15. Zullo F, Palomba S, Zupi E, et al. Effectiveness of presacral neurectomy in women with severe dysmenorrhea caused by endometriosis who were treated with laparoscopic conservative surgery: a 1-year prospective randomized double-blind study. *Am J Obstet Gynecol.* 2003, 189:5–10.
16. Curtis AH, Anson BJ, Ashley FL, Jones T. The anatomy of the pelvic autonomic nerves in relation to gynecology. *Surg Gynecol Obstet.* 1942;75:743.
17. Rosenshein NB, Rock JA. *Surgery in the Retroperitoneal Space.* Philadelphia: JB Lippincott; 1988:31–41.
18. Labate JS. The surgical anatomy of the superior hypogastric plexus-"presacral nerve." *Surg Gynecol Obstet.* 1938;67:199.
19. Cotte MG. Technique of presacral neurectomy. *Am J Surg.* 1949;78:50.
20. Meigs JV. Excision of the superior hypogastric plexus (presacral nerve) for primary dysmenorrhea. *Surg Gynecol Obstet.* 1939;68:723.
21. Lee RB, Stone K, Magelssen D, et al. Presacral neurectomy for chronic pelvic pain. *Obstet Gynecol.* 1986;68:517.
22. Nezhat C, Nezhat F. A simplified method of laparoscopic presacral neurectomy for the treatment of central pelvic pain due to endometriosis. *Br J Obstet Gynecol.* 1992;99:659.
23. Chen FP, Chang SD, Chu KK, et al. Comparison of laparoscopic presacral neurectomy and laparoscopic uterine nerve ablation for primary dysmenorrhea. *J Reprod Med.* 1996;41:463.
24. Jones HW, Rock JA. *Reparative and Constructive Surgery of the Female Generative Tract.* Baltimore: Williams & Wilkins; 1983.
25. Davis AA. The technique of resection of the presacral nerve (Cotte's operation). *Br J Surg* 1933;20:516.
26. Chen FP, Lo TS, Soong YK. Management of chylous ascites following laparoscopic presacral neurectomy. *Hum Reprod.* 1998;13: 880.
27. Yen CF, Wang CJ, Lin SL, Lee CL, Soong YK. Post-laparoscopic vulvar edema, a rare complication. *J Am Assoc Gynecol Laparosc.* 2003;10:123–126.
28. Nezhat C, Siegler A, Nezhat F, Nezhat C, Seidman D, Luciano A. *Operative Gynecologic Laparoscopy. Principles and Techniques.* 2nd Edition. New York: McGraw-Hill; 2000.

Section 15.2. Uterosacral Transection and Ablation

James E. Carter

Surgical methods for cutting off pain-conducting nerve pathways in the pelvis include:

1. Presacral neurectomy, involving cutting the T10-L1 sympathetic nerves on the anterior surface of the sacral bone
2. Paracervical uterine denervation, involving transection of the uterosacral ligament at its attachment to the uterus along with cutting the above-mentioned sympathetic nerves and the S1-S4 parasympathetic nerves, which transmit pain stimuli from the supravaginal region into the uterine cervix [1]

Uterosacral transection was developed and popularized as an alternative to presacral neurectomy with Doyle's vaginal approach, involving transection of the uterosacral ligaments.[1] As described by Sutton and Whitelaw [2]:

Doyle would place a suture through the posterior lip of the cervix at the apex of the vagina and place traction on this suture to increase the distance of the cervix from the ureter. The attachments of the uterosacral ligaments to the cervix were then divided between Heaney clamps. To prevent re-growth of the dissected nerve trunks, the posterior leaf of the peritoneal incision was interposed between them. An abdominal approach was recommended if endometriosis was suspected or any gross pathology such as fibroids was felt. The pathological tissue was then excised. The ligaments were divided between two clamps and the ligaments sutured together with stainless steel sutures to the isthmus of the cervix in the midline about 1 cm higher than the original attachment. Doyle reported complete pain relief in 63 out of 73 cases (86%); 35 had primary dysmenorrhea (85.7% success) and 33 had secondary dysmenorrhea (86.8% success).

A more recent technique involves not separation and transection, but ablation of the uterosacral ligaments to achieve pain control. Lichten and Bombard [3] reported relief of incapacitating primary dysmenorrhea in nine of 11 patients (81%) who underwent laparoscopic uterosacral nerve ablation (LUNA) with no cure in the control group, which had only diagnostic laparoscopy. However, 1 year later, fewer than half the patients who originally expressed improvement were pain-free. Gurgan and colleagues [4] reported that 17 of 23 patients had alleviation of dysmenorrhea, with a mean pain reduction of 33% based on pre- and postoperative pain scores. In a similar study, Sutton [5] reported a 63% reduction from the initial average pain score.

In a double-blind randomized, controlled trial of LUNA for women with chronic pelvic pain in the absence of endometriosis,

Johnson [6] reported a significant reduction in dysmenorrhea at 12-month follow-up. The median reduction on the visual analog scale (VAS) from baseline was 4.8 points for the LUNA group versus a reduction of 0.8 points for those who did not have LUNA. A total of 42.1% of the women experienced successful treatment for dysmenorrhea, defined as a 50% or greater reduction in VAS scores, versus 14.3% of those who did not undergo LUNA. There was no significant difference in pain scores in women with non-menstrual pelvic pain, deep dyspareunia, or dyschezia with no endometriosis who underwent LUNA versus those who did not undergo LUNA. The addition of LUNA to laparoscopic surgical treatment of endometriosis was not associated with a significant difference in pain outcome. Johnson concluded that LUNA is effective for dysmenorrhea in the absence of endometriosis and that there is no evidence for the effectiveness of LUNA for chronic pelvic pain without dysmenorrhea or for any type of pelvic pain associated with endometriosis.

Yen [7] performed an elegant study involving the addition of LUNA to laparoscopic bipolar coagulation of the uterine vessels. This study, which was performed for women with uterine myomas and dysmenorrhea, involved 85 patients. Forty of the 41 women (97.6%) underwent successful laparoscopic bipolar coagulation of uterine vessels with LUNA. Forty-three of the 44 women (97.7%) assigned to laparoscopic bipolar coagulation of uterine vessels only underwent successful surgery. Eighty women completed the 1-, 3-, and 6-month follow-ups. The frequency and severity of postoperative pain were less in the group that had LUNA than in the group receiving coagulation of the uterine arteries only ($P \leq 0.05$). At 3 months, dysmenorrhea improved 84.2% in the LUNA group versus 61.9% for the group that did not have LUNA, and improved 92.1% versus 73.8% at 6-month follow-up. The reduction was more significant in the group that received LUNA than in the group that did not ($P \leq 0.05$). The results suggest that LUNA may decrease postoperative ischemic pain and improve dysmenorrhea associated with uterine myomas treated with laparoscopic bipolar coagulation of uterine vessels.

ANATOMY

Uterine nerve ablation involves the cauterization resulting in transection of the uterosacral ligaments close to their point of insertion into the cervix. The procedure interrupts pelvic afferent sensory nerve fibers of the Lee–Frankenhäuser nerve plexus.[8] According to Counseller and Craig [8], the Th10-L1 sympathetic nerves are included in the hypogastric nerve and run along the inferior vena cava and the sacral bone. They enter the pelvic cavity and run inside the uterosacral ligaments before ultimately entering the uterus. The parasympathetic nerves from S1-S4 are included in the nervi erigentes, and they run inside the uterosacral ligament for a short distance in the lateral part of the pelvis and then form ganglia on each side of the uterus (Frankenhäuser ganglia). Johnson [6] elegantly summarized the anatomy important for an understanding of the LUNA procedure. He pointed out that "the ideal neuroablative surgical procedure for pelvic pain would transect all afferent sensory fibers from all the pelvic organs and leave all other nerves unaffected." Although pelvic neuroanatomy is complicated and still not completely understood, what is known makes it clear that no such "ideal neuroablative surgical procedure" exists (Figure 15.2.1). The body of the uterus is widely considered to be innervated only by sympathetic nerves.[9] The cervix has predominantly parasympathetic (but also sympathetic) innervation. The afferent sensory nerves from both the uterus and cervix traverse the cervical division of the Lee–Frankenhäuser plexus, which lies within and around the site of attachment of the uterosacral ligaments to the posterior aspect of the cervix.[10,11] From the uterosacral ligaments, the parasympathetic afferent nerves reach the dorsal root ganglia of

S1-S4 via the pelvic splanchnic nerves (nervi erigentes) and inferior hypogastric nerve plexus (also known as the pelvic plexus), and then the superior hypogastric nerve plexus (also known as the presacral nerve or hypogastric plexus).[12] The sympathetic afferent nerves emerging from the Lee–Frankenhäuser plexus accompany the uterine, iliac, and inferior mesenteric arteries to the sacral sympathetic trunk via the sacral splanchnic nerves, some of which bypass the superior hypogastric nerve plexus. Afferent nerves accompany both parasympathetic and sympathetic nerves from the ovary. Pain fibers bypass the uterosacral ligament and course through corresponding plexuses to their cells of origin in the dorsal root ganglia (T10-T11). Some of the afferent nerves of the upper ovarian plexus course directly via the renal and aortic plexuses and bypass the presacral nerve.[6]

It is no surprise that LUNA has not been known to be an effective adjunct to laparoscopic surgical removal of endometriosis.[6] The operation interrupts only some of the afferent sensory nerve fibers from the pelvis, and thus LUNA may be less effective for pelvic pain associated with more extensive pathology. Careful study of Figure 15.2.1 clarifies why transection of the

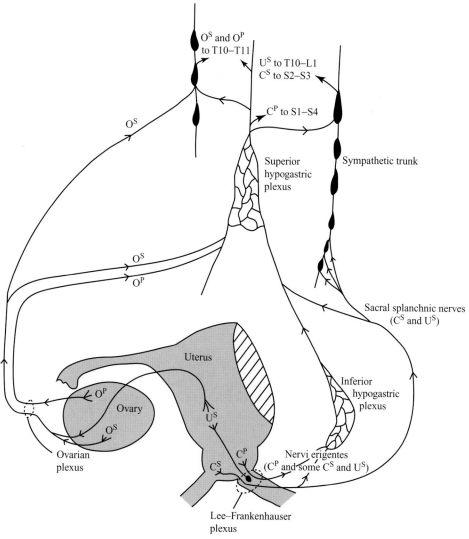

Figure 15.2.1. Sensory afferent nerve supply of the female pelvic organs. C, afferent nerve supply of cervix (illustrated on the right side of the diagram); O, afferent nerve supply of the ovary (illustrated on the left side of the diagram); U, afferent nerve supply of the uterus (illustrated on the right side of the diagram); P, parasympathetic nerve; S, sympathetic nerve. From Johnson NP et al.[6]

Lee–Frankenhäuser nerve plexus and LUNA could be particularly ineffective for pain arising from the ovary or adjacent tissues, as could be the case in ovarian or paraovarian endometriosis, because all ovarian afferent nerves bypass the Lee–Frankenhäuser plexus and many of the pain fibers also bypass the presacral nerve. Without performing a periarterial sympathectomy of the iliac, inferior mesenteric, and ovarian vessels, a number of afferent fibers will always be left intact. It has been argued persuasively that the effectiveness of a LUNA procedure for endometriosis-related pain could be due more to a debulking of endometriotic lesions. The most common site for endometriosis on the uterosacral ligament is the very site where the uterine nerve ablation is performed.[13]

Fujii et al. [14] investigated the localization of nerves in the uterosacral ligament to determine the optimal site for uterosacral nerve ablation. In their study, they found that the largest number of nerve fiber bundles and nerve cells were located 1.65 to 3.30 cm distal to the site of attachment of the uterosacral ligament to the uterine cervix at a depth of 0.3 to 1.5 cm. A relatively large number of nerve fiber bundles were found in horizontal sections at a depth of 1.0 cm. They concluded that this area is the most appropriate region anatomically for resection of the uterosacral ligament for the purpose of blocking the pain pathway.

TECHNIQUE

A standard three-puncture technique is suggested. The procedure is performed by placing the uterosacral ligaments on stretch by anteverting the uterus with the uterine manipulator. A CO_2 laser (40 to 60 W) or another cutting instrument is employed to transect the ligaments at the points of their insertion into the cervix using a vertical motion from medial to lateral (Figure 15.2.2).[15] Following the recommendation of Fujii [14], the tissue located approximately 1 to 3 cm along the uterosacral ligament should be treated to a depth of 1.5 cm. This segment of the uterosacral ligament is close to the uterine vessels and ureter. The suction–irrigator serves as a backstop to make the uterosacral ligament more prominent and protect the ureter. A relaxing incision may be made along the outer side of the ligament to retract the ureter laterally before the ligament is transected (Figure 15.2.3). The blood vessels run along the medial aspect of the uterosacral ligament, and bleeding in this area must be controlled carefully because of the proximity of the ureter and rectum. Some gynecologists also vaporize a path along the base of the cervix between the uterosacral ligaments (Figure 15.2.4). Interceed (Gynecare) may be placed over the transected area (Figure 15.2.5).

If the uterosacral ligaments are difficult to identify, uterosacral transection is not recommended. When the uterosacral ligament is cut, a blood vessel inside it tends to bleed. To ascertain if this has occurred, uterine traction should be released and pneumoperitoneum should be decreased.

The direction of the ureter should be identified from the pelvic brim to the bladder because ureteral injury is a serious complication associated with this procedure.[14] There is usually a distance of 2 to 3 cm between the ureter and the uterosacral ligaments; however, this varies.

If the ureter is close to the uterosacral ligaments, as mentioned above, a relaxing incision should be made as described. The ureter is retracted laterally before the ligament is transected. If uterosacral transection is unsuccessful, it is presumed that interruption of the nerve fibers was incomplete or the nerves regenerated. Lichten [16] reported that repeating the procedure did not relieve dysmenorrhea, implying that the course of the nerve

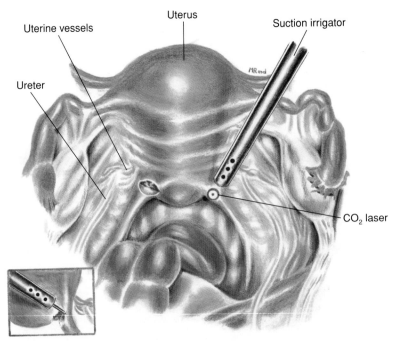

Figure 15.2.2. Transection at this location maximizes the number of nerve fibers transected because the fibers disperse as they pass along the uterosacral ligaments. Following the recommendation of Fujii [14], the tissue approximately 1 to 3 cm along the uterosacral ligament should be treated to a depth of 0.3 to 1.5 cm. From Nezhat C, Nezhat F.[15]

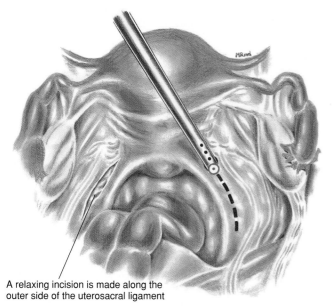

A relaxing incision is made along the
outer side of the uterosacral ligament

Figure 15.2.3. If the ureter is close to the uterosacral ligament, a relaxing incision is made along the outer side of the ligament. The ureter is retracted laterally before the ligament is transected. Occasionally, the rectum may appear similar to these ligaments. From Nezhat C, Nezhat F.[15]

fibers in these individuals may not be normal. Several patients with failed uterosacral transection have obtained relief from a subsequent presacral neurectomy.

COMPLICATIONS

Complications of the LUNA procedure include loss of uterine support, adhesions, and ureteral transections, with loss of uter-

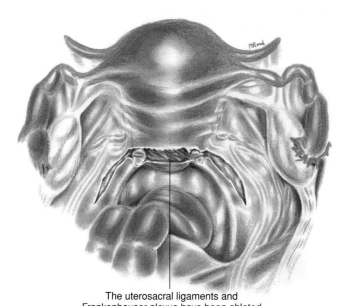

The uterosacral ligaments and
Frankenhauser plexus have been ablated

Figure 15.2.4. The ligaments have been transected with ablation of the combined nerves. From Nezhat C, Nezhat F.[15]

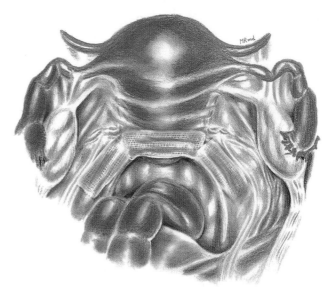

Figure 15.2.5. Interceed is placed over the transected area. From Nezhat C, Nezhat F.[15]

ine support deserving special mention. Davis [17] noted severe uterine prolapse in three young female soldiers during or after undergoing the rigors of airborne training. All three had previously undergone LUNA procedures. No other risk factors for uterine prolapse could be identified in these cases. He went on to state that although the etiology of uterine prolapse is complex, and no conclusions as to cause and effect can be made, these cases suggest that LUNA should be performed with caution on women whose occupation and lifestyle are associated with heavy physical labor or exercises producing marked increases in intra-abdominal pressure. Good [18] reported on uterine prolapse after laparoscopic uterosacral nerve transection in women who had previous vaginal delivery.

CONCLUSION

A randomized, controlled trial to assess the efficacy of LUNA in the treatment of chronic pelvic pain is ongoing through the LUNA trial collaborative study.[19] The principal objective of this multicenter prospective randomized, controlled study is to test the hypothesis that LUNA alleviates pain and improves life quality in women with chronic pelvic pain and no pathology or mild endometriosis (American Fertility Society score ≤5). Patients in the study are randomized to either diagnostic laparoscopy with LUNA or to no pelvic denervation. The site for the LUNA in this study is the Lee–Frankenhäuser plexus (Figure 15.2.6). Assessments are carried out in a blinded fashion, and the protocol calls for 12-month follow-up.

Latthe et al. [20] reported that among clinicians, there is widespread variation in the practice and use of LUNA for treatment of chronic pelvic pain. Additionally, they found wide variation in beliefs about the effectiveness of the procedure for pelvic pain, ranging from substantial benefit to slight harm. The majority of respondents stated that LUNA would benefit patients in terms of improved VAS scores, but expectations regarding the level of benefit varied widely.

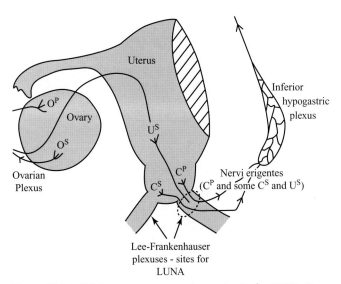

Figure 15.2.6. Pelvic sensory nerve pathways in site for LUNA. From LUNA Trial Collaboration.[19]

In a European survey, Latthe et al. [21] found variation in methods of performing the LUNA procedure. Noting that recent anatomic studies have demonstrated that the greatest numbers of nerve fiber bundles are found some distance from the site of the attachment of uterosacral ligament to the cervix [14], there is some controversy about the optimal site for LUNA. The effectiveness of LUNA may depend on the completeness of transection of the uterosacral ligaments. Latthe [21] found that compared to the U.K. group, the European group performed LUNA more frequently and transected the uterosacral ligament completely more often. The European group also transected the uterosacral ligament 2 cm or more from the point of cervical insertion more often. It is important to keep in mind the nerve plexus as described by Fujii [14] when performing LUNA. It is also helpful to keep in mind that the lateral nerves will not be affected (Figure 15.2.6). The studies of Johnson [6] and Yen [7] indicate that LUNA does have a role to play in the relief of central pelvic pain relief not related to endometriosis.

REFERENCES

1. Doyle EB. Paracervical uterine denervation by transection of the cervical plexus for the relief of dysmenorrhea. *Am J Obstet Gynecol.* 1955;70:11.
2. Sutton C, Whitelaw N. Laparoscopic uterine nerve ablation for intractable dysmenorrhea. In: Sutton C, Diamond M, eds. *Endoscopic Surgery for Gynaecologists.* London: WB Saunders; 1993: 159–168.
3. Lichten EM, Bombard J. Surgical treatment of primary dysmenorrhea with laparoscopic uterine nerve ablation. *J Reprod Med.* 1987;32:37–41.
4. Gurgan T, Urman B, Aksu T, et al. Laparoscopic CO_2 laser uterine nerve ablation for treatment of drug-resistant primary dysmenorrhea. *Fertil Steril.* 1992;58:422.
5. Sutton C. Laser uterine ablation. In: Donnez J, ed. *Laser Operative Laparoscopy and Hysteroscopy.* Leuven, Belgium: Nauwelaerts Printing; 1989:43–52.
6. Johnson NP, Farquhar CM, Crossley S, et al. A double-blind randomized controlled trial of laparoscopic uterine nerve ablation for women with chronic pelvic pain. *BJOG.* 2004;111:950–959.
7. Yen YK, Liu WM, Yuan CC, Ng HT. Addition of laparoscopic uterine nerve ablation to laparoscopic bipolar coagulation of uterine vessels for women with uterine myomas and dysmenorrhea. *J Am Assoc Gynecol Laparosc.* 2001;8:573–578.
8. Counseller VS, Craig W. The treatment of dysmenorrhea by resection of the presacral nerves: evaluation of end results. *Am J Obstet Gynecol.* 1934;28:161–167.
9. Owman C, Rosenbren E, Sjoberg NO. Adrenergic innervation of the human female reproductive organs: a histochemical and chemical investigation. *Obstet Gynecol.* 1967;30:763–773.
10. Frankenhauser G. Die Bewegungenerven der Gebarmutter. *Z Med Nat Wiss.* 1864;1:35.
11. Cleland JP. Paravertebral anesthesia in obstetrics. *Surg Gynecol Obstet.* 1933;57:51.
12. Williams PL, Warwick R. Reproductive organs of the female. In: Williams PL, Warwick R, eds. *Gray's Anatomy.* 36th ed. Edinburgh: Churchill Livingston; 1980:1423–1431.
13. Jones KD, Sutton C. Arcus Taurinus: the "mother and father" of all LUNAs. *Gynecol Endosc.* 2001;10:83–89.
14. Fujii M, Sagae S, Sato T, et al. Investigation of the localization of nerves in the uterosacral ligament: determination of the optimal site for uterosacral nerve ablation. *Gynecol Obstet Invest.* 2002;54(suppl 1):11–17.
15. Nezhat C, Siegler A, Nezhat F, Nezhat C, Seidman D, Luciano A. *Operative Gynecologic Laparoscopy. Principles and Techniques.* 2nd Edition. New York: McGraw-Hill; 2000.
16. Lichten E. Three years' experience with LUNA. *Am J Gynecol.* 1989;3:9.
17. Davis GD. Uterine prolapse after laparoscopic uterosacral transection in nulliparous airborne trainees. A report of three cases. *J Reprod Med.* 1996;41:279–282.
18. Good MC, Copas PR Jr, Voody MC. Uterine prolapse after laparoscopic uterosacral transection: a case report. *J Reprod Med.* 1992;37:995–996.
19. The LUNA trial collaboration, a randomized controlled trial to assess the efficacy of laparoscopic uterosacral nerve ablation (LUNA) in the treatment of chronic pelvic pain: the trial protocol (ISRCT In 41196151). Department of Obstetrics and Gynecology, Birmingham Clinical Trials Unit and Department of Public Health and Epidemiology, University of Birmingham B15 2TT, UK. *BMC Womens Health.* 2003;3:6.
20. Latthe PM, Braunholtz DA, Hills RK, et al. Measurement and beliefs about effectiveness of laparoscopic uterosacral nerve ablation. *BJOG.* 2005;112:243–246.
21. Latthe PM, Powell RJ, Daniels J, et al. Variation in practice of laparoscopic uterosacral nerve ablation: a European study. *J Obstet Gynecol.* 2004;24:547–551.

16 GYNECOLOGIC MALIGNANCY

Section 16.1. Introduction

Farr Nezhat

Laparoscopy has been used for second-look assessments in ovarian cancer since first described in 1973 by Bagley et al.[1] However, it was new developments in equipment and instrumentation, such as videolaparoscopy, high pressure insufflators, and energy sources, in the late 1980s to early 1990s – combined with the work of some of the pioneers of laparoscopic surgery – that made the use of operative laparoscopy in gynecologic oncology feasible. Dargent and Salvat [2], Querleu et al. [3], and Nezhat et al. [4] first established the safety and practicability of laparoscopic retroperitoneal and intraperitoneal lymphadenectomy and radical hysterectomy. An increasing number of surgeons have since used advanced operative techniques for evaluation and surgical management of gynecologic cancers.

Laparoscopy has the benefit of image magnification to aid in identification of metastatic or recurrent disease, especially in areas such as the upper abdomen, liver and diaphragm surfaces, posterior cul-de-sac, bowel, and mesenteric surfaces. In addition, challenging retroperitoneal spaces of the pelvis, such as the paravesical, pararectal, vesicovaginal, and especially the rectovaginal space, can be accessed laparoscopically. Additional benefits of laparoscopy in gynecologic oncology surgery include limited bleeding from small vessels due to the pressure established by pneumoperitoneum, elimination of large abdominal incisions, shortened hospital stay, and rapid recovery. The ease of recuperation from laparoscopic surgical management thus offers a smooth transition for patients to then undergo planned adjuvant therapies. Postoperative chemotherapy or radiation can be initiated earlier, and radiation complications from bowel adhesions are minimized.

For approximately two decades now, significant progress has been made in advancing the role of laparoscopy in the management of gynecologic malignancy, dealing with key issues such as minimizing radicality of a procedure, management of its complications, disease recurrence, and survival. As expected, these advanced endoscopic procedures must be carried out by surgeons who have the required skills, contemporary equipment, and trained ancillary staff. In this chapter, practiced surgeons address the utility of advanced operative laparoscopy in the management of various gynecologic malignancies.

REFERENCES

1. Bagley CM, Young RC, Schein PS, et al. Ovarian cancer metastatic to the diaphragm frequently undiagnosed at laparotomy: a preliminary report. *Am J Obstet Gynecol*. 1973;116:247.
2. Dargent D, Salvat J. *Lienvahissement Ganglionnaire Pelvien*. Paris: MEDSI; 1989.
3. Querleu D, Leblan E, Catelain B. Laparoscopic pelvic lymphadenectomy. *Am J Obstet Gynecol*. 1991;164:579.
4. Nezhat CR, Nezhat FR, Ramirez CE, et al. Laparoscopic radical hysterectomy and laparoscopic assisted radical vaginal hysterectomy with pelvic and paraaortic node dissection. *J Gynecol Surg* 1993;9:105.

Section 16.2. Laparoscopic Lymphadenectomy

Farr Nezhat and M. Shoma Datta

In patients with gynecologic cancer, prognosis correlates with the stage of disease according to the established Internation Federation of Gynecology and Obstetrics (FIGO) classification systems. Lymph node status is one of the most important prognostic factors in gynecologic cancer, and surgical removal of pelvic and/or para-aortic lymph nodes for histologic assessment is a crucial part of staging. Furthermore, cytoreduction of bulky lymph nodes may have therapeutic benefit.

Lymphadenectomy has generally been performed via laparotomy, using large incisions and often causing significant intra- and perioperative morbidity. Dargent and Salvat [1] in 1989 were the first to describe laparoscopic retroperitoneal pelvic lymphadenectomy for the management of gynecologic malignancies. In 1991, Querleu et al. [2] reported laparoscopic pelvic lymphadenectomy in 39 patients with cervical cancer. The first laparoscopic para-aortic lymphadenectomy was reported by Nezhat et al. [3–5] in 1991 through 1993 in a series of patients with cervical cancer undergoing laparoscopic radical hysterectomy with pelvic and para-aortic lymphadenectomy. Since that time, a number of other reports have described the safety and accuracy of laparoscopic lymphadenectomy for cervical, endometrial, and ovarian cancers, as well as for urologic malignancies and some lymphomas. Numerous reports describe better magnification, fewer complications, and superior visualization of the anatomy provided by the videolaparoscope in comparison with conventional techniques.

In recent years, an expanding literature has become available regarding outcomes and complications of the laparoscopic lymphadenectomy. Current reports, however, often reflect the developing skill set of the pioneering laparoscopists and the variable facility support for such advanced laparoscopic procedures.

TECHNIQUE

Pelvic and para-aortic lymphadenectomy can be accomplished before or after hysterectomy and bilateral salpingo-oophorectomy. Technically, there are many benefits of a laparoscopic approach specific to pelvic and para-aortic lymphadenectomy. The laparoscope provides a seven- to 10-fold magnification of the operative field, allowing identification of small tributary vessels. Furthermore, pneumoperitoneum facilitates development of the pelvic spaces and decreases venous bleeding, thereby maintaining a clean operative dissection with good visualization of the nodal bundles.

Pelvic Lymphadenectomy

The initial step to pelvic lymphadenectomy is to expose the anterior and posterior leaves of the broad ligament by incising the round ligament and dissecting the broad ligament in a cephalad fashion lateral and parallel to the infundibulopelvic ligament. An incision is made in the broad ligament lateral or parallel to the infundibulopelvic ligament to open the posterior peritoneum, allowing identification of the ureter. Using the suction–irrigator probe, grasper, and scissors, the paravesical space is created. It is bordered medially by the obliterated hypogastric artery, bladder, and vagina and laterally by the pelvic side wall. Creating the avascular paravesical space helps identify the obturator nerve and vessels and the distal portion of the pelvic wall vessels. The obliterated hypogastric artery and external iliac vein are landmarks to get to the paravesical space (Figure 16.2.1). The spaces lateral to this vessel and medial to the external iliac vein and obturator internus muscle are created with blunt and sharp dissection. Electrocoagulation should not be necessary as this space is generally avascular. Once this space is created, the bony lateral side wall, the levator plate laterally, and the obturator nerve and vessels anteriorly should be visible. The pelvic lymph nodes can now be safely removed. Starting laterally over the psoas muscle and proceeding medially provide a safe approach that avoids the genitofemoral nerve. The external iliac nodes along the external iliac artery and vein are excised caudally from common iliac vessels to the level of the deep circumflex iliac vein seen crossing over the distal portion of the external iliac artery (Figure 16.2.2).

The obturator space is then opened and the nerve is identified by blunt dissection below and between the obliterated umbilical artery and the external iliac vein (Figure 16.2.3). Although the majority of patients have both the obturator artery and vein dorsal to the obturator nerve, 10% will have an aberrant obturator vein anterior to the nerve, entering the midpoint of the external iliac vein. The obturator lymph nodes are grasped just under the external iliac vein, and traction is applied medially. The node chain is thereby separated from the obturator nerve and vessels, and the nodes are dissected cephalad to the hypogastric artery. The nodal tissue anterior and lateral to the nerve and medial and inferior to the external iliac vein is removed by blunt and sharp dissection. Venous anastomosis between the obturator and the external iliac veins is saved from injury. The obturator fossa lymph nodes are excised caudally to the pelvic side wall where the obturator nerve exits the pelvis through the obturator canal and cephalad up to the bifurcation of the common iliac artery. Before the removal of each nodal bundle, each pedicle is ligated by electrocoagulation, endoscopic hemoclips, or harmonic shears to prevent lymphocyst formation. The lymph node packets are removed in a bag through the largest trocar to avoid any contact between potentially malignant lymph node tissue and the abdominal wall. Using sharp and blunt dissection, the nodes between the external iliac vessels and the obliterated hypogastric artery are removed. The nodes along

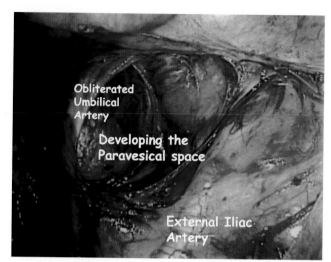

Figure 16.2.1. The paravesical space is developed to aid in identification of the obturator nerve, vessels, and pelvic vessels.

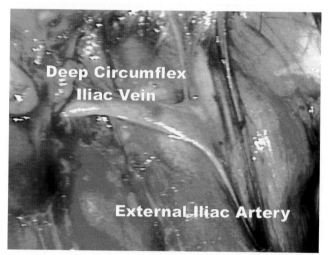

Figure 16.2.2. The nodes are dissected from the common iliac artery bifurcation to the circumflex iliac vein caudally.

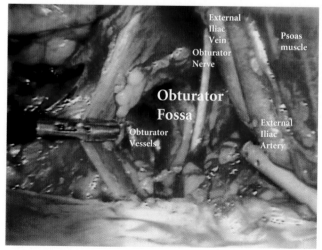

Figure 16.2.3. The obturator vessels and nerve are identified once the obturator space is opened.

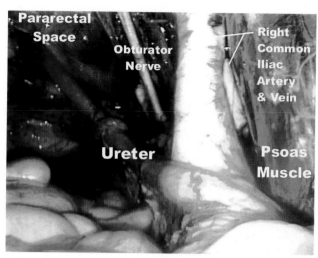

Figure 16.2.4. The ureter is identified crossing the common iliac artery at the pelvic brim.

the hypogastric vessels are excised up to the bifurcation of the common iliac vessels. Caution is necessary to avoid injury to the obturator nerve and hypogastric vein. To excise the lymph nodes around the common iliac artery, a plane is created between the posterior peritoneum and the adventitia overlying the common iliac artery. Another option is to extend the dissection over the common iliac vessels when removing the proximal portion of the external iliac nodes. Before the nodes are detached, the orientation of the ureter and ovarian vessels crossing the common iliac artery is identified (Figure 16.2.4). The uterine artery and vein can be isolated originating from the hypogastric vessels when necessary (Figure 16.2.5). When one is performing a left pelvic lymph node dissection, it may be necessary to take down rectosigmoid colon from the left pelvic side wall to allow visualization of the pelvic vessels.[3–5]

Para-aortic Lymphadenectomy

There are several ways to begin the para-aortic lymphadenectomy dissection: incising the peritoneum overlying the aorta, opening the peritoneum over the sacral promontory, or extending a

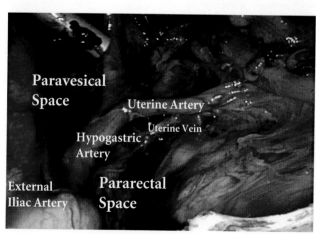

Figure 16.2.5. The uterine artery is identified at its origin from the hypogastric artery.

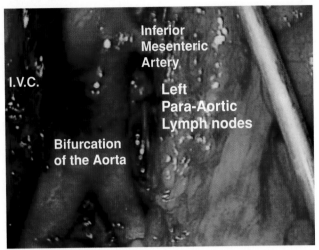

Figure 16.2.6. Para-aortic dissection seen here extends to the inferior mesenteric artery.

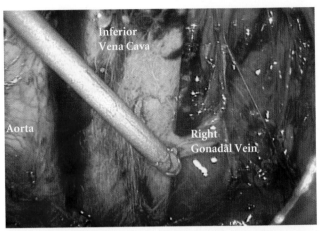

Figure 16.2.8. For para-aortic lymphadenectomy above the mesenteric artery, the peritoneal incision is extended to the level of the left renal vein and right ovarian vein.

preexisting incision over the common iliac artery toward the aorta. This incision is extended up to the inferior mesenteric artery (Figure 16.2.6) or up to the left renal vein in cases of ovarian or fallopian tube carcinoma. The underlying retroperitoneum is developed by blunt and sharp dissection. Next, the retroperitoneal space is created by using sharp and blunt dissection to develop the space lateral to the aorta. Before cutting, it is essential to identify the right ureter, separate it from underlying tissue, and retract it laterally. The nodal tissue overlying the aorta, right common iliac artery, and sacral promontory is removed laterally toward the psoas muscle. Fatty and nodal tissue overlying the sacral promontory is removed. This tissue may contain hypogastric nerves. The left common iliac vein must be observed before starting this dissection (Figure 16.2.7). This maneuver allows the nodal tissue anterior to the vena cava to be detached. The dissection is continued cephalad to the level of the inferior mesenteric artery, removing all lymphatic tissue anterior to and between the aorta and inferior vena cava. Again, it is essential to identify the

ureter along the inferior border of the dissection and the transverse duodenum along the superior margin of the dissection. Perforating vessels from the vena cava are electrocoagulated or ligated with hemoclips.

The removal of the left para-aortic nodes may be more difficult because of the location of the sigmoid colon. Attention is necessary to avoid injury to the inferior mesenteric artery, ovarian vessels, and ureter. The left common iliac vein lies at the bifurcation of the aorta. The dissection proceeds from the aorta laterally toward the psoas muscle, excising the lymph nodes from above the inferior mesenteric artery to below the left common iliac artery. This allows the surgeon to dissect laterally in a plane that is beneath the inferior mesenteric artery and the mesentery of the sigmoid colon. It is important not to dissect laterally until the adventitia of the aorta is incised to prevent entering the wrong plane.

When para-aortic lymphadenectomy above the mesenteric artery is being performed, the peritoneal incision is extended to the level of the left renal vein and right ovarian vein (Figure 16.2.8). If necessary, the ovarian vessels and the mesenteric artery are ligated for better exposure and to prevent bleeding. After the lymphadenectomy is completed, evaluation of the area under decreased pneumoperitoneal pressure is done to ensure hemostasis. As with pelvic lymphadenectomy, the peritoneum is not closed and drains are not placed. Adhesion barriers may be applied to decrease postoperative adhesions.[3–5]

COMPLICATIONS

Complications of laparoscopic lymphadenectomy can be divided into two general categories. The first includes complications that are inherent to laparoscopy itself, regardless of the specific procedure being performed. This category includes subcutaneous emphysema and trocar injuries to the bowel or the inferior epigastric vessels. The second group of complications includes those that are inherent to the procedure, regardless of the method by which it is performed. Obturator nerve injury, deep venous thrombosis, and postoperative lymphocele are all complications of a pelvic

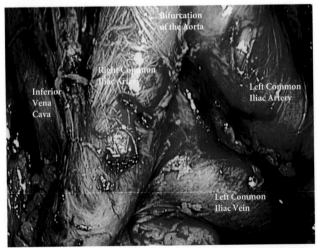

Figure 16.2.7. The left common iliac vein must be clearly identified during para-aortic lymphadenectomy.

Table 16.2.1: Complications of Laparoscopic Lymphadenectomy Performed for Gynecologic Malignancy [6–9]

	No. Pts.	Indication	Pelvic Nodes (n)	Aortic Nodes (n)	Major Intraoperative Complications	Postoperative Complications	Conversion
Possover et al., 1997	150	Various Gyn Cancers	26.8 (10–56)	7.3 (0–19)	vascular injury 7 small bowel injury 1	lymphedema 2 temporary obturator nerve impairment 1	4
Dottino et al., 1998	94	Various Gyn Cancers	11.9 (0–57)	3.7 (0–14)	vascular injury 1	UTI 1 fever 1	3
Renaud et al., 2000	102	Cervical Cancer	25	5.5	vascular injury 3 cystotomy 4	UTI 1 bladder atony 1 pelvic abscess 1 hematoma 1 lymphocele 2	6
Scribner et al., 2001	103	Endometrial and Ovarian Cancer	Pel + Comm Iliac 23.2	6.8	vascular injury 1 ureteral injury 1 bladder injury 1	DVT 1 PE 2 1 death wound infect 6	29% 30/103
TOTAL/MEAN	449	**Various Gyn Cancers**	21.7	5.8	**vascular 12 (2.6%) ureteral 1 (.2%) bladder 4 (.8%) bowel 1 (.2%)**	**Minor 16 (3.5%) Major 4 (1.81%)**	42 (9.3%)

and para-aortic lymphadenectomy. Initial studies indicate a low incidence of complications for laparoscopic lymphadenectomy (Tables 16.2.1, 16.2.2).[6–9]

To prevent complications, adequate exposure is critical to optimize surgical dissection. This is a basic surgical tenet for open abdominal surgery and is also a necessary component of effective laparoscopic technique. For a laparoscopic lymphadenectomy, adequate exposure requires a thorough preoperative bowel prep, steep Trendelenburg patient positioning, and adequate pneumoperitoneum. These steps are essential to effectively sweep the bowel away from the operative field and to reduce the opportunity for bowel injury. Bowel decompression with an orogastric or nasogastric tube and bladder decompression with a Foley catheter should be performed at the start of the procedure. The patient should be placed in lithotomy position with the thighs no higher than the level of the anterior abdominal wall. This allows free range of motion of the lower-quadrant laparoscopic instruments without interference from the legs. Full mobility of the lower quadrant instruments allows for optimal traction and countertraction of tissue planes for dissection.

Vascular Injuries

Vascular injuries related to lymphadenectomy are potentially life-threatening complications. Perhaps the most common vascular injury of laparoscopy in general, and laparoscopic lymphadenectomy in particular, is injury to the inferior epigastric and other superficial anterior abdominal wall vessels (Figure 16.2.9). Kavoussi et al. [10], in a series of laparoscopic lymphadenectomy, reported seven out of nine vascular complications occurred as a result of trocar injury to the anterior abdominal wall vasculature. Potential vascular compromise specific to a pelvic lymphadenec-

tomy includes injury to the obturator, internal iliac, external iliac, or the common iliac vessels. In the male, the testicular artery and vein should be carefully identified during a laparoscopic lymphadenectomy to maintain their integrity. Vessels at risk for injury during a para-aortic lymphadenectomy include the aorta and vena cava, as well as the common iliac, inferior mesenteric, lumbar, and renal vessels.

Fortunately, injury to major pelvic vessels during laparoscopic pelvic lymphadenectomy is an uncommon occurrence. In Kavoussi's series [10], seven of nine vascular injuries resulted from trocar injuries to the abdominal wall vessels as reported by the combined experience of eight institutions performing laparoscopic pelvic lymphadenectomy for early prostatic carcinoma. In the remaining cases, one patient sustained injury to the obturator vein and the other case involved interruption of the external iliac artery. Querleu et al. [2] reported their initial experience with laparoscopic lymphadenectomy in 39 women with cervical carcinoma. Although none of these patients suffered major vascular injury, one patient developed a large pelvic hematoma due to an unspecified vessel injury. This was managed conservatively and resolved spontaneously without any requirement for blood transfusion. Burney et al. [11] reported a combined experience with laparoscopic pelvic lymphadenectomy for prostatic carcinoma. One of these patients developed a pelvic hematoma that subsequently became infected after percutaneous drainage.

In Childers's experience [12,13] with more than 300 pelvic lymphadenectomies for gynecologic malignancy, injury to major pelvic vessels was a rare event. The vessel most likely to be injured is an aberrant obturator vein emerging from the obturator canal, across the nodal bundle, to empty into the external iliac vein. On one occasion, a 5-mm laceration in the external iliac vein was sustained with a lymphadenectomy during a second-look

Table 16.2.2: Selected Series of Laparoscopic Pelvic and Para-aortic Lymphadenectomy

Series	Modality	Patients, no.	PLND (mean)	PALND (mean)	Complications
Childers et al. [12]	Electrosurgery	29	Not indicated	Not indicated	1 ureteral, 1 cystotomy 1 pneumothorax, 3 minor
Chu et al.	Not indicated	67	26.7	8	1 vascular
Dottino et al. [7]	Electrosurgery	94	11.9	3.7	1 vascular, 2 minor
Vidaurreta et al. [27]	Electrosurgery	84	18.5	—	1 vascular, 2 lymphocele
Altgassen et al. [28]	Not indicated	99	21–24.3	5.1–10.6	3 vascular, 1 enterotomy 1 ureteral, 1 hemorrhage 2 nerve impairment 3 intestinal obstruction 5 minor
Scribner et al. [9]	Not indicated	103	23.2	6.8	1 vascular (fatal) 2 ureteral 1 bladder laceration 1 DVT 2 pulmonary embolus (1 fatal) 1 Richter's hernia
Schlaerth et al. [22]	Electrosurgery and ABC	67	32.1	12.1	7 vascular 1 ureteral, 8 infectious 2 hematomas 2 lymphoceles
Abu-Rustum et al. [29]	Monopolar and ABC	114	10.3	5.3	1 vascular, 1 enterotomy, 1 cystotomy, 1 uterine perforation, 3 intestinal 4 infectious 1 DVT
Kohler et al. [30]	Electrosurgery	650	18.8	10.8	19 (2.9%) intraoperative (7 vascular, 3 bowel). 35 (5.8%) postoperative (16 irritation of nerves, 6 lymphedema, 3 symptomatic lymphoceles, 3 chylocysts)
Holub et al. [26]	Ultrasonic shears (LCS)*	27	17.5	—	1 inflammation of obturator nerve, 1 febrile morbidity
	Electrosurgery	32	13.7[†]		1 injury to epigastric artery 1 fever
Nezhat et al. [15]	Ultrasonic shears (LCS)	100	20	15	2 vascular 1 cystotomy 1 trocar-site hernia 1 DVT 1 port-site metastasis 1 bowel obstruction (minor)

*Ethicon EndoSurgery.
†$P = 0.0008$.
ABC, argon beam coagulator; DVT, deep venous thrombosis; PLND, pelvic lymph node; PALND, para-aortic lymph node.

laparoscopic procedure. The patient had undergone a previous lymph node sampling at the time of ovarian cancer cytoreductive surgery. The external iliac vein was injured while opening the retroperitoneal space. The laceration was repaired laparoscopically with a clip applicator. The patient did not require transfusion or experience any postoperative complications.[14] Three other patients had vena cava injuries complicating their laparoscopic lymphadenectomy. The first required open laparotomy for vascular repair, was transfused with four units of packed red blood cells, and went on to develop a deep venous thrombosis. The remaining two cases were managed laparoscopically with endoscopic vascular clip applicators (Figure 16.2.10). Neither of these two patients

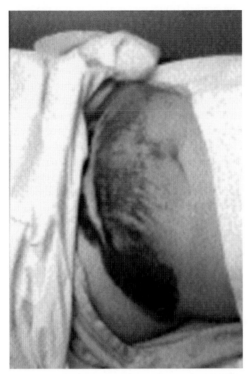

Figure 16.2.9. Extensive postoperative ecchymosis extending from the suprapubic port site.

activated shears, there were two vascular injuries.[15] The first was an injury to the branch of the inferior mesenteric artery during surgical staging of a cervical stage IIB cancer, which was controlled with bipolar forceps. The second vascular injury, involving the right hypogastric vein, occurred during a laparoscopically assisted radical hysterectomy and pelvic lymphadenectomy and was repaired laparoscopically without any postoperative sequelae.

A theoretic but nonetheless important concern is the possibility of an air embolus, especially with damage to larger vascular structures. This is especially a concern if the lymphadenectomy is performed using an argon beam coagulator because this gas is not readily absorbed into the circulation. The diagnosis of gas embolism is made via auscultation with a conventional or transesophageal stethoscope. A "wheel-mill" murmur is presumptive evidence of air entrapment in the right heart. Management consists of the placement of a central line into the right ventricle and subsequent aspiration of the embolized gas. Although such a complication has yet to be reported for laparoscopic lymphadenectomy, CO_2 embolism has been reported with other laparoscopic procedures.

Management of Vascular Injuries

Laparoscopic management of vascular injuries varies according to the type (artery or vein) and size of the vessel injured. The modalities used in managing these vascular injuries include pressure, monopolar and bipolar electricity, clips, and sutures. Depending on the caliber of the injured vessel, any one of these modalities may achieve hemostasis satisfactorily.

When a vessel is injured, it is important to control the bleeding as quickly as possible. This usually can be accomplished by using a laparoscopic grasper to occlude the bleeding vessel. If

received a transfusion or had any other postoperative complications. Experience with external iliac and vena cava injuries has revealed that bleeding in the presence of adequate pneumoperitoneum (i.e., 15 mm H_2O), even from large veins, is relatively limited. In our experience with 100 cases of laparoscopic lymphadenectomy for gynecologic malignancies using ultrasonically

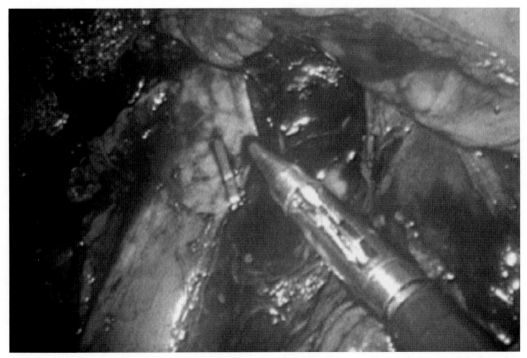

Figure 16.2.10. Endoscopic clip applied to the lower vena cava following a small venotomy created during a low right para-aortic laparoscopic lymphadenectomy.

visualization is obscured, or if the vessel is a large vein in which grasping may result in further laceration, pressure should be applied. Laparoscopic instruments, lymph node pads, 4- × 4-inch gauze, or minilaparotomy pads can be placed to achieve immediate control. To be prepared for any bleeding, a 4- × 4-inch gauze pad can be placed through a 10- to 12-mm port before beginning the lymph node dissection.

Small venous bleeds can be controlled with pressure alone. A minilaparotomy pad can be packed into the retroperitoneal space while the procedure is continued in another part of the surgical field. Later in the operative procedure, the packing can be removed and the area inspected for hemostasis. Placing pads into the abdomen laparoscopically may be a helpful technique; however, it also produces a new potential complication of retained laparotomy pads. Laparotomy rings, such as those used when a laparotomy is performed, cannot be used laparoscopically, so the surgeon must rely primarily on the operative pad count. If the count is incorrect, or if the surgeon wants to include an additional safety measure, a postoperative radiograph should be obtained. Figure 16.2.11 illustrates a radiograph of the abdomen demonstrating two retained retroperitoneal laparotomy pads. These pads were placed during a laparoscopic bilateral para-aortic lymphadenectomy.

Arterial bleeds should be quickly controlled, as blood loss may be rapid. Care should be taken to avoid arterial pumping of blood onto the laparoscope. When this occurs, visualization of the operative field is obscured and the laparoscope must be removed for cleaning, which expends valuable time and increases blood loss. Another common pitfall in controlling vascular injuries occurs during aspiration of pooled blood. While the pooled blood is being suctioned, the pneumoperitoneum frequently is suctioned

as well if the suction tip is not completely submerged. This may result in poor exposure of the operative site and can create a cascade of time-consuming events including inadequate pneumoperitoneum, bowel falling out of the upper abdomen, and the laparoscope lens becoming obscured by blood.

Monopolar electricity may be used to achieve control of small arterial and venous bleeds. Bipolar desiccation is especially useful to control venous and arterial bleeds of a larger caliber. The bipolar method may be used to coapt vessels or may be applied along the length of the instrument to provide surface cauterization over a friable area.[16] Bipolar electrocautery, however, is an unacceptable form of vascular injury control in vessels that should not be sacrificed or vessels of extremely large caliber, such as the iliac and the vena cava. In these situations, clips or suturing techniques should be used. Laparoscopically applied clips can control large venous bleeds adequately. Prefabricated slipknots may be used to control moderate-sized arterial bleeds. In these instances, a grasper is placed through the prefabricated loop and affixed to the injured vessel. The loop is slipped over the grasper and onto the vessel. Suturing techniques using needles most often require laparotomy. In certain conditions, in the hands of very experienced surgeons, small vascular injuries can be repaired using laparoscopic suturing. In the instance of vascular injury, consideration should be given to intraoperative consultation with a vascular surgeon.

Gastrointestinal Injuries

Bowel injury is a potential complication of any laparoscopic procedure. Bowel can be easily damaged at trocar insertion, adhesiolysis, or thermal injury during dissection (Figure 16.2.12). This complication can be avoided in all laparoscopic procedures by appropriate patient selection, preoperative preparation including a complete mechanical bowel preparation, and the intraoperative placement of an orogastric or nasogastric tube. The net effect is to keep the bowel flat and empty, resulting in easier "packing" into the upper abdomen, where it is less likely to enter the operative field.

Delayed bowel morbidity may occur throughout the postoperative period. Bowel herniation may result as a consequence of

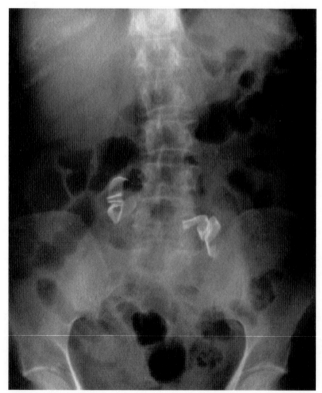

Figure 16.2.11. Radiograph demonstrating the radiolucent tags of a retained minilaparotomy pad. These pads were initially placed following a laparoscopic bilateral low para-aortic lymphadenectomy.

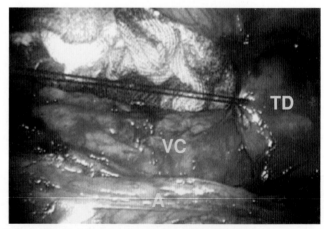

Figure 16.2.12. Laparoscopic photograph from the umbilical port. The surgeon is placing an imbricating silk suture on the transverse duodenum (t) to imbricate an area that was superficially burned during a para-aortic lymphadenectomy. TD, transverse duodenum; VC, vena cava; A, aorta.

absent or inadequate fascial closure of the trocar defects. In one report, two small bowel herniations occurred in a series of 35 laparoscopic pelvic and para-aortic lymphadenectomies performed for gynecologic malignancies.[17] These two small bowel herniations presented clinically with intestinal obstruction. It is notable that both occurred at lateral 12-mm trocar sites where stabilizing fascial screws were used followed by attempted fascial closure. Both cases were managed laparoscopically. Although not reported, bowel obstruction may occur as a result of post-laparoscopic adhesion formation.

Management of Gastrointestinal Injuries

Laparoscopic management of gastrointestinal injuries has been covered in previous chapters. Consideration of laparoscopic hernia reduction is not unreasonable, depending on the clinical situation, and has been accomplished and reported in the literature. Large and small bowel injuries can be repaired intracorporeally or extracorporeally through a slightly enlarged port site, particularly for small bowel. These techniques are discussed in detail in other chapters.

Genitourinary Injury

Laparoscopic injury to the urinary tract is well described in the literature. Cystotomy during trocar insertion, adhesiolysis, or dissection with endoscopic scissors with or without electrocautery has been described as a complication of laparoscopic lymphadenectomy, although not specific to this procedure. Cystotomy may occur during hysterectomy or when opening the obturator space, if the obliterated umbilical artery is not retracted medially. Meticulous surgical technique and decompression of the bladder with a Foley catheter are the cornerstones of the prevention of this type of injury. Ureterovaginal and vesicovaginal fistulae, as well as injury to the patent urachus, are other potential though as yet unreported complications.

Perhaps of most concern, and certainly germane to the laparoscopic lymphadenectomy, is the possibility of ureteral injury. Pelvic lymphadenectomy places the ureter at risk for sharp, crush, or thermal injury, which has been described in the urologic literature. The lumbar portion of the ureter is at risk during para-aortic lymphadenectomy; injury may occur if the lateral dissection overlying the psoas muscle is carried out above the ureter instead of in the correct surgical plane, thus incorporating the ureter into the nodal bundle. In our experience, injection of 10 mL of intravenous indigo carmine is very useful for recognition of ureteral perforation. If this injury occurs, management can be accomplished by placing a transureteral stent, oversewing the defect, and placing a retroperitoneal drain laparoscopically. Although it is an area of current investigation, there is no proven role for prophylactic ureteral stent placement before laparoscopic lymphadenectomy.

Neurologic Injury

Operative nerve injury can complicate any surgical procedure in the pelvis. There are, however, concerns that are particular to lymphadenectomy. Genitofemoral nerve injury is most likely to occur during removal of the lateral pelvic lymph nodes. Such an injury results in medial thigh numbness but is otherwise of little clinical consequence. It is arguably the most common injury encoun-

tered by the gynecologic oncologist. Injury of the obturator nerve is a more concerning, though extremely rare, complication that may occur during laparoscopic lymph node dissection.[10,11,18] Patients suffer from pain, weakness in leg adduction, and sensory loss of the medial thigh. This injury occurs only if the obturator nerve is not reliably identified before the resection of the obturator lymph node package. Theoretically, the femoral nerve, which lies within the body of the psoas muscle in the pelvis, is at risk during lymphadenectomy. This is particularly true if the nerve is not deep in the belly of the muscle and is exposed to extensive electrocautery during the dissection. Though not a direct operative injury, the ulnar nerve may also be traumatized if not properly padded in the course of tucking the arms for operative laparoscopy.

Other Complications

Various other injuries and complications may result as a consequence of this procedure. Both lymphocele and lymphedema have been reported to occur with laparoscopic lymphadenectomy [10,11,18], as they may also occur with open procedures. In Childers's experience [12,13] with more than 300 pelvic lymphadenectomies, there have been two symptomatic lymphoceles. As might be expected with any operative procedure, infectious complications have been reported with laparoscopic lymphadenectomy, including infected pelvic hematoma, *Clostridium difficile* infection, and wound complications.[10,11,19] Likewise, retained foreign bodies and equipment failure can complicate the conduct of this safe and effective procedure.

Perhaps of most concern are thromboembolic events, which can complicate any major operative procedure in the pelvis, especially in the cancer patient. Two separate series of laparoscopic lymphadenectomies performed for urologic malignancies reported three instances of deep venous thrombosis (1.5%) and no pulmonary emboli among 203 procedures.[17,18] Pomel et al. [20] reported a case of lower-extremity thrombophlebitis complicated by a subsequent pulmonary embolism following a staging laparoscopy for ovarian carcinoma.[19] More recently, Spirtos et al. [17] reported on a series of 40 patients who underwent bilateral pelvic and para-aortic lymphadenectomy for endometrial and ovarian cancer. Of the 35 patients whose operations were completed laparoscopically, two (5.7%) developed deep vein thrombosis during the postoperative period.

COMPLICATIONS REQUIRING LAPAROTOMY

Complications resulting in laparotomy have been related to damage to the ureter, bladder, bowel and vascular structures. Kavoussi et al. [10] reported a 4% (13/372) incidence of laparotomy related to laparoscopic pelvic lymphadenectomy. Complications were recognized at initial laparoscopic surgery in seven patients, and six individuals required secondary laparotomy. Reasons for laparotomy included transection of the ureter (two patients), cystotomy (two patients), bowel injuries or obstruction (four patients), vascular injury (four patients), and wound dehiscence (one patient).

Burney et al. [11] reported a laparotomy rate of 8% (4/54) for patients undergoing laparoscopic pelvic lymphadenectomy for urologic indications. One of four patients required laparotomy at the time of the procedure. Indications for laparotomy included ureteral damage (one patient), small bowel obstruction (two patients), and mesenteric hematoma (one patient). An overall major complication rate of 16.7% (9/54) was estimated, with the inclusion of a large fascial hematoma, two bladder perforations, and two patients requiring blood transfusion.

In a series reported by Boitke et al. [21], laparotomy was required in 10% of patients (3/29) undergoing laparoscopic pelvic and/or para-aortic lymphadenectomy for endometrial cancer. Two patients underwent secondary operations because of small bowel obstruction, and another patient had a vascular injury to a small branch of the aorta recognized intraoperatively and required minilaparotomy but no transfusion at the time of the primary surgery. In both patients with small bowel obstruction, the obstructions were related to herniations through trocar sites, both of which were greater than or equal to 10 mm. No complications directly resulting from the pelvic lymphadenectomy were observed, although two of 22 patients undergoing para-aortic lymphadenectomy had major complications. An additional patient required percutaneous nephrostomy 3 weeks postoperatively because of a leak in the left lumbar ureter; this was attributed to thermal injury from monopolar current during a left para-aortic lymphadenectomy.

Spirtos et al. [17] reported a series of 40 patients undergoing pelvic and para-aortic lymphadenectomy for gynecologic malignancies including 35 endometrial carcinomas, four ovarian cancers, and one tubal malignancy. Five patients required laparotomy at the time of the initial operation. In two cases, this was secondary to vascular injury to perforating branches of the vena cava and right iliac vessels, respectively. Two other patients required debulking at laparotomy for unsuspected intra-abdominal metastatic disease. A final patient was opened because of equipment failure.

Other authors reported significantly lower incidences of laparotomy consequent to laparoscopic lymphadenectomy. None of the 39 patients who underwent laparoscopic lymphadenectomy for cervical cancer in the series by Querleu et al. [2] required laparotomy. Pomel et al. [20] reported on 10 cases of pelvic and para-aortic laparoscopic lymphadenectomies performed for early-stage carcinoma of the ovary. They described one laparotomy at a second surgery, for postoperative hemoperitoneum. Childers et al. [12] reported a 1.7% (1/60) laparotomy rate for patients undergoing para-aortic lymphadenectomy for cervical, endometrial, and ovarian carcinoma. A single patient required laparotomy for an injury to the vena cava, which was created during a right-sided para-aortic lymphadenectomy. She required four units of blood and subsequently developed a deep venous thrombosis following surgery. In our experience of 100 cases of laparoscopic lymphadenectomy in gynecologic malignancy using ultrasonically activated shears, there were no unplanned conversions to laparotomy. Three intraoperative complications were all managed laparoscopically, and one postoperative trocar-site hernia and one small bowel obstruction were managed with a second laparoscopy.[15]

ADEQUACY OF NODE RETRIEVAL

Lymphadenectomy is performed primarily to evaluate for micrometastasis in the setting of a malignancy. It is therefore essential that the lymph node dissection achieve adequate node retrieval despite the operative approach, either by laparotomy or by laparoscopy. Gynecologic Oncology Group (GOG) protocol 9207 examined laparoscopic para-aortic lymph node sampling and therapeutic pelvic lymphadenectomy in women with stage IA, IB, and IIA cervical cancer. In 69 patients across seven institutions, the average lymph node retrieval was up to 70 (mean of 32) for pelvic nodes and up to 37 (mean of 12) for para-aortic nodes. The complication rate was 10% for major vascular injury and 1.4% for ureteral injury. The study thereby concluded that a laparoscopic approach is a feasible alternative for laparoscopic lymphadenectomy.[22] At our institution, in a series of 100 laparoscopic lymphadenectomies for gynecologic malignancy using the harmonic scalpel, up to 80 lymph nodes were retrieved and there were no conversions to laparotomy. Further, it is our experience that the nodal count is directly related to the surgical goals at the time of procedure. Cases are selected for full lymphadenectomy or for a more limited lymph node sampling depending on the indication for the procedure rather than on technical limitation.[15]

Patient outcomes and survival data support the utility of laparoscopic lymphadenectomy for gynecologic malignancy. Malur et al. [23] reported on a prospective randomized study comparing a laparoscopic approach with open laparotomy for the staging and treatment of endometrial cancer (Table 16.2.3). Notably, the operative time and the number of pelvic and para-aortic lymph nodes harvested were independent of the surgical approach; however, the estimated blood loss, transfusion

Table 16.2.3: Results Adapted from Malur et al. Reporting the Only Randomized Prospective Study Evaluating Laparoscopy versus Laparotomy for the Staging and Treatment of Endometrial Cancer

Variable	Laparoscopy	Laparotomy	
No. of Patients	37	33	
Mean age	68.3	67.7	NS
BMI	29.7	29.7	NS
Pelvic lymphadenectomy	25	24	NS
Pelvic lymph nodes (Mean)	16.1 ± 7.6	15.4 ± 7.6	NS
Para-aortic Lymph Nodes (Mean) (20 Pts.)	9.6 ± 4.7	8.4 ± 6.4	NS
OP. time	176.4 ± 85.4	166.1 ± 61	NS
EBL	229.2 ± 190.2	594.2 ± 629.9	0.003
Transfusion	1	11	0.005
LOS	8.6 ± 2.7	11.7 ± 3.8	<0.001
Complications	11 (29.7%)	13 (39.3%)	NS
Follow up (Mon.)	16.5 (2–43)	21.6 (2–48)	
Recurrences	1	2	NS
Recurrence related death	1	1	NS
Recurrence-Free Survival	97.3%	93.3%	NS
Overall Survival	83.9%	90.9%	NS

requirements, and length of hospital stay were significantly less for the patients who underwent a laparoscopic procedure.

THE LEARNING CURVE

Most surgeons report a decrease in the number and severity of complications, as well as operating times, as experience is gained with laparoscopic lymphadenectomy.[10,11,18,19,24] Eighty-eight percent (14/16) of aborted laparoscopic lymphadenectomies reported by Kavoussi et al. [10] occurred during the initial experience at each contributing institution. Lang et al. [18] reported a significantly higher complication rate for the first 50 laparoscopic lymphadenectomies (14%), as compared with the next 50 such surgeries (4%). In fact, five of the nine total complications occurred among the first 20 patients. The adequacy of the procedure also increases with experience. Fowler et al. [24] and Rukstalis et al. [19] reported a clear improvement in the adequacy of the dissection, as estimated by the percentage of lymph nodes removed, as operators gained experience with the technique. The experience of Melendez et al. [25] with laparoscopically assisted staging for endometrial carcinoma demonstrated a significant decrease in operating time with increasing experience. Notably, the major complication rate was unaffected, although the rate of conversion to laparotomy decreased significantly. With time, laparoscopic lymphadenectomy becomes a safer and more time-efficient procedure.

MODALITY

Various modalities, such as electrosurgery, laser, and argon beam coagulation, have been used for dissection and hemostasis during laparoscopic lymphadenectomy. Laser and electrical energies operate at 150°C to 400°C to desiccate and oxidize tissue, forming an eschar to seal bleeding vessels. Ultrasonic dissection occurs through conversion of mechanical vibration into thermal energy, breaking down tissue with high water content and sparing tissue with high collagen content, such as blood vessels and nerves. Ultrasonic techniques can be used to simultaneously cut and coagulate tissue at lower temperatures ($\leq100°C$), causing less thermal damage and smoke. Most studies of safety and efficacy employ electrosurgery. We analyzed the largest cohort in a single institution, 100 cases of lymphadenectomy using ultrasonically activated shears, and found lymph node retrieval rates and acceptable safety profiles similar to those of studies using electrosurgery (Table 16.2.3).[15] Interestingly, there were no lymphoceles, potentially because of effective sealing of small lymphatic channels with this instrumentation. Thus far, only Holub et al. [26] directly compared the two modalities of electrosurgery and ultrasonic shears for laparoscopic lymphadenectomy in a retrospective comparative study of 59 patients. This trial illustrated efficient coagulation, cutting, dissection, and grasping during laparoscopic lymphadenectomy in cervical and endometrial cancer cases.

CONCLUSION

Laparoscopic lymphadenectomy is an evolving technique that plays an increasingly important role in the management of gynecologic malignancies. Pelvic and para-aortic laparoscopic lymphadenectomy appears to be a safe, adequate, and feasible procedure, with a low complication rate. The risks include those traditionally attributed to laparoscopy, as well as those inherent to open lymphadenectomy. The use of simple preventive measures allows the patient to benefit from this technique while diminishing the likelihood of complication.

REFERENCES

1. Dargent D, Salvat J. *L'envahissement Ganglionnaire Pelvien: Place de la Pelviscopie Retroperitoneale.* Medsi, Paris: McGraw Hill; 1989.
2. Querleu D, Le Blanc E, Castelain B. Laparoscopic pelvic lymphadenectomy in the staging of early carcinoma of the cervix. *Am J Obstet Gynecol.* 1991;164:579–581.
3. Nezhat C, Nezhat F, Silfen SL. Video-laparoscopy: the CO_2 laser for advanced operative laparoscopy. *Obstet Gynecol Clin North Am.* 1991;18:585–604.
4. Nezhat C, Burell O, Nezhat FR, et al. Laparoscopic radical hysterectomy with para-aortic lymph node dissection. *Am J Obstet Gynecol.* 1992;166:864.
5. Nezhat CR, Nezhat FR, Ramirez CE, et al. Laparoscopic radical hysterectomy and laparoscopic assisted vaginal radical hysterectomy with pelvic and para-aortic node dissection. *J Gynecol Surg.* 1993;9:105.
6. Possover M, Krause N, Plaul K, Kuhne-Heid R, Schneider A. Laparoscopic para-aortic and pelvic lymphadenectomy: experience with 150 patients and review of the literature. *Gynecol Oncol.* 1998;71:19–28.
7. Dottino PR, Tobias DH, Beddoe A, Golden AL, Cohen CJ. Laparoscopic lymphadenectomy for gynecologic malignancies. *Gynecol Oncol.* 1999;73:383–388.
8. Renaud MC, Plante M, Roy M. Combined laparoscopic and vaginal radical surgery in cervical cancer. *Gynecol Oncol.* 2000;79:59–63.
9. Scribner DR, Walker JL, Johnson GA, McMeekin SD, Gold MA, Mannel RS. Laparoscopic pelvic and para-aortic lymph node dissection: analysis of the first 100 cases. *Gynecol Oncol.* 2001;82:498–503.
10. Kavoussi LR, Sosa E, Chandhoke P, et al. Complications of laparoscopic pelvic lymph node dissection. *J Urol.* 1993;149:322–325.
11. Burney TL, Campbell EC, Naslund MJ. Complications of staging laparoscopic pelvic lymphadenectomy. *Surg Laparosc Endosc.* 1993;3:184–190.
12. Childers JM, Hatch KD, Surwit EA. Laparoscopic para-aortic lymphadenectomy in gynecologic malignancies. *Obstet Gynecol.* 1993;82:741–747.
13. Childers JM, Lang JF, Surwit EA, et al. Laparoscopic staging of ovarian carcinoma. *Gynecol Oncol.* 1995;59:25–33.
14. Nezhat C, Childers J, Nezhat F, et al. Major retroperitoneal vascular injury during laparoscopic surgery. *Hum Reprod.* 1997;12:480.
15. Nezhat F, Yadav J, Rahaman J, Gretz H 3d, Gardner G, Cohen C. Laparoscopic lymphadenectomy for gynecologic malignancies using ultrasonically activated shears: analysis of first 100 cases. *Gynecol Oncol.* 2005;97:813–819.
16. Nezhat F, Brill A, Nezhat C. Traumatic hypogastric artery bleeding controlled with bipolar desiccation during operative laparoscopy. *J Am Assoc Gynecol Laparosc.* 1994;1:171.
17. Spirtos NM, Schaerth JB, Spirtos TW, et al. Laparoscopic bilateral pelvic and para-aortic lymph node sampling: an evolving technique. *Am J Obstet Gynecol.* 1995;173:105–111.
18. Lang GS, Ruckle HC, Hadley HR, et al. One hundred consecutive laparoscopic lymph node dissections: comparing complications of the first 50 cases to the second 50 cases. *Urology.* 1994;44:221–225.

19. Rukstalis DB, Gerber GS, Vogelzang NJ, et al. Laparoscopic pelvic lymph node dissection: a review of 103 consecutive cases. *J Urol.* 1994;151:670–674.

20. Pomel C, Provencher D, Dauplat J, et al. Laparoscopic staging of early ovarian cancer. *Gynecol Oncol.* 1995;58:301–306.

21. Boitke GM, Lurain JR, Burk JJ. A comparison of laparoscopic management of endometrial cancer with traditional laparotomy. Presented at: Society of Gynecologic Oncologists; February 1994; Orlando, Fla.

22. Schlaerth JB, Spirtos NM, Carson LF, Boike G, Adamec T, Stonebraker B. Laparoscopic retroperitoneal lymphadenectomy followed by immediate laparotomy in women with cervical cancer: a Gynecologic Oncology Group study. *Gynecol Oncol.* 2002;85:81–88.

23. Malur S, Possover M, Michels W, Schneider A. Laparoscopic-assisted vaginal versus abdominal surgery in patients with endometrial cancer: a prospective randomized trial. *Gynecol Oncol.* 2001;80:239–244.

24. Fowler JM, Carter J, Carlson J, et al. Lymph-node yield from laparoscopic lymphadenectomy in cervical cancer: a comparative study. *Gynecol Oncol.* 1993;51:187–192.

25. Melendez T, Childers JM, Nour M, Harrigill K, Surwit EA. Laparoscopic staging of endometrial cancer: the learning experience. *JSLS.* 1997;1:45–49.

26. Holub Z, Jabor A, Kliment L, Lukac J, Voracek J. Laparoscopic lymph node dissection using ultrasonically activated shears: comparison with electrosurgery. *J Laparoendosc Adv Surg Tech.* 2002;12:175–180.

27. Vidaurreta J, Bermudez A, Di Paola G, Sardi J. Laparoscopic staging in locally advanced cervical carcinoma: a new possible philosophy?, *Gynecol Oncol.* 1999;75(3):366–371.

28. Altgassen C, Possover M, Krause N, Plaul K, Michels W, Schneider A. Establishing a new technique of laparoscopic pelvic and para-aortic lymphadenectomy. *Obstet Gynecol.* 2000;95(3):348–352.

29. Abu-Rustum NR, Chi DS, Sonoda Y, DiClemente MJ, Bekker G, Gemignani M, et al., Transperitoneal laparoscopic pelvic and para-aortic lymph node dissection using the argon-beam coagulator and monopolar instruments: an 8-year study and description of technique. *Gynecol Oncol.* 2003;89(3):504–513.

30. Kohler C, Klemm P, Schau A, Passover M, Krause N, Tozzi R, et al., Introduction of transperitoneal lymphadenectomy in a gynecologic oncology center: analysis of 650 laparoscopic pelvic and/or para-aortic transperitoneal lymphadenectomies. *Gynecol Oncol.* 2004;95:52–61.

Section 16.3. Laparoscopic Sentinel Lymph Node Identification in Cervical Cancer

Pedro T. Ramirez, Charles Levenback, and Robert L. Coleman

In the United States, approximately 11,150 women will be diagnosed with cervical cancer in 2007. In that same year, nearly 3670 women will die of the disease.[1] In cervical cancer, the most important prognostic factor is the status of the lymph nodes. The primary lymphatic spread of cervical cancer is the pathologic and anatomic reason for therapeutic lymphadenectomy. Tumor cells reach the regional nodes at the pelvic wall, where they can metastasize via the lymphatics in the parametria. The frequency of regional lymph node involvement increases with increasing size of the primary tumor.

In patients with early-stage cervical cancer (stage IA2–IB1), lymph node status can influence treatment decisions. In general, early invasive carcinoma of the cervix is usually treated with either a modified or a radical hysterectomy. A thorough lymph node dissection is imperative because approximately 7% to 15% of all patients with early invasive disease have lymph node metastases. Pelvic radiotherapy alone is a reasonable alternative to lymph node dissection for patients who are not surgical candidates. For patients with stage IB1 cervical cancer, surgery in the form of radical hysterectomy or radiotherapy is equally effective. Typically, patients who are young and healthy opt for a radical hysterectomy and pelvic lymphadenectomy to prevent complete obliteration of ovarian function.

This section provides a brief review of the evolution of sentinel lymph node biopsy, illustrates challenges specific to sentinel lymph node biopsy for cervical cancer, describes the M. D. Anderson technique of laparoscopic sentinel node biopsy for cervical cancer, and reviews the results of the studies published to date on this procedure.

EVALUATION OF LYMPHATIC MAPPING AND SENTINEL NODE BIOPSY

Gould et al. [2] coined the term *sentinel lymph node* in 1960. The term next appeared in the literature in 1977, when Cabanas [3] pioneered the concept of sentinel lymph node in his work on penile carcinoma. He proposed that the metastatic status of the lymph nodes that first receive drainage from a tumor, the "sentinel" nodes, accurately reflects the cancer status of the remainder of the nodal basin, and he proposed that the sentinel nodes could be removed separately by limited surgery and examined to determine whether a more extensive lymphadenectomy should be performed. These concepts have been validated for both breast cancer [4] and melanoma.[5] In gynecologic malignancies, Levenback et al. [6] showed that intraoperative lymphatic mapping is technically feasible in vulvar cancer. In addition, Burke et al. [7] proposed that intraoperative lymphatic mapping might iden-

tify targets for selective nodal biopsy in women with high-risk endometrial cancer. More recently, the potential feasibility of this technique in cervical cancer has also been explored.

Initially, the sentinel lymph node was identified using lymphangiography. However, this method is technically difficult and poorly reproducible and may result in cellulitis and lymphangitis. Two different approaches are currently used. The first method, introduced by Morton et al. [5], is the use of isosulfan blue dye to identify the lymphatic ducts that drain into the sentinel nodes. The second method, described by Alex and Krag [8], is the use of radioactive tracers and a handheld gamma probe to directly visualize the sentinel nodes.

Blue-dye staining is the standard for determining whether a lymph node is a sentinel node: If a node and at least one afferent lymphatic channel entering the node are stained blue on intraoperative examination after injection of blue dye around the tumor, then this node is considered a sentinel node. The various dyes assessed as potential lymphatic mapping agents have included isosulfan blue, methylene blue, patent blue-V, phenyl oxalate ester (Cyalume, Cyalume Technologies, Inc.), and fluorescein.[9] Methylene blue was shown not to be ideal because it has very poor uptake and diffuses rapidly into the surrounding tissue, causing significant staining of the tissue without staining of the sentinel node. Cyalume, a fluorescent dye, allows ready identification of the lymphatic channels but is associated with significant background fluorescence. Fluorescein diffuses into the surrounding tissue, making it difficult to distinguish the sentinel node from the surrounding lymph nodes. The most useful mapping agents identified so far are isosulfan blue and patent blue-V. Of these two agents, isosulfan blue is the one most commonly used because it is rapidly transported through the lymphatics after intradermal injection and is not associated with diffusion into the surrounding tissue.

The introduction of radioactive tracer injection and lymphoscintigraphy has enhanced the accuracy of detection of the sentinel nodes. This technique consists of injecting a radioactive colloid around the tumor site and then obtaining lymphoscintigrams to track the movement of the colloid through the afferent lymphatic channels and the uptake of the colloid in sentinel nodes. The primary advantage of radiocolloid injection and lymphoscintigraphy is that this technique may permit detection of lymph nodes outside the routine anatomic boundaries of dissection and thus reduce the proportion of cases in which sentinel nodes cannot be identified. In addition, with intraoperative use of a gamma probe after radiocolloid injection, the surgeon may be able to identify sentinel nodes that might otherwise be missed, that is, sentinel nodes with poor uptake of blue dye or sentinel nodes not detected on lymphoscintigraphy.

The ideal radiocolloid for lymphatic mapping must enter the lumen of the initial lymphatic channel in sufficient quantity for the lymph vessels to be seen on lymphoscintigraphy, it must rapidly and predictably move toward the sentinel node, and it must be retained in the sentinel node. In the United States, the radiopharmaceutical most commonly used for lymphatic mapping is filtered technetium Tc-99m sulfur colloid. This agent has a particle size of less than 100 nm, is uniformly dispersed, is highly stable, and given that it is a gamma emitter, has a short half-life. This technique is a safe, reproducible, and noninvasive means of imaging the regional lymphatic drainage systems.

SAFETY OF LYMPHATIC MAPPING

A concern voiced about lymphatic mapping is the possibility that injection of blue dye around and into the tumor might cause iatrogenic tumor spread. Thus far, however, there have been no reports of this event in the literature. An issue of greater concern is the direct side effects caused by blue dyes. Evidence suggests that approximately 50% of isosulfan blue, in aqueous solution, is weakly bound to serum proteins, leading to its affinity for lymphatic channels. The primary excretion of isosulfan blue is biliary (90%), and thus patients with hepatobiliary insufficiency may be at increased risk for complications.[10] The overall complication rate is predicted not to exceed 1.5%.[11]

Allergic reactions with localized swelling at the site of administration and mild pruritus of the hands, abdomen, and neck have been described. Urticaria following administration of blue dyes was first reported by Collard and Collete in 1967.[12] Urticaria is an immediate type I hypersensitivity reaction that is immunoglobulin E dependent. The antigen from isosulfan blue reacts with preformed immunoglobulin E on the surface of dermal mast cells, causing degranulation. Vasoactive mediators, such as histamine, leukotrienes, and prostaglandins, are released and act on cutaneous venules to cause endothelial cell retraction and gap formation. This increased vascular permeability allows fluid and protein to leak into the superficial dermis, causing urticarial edema.[13] Anaphylaxis has also been reported following administration of blue dye, although the incidence of this side effect is low. In cases of anaphylactic reaction to blue dye, there may be a delay of 15 to 30 minutes between dye administration and anaphylaxis, reflecting the fact that the dye is administered intradermally rather than intravenously.

Another systemic manifestation seen after intradermal injections of isosulfan blue is an acute transient or longer-lasting decline in oxygen saturation as measured by pulse oximetry. Coleman et al. [14] provided a detailed review of the etiology of this phenomenon. Pulse oximetry is a noninvasive modality that provides continuous estimates of peripheral tissue oxygen saturation. The authors documented that the peak spectral absorption of isosulfan blue is similar to one of the hemoglobin species routinely measured by pulse oximetry algorithms. Competition at this wavelength can alter pulse oximetry measurements. The inaccuracy of the pulse oximeter after blue dye injection is transient and is confirmed when arterial blood sampling during the acute fall in spot oxygen saturation (SpO_2) documents adequate oxygen saturation. Surgeons and anesthesiologists involved in lymphatic mapping need to be aware of this effect.

There are two areas of concern regarding the use of radiocolloids: effects on the patient and effects on the surgical team. The radiation dose to which the patient is exposed is determined by the degree and speed of clearance from the site of injection and the lymph node. The clearance of radiocolloids from the interstitial space is very slow; therefore, the site that receives the highest radiation dose is the site of injection. According to the inverse square law, exposure to radiation diminishes with the square of the distance from the source. Hiller and Royal [15] showed that the doses per sentinel node mapping procedure to the surgeon's body and finger using 500 μm Tc-99m were 0.29 mrem and 6.60 mrem, respectively. The radiation dose to the pathologist is low compared with the dose to the surgeon because the pathologist has only a brief contact with the specimen. The dose to the pathologist's body in the study by Hiller and Royal was 0.052 mrem.

TECHNICAL CHALLENGES IN LYMPHATIC MAPPING FOR CERVICAL CANCER

Lymphatic drainage patterns of cervical cancer may pose technical challenges in lymphatic mapping for this disease. Plentl and Friedman [16] described a predictable pattern of lymphatic drainage from the cervix. This pattern includes a stepwise progression from the cervical stroma and serosal lymphatics to nodal groups in the parametrial, pelvic, pararectal, and para-aortic lymphatics. According to Leveuf and Godard [17], the main route of lymphatic drainage from the cervix follows the uterine artery, crosses the inferior vesical artery ventral to the point where the uterine artery arises from the internal iliac artery, crosses the obturator nerve, and stops in a lymph node located alongside the caudal, medial, or cephalic surface of the external iliac vein. There is overwhelming evidence that most sentinel nodes will be found in the pelvis. It would be rare to detect a sentinel node in the para-aortic area exclusively without evidence of a sentinel node in the pelvis. A detailed review of lymphatic anatomy can be found in other sources published from our institution.[18]

Pelvic lymph node metastases are found in 0% to 16% of patients with stage I cervical cancer and 24% to 31% of patients with stage II cervical cancer. Para-aortic lymph node metastases are found in 0% to 22% of patients with stage I disease and 11% to 19% of patients with stage II disease.[19]

M. D. ANDERSON TECHNIQUE FOR LAPAROSCOPIC LYMPHATIC MAPPING AND SENTINEL LYMPH NODE BIOPSY

Because hypothesis testing is critical to making an inference into the applicability of the technique in prospective trials and treatment algorithms, accurate false-negative rates must be established. At the University of Texas M. D. Anderson Cancer Center, cervical cancer patients who are considered candidates for radical hysterectomy and lymphadenectomy have the option of enrolling in a Gynecologic Oncology Group (GOG)-sponsored investigational protocol of lymphatic mapping and sentinel lymph node biopsy (GOG 206). The goal of this trial is to estimate the sensitivity of the sentinel lymph node in determination of the lymph node metastases in patients with invasive carcinoma of the cervix using combined preoperative and intraoperative lymphatic mapping.

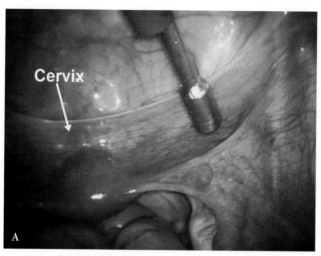
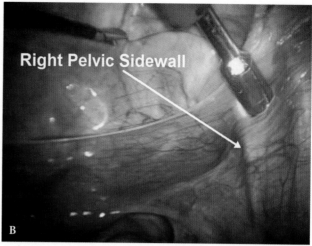

Figure 16.3.1. (**A**) Initial laparoscopic assessment is made with modified gamma probe. (**B**) Each of the lymphatic beds is evaluated for in vivo radioactivity. Blue dye can be seen infiltrating the cervical stroma. (Images provided by Michel Roy, MD.)

In addition, it also aims to evaluate the false negative predictive value of the sentinel lymph node. The trial allows for either a laparotomy or laparoscopy to perform the sentinel lymph node identification. The procedure for patients who undergo laparoscopic sentinel node identification is described in the following paragraphs.

The day before surgery, the patient reports to the nuclear medicine suite. Under direct visualization, while the patient is in the lithotomy position, Tc-99m–labeled sulfur colloid is injected in four quadrants of the cervix. Immediately after the injection, dynamic lymphoscintigraphy is performed using a gamma camera. The next morning, before surgery, Tc-99m–labeled sulfur colloid is once again injected in four quadrants of the cervix. After induction of general anesthesia, while the patient is in the lithotomy position, a sterile speculum is used to expose the cervix for full visualization. A short 25-gauge needle attached to a needle extender is used to inject a total of 5 mL of Lymphazurin 1% (isosulfan blue, United States Surgical Corp.) into the mucosa and cervical stroma midway between the cervical os and the rim of the exocervix, in four quadrants.

The laparoscopic exploration is then started by placing four bladeless trocars: one trocar in the umbilicus, two trocars in the right and left lower quadrants, and one trocar in the suprapubic area. The retroperitoneum is opened and explored very carefully to avoid bleeding, which may prevent adequate visualization of the lymphatic channels. Nodes with increased radioactivity ("hot" nodes) are identified using a laparoscopic gamma probe (Navigator, Autosuture, Norwalk, CT). The laparoscopic gamma probe is inserted through either of the lower-quadrant trocars. Sentinel nodes are also identified by searching the lymph node basins for nodes stained bright blue. Once a sentinel node is identified, its anatomic location is noted. The node is subsequently excised separately and sent to a pathologist for immediate frozen section evaluation. The laparoscopic gamma probe is then reinserted to ensure that there are no other hot nodes, and once this is confirmed, the lymphadenectomy is completed. The same laparoscopic sentinel node biopsy procedure is then performed on the opposite side.

At our institution, serial sectioning is performed on sentinel nodes that are negative for metastatic disease on routine hematoxylin–eosin (H&E) staining. Nodes that are negative on routine H&E staining may also be sent for immunohistochemical staining for cytokeratin antigen. The protocol in our institution is to include step sectioning at five levels with an interval of 250 μm with H&E and immunohistochemistry when the first-level H&E section is negative. The findings on frozen section evaluation are used to determine how to proceed. If pelvic nodes are found to contain metastatic disease, a para-aortic lymph node sampling is performed to determine what type of radiation field will be required and the radical hysterectomy is abandoned (Figures 16.3.1–16.3.3).

RATIONALE FOR LAPAROSCOPIC SENTINEL LYMPH NODE IDENTIFICATION IN CERVICAL CANCER AND RESULTS OF STUDIES TO DATE

Gynecologists first used laparoscopic surgery in the 1960s as a tool for the evaluation of the abdominal and pelvic cavity. Approximately 10 years later, laparoscopic surgery was used in performing bilateral tubal ligation. It was not until the 1980s that laparoscopic surgery was first used in the treatment of cancer – specifically, testicular cancer.

A large number of publications in the literature describe the potential benefits of laparoscopic surgery. Among the most common are improved quality of life, faster return to daily activities, decreased requirements for pain medication in the immediate postoperative period, faster return of bowel function, and shorter length of hospitalization.

According to Plante et al. [20], a number of factors support a laparoscopic approach to lymphatic mapping in cervical cancer. First, the laparoscopic approach allows for a more delicate and bloodless dissection of the retroperitoneum. Second, the laparoscope allows magnification, which facilitates visualization of the blue lymphatic vessels. Third, if positive nodes are identified, the surgeon has the opportunity to end the procedure and offer patients chemotherapy and radiotherapy with only minor delays, thus reducing morbidity in comparison to laparotomy.

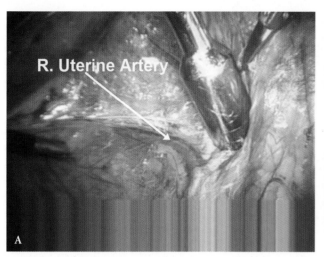
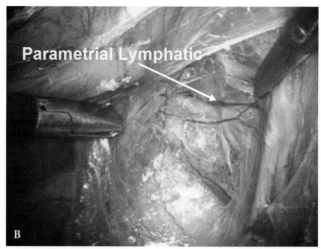

Figure 16.3.2. (**A**) Once the retroperitoneal spaces are carefully opened, a reassessment of radioactivity and blue dye is made. (**B**) The path of a blue dye lymphatic channel is easily seen traversing the parametrial tissue to the external iliac chain. (Images generously provided by Michel Roy, MD.)

A number of studies have been published on the use of laparoscopic surgery in the detection of sentinel nodes. In the following paragraphs, we summarize the findings of the largest studies to date (see Table 16.3.1). Daniel Dargent was one of the pioneers in exploring laparoscopic sentinel lymph node identification in cervical cancer. In 2000, Dargent et al. [21] reported on a series of 35 patients with early cervical cancer who underwent laparoscopic sentinel node identification using patent blue violet. In that study, the authors made a series of very important observations. First, the rate of failure to identify a sentinel node depended on the amount of blue dye injected: The failure rate was 50% when 1.5 mL or less of blue dye was used and only 10% when 4 mL of blue dye was used. Second, the detection rate was improved by injecting the blue dye directly into the cervix rather than into the cervicovaginal junction, as these authors had previously done. Third, the rate of false-negative sentinel nodes was zero. Fourth, prior conization, tumor volume, and stage did not affect the failure rate. Dargent et al. found that the overall failure rate was 14.5%. However, one should note that these authors used only blue dye and not the combination of blue dye and a radiocolloid.

In a 2001 report, Malur et al. [22] described their experience with laparoscopic sentinel node identification using a radioactive isotope, blue dye (patent blue), or both. This group was the first to report on the use of a laparoscopic gamma probe in sentinel node identification. In their series of 50 patients, 46 of whom underwent sentinel node identification by laparoscopy, the authors reported a sentinel node detection rate of 78%. In addition, the investigators found that the combination of isotope and blue dye led to the highest detection rate: The detection rate was 55% with blue dye alone, 76% with radiolabeled albumin alone, and 90% when both techniques were used. The false-negative rate in that study was 16.6%. The high false-negative rate may reflect the use of blue dye alone in some patients; the amount of blue dye injected (2 mL) also may not have been ideal. Finally, Malur et al. found that the majority of para-aortic sentinel nodes

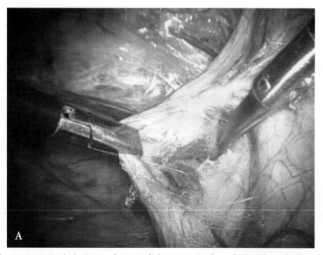
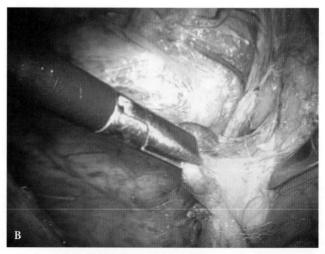

Figure 16.3.3. (**A**) Once the candidate sentinel node is identified, great care is used to isolate the node and (**B**) resect it. Ex vivo radioactivity along with the blue characteristic and location are recorded for pathologic assessment. (Images generously provided by Michel Roy, MD.)

Table 16.3.1: Laparoscopic Sentinel Lymph Node Identification

Study	Patients, no.	Stage	Tc-99m	Blue Detection	Detection Rate	False Negative Rate, %
Dargent et al. [21]	35	IA2–IB2	No	Yes	86	0
Malur et al. [22]	46	I–IV	Yes	Yes	90	17%
Lambaudie et al. [26]	12	IA–IB1	Yes	No	92	0
Buist et al. [23]	25	IB1–IIA	Yes	Yes	100	11%
Barrenger et al. [24]	13	IA2–IIA	Yes	Yes	92	0
Plante et al. [20]	70	IA–IIA	Yes	Yes	93	0
Gil-Moreno et al. [27]	12	IA2–IB1	Yes	Yes	100	0

identified (66%) were located in the precaval region. Interestingly, no patient had evidence of isolated para-aortic sentinel nodes.

In another study, Buist et al. [23] evaluated the utility of laparoscopic sentinel node identification in patients with early cervical cancer. In that study, the investigators reported on 25 patients who underwent lymphatic mapping before radical hysterectomy using intracervical radiocolloid injection as well as blue dye. The authors noted that one or more sentinel nodes could be detected via laparoscopy in 100% of patients. The investigators also evaluated the accuracy of frozen section of sentinel nodes at the time of surgery. They noted that frozen section sensitivity per sentinel node was 97% and per patient, 96%. Another interesting observation noted by the investigators was that sentinel node identification might be a time-consuming procedure. The median time from first incision to detection of the first sentinel node was 55 ± 17 minutes (range, 15 to 80 minutes). This was not significantly different between the first and second half of their learning curve.

In the largest series published to date on laparoscopic sentinel node identification, Plante et al. [20], in 2003, reported on 70 patients undergoing radical surgery for early-stage (stage IA–IIA) cervical cancer. The combination of preoperative lymphoscintigraphy and intracervical blue dye injection was used in 42% of those patients. In the remaining patients, sentinel node identification was performed using intracervical blue dye injection only. Sentinel node detection rates were 87% overall, 79% with blue dye alone, and 93% with blue dye plus lymphoscintigraphy. Among patients with macroscopically involved nodes at laparoscopy, the sentinel node identification rate was only 56%. This finding may reflect blockage of the lymphatic channels by tumor cells, prohibiting the blue dye or radiocolloid from reaching the sentinel node. The authors reported that the majority of the sentinel nodes (88%) were located in the external iliac area, the obturator area, or the bifurcation of the iliac vessels. Seventy-five percent of the patients had two or more sentinel nodes identified. The false-negative rate was zero. Only two patients (3%) suffered an allergic reaction. One patient had the characteristic skin reaction with development of blue hives. Another patient developed a more severe reaction with profound vasomotor shock after injection of the blue dye. Although that patient recovered without any major sequelae, she did require use of vasopressors and admission to the intensive care unit.

Also in 2003, Barranger et al. [24] published their experience with laparoscopic sentinel node identification using a combined approach with radioisotopes and patent blue dye. Although their series was small, including only 13 patients, their study is important because it was the first to show that laparoscopic sentinel node detection was possible in patients who had undergone neoadjuvant chemotherapy and radiotherapy.

CONCLUSIONS

Several conclusions can be drawn from these studies of laparoscopic sentinel node identification for cervical cancer. First, the overall sentinel node detection rate ranges between 60% and 100%. Second, the majority of studies published to date show that the sentinel node identification rate is higher when both preoperative lymphoscintigraphy and blue dye injection are used than when just one technique is used. Third, there is strong evidence in the literature that in patients with macroscopically suspicious nodes, the sentinel node detection rate is decreased. The explanation that has been proposed is that blockage of the lymphatic channels by tumor cells prohibits the blue dye or radiocolloid from reaching the sentinel node. In the prospective trial being conducted by the GOG (GOG 206), any patient with evidence of suspicious lymph nodes on preoperative evaluation is excluded from entry. Fourth, the overall false-negative rate is relatively low. This is important because for sentinel node identification to be accepted in the routine management of patients with cervical cancer, there needs to be definitive evidence that the sentinel node status accurately represents the status of all lymph nodes in the pelvis and para-aortic region. Fifth, the procedure is safe, with only rare cases of allergic reactions, which are transient and easily manageable. Most of these reactions are caused by the blue dye and not the radioactive colloid. Some investigators have suggested that allergic reactions are generally more common when larger amounts of blue dye ($\geq$4 mL) are used.

UNRESOLVED QUESTIONS

Among the questions that remain unresolved regarding laparoscopic sentinel lymph node identification is the number of cases required to master the technique. Some authors have suggested that about 30 cases will be required because the intracervical injection is technically difficult and the lymphatic drainage of the cervix is much more complex, involving three main trunks per side.[20] In the current GOG trial, an attempt at standardizing surgical acumen for lymphatic mapping is incorporated – investigators contributing patients to the trial must successfully perform the procedure in three cases. The outcome in these patients will not be used in the statistical design.

In addition, it remains to be determined whether immunohistochemical staining should routinely be performed on sentinel nodes. There is increasing information in the literature suggesting that immunohistochemical staining in addition to serial sectioning may improve the rate of detection of metastatic disease in the lymph nodes. Finally, we do not know the clinical implications of detecting occult micrometastases in patients with cervical cancer.

The combination of laparoscopic sentinel node identification and fertility-preserving options in patients with cervical cancer is already being explored.[25] In addition, future studies will need to explore the correlation of sentinel node findings with novel imaging technologies, such as positron emission tomography–computed tomography (PET-CT) scanning and high-resolution magnetic resonance imaging. We also look forward to the results of the prospective trial currently being conducted by the GOG to determine the ultimate role of sentinel node identification in patients with cervical cancer.

REFERENCES

1. American Cancer Society. Cancer facts & figures 2007. www.cancer.org. Atlanta; 2007.
2. Gould EA, Winship T, Philbin PH, et al. Observations on a "sentinel node" in the parotid. *Cancer*. 1960;13:77–78.
3. Cabanas R. An approach for the treatment of penile carcinoma. *Cancer*. 1977;39:456–466.
4. Krag D, Weaver D, Ashikaga T, et al. The sentinel node in breast cancer. *N Engl J Med*. 1998;339:941–946.
5. Morton DL, Wen D-R, Wong JH, et al. Technical details of intraoperative lymphatic mapping for early stage melanoma. *Arch Surg*. 1992;127:392–399.
6. Levenback C, Burke TW, Gershenson DM, Morris M, Malpica A, Ross MI. Intraoperative lymphatic mapping for vulvar cancer. *Obstet Gynecol*. 1994;84:163–167.
7. Burke TW, Levenback C, Tornos C, Morris M, Wharton JT, Gershenson DM. Intraabdominal lymphatic mapping to direct selective pelvic and paraaortic lymphadenectomy in women with high-risk endometrial cancer: results of a pilot study. *Gynecol Oncol*. 1996;62:169–173.
8. Alex JC, Krag DN. Gamma-probe guided localization of lymph nodes. *Surg Oncol*. 1993;2:137–143.
9. Bostick PJ, Giuliano AE. Vital dyes in sentinel node localization. *Semin Nucl Med*. 2000;30:18–24.
10. Ramirez PT, Levenback C. Sentinel nodes in gynecologic malignancies. *Curr Opin Oncol*. 2001;13:403–407.
11. Lymphazurin [package insert]. Norwalk, CT: United States Surgical Corp.
12. Collard M, Collete J. Les modalites cliniques de l'allergie au bleu patente violet. *J Belge Radiologie*. 1967;50:407–410.
13. Sadiq TS, Burns WW 3d, Taber DJ, Damitz L, Ollila DW. Blue urticaria: a previously unreported adverse event associated with isosulfan blue. *Arch Surg*. 2001;136:1433–1435.
14. Coleman RL, Whitten CW, O'Boyle J, Sidhu B. Unexplained decrease in measured oxygen saturation by pulse oximetry following injection of Lymphazurin 1% (isosulfan blue) during a lymphatic mapping procedure. *J Surg Oncol*. 1999;70:126–129.
15. Hiller DA, Royal HD. Intraoperative gamma radiation detection and radiation safety. Radioguided surgery. In: Whitman ED, Reintgen D, eds. *Handbook of Sentinel Lymph Node Mapping and Biopsy*. Austin, TX: Landes Bioscience; 1999:23–38.
16. Plentl AA, Friedman EA, eds. *Lymphatic System of the Female Genitalia: The Morphologic Basis of Oncologic Diagnosis and Therapy*. Philadelphia: Saunders; 1971:75–84.
17. Leveuf J, Godard H. Les lymphatiques de l'uterus. *Rev Chir*. 1923;219–248.
18. Coleman RL, Levenback C. Lymphatics of the cervix. In: Levenback C, van der Zee AGJ, Coleman RL, eds. *Clinical Lymphatic Mapping in Gynecologic Cancers*. New York: Taylor and Francis; 2004:41–49.
19. Hatch KD: Cervical cancer. In: Berek JS, Hacker NF, eds. *Practical Gynecologic Oncology*. Baltimore: Williams & Wilkins; 1994:243–283.
20. Plante M, Renaud MC, Tetu B, Harel F, Roy M. Laparoscopic sentinel node mapping in early-stage cervical cancer. *Gynecol Oncol*. 2003;91:494–503.
21. Dargent D, Martin X, Mathevet P. Laparoscopic assessment of the sentinel lymph node in early stage cervical cancer. *Gynecol Oncol*. 2000;79:411–415.
22. Malur S, Krause N, Kohler C, Schneider A. Sentinel lymph node detection in patients with cervical cancer. *Gynecol Oncol*. 2001;80:254–257.
23. Buist MR, Pijpers RJ, van Lingen A, et al. Laparoscopic detection of sentinel lymph nodes followed by lymph node dissection in patients with early stage cervical cancer. *Gynecol Oncol*. 2003;90:290–296.
24. Barranger E, Grahek D, Cortez A, Talbot JN, Uzan S, Darai E. Laparoscopic sentinel lymph node procedure using a combination of patent blue and radioisotope in women with cervical carcinoma. *Cancer*. 2003;97:3003–3009.
25. Plante M, Renaud MC, Francois H, Roy M. Vaginal radical trachelectomy: an oncologically safe fertility-preserving surgery. An updated series of 72 cases and review of the literature. *Gynecol Oncol*. 2004;94:614–623.
26. Lambaudie E, Collinet P, Narducci F, et al. Laparoscopic identification of sentinel lymph nodes in early stage cervical cancer. Prospective study using a combination of patent blue dye injection and technetium radiocolloid injection. *Gynecol Oncol*. 2003;89:84–87.
27. Gil-Moreno A, Diaz-Feijoo B, Roca I, et al. Total laparoscopic radical hysterectomy with intraoperative sentinel node identification in patients with early invasive cervical cancer. *Gynecol Oncol*. 2005;96:187–193.

Section 16.4. Schauta Radical Vaginal Hysterectomy and Total Laparoscopic Radical Hysterectomy

Yukio Sonoda and Nadeem R. Abu-Rustum

HISTORICAL BACKGROUND

The vaginal radical hysterectomy was initially described by the surgeon Anton Pawlik [1], but it was popularized by the Austrian Frederik Schauta [2], who described this surgical treatment option for patients with cervical cancer. The procedure was associated with a decreased postoperative mortality when compared with the abdominal route that was championed by Wertheim.[3] Schauta's technique was eventually modified by Peham and Amreich [4] and Stoeckel.[5] As pelvic lymphadenectomy became incorporated into the surgical treatment of this disease, however, the vaginal approach gave way to the abdominal radical hysterectomy, which allowed for both procedures to be performed through one incision. To counter this return to the abdominal approach, the extraperitoneal pelvic lymphadenectomy was introduced into the management scheme [6], but this still required multiple incisions. The laparoscopic lymphadenectomy was introduced by Dargent in 1987.[7] This allowed the vaginal approach to be used without sacrificing the benefits of a minimally invasive approach. Over time, the extent of the laparoscopic dissection expanded. The first laparoscopic radical hysterectomy, para-aortic and pelvic lymphadenectomy was performed by the Nezhats in 1989 and was reported in 1990, 1991 and 1992.[8–10] Now, many peform, such procedures routinely.

THE SCHAUTA–AMREICH RADICAL VAGINAL HYSTERECTOMY

The Schauta–Amreich is the more radical form of radical vaginal hysterectomy. Once the patient is positioned properly for radical vaginal surgery, a diluted solution of epinephrine is injected into the left mediolateral perineum in preparation for a Schuchardt incision. This is a type of enlarged mediolateral episiotomy that is made at the junction of the posterior and left lateral walls of the vagina. It enlarges the operative field and provides access to the left pararectal space. The incision extends from the most cranial point, which is at the level of the expected vaginal cuff incision, to the distal point, which is on the perineum (Figure 16.4.1). At the apex of this incision is the left pararectal space, which provides access for the surgeon to bluntly displace the rectum medially. The levator ani muscle can now be divided, except for the most proximal portion, to fully expose the left pararectal space.

The vaginal margin is now delineated. A series of Kocher forceps are put circumferentially onto the vaginal mucosa at the level of the junction between the upper and the middle thirds. Traction is exerted on the forceps, which results in an internal prolapse of the vaginal wall. The two walls of the vaginal fold raised by the traction are separated from each other by injecting the epinephrine solution along the edge of the fold midway between each traction forceps (Figure 16.4.2). The outer wall of the vagina is then incised circumferentially just beyond the tips of the Kocher forceps (Figure 16.4.3). The pressure on the scalpel blade must be released as soon as the outer wall of the vagina is incised so as not to incise the inner vaginal wall. This full-thickness incision (incision of the three layers of the vaginal wall) is made only on the anterior and posterior aspects of the developed vaginal cuff. Only the mucosa layer is incised on the dorsolateral aspects (between 3 and 4 o'clock and between 8 and 9 o'clock), so that the relationship between the vaginal cuff and the paracervical ligaments is maintained.

Once separated from the remainder of the vagina, the vaginal cuff is folded over the cervix to cover it by using strong grasping forceps that are aligned in a frontal plane (Figure 16.4.4). It is retracted dorsally in order to free the ventral aspect of the vaginal cuff at the same time the ventral aspect of the uterus and surrounding tissues (i.e., paracervical and parametrial ligaments) is freed. The bladder floor and terminal ureter are attached to these structures and must be separated from them. The vesicovaginal space is carefully developed in the midline so as not to injure the bladder, which is very close to the tips of the grasping forceps. Caution must be taken because of the condensation of the cellular tissue joining the bladder floor to the vagina. This condensation raises a pseudo-aponeurotic coronal structure named the supravaginal septum, which must be perforated (Figure 16.4.5) to reach the appropriate space. Once the vesicovaginal space has been opened, dissection of the bladder pillars can be approached. This is where the knee of the ureter lies (Figure 16.4.6).

The left paravesical space can be opened by using curved Metzenbaum scissors with closed tips pointed upward and outward (Figure 16.4.7). The scissors are introduced at the apex of the Schuchardt incision just medial to the apex of the remaining intact levator ani and lateral to the bladder pillar. The scissors are opened to spread the loose connective tissue of the paravesical space. The surgeon's fingers are successively introduced into the space and the bladder is mobilized medially.

Once the vesicovaginal and left paravesical spaces are developed, the left bladder pillar is divided and the ureter can be isolated. The bladder pillars are divided in two steps. Initially, the pillar is separated into the lateral and medial parts by opening the caudal brim of the pillar at an equal distance from its two sides and two extremities. After opening, the scissors are pushed laterally. One ensures that the instrument is placed lateral to the ureter by palpating and feeling the "click" (Figure 16.4.8).[11] Once these fibers are divided by clamping and tying or bipolar cauterization, the paravesical space becomes wider. A bigger retractor is put

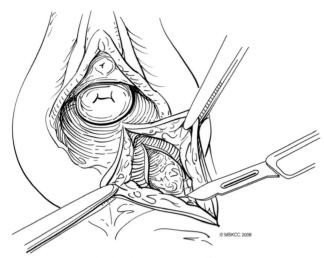

Figure 16.4.1. A Schuchardt incision is used to improve exposure and provide access to the pararectal space.

in place and the knee of the ureter appears in the deepest part. Once the knee of the ureter has been identified, the medial fibers (Figure 16.4.9) of the pillar can be divided. This division exposes the ventral aspect of the juxta-uterine part of the paracervical ligament. The para-isthmic window (the inferior brim of which is the superior brim of the paracervical ligament) is identified by palpation. The arch of the uterine artery is located inside it. The afferent branch of the arch is isolated and dissected upward as far as the level of the knee of the ureter. Then the dissection is pushed further laterally inside the knee of the ureter, and the artery is cut close to its origin (Figure 16.4.10).

The right paravesical space can be opened in a similar fashion, and the same procedure performed to isolate the right ureter.

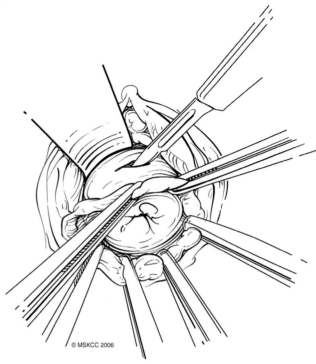

Figure 16.4.3. The vaginal incision is made circumferentially. The lateral portions of the incision are made through the vaginal mucosa only.

Next, the posterior peritoneal fold can be opened (Figure 16.4.11). The intestines are packed away with a packing tape, and the rectum is displaced posteriorly with a retractor. The rectal pillars can now be viewed. The peritoneum overlying the rectal pillars and rectum is first incised carefully as the ureters are adherent to this peritoneum. The rectal pillars are now isolated and divided close to the rectum (Figure 16.4.12).

Once the rectal pillars are divided, the cardinal ligaments can be divided. An anterior retractor pushes the bladder away, and

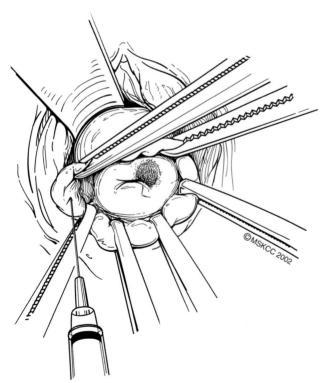

Figure 16.4.2. An epinephrine solution is injected circumferentially to separate the layers of the vagina.

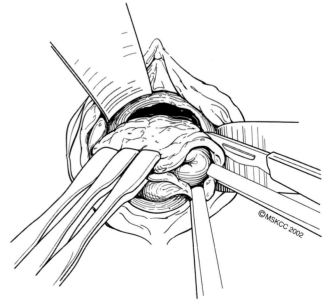

Figure 16.4.4. Chrobak forceps are used to fold the vagina over the cervix.

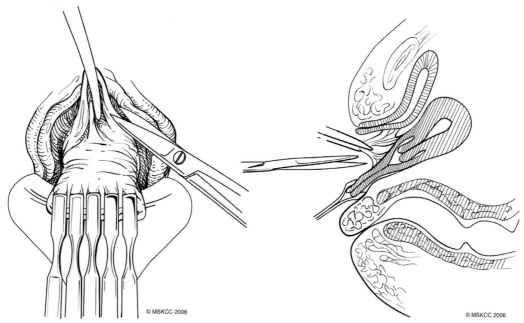

Figure 16.4.5. The vesicovaginal space is developed sharply. Note the relationship of the bladder to the plane of dissection.

two large clamps are placed across the left cardinal ligament close to the pelvic side wall (Figure 16.4.13). This is then divided and the pedicle secured. The identical maneuver is repeated on the right cardinal ligament.

The anterior peritoneum is now opened, and the uterine fundus can be delivered through it. At this point, the round ligaments and infundibulopelvic ligaments can be divided if the ovaries are to be removed. The peritoneum and vaginal cuff can be closed according to surgeon's preference. The Schuchardt

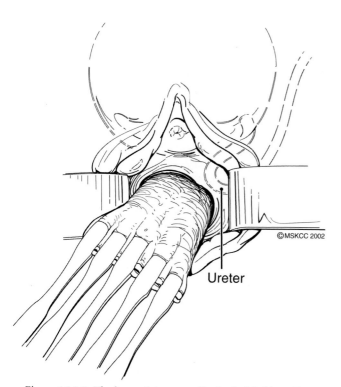

Figure 16.4.6. The knee of the ureter lies in the bladder pillar.

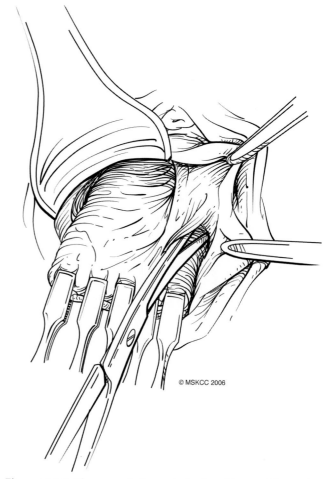

Figure 16.4.7. The paravesical space is developed by careful spreading of the tissue.

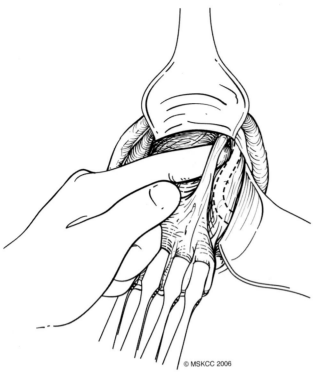

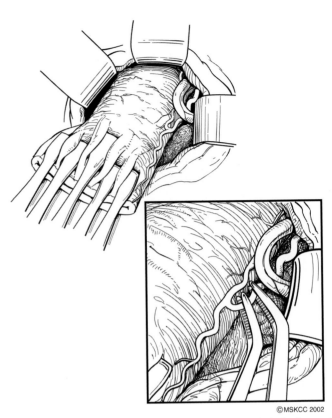

Figure 16.4.8. The knee of the ureter is palpated in the bladder pillar using the surgeon's opposite index finger.

Figure 16.4.10. After the bladder pillar has been divided, the knee of the ureter can be pushed laterally and the uterine artery can be clamped and ligated.

incision is closed by first reapproximating the levator ani muscles and then closing the subcutaneous tissues and skin.

THE SCHAUTA–STOECKEL RADICAL VAGINAL HYSTERECTOMY

The Schauta–Stoeckel is less radical than the abovementioned Schauta–Amreich technique. Many of the steps are similar, but the major differences are that the Schuata–Stoeckel operation does

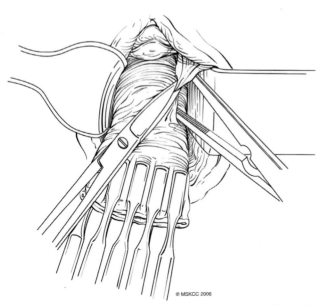

Figure 16.4.9. Once the knee of the ureter is located, the fibers of the bladder pillar can be divided.

not employ a Schuchardt incision and the cardinal ligaments are divided at an intermediate level.

The Schauta–Stoeckel begins with the formation of the vaginal cuff. This is performed in similar fashion to the Schauta–Amreich procedure, with a series of Kocher forceps placed circumferentially onto the vaginal mucosa at the level of the junction between the upper and the middle thirds. The vagina is incised and closed over the cervix as mentioned above. The vesicovaginal space is opened in similar fashion as previously mentioned. The paravesical space is then opened by placing two Kocher forceps on the free edge of the vaginal cuff at 1 o'clock and 3 o'clock. As outward traction is applied to these forceps, a small depression becomes visible between them. This marks the entrance to the left paravesical space, which is further developed by introducing curved Metzenbaum scissors in an outward and lateral direction. The left pararectal space is opened in a similar fashion by placing two Kocher forceps on the free vaginal edge at the 3 o'clock and 5 o'clock positions. As outward traction is placed on these forceps, a small depression becomes evident. This is the opening to the left pararectal space. This opening is further expanded by introducing curved Metzenbaum scissors in a downward and outward direction (Figure 16.4.14). The right paravesical and pararectal spaces can be opened by mirroring the technique on the opposite side. The bladder pillars are divided in two steps as previously described for the Schauta–Amreich procedure.

The pouch of Douglas is opened in the midline, and the rectal pillars are divided, that is, the uterosacral ligaments or more precisely, the medial part of them (i.e., the rectouterine peritoneal folds). Once these ligaments have been divided, the dorsal aspects

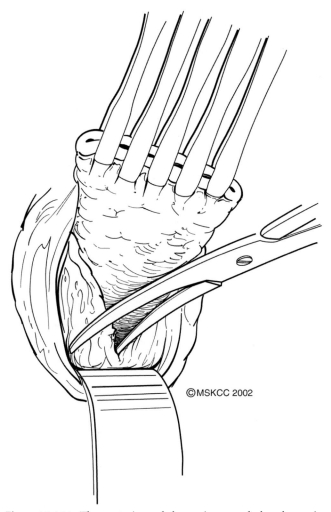

Figure 16.4.11. The posterior cul-de-sac is opened sharply, paying careful attention to the location of the rectum.

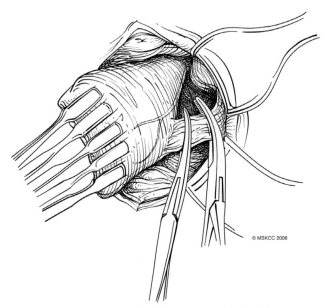

Figure 16.4.13. The cardinal ligaments are divided laterally.

of the para-isthmic windows are palpated. Their inferior brim corresponds to the superior brim of the paracervical ligaments.

A right-angle dissector is pushed from back to front through the parauterine ligament. Opening the dissector frees the upper brim of the paracervical ligament. This is done while dividing the paracolpos (i.e., the expansion that the paracervix sends to the vagina). This division is done by deepening the dorsolateral incision in the vagina and pushing it laterally while controlling the bleeders encountered during this action.

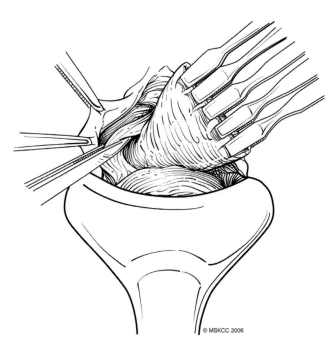

Figure 16.4.12. The rectal pillars are divided.

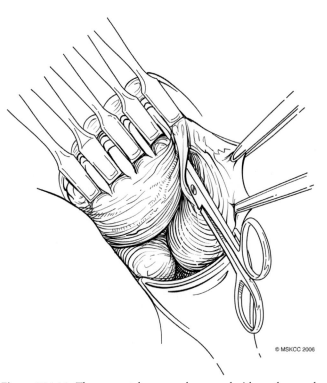

Figure 16.4.14. The pararectal space can be opened with gentle spreading of the tissue in a downward and outward direction.

Once the dorsal and ventral aspects of the paracervical ligaments are both exposed with the superior and inferior brims, they can be divided. Two clamps are placed on each ligament, the most lateral being just at the contact of the tip of the knee of the ureter.

With the two paracervical ligaments divided, the anterior peritoneum is opened and the uterine fundus is delivered. Any remaining peritoneal attachments are divided while assuring that the ureters are pushed away. The closure of the cuff and vagina are performed according to surgeon's preference.

EVOLUTION OF TWO TECHNIQUES

The inability to perform a pelvic lymphadenectomy diminished the popularity of the radical vaginal hysterectomy. The introduction of the laparoscopic lymphadenectomy provided the means to overcome this shortcoming of radical vaginal surgery. As surgeons became more adept with the use of laparoscopy, the two procedures of laparoscopic lymphadenectomy followed by vaginal radical hysterectomy eventually evolved into laparoscopically assisted radical vaginal hysterectomy and total laparoscopic radical hysterectomy.

Laparoscopic Lymphadenectomy Followed by Radical Vaginal Hysterectomy

Dargent's initial experience was based on a two-step procedure using laparoscopic surgery to perform a pelvic lymphadenectomy to be followed by radical vaginal hysterectomy. From 1986 to 1992 he performed 95 cases using such an approach (unpublished data). The mean duration of the laparoscopic staging was 60.4 ± 25.8 minutes. The Schauta–Stoeckel technique (less radical) was used in 28 cases, and the Schauta–Amreich technique (more radical) was used in 67 cases. The mean duration of the surgery was 74 ± 31 minutes and 89 ± 26 minutes, respectively. No perioperative complication was observed with the Schauta–Stoeckel technique, whereas six complications were observed with the Schauta–Amreich technique: one cystotomy, four ureterotomies, and one proctotomy (all repaired immediately with no postoperative complication). Only one patient required reoperation for postoperative bleeding after a Schauta–Amreich procedure. Only 14 patients received transfusions. Among the 28 patients who underwent the Schauta–Stoeckel operation, eight suffered from urinary bladder problems but only one had persistent dysuria after 6 months. Among the 67 patients who underwent the Schauta–Amreich procedure, 27 suffered the same bladder problems and 10 had persistent dysuria after 6 months.

Laparoscopically Assisted Vaginal Radical Hysterectomy

As surgeons became more familiar with laparoscopic surgery, new techniques were developed. In addition to performing a laparoscopic lymphadenectomy, surgeons began using the laparoscope to perform some of the dissection before performing the radical vaginal hysterectomy. This allowed the resection to be comparable to that of a classic abdominal radical hysterectomy.

One of the technical difficulties of the radical vaginal approach is obtaining a large amount of parametrium. This is in large part a result of the oblique angles that the vaginal surgeon is faced with, which can make the lateral placement of a clamp at the pelvic side wall difficult. However, because laparoscopic instruments are introduced transabdominally, placement can be adjusted to operate with an instrument in the plane of the pelvic side wall. Endoscopic staplers, vessel sealers, and argon beam coagulators are some examples of instruments that the surgeon can employ to divide the lateral parametrium at the pelvic side wall. There have been several reports since 1992 [12–20] of series describing the laparoscopically assisted vaginal radical hysterectomy (LAVRH) during which the surgeon divided the parametrium during the laparoscopic step. The common feature of the techniques described therein was the use of the laparoscope to increase the resection of the parametrium. Once this is performed, the remainder of the procedure can be performed using either a Schauta–Amreich or Stoeckel approach. As a consequence, the operative specimen is very large (i.e., identical to the type III abdominal radical hysterectomy).

The concept of the "paracervical cellulolymphadenectomy" has been combined with a modified radical vaginal hysterectomy, thereby accomplishing the oncologic goals of the radical hysterectomy.[17] The paracervical cellulolymphadenectomy consists of removing all the lymph node–bearing tissues located in the lateral part of the paracervical ligament in a multistep procedure.

First, the obturator nodes below the obturator nerve are removed to identify the origin of the obturator vessels and expose the ventral surface of the paracervical ligament. In the second step, the dorsal aspect of the paracervix is exposed. The pararectal space opens when pushing the posterior sheet of the broad ligament, to which the ureter is attached, medially. Following the ureter ventrally, one arrives at the point where the ureter crosses the uterine artery. Starting from this point, the pararectal space is developed as far as the sacrospinous muscle. The node-bearing tissues lying anterior to the sacrum, lateral to the rectum, and medial to the pelvic side wall are removed. During this step, the dissection must proceed with caution, particularly on the left side, where the left common iliac vein is encountered. Once the two aspects of the paracervical ligament are exposed, the fatty tissue among the paracervical vascular network must be carefully removed.

Hertel et al. [12] have reported the largest series of LAVRH to date. Over an 8-year period, 200 patients underwent the procedure. One patient required conversion to laparotomy and was not included in the evaluation. The mean Quetelet index was 25 (14 to 38). The average duration of the surgery was 333 (151 to 556) minutes. A mean of 22 (three to 57) pelvic nodes were removed. Major intraoperative injuries included 14 bladder, seven ureteral, four blood vessel, and one bowel injury. With a median follow-up of 40 months, the estimated 5-year survival was 83%. The larger series of LAVRH reported in the literature are listed in Table 16.4.1.[12–20]

TECHNIQUE OF TOTAL LAPAROSCOPIC RADICAL HYSTERECTOMY WITH PELVIC LYMPHADENECTOMY

For many surgeons more familiar with abdominal surgery, the laparoscope may be used to perform the radical hysterectomy

Table 16.4.1: Summary of the Larger Series of Laparoscopically Assisted Vaginal Radical Hysterectomy

Study	Patients, no.	PLN	ORT, min.	EBL, mL	LOS, days	Complications	Recurrences, no.
Hertel et al. [12]	200	22	333	—	—	7 ureter, 4 vascular, 1 bowel, 14 bladder	37
Hallum et al. [13]	37	35	225	525	5	2 bladder, 1 fistula, 1 bowel	—
Jackson et al. [14]	57		180	350	5	3 bladder, 1 bowel	2
Nam et al. [15]	47	33	232	—	15	1 bladder, 1 hernia, 1 fistula, 1 obstruction	4
Steed et al. [16]	71		210			7 bladder, 1 ureter, 1 bowel, 2 fistulas	4
Querleu et al. [17]	47	25	228	391	—	2 ureter	3
Park et al. [18]	52	27	380	—	—	4 ureter, 1 hematoma, 2 conversions	2
Sardi et al. [19]	56	17	267	—	4	2 bladder, 3 ureter, 2 technical, 1 abscess	4
Renaud et al. [20]	57	27	270	300	5	3 cystotomies, 1 vascular	2

PLN, mean pelvic lymph nodes; ORT, mean operating room time; EBL, mean estimated blood loss; LOS, mean hospital stay.

by mimicking the same steps used at abdominal radical hysterectomy. The laparoscopic radical hysterectomy with pelvic and aortic lymph node dissection was first reported in 1990.[8] This technique can be appealing to the abdominal surgeon in that one needs to master only the laparoscopic skills required to perform this procedure, compared with LAVRH, which requires expertise in both laparoscopic and vaginal surgery. Once the technique was standardized, this operation became popular in the United States because it complies with oncologic principles while maintaining a minimally invasive approach.

Before beginning the laparoscopic radical hysterectomy, the surgeon can perform cystourethroscopy and place ureteral catheters. This decision depends on the surgeon's preference but may be helpful during ureteral dissection.

A variety of endoscopic dissecting instruments, clip appliers, staplers, and specimen-retrieval devices, as well as monopolar current attached to a dissector or scissors, may be used. The gas flow is set to manual at 3 to 4 L/minute, which contributes to increased pneumoperitoneum, necessitating continuous monitoring of intra-abdominal pressure and active venting during the procedure via one of the laparoscopic trocar valves to keep the intra-abdominal pressure under 16 mm Hg.

A four-trocar transperitoneal approach is usually used for these procedures (Figure 16.4.15), with the initial incision made in the periumbilical area. A carbon dioxide pneumoperitoneum is then generated, keeping the intra-abdominal pressure under 16 mm Hg. A 0° laparoscope is then introduced via the umbilical port, and the peritoneal cavity is inspected. Three accessory 5- to 12-mm trocars are then placed under direct visualization medial to the iliac crest and in the suprapubic area.

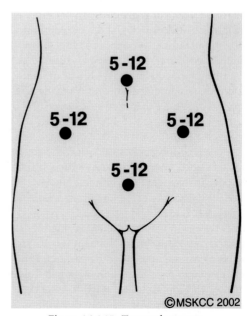

Figure 16.4.15. Trocar placement.

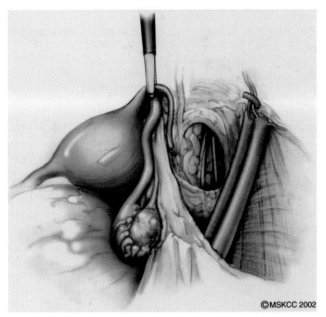

Figure 16.4.16. Opening of the right paravesical space.

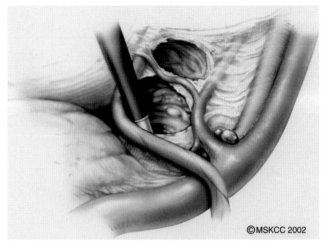

Figure 16.4.17. Opening of the right pararectal space.

Transperitoneal pelvic lymphadenectomy is performed with the patient in a 30° to 45° Trendelenburg position to facilitate retroperitoneal exposure by retaining the small intestine in the mid- and upper abdomen using gravity and gentle instrumentation. The use of intraoperative epidural anesthesia is surgeon dependent and may facilitate exposure by contracting the intestine, as the result of sympathetic blockade.

The pelvic lymphadenectomy is started by developing the paravesical and pararectal space. We routinely use the laparoscopic 10-mm argon beam coagulator (ABC) foot-switching probe (ConMed Electrosurgery System 7500, Utica, NY), set at 70 W, for these laparoscopic procedures. The 10-mm ABC probe replaces multiple laparoscopic instruments by working as a dissector, cutter, and coagulator. It also functions as a rigid probe to allow transfer of tactile sensation from tissues to the surgeon's hand. The round ligament is divided with the ABC. The umbilical ligament is isolated medially, and a retroperitoneal incision between the round ligament and the umbilical ligament, parallel to the umbilical ligament, is performed and extended just to the reflection of the interior abdominal wall. The umbilical ligament is then placed on traction medially, and using the ABC, the paravesical space is developed to expose the external iliac vessels, the obturator area and the obturator internus muscle, and the pubic bone (Figure 16.4.16).

After developing the paravesical space, the retroperitoneal incision is extended over the psoas muscle parallel to the infundibulopelvic ligament. The infundibulopelvic ligament is pulled medially. The ureter is visualized medially, and the hypogastric vessel is identified laterally. The pararectal space is developed between these two structures using blunt dissection on the posterior leaf of the broad ligament (Figure 16.4.17).

After complete development of the pararectal and paravesical spaces, the lymph node dissection is started. This dissection can begin over the common iliac artery on the right side and may be carried to the level of the deep circumflex iliac vessels (Figure 16.4.18). Leaving the ureter attached to the peritoneum

allows it to be retracted away with medial traction on the peritoneal edge and infundibulopelvic ligament. The psoas muscle is identified, the genitofemoral nerve is protected, and the lymph nodes between the genitofemoral nerve and the surface of the right external iliac artery and vein are removed.

The obturator nerve is then identified, the obturator vessels are protected, and the lymph node package between the external iliac vein and obturator nerve is dissected. Lymph nodes around and below the obturator nerve are removed. Hypogastric nodes can now be removed from the proximal part of the umbilical ligament and near the uterine artery origin. The iliac vessels can then be dissected from the psoas muscle and pulled medially, and the obturator space is exposed through the lateral approach to

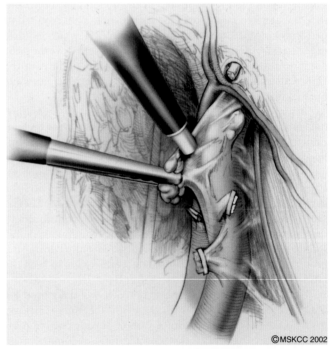

Figure 16.4.18. The removal of the right external iliac lymph nodes.

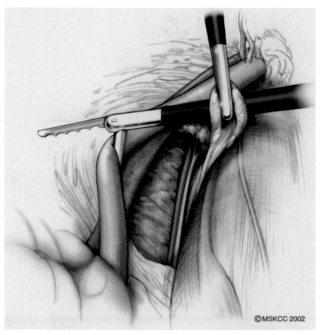

Figure 16.4.19. Right iliac and obturator lymphadenectomy using the lateral approach between the psoas muscle and right external iliac vessels.

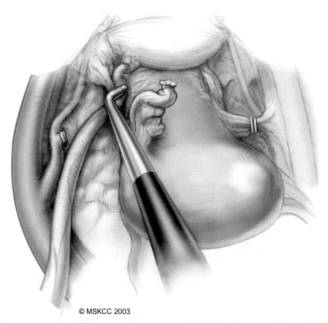

Figure 16.4.21. The medial edge of the divided uterine vessels is pulled medially, and the ureter is unroofed with the argon beam coagulator and endoscopic right angle dissector, with clips placed as needed.

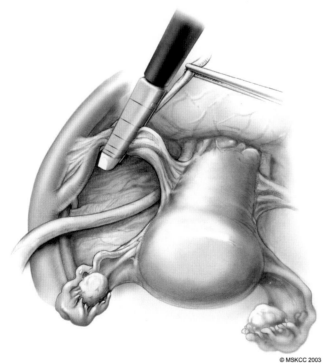

Figure 16.4.20. The uterine vessels are stapled with a vascular endoscopic stapler at the origin from the hypogastric vessels.

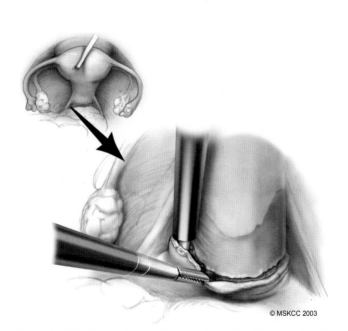

Figure 16.4.22. A posterior cul-de-sac peritoneal incision is made with the argon beam coagulator, and the rectovaginal septum is developed.

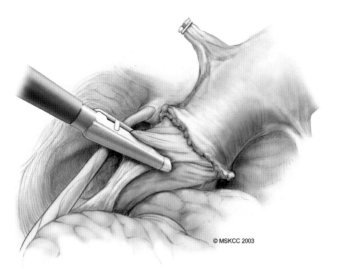

Figure 16.4.23. The uterosacral ligaments are divided or stapled.

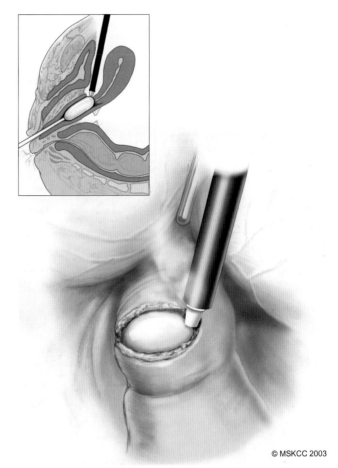

Figure 16.4.25. Anterior colpotomy is performed using the argon beam coagulator, guided by the nonconducting vaginal probe and the incision extended circumferentially.

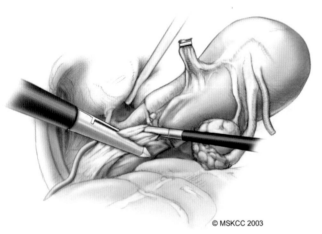

Figure 16.4.24. The remaining parametria and paracolpos are divided by the endoscopic stapler.

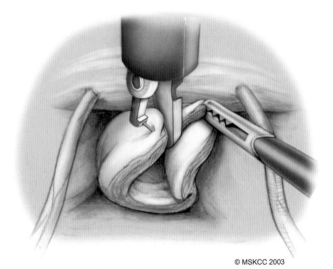

Figure 16.4.26. The vaginal cuff is closed anterior to posterior using the Endo Stitch (United States Surgical Corporation, Norwalk, CT) in a running manner.

Table 16.4.2: Summary of Reports on Laparoscopic Radical Hysterectomy and Pelvic Lymphadenectomy with or without Para-aortic Aortic Lymphadenectomy

Author Group	Year	Patients, no.*	PLN	ORT, min.	EBL, mL	LOS, days	Complications
Nezhat	1992 [10] 1993 [22]	7	22.0	315	30–250	2.1	None
Sedlacek	1994 [23] 1995 [24]	14	16.0	420	334	5.5	1 VVF, 1 ureteral injury
Ting	1994 [25]	4	8.0	330–480	150–500	—	None
Ostrzenski	1996 [26]	6	—	280	—	2.0–6.0	1 hydronephrosis
Kim	1998 [27]	18	22.0	363	619	—	None
Hsieh	1998 [28]	8	—	—		6.5	None
Spirtos	2002 [21]	78	23.8	205	250	2.9	1.3% transfusion, 3 cystotomies, 1 UVF, 1 DVT, 5 conversions
Lee	2002 [29]	12	19.2	235	428	6.8	2 transfusions
Lin	2003 [30]	10	16.8	159	250	4.1	None
Obermair	2003 [31]	55	—	210	200	5.0	3 vascular, 1 nerve
Pomel	2003 [32]	50	13.2	258	200	7.5	1 bladder, 1 ureter, 1 hernia
Abu-Rustum	2003 [33]	19	25.5	371	301	4.5	1 transfusion, 2 conversions 1 fever
Gil-Moreno	2005 [34]	27	19.1	285	400	5.0	None

*Some patients may be reported more than once.

PLN, mean pelvic lymph nodes; ORT, mean operating room time; EBL, mean estimated blood loss; LOS, mean hospital stay; VVF, vesicovaginal fistula; UVF, ureterovaginal fistula; DVT, deep venous thrombosis.

ensure removal of all nodal tissue, particularly in the proximal part just lateral to the common iliac artery (Figure 16.4.19). The same steps are performed on the contralateral side.

For the total laparoscopic radical hysterectomy, the bladder flap is dissected sharply and pushed caudally using the ABC. A vaginal probe (Apple Medical Corporation, Marlboro, MA) facilitates the dissection by stretching the vaginal fornix. The uterine vessels are either divided with a vascular endoscopic stapler (Autosuture Multifire Endo GIA 30-2.0; United States Surgical Corporation, Norwalk, CT) at their origin from the hypogastric vessels (Figure 16.4.20), or sealed with the endoscopic vessel sealing system (LigaSure; Valleylab, Boulder, CO). The medial edge of the divided uterine vessels is then pulled medially, and the ureter is unroofed with the ABC and endoscopic right-angle dissector, with clips placed as needed (Figure 16.4.21). A posterior cul-de-sac peritoneal incision is then made and the rectovaginal septum developed (Figure 16.4.22). The uterosacral ligaments are divided or stapled, and the remaining parametria and paracolpos are divided (Figures 16.4.23 and 16.4.24). Anterior colpotomy is then performed using the ABC, guided by the vaginal probe, and the incision is extended circumferentially (Figure 16.4.25). The specimen is removed vaginally. The vaginal cuff is then closed from anterior to posterior using the Endo Stitch (United States Surgical Corporation, Norwalk, CT) with absorbable suture in a running manner (Figure 16.4.26). The ureteral catheters are usually removed at the completion of the operation or before discharge.

The largest series reported so far, by Spirtos et al. [21], describes 78 consecutive patients, all with early cervical cancer and a Quetelet body mass index greater than 35, who underwent this procedure. In all, 94% of the procedures were completed laparoscopically, with an average operative time of 205 minutes and an average blood loss of 225 mL, with only one patient (1.3%) requiring transfusion. There was one ureterovaginal fistula documented. The average lymph node count was 34, with 11.5% of patients having positive lymph nodes. Three patients (3.8%) had close or positive surgical margins, and eight patients (10.3%) had a recurrence with a minimum of 3-year follow-up. The estimated 5-year disease-free interval for those patients was 89.7%. Table 16.4.2 summarizes published reports on laparoscopic radical hysterectomy and pelvic lymphadenectomy with or without para-aortic lymphadenectomy.[10, 21–34]

CONCLUSIONS

Laparoscopy has revived interest in the minimally invasive surgical approach to the management of early cervical cancer. In addition to allowing the vaginal radical hysterectomy to remain a surgical option, it has provided a means of facilitating the vaginal dissection while also increasing the extensiveness of the dissection. Furthermore, total laparoscopic radical hysterectomy has also opened the world of minimally access surgery to surgeons more accustomed to abdominal surgery. As more data are accumulated, the exact role of these procedures in the surgical management of cervical cancer will be determined.

REFERENCES

1. Novak F. *Gynakologische Operationstechnik*. New York: Springer-Verlag; 1978.
2. Schauta F. *Die enveiterte vaginale Totalextirpation der Uterus beim Collumcarzinom*. Wien Seipzig: J. Safar; 1908.
3. Wertheim E. The extended abdominal operations for carcinoma uteri (based on 5000 operative cases). *Am J Obstet Gynecol*. 1912;66:169.
4. Amreich I. Zur anatomie und technik der erweiterten vaginalen carcinoperation. *Arch Gynakol*. 1924;122:497.
5. Stoeckel W. Die vaginale radikaloperation des kollumcarzinom. *Zentralbl Gynakol*. 1928;39.
6. Mitra S. *Mitra Operation for Cancer of the Cervix*. Springfield: Ch Thomas; 1960.
7. Dargent D. A new future for Schauta's operation through pre-surgical retroperitoneal pelviscopy. *Eur J Gynecol Oncol*. 1987;8:292.
8. Nezhat C, Nezhat F. Videolaseroscopy for the treatment of upper, mid, and lower peritoneal cavity pathology. *Annual Meeting of AAGL, Nov.* 1990.
9. Nezhat C, Nezhat F, Silfen S. Videolaseroscopy: the CO_2 laser for advanced operative laparoscopy. *Obstet Gynecol Clin North Am*. 1991;18(3):585–604.
10. Nezhat CR, Burrell MO, Nezhat FR, Benigno BB, Welander CE. Laparoscopic radical hysterectomy with paraaortic and pelvic node dissection. *Am J Obstet Gynecol*. 1992;166:864.
11. Possover M, Krause N, Schneider A. Identification of the ureter and dissection of the bladder pillar in laparoscopic-assisted radical vaginal hysterectomy. *Obstet Gynecol*. 1998;91:139–143.
12. Hertel H, Kohler C, Michels W, Possover M, Tozzi R, Schneider A. Laparoscopic-assisted radical vaginal hysterectomy (LARVH): prospective evaluation of 200 patients with cervical cancer. *Gynecol Oncol*. 2003;90:505–511.
13. Hallum AV, Hatch KD, Nour M, Saucedo M. Comparison of radical abdominal hysterectomy with laparoscopic-assisted radical vaginal hysterectomy for treatment of early cervical cancer. *J Gynecol Tech*. 2000;6:2–6.
14. Jackson KS, Das N, Naik R, et al. Laparoscopically assisted radical vaginal hysterectomy vs. radical abdominal hysterectomy for cervical cancer: a match controlled study. *Gynecol Oncol*. 2004;95:655–661.
15. Nam JH, Kim JH, Kim DY, et al. Comparative study of laparoscopico-vaginal radical hysterectomy and abdominal radical hysterectomy in patients with early cervical cancer. *Gynecol Oncol*. 2004;92:277–283.
16. Steed H, Rosen B, Murphy J, Laframboise S, De Petrillo D, Covens A. A comparison of laparoscopic-assisted radical vaginal hysterectomy and radical abdominal hysterectomy in the treatment of cervical cancer. *Gynecol Oncol*. 2004;93:588–593.
17. Querleu D, Narducci F, Poulard V, et al. Modified radical vaginal hysterectomy with or without laparoscopic nerve-sparing dissection: a comparative study. *Gynecol Oncol*. 2002;85:154–158.
18. Park CT, Lim KT, Chung HW, et al. Clinical evaluation of laparoscopic-assisted radical vaginal hysterectomy with pelvic and/or paraaortic lymphadenectomy. *J Am Assoc Gynecol Laparosc*. 2002;9:49–53.
19. Sardi J, Vidaurreta J, Bermudez A, di Paola G. Laparoscopically assisted Schauta operation: learning experience at the Gynecologic Oncology Unit, Buenos Aires University Hospital. *Gynecol Oncol*. 1999;75:361–365.
20. Renaud MC, Plante M, Roy M. Combined laparoscopic and vaginal radical surgery in cervical cancer. *Gynecol Oncol*. 2000;79:59–63.
21. Spirtos NM, Eisenkop SM, Schlaerth JB, Ballon SC. Laparoscopic radical hysterectomy (type III) with aortic and pelvic lymphadenectomy in patients with stage I cervical cancer: surgical morbidity and intermediate follow-up. *Am J Obstet Gynecol*. 2002;187:340–348.
22. Nezhat CR, Nezhat FR, Burrell MO, et al. Laparoscopic radical hysterectomy and laparoscopically assisted vaginal radical hysterectomy with pelvic and paraaortic node dissection. *J Gynecol Surg*. 1993;9:105–120.
23. Sedlacek TV, Campion MJ, Hutchins RA, Reich H. Laparoscopic radical hysterectomy: a preliminary report. *J Am Assoc Gynecol Laparosc*. 1994;1(4 pt 2):S32.
24. Sedlacek TV, Campion MJ, Reich H, Sedlacek T. Laparoscopic radical hysterectomy: a feasibility study [abstract]. *Gynecol Oncol*. 1995;56:126.
25. Ting HC. Laparoscopic radical hysterectomy: a preliminary experience. *J Am Assoc Gynecol Laparosc*. 1994;1(4 pt 2):S36.
26. Ostrzenski A. A new laparoscopic abdominal radical hysterectomy: a pilot phase trial. *Eur J Surg Oncol*. 1996;22:602–606.
27. Kim DH, Moon JS. Laparoscopic radical hysterectomy with pelvic lymphadenectomy for early, invasive cervical carcinoma. *J Am Assoc Gynecol Laparosc*. 1998;5:411–417.
28. Hsieh YY, Lin WC, Chang CC, Yeh LS, Hsu TY, Tsai HD. Laparoscopic radical hysterectomy with low paraaortic, subaortic and pelvic lymphadenectomy. Results of short-term follow-up. *J Reprod Med*. 1998;43:528–534.
29. Lee CL, Huang KG. Total laparoscopic radical hysterectomy using Lee-Huang portal and McCartney transvaginal tube. *J Am Assoc Gynecol Laparosc*. 2002;9:536–540.
30. Lin YS. Preliminary results of laparoscopic modified radical hysterectomy in early invasive cervical cancer. *J Am Assoc Gynecol Laparosc*. 2003;10:80–84.
31. Obermair A, Ginbey P, McCartney AJ. Feasibility and safety of total laparoscopic radical hysterectomy. *J Am Assoc Gynecol Laparosc*. 2003;10:345–349.
32. Pomel C, Atallah D, Le Bouedec G, et al. Laparoscopic radical hysterectomy for invasive cervical cancer: 8-year experience of a pilot study. *Gynecol Oncol*. 2003;91:534–539.
33. Abu-Rustum NR, Gemignani ML, Moore K, et al. Total laparoscopic radical hysterectomy with pelvic lymphadenectomy using the argon-beam coagulator: pilot data and comparison to laparotomy. *Gynecol Oncol*. 2003;91:402–409.
34. Gil-Moreno A, Puig O, Perez-Benavente MA, et al. Total laparoscopic radical hysterectomy (type II-III) with pelvic lymphadenectomy in early invasive cervical cancer. *J Minim Invasive Gynecol*. 2005;12:113–120.

Section 16.5. Laparoscopy for Endometrial Cancer

Javier F. Magrina, Andrea Mariani, and Paul M. Magtibay

Reports on the outcomes of laparoscopy or laparotomy for benign gynecologic conditions have shown superior benefits for patients treated laparoscopically. Laparoscopy offers three main advantages: (1) reduced operative blood loss, (2) shorter hospitalization, and (3) a faster resumption to normal activities and return to work.

Some gynecologic oncologists, encouraged by these findings, have applied these techniques to patients with gynecologic malignancies. Not surprisingly, similar benefits were noted for laparoscopically treated patients compared with laparotomy-treated patients.

Numerous literature reports have addressed the feasibility, perioperative morbidity, conversion rates, quality-of-life measures, cost, recurrence, and survival results of laparoscopic techniques in patients with endometrial, cervical, ovarian, vaginal, or vulvar cancers. For patients with endometrial cancer, laparoscopy has been shown to provide additional benefits to laparotomy. These findings are reviewed in this section.

LAPAROSCOPY APPLICATIONS FOR ENDOMETRIAL CANCER

Laparoscopic techniques are applicable to patients with primary endometrial cancer clinically localized to the uterus, for the staging of posthysterectomy patients with previously undiagnosed endometrial cancer, and for patients with pelvic recurrences amenable to surgical resection or irradiation.

Primary Endometrial Cancer

Gynecologic oncologists who complete a comprehensive review of the multiple studies addressing the application of laparoscopy for the surgical treatment of primary endometrial carcinoma will easily conclude that a total abdominal hysterectomy with bilateral salpingo-oophorectomy is a viable alternative to treatment for patients with endometrial cancer and that laparoscopy should be the primary surgical approach.

Surgical Technique

Trocar placement for laparoscopic pelvic surgery is shown in Figure 16.5.1. Exploration of the peritoneal surface of the abdominal and pelvic cavities from the diaphragm to the pelvic cul-de-sac is carried out, and pelvic peritoneal cytology is obtained. A total laparoscopic hysterectomy with bilateral salpingo-oophorectomy is performed. We routinely remove the appendix when it is present. The uterus, tubes, ovaries, and appendix are extirpated through the open vaginal cuff before closure. The uterus is submitted for frozen histologic section. When indications for lymphadenectomy are present (see below), we conduct a bilateral pelvic lymphadenectomy and, if indicated, an aortic lymphadenectomy to the renal vessels. A pelvic lymphadenectomy includes the obturator, external, internal, and common iliac nodes. The aortic nodes include right- and left-sided nodes and lower (to inferior mesenteric artery) and higher (to left renal vein) groups. For the right aortic lymphadenectomy, a bowel retractor is inserted through the left lower pelvic trocar to retract the small-bowel mesentery and duodenum ventrally. For the left aortic nodes, an additional trocar is then inserted 7 to 10 cm craniad to the left lower quadrant trocar (Figure 16.5.2). It is used to retract sigmoid mesentery, the left ureter, and the left gonadal vein laterally. The inferior mesenteric artery is routinely divided to provide ample access to the higher group of the left aortic nodes. The peritoneum of the pelvis and the aortic area are left open, and drains are not routinely used.

Since March 2003, we have used a robotic surgical interface system (da Vinci Surgical System; Intuitive Surgical, Inc., Sunnyvale, CA) in the treatment of patients with endometrial cancer. The robotic column is situated between the patient's lower extremities for the hysterectomy and pelvic node dissection. For the aortic lymphadenectomy, it is positioned at the patient's head. To expedite the change of positions, we prefer to rotate the patient on the operating room table 180° instead of moving the robotic column cephalad.

The articulated instruments facilitate tissue dissection by allowing the dissecting instrument to be directed in the correct tissue plane and in the appropriate direction, instead of forcing the tissues to accommodate the direction of rigid conventional laparoscopic instruments. Because the articulated robotic instruments can be directed in the correct tissue plane following the path of large vessels, nerves, ureters, and any other pelvic structures, the robotic surgical system is most helpful for the performance of pelvic surgery and, in particular, for treatment of gynecologic malignancies. The system's ability to downsize the surgeon's movements (3:1 or 5:1), its lack of tremor, and its three-dimensional visualization screen provide increased accuracy of tissue dissection and suturing. The surgeon, the physician's assistant, and the scrub nurse are also able to sit down comfortably during surgery, which reduces their physical fatigue. Because robotic systems are limited to a few institutions at the present, most gynecologic oncologists routinely perform the hysterectomy and lymphadenectomy through a laparoscopic approach, a technique commonly used in Europe, Asia, Australia, and the United States.

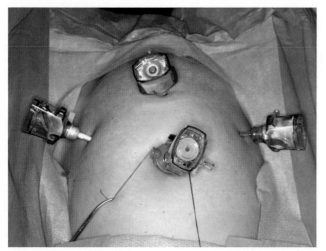

Figure 16.5.1. Trocar placement for pelvic lymphadenectomy and hysterectomy.

Surgical Staging

Lymph node dissection is an integral part of the management of patients with endometrial cancer. The value of a lymphadenectomy (pelvic or aortic or both) is multiple: (1) staging – to define the extent of the spread of disease, to provide an estimate of prognosis, and to facilitate comparative evaluations among institutions; (2) therapeutic – our retrospective data and that of others indicate a therapeutic role for both pelvic [1–3] and aortic [4] lymphadenectomy; and (3) diagnostic – to determine the need and extent of adjuvant therapy. In fact, patients with negative lymph nodes as determined by systematic surgical staging do not benefit from adjuvant pelvic or aortic external irradiation.[5]

SELECTION OF PATIENTS TO AVOID PELVIC AND AORTIC LYMPHADENECTOMY

Microinvasive Endometrial Cancer

At Mayo Clinic, pelvic lymphadenectomy is routinely performed in all patients with the exception of a select group of patients

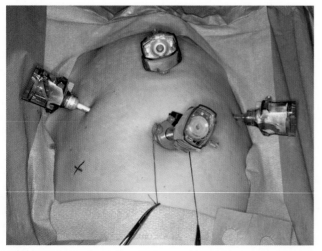

Figure 16.5.2. For aortic lymphadenectomy, a fifth trocar is inserted 7 to 10 cm above the left lateral trocar to retract the sigmoid mesentery.

considered to be at extremely low risk for lymphatic spread. These low-risk patients have endometrioid tumors localized to the uterus (no spread to peritoneal surfaces, cervix, or adnexa) with (1) no myometrial invasion (regardless of grade or tumor diameter) or (2) grade 1 or grade 2 tumors 2 cm or less in diameter with less than 50% of myometrial invasion.

One review of 123 patients with such histologic findings found a 0% incidence of nodal metastases or nodal recurrence.[6] At 5-year follow-up, all 123 patients(100%) were alive with no evidence of disease. The absence of lymph nodal metastases in such patients, reported also in other studies [7], confirms the superiority of primary tumor diameter over grade in predicting lymph node invasion in the above-defined low-risk group, which could be addressed as microinvasive endometrial cancer. Patients with such histologic findings (approximately one fourth of all endometrial cancer patients operated on at our institution) do not benefit from surgical staging.

PELVIC DISSEMINATION: WHICH PELVIC NODAL SITES ARE MOST LIKELY TO CONTAIN METASTATIC DISEASE?

A review of our experience with endometrial cancer revealed the external iliac region as the most frequently observed site of nodal metastases, either isolated or in association with other positive nodal groups.[8] The second most common sites of nodal metastases were the obturator nodes in patients without cervical involvement and the common iliac nodes for patients with cervical involvement.[8]

INDICATIONS FOR PELVIC LYMPHADENECTOMY

Pelvic lymphadenectomy is routinely performed in all patients who do not fit the criteria for microinvasive endometrial cancer. Such patients include all those with histologic types other than endometrioid, regardless of the degree of myometrial invasion or tumor size.

AORTIC NODAL DISSEMINATION

Tumor invasion of the pelvic lymph nodes together with lymphovascular invasion is the strongest predictor of cancer dissemination in the aortic area.[9] In previous reports from our institution [8] and others [10], positive aortic nodes were observed in 55% to 75% of patients with pelvic node metastases. In a more recent analysis from Mayo Clinic, positive aortic nodes were detected in 47% of patients with positive pelvic nodes, found either by staging or as a subsequent relapse in the aortic area.[9]

AORTIC LYMPHADENECTOMY

Indications

Two of us (A.M. and P.M.) prefer to perform an aortic lymphadenectomy to renal vessels in all patients who do not fit the criteria for microinvasive endometrial cancer. The rationale for this approach is the fact that, in spite of a low frequency of isolated aortic metastases, it is not always feasible or accurate to use either frozen section analysis for definition of pelvic lymph node status or lymphovascular invasion as a possible surrogate of para-aortic dissemination.[9] Furthermore, systematic aortic lymphadenectomy has therapeutic value in patients with histologically detected aortic metastases and in those with negative aortic nodes but histologically undetected micrometastases.[4]

For the other author (J.F.M.), aortic lymphadenectomy to renal vessels is indicated (1) in the presence of positive pelvic nodes and (2) in patients with negative pelvic nodes but lymphovascular invasion and outer third myometrial involvement, as explained later.

Most gynecologic oncologists concur that aortic lymphadenectomy is indicated in all patients with positive pelvic nodes because of the high frequency of positive aortic nodes in the presence of pelvic node metastases. Aortic nodal dissection should be extended to the renal vessels because of the frequent involvement of the high aortic nodal groups and because of skip metastases to the high aortic group. In fact, more than 80% of patients operated on at Mayo Clinic who had positive aortic nodes had involvement of the nodes above the inferior mesenteric artery, with a high rate of skipping the lower aortic nodes. The high aortic nodes were involved in nine of 11 patients (81.8%) who had positive aortic nodes. Among these nine patients, skipping of the ipsilateral nodes below the inferior mesenteric artery (low aortic nodes) was observed in six (66.7%) patients (unpublished data from Mayo Clinic).

In the absence of positive pelvic nodes, aortic lymphadenectomy is indicated in patients with lymphovascular invasion and invasion of the outer third of the myometrium. The presence of positive aortic nodes in the absence of pelvic node metastases is uncommon and was observed in only 2% of patients (range, 0% to 3%) (Table 16.5.1).[9–14] However, in patients with negative nodes but lymphovascular invasion, this rate is much higher. In our experience, three of 181 patients (1.7%) who underwent systematic pelvic and aortic lymphadenectomy had isolated aortic invasion. In the presence of lymphovascular invasion, positive aortic nodes were observed in as many as 9% of patients with negative pelvic nodes.[9] A common risk factor for all three patients with negative pelvic but positive aortic nodes was invasion of the outer third of the myometrium associated with lymphovascular invasion (unpublished data).

Intraoperative Complications

A review of four studies comparing intraoperative complications between laparoscopy and laparotomy patients showed reduced complication rates for laparoscopy patients (Table 16.5.2). [15–18] In 187 laparoscopy patients, the intraoperative complication rate was 4.2%, whereas it was 11.1% for 164 laparotomy patients.

Perioperative Data and Morbidity

A review of 17 studies addressing results of perioperative data (e.g., operating room time, estimated blood loss, number of retrieved lymph nodes, length of hospitalization, and conversion rates to laparotomy) between 945 laparoscopy and 1039 laparotomy patients with endometrial cancer is shown

Table 16.5.1: Presence of Positive Aortic Lymph Nodes in Patients with and without Pelvic Node Metastases

Study	Cancer Stage	Patients with Negative Pelvic Nodes, N + Aortic LNs (%)	Patients with Positive Pelvic Nodes, N + Aortic LNs (%)
Mariani et al. (2004) [9]	I–IV	90* + 2 (2)	51* + 2 (4)
McMeekin et al. (2001) [10]	I–IV	NA	47 + 8 (17)
Ayhan et al. (1995) [11]	Clinical I	209 + 6 (3)	36 + 6 (17)
Fanning et al. (1996) [12]	I–III	60 + 0 (0)	5 + 0 (0)
Hirahatake et al. (1997) [13]	I–IV	200 + 2 (1)	42 + 2 (5)
Larson and Johnson (1993) [14]	I–IV	50 + 0 (0)	10 + 0 (0)
Total		1647 + 34 (2)	350 + 42 (12)

*We excluded the three patients who had positive para-aortic nodes but for whom no data were available about the pelvis.
LN, lymph node; NA, not available.

in Table 16.5.3.[15–17,19–32] Laparoscopy patients experienced less blood loss (216 vs. 284 mL), reduced hospitalization (3.5 vs. 6.8 days), a similar number of retrieved lymph nodes (16.2 vs. 14.5), and a longer operating time (171 vs. 133 minutes). Major differences were found in operating times, number of nodes, and days of hospitalization, depending on the surgeon's experience; whether patients had lymphadenectomy and, if so, whether it was pelvic or aortic or both; the extent of the lymphadenectomy; and the usual length of hospitalization for different countries.

Conversion to Laparotomy

Conversion to laparotomy may be necessary because of anesthesia complications or difficulties with ventilation, intolerance to the Trendelenburg position, intraoperative complications not amenable to laparoscopic correction, or advanced disease. Conversion rates to laparotomy from all causes range from 0% to 12.4%.[33] However, the rate is lower (0% to 5.3%) when all conversions due to operative complications are considered.[33] In 14 studies, the conversion rate due to complications was 2% (Table 16.5.2).

Various operative reasons (e.g., dense adhesions, uncontrolled bleeding, difficult exposure, inadequate instrumentation, or equipment failure) may result in a determination by the surgeon to proceed with a laparotomy approach. At Mayo Clinic, the expertise of the surgeon and the assistant, as well as available instrumentation, plays a major role and may result either in continuation or in completion of the operation laparoscopically. These factors may also explain the wide range of reported conversion rates.

Table 16.5.2: Comparison of Intraoperative Complications of Laparoscopy versus Laparotomy in Patients with Endometrial Cancer

| | Intraoperative Complications | | | |
| | Laparoscopy | | Laparotomy | |
Study	Patients, no.	Complications, %	Patients, no.	Complications, %
Kuoppala et al. (2004) [15]	40	0	40	0
Magrina et al. (1995) [16]	15	6.6	15	6.6
Occelli et al. (2003) [17]	69	5.6	50	22.4
Tozzi et al. (2005) [18]	63	4.7	59	15.2
Total	187	4.2	164	11.1

There is no doubt that many anesthesiologists look unfavorably on positioning the patient in a deep Trendelenburg tilt because it results in increased ventilation requirements. However, such patient positioning is necessary for performance of some gynecologic oncology procedures (e.g., aortic lymphadenectomy) and for execution of a safe and an expeditious pelvic operation. This is particularly true in patients with dilated loops of small bowel or redundant sigmoid that obstruct the view of, or access to, the pelvic organs.

Inadvertent injury to the major pelvic veins and vena cava that results from scissors, cautery, or avulsion of the small tributaries is a common reason for laparotomy. However, this type of injury can be repaired laparoscopically as long as adequate visualization can be obtained by proper efferent pressure and effective suction. One of us (J.F.M.) has effectively repaired injuries to the vena cava, the left common iliac, and the right external iliac veins using the following laparoscopic technique. First, a 5-cm precut 4-0 polypropylene suture (Prolene; Ethicon Endo-Surgery, Inc., Cincinnati, OH) or similar nonabsorbable suture with a Vicryl clip (Lapra-Ty; Ethicon Endo-Surgery, Inc.) fastened at the distal end is introduced. Opposite edges of the injury site are brought together with a single pass of the needle. The suture is then pulled upward. In most instances, pulling the edges together will stop the bleeding of minor defects. A second or third pass of the needle will occlude most injury sites. After the defect is closed, another Lapra-Ty is fastened to the suture, flush with the vein wall. When feasible, such as with bleeding secondary to injury to the external or common iliac veins, a caudal tourniquet applied with a vessel loop introduced through an additional port will control the bleeding and allow an unhurried repair.

Adhesions among bowel loops that result in distorted anatomy can be managed laparoscopically when they are limited to a portion of the abdominal or pelvic cavity and when proper tissue planes can be identified, dissected, and separated. The insertion of additional trocars may be necessary to obtain proper traction and countertraction, or to place the dissecting scissors in the proper direction. The da Vinci robotic surgical interface system has articulated instruments that facilitate dissection of problematic adhesions. To prevent thermal intestinal injury, we use cautery minimally or not at all. The bowel and colon must always be thoroughly inspected for any injury after adhesiolysis.

Postoperative Complications

Because the type of annotated postoperative complication varies among different studies, there is a wide range of reported complication rates for patients with endometrial cancer treated either by laparoscopy or by laparotomy. Some studies address all minor and major complications, whereas others address only major complications and still others do not indicate what deviances from a normal postoperative course should be considered complications. Reduced postoperative complication rates are observed among laparoscopy patients compared with laparotomy patients.

We reviewed 12 reports published between 1995 and 2005 to compare postoperative complications between laparoscopy and laparotomy patients (Table 16.5.4).[15–17,20,21,23,25–27,30,34,35] For laparoscopy patients, the range of complications was 0% to 23.8%, whereas it was 0% to 58% for laparotomy patients. An increased rate of complications was observed among laparotomy-treated patients in 10 studies, whereas in the remaining two it was similar (0% and 20%, respectively), with no major differences observed.

Late complications (≥42 days) are either reduced with laparoscopy or similar to those of laparotomy patients. In one study, late complications were observed in only five of 63 laparoscopy patients (7.9%) compared with 21 of 59 laparotomy patients (35.6%).[35] In another study, late postoperative complications were similar between both groups (20% vs. 22.5%).[15]

Univariate analysis of risk factors for postoperative complications showed that weight of more than 80 kg, Quetelet index (body mass index; weight [kg]/height [m^2]) of more than 30, and age of more than 65 years were highly predictive of complications both for laparoscopy and for laparotomy patients.[35] Patients who met these parameters experienced 60% of all complications. This group of patients appeared to benefit even more from a laparoscopic approach. Interestingly, multivariate analysis identified the surgical approach as the only significant risk factor predictive of complications.

Recurrence

Recurrence rates for patients treated laparoscopically are low and comparable to those of patients treated by laparotomy. A review of six comparison studies showed the mean rate of recurrence

Table 16.5.3: Comparison of Perioperative Laparoscopy and Laparotomy Data for Endometrial Cancer

Study	Patients, no.	Mean Operating Time, min	Mean Blood Loss, mL	Mean Lymph Nodes, no.	Mean Hospital Stay, days	Conversion to Laparotomy,%
Laparoscopy						
Kuoppala et al. (2004) [15]	40	145	171	11.1	2.7	0
Magrina et al. (1995) [16]	15	174	272	18.5	3.4	3.4
Occelli et al. (2003) [17]	69	164.5	NA	15.8	4.0	1.2
Boike et al. (1994) [19]	33	217	NA	18.9	2.5	5.3
Eltabbakh (2002) [20]	100	NA	200	13.5	2	1.0
Eltabbakh et al. (2000) [21]*	40	195	318	11.3	2.5	2.5
Gemignani et al. (1999) [22]	69†	214	211	7 (0–14)	2.9	3.0
Holub et al. (2002) [23]	177	163.1	211.2	16.8	3.9	3.4
Holub et al. (1998) [24]	11	153	130	NA	4.7	NA
Langebrekke et al. (2002) [25]	27	143	NA	6.8	4.3	3.7
Litta et al. (2003) [26]	29	186	125	14.2	2.5	0
Manolitsas et al. (2002) [27]	161	138	NA	NA	4.3	NA
Moore et al. (1999) [28]	80	170	223	20.1	2.5	1.3
Peng et al. (2004) [29]	24	97	163	13.6	6.3	NA
Scribner et al. (1999) [30]	19	237	350	34	3.7	0
Spirtos et al. (1995) [31]	13	NA	NA	28	2.4	0
Zapico et al. (2005) [32]	38	165	NA	13.5	5.0	0
	945	171	216	16.2	3.5	1.8
Laparotomy						
Kuoppala et al. (2004) [15]	40	96	238	7.3	7.6	
Magrina et al. (1995) [16]	15	142	502	23.5	6.6	
Occelli et al. (2003) [17]	58	122.9	NA	11	9.0	
Boike et al. (1994) [19]	37	194.0	NA	18.7	5	
Eltabbakh (2002) [20]	40	138	303	5.3	6.5	
Eltabbakh et al. (2000) [21]*	86	NA	250	10.5	5	
Gemignani et al. (1999) [22]	251‡	144	209	6 (0–30)	6.7	
Holub et al. (2002) [23]	44	114.7	245.7	14.3	7.3	
Holub et al. (1998) [24]	26	127	150	NA	7.7	
Langebrekke et al. (2002) [25]	24	87	NA	5.6	6.2	
Litta et al. (2003) [26]	30	152	153	13.4	6.4	
Manolitsas et al. (2002) [27]	230	121	NA	NA	8.5	
Moore et al. (1999) [28]	45	140	474	11.7	4.1	
Peng et al. (2004) [29]	41	134	259	19.6	9.6	
Scribner et al. (1999) [30]	17	157	344	30	5.2	
Spirtos et al. (1995) [31]	17	NA	NA	29.0	6.4	
Zapico et al. (2005) [32]	38	130	NA	15.0	7.0	
	1039	133	284	14.5	6.8	

*Only patients with a body mass index of 28 to 60.
†Only 11 patients with lymphadenectomy.
‡Only 113 patients with lymphadenectomy.
NA, not available.

Table 16.5.4: Comparison of Postoperative Complications between Laparoscopy and Laparotomy Treatments for Endometrial Cancer

Study	Postoperative Complications, %	
	Laparoscopy	Laparotomy
Kuoppala et al. (2004) [15]	17.5	32.5
Magrina et al. (1995) [16]	20.0	20.0
Occelli et al. (2003) [17]	1.4	6.9
Eltabbakh (2002) [20]	9.0	18.6
Eltabbakh et al. (2000) [21]	7.5	10.0
Holub et al. (2002) [23]	15.2	20.4
Langebrekke et al. (2002) [25]	3.7	4.1
Litta et al. (2003) [26]	0	0
Manolitsas and McCartney (2002) [27]	17.0	43.0
Scribner et al. (1999) [30]	10.5	17.6
Obermair et al. (2005) [34]	21.2	58.0
Tozzi et al. (2005) [35]	23.8	47.4

Table 16.5.5: Comparison of Recurrences after Treatment for Endometrial Cancer by Laparoscopy and Laparotomy

Study	Laparotomy		Laparoscopy	
	Patients, no.	Recurrence, %	Patients, no.	Recurrence, %
Kuoppala et al. (2004) [15]	40	2.0	50	2.5
Eltabbakh (2002) [20]	86	10.5	100	7.0
Holub et al. (2002) [23]	44	6.8	177	6.2
Langebrekke et al. (2002) [25]	22	4.1	26	0
Tozzi et al. (2005) [35]	59	8.5	63	12.6
Obermair et al. (2004) [36]	226	14.9	248	4.0
Total	477	11.7	654	5.4

for 654 laparoscopy patients to be 5.4% (range, 0% to 12.6%) compared with 11.7% (range, 2% to 14.9%) for 477 patients treated by laparotomy (Table 16.5.5).[15,20,23,25,35,36] Analysis of patterns of recurrence demonstrated similar sites of recurrence for laparoscopy and laparotomy.[25,36] We observed no vaginal cuff recurrences, and no vaginal suture line recurrences in patients undergoing vaginal repairs or anti-incontinence procedures.[37] There was not a single instance of trocar site recurrence in any patient in the series we reviewed and report on herein.

Survival

A review of 11 studies of survival rates for endometrial carcinoma patients treated by a laparoscopic approach with a mean length of follow-up of 31.6 months (range, 12 to 76 months) showed the mean disease-free survival rate to be 95.3% (range, 91.2% to 100%) (Table 16.5.6).[15,18,20,23,25,36,38–42]

When endometrial cancer patients treated by laparoscopy or laparotomy are compared, similar disease-free survival rates are observed among both groups of patients. The mean disease-free survival rate for 468 patients treated by laparoscopy was 96% (range, 91.2% to 100%) compared with 94.3% (range, 92% to 95.9%) for 331 laparotomy patients (Table 16.5.7). A review of factors influencing survival showed independent impact by advanced age, higher stage, higher grade, and degree of myometrial invasion. The type of surgical approach (laparoscopy or laparotomy) did not influence survival.[36]

Quality-of-Life Measures

An analysis of quality-of-life measures comparing patients treated by laparoscopy and laparotomy [20] showed a favorable trend for

patients treated laparoscopically. In particular, a mean difference of 21 days was noted for resumption to full activity and of 31.7 days for return to work. Other studies also noted an earlier return to full activity in patients treated laparoscopically.[43] However, no differences were noted for recall of pain control in the two groups of patients (2.4 vs. 2.4), although the laparoscopy patients required a lower mean dose (32.3 mg) of intravenous morphine postoperatively compared with 124.1 mg for laparotomy-treated patients. Nonetheless, no differences were noted for satisfaction with disease management by laparoscopy or laparotomy (2.5 vs. 2.6).

Cost

Cost analyses have indicated similar or reduced costs for the laparoscopic approach compared with the standard open abdominal technique. Of four published studies addressing cost analysis, two reported lower costs for patients in the laparoscopic group [22,31] and two reported similar costs for the two procedures (Table 16.5.8).[21,30] The mean cost for laparoscopy was $10,959 compared with $12,379 for laparotomy, for a $1420 difference. The range of costs for laparoscopy was $5198 to $13,809, compared with $5331 to $17,119 for laparotomy.[21,22,30,31]

In the former two reports [22,31], operating room charges were higher for the laparoscopy group, but the shorter hospitalization resulted in an overall lower cost. In the latter two studies [21,30], similarly increased operative costs were noted for laparoscopy patients, but these were offset by shorter hospitalization. In particular, increased fees for surgeons and anesthesiologists and increased operating room charges were noted for laparoscopy patients, whereas the laparotomy patients incurred increased hospitalization and pharmacy charges.

Contraindications

A laparoscopic approach is contraindicated in any patient with a large uterus that cannot be removed intact through the vagina

Table 16.5.6: Disease-free Survival (DFS) for Laparoscopy-Treated Patients with Endometrial Cancer

Study	Patients, no.	Mean Follow-up, mo.	DFS,%
Kuoppala et al. (2004) [15]	40	34	100
Tozzi et al. (2005) [18]	63	44	91.2
Eltabbakh (2002) [20]	100	27	93
Holub et al. (2002) [23]	177	33.6	93.7
Langebrekke et al. (2002) [25]	27	12	100
Obermair et al. (2004) [36]	226	29.4	98.2
Liauw et al. (2003) [38]	30	15.5	100
Lim et al. (2000) [39]	40	29.5	92.5
Magrina et al. (2004) [40]	45	76	94.7
Malur et al. (2001) [41]	37	16.5	97.3
Siow et al. (2003) [42]	16	20–60	100
Total	801	31.6*	95.3

*Excluding Siow et al. (2003).

Table 16.5.7: Comparison of Disease-free Survival between Laparoscopy- and Laparotomy-Treated Patients with Endometrial Cancer

Reference	Disease-free Survival	
	Laparoscopy, no. (%)	Laparotomy, no. (%)
Kuoppala et al. (2004) [15]	40 (100)	40 (95)
Eltabbakh (2002) [20]	100 (90)	86 (92)
Holub et al. (2002) [23]	177 (93.7)	44 (93.2)
Langebrekke et al. (2002) [25]	27 (100)	24 (95.9)
Peng et al. (2004) [29]	24 (100)	41 (97)
Tozzi et al. (2005) [35]	63 (91.2)	59 (93.8)
Malur et al. (2001) [41]	37 (97.3)	37 (93.3)
Total	468 (96)	331 (94.3)

Table 16.5.8: Overall Cost Analysis Comparison between Laparoscopy and Laparotomy for Endometrial Cancer

Study	Laparoscopy cost, US $	Laparotomy cost, US $
Eltabbakh (2002) [20]	13,003	11,878
Gemignani et al. (1999) [22]	11,826	15,189
Scribner et al. (1999) [30]	5198	5331
Spirtos et al. (1996) [43]	13,809	17,119

and also in medically compromised patients for whom a laparoscopic approach might not be safe. In our experience, medically compromised patients are almost exclusively obese patients with respiratory compromise. Although no reports have attested to the risks of morcellating a uterus containing malignancy, it violates the elemental principle of cancer surgery of extirpating an intact tumor site whenever possible. Obesity, in the absence of respiratory deficit, should not be a contraindication in the hands of an expert anesthesiologist and gynecologic oncologist. Nor does a history of adhesions contraindicate laparoscopy. If thick, dense adhesions preventing laparoscopy are noted on entry, the surgeon would soon realize a laparotomy is necessary. However, many patients with a history of previous pelvic surgeries may have a paucity of adhesions or those they do have may be easily lysed so the planned procedure can be carried out. In such instances, a different placement or additional insertion of trocars may be necessary.

SPECIAL CLINICAL SITUATIONS

Morbidly Obese Patients

As the body mass index increases and the thickness of the subcutaneous tissue increases, so do the difficulty of the operation and the risk of postlaparotomy wound infection, respectively. Laparoscopy is and should continue to be the preferred approach for morbidly obese patients, even if only to eliminate or reduce the risk of wound infection, evisceration, or subsequent ventral hernia formation.

There are no major contraindications to use of the Trendelenburg position for morbidly obese patients. It does, however, require a more labor-intensive anesthesia because prompt ventilation adjustments are needed throughout the operation and the anesthesiologist must maintain a watchful eye for hypercarbia.

The feasibility of the laparoscopic approach in obese patients has been demonstrated. Endometrial cancer can be treated successfully in the majority of obese and morbidly obese patients. Of 91 morbidly obese patients treated by laparoscopy in three studies, 83 (91.2%) had a successful procedure. [21,34, 44] When conversions due to advanced disease or other anatomic or abnormal surgical findings are excluded, the success rate is 95.7% for conversions due only to intraoperative complications.[15,20,23,25,29,35,41]

Perioperative differences noted between the two groups are similar to those observed between lower-weight patients (Table 16.5.2). Compared with the laparotomy group, the laparoscopy patients had similar or longer operating times, similar or reduced blood loss, and shorter hospitalization.[21,34,44] Other authors have noted similar findings among obese patients.[27]

Obese laparotomy patients experienced a wound infection rate 28 times higher than that of laparoscopy patients (54.2% vs. 1.9%; Table 16.5.9) [21,34,44], securing an important reason for selection of a laparoscopic approach in such patients. In one small study, all four of four laparotomy patients had wound infection whereas none of the four laparoscopy patients experienced wound infection.[44] In another study, wound infections occurred in 15 of 31 laparotomy patients (48.4%) but in only one of 47 laparoscopy patients (2.1%) converted to laparotomy.[34]

In the presence of a markedly thick and redundant abdominal pannus, the laparoscopic trocar may not be long enough to

Table 16.5.9: Comparison of Perioperative Laparoscopy and Laparotomy Data for Obese Patients with Endometrial Cancer

Study	Patients, no.	Mean Operating Time, min.	Mean Blood Loss, mL	Mean Lymph Nodes, no.	Mean Hospital Stay, days	Conversion to Laparotomy,%	Wound Infection,%
Laparoscopy							
Eltabbakh et al. (2000) [21]*	40	195	318	11.3	2.5	2.5	NA
Obermair et al. (2005) [34]†	47	139	279	7.9	4.4	6.3	2.5‡
Yu et al. (2005) [44]	4	154	325	NA	4	0	0
Total	91	163	307	9.6	3.6	4.4	1.3
Laparotomy							
Eltabbakh et al. (2000) [21]*	86	138	303	5.3	5.6	—	NA
Obermair et al. (2005) [34]§	31	127	320	20.0	7.9		48.4
Yu et al. (2005) [44]	4	143	700	NA	11.5		100.0
Total	121	136	441	12.7	8.3		74.2

*Body mass index between 28 and 60 (weight [kg]/height [m^2]).
†Mean weight, 121.6 kg.
‡The only patient with wound infection had a laparotomy conversion.
§Mean weight, 113.7 kg.
NA, not available.

reach or penetrate sufficiently into the abdominal cavity. With such patients, the torque necessary to manipulate the laparoscopic instruments may also result in arm fatigue or detract from precision. Removal of the pannus, a medically indicated panniculectomy, not an abdominoplasty, allows direct placement of the trocars on the anterior abdominal wall fascia and facilitates the performance of the laparoscopic approach. The postpanniculectomy wound infection rate is lower than that after a conventional laparotomy incision in similarly obese patients.[45] In a series of 87 noncosmetic panniculectomy patients with endometrial cancer operated on at the Mayo Clinic, the wound infection rate was 2.3%. This finding compares favorably with the wound infection rate of 2.3% observed in 1179 gynecologic inpatients operated on at the same institution.[45]

In morbidly obese patients, our approach is to perform a vaginal hysterectomy and a bilateral salpingo-oophorectomy in select patients with endometrioid, low-grade tumors and then to proceed with staging if indicated by frozen section. This approach shortens the laparoscopic operating time, if it is indicated on the basis of prognostic factors by the frozen section, and it also eliminates the demands of a more challenging laparoscopic hysterectomy or panniculectomy.

SURGICAL STAGING AFTER UNEXPECTED ENDOMETRIAL CANCER IN A HYSTERECTOMY SPECIMEN

Laparoscopy is useful for completion of disease treatment and for surgical staging in patients found to have an unexpected endometrial cancer after a hysterectomy performed for benign indications. In a series of 13 such patients, laparoscopic staging was useful in removing the remaining adnexa and in detecting extrauterine disease in three patients (23%; one with positive peritoneal cytologic findings and two with positive pelvic nodes).[46] These patients had no intraoperative complications, had a mean operative blood loss of 50 mL, and had a mean hospital stay of 1.5 days (range, 0 to 3 days). The mean interval from hysterectomy to laparoscopy was 47 days (range, 14 to 63 days). One patient who experienced deep venous thrombosis after being discharged was readmitted for anticoagulation treatment.

Recurrent Endometrial Cancer

Patients with a pelvic recurrence of endometrial carcinoma after initial surgery or after surgery followed by irradiation are candidates for salvage therapy, in particular those with involvement of the vaginal cuff. Some patients with clinically apparent isolated pelvic or vaginal recurrence have concomitant metastatic disease at additional abdominal sites, which may go undetected even with advanced imaging techniques. In a series of eight patients with pelvic recurrence explored by laparotomy, three (37.5%) had upper abdominal disease. In patients with central pelvic recurrence who are candidates for pelvic exenteration, the procedure is abandoned at laparotomy about one third of the time.[47] Reasons for unresectability are direct peritoneal involvement by tumor, intra-abdominal peritoneal disease, retroperitoneal nodal disease, and involvement of the lateral pelvic wall.[47] In a series of 31 patients with recurrent endometrial carcinoma who were candidates for exenteration, the procedure was abandoned in four (12.9%).[48] Reasons included intraperitoneal metastases, positive retroperitoneal nodes (pelvic or aortic), and lung metastases. Laparoscopic peritoneal and retroperitoneal exploration before pelvic irradiation, upper vaginectomy, or exenteration affords detection of intraperitoneal and retroperitoneal metastatic sites. These patients obviously require a different therapeutic approach, and their recurrent disease carries a much worse prognosis. In our experience with two patients with recurrent endometrial cancer after irradiation, pre-exenteration laparoscopy revealed the presence of an unresectable tumor affixed to the common iliac vessels and sacral promontory in one patient and peritoneal invasion by a tumor in the other patient. A laparotomy was avoided in both patients. In two series that included 21 pre-exenteration laparoscopic explorations for recurrent cervical cancer, laparotomy was avoided in 12 patients (57.1%) who had contraindications because of metastases.[49,50] The mean operating time was 112 to 150 minutes.[49,50] Patients were hospitalized for 3 days and were able to initiate chemotherapy on the second postoperative day.[49]

Pre-exenteration laparoscopy is a valuable tool for potential candidates because it eliminates unnecessary laparotomies, decreases surgical morbidity in already compromised patients, reduces unused operating room time, and alleviates the emotional burden on patients in whom it is not performed. The overall exenteration time is reduced because of the previous exploration, because patients are aware of the extent of the operation, and because operating room efficiency is increased because none of the planned exenterations is aborted.

CONCLUSION

When perioperative results for endometrial cancer patients treated by laparoscopy or laparotomy are analyzed, patients treated by laparoscopy are found to have reduced operative blood loss and hospitalization, increased operating time, a similar or reduced number of lymph nodes, and a similar or reduced number of postoperative complications. Tumor recurrence and disease-free survival rates are similar for both groups of patients, whereas costs remain reduced for laparoscopy-treated patients because of their shorter hospitalization.

The type of surgical approach (laparoscopy or laparotomy) was the only identified significant risk factor predictive of intra- and postoperative complications for patients 65 years of age or older, weighing more than 80 kg, and with a Quetelet index of more than 30. In this particular group of patients, laparoscopy is associated with a significantly lower risk of complications. Obese or morbidly obese patients have similar results and advantages compared with lower-weight patients, and they are ideal candidates for laparoscopy. In such patients, the risk of wound infection is reduced 39 times when the procedure is performed laparoscopically.

If either of two cancer treatments provides similar survival and recurrence rates and is associated with a lower morbidity, it should be the preferred therapeutic approach. Such is the case for the primary surgical treatment of patients with endometrial cancer when considering whether to treat them with laparoscopy or laparotomy. Unfortunately, it will take a new generation of gynecologic oncologists trained in advanced laparoscopic techniques before the laparoscopic approach will become universal for treatment of endometrial cancer.

REFERENCES

1. Cragun J, Havrilesky L, Calingaert B, et al. Retrospective analysis of selective lymphadenectomy in apparent early-stage endometrial cancer. *J Clin Oncol.* 2005;23:3668–3675.

2. Kilgore L, Partridge E, Alvarez R, et al. Adenocarcinoma of the endometrium: survival comparisons of patients with and without pelvic node sampling. *Gynecol Oncol.* 1995;56:29–33.

3. Onda T, Yoshikawa H, Maizutani K, et al. Treatment of node-positive endometrial cancer with complete node dissection, chemotherapy and radiation therapy. *Br J Cancer.* 1997;75:1836–1841.

4. Mariani A, Webb M, Galli L, Podratz K. Potential therapeutic role of para-aortic lymphadenectomy in node-positive endometrial cancer. *Gynecol Oncol.* 2000;76:348–356.

5. Podratz K, Mariani A, Webb M. Staging and therapeutic value of lymphadenectomy in endometrial cancer [editorial]. *Gynecol Oncol.* 1998;70:163–164.

6. Mariani A, Webb M, Keeney G, Haddock M, Calori G, Podratz K. Low-risk corpus cancer: is lymphadenectomy or radiotherapy necessary? *Am J Obstet Gynecol.* 2000;182:1506–1519.

7. Schink J, Rademaker A, Miller D, Lurain J. Tumor size in endometrial cancer. *Cancer.* 1991;67:2791–2794.

8. Mariani A, Webb M, Keeney G, Podratz K. Routes of lymphatic spread: a study of 112 consecutive patients with endometrial cancer. *Gynecol Oncol.* 2001;81:100–104.

9. Mariani A, Webb M, Galli L, Podratz K. Endometrial carcinoma: paraaortic dissemination. *Gynecol Oncol.* 2004;92:833–838.

10. McMeekin D, Lashbrook D, Gold M, Johnson G, Walker J, Mannel R. Analysis of FIGO Stage IIIc endometrial cancer patients. *Gynecol Oncol.* 2001;81:273–278.

11. Ayhan A, Tuncer Z, Tuncer R, Yuce K, Kucukali T. Tumor status of lymph nodes in early endometrial cancer in relation to lymph node size. *Eur J Obstet Gynecol Reprod Biol.* 1995;60:61–63.

12. Fanning J, Nanavati P, Hilgers R. Surgical staging and high dose rate brachytherapy for endometrial cancer: limiting external radiotherapy to node-positive tumors. *Obstet Gynecol.* 1996;87:1041–1044.

13. Hirahatake K, Hareyama H, Sakuragi N, Nishiya M, Makinoda S, Fujimoto S. A clinical and pathologic study on para-aortic lymph node metastasis in endometrial carcinoma. *J Surg Oncol.* 1997;65:82–87.

14. Larson D, Johnson K. Pelvic and para-aortic lymphadenectomy for surgical staging of high-risk endometrioid adenocarcinoma of the endometrium. *Gynecol Oncol.* 1993;51:345–348.

15. Kuoppala T, Tomas E, Heinonen P. Clinical outcome and complications of laparoscopic surgery compared with traditional surgery in women with endometrial cancer. *Arch Gynecol Obstet.* 2004;270:25–30.

16. Magrina J, Serrano L, Cornella J. Laparoscopic lymphadenectomy and radical or modified radical vaginal hysterectomy for endometrial and cervical carcinoma – preliminary experience. *J Gynecol Surg.* 1995;11:147–151.

17. Occelli B, Samouelian V, Narducci F, Leblanc E, Querleu D. The choice of approach in the surgical management of endometrial carcinoma: a retrospective series of 155 cases [in French]. *Bull Cancer.* 2003;90:347–355.

18. Tozzi R, Malur S, Koehler C, Schneider A. Laparoscopy versus laparotomy in endometrial cancer: first analysis of survival of a randomized prospective study. *J Minim Invasive Gynecol.* 2005;12:130–136.

19. Boike G, Lurain J, Burke J. A comparison of laparoscopic management of endometrial cancer with traditional laparotomy. *Gynecol Oncol.* 1994;52:105.

20. Eltabbakh G. Analysis of survival after laparoscopy in women with endometrial carcinoma. *Cancer.* 2002;95:1894–1901.

21. Eltabbakh G, Shamonki M, Moody J, Garafano L. Hysterectomy for obese women with endometrial cancer: laparoscopy or laparotomy? *Gynecol Oncol.* 2000;78:329–335.

22. Gemignani M, Curtin J, Zelmanovich J, Patel D, Venkatraman E, Barakat R. Laparoscopic-assisted vaginal hysterectomy

for endometrial cancer: clinical outcomes and hospital charges. *Gynecol Oncol.* 1999;73:5–11.

23. Holub Z, Jabor A, Bartos P, Eim J, Urbanek S, Pivovarnikova R. Laparoscopic surgery for endometrial cancer: long-term results of a multicentric study. *Eur J Gynaecol Oncol.* 2002;23:305–310.

24. Holub Z, Voracek J, Shomani A. A comparison of laparoscopic surgery with open procedure in endometrial cancer. *Eur J Gynaecol Oncol.* 1998;19:294–296.

25. Langebrekke A, Istre O, Hallqvist A, Hartgill T, Onsrud M. Comparison of laparoscopy and laparotomy in patients with endometrial cancer. *J Am Assoc Gynecol Laparosc.* 2002;9:152–157.

26. Litta P, Fracas M, Pozzan C, et al. Laparoscopic management of early stage endometrial cancer. *Eur J Gynaecol Oncol.* 2003;24:41–44.

27. Manolitsas T, McCartney A. Total laparoscopic hysterectomy in the management of endometrial carcinoma. *J Am Assoc Gynecol Laparosc.* 2002;9:54–62.

28. Moore J, Hatch K, Hallum A 3d, Magdy N. Comparison of laparoscopic assisted vaginal hysterectomy with total abdominal hysterectomy for the management of endometrial cancer. Abstract presented at: the 30th Annual Meeting of the Society of Gynecologic Oncologists; March 20–24; San Francisco, CA.

29. Peng P, Huang H, Shen K, et al. Comparative analysis of laparoscopic surgery and laparotomy for early stage endometrial cancer. *Chinese J Obstet Gynecol.* 2004;39:165–168.

30. Scribner D, Mannel R, Walker J, Johnson G. Cost analysis of laparoscopy versus laparotomy for early endometrial cancer. *Gynecol Oncol.* 1999;75:460–463.

31. Spirtos N, Schlaerth J, Spirtos T, Schlaerth A, Indman P, Kimball R. Laparoscopic bilateral pelvic and paraaortic lymph node sampling: an evolving technique. *Am J Obstet Gynecol.* 1995;173:105–111.

32. Zapico A, Fuentes P, Grassa A, Arnanz F, Otazua J, Cortes-Prieto J. Laparoscopic-assisted vaginal hysterectomy versus abdominal hysterectomy in stages I and II endometrial cancer. Operating data, follow up and survival. *Gynecol Oncol.* 2005;98:222–227.

33. Magrina J. Laparoscopic surgery for gynecologic cancers. *Clin Obstet Gynecol.* 2000;43:619–640.

34. Obermair A, Manolitsas T, Leung Y, Hammond I, McCartney A. Total laparoscopic hysterectomy versus total abdominal hysterectomy for obese women with endometrial cancer. *Int J Gynecol Cancer.* 2005;15:319–324.

35. Tozzi R, Malur S, Koehler C, Schneider A. Analysis of morbidity in patients with endometrial cancer: is there a commitment to offer laparoscopy? *Gynecol Oncol.* 2005;97:4–9.

36. Obermair A, Manolitsas T, Leung Y, Hammond I, McCartney A. Total laparoscopic hysterectomy for endometrial cancer: patterns of recurrence and survival. *Gynecol Oncol.* 2004;92:789–793.

37. Magrina J, Mutone N, Weaver A, Magtibay P, Fowler R, Cornella J. Laparoscopic lymphadenectomy and vaginal or laparoscopic hysterectomy with bilateral salpingo-oophorectomy for endometrial cancer: morbidity and survival. *Am J Obstet Gynecol.* 1999;181:376–381.

38. Liauw L, Chung Y, Tsoi C, Cheung K. Laparoscopy for the treatment of women with endometrial cancer. *Hong Kong Med J.* 2003;9:108–112.

39. Lim B, Lavie O, Bolger B, Lopes T, Monaghan J. The role of laparoscopic surgery in the management of endometrial cancer. *BJOG.* 2000;107:24–27.

40. Magrina J, Weaver A. Laparoscopic treatment of endometrial cancer: five-year recurrence and survival rates. *Eur J Gynaecol Oncol.* 2004;25:439–441.

41. Malur S, Possover M, Michaels W, Schneider A. Laparoscopic-assisted vaginal versus abdominal surgery in patients with endometrial cancer – a prospective randomized trial. *Gynecol Oncol.* 2001;80:239–244.

42. Siow A, Beh S, Tay E. Initial experience of laparoscopic management of apparent early endometrial cancer. *Singapore Med J.* 2003;44:288–292.

43. Spirtos N, Schlaerth J, Bross G, Spirtos T, Schlaerth A, Ballon S. Cost and quality-of-life analyses of surgery for early endometrial cancer: laparotomy versus laparoscopy. *Am J Obstet Gynecol.* 1996;174:1795–1800.

44. Yu C, Cutner A, Mould T, Olaitan A. Total laparoscopic hysterectomy as a primary surgical treatment for endometrial cancer in morbidly obese women. *BJOG.* 2005;112:115–117.

45. Stanhope C, Winburn K, Silverman M. Indicated noncosmetic panniculectomy in gynecologic surgery. *J Pelvic Surg.* 2002;8:197–201.

46. Childers J, Brzechffa P, Hatch K, Surwit E. Laparoscopically assisted surgical staging (LASS) of endometrial cancer. *Gynecol Oncol.* 1993;51:33–38.

47. Miller B, Morris M, Rutledge F, et al. Aborted exenterative procedures in recurrent cervical cancer. *Gynecol Oncol.* 1993;50:94–99.

48. Morris M, Alvarez R, Kinney W, Wilson T. Treatment of recurrent adenocarcinoma of the endometrium with pelvic exenteration. *Gynecol Oncol.* 1996;60:288–291.

49. Dargent D, Ansquer Y, Mathevet P. Can laparoscopic para-aortic lymphadenectomy help to select patients with pelvic relapse of cervical cancer patients eligible for pelvic exenteration [letter to the editor]? *Gynecol Oncol.* 1999;73:172.

50. Plante M, Roy M. Operative laparoscopy prior to a pelvic exenteration in patients with recurrent cervical cancer. *Gynecol Oncol.* 1998;69:94–99.

Section 16.6. Laparoscopic Management of Ovarian Cancer

Ali Mahdavi and Farr Nezhat

The American Cancer Society estimates that more than 22,000 women will be diagnosed with ovarian cancer in 2007.[1] Of these 22,000 patients, 25% will have stage I disease, for which 5-year survival rates approach 90%. However, numerous studies have shown that a significant percentage of patients with apparent early-stage (stage I) ovarian cancer actually harbor microscopic metastatic disease. Consequently, the benefits of surgical staging for epithelial ovarian carcinoma have been well established.[2] Traditionally, it has been recommended that a comprehensive surgical staging procedure for epithelial ovarian and fallopian tube cancers include a total abdominal hysterectomy, bilateral salpingo-oophorectomy, peritoneal cytologic washings, biopsies of adhesions and peritoneal surfaces, omentectomy, and retroperitoneal lymph node sampling from the pelvic and para-aortic regions through a generous vertical midline laparotomy incision.[2] With the advent of minimally invasive surgical techniques, surgeons are now able to perform all of the necessary procedures for comprehensive surgical staging laparoscopically, including laparoscopic pelvic and para-aortic lymphadenectomies and omentectomies, in selected patients. Small series of laparoscopic staging of early ovarian cancer (EOC) have been reported, and preliminary data suggest that the minimally invasive approach in experienced hands is adequate to perform comprehensive surgical staging.[3]

Querleu and Leblanc [4] in 1994 reported complete laparoscopic surgical staging procedures for ovarian or fallopian tube cancer. Eight referred patients with ovarian and fallopian tube cancers underwent complete laparoscopic staging after inadequate initial surgical staging. Since this initial series, others have confirmed the feasibility of comprehensive laparoscopic surgical staging of ovarian or fallopian tube cancers.[5]

Recently, the results of a GOG study [6] to determine the feasibility of laparoscopic completion staging in patients with incompletely staged gynecologic cancers were reported. Of 95 eligible patients, 73 had incompletely staged ovarian, fallopian tube, or primary peritoneal cancer. Eleven patients were later excluded based on pathology review, progression of the disease, or incomplete documentation. Fifty-eight (69%) of these 84 patients were successfully completely staged with photographic documentation. Nine (10%) and 17 (20%) of 84 patients were incompletely staged or required conversion to laparotomy, respectively. In patients undergoing laparoscopy, 6% had bowel complications and 11% were found to have more advanced disease. Hospital stay was significantly shorter with laparoscopy alone (3 vs. 6 days, $P = 0.04$). The investigators concluded that interval laparoscopic staging of gynecologic malignancies can be successfully undertaken in selected patients, but laparotomy for adhesions or metastatic disease and risk of visceral injury should be anticipated.

One of the largest and most recent reports is by Tozzi and colleagues [7], who described 24 cases of ovarian cancer in which laparoscopic staging was performed. In this series, all surgical specimens, except for the primary ovarian tumor(s), were free of disease. One patient (4%) developed a postoperative complication, and no long-term complications were noted. Seven patients (29%) had tumors of low malignant potential, and six (25%) had stromal or germ cell tumors. Five (21%) of the 24 patients received postoperative chemotherapy. With a median follow-up of 46 months, the disease-free survival rate was 92% and the overall survival rate was 100%. Although these survival results are difficult to interpret in a patient cohort in which less than half the patients (11/24) had invasive carcinomas, the average of 38 lymph nodes per patient compares favorably with series of both laparoscopic staging and staging performed via laparotomy. Moreover, this study demonstrates that with proper training and experience, extensive laparoscopic lymphadenectomies can be performed with minimal morbidity. The major advantages in patients with EOC treated by laparoscopy were the lower rate of intra- and postoperative complications and the shorter length of hospitalization. A reported rate of complications ranging between 10% and 30% in patients with EOC staged or restaged by laparotomy exceeds the 3% to 7% rate reported in patients who underwent laparoscopy. A faster recovery may be relevant for the administration of chemotherapy in patients upstaged as a result of the restaging procedure. Whether delay in starting the adjuvant chemotherapy has a prognostic impact is yet to be demonstrated, but because clear data are lacking, the procedure associated with less morbidity should be followed. Survival outcomes, such as disease-free and overall survival, were in the range of 90% to 100% for laparoscopy and did not differ in patients managed by laparotomy. The number of patients was probably too small to definitively rule out an influence of laparoscopy on tumor growth. However, the absence of trocar metastasis and the favorable prognosis indicated that laparoscopy did not promote or induce tumor dissemination as postulated in some case reports.[8]

BORDERLINE OVARIAN TUMORS

Borderline ovarian tumors (BOTs) do not invade the basal membrane but may spread widely across peritoneal surfaces. They tend to occur in patients younger than those with invasive epithelial ovarian cancer, and their prognosis is better than the latter. Fifteen percent to 40% of serous BOTs are associated with peritoneal disease. The prognosis for such patients with advanced-stage disease is perceptibly different from those with stage I disease. The most important prognostic factor is the type of peritoneal implants (invasive or noninvasive). Prognosis of patients with noninvasive implants remains good if the totality of peritoneal implants is removed. The treatment is exclusively surgical, without adjuvant treatment. In selected cases of young patients with advanced-stage disease, a conservative surgery could be proposed to maintain fertility.[9]

The use of the laparoscopic approach to conservatively treat BOTs appears attractive because such management theoretically reduces postoperative adhesions and therefore could increase fertility results. There are few data on the laparoscopic management of BOTs. Three series were published and one was reported in abstract.[10–12] These papers demonstrated that laparoscopic treatment of BOTs is feasible and safe in patients with early-stage disease (apparent "stage I" disease). In addition, pregnancies after laparoscopic staging have been reported. Seracchioli et al. [11] reported six pregnancies among 19 patients, Camatte et al. [10] described 17 pregnancies in 34 patients, and 12 pregnancies were reported in the series of Donnez et al.[12] Therefore, laparoscopic staging of BOTs is attractive, particularly in young patients desiring pregnancy.

There are very few data on the laparoscopic management of advanced-stage borderline tumors. Deffieux et al. [13] reported nine patients who underwent a laparoscopic treatment of stage II/III serous borderline tumor. Laparoscopic treatment of peritoneal implants included omentectomy (or omental biopsies) in four patients and/or large peritoneal resection in five patients. Each implant was less than 5 mm. Four patients recurred; three of them had a borderline ovarian recurrence after conservative management. Two patients had peritoneal disease found during a second-look surgery (associated with ovarian recurrence in one). Three spontaneous pregnancies were observed. All patients were alive without evidence of disease with a median time of follow-up of 35 months following the laparoscopic treatment. This series suggests that laparoscopic treatment of patients with BOTs associated with small-size noninvasive implants is feasible, seems to be safe, and remains an attractive alternative for young patients wishing to preserve their fertility.

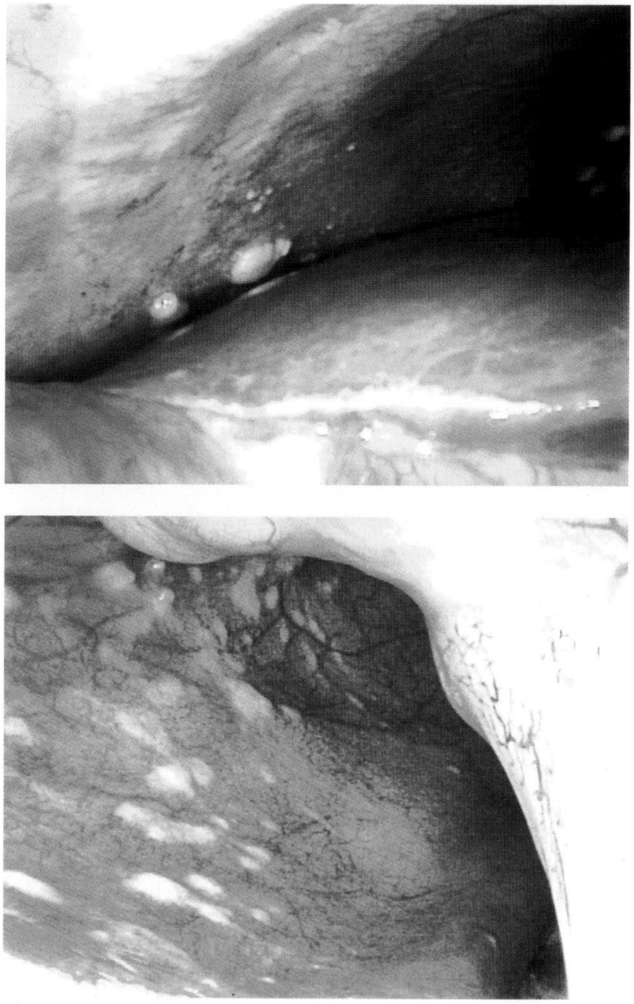

SURGICAL TECHNIQUE

A multipuncture operative laparoscopic approach is used as previously described.[14] A 0° 5- or 10-mm transumbilical videolaparoscope is used. Pelvic washings are collected for cytology, and parietal and visceral peritoneal surfaces of the deep pelvis and middle and upper abdominal cavities are thoroughly inspected (Figure 16.6.1). Any suspicious growth is biopsied. In the case of normal visual exploration, eight to 10 random peritoneal biopsies are performed in the Douglas pouch, pelvic and abdominal parietal peritoneum, paracolic gutters, hemidiaphragms, and mesentery. Small and large bowel can also be carefully inspected laparoscopically. "Running" the small bowel can be accomplished from the ileocecal valve to the ligament of Treitz using two atraumatic bowel graspers (Figure 16.6.2). When conservative treatment is considered, biopsy of the contralateral ovary is performed only in the case of suspicious growth. In this context, dilatation and curettage are performed so as not to miss a possible endometrial spread or a synchronous tumor. Every attempt should be made to avoid the rupture of a suspicious adnexal mass in the abdomen, including choosing unilateral adnexectomy over ovarian cystec-

Figure 16.6.1. Metastatic lesions of the right hemidiaphragm and cul-de-sac are noted in the upper abdomen and deep pelvis upon initial inspection.

tomy, limited manipulation of the mass, use of nontraumatic graspers, and preventive coagulation to avoid bleeding, which may obscure the identification of the cleavage planes. Additional safety measures are the removal of the specimen exclusively via a laparoscopic bag and control of the bag integrity once extracted (Figure 16.6.3). Laparoscopy is intrinsically limited by the size of the trocar incisions. Even when the incision is enlarged, a puncture is required to remove large masses. If the puncture can be located within an Endobag (United States Surgical), and the Endobag's integrity is preserved, the procedure is safe according to previous findings.

To achieve an infracolic omentectomy, the patient is placed in a straight supine position and the omentum is excised from the inferior margin of the transverse colon using a harmonic scalpel, a bipolar forceps and Endoshears (United States Surgical), a linear stapler, endoligature, or sutures. The harmonic scalpel and endoligature are superior for omentectomy because of minimal plume formation, ease and speed of use, and lack of protruding staple edges (Figure 16.6.4). The omentum specimen can also be removed with an Endobag (Figure 16.6.5).

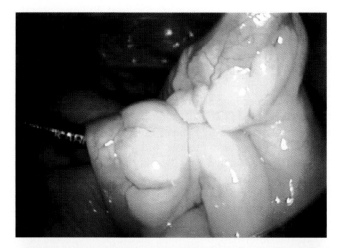

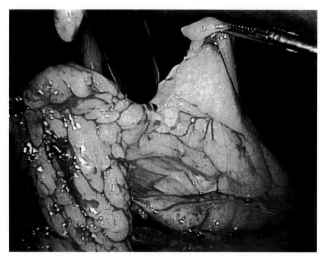

Figure 16.6.4. Laparoscopic omentectomy using the harmonic scalpel.

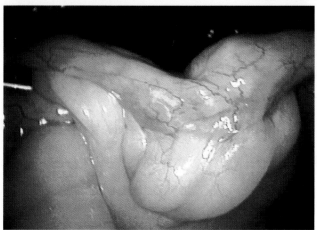

Figure 16.6.2. "Running" the small bowel using atraumatic bowel graspers.

surgeon while the second assistant is at the bottom of the table, between the patient's legs. The peritoneum overlying the psoas muscle is incised from the round ligament to the base of the infundibular pelvic ligament. External and internal iliac vessels, their major branches, and the ureter are delineated and the avascular spaces developed. Following delineation of the anatomy of the pelvic side wall, sampling or complete removal of all nodal packets along the external and internal iliac vessels and the obturator fossa is performed. While held with a grasper, the lymphatic tissue is teased off the underlying vessels using either a suction–irrigator probe or ultrasonic shears. The feeding lymphatic and vascular channels are isolated and then coagulated and divided using low and high ultrasonic power, respectively. Lymph nodes are retrieved through the suprapubic trocar sleeve (10/12 mm) avoiding contamination of the abdominal wall.

For para-aortic lymph node dissection, the room setup and trocar placement is similar to that for pelvic lymphadenectomy with the laparoscope introduced through the umbilical port. An additional 5-mm port is placed in the left or right mid-abdomen

Transperitoneal pelvic and/or para-aortic lymph node dissection is performed as previously described.[14] For pelvic lymph node retrievals, the primary surgeon stands on either side of the patient facing the monitors, which are positioned on both sides of the patient's legs. The first assistant stands across from the

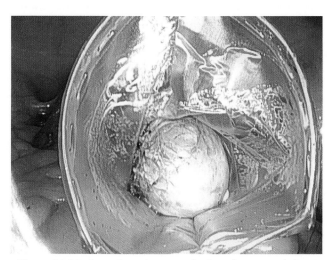

Figure 16.6.3. A specimen is removed using a laparoscopic bag.

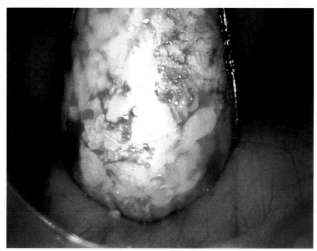

Figure 16.6.5. The omentum specimen is removed using an endoscopic specimen bag.

lateral to the rectus muscle for introduction of the ultrasonic shears. When para-aortic lymphadenectomy is extended to the level of the left renal vein, the laparoscope is moved from the transumbilical port to another port placed approximately 3 to 5 cm higher in the midline. The patient is placed in steep Trendelenburg position; the bowel is directed toward the upper abdomen and is held in that position with a grasper or laparoscopic fan. The peritoneum is incised over the right common iliac artery, and the incision is extended cephalad over the inferior vena cava and lower abdominal aorta to the level of the duodenum, exposing the ureters, ovarian vessels, and inferior mesenteric artery. The nodal packets are removed using the technique described for the pelvic lymphadenectomy using the ultrasonic shears. All precaval and para-aortic nodes are removed from the bifurcation of the common iliac arteries up to the level of the renal vein. Following the procedure, no drains are placed and all retroperitoneal spaces are left open.

ASSESSMENT OF THE FEASIBILITY OF LAPAROSCOPIC OPTIMAL CYTOREDUCTIVE SURGERY IN OVARIAN CANCER

Residual disease after surgery is one of the most important prognostic factors for patients with advanced ovarian cancer [15], and the complete excision of all measurable disease has been shown to provide better survival compared with leaving small amounts (1 to 2 cm) of residual tumor. However, depending on individual institutions, surgical skills, and aggressiveness, the percentage of patients with no measurable tumor following debulking surgery ranges from 8% to 85%.[16] Furthermore, some patients originally selected for debulking treatment will be able to undergo only explorative laparotomy because of extremely advanced disease.

An accurate and reliable method should be pursued to avoid unnecessary explorative laparotomies and to better select patients for surgical and/or medical specific treatments. Bristow et al. [17] elaborated a "predictive index model" based on preoperative CT scanning, which is highly accurate in recognizing patients with advanced epithelial ovarian carcinoma unlikely to undergo optimal primary cytoreductive surgery. However, the study did not address the appropriateness of extensive open surgical staging, a keystone in the management of patients with advanced ovarian cancer.

Recently, Fagotti et al. [18] compared the power of laparoscopy with the standard explorative laparotomy in predicting optimal cytoreduction in the same group of advanced ovarian cancer patients. The few well-known indicators of unresectability (i.e., extensive bulky carcinomatosis, agglutinated bowel/mesentery, diaphragm bulky disease, and unresectable upper abdominal metastases) were investigated by laparoscopy. The accuracy rate of laparoscopy in predicting the laparotomic probability of each one of these parameters ranged from 80% to 100%. In particular, all cases with peritoneal and/or diaphragmatic carcinomatosis and/or mesentery disease were correctly identified by laparoscopy (positive predictive value [PPV] = 100%, 82%, and 100%, respectively), resulting in an overall predictive judgment of unresectability, or negative predictive value (NPV) of 100%. In this context, NPV represents a very important clinical parameter, that is, the rate of inappropriate nonexploration or the ratio of patients thought to have unresectable disease but who will in fact undergo optimal surgery if operated on. This measure corresponds to the false-negative rate and in this study was zero, because in no case was the laparoscopic decision changed by the immediately following laparotomy. In this study, an optimal debulking was achievable in 34 of 39 cases (87%) selected as completely resectable by explorative laparoscopy.

In the recent paper, Bristow et al. [17] described the combination of clinical and radiologic parameters that can provide a very accurate score to identify patients unlikely to undergo primary cytoreductive surgery. In Fagotti's study [18], laparoscopy showed a higher NPV compared with the clinical–radiologic evaluation (100% vs. 73%) whereas the PPV is superimposable between the two techniques. As a consequence, those patients considered resectable by preoperative clinical–radiologic assessment would probably not benefit from laparoscopy, which seems not to add any further information regarding the surgical outcome of the patients. On the contrary, cases judged unresectable by clinical–radiologic evaluation could really benefit from a laparoscopic approach that can improve the predicted surgical outcome and provide a histologic diagnosis by a less traumatic access.

SECOND-LOOK LAPAROSCOPY AND INSERTION OF INTRAPERITONEAL CATHETERS

The role of second-look surgery in the management of advanced epithelial ovarian cancer is controversial. High recurrence rates after negative histologic findings, the lack of consistently effective salvage therapy, and the absence of data showing improved survival benefits have diminished acceptance of the routine use of second-look surgery. Nevertheless, patients with suboptimal initial cytoreductive surgery for stage III ovarian cancer who have a complete clinical response to platinum-based combination chemotherapy appear to achieve a distinct survival benefit from second-look surgical procedures.[19] The management of advanced epithelial ovarian cancer includes surgical staging and aggressive debulking by laparotomy followed by intravenous chemotherapy. Nevertheless, even in cases of a good response after optimal debulking surgery and intravenous chemotherapy, 50% of the patients with no clinical evidence of residual disease will suffer a recurrence because of the presence of microscopic peritoneal implants. In those patients, the failure of second-line intravenous chemotherapy to control residual disease has led to the use of intraperitoneal chemotherapies for small microscopic residual disease.

Until recently, second-look procedures and insertion of intraperitoneal catheters were almost always carried out by laparotomy or "blind" surgical technique. With the improvement of instrumentation and surgical techniques, we are now able to perform these procedures by laparoscopy.

Considering that all patients were previously operated on by laparotomy, we prefer to introduce the trocar in the left upper quadrant as previously discussed. Three 5- or 10-mm trocars are then inserted in places free of any adhesion. The sites of the trocars are chosen according to the site of planned adhesiolysis.

Peritoneal washings are performed for cytologic evaluation. Subsequently, adhesiolysis between the small or large bowel and the abdominal wall is first performed with the help of laparoscopic scissors and harmonic shears. Every aspect of the abdominal cavity, the entire surface of the parietal peritoneum, and the surfaces of the intraperitoneal organs are observed. Biopsies from the pelvic side walls, the pelvic cul-de-sac, the bladder, the paracolic gutters, and the diaphragm are taken. Small peritoneal tumors may also be resected and put into an intraperitoneal bag for abdominal extraction. A 5-mm polyurethane catheter (Sims Deltec, Inc., St Paul, MN) is then inserted into the abdomen via a 5-mm trocar transfixing the left rectus abdominis muscle. A laparoscopic forceps holds the intraperitoneal part of the catheter, and the 5-mm trocar is then withdrawn. The laparoscopic entry incision is then prolonged vertically and cranially over the ninth and eighth ribs on the mid-clavicular line. The laparoscope entry site is closed layer by layer and carefully flushed. A peritoneal pocket is then created by dissecting the tissue over the eighth and ninth ribs. A laparoscopic forceps is introduced through this incision, running on the aponeurosis toward the catheter entry. The extraperitoneal extremity of the catheter is grasped with this forceps and brought to the portal. The catheter is cut to the required length and connected to the portal chamber. The portal chamber and the catheter are then flushed with heparinized saline (50 IU/mL). The four corners of the portal are sutured to the underlying fascia using permanent sutures (Silk O; Sherwood, Davis & Geck). After disinfection of the sites, the subcutaneous tissue and the skin are closed over the catheter entry site and the portal. The other trocar entry sites are then closed.

Using this technique, Anaf et al. [20] showed that laparoscopy was possible in all of their eight patients and the catheters were easily inserted. All patients received intraperitoneal chemotherapy on the second postoperative day. The authors did not observe any complication after a mean follow-up of 12 months.

HAND-ASSISTED LAPAROSCOPY IN OVARIAN CANCER

Hand-assisted laparoscopic surgery (HALS) is a unique surgical approach that combines traditional laparoscopy with the ability to place a hand intraperitoneally, thus retaining tactile sensation for the surgeon. General surgeons and urologists already use hand-assisted laparoscopy for a wide range of surgical procedures on a variety of organ systems, including the kidney, spleen, liver, prostate, and gastrointestinal tract.[21]

There are few reports to date using HALS in gynecologic oncology. The first report using this surgical approach for treating patients with gynecologic malignancies was by Klingler et al.[22] The authors reported using HALS to perform a splenectomy in a patient with an isolated ovarian cancer recurrence. Pelosi et al. [23] used HALS to stage two patients, one with an ovarian dysgerminoma and the other with a grade 3 endometrial adenocarcinoma. The authors also used HALS to repair a small bowel herniation through the vaginal cuff after a cytoreductive procedure.

Krivak et al. [21] recently managed 25 ovarian cancer patients with hand-assisted laparoscopy. Six patients had apparent advanced-stage ovarian cancer at the time of referral, and 19 patients had apparent early-stage ovarian cancer. Of the 19 patients with presumed early-stage disease, five patients were upstaged based on retroperitoneal lymph node involvement, three had disease in other pelvic structures, and two had microscopic disease in the omentum. Twenty-two patients had their

surgeries completed via hand-assisted laparoscopy, and three cases required conversion to laparotomy for completion of debulking surgery. Complication rates were low, with three complications requiring reoperation or hospitalization. The mean hospital stay was 1.8 days for the 22 patients who had a successful hand-assisted laparoscopic evaluation. Operating times were variable and ranged from 81 to 365 minutes.

For HALS, all patients are consented for laparoscopy as well as laparotomy and are admitted on the day of surgery following mechanical bowel prep. In patients with suspected early-stage disease, a 10-mm laparoscopic intraumbilical trocar is placed intraperitoneally using a direct-entry technique. A pneumoperitoneum is obtained and a thorough review of the abdomen and pelvis performed. Two 5-mm lateral ports and a 5- or 10-mm suprapubic midline port are placed under direct visualization. If HALS is deemed necessary for completion of the surgery, a 6- to 7-cm periumbilical or suprapubic vertical midline incision is made depending on the site of disease. The length of the hand port incision is equal to the surgeon's glove size (e.g., 7 cm for glove size 7). A hand-assisted device (Lap Disc; Ethicon Endo-Surgery, Cincinnati, OH) is placed to permit free insertion and withdrawal of the surgeon's hand from the abdomen while maintaining an intact pneumoperitoneum. After the hand port is placed, and with the assistance of the laparoscope, the surgeon has the ability to visualize and palpate all peritoneal surfaces and retroperitoneal structures. Staging biopsies and washings are performed as indicated. If an extensive dissection and resection are necessary, standard minimally invasive techniques are augmented with the hand placed intraperitoneally. Small bowel, colon, or omentum can be elevated out of the peritoneal cavity and the dissection performed extracorporeally using standard techniques.[21]

Although the role of HALS in the primary surgical management of gynecologic malignancies requires further investigation, it appears that select patients with early- and advanced-stage ovarian cancer may be treated appropriately and successfully with HALS. Patients treated via this approach appear to benefit from the advantages associated with traditional minimally invasive surgery.

CONCERNS ABOUT LAPAROSCOPY AND OVARIAN CANCER

The occurrence of port-site metastases has raised significant concern about the use of laparoscopic surgery for procedures associated with malignant disease. The actual incidence of port-site metastases is unknown; however, estimates range from 0% to 2.3%. The overall incidence of port-site metastases in gynecologic cancers in a study by Nagarsheth et al. [24] was 2.3%. The risk of port-site metastases was highest (5%) in patients with recurrence of ovarian or primary peritoneal malignancies undergoing procedures in the presence of ascites. A recent paper by Abu-Rustum et al. [25] demonstrated that CO_2 pneumoperitoneum does not affect the overall survival of women with persistent metastatic ovarian cancer. Some techniques, such as deflation of the abdomen with trocars in place, irrigation of the trocar site with 5% povidone–iodine, and closure of the peritoneal trocar sites (10- to 12-mm trocars), have been suggested to decrease the risk of port-site metastases; however, their effectiveness has not been shown in clinical studies.

To date, the available retrospective data are conflicting, and there are no prospective clinical trials showing that intraoperative cyst rupture in early-stage ovarian cancer will worsen prognosis. However, if spillage of cyst contents occurs, massive irrigation and immediate surgical treatment and staging are prudent because there is also no evidence to support the safety of delayed definitive management after capsular rupture.[26]

When intraoperative cyst rupture and spillage of tumor cells occur with the resulting upstaging from stage IA to stage IC, there are no data to answer the question of whether adjuvant chemotherapy should be administered. Should a patient be treated postoperatively with chemotherapy based on cyst rupture if she otherwise would have not been recommended for any postoperative therapy? Although many experts would recommend treatment for such patients, there are no good studies that address the problem.[26]

In one of the largest series of laparoscopic staging for early-stage ovarian and fallopian tube cancers at Mount Sinai Medical Center in New York City, 27 staging procedures by a gynecologic oncology service were reviewed. There were no intraoperative complications, and there was only one postoperative complication of small bowel obstruction, which resolved with conservative management. One patient was upstaged to advanced disease secondary to microscopic metastasis to the omentum, and there have been three cases of recurrence. Overall, this experience shows that laparoscopic staging of these cancers appears to be comprehensive when performed by gynecologic oncologists experienced with advanced laparoscopy.[27]

SURGICAL TRAINING AND PATIENT REFERRAL

Although laparoscopy provides excellent outcomes, its integration into gynecologic cancer surgery is hampered by a significant learning curve and lack of training at the subspecialty level. Because large prospective trials are lacking, the route used to perform staging or restaging will mainly depend on the surgeon's training. As shown in a series on other gynecologic malignancies [28], all patients undergoing laparoscopy have a better surgical outcome in terms of morbidity when compared with patients undergoing laparotomy. However, the group of patients with ovarian cancer most likely to benefit from a laparoscopic approach are young patients with early-stage disease wishing to retain their fertility. In fact, laparoscopy has been shown to be associated with a lower rate of adhesion formation than laparotomy and therefore may impinge less on a patient's fertility. When a physician is confronted with this latter situation, referral to oncologic centers with adequate skills in laparoscopic management of ovarian cancer would probably be in the best interest of the patient.

REFERENCES

1. American Cancer Society. *Cancer Facts & Figures, 2007*. Atlanta, GA: ACS; 2007.
2. Moore DH. Primary surgical management of early epithelial ovarian carcinoma. In: Rubin SC, Sutton GP, eds. *Ovarian Cancer*. 2nd ed. Philadelphia: Lippincott Williams & Wilkins; 2001:201–218.
3. Chi DS, Abu-Rustum NR, Sonoda Y, et al. The safety and efficacy of laparoscopic surgical staging of apparent stage I ovarian and fallopian tube cancers. *Am J Obstet Gynecol*. 2005;192:1614–1619.
4. Querleu D, Leblanc E. Laparoscopic infrarenal para-aortic lymph node dissection for restaging of carcinoma of the ovary or fallopian tube. *Cancer*. 1994;73:1467–1471.
5. Childers JM, Lang J, Surwit EA, Hatch KD. Laparoscopic surgical staging of ovarian cancer. *Gynecol Oncol*. 1995;59:25–33.
6. Spirtos NM, Eisekop SM, Boike G, Schlaerth JB, Cappellari JO. Laparoscopic staging in patients with incompletely staged cancers of the uterus, ovary, fallopian tube, and primary peritoneum: a Gynecologic Oncology Group (GOG) study. *Am J Obstet Gynecol*. 2005;193:1645–1649.
7. Tozzi R, Kohler C, Ferrara A, Schneider A. Laparoscopic treatment of early ovarian cancer: surgical and survival outcomes. *Gynecol Oncol*. 2004;93:199–203.
8. Tozzi R, Schneider A. Laparoscopic treatment of early ovarian cancer. *Curr Opin Obstet Gynecol*. 2005;17:354–358.
9. Camatte S, Morice P, Pautier P, Atallah D, Lhommé C, et al. Fertility results after conservative treatment of advanced stage serous borderline tumors of the ovary. *BJOG*. 2002;109:373–380.
10. Camatte P, Morice P, Atallah D et al. Clinical outcome after laparoscopic pure management of borderline ovarian tumors: results of a series of 34 patients. *Ann Oncol*. 2004;15:605–609.
11. Seracchioli R, Venturoli S, Colombo FM, Govoni F, Missiroli S, Bagnoli A. Fertility and tumor recurrence rate after conservative laparoscopic management of young women with early-stage borderline ovarian tumors. *Fertil Steril*. 2001;76:999–1004.
12. Donnez J, Munschke A, Berliere M et al. Safety of conservative management and fertility outcome in women with borderline tumors of the ovary. *Fertil Steril*. 2003;79:1216–1221.
13. Deffieux X, Morice P, Camatte S, Fourchotte V, Duvillard P, Castaigne D. Results after laparoscopic management of serous borderline tumor of the ovary with peritoneal implants. *Gynecol Oncol*. 2005;97:84–89.
14. Nezhat F, Yadav J, Rahaman J, Gretz H 3rd, Gardner GJ, Cohen CJ. Laparoscopic lymphadenectomy for gynecologic malignancies using ultrasonically activated shears: analysis of first 100 cases. *Gynecol Oncol*. 2005;97:813–819.
15. Hoskins WJ, Bundy BN, Thigpen JT, Omura GA. The influence of cytoreductive surgery on recurrence-free survival in small volume stage III epithelial ovarian cancer: a gynecologic oncology group study. *Gynecol Oncol*. 1992;47:159–166.
16. Bristow RE, Tomacruz SR, Armstrong DK, Trimble EL, Montz FJ. Survival effect of maximal cytoreductive surgery for advanced ovarian carcinoma during the platino-era: a meta analysis, *J Clin Oncol*. 2002;20:1248–1259.
17. Bristow RE, Duska LR, Lambrou NC, et al. A model for predicting surgical outcome in patient with advanced ovarian carcinoma using computed tomography. *Cancer*. 2000;89:1532–1540.
18. Fagotti A, Fanfani F, Ludovisi M, et al. Role of laparoscopy to assess the chance of optimal cytoreductive surgery in advanced ovarian cancer: a pilot study. *Gynecol Oncol*. 2005;96:729–735.
19. Rahaman J, Dottino P, Jennings TS, Holland J, Cohen CJ. The second-look operation improves survival in suboptimally debulked stage III ovarian cancer patients. *Int J Gynecol Cancer*. 2005;15:19–25.
20. Anaf V, Gangji D, Simon P, Saylam K. Laparoscopical insertion of intraperitoneal catheters for intraperitoneal chemotherapy. *Acta Obstet Gynecol Scand*. 2003;82:1140–1145.
21. Krivak TC, Elkas JC, Rose GS, et al. The utility of hand-assisted laparoscopy in ovarian cancer. *Gynecol Oncol*. 2005;96:72–76.
22. Klingler PJ, Smith SL, Abendstein BJ, Hinder RA. Hand assisted laparoscopic splenectomy for isolated splenic metastasis from an ovarian carcinoma. *Surg Laparosc Endosc*. 1997;8:49–54.

23. Pelosi MA, Pelsoi MA 3rd, Eim J. Hand assisted laparoscopy for pelvic malignancy. *J Laparoendosc Adv Surg Tech*. 2000;10:143–150.

24. Nagarsheth NP, Rahaman J, Cohen CJ, Gretz H, Nezhat F. The incidence of port-site metastases in gynecologic cancers. *JSLS*. 2004;8:133–139.

25. Abu-Rustum NR, Sonoda Y, Chi DS, et al. The effects of CO_2 pneumoperitoneum on the survival of women with persistent metastatic ovarian cancer. *Gynecol Oncol*. 2003;90:431–434.

26. Vaisbuch E, Dgani R, Ben-Arie A, Hagay Z. The role of laparoscopy in ovarian tumors of low malignant potential and early-stage ovarian cancer. *Obstet Gynecol Surv*. 2005;60:326–330.

27. Prasad M, Shamshirsaz, Rahaman J, Nezhat F. Laparoscopic staging of early stage ovarian and fallopian tube neoplasms. Presented at: the Biennial Meeting of the International Gynecologic Cancer Society; October 2006; Santa Monica, CA.

28. Chi DS, Curtin JP. Gynecologic cancer and laparoscopy. *Obstet Gynecol Clin North Am*. 1999;26:201–215.

Section 16.7. Second-Look Surgery for Gynecologic Malignancy

Sharyn N. Lewin and Thomas Herzog

HISTORY

Second-look procedures were first introduced into the surgical community in 1951 by Wangensteen et al. [1] in the surgical reevaluation of colon cancer patients. From a landmark *Lancet* publication in 1957, Wangensteen wrote, "While the patients are asymptomatic and without clinical evidence of residual cancer, they are re-operated upon. A thorough search for any suggestion of residual is made; any suspicious nodule is removed, together with any remaining lymph node-bearing tissue. . . ."[2] The concept of second-look operations in ovarian cancer treatment began in the 1960s after reports described clinically occult but surgically demonstrable disease following adjuvant chemotherapy.[3–5] Additionally, the substantial risk of hematologic malignancies following the use of alkylating agents further propagated the need for surgical reassessment and early discontinuation of cytotoxic therapy.[6,7] Today, the role of second-look surgical procedures in ovarian cancer treatment remains highly controversial. Supporting literature describing the advantages and disadvantages will be discussed as well as the current use of laparoscopy in this procedure.

DEFINITION

The second-look procedure has been falsely used to describe various secondary surgical procedures in ovarian cancer management. The appropriate definition is a surgical exploration in ovarian cancer patients with no clinical evidence of disease after a completed course of chemotherapy. This procedure should not be confused with secondary cytoreduction, which entails the excision of clinically apparent recurrent or persistent disease. The surgical procedure itself incorporates a thorough evaluation of the pelvic and abdominal cavities. (See Table 16.7.1.) Multiple cytologic washings are obtained from the pelvis, the paracolic gutters, and under the hemidiaphragms. Numerous systematic biopsies should be sampled from the peritoneal cavity, including the pelvic cul-de-sac, the pedicles of the infundibulopelvic ligaments, the bladder, the pelvic side walls, the paracolic gutters, and both hemidiaphragms. A pelvic and para-aortic lymph node dissection should be performed if not done previously, and any residual omentum should be removed. If tumor is not readily apparent, a standard second-look procedure should generate 20 to 30 biopsy specimens.[8] Adhesions should be removed and sent for histologic evaluation along with any surface abnormalities. Particular attention should be paid toward areas of previously documented tumor. If residual tumor is found, resecting as much as possible is preferred.

Obtaining at least 20 to 30 biopsy specimens along with multiple cytologic washings is necessary to reduce the "false-negative rate" of second-look surgery. Several studies have reported between 14% and 24% of patients with microscopic persistence but no evidence of gross disease.[8–11] Furthermore, these studies have shown microscopic disease in only one or two specimens.

ADVANTAGES OF SECOND LOOK

Overview

Throughout the literature, the benefits or advantages of second-look procedures fall into three broad categories. The histologic evidence of disease status obtained in this procedure historically (1) provides highly prognostic information; (2) prevents discontinuation of cytotoxic therapy in patients with occult disease, particularly in centers with active second-line clinical trials; and (3) allows timely cessation of chemotherapeutic agents to decrease adverse side effects.[12,13] The third point was more relevant historically when patients were treated with alkylating agents and concern arose over prolonged exposure leading to hematologic malignancies.[6,7] This issue may no longer be as relevant given primary cytotoxic therapy with paclitaxel and platinum-based agents; however, the cumulative toxicities of neuropathy still are important considerations that accompany paclitaxel and platinum-based regimens.[14] (See Table 16.7.2.)

Best Predictor of Disease Status

The second-look procedure is purely a diagnostic modality. Proponents argue this procedure " . . . remains the single most specific and sensitive means available for determining the status of the cancer before, during, or after chemotherapy."[13] Noninvasive modalities, such as CT scans and serum CA-125 measurements, have only modest sensitivity in detecting recurrent disease. Reports describe sensitivity with CT scans of only 40% to 61% in this setting – especially low because of the lack of sensitivity in detecting small-volume disease.[15,16] Recent studies have addressed the value of PET in detecting advanced ovarian cancer. One timely article compared PET with second-look procedure results.[17] These authors divided 55 advanced ovarian cancer patients into two groups, PET versus second-look procedure, following primary cytoreductive surgery and six cycles of adjuvant chemotherapy. The cohort evaluated with PET for recurrent and/or persistent disease revealed a sensitivity of 82%, specificity of 88%, and accuracy of 84% in detecting the presence of disease. The positive and negative predictive values of the PET scans were 93% and 70%, respectively. No significant

Table 16.7.1: Key Components in Second-Look Procedures

Midline laparotomy or laparoscopy

Thorough inspection and palpation

Cytologic saline washings

Pelvis

Bilateral paracolic gutters

Below both hemidiaphragms

Systematic peritoneal biopsies (20–30)

Pelvic cul-de-sac

Infundibulopelvic ligament pedicles

Bladder dome

Bilateral pelvic side walls

Paracolic gutters bilaterally

Hemidiaphragms bilaterally

Pelvic and para-aortic lymph node dissection

Omentectomy

Lysis and pathologic assessment of adhesions

Surface irregularities

Prior disease sites

± Secondary cytoreduction

Table 16.7.2: Advantages and Disadvantages of Second Look

Advantages

Most sensitive predictor of disease status

Prevents premature discontinuation of cytotoxic therapy

Allows timely cessation of chemotherapeutic agents

Provides highly prognostic information

Excellent clinical trial end point

Disadvantages

Lack of prospective data demonstrating a survival advantage

Perioperative morbidity

Decreased quality of life

Pain

Adhesions

Cost

To patient

To health care system/society

High recurrence rate despite negative findings

Relative lack of cure with current second-line therapies

Table 16.7.3: Second-Look Procedures: Most Sensitive Predictor of Disease Status

Diagnostic Modality	Sensitivity, %	Specificity, %	PPV, %	NPV, %
Second-look procedure [11]	85.7	90.9		
CT scan [15,16]	40–61	46–84		
PET [17]	82	88	93	70
CA-125 [18,19]				
<35 U/mL			43–62	38–57
>35 U/mL	78.5		100	0

PPV, positive predictive value; NPV, negative predictive value.

difference in progression-free interval or disease-free survival was seen between the PET and second-look procedure groups. The authors' results coincide with previously reported data regarding the sensitivity (83% to 91%) and specificity (66% to 93%) of PET scans in detecting recurrent ovarian cancer compared with those of CT scans (sensitivity, 45% to 91%; specificity, 46% to 84%).[16] Further investigations are necessary to assess and validate the role of PET scans in recurrent ovarian cancer. (See Table 16.7.3.)

Although serum CA-125 measurements have a sensitivity of 75% to 80% in detecting advanced and recurrent disease, a negative value does not exclude the presence of microscopic disease.[15,18] In fact, several studies have addressed the predictive value of serum CA-125 measurements in patients undergoing second-look procedures. Berek et al. [18] reported the correlation of CA-125 measurements with findings at second-look procedure in 55 patients clinically free of disease after a prescribed course of chemotherapy. The predictive value of a CA-125 level less than or equal to 35 U/mL was 56%.[18] In other words, 44% of patients with a negative CA-125 serum measurement had disease at second-look procedure. Conversely, 100% of patients with values greater than or equal to 35 U/mL had macroscopic or microscopic evidence of disease.[18]

In another study comparing CA-125 levels and findings at second laparotomies, Rubin et al. [19] reported data on 96 prospectively studied procedures. Sixty-two percent of cases (18 of 29) with CA-125 measurements less than or equal to 35 U/mL had documented disease upon exploration. Additionally, of the 84 patients with persistent disease at secondary laparotomy, 22% had normal CA-125 values. Furthermore, 98% of patients with elevated CA-125 measurements had disease detected at exploration. The authors noted " . . . the accuracy of the marker in predicting disease was significantly related to the volume of residual disease as determined by the maximum diameter of the largest tumor mass."[19] Given the high percentage of patients with disease at exploration despite normal serum CA-125 measurements in both studies (44% and 62%), proponents argue that other modalities are necessary to definitely determine disease recurrence, namely second-look procedures. Similar findings have been shown in other studies as well.

Variables Predicting Second-Look Findings

Numerous studies have shown that second-look procedures provide highly prognostic information. This is the most frequently cited advantage to second-look surgeries as the findings at exploration can correlate with clinical outcomes and overall survival. Additionally, several histologic and clinical variables have been associated with second-look findings and can broadly be discussed under the following headings: histologic grade, initial stage, residual tumor size, and chemotherapy type. Several reports have described a higher negative second-look procedure rate (i.e., no macroscopic or microscopic disease) in patients with well- to moderately differentiated original tumors (grades 1 and 2) compared with those with poorly differentiated tumors (grades 3 and 4).[8,20,21] Approximately 60% to 70% of patients with grade 1 tumors will have negative second-look procedures. The percentages for grades 2 and 3 are 50% and 40%, respectively.[8,20,21]

Likewise, several studies have documented that patients with original stage I and II tumors have a higher chance of a negative second-look procedure than do patients with stage III and IV tumors.[8,20,21] Various studies have documented the incidence of a negative second-look procedure in patients with stage I disease as 80% to 95%, stage II as 70% to 80%, and stages III to IV as 30% to 40%.[8,20,21] In fact, a study from Memorial Sloan-Kettering Cancer Center (MSKCC) evaluated second-look laparotomy results in 54 women with comprehensively staged stage I epithelial ovarian cancer.[22] Five percent of the women in this study had disease present at second-look procedure. The authors concluded that among women with comprehensively staged stage I epithelial ovarian cancer, those who are disease-free following surgical staging and chemotherapy should not undergo a second-look procedure.[22] Evaluating the clinical and histologic variables that make patients more likely to have occult disease would better define which patients may be best suited for second-look procedures from those who do not need an additional invasive surgical procedure.

One of the strongest predictors of negative second-look procedure findings, and of overall survival and clinical outcomes in general, is the amount of residual disease following primary cytoreduction. Numerous studies have reinforced the benefits of optimal debulking, and although the subject of debulking is beyond the scope of this section, the benefits of this procedure can be broadly summarized into the following categories: improved response to chemotherapy; improved clinical disease-free status and, therefore, a higher second-look procedure rate; more negative findings at the second-look procedure; longer progression-free interval; and improved overall disease survival.[8,20,21,23] Approximately a dozen studies have shown that the completeness of the initial cytoreductive effort correlates with the negative second-look procedure rate.[8,20,21,23] In a pooled analysis of these retrospective studies, a negative second-look procedure rate was most likely in patients with no residual disease following primary cytoreduction (77%) compared with optimal (45% to 50%) and suboptimal residual (25%).[8,20,21,23]

Over the years, as retrospective studies have been published on the variables associated with second-look procedures, several chemotherapy regimens have been used with similar rates of negative second-look results.[22] With the advent of a platinum- and paclitaxel-based primary chemotherapeutic regimen, the incidence of a negative second-look procedure is approximately 50%.[24] Although not an end point of the study, this finding was described in a randomized GOG study (GOG 158) evaluating the efficacy of carboplatin/paclitaxel versus cisplatin/paclitaxel in optimally resected stage III ovarian cancer patients.[24] In an earlier study by Berek et al. [8], findings from second-look laparotomies in advanced ovarian cancer patients revealed the same probability of negative findings in patients treated with six to nine cycles of cisplatin-containing combination chemotherapy as that found in patients treated with 10 to 12 cycles. In this instance, second-look procedures tailored and decreased the number of chemotherapy cycles needed for clinical remission.[8]

Prognostic Value

As previously described, many retrospective studies have described the clinical and histologic variables associated with second-look findings. Multiple studies have also reviewed the prognostic significance of findings at second-look procedures in terms of overall disease survival. For example, Gershenson et al. [25] described the experience at M. D. Anderson over a 10-year period in 246 patients who underwent second-look procedures. Of 246 patients with advanced ovarian cancer who were clinically disease-free, 85 (35%) had no surgical evidence of disease at laparotomy whereas 111 (45%) had macroscopic disease and 50 (20%) had microscopic disease. Of the 85 patients without histologic or cytologic evidence of disease, 24% developed a recurrence, with a median interval of 18.5 months (5 to 47 months). Of a dozen variables studied, only histologic grade and type had a significant link to recurrence. Patients with mixed histologies and grade 3 tumors were most likely to have a recurrence. These variables, along with residual tumor mass following the second-look procedure, had a statistically significant correlation with progression-free interval.

In another key study, a negative procedure (38% occurrence rate) was associated with the original tumor stage and completeness of the surgical cytoreduction.[20] A worsened prognosis was correlated with a higher histologic grade of the residual tumor, a larger size of the occult tumor found, positive cytologic washings, and the amount and size of the residual tumor following the second-look procedure.[20] Overall, the prognostic significance of findings at second-look procedure can be broadly categorized into disease status at three levels: no residual, microscopic disease, and gross tumor. Patients with no histologic evidence of disease have a longer survival, with recurrence rates of 26% for patients with advanced disease.[8,20,21,23]

DISADVANTAGES OF SECOND LOOK

Overview

Although the preceding text discusses the advantages of second-look procedures, a compelling number of disadvantages have been heavily contested in the literature. (See Table 16.7.2.) Broadly, the cited disadvantages are (1) a lack of randomized, prospective trials documenting improved survival with second-look procedures, (2) perioperative morbidity associated with an invasive surgical procedure, (3) the cost to the health care system for utilization of resources, (4) recurrence in approximately 50% of patients despite negative findings, and (5) ineffective second-line therapies in ovarian cancer management.[12,26] The majority of literature surrounding the second-look procedure is retrospective in nature and addresses prognostic variables associated with findings from the procedure.[27] Studies addressing the survival impact of this procedure remain sparse. Cohen et al. [28] were the first to describe a lack of survival difference in patients who underwent second-look procedures compared with their matched counterparts who declined. The only prospective, randomized studies are two European multicenter trials, both of which failed to show a survival advantage with second-look operations, but indeed have their own study design limitations.[29,30] Nicoletto et al. [29] reported the results of 102 patients who had achieved a clinical complete response after primary cytoreduction and chemotherapy (as documented by clinical examination, serum CA-125 measurements, CT scans, and laparoscopy). Patients were randomized to one of two arms, either clinical follow-up only (48 patients) or surgical second look (54 patients). Eight of the patients in the second-look group subsequently refused surgery. Patients found with disease at their second-look procedure were then treated with second-line therapy. After a 5-year follow-up period, no difference in survival was noted between the two groups. The authors concluded that (1) second-look procedures did not prolong survival but did define complete responders to first-line therapy and (2) second-line therapies were essentially ineffective.

In the second European prospective randomized, controlled trial, 166 patients were randomized to one of three arms following primary cytoreduction and chemotherapy with cisplatin.[30] Two groups of patients underwent second-look laparotomy followed by either oral chlorambucil (53 patients) or whole abdomen and pelvic irradiation (56 patients), and one group received oral chlorambucil only without surgical intervention (57 patients). The authors found no difference in survival among the three groups and therefore concluded that second-look laparotomy did not provide any survival advantage. It is noteworthy that these studies have been criticized because of the chemotherapy regimens used, but they remain the only randomized prospective studies to date.

Of interest is the previously mentioned GOG 158 study, in which patients chose whether or not to undergo a second-look procedure following their completed chemotherapy course.[14] Although this aspect of the study was nonrandomized and was not a primary end point of the study, it does provide a prospective comparison of outcomes in patients who elected second-look laparotomy versus those who did not. Essentially, no difference in overall survival was noted between optimally resected stage III ovarian cancer patients treated with a course of platinum plus paclitaxel who subsequently underwent second-look laparotomy and those who then chose clinical follow-up (median 53.5 vs. 56.6 months). The authors concluded that "although second-look laparotomy remains the best means available for determining the post-treatment status of ovarian cancer . . . its current use should be limited to research until additional adjuvant therapy, initiated on the basis of second-look laparotomy findings, have been shown to improve survival."[14]

In an interesting single-institution retrospective cohort study, Rahaman et al. [27] described Mount Sinai Medical Center's experience with patients eligible for second-look operations over a 9-year period. The study's global objective was to identify a subgroup of patients most likely to benefit from second look by comparing the survival of stage III ovarian cancer patients who underwent second-look procedures with that of patients who declined. Among patients who had optimal cytoreduction during their primary surgery, there was no survival advantage to a second-look procedure. In contrast, patients who initially had suboptimal resection, achieved a complete clinical response to chemotherapy, and subsequently chose a second-look procedure had an improved 5-year survival rate compared with those who declined (36% vs. 13%; $P \leq 0.05$). This finding was solely the result of the second-look procedure itself, with identification and treatment of persistent disease. This further illustrates that selective groups of ovarian cancer patients may benefit more than others from second-look procedures, but larger, randomized trials are still needed to explore and validate these points.

Morbidity

Several publications described the morbidity associated with second-look laparotomies. One study reported the incidence of the following complications: prolonged ileus, 13%; wound infection, 12%; urinary tract infection, 13%; pulmonary events, 5%; and bowel injury, 4%.[31] Other studies reported similar findings and noted bowel dysfunction is the most common morbidity. For example, Luesley et al. [9] evaluated the findings and outcomes in 50 patients who underwent second-look laparotomies. Within this series, the most frequent complication was a postoperative ileus, which occurred in 70% of the patients. Other less common morbidities included infections, 24%, and deep venous thrombosis, 4%. Interestingly, 54% of patients required intraoperative blood transfusions whereas 16% were transfused postoperatively. The average length of inpatient hospitalization was 12 days (range, 6 to 21 days). Although the morbidities listed are not uncommon following gynecologic oncology surgery, an added invasive surgical procedure does have an impact on patients' quality of life. Even without morbidity, additional surgical procedures cause discomfort, increased costs, and additional time in the hospital.

ROLE OF LAPAROSCOPY IN SECOND LOOK

Literature over the past 30 years has reported the use of laparoscopy to detect recurrent or persistent disease, thereby eliminating the need for laparotomy in selected patients. These studies reported between 36% and 50% of patients with disease detectable by laparoscopy who may be spared the need for abdominal exploration.[32–34] The earlier studies reported a higher complication rate (2% to 14%) and inadequate visualization leading to increased false-negative rates (12% to 55%), so acceptance and subsequent use of laparoscopy were initially limited.[34,35] With advances in minimally invasive surgery, a renewed interest has been seen over the past decade in laparoscopic procedures in general. More contemporary reports regarding the role of laparoscopy in second-look procedures have shown less morbidity, reduced costs, and equivalent disease detection rates and survival with laparoscopic compared with open procedures.[36–38] Several sentinel publications in this regard are reviewed below. (See Table 16.7.4.)

In the early 1980s, Berek et al. [35] reported the results of 119 consecutive laparoscopies performed on 57 ovarian cancer patients to determine disease status and response to chemotherapy. Fourteen percent of patients had a major complication

Table 16.7.4: Laparoscopy in Second-Look Procedures

Study	Patients, no.	False Negative, %	Spared Laparotomy, %
Clough (1999) [40]	20	14	
Nicoletto (1997) [29]	35	24	
Ozols (1981) [32]	99	55	36
Piver (1980) [33]	22	20	55
Quinn (1980) [41]	62	77	
Xygakis (1984) [34]	46	12	43

Study	Patients, no.	% +	Exlap	TTR, mo.	Complications, %
Abu-Rustum [36]	39	44	No	NA	0
Berek [35]	57	38	No	22	14
Casey [37]	93	47	No	NA	8.6
Childers [38]	44	56	No	NA	14
Clough [40]	20	30	Yes	NA	15.7
Husain [39]	150	54	No	16	2.7
Ozols [32]	99	50	No	NA	2.5

Author	Outcome Variable	Laparotomy	Laparoscopy
Casey	Estimated blood loss, mL	158.3	30.5
Abu-Rustum	Estimated blood loss, mL	208	27
Casey	Biopsies, no.	23	12.5
Abu-Rustum	Biopsies, no.	15.9	9.5
Casey	OR time, min.	145	84.75
Abu-Rustum	OR time, min.	153	129
Casey	Hospital stay, days	7.2	0.7
Abu-Rustum	Hospital stay, days	6.8	1.6
Casey	Cost, $	5345	2393
Abu-Rustum	Cost, $	17,969	9448
Casey	Disease detection, %	47.3	55.7
Abu-Rustum	Disease detection, %	61.4	54.8

Data from Casey et al. [37] and Abu-Rustum et al. [36].
Exlap, comparative laparotomy performed; TTR, time to recurrence; NA, not available; OR, operating room.

requiring laparotomy, mostly as a result of bowel perforation. By changing the technique and using a 14-gauge fiberoptic endoscope, or needlescope, to visualize Veress needle insertion, the complication rate was decreased to 1.2%. Reduced complication rates have also been seen in other studies as improvements in laparoscopic techniques and instruments have been made.

In a more recent study from MSKCC, 150 patients who underwent laparoscopic second-look procedures were retrospectively reviewed.[39] The majority of patients had advanced disease, and the optimal rate of primary cytoreduction was 54%. Forty-six percent were pathologically disease-free, whereas 54% were noted to have persistent disease. Twelve percent of patients required conversion to laparotomy for the following reasons: tumor cytoreduction in 11 patients, lysis of adhesions in three patients, enterotomy repair in three patients, and cystotomy repair in one patient. The overall reported complication rate was 2.7%. These authors described their technique to include an "open" insertion, in which a periumbilical incision was made and a Hasson-type, 10-mm blunt trocar was inserted under direct visualization.

Overall, reports have shown laparoscopy is a safe option in second-look surgery. Complications of laparoscopy in this setting include subcutaneous hematomas and emphysema as well as vascular injuries, superficial wound infections, and most commonly, bowel injuries.[37] In studies comparing laparoscopy with laparotomy, more complications were found in the laparotomy groups compared with the laparoscopy groups.[36,37] The cited complication rates in recent studies for second-look laparoscopy and laparotomy are 3% to 15% and 9% to 27%, respectively.[40]

Laparoscopy affords magnification and illumination that, at least in theory, may improve visualization of peritoneal surfaces, a factor that is especially important during a second-look procedure.[38] Laparoscopic assessment should include diaphragmatic peritoneum, adhesion bands, residual pelvic and para-aortic lymph nodes, residual omentum, and cytologic washings (see Figure 16.7.1.). Laparoscopy is still limited, however, by the inability to palpate and visualize certain anatomic areas, such as the mesentery and small bowel serosa.[36,38,40] Although laparoscopy missed occult disease in the past, with improved skills and equipment, the outcomes and results are now equivalent to those of laparotomy. Casey et al. [37] found no difference in disease detection rates between patients undergoing laparoscopy versus laparotomy in advanced ovarian cancer. Furthermore, the overall survival between the two groups was the same. Others have confirmed these findings.[36,39,40]

In another series from MSKCC, the outcomes of second-look laparoscopy versus laparotomy in a rather homogeneous group of advanced ovarian cancer patients were retrospectively reviewed.[36] Of 109 patients who underwent second-look procedures, 64.2% underwent laparotomy, 28.4% underwent laparoscopy, and 7.3% underwent both procedures. Patients in the laparoscopy group had a significantly lower mean blood loss and shorter mean operating times as well as reduced hospital stays.[39] This translated into significantly lower hospital charges in the laparoscopy versus the laparotomy group ($9448 vs. $17,969; $P \leq 0.01$). The authors noted that all the complications were in the laparotomy group and that the most common was postoperative ileus (eight of 11 patients, or 11.4%).[39] Disease detection rates and overall survival were similar between the two groups. Casey et al. [37] essentially replicated these findings in another comparative study. (See Table 16.7.5.)

The inability to complete a thorough laparoscopic second-look procedure has been attributed to dense adhesions.[37,40] In one of the few prospective series, by Clough et al. [40], 20 patients underwent a laparoscopic second look followed by a comparative laparotomy. In the majority of cases, intraperitoneal adhesions were the limiting factor preventing a thorough and complete laparoscopic evaluation. As such, only 41% of patients underwent a complete laparoscopic exploration. However, significantly higher completion rates using the laparoscope have been reported in other studies, with up to a 90% adequate completion rate.[38,40] Interestingly, Clough et al. [40] noted that the

Table 16.7.5: Advantages and Disadvantages of Laparoscopic Second Look

Advantages

Decreased blood loss

Reduced length of hospital stay

Decreased costs

Decreased operating times in selected studies

Equivalent disease detection rates

Equivalent survival rates

Improved visualization of certain peritoneal surfaces

Disadvantages

Inability to palpate anatomic structures

Decreased visualization of bowel serosa and mesentery

Acquired technical skills

Lack of standardized training

Increased operative time in low-volume laparoscopic centers

High false-negative rate

Complications

Port-site recurrences

---

negative predictive value of laparoscopy for diagnosing residual disease was 86%, owing to microscopic disease that was detected only via comparative laparotomy. Although similar disease detection and overall survival rates have been seen retrospectively between these two modalities, randomized clinical trials may be necessary to further support these findings. The need for randomized data is reinforced by the fact that many of the published data are from selected centers that perform numerous laparoscopic procedures, and thus the applicability of the results to the general medical community remain unclear. Nonetheless, the continued improvement in minimally invasive surgical techniques should facilitate further interest in developing laparoscopy as the mode of choice in performing second-look procedures.

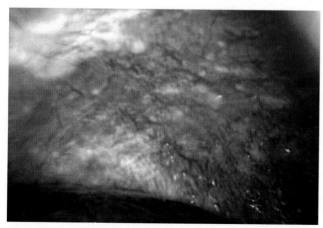

Figure 16.7.1. Diaphragm of a patient with ovarian cancer undergoing second-look laparoscopy.

CONCLUSIONS

The second-look procedure for ovarian cancer is a tool, and as such, it can be a valuable asset when correctly used. Alternatively, improper use may be problematic and may cause patients direct harm and unnecessary expense, pain, and inconvenience. Currently, the strongest indication for performing a second look is in the context of a clinical trial to confirm complete pathologic responses after initial surgery and adjuvant treatment. Complete pathologic response confirmation may be the gold standard for assessing efficacy of novel chemotherapeutics as well as biologics and novel targeted therapies. Outside of clinical trials, the use of this procedure must be individualized as the therapeutic index appears to be decreased because of the lack of prospective data to support second look. The expanding role of minimally invasive surgery conversely may increase the therapeutic index in that the majority of patients can have second look performed via laparoscopy. As novel treatments and imaging modalities evolve, so too shall the role of the second-look procedure in the treatment of ovarian cancer.

REFERENCES

1. Wangensteen OH, Lewis FJ, Tongen LA. The "second-look" in cancer surgery; a patient with colic cancer and involved lymph nodes negative on the "sixth-look." *J Lancet.* 1951;71:303–307.
2. Arhelger SW, Jensen CB, Wangensteen OH. Experiences with the "second-look" procedure in the management of cancer of the colon and rectum: with special reference to site of residual cancer. *Lancet.* 1957;77:412–417.
3. Rutledge F, Burns BC. Chemotherapy for advanced ovarian cancer. *Am J Obstet Gynecol.* 1966;96:761–772.
4. Wallach RC, Blinick G. The second look operation for carcinoma of the ovary. *Surg Gynecol Obstet.* 1970;131:1085–1089.
5. Smith JP, Delgado G, Rutledge R. Second-look operation in ovarian carcinoma: postchemotherapy. *Cancer.* 1976;38:1438–1442.
6. Reimer RR, Hoover R, Fraumeni JF, Young RC. Acute leukemia after alkylating-agent therapy of ovarian cancer. *N Engl J Med.* 1977;297:177–181.
7. Einhorn N. Acute leukemia after chemotherapy (melphalan). *Cancer.* 1978;41:444–447.
8. Berek JS, Hacker NF, Lagasse LD, Poth T, Resnick B, Neiberg RK. Second-look laparotomy in stage III epithelial ovarian cancer: clinical variables associated with disease status. *Obstet Gynecol.* 1984;64:207–212.
9. Luesley DM, Cahn KK, Fielding JWL, Hurlow R, Blackledge GR, Jordon JA. Second-look laparotomy in the management of epithelial ovarian carcinoma: an evaluation of fifty cases. *Obstet Gynecol.* 1984;64:421–426.
10. Smirz LR, Stehman FB, Ulbright TM, Sutton GP, Ehrlich CE. Second-look laparotomy after chemotherapy in the management of ovarian malignancy. *Am J Obstet Gynecol.* 1985;152:661–668.
11. Ballon SC, Portnuff JC, Sikic BI, Turbow MM, Teng NNH, Soriero OM. Second-look laparotomy in epithelial ovarian carcinoma: precise definition, sensitivity and specificity of the operative procedure. *Gynecol Oncol.* 1984;17:154–160.
12. Podratz KC, Cliby WA. Second-look surgery in the management of epithelial ovarian carcinoma. *Gynecol Oncol.* 1994;55:S128–S133.
13. Morrow CP. An opinion in support of second-look surgery in ovarian cancer. *Gynecol Oncol.* 2000;79:341–343.
14. Greer BE, Bundy BN, Ozols RF, et al. Implications of second-look laparotomy in the context of optimally resected stage III ovarian

cancer: a non-randomized comparison using an explanatory analysis: a Gynecologic Oncology Group study. *Gynecol Oncol.* 2005;99:71–79.

15. Baram A, Kovner F, Lessing JB. A second thought on second look laparotomy. *Acta Obstet Gynecol Scand.* 1993;72:386–390.

16. Delbeke D, Martin WH. Positron emission tomography imaging in oncology. *Radiol Clin North Am.* 2001;39:883–917.

17. Kim S, Chung JK, Kang SM, et al. [18F]FDG PET as a substitute for second-look laparotomy in patients with advanced ovarian carcinoma. *Eur J Nucl Med Mol Imaging.* 2004;31:196–201.

18. Berek JS, Knapp RC, Malkasian GD, et al. CA 125 serum levels correlated with second-look operations among ovarian cancer patients. *Obstet Gynecol.* 1986;67:685–689.

19. Rubin SC, Hoskins WJ, Hakes TB, et al. Serum CA 125 levels and surgical findings in patients undergoing secondary operations for epithelial ovarian cancer. *Am J Obstet Gynecol.* 1989;160:667–671.

20. Podratz KC, Malkasian GD, Hilton JF, Harris EA, Gaffey TA. Second-look laparotomy in ovarian cancer: evaluation of pathologic variables. *Am J Obstet Gynecol.* 1985;152:230–238.

21. Rubin SC, Hoskins WJ, Saigo PE, et al. Prognostic factors for recurrence following negative second-look laparotomy in ovarian cancer patients treated with platinum-based chemotherapy. *Gynecol Oncol.* 1991;42:137–141.

22. Rubin SC, Jones WB, Curtin JP, Barakat RR, Hakes TB, Hoskins WJ. Second-look laparotomy in stage I ovarian cancer following comprehensive surgical staging. *Obstet Gynecol.* 1993;82:139–142.

23. Rubin SC, Lewis JR. Second-look surgery in ovarian cancer. *Crit Rev Oncol Hematol.* 1988;88:75–91.

24. Ozols RF, Bundy BN, Greer BE, et al. Phase III trial of carboplatin and paclitaxel compared with cisplatin and paclitaxel in patients with optimally resected stage III ovarian cancer: a Gynecologic Oncology Group study. *J Clin Oncol.* 2003;21:3194–3200.

25. Gershenson DM, Copeland LJ, Wharton JT, et al. Prognosis of surgically determined complete responders in advanced ovarian cancer. *Cancer.* 1985;55:1129–1135.

26. Berek JS. Second-look versus second-nature. *Gynecol Oncol.* 1992;44:1–2.

27. Rahaman J, Lottino P, Jennings TS, Holland J, Cohen CJ. The second-look operation improves survival in suboptimally debulked stage III ovarian cancer patients. *Int J Gynecol Cancer.* 2005;15:19–25.

28. Cohen CJ, Bruckner HW, Goldberg JD, Holland JF. Improved therapy with cisplatin regimens for patients with ovarian carcinoma (FIGO III and IV) as measured by surgical end-staging (second-look surgery) – the Mount Sinai experience. *Clin Obstet Gynaecol.* 1983;10:307–324.

29. Nicoletto MO, Tumolo S, Talamini R, et al. Surgical second look in ovarian cancer: a randomized study in patients with laparoscopic complete remission – a Northeastern Oncology Cooperative Group–Ovarian Cancer Cooperative Group study. *J Clin Oncol.* 1997;15:994–999.

30. Luesley D, Lawton F, Blackledge G, et al. Failure of second-look laparotomy to influence survival in epithelial ovarian cancer. *Lancet.* 1988;2:599–603.

31. Janisch H, Schieder K, Koelbl H. Diagnostic versus therapeutic second-look surgery in patients with ovarian cancer. *Baillieres Clin Obstet Gynaecol.* 1989;3:191–200.

32. Ozols RF, Fisher RI, Anderson T, Makuch R, Young RC. Peritoneoscopy in the management of ovarian cancer. *Am J Obstet Gynecol.* 1981;140:611–619.

33. Piver MS, Lele SB, Barlow JJ, Gamarra M. Second-look laparoscopy prior to proposed second-look laparotomy. *Obstet Gynecol.* 1980;55:573–571.

34. Xygakis AM, Politis GS, Michalas SP, Kaskarelis DB. Second-look laparoscopy in ovarian cancer. *J Repro Med.* 1984;29:583–585.

35. Berek JS, Griffiths CT, Leventhal JM. Laparoscopy for second-look evaluation in ovarian cancer. *Obstet Gynecol.* 1981;58:193–198.

36. Abu-Rustum NR, Barakat RR, Diegel PL, Venkatraman E, Curtin JP, Hoskins WJ. Second-look operation for epithelial ovarian cancer: laparoscopy or laparotomy? *Obstet Gynecol.* 1996;88:549–553.

37. Casey AC, Farias-Eisner R, Pisani AL, et al. What is the role of reassessment laparoscopy in the management of gynecologic cancers in 1995? *Gynecol Oncol.* 1996;60:454–461.

38. Childers JM, Lang J, Surwit EA, Hatch KD. Laparoscopic surgical staging of ovarian cancer. *Gynecol Oncol.* 1995;59:25–33.

39. Husain A, Chi DS, Prasad M, et al. The role of laparoscopy in second-look evaluations for ovarian cancer. *Gynecol Oncol.* 2001;80:44–47.

40. Clough KB, Ladonne JM, Nos C, Renolleau C, Validire P, Durand JC. Second look for ovarian cancer: laparoscopy or laparotomy? A prospective comparative study. *Gynecol Oncol.* 1999;72:411–417.

41. Quinn MA, Bishop GJ, Campbell JJ, Rodgerson J, Pepperell RJ. Laparoscopic follow-up of patients with ovarian carcinoma. *Br J Obstet Gynaecol.* 1980;87:1132–1139.

Section 16.8. Port-Site Metastasis and Pneumoperitoneum

Chandrakanth Are and Nadeem R. Abu-Rustum

The success of laparoscopic surgery in treating benign disorders is well documented and has been adapted as the gold standard in certain conditions, such as in gallbladder disease and gastroesophageal reflux disease. This success led to the incorporation of laparoscopy in the treatment algorithm of malignant disorders. The initial enthusiasm was tempered by the steep learning curve, lack of randomized controlled trials, and the high incidence of port-site metastasis (PSM; Figure 16.8.1).[1–7] Superior instrumentation, easy access to training, and a wider acceptance of the laparoscopic approach have helped surmount the learning curve. The recent publications of landmark randomized controlled trials with large numbers of patients have established that laparoscopy is justifiable in the treatment of malignancy as long as the same oncologic principles are adhered to.[8,9] What remains at controversial stake is the actual incidence, effect, and possible negative effects of PSM on the overall efficacy of laparoscopic oncologic surgery.

First, one has to clarify the actual definition of *port-site metastasis*. PSM may occur as an isolated event (true PSM) or as part of the general carcinomatosis, in which case it should not be reported as PSM. Second, metastasis in itself implies that the tumor has spread to this location either by the hematogenous route or via the lymphatic system. This does not seem to be the case with the majority of PSM, in which the most common likely cause is direct implantation of malignant cells. Therefore, the more appropriate term would be *port-site implants*, although for convenience, we will retain the term *PSM* for this review. PSM should be defined as early tumor recurrences that develop in the abdominal wall within the wound or scar tissues of one or more port sites and is not associated with peritoneal carcinomatosis.

The high incidence of PSM in early reports stimulated extensive research into the pathogenesis of PSM. The majority of this work, by various authors, was performed in different animal models using variable cancer cell lines administered via equally divergent routes.[10–15] In addition to providing conflicting evidence, these studies had various flaws, and the results could not be extrapolated to human subjects. In the late 1990s, with increasing clinical experience in human subjects, it became clear that the incidence of PSM was similar to wound recurrences following open surgery.[16–18] We now have randomized controlled trials that have shown similar wound recurrence rates between laparoscopic and open approaches.[8,9]

In summary, the early reported high incidence of PSM and the results of animal studies have not been confirmed by the recent publication of clinical data. Several large-volume clinical reports have conclusively shown that incidence of PSM is no higher than that of open surgery.[9,19–22] This is the result of increased awareness of the condition and adherence to strict oncologic principles similar to those practiced with open surgery. With meticulous oncologic technique, this low incidence of PSM should therefore be able to be reproduced and thereby help in retaining the beneficial contribution of laparoscopy. In this chapter, we review the early reports, etiology, and pathogenesis; summarize the animal studies; analyze the clinical studies relating to PSM; and suggest methods to prevent PSM. This should enable the reader to obtain a current view of PSM and its prevention.

EARLY REPORTS AND INCIDENCE

PSM was first reported in 1978, when Dobronte et al. [23] reported PSM within 2 weeks after laparoscopy in a patient with advanced ovarian cancer (Figure 16.8.1). In 1984, Umpleby et al. [24] reported an incidence of 16% in patients undergoing laparoscopy for advanced ovarian cancer. In the current era of broader application of laparoscopy, Alexander et al. [25] were the first to report PSM in patients with Duke's B and C colon cancer treated with curative intent. This was followed by the alarming report of Berends et al. [1] that documented a 21% incidence of PSM in patients undergoing laparoscopy for colon cancer. This rate of PSM is unfavorably high when compared with wound recurrence rates of 0.7% [26] and 0.6% [27] following open surgery (Figure 16.8.1). A thorough analysis of the literature by Wexner et al. [28] in 1995 found an incidence of PSM ranging from 1.5% to 21%, with an overall incidence of 4%. Another report by Paolucci et al. [29] in 1999, which analyzed a large number of patients with gallbladder cancer, documented the incidence of PSM to be 17%.

The more recently published reports of laparoscopic surgery on various organ systems have consistently noted rates of PSM comparable to wound recurrence rates after open surgery.[19–22,30] Santoro et al. [31] reported an incidence of 0.7% in patients undergoing laparoscopy for gastrointestinal malignancies. In 533 patients subjected to laparoscopy for intra-abdominal malignancy, Pearlstone et al. [32] noted an incidence of 0.19%. In another large series consisting of 1548 patients with upper gastrointestinal malignancies, the incidence of PSM was 0.79%.[33] Rassweiler et al. [34] documented an incidence of PSM ranging from 0.18% (in 1098 patients undergoing urologic procedures) to 0% (500 patients undergoing laparoscopic radical prostatectomy). In a 12-year period that included 1288 patients with gynecologic malignancies subjected to laparoscopy, the incidence of PSM was 0.97%.[19] Similarly, Nezhat et al. [35] documented a rate of 1% in patients with gynecologic malignancies undergoing laparoscopic lymphadenectomy.

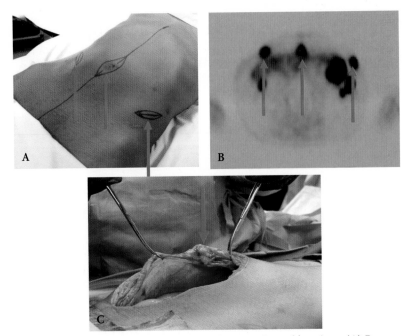

Figure 16.8.1. Recurrent cervical cancer in trocar site and intraperitoneal locations. (**A**) Recurrences at trocar sites. (**B**) PET scan documenting recurrence at port sites and intra-abdominal locations. (**C**) Tumor deposit at port site at surgery.

This trend shows that the early high incidence of PSM was reported during the learning curve from centers with small numbers of patients. The recent reports showing low incidence of PSM are from large-volume, specialized centers with greater experience in proper oncologic technique. This trend reflects the current thinking that experience and good oncologic technique are crucial to maintain the low incidence of PSM.

ETIOLOGY, PATHOGENESIS, AND ANIMAL STUDIES

Various theories have been put forward to explain the early high incidence of PSM. These theories generated an enormous body of conflicting research into the numerous probable causes of PSM. These conflicting results could be due to several drawbacks inherent to the animal models. The most common drawback is injecting cancer cells into nonorthotopic locations, such as mammary adenocarcinoma cells into the peritoneum [36] or colon cancer cells into the renal capsule.[37] The method of delivery is not standardized, and the various routes (cecal mesentery, intraperitoneal, into the portal vein, into the renal capsule, and transanal) may have a bearing on the results as well. Similarly, the volume of tumor cells injected is not uniform; neither are the end points, which are equally different.[38] Finally, analyzing the effects of CO_2 pneumoperitoneum on tumors (located at sites distant from the abdomen not directly exposed to CO_2 pneumoperitoneum) may be misleading. These results are therefore to be interpreted with a measure of caution and may not exactly be extrapolated to the clinical situation.

Although any, none, or all of these could be the cause of PSM, it is worthwhile to have an understanding of the possible causes as it will help in preventing PSM. These causes may be divided

broadly into mechanical and metabolic aspects of pneumoperitoneum [38,39] as summarized in Table 16.8.1.

Aerosolization and Chimney Effect

Umpleby et al. [24] showed that free cancer cells inhabit the peritoneal cavity in 70% of the patients. Allardyce et al. [40] noted uniform distribution of chromium-51 (^{51}Cr)-labeled HeLa cells throughout the abdomen after intraperitoneal injection. It is likely that increasing the intra-abdominal pressure in these patients can aerosolize the cancer cells. This aerosolization under pressure can leak around the port sites to cause a chimney effect whereby cancer cells may come in direct contact and cause PSM. Mathew et al. [41] reported that CO_2 pneumoperitoneum causes significant dissemination of radiolabeled adenocarcinoma cells when compared with gasless laparoscopy. Knolmayer et al. [42] found an ongoing egress of malignant cells in swine subjected to CO_2 pneumoperitoneum. Champault et al. [43] allowed CO_2 to leak during laparoscopy to mimic the chimney effect and by using immunohistochemistry, found cancer cells in six out of nine patients.

Other authors have shown that aerosolization and chimney effect are not responsible for PSM. In Wistar-Agouti rats injected with CC 531 cancer cells, Wittich et al. [44] concluded that aerosolization is not a relevant factor in the pathogenesis of PSM. By using B16 melanoma and colon cancer cells in both in vitro (19L plastic vessels) and in vivo (Sprague-Dawley rats) experiments, Whelan et al. [45] were unable to demonstrate any aerosolization of cancer cells. In patients undergoing elective laparoscopy, Ikramuddin et al. [46] concluded that tumor cell aerosolization is unlikely to contribute to PSM. Kim et al. [47] noted that laparoscopy is not associated with increased tumor spillage when compared with open procedures if strict oncologic

Table 16.8.1: Causes of PSM

Mechanical Aspects	Metabolic Aspects
Aerosolization and chimney effect	Effect of CO_2 on systemic immune response
Direct wound implantation and instrument contamination	Effect of CO_2 on peritoneal immune response
Pneumoperitoneum pressure	Effect of CO_2 on tumor growth
Tissue trauma and tumor manipulation	Effect of type of gas

principles are adhered to. Similarly, other studies have failed to demonstrate aerosolization of viable tumor cells in both in vivo and in vitro experiments.[44,45,48,49]

Direct Wound Implantation and Instrument Contamination

Direct wound implantation and instrument contamination usually lead to PSM at the extraction site or the operating port (Figures 16.8.2, 16.8.3). Bouvy et al. [50] noted that the size of abdominal wall metastasis was greater at the tumor extraction sites than at the other sites. Other authors have shown increasing incidence of PSM at the operating ports or at port sites associated with increasing manipulation.[40,51] In human subjects, Reymond et al. [52] detected K-ras genetic material on instruments, suction devices, and trocar sites in patients undergoing staging laparoscopy for pancreatic cancer. In an in vitro model, Thomas et al. [53] noted contamination of all instruments with malignant cells. Similarly, in a swine model, Hewett et al. [54] concluded

that movement of cancer cells occurs via contaminated instruments. This probably was an important cause when specimens were retrieved through small port incisions without using protective specimen Endobags (United States Surgical). With universal usage of Endobags, the incidence has been reduced dramatically. In addition, better instrumentation and port retaining devices help prevent dislodgement and decrease the incidence of direct contact or repeated manipulation at port sites.

Pneumoperitoneum Pressure

Moreira et al. [55] noted that increasing pressure of pneumoperitoneum in a hamster model increased the incidence of instrument contamination and port-site recurrences, although it was not associated with increased aerosolization. Bouvy et al. [50] reported that laparoscopy was associated with a greater rate of PSM when compared with gasless laparoscopy in a solid tumor animal model. On the other hand, Jacobi et al. [56] and Gutt et al. [57] reported differential and discordant rates of PSM with varying levels of CO_2 pneumoperitoneum and different cell lines. These conflicting results could be due to the variation in animal models used. In any case, in human subjects, it is now accepted that the pressure is maintained at the lowest permissible level that does not compromise visibility.

Tissue Trauma and Tumor Manipulation

Regardless of the operative approach, strict oncologic principles dictate minimal tumor handling and minimize operative trauma. Laparoscopy is associated with tumor handling with unyielding instruments without any tactile feedback compared with open surgery, in which tumor handling can be kept to a minimum. This excessive tumor manipulation is accentuated during the learning

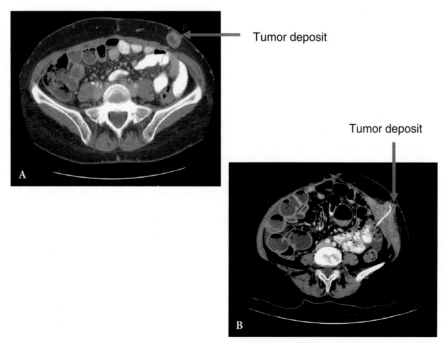

Figure 16.8.2. (**A**) Port site recurrence after operative intervention for ovarian cancer-Stage III C. (**B**) Port site recurrence at site of intra-peritoneal catheter for patient with Stage III C ovarian cancer.

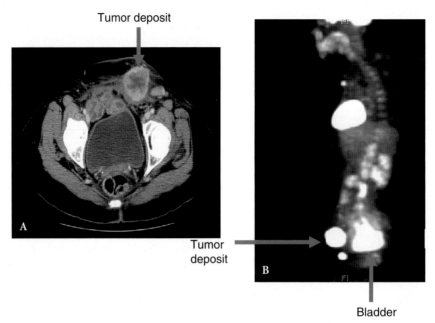

Figure 16.8.3. Wound site matastasis after operative intervention via laparotomy (transverse incision). (**A**) CT scan demonstrating metastatic deposit at wound site after laparotomy. (**B**) PET scan demonstrating increased FDG activity at wound site after laparotomy.

curve, which could account for the high early incidence of PSM. A correlation between tumor manipulation and PSM has been demonstrated in various animal models. Tseng et al. [58] noted a difference in the weight of tumor deposits in port sites without any induced trauma (22 mg) compared with sites subjected to additional crushing injury (316 mg). In a rat model, Mutter et al. [59] demonstrated that tumor manipulation is the main factor behind tumor cell dissemination and seeding of port sites. Similarly, purposeful crushing of splenic tumors before resection in Balb C mice resulted in an increase in the incidence of PSM.[60] With increasing experience, better tissue handling, and minimal tumor manipulation, the incidence of PSM has been reduced to rates comparable to those of open surgery.

Effect of CO_2 on Systemic Immune Response

It is well known that any type of trauma is associated with a degree of reversible posttraumatic immunosuppression. These changes affect both the cellular and humoral aspects of the immune system. Laparoscopy has been shown to be associated with a lesser magnitude of postoperative immunosuppression when compared with laparotomy.[61,62] Interleukin-6 (IL-6), a cytokine produced by macrophages, is a sensitive marker of the degree of trauma, and its levels correlate with the development of postoperative complications. It has been shown that laparoscopy is associated with lower levels of IL-6 when compared with laparotomy.[63–65] Hansbrough et al. [66] reported that the count of lymphocyte subpopulations (CD4 and CD8) are reduced more with laparotomy when compared with laparoscopy. Similarly, delayed-type hypersensitivity has been shown to be better preserved with laparoscopy.[67] This better preservation of the immune response should theoretically confer benefits to the patients. This further reiterates the pos-

sibility that PSM could be caused by factors other than effects of CO_2.

Effect of CO_2 on Peritoneal Immune Response

The effect of CO_2 on the peritoneal immune mechanism differs from its effect on systemic immune mechanisms. Macrophages (tumor-associated macrophages [TAMs]) constitute a significant part and play a major role in the peritoneal immune mechanisms.[38] TAMs represent the first line of local cellular defense in the abdomen. TAMs play a significant role by undertaking several functions, such as antigen presentation, phagocytosis, and secretion of various cytokines that affect angiogenesis.[68–75] It has been shown that TAMs exposed to CO_2 do not function properly.[76–79] Carozzi et al. [77] reported a decreased release of IL-1, IL-6, IL-8, and tumor necrosis factor-α (TNF-α) from macrophages incubated at a pH of 5.5 compared with a pH of 7.4. West et al. [76] noted that macrophages exposed to CO_2 produced less IL-1 and TNF-α. Gutt et al. [79] noted that exposure to CO_2 significantly reduces the phagocytic potential of macrophages. It is not known whether these negative effects on local peritoneal defense mechanisms increase the incidence of PSM.

Effect of CO_2 on Tumor Growth

The effect of CO_2 pneumoperitoneum on tumor growth is controversial. Some authors have suggested that CO_2 pneumoperitoneum increases the incidence of PSM as well as the aggressiveness of tumor growth.[11,12,36,80–87] By using MAT B III mammary adenocarcinoma cells in a rat model, Hopkins et al. [36] showed a lower incidence of implantation with laparotomy when compared with CO_2 pneumoperitoneum. Similarly, in rabbits, injection of VX2 cancer cells into the portal vein was associated with an increased incidence of tumors in the laparoscopy group.[80] Ridgway et al. [88] reported that the invasiveness of pancreatic cancer in vitro is augmented with CO_2, which could be the result of up-regulation of gelatinase and matrix metalloproteinase (MMP) activity and down-regulation of tissue inhibitors of matrix metalloproteinase (TIMP). On the other hand, some authors have demonstrated that CO_2 pneumoperitoneum reduces tumor growth when compared with laparotomy. In a rat model, Mutter et al. [59] noted a beneficial effect of CO_2 pneumoperitoneum on intrapancreatic tumor growth. Gutt et al. [15] noted that laparotomy is associated with greater tumor growth compared with laparoscopy after murine transanal injection with cancer cells. The precise role of CO_2 pneumoperitoneum on tumor biology is unknown and depends on a balance of its protective and deleterious effects on the systemic and peritoneal defense mechanisms, respectively.

Effect of Different Gases

CO_2 is the ideal gas for laparoscopy as it is cheap, easily available, dissolves rapidly in the blood, is not flammable, and is actively excreted by the body. Some studies have reported that CO_2 increases tumor compared with other gases, such as helium and nitrous oxide.[89] In Dark Agouti rats, Neuhaus et al. [89] noted that helium was associated with reduced tumor growth when compared with CO_2 and N_2O. In another study, Gupta et al. [90] reported that helium was associated with the least number of PSMs and the least amount of intraperitoneal tumor growth. Interestingly, in the same study, CO_2 was associated with a lesser growth rate when compared with argon and N_2O. These findings also cannot explain why PSMs develop in patients undergoing thoracoscopic surgery, in which no CO_2 is used.

In summary, it is impossible to deduce the precise cause of PSM from the animal studies. Because of several inherent drawbacks, the multitude of animal experiments provide very conflicting evidence. Suffice it to say, they do point to possible causes of PSM. The ability to prevent, minimize, or avoid some of the aforementioned causes with increasing experience and strict adherence to safe oncologic principles may account for the favorable decrease in the incidence of PSM.

CLINICAL DATA AND CURRENT UPDATE ON PSM

The clinical data from recent years have demonstrated that the incidence of PSM is comparable to wound recurrences after open procedures (Tables 16.8.2–16.8.5). The early reporting of a high incidence of PSM has been overcome by increased experience; concentration of care at high-volume, specialized centers; and fastidious adherence to strict oncologic principles. This trend is true for almost every organ system to which laparoscopy has been applied. The following paragraphs summarize the current data based on individual organ systems.

Gynecologic Malignancy

A selective list of PSMs reported in patients with gynecologic malignancies is summarized in Table 16.8.2. It is clear from the

Table 16.8.2: Selected Reports of PSM

Author/Year	Number of patients	Number of port site metastases
Dobronte et al. (1978) [23]	1	1
Stockdale et al. (1985) [91]	1	1
Kruitwagen et al. (1996) [92]	43	7
Kadar et al. (1997) [93]	25	4
van Dam et al. (1999) [94]	104	9
Hopkins et al. (2000) [7]	3	3
Lecuru et al. (2000) [95]	2	2

table that most cases of PSM were reported early on in the learning curve and consisted of a small number of patients, some of whom had very advanced disease. In a series of 25 patients that documented a 16% incidence of PSM, 24 patients had advanced disease; this included metastatic disease and would therefore make it difficult to assess the incidence of true PSM.[93] In a survey sent to 127 German hospitals during the period from 1991 to 1994, it was noted that laparoscopy was frequently used to treat gynecologic malignancies.[114] In an analysis of the laparoscopic trends among this large group of surgeons, it was noted that in 92% of the patients, there was evidence of tumor rupture and morcellement with intra-abdominal spilling of tumor cells. In addition, it was noted that an Endobag was used in only 7.5% of the patients. These studies show that the indications and contraindications for laparoscopy were not clearly defined early on and that strict oncologic principles were not followed.

The more recent selective data on the application of laparoscopy to the management of gynecologic malignancy are shown in Table 16.8.3. Several observations are evident from this table. The referral of patients to high-volume centers with expertise in oncology and laparoscopy has helped decrease the incidence of PSM. Unlike early reports in which the majority of patients underwent only diagnostic laparoscopy, some of the recent studies include complete staging lymphadenectomy as well.[96,98,100] Despite the increasing complexity of

Table 16.8.3: Recent Publications of PSM in Patients with Gynecologic Malignancies

Author/Year	Number of patients	Percent of port site metastases
Scribner et al. (2001) [96]	125	0
Chi et al. (2004) [97]	724	0
Nagarseth et al. (2004) [30]	83	2.30
Leblanc et al. (2004) [98]	53	0
Abu-Rustum et al. (2004) [19]	1288	0.97
Tozzi et al. (2004) [99]	24	0
Chi et al. (2005) [100]	20	0
Nezhat et al. (2005) [35]	100	0

Table 16.8.4: Recent Publications of PSM in Patients with Gastrointestinal Malignancies

Author/Year	Number of patients	Percent of port site metastases
Lacy et al. (1998) [101]	44	0
Santoro et al. (1998) [31]	131	0.70
Milsom et al. (1998) [102]	55	0
Poulin et al. (1999) [17]	172	0
Pearlstone et al. (1999) [18]	533	0.80
Shoup et al. (2002) [33]	1548	0.79
Lacy et al. (2002) [8]	111	0.90
Morino et al. (2003) [103]	100	1.40
COST study (2004) [9]	435	0.50

COST, Clinical Outcomes of Surgical Therapy Study Group.

therapeutic procedures compared with diagnostic laparoscopy only, the incidence of PSM has been comparable to recurrence rates after open surgery.[96,98,100] In addition, PSM seems to occur mainly in patients with advanced cancer, as reported in the study of Leblanc et al.[98] In their series of 53 patients, the two patients who had PSM also had ascites, which underlies the fact that laparoscopy should be performed with caution in this group of patients. Lastly, the laparoscopic procedures have been shown to be oncologically adequate in terms of number of lymph nodes harvested, recurrence patterns, and overall survival when compared with open procedures.[35,98,100] These studies show that by following strict oncologic principles and keeping the inci-

Table 16.8.5: Recent Publications of PSM in Patients with Urologic Malignancies

Author/Year	Number of patients	Port-Site Percent of port site metastases
Gill et al. (2000) [104]	77	0
Cicco et al. (2000) [105]	56	0
Guillonneau and Vallancien (2000) [106]	120	0
Rassweiler et al. (2003) [34]	1098	0.18
Klingler et al. (2003) [107]	19	0
Guillonneau et al. (2003) [108]	1000	0
Makhoul et al. (2004) [109]	39	0
Wille et al. (2004) [110]	125	0
Micali et al. (2004; survey of 50 international urology departments) [111]	10,912	0.09
Moinzadeh et al. (2005) [112]	31	0
Rassweiler et al. (2005) [113]	500	0

dence of PSM at an acceptable rate, one can garner the benefits of laparoscopy.

Gastrointestinal Malignancy

The earliest report of PSM in the treatment of gastrointestinal malignancy was reported by Alexander et al. [25] in 1993. This was the stimulus for several well-fashioned randomized controlled trials commencing in 1993.[9,33,101] The first randomized controlled trial to analyze PSM was by Lacy et al. [101] in 1998. In their series of 91 patients divided into laparoscopy (44 patients) and open (47 patients) groups, the incidence of PSM was zero in both. The results of the first single-center, large-volume randomized controlled trial confirmed that laparoscopic colectomy can be performed with a PSM rate of less than 1%.[8] This was followed by the Clinical Outcomes of Surgical Therapy (COST) study that included results from 68 credentialed surgeons from 48 institutions.[9] Participating surgeons had to have performed at least 20 laparoscopic operations and were credentialed after a video of their operation was reviewed by an expert committee. The video was reviewed to assess proper oncologic technique, such as minimal handling of tumor, level of mesenteric ligation, identification of critical structures, and thoroughness of abdominal exploration. This large-volume multicenter study again showed that laparoscopic colectomy can be performed with acceptable rates of PSM as long as strict oncologic principles are followed.[9]

Genitourinary Malignancy

Laparoscopy was already extensively being used to perform donor nephrectomies before its application to treating urologic malignancies. This prior experience with laparoscopy enabled a smooth transition for urologists in dealing with genitourinary malignancies. The recent studies using a large number of patients again demonstrate that laparoscopy can be performed with rates of PSM comparable to those of open surgery.

In summary, the early reports of a high incidence of PSM do not translate to the more recently published data. Recently published data have consistently shown that with strict adherence to oncologic principles, the incidence of PSM can be kept low, at levels comparable to those following open surgery.

PREVENTION

Several precautions need to be taken to reduce the incidence of PSM. These precautions are similar those taken during open surgery for malignant disorders to reduce the incidence of wound recurrence and include the following:

1. Maintain tumor manipulation at a minimum
2. Avoid tumor rupture
3. Perform high ligation of vasculature
4. Avoid excessive manipulation of the port sites
5. Prevent dislodgement of the trocars by securing them
6. Keep pneumoperitoneum at the lowest pressure possible to maintain visibility
7. Avoid leaks around the port sites
8. Retrieve specimens in Endobags

9. Deflate the pneumoperitoneum with the trocars in place
10. Drain all fluid with trocars in place to avoid contact with port sites
11. Use wound protectors for wounds used for extracorporeal anastomoses, when necessary
12. Close the peritoneum when possible

Other studies have shown that topical application of certain agents, such as heparin [115], MMP inhibitor [116], taurolidine [117], and doxorubicin [118], can reduce the incidence of PSM. These studies also have inherent flaws, and the findings cannot be extrapolated to the true clinical situation. What is more important and imperative is the application of sound oncologic principles, which cannot be substituted or replaced by newer techniques or agents.

SUMMARY

The success of laparoscopy in the treatment of malignant disorders depends solely on the application of the oncologic principles that have been tested and used in open surgery. The availability of new technology should not broaden the indications for cancer surgery nor should laparoscopy be undertaken when contraindications exist. The application of laparoscopy in treating cancer of any organ system demands the performance of a minimum number of procedures for benign conditions of the same organ. Only then can one embark on treating malignant conditions via the laparoscope. The benefits of any new technology are substantiated only when its application results in similar or better disease-free and overall survival rates when compared with the established gold standard. We know that laparoscopy has several benefits, such as less pain, faster recovery, and earlier return to work. With strict application of sound oncologic principles and adequate training in minimally invasive surgery, we can hope to avoid complications such as PSM and obtain long-term survival rates similar to those for open surgery.

REFERENCES

1. Berends FJ, Kazemier G, Bonjer HJ, Lange JF. Subcutaneous metastases after laparoscopic colectomy. *Lancet.* 1994;344:58.
2. Lundberg O. Port site metastases after laparoscopic cholecystectomy. *Eur J Surg Suppl.* 2000;(585):27–30.
3. Siriwardena A, Samarji WN. Cutaneous tumor seeding from a previously undiagnosed pancreatic carcinoma after laparoscopic cholecystectomy. *Ann R Coll Surg Engl.* 1993;75:199–200.
4. Jorgensen JO, McCall JL, Morris DL. Port site seeding after laparoscopic ultrasonographic staging of pancreatic carcinoma. *Surgery.* 1995;117:118–119.
5. Freeman RK, Wait MA. Port site metastasis after laparoscopic staging of esophageal carcinoma. *Ann Thorac Surg.* 2001;71:1032–1034.
6. Cava A, Roman J, Gonzalez Quintela A, Martin F, Aramburo P. Subcutaneous metastasis following laparoscopy in gastric adenocarcinoma. *Eur J Surg Oncol.* 1990;16:63–67.
7. Hopkins MP, von Gruenigen V, Gaich S. Laparoscopic port site implantation with ovarian cancer. *Am J Obstet Gynecol.* 2000;182:735–736.
8. Lacy AM, Garcia-Valdecasas JC, Delgado S, et al. Laparoscopy-assisted colectomy versus open colectomy for treatment of non-metastatic colon cancer: a randomised trial. *Lancet.* 2002;359: 2224–2229.
9. Clinical Outcomes of Surgical Therapy Study Group. A comparison of laparoscopically assisted and open colectomy for colon cancer. *N Engl J Med.* 2004;350:2050–2059.
10. Jones DB, Guo LW, Reinhard MK, et al. Impact of pneumoperitoneum on trocar site implantation of colon cancer in hamster model. *Dis Colon Rectum.* 1995;38:1182–1188.
11. Jacobi CA, Ordemann J, Bohm B, et al. The influence of laparotomy and laparoscopy on tumor growth in a rat model. *Surg Endosc.* 1997;11:618–621.
12. Le Moine MC, Navarro F, Burgel JS, et al. Experimental assessment of the risk of tumor recurrence after laparoscopic surgery. *Surgery.* 1998;123:427–431.
13. Bouvy ND, Marquet RL, Jeekel J, Bonjer HJ. Laparoscopic surgery is associated with less tumor growth stimulation than conventional surgery: an experimental study. *Br J Surg.* 1997;84:358–361.
14. Southall JC, Lee SW, Allendorf JD, Bessler M, Whelan RL. Colon adenocarcinoma and B-16 melanoma grow larger following laparotomy vs. pneumoperitoneum in a murine model. *Dis Colon Rectum.* 1998;41:564–569.
15. Gutt CN, Riemer V, Kim ZG, Jacobi CA, Paolucci V, Lorenz M. Impact of laparoscopic colonic resection on tumor growth and spread in an experimental model. *Br J Surg.* 1999;86:1180–1184.
16. Bohm B, Schwenk W, Muller JM. Long-term results after laparoscopic resection of colorectal carcinoma [in German]. *Chirurg.* 1999;70:453–455.
17. Poulin EC, Mamazza J, Schlachta CM, Gregoire R, Roy N. Laparoscopic resection does not adversely affect early survival curves in patients undergoing surgery for colorectal adenocarcinoma. *Ann Surg.* 1999;229:487–492.
18. Pearlstone DB, Mansfield PF, Curley SA, Kumparatana M, Cook P, Feig BW. Laparoscopy in 533 patients with abdominal malignancy. *Surgery.* 1999;125:67–72.
19. Abu-Rustum NR, Rhee EH, Chi DS, Sonoda Y, Gemignani M, Barakat RR. Subcutaneous tumor implantation after laparoscopic procedures in women with malignant disease. *Obstet Gynecol.* 2004;103:480–487.
20. De Mulder W, Gillardin JP, Hofman P, Van Molhem Y. Laparoscopic colorectal surgery. Analysis of the first 237 cases. *Acta Chir Belg.* 2001;101:25–30.
21. Hong D, Tabet J, Anvari M. Laparoscopic vs. open resection for colorectal adenocarcinoma. *Dis Colon Rectum.* 2001;44:10–18; discussion 18–19.
22. Lauter DM, Froines EJ. Initial experience with 150 cases of laparoscopic assisted colectomy. *Am J Surg.* 2001;181:398–403.
23. Dobronte Z, Wittmann T, Karacsony G. Rapid development of malignant metastases in the abdominal wall after laparoscopy. *Endoscopy.* 1978;10:127–130.
24. Umpleby HC, Fermor B, Symes MO, Williamson RC. Viability of exfoliated colorectal carcinoma cells. *Br J Surg.* 1984;71:659–663.
25. Alexander RJ, Jaques BC, Mitchell KG. Laparoscopically assisted colectomy and wound recurrence. *Lancet.* 1993;341:249–250.
26. Hughes ES, McDermott FT, Polglase AL, Johnson WR. Tumor recurrence in the abdominal wall scar tissue after large-bowel cancer surgery. *Dis Colon Rectum.* 1983;26:571–572.
27. Reilly WT, Nelson H, Schroeder G, Wieand HS, Bolton J, O'Connell MJ. Wound recurrence following conventional treatment of colorectal cancer. A rare but perhaps underestimated problem. *Dis Colon Rectum.* 1996;39:200–207.
28. Wexner SD, Cohen SM. Port site metastases after laparoscopic colorectal surgery for cure of malignancy. *Br J Surg.* 1995;82:295–298.

29. Paolucci V, Schaeff B, Schneider M, Gutt C. Tumor seeding following laparoscopy: international survey. *World J Surg.* 1999;23: 989–995; discussion 996–997.

30. Nagarsheth NP, Rahaman J, Cohen CJ, Gretz H, Nezhat F. The incidence of port-site metastases in gynecologic cancers. *JSLS.* 2004;8:133–139.

31. Santoro R, Barrat C, Catheline JM, Faranda C, Champault G. Port site metastasis. Prospective study of 131 cases [in Italian]. *Chir Ital.* 1998;50:15–22.

32. Pearlstone DB, Feig BW, Mansfield PF. Port site recurrences after laparoscopy for malignant disease. *Semin Surg Oncol.* 1999;16: 307–312.

33. Shoup M, Brennan MF, Karpeh MS, Gillern SM, McMahon RL, Conlon KC. Port site metastasis after diagnostic laparoscopy for upper gastrointestinal tract malignancies: an uncommon entity. *Ann Surg Oncol.* 2002;9:632–636.

34. Rassweiler J, Tsivian A, Kumar AV, et al. Oncological safety of laparoscopic surgery for urological malignancy: experience with more than 1000 operations. *J Urol.* 2003;169:2072–2075.

35. Nezhat F, Yadav J, Rahaman J, Gretz H 3rd, Gardner GJ, Cohen CJ. Laparoscopic lymphadenectomy for gynecologic malignancies using ultrasonically activated shears: analysis of first 100 cases. *Gynecol Oncol.* 2005;97:813–819.

36. Hopkins MP, Dulai RM, Occhino A, Holda S. The effects of carbon dioxide pneumoperitoneum on seeding of tumor in port sites in a rat model. *Am J Obstet Gynecol.* 1999;181:1329–1333; discussion 1333–1334.

37. Dore F, Melis GC, Fumu E, et al. Role of densitometry and scintigraphy in post-traumatic algodystrophy of the arms. Initial diagnosis and monitoring during treatment with carbocalcitonin [in Italian]. *Radiol Med (Torino).* 1991;81:114–117.

38. Are C, Talamini MA. Laparoscopy and malignancy. *J Laparoendosc Adv Surg Tech A.* 2005;15:38–47.

39. Are C, Talamini MA. Current knowledge regarding the biology of pneumoperitoneum based surgery. *Curr Probl Gen Surg.* 2001;18:52–63.

40. Allardyce R, Morreau P, Bagshaw P. Tumor cell distribution following laparoscopic colectomy in a porcine model. *Dis Colon Rectum.* 1996;39(suppl):S47–S52.

41. Mathew G, Watson DI, Ellis T, De Young N, Rofe AM, Jamieson GG. The effect of laparoscopy on the movement of tumor cells and metastasis to surgical wounds. *Surg Endosc.* 1997;11:1163–1166.

42. Knolmayer TJ, Asbun HJ, Shibata G, Bowyer MW. An experimental model of cellular aerosolization during laparoscopic surgery. *Surg Laparosc Endosc.* 1997;7:399–402.

43. Champault G, Taffinder N, Ziol M, Riskalla H, Catheline JM. Cells are present in the smoke created during laparoscopic surgery. *Br J Surg.* 1997;84:993–995.

44. Wittich P, Marquet RL, Kazemier G, Bonjer HJ. Port-site metastases after CO(2) laparoscopy. Is aerosolization of tumor cells a pivotal factor? *Surg Endosc.* 2000;14:189–192.

45. Whelan RL, Sellers GJ, Allendorf JD, et al. Trocar site recurrence is unlikely to result from aerosolization of tumor cells. *Dis Colon Rectum.* 1996;39(10 suppl):S7–S13.

46. Ikramuddin S, Lucus J, Ellison EC, Schirmer WJ, Melvin WS. Detection of aerosolized cells during carbon dioxide laparoscopy. *J Gastrointest Surg.* 1998;2:580–583; discussion 584.

47. Kim SH, Milsom JW, Gramlich TL, et al. Does laparoscopic vs. conventional surgery increase exfoliated cancer cells in the peritoneal cavity during resection of colorectal cancer? *Dis Colon Rectum.* 1998;41:971–978.

48. Nduka CC, Poland N, Kennedy M, Dye J, Darzi A. Does the ultrasonically activated scalpel release viable airborne cancer cells? *Surg Endosc.* 1998;12:1031–1034.

49. Sellers GJ, Whelan RL, Allendorf JD, et al. An in vitro model fails to demonstrate aerosolization of tumor cells. *Surg Endosc.* 1998;12:436–439.

50. Bouvy ND, Marquet RL, Jeekel H, Bonjer HJ. Impact of gas(less) laparoscopy and laparotomy on peritoneal tumor growth and abdominal wall metastases. *Ann Surg.* 1996;224:694–700; discussion 700–701.

51. Allardyce RA, Morreau P, Bagshaw PF. Operative factors affecting tumor cell distribution following laparoscopic colectomy in a porcine model. *Dis Colon Rectum.* 1997;40:939–945.

52. Reymond MA, Wittekind C, Jung A, Hohenberger W, Kirchner T, Kockerling F. The incidence of port-site metastases might be reduced. *Surg Endosc.* 1997;11:902–906.

53. Thomas WM, Eaton MC, Hewett PJ. A proposed model for the movement of cells within the abdominal cavity during CO_2 insufflation and laparoscopy. *Aust N Z J Surg.* 1996;66:105–106.

54. Hewett PJ, Thomas WM, King G, Eaton M. Intraperitoneal cell movement during abdominal carbon dioxide insufflation and laparoscopy. An in vivo model. *Dis Colon Rectum.* 1996;39(10 suppl):S62–S66.

55. Moreira H Jr, Yamaguchi T, Wexner S, et al. Effect of pneumoperitoneal pressure on tumor dissemination and tumor recurrence at port-site and midline incisions. *Am Surg.* 2001;67:369–373.

56. Jacobi CA, Wenger FA, Ordemann J, Gutt C, Sabat R, Muller JM. Experimental study of the effect of intra-abdominal pressure during laparoscopy on tumor growth and port site metastasis. *Br J Surg.* 1998;85:1419–1422.

57. Gutt CN, Kim ZG, Hollander D, Bruttel T, Lorenz M. CO_2 environment influences the growth of cultured human cancer cells dependent on insufflation pressure. *Surg Endosc.* 2001;15:314–318.

58. Tseng LN, Berends FJ, Wittich P, et al. Port-site metastases. Impact of local tissue trauma and gas leakage. *Surg Endosc.* 1998;12:1377–1380.

59. Mutter D, Hajri A, Tassetti V, Solis-Caxaj C, Aprahamian M, Marescaux J. Increased tumor growth and spread after laparoscopy vs laparotomy: influence of tumor manipulation in a rat model. *Surg Endosc.* 1999;13:365–370.

60. Lee SW, Southall J, Allendorf J, Bessler M, Whelan RL. Traumatic handling of the tumor independent of pneumoperitoneum increases port site implantation rate of colon cancer in a murine model. *Surg Endosc.* 1998;12:828–834.

61. Redmond HP, Watson RW, Houghton T, Condron C, Watson RG, Bouchier-Hayes D. Immune function in patients undergoing open vs laparoscopic cholecystectomy. *Arch Surg.* 1994;129:1240–1246.

62. Trokel MJ, Bessler M, Treat MR, Whelan RL, Nowygrod R. Preservation of immune response after laparoscopy. *Surg Endosc.* 1994;8:1385–1387; discussion 1387–1388.

63. Cho JM, LaPorta AJ, Clark JR, Schofield MJ, Hammond SL, Mallory PL 2nd. Response of serum cytokines in patients undergoing laparoscopic cholecystectomy. *Surg Endosc.* 1994;8:1380–1383; discussion 1383–1384.

64. Glaser F, Sannwald GA, Buhr HJ, et al. General stress response to conventional and laparoscopic cholecystectomy. *Ann Surg.* 1995;221:372–380.

65. Maruszynski M, Pojda Z. Interleukin 6 (IL-6) levels in the monitoring of surgical trauma. A comparison of serum IL-6 concentrations in patients treated by cholecystectomy via laparotomy or laparoscopy. *Surg Endosc.* 1995;9:882–885.

66. Hansbrough JF, Bender EM, Zapata-Sirvent R, Anderson J. Altered helper and suppressor lymphocyte populations in surgical patients. A measure of postoperative immunosuppression. *Am J Surg.* 1984;148:303–307.

67. Christou NV, Ing AF, Larson DL, Meakins JL. A reliable rat model of the delayed hypersensitivity skin test response. *J Surg Res*. 1984;37:264–268.

68. Ribeiro-Dias F, Russo M, Nascimento FR, Barbuto JA, Timenetsky J, Jancar S. Thioglycollate-elicited murine macrophages are cytotoxic to *Mycoplasma arginini*–infected YAC-1 tumor cells. *Braz J Med Biol Res*. 1998;31:1425–1428.

69. Kumar R, Yoneda J, Fidler IJ, Dong Z. GM-CSF-transduced B16 melanoma cells are highly susceptible to lysis by normal murine macrophages and poorly tumorigenic in immune-compromised mice. *J Leukoc Biol*. 1999;65:102–108.

70. Hennemann B, Rehm A, Kottke A, Meidenbauer N, Andreesen R. Adoptive immunotherapy with tumor-cytotoxic macrophages derived from recombinant human granulocyte-macrophage colony-stimulating factor (rhuGM-CSF) mobilized peripheral blood monocytes. *J Immunother*. 1997;20:365–371.

71. Pujade-Lauraine E, Guastalla JP, Colombo N, et al. Intraperitoneal recombinant interferon gamma in ovarian cancer patients with residual disease at second-look laparotomy. *J Clin Oncol*. 1996;14:343–350.

72. Macfarlan RI, Burns WH, White DO. Two cytotoxic cells in peritoneal cavity of virus-infected mice: antibody-dependent macrophages and nonspecific killer cells. *J Immunol*. 1977;119:1569–1574.

73. Greenberg AH, Shen L, Medley G. Characteristics of the effector cells mediating cytotoxicity against antibody-coated target cells. I. Phagocytic and non-phagocytic effector cell activity against erythrocyte and tumor target cells in a 51Cr release cytotoxicity assay and [125I]IUdR growth inhibition assay. *Immunology*. 1975;29:719–729.

74. Bingle L, Brown NJ, Lewis CE. The role of tumor-associated macrophages in tumor progression: implications for new anticancer therapies. *J Pathol*. 2002;196:254–265.

75. Chen JJ, Lin YC, Yao PL, et al. Tumor-associated macrophages: the double-edged sword in cancer progression. *J Clin Oncol*. 2005;23:953–964.

76. West MA, Hackam DJ, Baker J, Rodriguez JL, Bellingham J, Rotstein OD. Mechanism of decreased in vitro murine macrophage cytokine release after exposure to carbon dioxide: relevance to laparoscopic surgery. *Ann Surg*. 1997;226:179–190.

77. Carozzi S, Caviglia PM, Nasini MG, Schelotto C, Santoni O, Pietrucci A. Peritoneal dialysis solution pH and Ca2+ concentration regulate peritoneal macrophage and mesothelial cell activation. *ASAIO J*. 1994;40:20–23.

78. Kopernik G, Avinoach E, Grossman Y, et al. The effect of a high partial pressure of carbon dioxide environment on metabolism and immune functions of human peritoneal cells – relevance to carbon dioxide pneumoperitoneum. *Am J Obstet Gynecol*. 1998;179(6 pt 1):1503–1510.

79. Gutt CN, Heinz P, Kaps W, Paolucci V. The phagocytosis activity during conventional and laparoscopic operations in the rat. A preliminary study. *Surg Endosc*. 1997;11:899–901.

80. Ishida H, Murata N, Yamada H, et al. Pneumoperitoneum with carbon dioxide enhances liver metastases of cancer cells implanted into the portal vein in rabbits [erratum in: *Surg Endosc*. 2000;14:411]. *Surg Endosc*. 2000;14:239–242.

81. Mathew G, Watson DI, Rofe AM, Ellis T, Jamieson GG. Adverse impact of pneumoperitoneum on intraperitoneal implantation and growth of tumor cell suspension in an experimental model. *Aust N Z J Surg*. 1997;67:289–292.

82. Cavina E, Goletti O, Molea N, et al. Trocar site tumor recurrences. May pneumoperitoneum be responsible? *Surg Endosc*. 1998;12:1294–1296.

83. Targarona EM, Martinez J, Nadal A, et al. Cancer dissemination during laparoscopic surgery: tubes, gas, and cells. *World J Surg*. 1998;22:55–60; discussion 60–61.

84. Volz J, Koster S, Spacek Z, Paweletz N. The influence of pneumoperitoneum used in laparoscopic surgery on an intraabdominal tumor growth. *Cancer*. 1999;86:770–774.

85. Koster S, Melchert F, Volz J. Effect of CO$_2$ pneumoperitoneum on intraperitoneal tumor growth in the animal model [in German]. *Geburtshilfe Frauenheilkd*. 1996;56:458–461.

86. Mathew G, Watson DI, Rofe AM, Baigrie CF, Ellis T, Jamieson GG. Wound metastases following laparoscopic and open surgery for abdominal cancer in a rat model. *Br J Surg*. 1996;83:1087–1090.

87. Canis M, Botchorishvili R, Wattiez A, Mage G, Pouly JL, Bruhat MA. Tumor growth and dissemination after laparotomy and CO$_2$ pneumoperitoneum: a rat ovarian cancer model. *Obstet Gynecol*. 1998;92:104–108.

88. Ridgway PF, Smith A, Ziprin P, et al. Pneumoperitoneum augmented tumor invasiveness is abolished by matrix metalloproteinase blockade. *Surg Endosc*. 2002;16:533–536.

89. Neuhaus SJ, Ellis T, Rofe AM, Pike GK, Jamieson GG, Watson DI. Tumor implantation following laparoscopy using different insufflation gases. *Surg Endosc*. 1998;12:1300–1302.

90. Gupta A, Watson DI, Ellis T, Jamieson GG. Tumor implantation following laparoscopy using different insufflation gases. *ANZ J Surg*. 2002;72:254–257.

91. Stockdale AD, Pocock TJ. Abdominal wall metastasis following laparoscopy: a case report. *Eur J Surg Oncol*. 1985;11:373–375.

92. Kruitwagen RF, Swinkels BM, Keyser KG, Doesburg WH, Schijf CP. Incidence and effect on survival of abdominal wall metastases at trocar or puncture sites following laparoscopy or paracentesis in women with ovarian cancer. *Gynecol Oncol*. 1996;60:233–237.

93. Kadar N. Port-site recurrences following laparoscopic operations for gynaecological malignancies. *Br J Obstet Gynaecol*. 1997;104:1308–1313.

94. van Dam PA, DeCloedt J, Tjalma WA, Buytaert P, Becquart D, Vergote IB. Trocar implantation metastasis after laparoscopy in patients with advanced ovarian cancer: can the risk be reduced? *Am J Obstet Gynecol*. 1999;181:536–541.

95. Lecuru F, Darai E, Robin F, Housset M, Durdux C, Taurelle R. Port site metastasis after laparoscopy for gynecological cancer: report of two cases. *Acta Obstet Gynecol Scand*. 2000;79:1021–1023.

96. Scribner DR Jr, Walker JL, Johnson GA, McMeekin SD, Gold MA, Mannel RS. Surgical management of early-stage endometrial cancer in the elderly: is laparoscopy feasible? *Gynecol Oncol*. 2001;83:563–568.

97. Chi DS, Abu-Rustum NR, Sonoda Y, et al. Ten-year experience with laparoscopy on a gynecologic oncology service: analysis of risk factors for complications and conversion to laparotomy. *Am J Obstet Gynecol*. 2004;191:1138–1145.

98. Leblanc E, Querleu D, Narducci F, Occelli B, Papageorgiou T, Sonoda Y. Laparoscopic restaging of early stage invasive adnexal tumors: a 10-year experience. *Gynecol Oncol*. 2004;94:624–629.

99. Tozzi R, Kohler C, Ferrara A, Schneider A. Laparoscopic treatment of early ovarian cancer: surgical and survival outcomes. *Gynecol Oncol*. 2004;93:199–203.

100. Chi DS, Abu-Rustum NR, Sonoda Y, et al. The safety and efficacy of laparoscopic surgical staging of apparent stage I ovarian and fallopian tube cancers. *Am J Obstet Gynecol*. 2005;192:1614–1619.

101. Lacy AM, Delgado S, Garcia-Valdecasas JC, et al. Port site metastases and recurrence after laparoscopic colectomy. A randomized trial. *Surg Endosc*. 1998;12:1039–1042.

102. Milsom JW, Bohm B, Hammerhofer KA, Fazio V, Steiger E, Elson P. A prospective, randomized trial comparing laparoscopic versus

conventional techniques in colorectal cancer surgery: a preliminary report. *J Am Coll Surg*. 1998;187:46–54; discussion 54–55.

103. Morino M, Parini U, Giraudo G, et al. Laparoscopic total mesorectal excision: a consecutive series of 100 patients. *Ann Surg*. 2003;237:335–342.

104. Gill IS, Sung GT, Hobart MG, et al. Laparoscopic radical nephroureterectomy for upper tract transitional cell carcinoma: the Cleveland Clinic experience. *J Urol*. 2000;164:1513–1522.

105. Cicco A, Salomon L, Hoznek H, et al. Carcinological risks and retroperitoneal laparoscopy. *Eur Urol*. 2000;38:606–612.

106. Guillonneau B, Vallancien G. Laparoscopic radical prostatectomy: the Montsouris experience. *J Urol*. 2000;163:418–422.

107. Klingler HC, Lodde M, Pycha A, Remzi M, Janetschek G, Marberger M. Modified laparoscopic nephroureterectomy for treatment of upper urinary tract transitional cell cancer is not associated with an increased risk of tumor recurrence. *Eur Urol*. 2003;44:442–447.

108. Guillonneau B, el-Fettouh H, Baumert H, et al. Laparoscopic radical prostatectomy: oncological evaluation after 1000 cases at Montsouris Institute. *J Urol*. 2003;169:1261–1266.

109. Makhoul B, De La Taille A, Vordos D, et al. Laparoscopic radical nephrectomy for T1 renal cancer: the gold standard? A comparison of laparoscopic vs open nephrectomy. *BJU Int*. 2004;93:67–70.

110. Wille AH, Roigas J, Deger S, Tullmann M, Turk I, Loening SA. Laparoscopic radical nephrectomy: techniques, results and oncological outcome in 125 consecutive cases. *Eur Urol*. 2004;45:483–488; discussion 488–489.

111. Micali S, Celia A, Bove P, et al. Tumor seeding in urological laparoscopy: an international survey. *J Urol*. 2004;171(6 pt 1):2151–2154.

112. Moinzadeh A, Gill IS. Laparoscopic radical adrenalectomy for malignancy in 31 patients. *J Urol*. 2005;173:519–525.

113. Rassweiler J, Schulze M, Teber D, et al. Laparoscopic radical prostatectomy with the Heilbronn technique: oncological results in the first 500 patients. *J Urol*. 2005;173:761–764.

114. Kindermann G, Maassen V, Kuhn W. Laparoscopic preliminary surgery of ovarian malignancies. Experiences from 127 German gynecologic clinics [in German]. *Geburtshilfe Frauenheilkd*. 1995;55:687–694.

115. Jacobi CA, Peter FJ, Wenger FA, Ordemann J, Muller JM. New therapeutic strategies to avoid intra- and extraperitoneal metastases during laparoscopy: results of a tumor model in the rat. *Dig Surg*. 1999;16:393–399.

116. Hase K, Ueno H, Kuranaga N, Utsunomiya K, Kanabe S, Mochizuki H. Intraperitoneal exfoliated cancer cells in patients with colorectal cancer [erratum in: *Dis Colon Rectum*. 1998;41:1249]. *Dis Colon Rectum*. 1998;41:1134–1140.

117. Jacobi CA, Ordemann J, Bohm B, Zieren HU, Sabat R, Muller JM. Inhibition of peritoneal tumor cell growth and implantation in laparoscopic surgery in a rat model. *Am J Surg*. 1997;174:359–363.

118. Hamilton RE. Opposition to NH1 urged [letter]. *J Oral Surg*. 1975;33:487.

17 | LAPAROSCOPY IN THE PREGNANT PATIENT

Maureen M. Tedesco and Myriam J. Curet

Since the advent of laparoscopic surgery in the 1980s, laparoscopic surgery has been popularized by surgeons throughout the world. However, routine laparoscopic surgery has been slow to catch on in one group of patients, that is, the pregnant patient. The responsibility of caring for two patients during one operation and the concern over potential harm to the unborn fetus due to the pneumoperitoneum and/or instrumentation are factors that have played a role in the delay of adapting laparoscopic surgery to the pregnant patient. However, recent evidence suggests that not only is laparoscopic surgery safe in the pregnant patient in all three trimesters, but it is also often preferable.

This chapter reviews several aspects of laparoscopic surgery in the pregnant patient.

PHYSIOLOGIC CHANGES OF PREGNANCY

One must consider the many physiologic changes that occur during pregnancy when discussing any surgery in a pregnant patient. From a respiratory standpoint, the minute ventilation is 50% higher than normal, resulting in a marked decrease in arterial concentration of carbon dioxide, and mild respiratory alkalosis.[1] In contrast, the fetus has a normal mild respiratory acidosis, which is thought to facilitate delivery of oxygen.[2] It has also been shown that the normal pregnant patient has a mild anemia, increased cardiac output, increased heart rate, and an increased oxygen consumption to support two circulatory systems and provide adequate oxygenation to both the mother and fetus. These factors must be taken into account when planning general anesthesia.

In addition to the respiratory changes, there are mild hematologic abnormalities in the pregnant patient. Levels of fibrinogen, factor VII, and factor XII are increased, whereas there are decreased levels of antithrombin III, all of which result in an increased risk of venous thromboembolism. [3,4]

When considering the acute abdomen in a pregnant patient, making the correct diagnosis may often be difficult. Nausea and vomiting, leukocytosis, low-grade fever, mild hypotension, and anorexia are common. The gravid uterus pushes the abdominal contents cephalad, displacing organs and inhibiting the migration of the omentum, causing altered landmarks and often distorting the clinical picture.[5] During the second and third trimesters, the gravid uterus may cause decreased gastric motility and may lead to an increased risk of gastroesophageal reflux disease (GERD) and aspiration as well.[1]

ABDOMINAL SURGERY IN PREGNANCY

Surgery in pregnancy is not uncommon, nor is it without risk. It is estimated that 0.2% of pregnancies require nongynecologic surgery.[3] The most common general surgery emergencies during pregnancy are appendicitis, intestinal obstruction, and cholecystitis.[5]

There are multiple concerns about abdominal operations during pregnancy, as the life of both the mother and the fetus must be taken into consideration. Direct uterine trauma, changes in uteroplacental blood flow and oxygen delivery, teratogenic effects of anesthetics, effects of anesthetics on maternal hemostasis, exacerbation of the impaired ventilatory mechanics common in pregnancy, effects of postoperative medications such as analgesics and antiemetics, and a risk of incisional hernias are a few of the concerns the surgeon has when planning an abdominal operation in a pregnant patient.[6]

It has been shown that abdominal surgery during the first trimester has been associated with a 12% spontaneous abortion rate, which is significantly reduced to 0% during the third trimester. Abdominal surgery during pregnancy also increases the rate of preterm labor; during the second trimester, the rate is estimated to be 5% to 8%, which increases to 30% to 40% during the third trimester.[4,7] As a result, the safest time to perform surgery in pregnancy is during the second trimester, when spontaneous abortion and preterm labor rates are at their lowest.

Mazze and Kallen [8] reported a large study on adverse outcomes of nonobstetric operations during pregnancy, obtaining data from three Swedish Health Care registries in which 5405 operative cases were evaluated, 16.1% of which were laparoscopic. In this report, the incidence of stillbirths or congenital anomalies in the pregnant patient who underwent an operation was not increased, even when the operation was performed in the first trimester. There was an increase in low–birth-weight infants (due to intrauterine growth retardation and premature delivery) and infants who died within 7 days of delivery, though, compared with women who had not undergone an operation. In addition, there was no increase in adverse outcomes when the laparoscopic group was compared with those undergoing other surgical procedures.

Appendicitis in Pregnancy

Appendicitis is the most common acute general surgical condition during pregnancy.[9] Approximately one in 15,000 or 0.05% to 0.1% of pregnant women will have acute appendicitis, which is evenly distributed through all three trimesters.[3,5]

Compared with the nonpregnant patient, there is a high negative appendicitis rate because of anatomic and physiologic changes of pregnancy, which were discussed earlier. There is a 35% to 55% negative appendicitis rate in the pregnant patient compared with a 5% to 10% negative appendicitis rate in the nonpregnant patient.[10,11] Specifically, the presence of leukocytosis, nausea, vomiting, and abdominal pain in the pregnant patient can make the diagnosis of acute appendicitis difficult.[7] The length of gestation also plays a role in the accuracy of the preoperative diagnosis of appendicitis in pregnancy. The preoperative diagnosis is correct in the first trimester 85% of the time, whereas it is correct only 30% to 50% of the time in the third trimester.[3]

The rate of fetal loss is 1.5% with uncomplicated appendicitis, and increases significantly to 35% with perforated appendicitis.[9] A delay in the diagnosis of acute appendicitis can have life-threatening consequences for the fetus. A delay in diagnosis of appendicitis leads to a 10% to 15% perforation rate, which leads to increases in fetal mortality of 5% to 35% and a premature delivery rate of 40% in all three trimesters.[3] Therefore, it is recommended that a pregnant patient with acute appendicitis be treated as a nonpregnant patient, with rapid resuscitation with intravenous fluids, antibiotics, and prompt surgical treatment.

Biliary Disease in the Pregnant Patient

Like appendicitis, gallstones are also common in pregnancy and can be found in 12% of all pregnancies.[3] It is estimated that 4.5% to 12% of pregnant women have asymptomatic cholelithiasis whereas 0.05% of pregnant women will experience symptomatic cholelithiasis [4] (30% to 40% higher than the general population [12]). Forty percent of those who have symptomatic cholelithiasis will ultimately receive surgical intervention, resulting in three to eight out of 10,000 pregnancies requiring a cholecystectomy.[3] The cholecystectomy is the most common general surgical procedure performed during pregnancy.[11,13]

Pregnancy predisposes women to biliary disease and gallstone formation. Multiparity carries with it an increased risk of gallstone disease because of increased secretion of cholesterol compared with bile acids, and increased secretion of phospholipids.[14] During pregnancy, there is increased gallbladder size during fasting, increased residual volume after emptying, increased saturation of bile with cholesterol, and a decreased circulating pool of bile salt that also contributes to the large number of pregnant women with cholelithiasis.[4]

Delay in adequate treatment of biliary disease may be life threatening to both the mother and the fetus. The rate of spontaneous abortion is 5% in uncomplicated cholecystectomies and as high as 60% in those associated with gallstone pancreatitis.[5] There is a 12% risk of spontaneous abortion with nonoperative management of symptomatic cholelithiasis during the first trimester.[13] In addition, nonoperative management of symptomatic cholelithiasis increases the risk of gallstone pancreatitis up to 13% [11] and gallstone pancreatitis increases maternal mortality to 15% and fetal mortality to 60%.[3,4]

The recommended initial management of symptomatic cholelithiasis is conservative: Restrict the patient from oral intake, rehydrate with intravenous fluids, manage pain appropriately, and initiate antibiotic therapy if needed.[4,14] As many as 70% of patients treated conservatively will relapse, of which 90% will require rehospitalization. The risk of relapse is greatest, at 92%, in the first trimester, 64% in the second trimester, and 44% in the third trimester.[4] Muench et al. [12] found that of those patients diagnosed with biliary disease who were treated nonoperatively, 12% had spontaneous abortion and 30% failed medical management, resulting in a cholecystectomy.

Indications for surgery in the pregnant patient are failed medical therapy, acute cholecystitis, obstructive jaundice, gallstone pancreatitis, and peritonitis.[14] The same indications for intraoperative cholangiography exist for the pregnant patient and include a total bilirubin greater than or equal to 1.5 ng/dL, a dilated common bile duct greater than or equal to 8 mm, and the presence of gallstone pancreatitis.[5]

LAPAROSCOPIC SURGERY IN PREGNANCY

Despite the explosion of laparoscopic surgery since the 1980s, the application of laparoscopic surgery in the pregnant patient has been slower to progress. In addition to the above-mentioned risks of abdominal surgery during pregnancy, there are specific risks and special factors to consider when discussing laparoscopic surgery during pregnancy. These include the potential mechanical problems of laparoscopic surgery with the pregnant uterus, and concern over fetal injury from instrumentation and/or the pneumoperitoneum.[15]

Until recently, pregnancy had been considered a contraindication to laparoscopic surgery. Weber et al. [16] published the first data on successful laparoscopic cholecystectomy during pregnancy, and since then there have been numerous reports of successful laparoscopic appendectomies and cholecystectomies in the pregnant patient.

More than 100 cases of laparoscopic appendectomies during pregnancy have been reported in the literature. Table 17.1 summarizes these data and includes published series including four or more cases. Rollins et al. [11] published the largest study of laparoscopic appendectomies, with 28 cases reported. The rate of preterm delivery was 21.4%, statistically significantly higher than the rate of preterm delivery for those not undergoing surgery. However, there were no fetal losses reported. It is interesting to note that in this report, both the Hasson and Veress needle techniques of abdominal cannulation were used in all three trimesters without any increase in maternal or fetal mortality. Lyass et al. [17] observed no abnormal fetal organogenesis in the laparoscopic appendectomies performed during the first trimester, which was previously thought unsafe. They also noted a shorter length of stay when comparing the laparoscopic group to the open group.

More than 290 cases of laparoscopic cholecystectomies in pregnant women have been reported in the literature. Table 17.2 summarizes the data on the series that included four or more cases. Most authors reported success with the procedure, with good outcomes with regard to full-term delivery rates, rates of spontaneous abortions, preterm delivery, and teratogenesis. Affleck et al. [18] published the largest case series of laparoscopic cholecystectomies and found no fetal losses, no birth defects, and no uterine injuries. Amos et al. [2] published a frequently cited report in which four out of seven laparoscopic cases resulted in adverse outcomes (two intrauterine fetal deaths and two incomplete abortions). Three of the four patients who experienced adverse outcomes in this report suffered from gallstone

Table 17.1: Laparoscopic Appendectomy*

Author	Year	LA, no.	EGA, weeks	Trimester: no. of patients	Pneumo mm Hg	LOS, days	Tocolytics, no.	OR Time, min.	# Delivered	Adverse Outcome
Schreiber [25]	1990	6							NA	
Curet [7]	1996	4	≤28	1st or 2nd	10–15				4	
Gurbuz [5]	1997	5	26			1.2		64	5	
Lemaire[10]	1997	4	12–26		12	1–6	1	35	4	
Affleck [18]	1999	19		1st: 6 2nd: 9 3rd: 4		1–4	4		19	3 delivered preterm, 1 before 35 weeks 15.8% preterm delivery rate
Andreoli[26]	1999	5	18.4			2.6		45–85 (mean 66)		1 preterm delivery at 35 weeks†
de Perrot [27]	2000	6		1st: 2 2nd: 3 3rd: 1					3	2 patients developed uterine infections and had spontaneous abortion
Lyass [17]	2001	11	16 (7–34)						11	
Rizzo [9]	2003	4	16–24		10			25–90	4	
Rollins [11]	2004	28	20.7	1st: 6 2nd: 13 3rd: 9	12.6 ± 1.6		6	46.3	28	21.4% delivered preterm (≤37 weeks); 10.7% early preterm delivery (≤35 weeks)
Total		92								

*Reported cases of four or more are included.
†Author did not identify laparoscopic procedure that resulted in preterm delivery.
LA, laparoscopic appendectomies; EGA, estimated gestational age; Pneumo, pneumoperitoneum pressure; LOS, length of stay postoperatively; NA, data not available; OR, operating room.

pancreatitis or perforated appendicitis, both of which are associated with high fetal mortality as discussed earlier. In addition, the operating time for these reported procedures was significantly longer than those in similar reports by other authors. Therefore, it has been argued that the underlying maternal disease process could have contributed to the fetal demise and not necessarily the procedure itself.[19]

Some authors have compared laparoscopic procedures to open procedures in the pregnant patient, comparing various outcomes such as hospital length of stay, use of tocolytics, need for postoperative analgesics, and time of return to a regular diet and mobilization (see Table 17.3). Curet et al. [7] compared 16 pregnant patients undergoing laparoscopic procedures with 18 pregnant patients undergoing open procedures (with both groups comparable in age, trimester, intraoperative oxygenation, and end-tidal CO_2) and found that the gestational age at delivery, birth weight, and Apgar scores were not statistically different between the groups.[7] In addition, the laparoscopic group had a shorter length of stay, required postoperative narcotics for fewer days, and resumed a regular diet sooner post surgery compared with the laparotomy group. These differences are statistically significant.

Reedy et al. [20] published the results of a survey in which surgeons from the Society of Laparoscopic Surgeons were queried about their unpublished experiences with pregnant patients. The authors reported data (199 laparoscopic cholecystectomies and 67 laparoscopic appendectomies) demonstrating an overall trend toward increased usage of laparoscopic surgery in the pregnant patient.

It is clear that the use of laparoscopic surgery has become more widespread. Thus, it is important to discuss the specifics of laparoscopic surgery in the pregnant patient and the varying opinions concerning method and location of abdominal cannulation, the pneumoperitoneum pressure, fetal monitoring, and perioperative care in the pregnant patient.

There are well-known hemodynamic changes that occur during laparoscopic surgery. First, CO_2 pneumoperitoneum causes a decrease in the cardiac index, an increase in the mean arterial pressure, and an increase in the systemic vascular resistance.[21] Although these hemodynamic changes are usually transient, they must be considered given the normal physiologic changes of pregnancy as mentioned earlier. The increased intra-abdominal pressure decreases venous return and cardiac output, which may lead to decreased uterine blood flow, increased intrauterine pressure, and ultimately decreased fetal perfusion. The decreased venous return seen during laparoscopic surgery due to increased intra-abdominal pressure is volume dependent; in adequately resuscitated pregnant women, increased intra-abdominal pressure should not lead to decreased CO_2 and fetal blood flow.[17]

Table 17.2: Laparoscopic Cholecystectomy*

Author	Year	LC, no.	EGA, weeks	Trimester: no. of patients	Pneumo, mm Hg	LOS, days	Tocolytics, no.	OR Time, min.	# Delivered	Adverse Outcomes
Morrell [28]	1992	5	13–23						4	
Soper [23]	1992	5		2nd		1–2	2		3	
Elerding [29]	1993	5		1st :1 2nd: 3 3rd: 1			5		5	
Comitalo [30]	1994	4		2nd					4	1 hyaline membrane disease
Ronaghan [31]	1994	10								
Lanzafame [32]	1995	5		2nd: 3 3rd: 2			2		5	
Steinbrook [33]	1996	10	9–30	1st: 3 2nd: 6 3rd: 1			1		10	
Wishner [34]	1996	6		2nd: 5 3rd: 1					6	
Eichenberg [35]	1996	4		3rd	8–10	1–4	1	40–125	4	
Curet [7]	1996	12		1st or 2nd	10–15				12	
Abuabara [15]	1997	22	5–31	1st: 2 2nd: 16 3rd: 4					22	
Gurbuz [5]	1997	10	16.8	1st: 2 2nd: 7 3rd: 1		1.3		68	10	
Reyes-Tineo [36]	1997	5		2nd					5?	
Glasgow [6]	1998	14	18.6	1st: 3 2nd: 11	6–15	1–3	7	40–120	11	
Gouldman [37]	1998	8		1st: 1 2nd: 7	12	3 (1–7)	4	Mean 59 (40–86)	7	
Geisler [38]	1998	6	25				5		6	
Graham [4]	1998	6		1st: 2 2nd: 4	Up to 15	1–3	0		4	2 elective abortions
Thomas [39]	1998	4	10–30							1 elective abortion, 1 premature delivery, healthy infant

502

Author	Year	LC, no.	EGA, weeks	Trimester: no. of patients	Pneumo, mm Hg	LOS, days	Tocolytics, no.	OR Time, min.	# Delivered	Adverse Outcomes
Affleck [18]	1999	42		1st: 3 2nd: 28 3rd: 11					42	5 delivered preterm, 2 delivered before 35 weeks (11.9% preterm delivery)
Andreoli [26]	1999	5	24.8			1.4		Mean 63 (10–90)		1 preterm delivery at 35 weeks[†]
Barone [1]	1999	20	18.4				1	82.8	19	Maternal–fetal mortality due to intra-abdominal hemorrhage 2 weeks postoperatively
Cosenza [40]	1999	10	20.5		12			85	NA	
Sungler [13]	2000	9	13–32	2nd: 8 3rd: 1	10 (gasless in 1 procedure)		2		9	1 conversion to open
Muench [12]	2001	6	19.3	1st: 3 2nd: 11 3rd: 2	12–15	2.6 ± 1.7	4	67	11	2 procedures converted to open
Steinbrook [21]	2001	4		17, 20, 23, 24 weeks	15					
Buser [41]	2002	10		1st: 2 2nd: 5 3rd: 4						1 uterine perforation with blunt port 1 premature labor and cesarean delivery
Rizzo [9]	2003	5	10–27		10			25–90	5	
Lu [42]	2004	6		2nd: 6			1		6	
Rollins [11]	2004	31	20.8	1st: 3 2nd: 19 3rd: 9	13.1 ± 1.7		9	61.2	29	20.0% delivered preterm (≤37 weeks) 6.7% early preterm delivery (≤35 weeks) 1 fetal death 9.4 weeks after procedure 1 (23.4 week EGA) delivery of nonviable fetus
Total		294								

*Reported cases of four or more are included.
[†]Author did not identify laparoscopic procedure that resulted in preterm delivery.
LC, laparoscopic cholecystectomies; EGA, estimated gestational age; Pneumo, pneumoperitoneum pressure; LOS, length of stay postoperatively; NA, data not available; OR, operating room.

Table 17.3: Laparoscopic versus Open Surgery

Author	Year	Lap	Open	EGA	Trimester: no. of patients	OR Time, min. (lap/ open)	LOS (lap/ open)	Days to RD (lap/ open)	Duration of NU (lap/ open)	GA, weeks (lap/ open)	# Delivered	Adverse Outcomes
Curet [7]	1996	4 LA 12 LC	7 OA 10 OC 1 ex lap		Lap 1st: 7 2nd: 9 Open 1st: 8 2nd: 10	82/49	1.5 days/2.8 days	1.0/2.4	1.2 days/ 2.6 days	38.2/ 39.2	34	
Amos [2]	1996	3 LA 4 LC	5 open (4 resection of adnexal mass, 1 laparotomy for ovarian cancer)	Lap: 18.9 Open: NA		107/NA					Lap: 2 Open: 4	Open: 1 lost to f/u Lap: 2 incomplete abortions, 2 intrauterine fetal deaths, 1 lost to f/u
Gurbuz [5]	1997	5 LA 10 LC	4 OA	OA: 17 LA: 26		64/58	1.2 days/1.8 days				19	
Glasgow [6]	1998	14 LC	3 OC		OC 2nd: 2 3rd: 1 LC 1st: 3 2nd: 11 3rd: 0						3 OC, 11 LC	Open: transient postoperative preterm labor in 1 patient and 1 preterm delivery
Affleck [18]	1999	45 LC 22 LA	13 OC 18 OA								98	Open: 11.1% PTD Lap: 14.0% PTD

Author	Year	Lap	Open	EGA	Trimester: no. of patients	OR Time, min. (lap/open)	LOS (lap/open)	Days to RD (lap/open)	Duration of NU (lap/open)	GA, weeks (lap/open)	# Delivered	Adverse Outcomes
Barone [1]	1999	20 LC	26 OC	LC: 18.4 OC: 23.7		82.8/18.5				39.3/ 38.3	44	Open: fetal demise in OC group at 21 weeks, 5 weeks postop; 8 premature contractions in OC; 1 premature birth in the OC group Lap: maternal–fetal mortality due to intra-abdominal hemorrhage 2 weeks postop in LC group; 1 premature contraction in LC
Conron [43]	1999	12 Lap	9 Open				34 hours/ 90.7 hours		5.2 hours/ 29.4 hours	39.2/ 38.4	Lap: 9 Open: 9	Lap: 1 tubal pregnancy, 2 spontaneous abortion
Cosenza [40]	1999	10 LC	15 OC	LC: 20.5 OC: 21		85/90				38.5/ 38.5	29	Open: 1 fetal demise in OC during 14th week; preterm delivery at 31 weeks after OC
Lyass [17]	2001	11 LA	11 OA	LA: 16 (7–34) OA: 24 (11–37)			3.6 days/5.2 days				22	

LA, laparoscopic appendectomy; LC, laparoscopic cholecystectomy; LOS, length of stay; OA, open appendectomy; OC, open cholecystectomy; ex lap, exploratory laporotomy; RD, regular diet; NU, narcotic use; GA, gestational age at delivery; PTD, preterm delivery; f/u, follow-up; Lap, laparoscopy; Open, open surgery.
Reprinted from Gurbuz AT, Peetz ME [5] with kind permission of Springer Science and Business Media.

However, although the average pneumoperitoneum in the non-pregnant patient is 15 mm Hg, low-pressure pneumoperitoneum should be used in the pregnant patient, at 8 to 12 mm Hg, to minimize any adverse effect on fetal perfusion. (It is interesting to note, however, that intrauterine pressure during coughing and contractions is much higher than 15 mm Hg.[10])

For the pregnant patient, there is also concern that CO_2 insufflation may lead to maternal hypercapnia, which may cause fetal hypercapnia, tachycardia, and hypertension. This was documented in pregnant ewes in a study performed by Hunter et al. [22]; however, this was a transient effect, with no long-term sequelae. The investigators found no fetal tachycardia or fetal hypertension when nitrous oxide (NO) was used to insufflate the abdomen in pregnant ewes, which led to the conclusion that the increased intra-abdominal pressure was not the cause of the hemodynamic changes seen in the fetus. Instead, the CO_2 was thought to be detrimental to the ewe fetus. However, no abnormal fetal organogenesis has been observed in laparoscopic appendectomies performed in humans in the first trimester with CO_2 as the insufflation agent.[17] Some thought has been given to the use of NO as an insufflation agent; however, most hospitals are resistant to using NO because of its flammability and the increased risk of fire.[1] As there is a risk of hypercapnia with a CO_2 pneumoperitoneum, the authors recommend monitoring the end-tidal CO_2, with a goal of less than 35 mm Hg. It has also been recommended to hyperventilate the mother to keep end-tidal CO_2 concentration in expired air ($ETCO_2$) less than or equal to 35 mm Hg and to convert the procedure to open if maternal hypercarbia or acidosis develops.[2] Following serial arterial blood gases to monitor arterial CO_2 partial pressure ($PaCO_2$) in women predisposed to hypercarbia is controversial.

The risk of trocar injury to the uterus increases with increased estimated gestational age.[1] As a result, trocar placement should be adjusted given the patient's estimated gestational age (Figures 17.1). There is also some debate over the method of placement of the first trocar. Most authors support the Hasson technique, as this is done under direct visualization and there is a decreased theoretical risk of injury to the uterus.[12,23] However, many authors have reported success with the Veress technique in the upper abdomen without any reported injuries to the gravid uterus, even late in the third trimester.[11,18] It is recommended that with either technique, the location of abdominal entry should be appropriate for the trimester, and one should choose alternative sites for Hasson or Veress needle entry. During the first trimester, umbilical access is safe; however, later in pregnancy, the left upper quadrant, right upper quadrant, or midclavicular line should be used.[10] The gravid uterus also predisposes the patient to an increased risk of GERD. As a result, changes in position during the operation should be done gradually for the pregnant patient.

Transabdominal monitoring of the fetal heart rate is not feasible in laparoscopic surgery as it contaminates the operative field. Instead, transvaginal monitoring in all patients, especially high-risk patients, even in second- and early third-trimester pregnancies in which the fetus is nonviable, is recommended. In the event that fetal distress is detected, the surgeon can release the pneumoperitoneum and deflate the abdomen to potentially reverse the distress. Pre- and postoperative fetal heart tones should be documented as well. There has been no evidence to support the routine use of prophylactic tocolytics.[4]

Given the increased risk of venous thromboembolism in pregnancy, encouraging rapid mobilization, administering subcutaneous heparin injections twice daily, using sequential compression devices and left-side-down positioning, and minimizing reverse Trendelenburg positioning are useful prophylaxis for deep venous thrombosis.[4] Lemaire and van Erp [10] recommend beginning heparin therapy 2 hours preoperatively and continuing until the patient ambulates.

The Society of American Gastrointestinal Endoscopic Surgeons (SAGES) has published guidelines for laparoscopic surgery

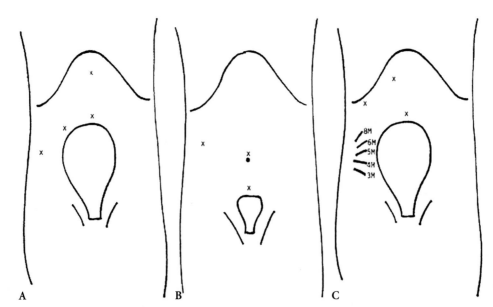

Figure 17.1. Trocar placement is adjusted given the patient's estimated gestational age. M = month of gestation. (**A**) Port placement for laparoscopic cholecystectomy in third trimester. (**B**) Port placement for laparoscopic appendectomy in early pregnancy. (**C**) Port placement for laparoscopic appendectomy in late second or third trimester.

during pregnancy.[24] Preoperative obstetric consultation is advised, and any operative intervention should be deferred if possible until the second trimester, when fetal risk is lowest. Intraoperatively, pneumatic compression devices should be used whenever possible, and fetal and uterine status as well as maternal end-tidal CO_2 and/or arterial blood gases should be monitored. The uterus should be protected with a lead shield if intraoperative cholangiography is a possibility, and fluoroscopy should be used selectively. SAGES also recommends obtaining access to the abdomen through an open technique, using left-side-down positioning, and minimizing the pneumoperitoneum pressure to 8 to 12 mm Hg, not to exceed 15 mm Hg.

There are many advantages to performing laparoscopic surgery instead of an open procedure in the pregnant patient, just as there are in the nonpregnant patient. An earlier return of gastrointestinal function and ambulation; decreased hospital length of stay, postoperative pain, and incisional hernia rate; and a quicker return to normal activity have been shown when comparing laparoscopic surgery with open procedures.[3,4,12] Laparoscopy also helps in providing the correct diagnosis.[17] There are some added benefits for the pregnant patient in particular. Less manipulation of the uterus and a decreased delay in diagnosis can decrease maternal and infant mortality.[3,12] Decreased costs, decreased postoperative adhesions, and early mobilization, which theoretically reduces the incidence of venous thromboembolism, can also be enjoyed by the pregnant patient.

SUMMARY

There have been many advances in laparoscopic surgery since the advent of minimally invasive surgery in the early 1980s. The application of laparoscopic surgery in the pregnant patient has been slower to progress, given the risk of injury to both the mother and the fetus. However, recent data have overwhelmingly shown that laparoscopic abdominal surgery in the pregnant patient is safe in all three trimesters and has many benefits.

REFERENCES

1. Barone JE, Bears S, Chen S, Tsai J, Russell JC. Outcome study of cholecystectomy during pregnancy. *Am J Surg.* 1999;177:232–236.

2. Amos JD, Schorr SJ, Norman PF, et al. Laparoscopic surgery in pregnancy. *Am J Surg.* 1996;171:435–437.

3. Curet MJ. Special problems in laparoscopic surgery. Previous abdominal surgery, obesity, and pregnancy. *Surg Clin North Am.* 2000;80:1093–1110.

4. Graham G, Baxi L, Tharakan T. Laparoscopic cholecystectomy during pregnancy: a case series and review of the literature. *Obstet Gynecol Surv.* 1998;9:566–574.

5. Gurbuz AT, Peetz ME. The acute abdomen in the pregnant patient. Is there a role for laparoscopy? *Surg Endosc.* 1997;11:98–102.

6. Glasgow RE, Visser BC, Harris HW, et al. Changing management of gallstone disease during pregnancy. *Surg Endosc.* 1998;12:241–246.

7. Curet MJ, Allen D, Josloff RK, et al. Laparoscopy during pregnancy. *Arch Surg.* 1996;131:546–551.

8. Mazze RI, Kallen B. Reproductive outcome after anesthesia and operation during pregnancy: a registry of 5405 cases. *Am J Obstet Gynecol.* 1989;161:1178–1185.

9. Rizzo AG. Laparoscopic surgery in pregnancy: long-term follow-up. *J Laparoendosc Adv Surg Tech A.* 2003;13:11–15.

10. Lemaire BM, van Erp WF. Laparoscopic surgery during pregnancy. *Surg Endosc.* 1997;11:15–18.

11. Rollins MD, Chan KJ, Price RR. Laparoscopy for appendicitis and cholelithiasis during pregnancy. A new standard of care. *Surg Endosc.* 2004;8:237–241.

12. Muench J, Albrink M, Serafini F, et al. Delay in treatment of biliary disease during pregnancy increases morbidity and can be avoided with safe laparoscopic cholecystectomy. *Am Surg.* 2001;67:539–542; discussion 542–543.

13. Sungler P, Heinerman PM, Steiner H, et al. Laparoscopic cholecystectomy and interventional endoscopy for gallstone complications during pregnancy. *Surg Endosc.* 2000;14:267–271.

14. Sen G, Nagabhushan JS, Joypaul V. Laparoscopic cholecystectomy in 3rd trimester of pregnancy. *J Obstet Gynaecol.* 2002;22:556–557.

15. Abuabara SF, Gross GWW, Sirinek KR. Laparoscopic cholecystectomy during pregnancy is safe for both mother and fetus. *J Gastrointest Surg.* 1997;1:48–52.

16. Weber AM, Bloom GP, Allan TR, Curry SL. Laparoscopic cholecystectomy during pregnancy. *Obstet Gynecol* 1991;78:958–959.

17. Lyass S, Pikarsky A, Eisenberg H, et al. Is laparoscopic appendectomy safe in pregnant women? *Surg Endosc.* 2001;15:377–379.

18. Affleck DG, Handrahan DL, Egger MJ, Price RR. The laparoscopic management of appendicitis and cholelithiasis during pregnancy. *Am J Surg.* 1999;178:523–528.

19. Steinbrook RA, Brooks DC, Datta S. Laparoscopic surgery during pregnancy. *Am J Surg.* 1997;174:222–223.

20. Reedy MB, Galan HL, Richards WE, et al. Laparoscopic surgery during pregnancy. a survey of laparoscopic surgeons. *J Reprod Med.* 1997;42:33–38.

21. Steinbrook RA, Bhavani-Shankar K. Hemodynamics during laparoscopic surgery in pregnancy. *Anesth Analg.* 2001;93:1570–1571.

22. Hunter JG, Svantstrom L, Thornburg K. Carbon dioxide pneumoperitoneum induces fetal acidosis in a pregnant ewe model. *Surg Endosc.* 1995;9:272–277.

23. Soper NJ, Hunter JG, Petrie RH. Laparoscopic cholecystectomy during pregnancy. *Surg Endosc.* 1992;6:115–117.

24. The Society of Gastrointestinal and Endoscopic Surgeons. *SAGES Guidelines for Laparoscopic Surgery during Pregnancy.* Los Angeles: SAGES; 2000.

25. Schreiber JH. Laparoscopic appendectomy in pregnancy. *Surg Endosc.* 1990;4:100–102.

26. Andreoli M, Servakov M, Meyers P, Mann WJ Jr. Laparoscopic surgery during pregnancy. *J Am Assoc Gynecol Laparosc.* 1999;6:229–233.

27. de Perrot M, Jenny A, Morales M, et al. Laparoscopic appendectomy during pregnancy. *Surg Laparosc Endosc Percutan Tech.* 2000;10:368–371.

28. Morrell DG, Mullins JR, Harrison PB. Laparoscopic cholecystectomy during pregnancy in symptomatic patients. *Surgery.* 1992;112:856–859.

29. Elerding SC. Laparoscopic cholecystectomy in pregnancy *Am J Surg.* 1993;165:625–627.

30. Comitalo JB, Lynch D. Laparoscopic cholecystectomy in the pregnant patient. *Surg Laparosc Endosc.* 1994;4:268–271.

31. Ronaghan JE. Discussion on paper on biliary disease during pregnancy: 10 cases of laparoscopic cholecystectomy. *Am J Surg.* 1994;168:580.

32. Lanzafame RJ. Laparoscopic cholecystectomy during pregnancy. *Surgery.* 1995;118:627–631.

33. Steinbrook RA, Brooks DC, Datta S. Laparoscopic cholecystectomy during pregnancy. Review of anesthetic management, surgical considerations. *Surg Endosc.* 1996;10:511–515.

34. Wishner JD, Zolfaghari D, Wohlgemuth SD, et al. Laparoscopic cholecystectomy in pregnancy. A report of 6 cases and review of the literature. *Surg Endosc.* 1996;10:314–318.

35. Eichenberg BJ, Vanderlinden J. Laparoscopic cholecystectomy in the third trimester of pregnancy. *Am Surg.* 1996;62:874–877.

36. Reyes-Tineo R. Laparoscopic cholecystectomy in pregnancy. *Bol Asoc Med P R.* 1997;89:9–11.

37. Gouldman J, Sticca RP, Rippon MB, McAlhany JC. Laparoscopic cholecystectomy in pregnancy. *Am Surg.* 1998;64:93–98.

38. Geisler JP, Rose SL, Mernitz CS, Warner JL, Hiett AK. Nongynecologic laparoscopy in second and third trimester pregnancy: obstetric implications. *JSLS.* 1998;2:235–238.

39. Thomas SJ, Brisson P. Laparoscopic appendectomy and cholecystectomy during pregnancy: six case reports. *JSLS.* 1998;2:41–46.

40. Cosenza CA, Saffari B, Jabbour N, et al. Surgical management of biliary gallstone disease during pregnancy. *Am J Surg.* 1999;178:545–548.

41. Buser KB. Laparoscopic surgery in the pregnant patient – one surgeon's experience in a small rural hospital. *JSLS.* 2002;6:121–124.

42. Lu EJ, Curet MJ, El-Sayed YY, Kirkwood KS. Medical versus surgical management of biliary tract disease in pregnancy. *Am J Surg.* 2004;188:755–759.

43. Conron RW, Abbruzzi K, Cochrane SO, et al. Laparoscopic procedures in pregnancy. *Am Surg.* 1999;65:259–263.

18 | MINIMAL ACCESS PEDIATRIC SURGERY

Venita Chandra, Sanjeev Dutta, and Craig T. Albanese

The rapid co-evolution of instrumentation and surgical technique has allowed for an ever-growing number of pediatric procedures to be performed using minimal access surgery (MAS). Presently, patients of any size or age (i.e., from fetus to adolescent) can benefit from MAS. This chapter discusses current applications of MAS in infants and children and explores new developments and future directions in the field. Throughout this chapter, the term *MAS* is defined as procedures that are performed with tiny ($\leq$12-mm) incisions, those performed percutaneously, or those performed endoluminally. It encompasses the field of robotic surgery and image-guided therapy. Common synonyms are *laparoscopic surgery* (abdominal MAS), *thoracoscopic surgery* (thoracic MAS), *videoscopic surgery*, and *endosurgery*.

WHY MINIMAL ACCESS PEDIATRIC SURGERY?

To date, there is only one randomized controlled trial of MAS in the pediatric population [1]; however, many large retrospective studies in adults have demonstrated decreased postoperative pain, earlier return to feeds, shorter hospital stays, and improved cosmetic results [2–7] when compared with open surgery. Despite these advantages, a number of concerns limited early widespread adoption of minimal access techniques in children. Appropriately sized instruments were slow to develop as the manufacturers focused on the adult population. The cost of these instruments was believed to be too high and the length of setup too long. Further, perioperative pain and stress have historically been underappreciated in children [8], and the benefit of smaller incisions was not seen to be substantial as many pediatric surgeons believed they had already made "small incisions." Finally, the advanced techniques required for pediatric minimal access procedures are associated with variable learning curves. Loss of depth perception and tactile sensation necessitates major changes in operative technique, requiring "retraining" of many established senior surgeons.[9,10] Nevertheless, despite these obstacles, recognition of the many potential advantages of MAS has resulted in widespread acceptance and growth in the use of MAS techniques in pediatric populations.

PEDIATRIC MAS INSTRUMENTS

The small pediatric surgery patient initially presented significant technical challenges related, in part, to the smaller operative area and restricted surface area for trocar placement. Early attempts to make telescopes smaller than the standard 10-cm diameter/36-cm length merely resulted in suboptimal optics and poor vision. With the advent of improved fiberoptic light sources, lens systems, and video cameras, angled telescopes with a diameter from 2.7 to 4 mm (lengths of 18 to 22 cm) were created, allowing for the expansion of MAS application to patients as small as 1 kg in weight.

Pediatric MAS surgeons today have a wide array of sophisticated and delicate instruments to choose from, usually 3 or 5 mm in diameter (lengths, 18 to 32 cm), to perform the operative manipulations needed, including fine dissection and suturing (Figure 18.1). Similarly, electrosurgical devices and surgical clips have been downsized to 5-mm diameter, giving the surgeon a wide array of choices to provide hemostasis (e.g., monopolar and bipolar cautery, argon beam coagulation, radiofrequency coagulation [LigaSure; Valleylab, Boulder, CO]). A variety of disposable and reusable ports (3- and 5-mm diameter) exist in both short (70-mm) and long (100- to 120-mm) lengths. Radially expanding ports (STEP; United States Surgical, Norwalk, CT) are particularly useful for thin abdominal or chest walls as they spread tissue rather than cut it, giving a more secure anchor for the pediatric patient.

ANESTHESIA FOR PEDIATRIC MINIMAL ACCESS SURGERY

It is important to limit bag–mask ventilation before intubation in small children undergoing laparoscopic procedures because intraluminal bowel gas can quickly accumulate, reducing workspace and potentially making some procedures nearly impossible due to the distended small and large bowel. Nitrous oxide is best avoided for the same reason. Insufflation of the abdomen or thorax results in changes in P_{CO_2} and cardiac output, the clinical significance of which is unknown.[11–13] Although children with cardiopulmonary pathology have significantly less reserve than a healthy patient, they tend to tolerate MAS and stand to benefit the most by the smaller incisions (i.e., reduced narcotic requirement seen with MAS, resulting in decreased postoperative pulmonary dysfunction).[14,15] Although endotracheal intubation is preferred for all MAS, some brief pelvic procedures may be done with the use of laryngeal mask airway.

Thoracoscopic procedures are accomplished using valved trocars and single-lung ventilation. The ipsilateral lung is isolated by any of the following methods, depending on patient size: double-lumen endotracheal tube, mainstem intubation, or bronchial blocker. Low-pressure (4 to 6 torr), low-flow (1 L/min) insufflation further collapses the ipsilateral lung, obviating the need for manual lung retraction.

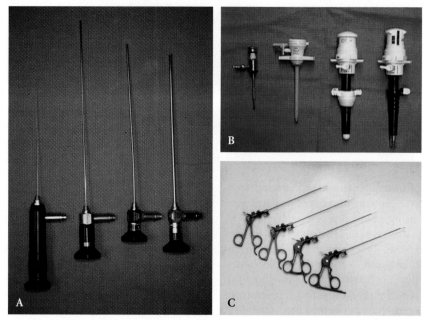

Figure 18.1. (**A**) 1.2-, 2.7-, and 4-mm telescopes useful for procedures in infants. (**B**) Reusable and disposable laparoscopic ports. A section of red rubber catheter placed around the shaft of the reusable 3-mm port is used to secure the port into the skin with a suture to avoid displacement. (**C**) 3-mm short (18-cm) instruments that are more appropriately sized for use in infants as opposed to adult-sized instrumentation.

POSITIONING

As opposed to open surgery, the minimal access surgeon needs to stand in-line with the video monitor and the operative area. Therefore, patients are often placed in unconventional locations/positions on the operating table. For example, procedures like infantile pyloromyotomy and intestinal pull-through for Hirschsprung's disease or imperforate anus are best performed with the child positioned sideways on the table. Fundoplication is performed with a small child at the very end of the table in a frog-legged position, whereas the older child/adolescent is in stirrups.

Unlike the conventional lateral decubitus position used for nearly all open thoracotomy procedures, positioning during thoracoscopy is highly dependent on where in the mediastinum the surgeon is operating. For anterior mediastinal procedures (e.g., thymectomy), the patient is positioned semi-supine, elevated about 30° off the table. Middle mediastinal procedures require lateral decubitus position, whereas posterior mediastinal procedures require the patient to be virtually prone with approximately 30° elevation off the table. Low-pressure insufflation, lung isolation, and these positions allow the lung to "fall away" from the operative field – a lung retractor is virtually never necessary. Similarly, laparoscopic procedures are best accomplished with a combination of table tilt up/down or left/right in order to displace the viscera from the operative field, again obviating the need for manual retraction.

TROCAR INSERTION

After intubation, the stomach is suctioned and a Credé maneuver (manual compression) decompresses the urinary bladder. Only for long (≥2-hour) procedures are indwelling bladder catheters considered. Because children have significantly thinner abdominal walls and shorter anteroposterior distance than do adolescents and adults, care must be taken not to accidentally injure the underlying structures, including the aorta, vena cava, mesenteric vessels, urinary bladder, bowel, and occasionally patent urachus or umbilical vessels.[16–18] One must remember that in babies and children, the urinary bladder is an intraperitoneal organ that, when filled with urine, can extend to the level of the umbilicus. Insufflation is achieved by either the Veress needle technique or an open (Hasson) technique, based principally on surgeon comfort and experience.

Most pediatric surgeons place the initial (telescopic) trocar in the center of the umbilicus. This necessitates thorough cleansing of this area and a prophylactic anti-staphylococcal antibiotic (e.g., cephazolin). All other trocars are placed under direct vision.

SELECTED PEDIATRIC SURGERY PROCEDURES

Over the past decade, minimal access pediatric surgery has proliferated at an incredible rate. The current number and types of surgical procedures being performed are expansive (Table 18.1). This section highlights a few of these procedures, focusing on unique technical advancements to accomplish operations in the abdomen, thorax, subcutaneous space, and uterus. Examples include the fetus, newborn, child, and adolescent.

Pyloromyotomy for Pyloric Stenosis

The Ramstedt pyloromyotomy, first described in 1912, involves splitting the pyloric muscle in newborns and has been the treatment of choice for more than 100 years. The laparoscopic approach also splits the muscle but in a very unique way. The

Table 18.1: Minimal Access Procedures Performed in Pediatric Patients

Laparoscopic	Thoracoscopic	Other
Fundoplication	Lung biopsy	Subcutaneous endoscopically assisted ligation of the internal ring (SEAL) for inguinal hernia
Gastrostomy tube	Lobectomy	Nuss procedure for pectus excavatum
Pyloromyotomy	Sequestration resection	Endoscopic subcutaneous mass excision
Ladd's procedure	Thymectomy	
Cholecystectomy	Decortication	
Heller myotomy	Foregut duplication resection	
Liver biopsy	Diagnostic	
Ovarian cystectomy	PDA ligation	
Oophorectomy	Thoracic duct ligation	
Choledochal cystectomy	Esophageal atresia repair	
Adrenalectomy	Sympathectomy	
Kasai procedure	Aortopexy	
Diaphragmatic plication	Mediastinal mass excision	
Diaphragmatic hernia repair		
Bowel resection		
Nephrectomy		
Pull-through procedure		
Imperforate anus repair		
Inguinal hernia repair		
Umbilical, epigastric hernia repair		
Duodenal atresia		
Orchiopexy		
Splenectomy		
Gastric bypass		

PDA, patent ductus arteriosus.

child is placed sideways on the operating table. Only one umbilical trocar is used for a 2.7-mm, 30° telescope. Two operating instruments are placed percutaneously through two 2-mm stab wounds in the upper quadrants. A disposable, retractable blade is used to incise the pylorus (Figure 18.2). This instrument is the Arthro-Knife (ConMed Linvatec, Largo, FL) used by our orthopedic colleagues. The other instrument is an endoscopic Babcock grasper. The procedure takes 5 to 10 minutes to perform, and the patients are discharged the same evening or the next morning.

Fundoplication for Gastroesophageal Reflux Disease

Gastroesophageal reflux disease is a common problem in the pediatric population and is reportedly one of the three most common indications for major surgical procedures performed in infants and children by pediatric surgeons in the United States.[19] Similar to splenectomy, the laparoscopic procedure for fundoplication has virtually replaced the open procedure, even for reoperations (Figure 18.3).[20,21] Compared with open surgery, the minimal access approach enhances visualization of the hiatus and retroesophageal regions, significantly reduces pain and narcotic requirement, and is associated with less postoperative ileus and quicker hospital discharge.[22–24]

Roux-en-Y Gastric Bypass for Adolescent Morbid Obesity

Nearly 20% of children in the United States meet body mass index criteria for obesity.[25] In 2004, Inge and colleagues [26]

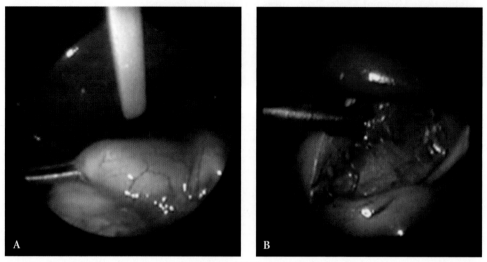

Figure 18.2. Laparoscopic view of a pyloromyotomy. (**A**) Sheathed blade (blade still retracted) about to be used to split the pylorus. (**B**) Split and spread of pyloric muscle.

reviewed current issues regarding bariatric surgery in adolescents. They concluded that bariatric surgery is in fact a viable treatment option for adolescents who fit certain stringent requirements, including failure of organized weight loss programs in adolescents with obesity-related comorbidities.

The treatment of choice for morbid obesity is now the laparoscopic Roux-en-Y gastric bypass, which involves creation of a very small proximal gastric reservoir that is drained with a Roux limb. The procedure involves the use of five trocars, sized from 5 to 12 mm. The procedure takes approximately 2 hours, and the hospital stay is 2 to 3 days. The laparoscopic adjustable gastric band, which creates a small gastric reservoir in an adjustable manner, is an alternative to the gastric bypass. This device, though appealing because of its reversibility and low rate of complications, is not currently approved for use in the pediatric population; however, it is available off-label and is currently being assessed in a clinical trial.[27,28]

Pulmonary Lobectomy

The majority of children requiring pulmonary resections have congenital lung lesions or infectious complications, such as cystic

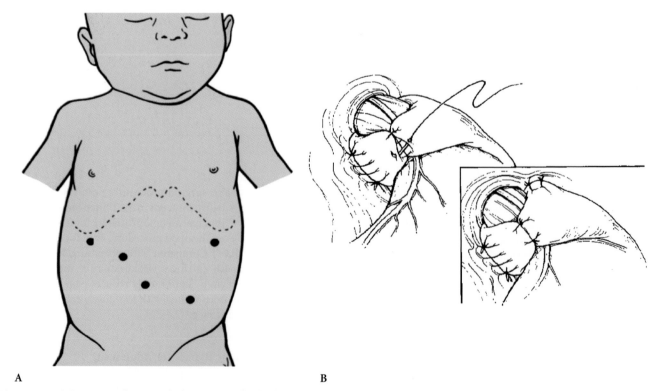

A   **B**

Figure 18.3. (**A**) Port-site placement for laparoscopic fundoplication in children. (**B**) Demonstration of a 360° fundal wrap (Nissen fundoplication) around the distal esophagus.

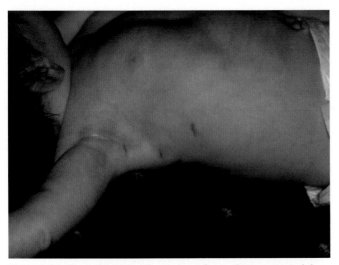

Figure 18.4. Typical incisional scarring after a thoracoscopic lobectomy. The lower trocar site is lengthened slightly to allow the removal of the resected lobe.

thoracotomy, which may lead to shoulder girdle muscle weakness later in life (Figure 18.4).[34]

Esophageal Atresia Repair

Esophageal atresia is a condition in which the proximal and distal portions of the esophagus do not communicate. It is usually associated with a tracheoesophageal fistula most commonly occurring between the distal esophageal segment and the distal third of the trachea. Minimal access repair using a thoracoscopic approach to this disorder is still in its infancy; however, it has the advantage of avoiding the traditional right thoracotomy and its postoperative sequelae, including pain, scoliosis, and chest wall deformity.[34] This procedure is performed using three ports and involves single-lung ventilation and low-flow insufflation. Several recent reports describe thoracoscopic esophageal atresia repair, including a multicenter review by Holcomb and colleagues [35] that found the procedure to be safe and efficacious, with the added advantages of improved intraoperative fistula visualization and less postoperative morbidity.[36–38]

adenomatoid malformation, sequestration, and bronchiectasis. As outlined in previous sections, the use of valved trocars, low-pressure insufflation, and unique positioning has allowed the field of operative pediatric thoracoscopy to blossom. A major advance has been the availability of a 5-mm coagulation device called the LigaSure. This bipolar device uses radiofrequency energy to coagulate vessels up to 7 mm in diameter. Thus, all the pulmonary vessel branches in small children – both artery and vein – can be sealed without the use of sutures, staples, or clips. The device does not, however, seal bronchial tissue; this tissue still must be sutured closed in small children and stapled closed in patients whose hemithorax is of sufficient size to accept the large, 12-mm/36 cm–long laparoscopic staplers.[29–33] Three small incisions to perform a lobectomy obviate the need for a large posterolateral

Endoscopic Subcutaneous Procedures for Excision of Benign Lesions

Traditional open techniques used by pediatric general surgeons for excision of benign forehead tumors, such as dermoid cysts and pilomatrixomas, may have significant adverse cosmetic consequences. Dutta and colleagues [39] recently described a novel minimal access technique based on the endoscopic brow-lift procedure performed by plastic surgeons. Using a specially designed telescope with a retractor on its end, masses in the lateral brow, mid-forehead, and nasal bridge areas of the face are removed via a 1.5-cm incision well hidden behind the hairline (Figure 18.5). This technique, although not yet widespread in the general surgery community, has the advantage of markedly superior cosmesis and decreased wound infection risk in children with

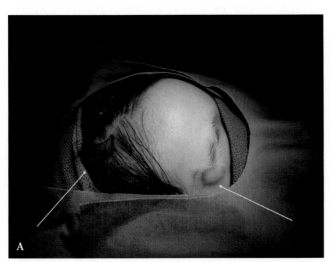

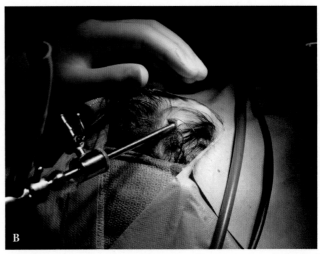

Figure 18.5. (A) Preoperative appearance of a lateral brow dermoid cyst. The *left arrow* points to the planned incision 1.5 cm posterior to the hairline on the parietal scalp to approach the lateral brow dermoid cyst (*right arrow*). (B) Scalp incision and endoscope placement in the dissected subperiosteal tunnel.

facial acne. Endoscopic subcutaneous techniques may potentially be applied to the excision of benign tumors in other cosmetically sensitive areas of the body.

Fetal Surgery

In utero minimal access procedures can be performed with a telescope ("fetoscopic" surgery) or with percutaneously placed catheters. The development of these techniques was stimulated by the complications of open hysterotomy for fetal surgery, namely preterm labor, premature rupture of membranes, and maternal complications from tocolytic therapy.[40] A rapidly expanding list of procedures are being performed using these techniques, including treatment of severe twin–twin transfusion syndrome, division of amniotic bands, bladder decompression for fetal obstructive uropathy (e.g., posterior urethral valves), and valvuloplasty for hypoplastic left heart syndrome.[40–45]

FUTURE DIRECTIONS

Robotics and image-guided therapy hold great promise for pediatric surgical disease therapy. These are rapidly evolving therapy delivery systems that have developed out of a union of imaging and minimal access techniques. Originally conceived as a military tool for remote surgical care of the injured soldier, surgical robots were introduced into clinical practice to overcome the limits of conventional laparoscopy. Robotic technology assists the pediatric surgeon by (1) increasing dexterity and precision of movements, (2) restoring proper hand–eye coordination in an ergonomic position, and (3) improving visualization via three-dimensional stereoscopic optics.[46] These benefits of computer-enhanced robotic surgical systems enable surgeons of both adults and children to perform an increasing number of complex minimal access surgical procedures and are now being effectively used for a broad spectrum of disease processes.[47–51]

Image-guided therapy involves the use of imaging modalities such as ultrasound, computed tomography, and magnetic resonance imaging in combination with sophisticated interactive computer applications to directly guide surgical procedures. Imaging data provide surgeons with detailed spatial information, allowing regions of interest in the body to be targeted with great precision, enabling many traditionally open or laparoscopic procedures to be done with decreased need of general anesthesia and with greater accuracy.[52–54]

Robotics and image-guided therapy are each playing an increasing role in the developing landscape of modern minimal access pediatric surgical procedures. Although both technologies are rapidly advancing independently, their convergence promises exciting future innovations in the form of sophisticated therapy delivery systems, potentially giving rise to operative techniques that transcend human capability.

REFERENCES

1. St. Peter SD, Holcomb GW, Calkins CM, et al. Open versus laparoscopic pyloromyotomy for pyloric stenosis: a prospective randomized trial. *Ann Surg*. 2006;244:363–370.

2. Wenner J, Nilsson G, Oberg S, et al. Short-term outcome after laparoscopic and open 360 degrees fundoplication. A prospective randomized trial. *Surg Endosc*. 2001;15:1124.

3. Rangel SJ, Henry MCW, Brindle M, et al. Small evidence for small incisions: pediatric laparoscopy and the need for more rigorous evaluation of novel surgical therapies. *J Pediatr Surg*. 2003;38:1429.

4. Nilsson G, Larsson S, Johnsson F. Randomized clinical trial of laparoscopic versus open fundoplication: blind evaluation of recovery and discharge period. *Br J Surg*. 2000;87:873.

5. Sauerland S, Lefering R, Neugebauer EAM. Laparoscopic versus open surgery for suspected appendicitis. *Cochrane Database Syst Rev*. 2004;CD001546.

6. Golub R, Siddiqui F, Pohl D. Laparoscopic versus open appendectomy: a metaanalysis. *J Am Coll Surg*. 1998;186:545.

7. Katkhouda N, Mason RJ, Towfigh S, et al. Laparoscopic versus open appendectomy: a prospective randomized double-blind study. *Ann Surg*. 2005;242:439.

8. Schechter NL. The undertreatment of pain in children: an overview. *Pediatr Clin North Am*. 1989;36:781.

9. Chang JH, Rothenberg SS, Bealer JF, et al. Endosurgery and the senior pediatric surgeon. *J Pediatr Surg*. 2001;36:690.

10. Meehan JJ, Georgeson KE. The learning curve associated with laparoscopic antireflux surgery in infants and children. *J Pediatr Surg*. 1997;32:426.

11. Sakka SG, Huettemann E, Petrat G, et al. Transoesophageal echocardiographic assessment of haemodynamic changes during laparoscopic herniorrhaphy in small children. *Br J Anaesth*. 2000;84:330.

12. Gueugniaud PY, Abisseror M, Moussa M, et al. The hemodynamic effects of pneumoperitoneum during laparoscopic surgery in healthy infants: assessment by continuous esophageal aortic blood flow echo-Doppler. *Anesth Analg*. 1998;86:290.

13. Siedman L. Anesthesia for pediatric minimal access surgery. In: Langer JC, Albanese CT, eds. *Pediatric Minimal Access Surgery*. Boca Raton, FL: Taylor & Francis; 2005:15–27.

14. Meehan JJ, Georgeson KE. Laparoscopic fundoplication yields low postoperative pulmonary complications in neurologically impaired children. *Pediatr Endosurg Innov Tech*. 1997;1:11–14.

15. Powers CJ, Levitt MA, Tantoco J, et al. The respiratory advantage of laparoscopic Nissen fundoplication. *J Pediatr Surg*. 2003;38:886.

16. Dutta S, Langer JC. Minimal access surgical approaches in infants and children. *Adv Surg*. 2004;38:337.

17. Sharp HT. Laparoscopy in children. *Clin Obstet Gynecol*. 1997; 40:210.

18. Mansuria SM, Sanfilippo JS. Laparoscopy in the pediatric and adolescent population. *Obstet Gynecol Clin North Am*. 2004;31:469.

19. Di Lorenzo C, Orenstein S. Fundoplication: friend or foe? *J Pediatr Gastroenterol Nutr*. 2002;34:117.

20. Dutta S, Price VE, Blanchette V, Langer JC. A laparoscopic approach to partial splenectomy in children with hereditary spherocytosis. *Surg Endosc*. 2006;20:1719–1724.

21. Zitsman JL. Current concepts in minimal access surgery for children. *Pediatrics*. 2003;111:1239.

22. Ostlie DJ, Holcomb GW. Laparoscopic fundoplication in infants and children. In: Langer JC, Albanese CT, eds. *Pediatric Minimal Access Surgery*. Boca Raton, FL: Taylor & Francis; 2005:165–186.

23. Mattioli G, Repetto P, Leggio S, et al. Laparoscopic Nissen-Rossetti fundoplication in children. *Semin Laparosc Surg*. 2002;9:153.

24. Georgeson KE. Laparoscopic fundoplication. *Curr Opin Pediatr*. 1998;10:318.

25. Ogden CL, Carroll MD, Curtin LR, et al. Prevalence of overweight and obesity in the United States, 1999–2004. *JAMA*. 2006;295:1549.

26. Inge TH, Krebs NF, Garcia VF, et al. Bariatric surgery for severely overweight adolescents: concerns and recommendations. *Pediatrics*. 2004;114:217.

27. O'Brien PE, Dixon JB, Brown W, et al. The laparoscopic adjustable gastric band (Lap-Band): a prospective study of medium-term effects on weight, health and quality of life. *Obes Surg*. 2002;12: 652.

28. Parikh MS, Laker S, Weiner M, et al. Objective comparison of complications resulting from laparoscopic bariatric procedures. *J Am Coll Surg*. 2006;202:252.

29. Rothenberg SS. Experience with thoracoscopic lobectomy in infants and children. *J Pediatr Surg*. 2003;38:102.

30. Albanese CT, Sydorak RM, Tsao K, et al. Thoracoscopic lobectomy for prenatally diagnosed lung lesions. *J Pediatr Surg*. 2003;38:553.

31. Rothenberg SS. Thoracoscopic lung resection in children. *J Pediatr Surg*. 2000;35:271.

32. de Lagausie P, Bonnard A, Berrebi D, et al. Video-assisted thoracoscopic surgery for pulmonary sequestration in children. *Ann Thorac Surg*. 2005;80:1266.

33. Mattioli G, Buffa P, Granata C, et al. Lung resection in pediatric patients. *Pediatr Surg Int*. 1998;13:10.

34. Jaureguizar E, Vazquez J, Murcia J, et al. Morbid musculoskeletal sequelae of thoracotomy for tracheoesophageal fistula. *J Pediatr Surg*. 1985;20:511.

35. Holcomb GW, Rothenberg SS, Bax KMA, et al. Thoracoscopic repair of esophageal atresia and tracheoesophageal fistula: a multi-institutional analysis. *Ann Surg*. 2005;242:422.

36. Rothenberg SS. Thoracoscopic repair of tracheoesophageal fistula in newborns. *J Pediatr Surg*. 2002;37:869.

37. Rothenberg SS. Thoracoscopic repair of esophageal atresia and tracheo-esophageal fistula. *Semin Pediatr Surg*. 2005;14:2.

38. Tsao K, Lee H. Extrapleural thoracoscopic repair of esophageal atresia with tracheoesophageal fistula. *Pediatr Surg Int*. 2005; 21:308.

39. Dutta S, Lorenz HP, Albanese CT. Endoscopic excision of benign forehead masses: a novel approach for pediatric general surgeons. *J Pediatr Surg*. 2006;41:1874–1878.

40. Malladi P, Sylvester K, Albanese CT. Clinical outcomes in minimal access fetal surgery. In: Langer JC, Albanese CT, eds. *Pediatric Minimal Access Surgery*. Boca Raton, FL: Taylor & Francis; 2005:41–71.

41. Fowler SF, Sydorak RM, Albanese CT, et al. Fetal endoscopic surgery: lessons learned and trends reviewed. *J Pediatr Surg*. 2002;37:1700.

42. Sydorak RM, Albanese CT. Minimal access techniques for fetal surgery. *World J Surg*. 2003;27:95.

43. McLean KM, Lorts A, Pearl JM. Current treatments for congenital aortic stenosis. *Curr Opin Cardiol*. 2006;21:200.

44. Gardiner HM. Progression of fetal heart disease and rationale for fetal intracardiac interventions. *Semin Fetal Neonatal Med*. 2005;10:578.

45. Crombleholme TM. The treatment of twin–twin transfusion syndrome. *Semin Pediatr Surg*. 2003;12:175.

46. Hollands CM, Dixey LN. Applications of robotic surgery in pediatric patients. *Surg Laparosc Endosc Percutan Tech*. 2002;12:71.

47. Camarillo DB, Krummel TM, Salisbury JK. Robotic technology in surgery: past, present, and future. *Am J Surg*. 2004;188:2S.

48. Gutt CN, Markus B, Kim ZG, et al. Early experiences of robotic surgery in children. *Surg Endosc*. 2002;16:1083.

49. Gallagher AG, Smith CD. From the operating room of the present to the operating room of the future. Human-factors lessons learned from the minimally invasive surgery revolution. *Semin Laparosc Surg*. 2003;10:127.

50. Woo R, Le D, Krummel TM, et al. Robot-assisted pediatric surgery. *Am J Surg*. 2004;188:27.

51. Lanfranco AR, Castellanos AE, Desai JP, et al. Robotic surgery: a current perspective. *Ann Surg*. 2004;239:14.

52. Temple MJ, Langer JC. Image-guided surgery for the pediatric patient: ultrasound, computerized tomography, and magnetic resonance imaging. *Curr Opin Pediatr*. 2003;15:256.

53. Shlomovitz E, Amaral JG, Chait PG. Image-guided therapy and minimally invasive surgery in children: a merging future. *Pediatr Radiol*. 2006;36:398.

54. Tempany CM, McNeil BJ. Advances in biomedical imaging. *JAMA*. 2001;285:562.

19 | LAPAROSCOPIC VASCULAR SURGERY IN 2007

Jean Picquet, Oscar J. Abilez, Jérôme Cau, Olivier Goëau-Brissonnière, and Christopher K. Zarins

Vascular surgery has been one of the last fields in surgery to incorporate laparoscopy. This may largely be the result of the fact that laparoscopic control of bleeding remains challenging and vascular procedures inherently involve bleeding. However, recent improvements in laparoscopic approach, exposure, and instrumentation have resulted in an increase in the number of surgeons performing laparoscopic vascular surgery (LVS). Here, we present an overview of the current advantages, disadvantages, and special considerations of LVS and provide a description of the laparoscopic technique for aorto-bifemoral bypass.

CURRENT INDICATIONS AND LIMITATIONS

Laparoscopy is a surgical approach and must not change the indications or contraindications for surgery. This means that the same type of operation is performed laparoscopically as it is performed conventionally (e.g., the proximal and distal targets of a bypass are independent of the surgical approach). Currently, LVS is mainly performed for the treatment of aorto-iliac occlusive disease and abdominal aortic aneurysms. For aorto-iliac occlusive disease, LVS has become complementary to endovascular repair. The Transatlantic Society Consensus (TASC) has described the respective indications for conventional and endovascular repair for occlusive diseases. From these guidelines, patients not amenable to endovascular repair (TASC types C and D) [1], and with non-massive aortic calcifications, represent the most suitable candidates for LVS. It should be noted that major calcifications represent the largest limitation to laparoscopy. However, such barriers can be overcome with surgeon experience and skill, as has been the case for other newly introduced techniques. For example, the tortuous character of the iliac arteries was first considered a major limitation for endovascular aortic aneurysm repair, but this became less important with increasing operative volume.

ADVANTAGES OF LAPAROSCOPY

The specific advantages of laparoscopy have been demonstrated in comparison with open procedures. Greater magnification, less risk of adhesion formation, less abdominal wall injury, less risk of hernia development, better cosmetic outcome, less pain, shorter hospital stay, and faster recovery after major procedures are the main advantages.[2]

Furthermore, the same vascular grafts are used in laparoscopy and in open repair. Therefore, their long-term patency rates are expected to be similar.

SPECIFIC CONSIDERATIONS

Laparoscopy in vascular surgery presents special challenges when compared with laparoscopy in other specialties. Procedures in vascular surgery are about reconstruction instead of extirpation. Moreover, major bleeding risk (without the possibility of aspiration due to loss of pneumoperitoneum and visibility) is inherent to operating on large vessels. Special instrumentation is required and has been developed for LVS. The need for sutures and laparoscopic clamps to be safe and powerful enough to be used on calcified vessels has also been addressed.[3,4]

DISADVANTAGES OF LAPAROSCOPY

The history of LVS emphasizes the difficulties met by the pioneers. Dion and Gracia [5–7] were the first to perform and report total laparoscopic aorto-bifemoral bypass and abdominal aortic aneurysm repair and much is due to them and their team in this field. But before becoming a reliable technique, two kinds of problems arose: inadequate aortic exposure [8] and difficulty creating anastomoses.[9,10]

A direct intraperitoneal approach of the aorta was first used. The major difficulty was the management of the small bowel that blocked the operative field. Some surgeons created complex retractors that were never proven to be usable except by their designers.[11,12]

In addition, creating anastomoses presented a big challenge. Surgeons recorded their anastomoses-related times to determine their learning curve and tried to approach the conventional procedure standards. Some found other means to avoid these problems. Laparoscopic hand-assisted procedures allowed some surgeons to feel more comfortable with the time required for anastomosis; this came at the price of a minilaparotomy, which reduced the interest of laparoscopy.[13,14] Others used a minilaparotomy to perform the anastomosis with an open approach after laparoscopic dissection [15], also reducing significantly the advantages of laparoscopy.

Then the concept of the intraperitoneal plus extraperitoneal approach was introduced. This approach gives a large and stable aortic exposure without the need for any specific retractors, thus greatly improving the procedure.[16–18] This approach is described below for aorto-bifemoral bypass.

The tension of oversewing was also considered a problem because most vascular surgeons need an assistant to maintain good tension on the suture during a conventional open procedure. Specific sutures with fixed pledgets now help the surgeon perform

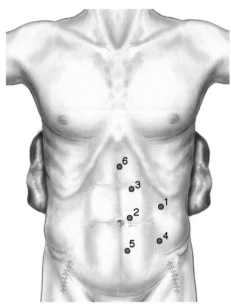

Figure 19.1. Port placement for laparoscopic aorto-bifemoral bypass.

anastomoses laparoscopically without requiring an assistant to maintain tension on the line.

The disadvantages of LVS have been addressed with better laparoscopic exposure along with improved anastomosis technique; these improvements have recently resulted in an increase in the number of surgeons performing LVS, and now larger series have been reported.[19]

CURRENT LAPAROSCOPIC TECHNIQUE FOR AORTO-BIFEMORAL BYPASS

The laparoscopic procedure begins with the patient placed in the supine position. All the ports are introduced as shown in Figure 19.1, and pneumoperitoneum is established up to 15 mm Hg. An inflated pillow placed under the left flank of the patient provides a 45° rotation and allows the surgeon to make an incision of the peritoneum along the left paracolic gutter from the sigmoid to the splenic flexure. A right rotation of the operative table adds 45° of rotation to the patient who is now in a complete right lateral decubitus position. While rotating the patient, the left arm is moved to the right, in front of the patient's face to avoid any brachial plexus injury (Figure 19.2). The descending colon is mobilized to the right by dissection along the avascular line of Toldt. The small bowel is then retracted safely out of the

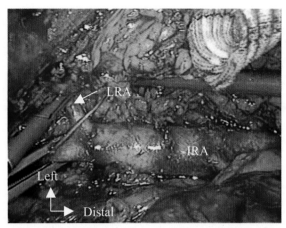

Figure 19.3. Suprarenal occlusion with laparoscopic clamps. LRA, left renal artery; IRA, infrarenal aorta.

operative field. The procedure then continues in the retroperitoneal space. Particular attention is given to staying anterior to the left kidney during the dissection. The left renal vein is identified as an important landmark to find the infrarenal aorta. Dissection of the aorta is performed down to its bifurcation. The operative field can be maintained by fixing the left colon to the mid-anterior abdominal wall by one or two stitches. The left kidney will tend to obscure the operative field and can be fixed by a stitch to the left abdominal wall. When complete exposure is achieved, a bifurcated graft is introduced inside the abdominal cavity through a trocar. The graft has been previously fashioned for an end-to-end or end-to-side anastomosis, and its left limb has been temporarily ligated at its end. The right limb of the graft is brought into the right groin region (which has been previously dissected free) alongside the right iliac arteries and under videoscopic control. The left limb is left inside the abdomen while performing the anastomosis, allowing the surgeon to rotate the graft during this time or, after declamping, to control any leak by adding other sutures. After systemic heparinization, the aorta is occluded proximally and distally by two laparoscopic clamps (Figure 19.3). The aorta is opened as required. An end-to-end or end-to-side anastomosis is performed with two semicircular running sutures beginning at the distal end of the aortic incision for an end-to-side anastomosis, and at the posterior aortic wall for an end-to-end anastomosis. Figure 19.4 shows the initial suture

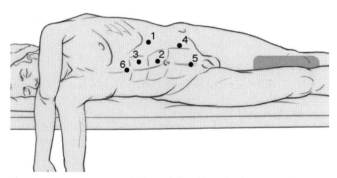

Figure 19.2. Patient in right lateral decubitus for laparoscopic aorto-bifemoral bypass.

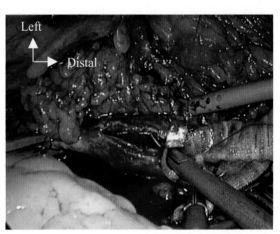

Figure 19.4. Initial suture being placed in an end-to-side anastomosis.

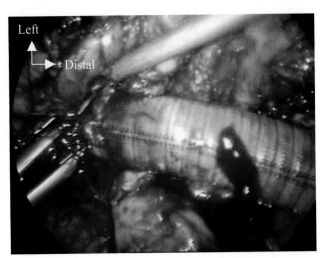

Figure 19.5. Aorto-bifemoral graft in place after declamping.

being placed in an end-to-side anastomosis. Pledgeted sutures make it possible to maintain good tension for creating a leak-free anastomosis. To complete the anastomosis, the two sutures are tied together at the proximal end of the aortic incision or at the anterior aortic wall. After declamping the aorta, the left limb is brought into the left groin region. The proximal anastomosis is inspected for leaks while returning the patient to the supine position under direct videoscopic observation. During rotation, the left colon falls into its anatomic position, covering the aorta and the graft. It is naturally maintained in place by the overlying small bowel. Figure 19.5 shows the graft in place after removal of the aortic clamps. Distal femoral anastomoses are then performed after flattening the table. The trocars are removed and the puncture sites are reapproximated.

THE ROLE OF LAPAROSCOPY IN VASCULAR SURGERY

As in any relatively new technique, laparoscopy's place in vascular surgery remains to be defined. We can hypothesize that it should not replace endovascular repair in the TASC A and B indications for aorto-iliac occlusive diseases as endovascular techniques have shown excellent results with minimal adverse events. However, laparoscopy competes with open repair for the treatment of TASC C and D occlusive diseases in select patients who are typically younger and at lower risk. For instance, a 60-year-old patient with complete aortic bifurcation occlusion without major operative risks would be a good candidate for LVS.

Laparoscopic aneurysm repair has also been demonstrated to be feasible and reliable.[20] However, with the emergence of endovascular repair as the standard for aneurysm disease, laparoscopy will face difficulty in finding its place.

More complex and varied laparoscopic vascular procedures have already been performed [21–23], demonstrating the potential for laparoscopy in replacing most conventional open procedures, as in other fields of surgery.[24] Over the last decade, endovascular repair has taken such an important place that all vascular surgeons absolutely have had to learn it, and it is now a part of most residency and fellowship programs. Specific training,

which remains particularly important to reach technical success in laparoscopy, now needs to conveyed to the young generation of vascular surgeons.[25]

REFERENCES

1. Management of peripheral arterial disease (PAD). TransAtlantic Inter-Society Consensus (TASC). *Eur J Vasc Endovasc Surg.* 2000;19(suppl A):Si–xxviii, S1–250.
2. Nezhat C, Nezhat F, Nezhat C. Operative laparoscopy (minimally invasive surgery): state of the art. *J Gynecol Surg.* 1992;8:111–141.
3. Geier B, Neuking K, Mumme A, Eggeler G, Barbera L. Comparison of laparoscopic aortic clamps in a pulsatile circulation model. *J Laparoendosc Adv Surg Tech A.* 2002;12:317–326.
4. Alimi YS. Laparoscopic aortic surgery: recent development in instrumentation. *Acta Chir Belg.* 2004;104:505–512.
5. Dion YM, Katkhouda N, Rouleau C, Aucoin A. Laparoscopy-assisted aortobifemoral bypass. *Surg Laparosc Endosc.* 1993;3:425–429.
6. Dion YM, Gracia CR, Estakhri M, et al. Totally laparoscopic aortobifemoral bypass: a review of 10 patients. *Surg Laparosc Endosc.* 1998;8:165–170.
7. Dion YM, Gracia CR, Ben El Kadi HH. Totally laparoscopic abdominal aortic aneurysm repair. *J Vasc Surg.* 2001;33:181–185.
8. Alimi YS, Hartung O, Orsoni P, Juhan C. Abdominal aortic laparoscopic surgery: retroperitoneal or transperitoneal approach? *Eur J Vasc Endovasc Surg.* 2000;19:21–26.
9. Berens ES, Herde JR. Laparoscopic vascular surgery: four case reports. *J Vasc Surg.* 1995;22:73–79.
10. Dion YM, Chin AK, Thompson TA. Experimental laparoscopic aortobifemoral bypass. *Surg Endosc.* 1995;9:894–897.
11. Alimi YS, Hartung O, Cavalero C, Brunet C, Bonnoit J, Juhan C. Intestinal retractor for transperitoneal laparoscopic aortoiliac reconstruction: experimental study on human cadavers and initial clinical experience. *Surg Endosc.* 2000;14:915–919.
12. Barbera L, Ludemann R, Grossefeld M, Welch L, Mumme A, Swanstrom L. Newly designed retraction devices for intestine control during laparoscopic aortic surgery: a comparative study in an animal model. *Surg Endosc.* 2000;14:63–66.
13. Arous EJ, Nelson PR, Yood SM, Kelly JJ, Sandor A, Litwin DE. Hand-assisted laparoscopic aortobifemoral bypass grafting. *J Vasc Surg.* 2000;31:1142–1148.
14. Kolvenbach R. Hand-assisted laparoscopic abdominal aortic aneurysm repair. *Semin Laparosc Surg.* 2001;8:168–177.
15. Alimi YS, De Caridi G, Hartung O, et al. Laparoscopy-assisted reconstruction to treat severe aortoiliac occlusive disease: early and midterm results. *J Vasc Surg.* 2004;39:777–783.
16. Dion YM, Gracia CR. A new technique for laparoscopic aortobifemoral grafting in occlusive aortoiliac disease. *J Vasc Surg.* 1997;26:685–692.
17. Coggia M, Bourriez A, Javerliat I, Goeau-Brissonniere O. Totally laparoscopic aortobifemoral bypass: a new and simplified approach. *Eur J Vasc Endovasc Surg.* 2002;24:274–275.
18. Coggia M, Di Centa I, Javerliat I, Colacchio G, Goeau-Brissonniere O. Total laparoscopic aortic surgery: transperitoneal left retrorenal approach. *Eur J Vasc Endovasc Surg.* 2004;28:619–622.
19. Coggia M, Javerliat I, Di Centa I, et al. Total laparoscopic bypass for aortoiliac occlusive lesions: 93-case experience. *J Vasc Surg.* 2004;40:899–906.
20. Coggia M, Javerliat I, Di Centa I, et al. Total laparoscopic infrarenal aortic aneurysm repair: preliminary results. *J Vasc Surg.* 2004;40:448–454.

21. Barbera L, Geier B, Kemen M, Mumme A. Laparoscopic thromben-darterectomy of the infrarenal aorta. *Surg Laparosc Endosc Percutan Tech*. 1999;9:426–429.

22. Coggia M, Bourriez A, Cerceau P, Di Centa I, Leschi JP, Goeau-Brissonniere O. Videoscopic approach to femoral bifurcation. *J Vasc Surg*. 2004;39:471–473.

23. Javerliat I, Coggia M, Di Centa I, Kitzis M, Mercier O, Goeau-Brissonniere O. Total laparoscopic abdominal aortic aneurysm repair with reimplantation of the inferior mesenteric artery. *J Vasc Surg*. 2004;39:1115–1117.

24. Nezhat C. Operative endoscopy will replace almost all open procedures. *JSLS*. 2004;8:101–102.

25. Goeau-Brissonniere O. What is the future for laparoscopic aortic surgery? *Ann Vasc Surg*. 2004;18:393–394.

20 COMPLICATIONS IN LAPAROSCOPY
Section 20.1. Major Vascular Injury

Oscar J. Abilez, Jean Picquet, and Christopher K. Zarins

INTRODUCTION

Laparoscopy is an accepted method of treatment in gynecology, general surgery, urology, and pediatric surgery. It is generally safe, is usually well tolerated by patients, and, when compared to its open surgical counterpart, offers the advantages of less postoperative pain, reduced surgical trauma, and a shortened postoperative hospital stay.[1–5] However, as with any surgical procedure, laparoscopy has technique-related complications. One of these complications is major vascular injury (MVI), of which consequences can be quite serious. Injuries to the large vessels (aorta, vena cava, iliac vessels, and mesenteric vessels) are commonly referred to as MVI and occur in a variety of laparoscopic fields (see Figure 20.1.1, Table 20.1.1). [4–11] Many of these injuries occur while inserting the Veress needle and/or trocars through the abdominal wall and, as a result, do not occur in conventional procedures.[5] While the reported incidence may be low, ranging from 0.05% to 0.14% [9,10,12–15], the mortality arising from these injuries is substantially higher and has been reported to reach up to 17% (see Table 20.1.2).[12–14,16] Therefore, the rare occurrence of MVI carries with it the risk of a potentially catastrophic outcome.

INCIDENCE

MVI can occur in laparoscopic surgery during the early maneuvers required to enter the peritoneal cavity, or during the surgical dissection required for the specific procedure.[4,5,11,14,16–19] Bleeding from the Veress needle or trocar insertion sites is specific to laparoscopic surgery, while bleeding from surgical dissection can also occur during conventional surgery (see Table 20.1.3).

MVI during diagnostic and therapeutic laparoscopy have been reported since the 1970s.[5–7,12,20–23] Though rare, the occurrence of MVI leads to mortality in a high proportion of cases. An analysis of more than 77,000 laparoscopic cholecystectomies identified 36 cases of retroperitoneal great vessel lesions (0.05% of all complications) and carried a mortality rate of 8%.[12] Another study involving more than 103,000 laparoscopic procedures confirmed the same incidence of MVI (0.05%), but with a higher mortality rate (13%).[13] In other studies, MVI have been reported with similar figures (see Table 20.1.2).[10,14–16,24–28]

Several reports have raised the possibility that the incidence of MVI is underreported and underestimated.[11,29–34] In addition, a review of MVI points out the inaccuracy of collected data.[5] In 1992, one study[12] reported 36 cases of MVI, and then 3 years later, in 1995, another study[4] cited only 20 reports in the literature. However, in 1995, a third study[13] reported that 47 MVI had occurred in over 103,000 laparoscopic procedures.

PRESENTATION

MVI can present in different manners, with rapid intra-operative evidence of hemodynamic instability, to the development of a retroperitoneal hematoma with no apparent clinical signs or symptoms. Some cases of MVI have also been identified during the postoperative course.[4,5,7,14,35]

Early diagnosis is important for reducing mortality and other morbidities.[4,7,17,20,35,36] A delay in diagnosis can be due to a number of reasons, such as absence of blood in the peritoneal cavity or the presence of a large undetected retroperitoneal hematoma. Several deaths due to delayed diagnosis of MVI have been reported.[7,17,33,37] In a handful of such cases diagnostic laparotomy was delayed because the condition was diagnosed as carbon dioxide (CO_2) gas embolism.[7,33,38] The probability of a CO_2 embolism has been estimated to be approximately 100 lower than the probability of having an MVI; therefore, MVI should be considered first.[5]

Injuries to multiple major vessels (such as to the aorta and iliac vessels, or to the aorta and vena cava) or even simultaneous anterior and posterior vessel wall injuries may occur. In general, these injuries are harder to manage and may necessitate the assistance of a vascular surgeon to place grafts and/or patches.[4,5,17,19]

ETIOLOGY

More than three quarters of MVI occur during insertion of the Veress needle and/or trocars at the beginning of a laparoscopic procedure.[5,9,13,25] The most frequently reported causes are inexperience of the surgeon [10,13,17,30,39]; insufficient acquaintance with anatomical landmarks [10,11,33,40]; the position of the patient during access to the peritoneal cavity [30,32,41]; and surgeon position in inserting the Veress needle and/or trocars.[5,16]

Surgeon Experience

The relevance of a surgeons experience in preventing the occurrence of MVI is mixed among published reports. Many studies consider experience to be an important factor [5,10,13,17,39] for preventing MVI, which occur more frequently during a surgeon's first 100 laparoscopic operations.[30] However, other

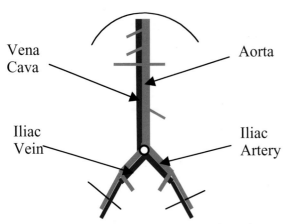

Figure 20.1.1. Most frequent major vessels injured during laparoscopy.

studies [32,42] claim that MVI occur sporadically, even throughout the careers of experienced laparoscopic surgeons. Therefore, care should be taken to avoid MVI, regardless of experience.

Anatomic Landmarks

Knowledge of anatomic landmarks and relationships is very important in helping to avoid MVI. In one study, the aortic bifurcation was found to be cephalad to the umbilicus in more than 50% of nonobese patients.[40] This percentage gradually decreased as the body mass index (BMI) increased; however, the aortic bifurcation remained cephalad to the umbilicus in less than or equal to 30% of obese patients. The same study demonstrated that the left iliac vein always crossed the median line cephalad to the umbilicus, regardless of the patient's physical characteristics.

Another important anatomic relationship concerns the distance between the skin and the retroperitoneal vascular structures.[5,16] In a study reporting an aortic lesion that occurred during the incision of the skin at the umbilicus, the distance between the umbilicus and the aorta was found to be reduced to around 2 cm.[33] This reduction in distance occurred after the induction of general anesthesia and the subsequent muscular relaxation and lateral displacement of the bowel.

Patient Position

The position of the patient on the operating table is also important.[5] In patients of medium height with an estimated distance of 6 cm between the skin and retroperitoneal vascular structures, the Trendelenburg position causes an anterior rotation of the sacral promontory, which shifts the aortic bifurcation nearer to the skin.[32,40,43] Therefore, this shift should be kept in mind when performing laparoscopy on patients with this body habitus.

Surgeon Position

Another important factor is the position of the surgeon. In one reported case of MVI [5], the right lateral trocar was inserted by a surgeon who was standing on the left side of the patient. This position prevented accurate control of the direction and force of insertion, a problem that was further enhanced by the strong resistance of the fascia. A simple but effective recommendation

Table 20.1.1: Surgical Fields with Reported Major Vascular Injuries (MVI), Non-Comprehensive

Surgical Field	Ref
GYNECOLOGIC SURGERY	6–10, 17, 19, 21, 22, 27, 32, 36, 38, 43, 55, 59–78
Adhesiolysis	63, 68, 76
Tubal sterilization	7, 19, 21, 36, 59, 76–78
Endometriosis excision	60, 63, 76
Lymphadenectomy	17, 75, 76
Laparoscopy-assisted vaginal hysterectomy (LAVH)	76
GENERAL SURGERY	4, 10, 12, 15, 16, 23–26, 28, 30, 35, 54, 58, 79–108
Cholecystectomy	10, 12, 15, 23–26, 28, 30, 35, 54, 58, 79–106
Appendectomy	16, 106
Hernia repair	4, 25, 107, 108
UROLOGIC SURGERY	44, 109–111, 112, 113
Nephrectomy	44, 109–111
Adrenalectomy	112
Prostatectomy	113
PEDIATRIC SURGERY	114
Diagnostic laparoscopy	114

is that the surgeon stand on the same side of the patient in which the trocar is being placed to avoid any loss of balance that may occur.

TREATMENT

Treatment usually consists of conversion to open repair, but laparoscopic repair has also been described. In either case, prompt recognition of a vascular injury is key in performing beneficial treatment.

Open

If blood is returned or seen at the needle/trocar insertion site or a retroperitoneal hematoma is identified with the laparoscope, preparation for immediate laparotomy should be made.[4] With a retroperitoneal hematoma, it is not uncommon to have minimal free blood in the intraperitoneal space. Initial control should be obtained with direct pressure on the bleeding site (with hands, packs, or vascular clamps) and then the peritoneum overlying the bleeding site should be opened.[17] At this point, atraumatic control of the injured vessel should be achieved, free blood should be suctioned, and repair accomplished. The bleeding site should be fully exposed and inspected to exclude injury to the back wall of the vessel.[14] For extensive or complicated injuries, it may be necessary to obtain the expertise of a vascular surgeon to assist in the repair.[4,5,17,19]

Table 20.1.2: Literature Reports of Laparoscopic Major Vascular Injuries (MVI)

Author	Year	Patients	MVI	% MVI	Deaths	% Deaths	Ref
Deziel	1993	77,604	36	0.05	3	8	12
Sigman	1993	1,028	1	0.10	0	0	29
Saville	1995	3,951	4	0.10	0	0	42
Geers	1996	2,201	3	0.14	0	0	15
Champault	1996	103,852	47	0.05	6	13	13
Fruhwirth	1997	–	–	0.08	–	–	10
Chapron	1997	–	17	–	2	12	9
Hashizume	1997	15,422	10	0.06	0	0	25
Usal	1998	2,589	2	0.08	0	0	26
Bhoyrul	2001	–	407	–	26	6	16
Schafer	2002	14,243	12	0.08	2	17	14
Roviaro	2002	3,545	2	0.06	0	0	5

Table 20.1.3: Vascular Injuries due to Laparoscopic Trocar Placement (from the Medical Device Reports (MDR) of the U.S. Food and Drug Administration (FDA), 1993–1996) [16]

Vascular Injury	n	%
Non-fatal		
Aorta or IVC	69	17
Iliac	151	37
Mesenteric	32	8
Other	129	32
Subtotal	381	94
Fatal		
Aorta or IVC	10	2
Iliac	3	1
Other	13	3
Subtotal	26	6
Total	407	100

Laparoscopic

MVI have been treated via a direct laparoscopic approach, although in many of these cases the injury occurred under direct laparoscopic vision.[9,17,19,44] This differs from the unwitnessed, but clinically suspected, MVI sustained during access to the peritoneal cavity; in the latter case, an open approach is recommended.[4,5,14,17,19] Several reports have shown that in instances where patients were not managed with laparotomy, a significant proportion resulted in death; the only survivor had a small hematoma located at the aortic bifurcation that was discovered intraoperatively.[33,43,44]

PREVENTION

Trocar Design

In attempts to avoid MVI, new designs for trocars and new techniques for access to the peritoneal cavity have been devised. The main improvements have been in the development of trocars with blunt tips, trocars with protective sleeves, and optical trocars that allow direct recognition of each layer of the abdominal wall during access to the peritoneal cavity.[45–53] However,

without good technique, none of these safety devices can eliminate the risk of an MVI.[10] In 1996, the Food and Drug Administration (FDA) advised manufacturers to avoid the term "safety trocar" when describing cannulas with a blunt tip or a retractable sleeve and use the term "shielded cannula" because a number of MVI had occurred despite the use of these instruments.[5,9,13,30,32] The FDA's advice was justified as subsequently there were several reports of MVI that had occurred despite the introduction of these shielded cannulas (see Table 20.1.3).[5,33,39,54,55]

Trocar Placement

Other precautions employed by surgeons to avoid MVI include applying clamps to the anterior abdominal wall and lifting anteriorly to increase the distance from the trocar insertion site to the iliac vessels.[9,16]

Another precaution is to incline the Veress needle in the sagittal plane caudally at 45 degrees with respect to the anterior abdominal wall to avoid the aortic bifurcation (see Figure 20.1.2).[4,10,11,16,33,56]

In a recent study based on computed tomography (CT) and ultrasonography, the recommendations for the primary trocar

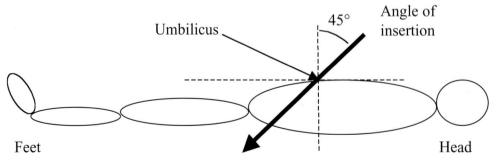

Figure 20.1.2. Angle of insertion of Veress needle and/or trocar to avoid aortic bifurcation. [4,10,11,16,33,56]

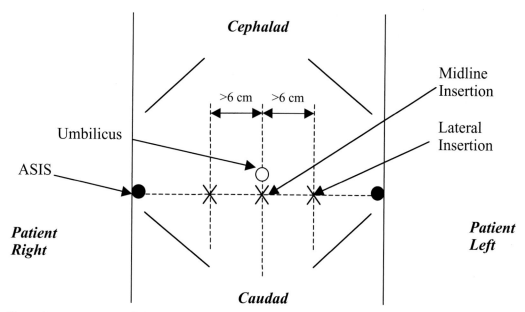

Figure 20.1.3. Recommended primary port site in anterior superior iliac spine (ASIS) plane in the midline and recommended lateral port site in the same plane greater than 6 cm from midline.[11]

(or Veress needle) entry site is at the anterior superior iliac spine (ASIS) plane in the midline, and the recommendation for lateral trocar entry is at the same plane, greater than 6 cm from the midline (see Figure 20.1.3).[11] These recommendations are based on the notion that the ASIS represents more of a fixed point when compared to the umbilicus.

Some surgeons induce a high pressure (25–30 mmHg) in the peritoneal cavity before inserting the first trocar; others prefer to use the open technique to gain access to the peritoneal cavity, with or without a Hasson trocar.[13,16,29,32,39,41] The Hasson trocar has gained the approval of many surgeons because it is simple to use and has yielded excellent results.[15,16] In addition, the combination of inducing pneumoperitoneum with the open technique has been effective in avoiding MVI.

The few cases of MVI that have occurred despite the use of an open technique and a Hasson trocar illustrates that the risk of MVI is always present, even when good technique and instruments with improved designs are used.[41,57,58]

Surgeon Position

The operating table should be at a height that allows slight abduction of the surgeon's elbow. The technique for inserting the trocar should rely on the force generated with the entire arm and shoulder. With a twisting motion, the hand, arm, and shoulder should advance the trocar as one unit. By going slowly, the strength of the entire upper extremity can be employed to stop penetration when fascial resistance ceases after the trocar enters the intraperitoneal space.[16] In all cases, the trocar should be directed away from the aorta and iliac vessels in the event the trocar penetrates more deeply than intended.

CONCLUSIONS

Major vascular injury (MVI) in laparoscopy commonly refers to injury of the large vessels (aorta, vena cava, iliac vessels, and mesenteric vessels). Although its reported incidence is low, the mortality arising from these injuries is significant. In addition, the true incidence of MVI may be underestimated due to under-reporting.

MVI can present in several ways, including, at the extremes, intraoperatively with abrupt hemodynamic instability or postoperatively with no initial accompaniment of clinical signs or symptoms. Whatever the presentation, it is important to identify MVI as soon as possible because delayed diagnosis has been shown to end in a high proportion of deaths.

The etiology of MVI is mainly due to the insertion of the Veress needle and/or trocars at the beginning of the laparoscopic procedure. The main treatment for MVI is conversion to open repair, although there have been successful descriptions of laparoscopic repair by experienced laparoscopic surgeons. The important point in either treatment is identifying the MVI as soon as possible. In some instances it may be necessary to obtain the expertise of a vascular surgeon to assist in the repair.

Prevention of MVI has been aided by trocar design, specific techniques for trocar placement, establishment of pneumoperitoneum, and the use of an open technique to gain access to the peritoneum. However, despite these improvements, new cases of MVI still occur.

Although no single factor has been shown to eliminate MVI, knowledge of its presentation, etiology, treatment, and steps for prevention gives insight on how to avoid this potentially catastrophic event.

REFERENCES

1. Reddick EJ, Olsen DO. Outpatient laparoscopic laser cholecystectomy. *Am J Surg.* 1990;160(5):485–487; discussion 488–489.
2. Cuschieri A, Dubois F, Mouiel J, et al. The European experience with laparoscopic cholecystectomy. *Am J Surg.* 1991; 161(3):385–387.

3. Scott TR, Zucker KA, Bailey RW. Laparoscopic cholecystectomy: a review of 12,397 patients. *Surg Laparosc Endosc.* 1992;2(3):191–198.

4. Nordestgaard AG, Bodily KC, Osborne RW, Jr., Buttorff JD. Major vascular injuries during laparoscopic procedures. *Am J Surg.* 1995;169(5):543–545.

5. Roviaro GC, Varoli F, Saguatti L, Vergani C, Maciocco M, Scarduelli A. Major vascular injuries in laparoscopic surgery. *Surg Endosc.* 2002;16(8):1192–1196.

6. Katz M, Beck P, Tancer ML. Major vessel injury during laparoscopy: anatomy of two cases. *Am J Obstet Gynecol.* 1979;135(4):544–545.

7. Peterson HB, Greenspan JR, Ory HW. Death following puncture of the aorta during laparoscopic sterilization. *Obstet Gynecol.* 1982;59(1):133–134.

8. Baadsgaard SE, Bille S, Egeblad K. Major vascular injury during gynecologic laparoscopy. Report of a case and review of published cases. *Acta Obstet Gynecol Scand.* 1989;68(3):283–285.

9. Chapron CM, Pierre F, Lacroix S, Querleu D, Lansac J, Dubuisson JB. Major vascular injuries during gynecologic laparoscopy. *J Am Coll Surg.* 1997;185(5):461–465.

10. Fruhwirth J, Koch G, Mischinger HJ, Werkgartner G, Tesch NP. Vascular complications in minimally invasive surgery. *Surg Laparosc Endosc.* 1997;7(3):251–254.

11. Sriprasad S, Yu DF, Muir GH, Poulsen J, Sidhu PS. Positional anatomy of vessels that may be damaged at laparoscopy: new access criteria based on CT and ultrasonography to avoid vascular injury. *Journal of Endourology.* 2006;20(7):498–503.

12. Deziel DJ, Millikan KW, Economou SG, Doolas A, Ko ST, Airan MC. Complications of laparoscopic cholecystectomy: a national survey of 4,292 hospitals and an analysis of 77,604 cases. *Am J Surg.* 1993;165(1):9–14.

13. Champault G, Cazacu F, Taffinder N. Serious trocar accidents in laparoscopic surgery: a French survey of 103,852 operations. *Surgical Laparoscopy & Endoscopy.* 1996;6(5):367–370.

14. Schafer M, Lauper M, Krahenbuhl L. A nation's experience of bleeding complications during laparoscopy. *Am J Surg.* 2000;180(1):73–77.

15. Geers J, Holden C. Major vascular injury as a complication of laparoscopic surgery: a report of three cases and review of the literature. *Am Surg.* 1996;62(5):377–379.

16. Bhoyrul S, Vierra MA, Nezhat CR, Krummel TM, Way LW. Trocar injuries in laparoscopic surgery. *J Am Coll Surg.* 2001;192(6):677–683.

17. Nezhat C, Childers J, Nezhat F, Nezhat CH, Seidman DS. Major retroperitoneal vascular injury during laparoscopic surgery. *Hum Reprod.* 1997;12(3):480–483.

18. Schafer M, Lauper M, Krahenbuhl L. Trocar and Veress needle injuries during laparoscopy. *Surgical Endoscopy.* 2001;15(3):275.

19. Jacobson MT, Oesterling S, Milki A, Nezhat C. Laparoscopic control of a leaking inferior mesenteric vessel secondary to trocar injury. *JSLS.* 2002;6(4):389–391.

20. McDonald PT, Rich NM, Collins GJ, Jr., Andersen CA, Kozloff L. Vascular trauma secondary to diagnostic and therapeutic procedures: laparoscopy. *Am J Surg.* 1978;135(5):651–655.

21. Lynn SC, Jr., Katz AR, Ross PJ. Aortic perforation sustained at laparoscopy. *J Reprod Med.* 1982;27(4):217–219.

22. Bergqvist D, Bergqvist A. Vascular injuries during gynecologic surgery. *Acta Obstet Gynecol Scand.* 1987;66(1):19–23.

23. Buell JF, Cronin DC, Funaki B, et al. Devastating and fatal complications associated with combined vascular and bile duct injuries during cholecystectomy. *Arch Surg.* 2002;137(6):703–708; discussion 708–710.

24. Fried GM, Barkun JS, Sigman HH, et al. Factors determining conversion to laparotomy in patients undergoing laparoscopic cholecystectomy. *Am J Surg.* 1994;167(1):35–39; discussion 39–41.

25. Hashizume M, Sugimachi K. Needle and trocar injury during laparoscopic surgery in Japan. *Surg Endosc.* 1997;11(12):1198–1201.

26. Usal H, Sayad P, Hayek N, Hallak A, Huie F, Ferzli G. Major vascular injuries during laparoscopic cholecystectomy – an institutional review of experience with 2589 procedures and literature review. *Surgical Endoscopy-Ultrasound and Interventional Techniques.* 1998;12(7):960–962.

27. Vasquez JM, Demarque AM, Diamond MP. Vascular complications of laparoscopic surgery. *J Am Assoc Gynecol Laparosc.* 1994;1(2):163–167.

28. Wherry DC, Marohn MR, Malanoski MP, Hetz SP, Rich NM. An external audit of laparoscopic cholecystectomy in the steady state performed in medical treatment facilities of the Department of Defense. *Ann Surg.* 1996;224(2):145–154.

29. Sigman HH, Fried GM, Garzon J, et al. Risks of blind versus open approach to celiotomy for laparoscopic surgery. *Surg Laparosc Endosc.* 1993;3(4):296–299.

30. Apelgren KN, Scheeres DE. Aortic injury. A catastrophic complication of laparoscopic cholecystectomy. *Surg Endosc.* 1994;8(6):689–691.

31. Nault P, Beaulieu RC. Major vascular injury secondary to laparoscopy. *Vascular Surgery.* 1996;30(5):413–416.

32. Pasic R, Mullins F, Gable DR, Levine RL. Major vascular injuries in laparoscopy. *Journal of Gynecologic Surgery.* 1998;14(3):123–128.

33. Hanney RM, Carmalt HL, Merrett N, Tait N. Use of the Hasson cannula producing major vascular injury at laparoscopy. *Surg Endosc.* 1999;13(12):1238–1240.

34. Leggett PL, Bissell CD, Churchman-Winn R. Aortic injury during laparoscopic fundoplication: an underreported complication. *Surg Endosc.* 2002;16(2):362.

35. Mases A, Montes A, Ramos R, Trillo L, Puig MM. Injury to the abdominal aorta during laparoscopic surgery: an unusual presentation. *Anesth Analg.* 2000;91(3):561–562.

36. Oza KN, O'Donnell N, Fisher JB. Aortic laceration: a rare complication of laparoscopy. *J Laparoendosc Surg.* 1992;2(5):235–237.

37. Witz M, Lehmann JM. Major vascular injury during laparoscopy. *British Journal of Surgery.* 1997;84(6):800.

38. Seidman DS, Nasserbakht F, Nezhat F, Nezhat C, Nezhat C. Delayed recognition of iliac artery injury during laparoscopic surgery. *Surgical Endoscopy-Ultrasound and Interventional Techniques.* 1996;10(11):1099–1101.

39. Dixon M, Carrillo EH. Iliac vascular injuries during elective laparoscopic surgery. *Surg Endosc.* 1999;13(12):1230–1233.

40. Hurd WW, Bude RO, DeLancey JO, Pearl ML. The relationship of the umbilicus to the aortic bifurcation: implications for laparoscopic technique. *Obstet Gynecol.* 1992;80(1):48–51.

41. Bonjer HJ, Hazebroek EJ, Kazemier G, Giuffrida MC, Meijer WS, Lange JF. Open versus closed establishment of pneumoperitoneum in laparoscopic surgery. *British Journal of Surgery.* 1997;84(5):599–602.

42. Saville LE, Woods MS. Laparoscopy and major retroperitoneal vascular injuries (MRVI). *Surg Endosc.* 1995;9(10):1096–1100.

43. Soderstrom RM. Injuries to major blood vessels during endoscopy. *J Am Assoc Gynecol Laparosc.* 1997;4(3):395–398.

44. Thiel R, Adams JB, Schulam PG, Moore RG, Kavoussi LR. Venous dissection injuries during laparoscopic urological surgery. *J Urol.* 1996;155(6):1874–1876.

45. Kaali SG, Barad DH, Merkatz IR. Comparison of visual and tactile localization of the trocar tip during abdominal entry. *J Am Assoc Gynecol Laparosc.* 1994;2(1):75–77.

46. Schaller G, Kuenkel M, Manegold BC. The optical "Veress-needle" – initial puncture with a miniopic. *Endosc Surg Allied Technol.* 1995;3(1):55–57.

47. Melzer A, Kipfmuller K, Groenemeyer D, Seibel R, Buess G. Ports, trocars/cannulae, and access techniques. *Semin Laparosc Surg.* 1995;2(3):179–204.

48. Kaali SG, Barad DH, Merkatz IR. Visually guided trocar entry: experience with the optical trocar. *Surg Technol Int.* 1996;5:153–156.

49. Mettler L, Ibrahim M, Vinh VQ, Jonat W. Clinical experience with an optical access trocar in gynecological laparoscopy-pelviscopy. *JSLS.* 1997;1(4):315–318.

50. Wolf JS, Jr. Laparoscopic access with a visualizing trocar. *Tech Urol.* Spring 1997;3(1):34–37.

51. Hallfeldt KK, Trupka A, Kalteis T, Stuetzle H. Safe creation of pneumoperitoneum using an optical trocar. *Surg Endosc.* 1999;13(3):306–307.

52. Schoonderwoerd L, Swank DJ. The role of optical access trocars in laparoscopic surgery. *Surg Technol Int.* 2005;14:61–67.

53. Berch BR, Torquati A, Lutfi RE, Richards WO. Experience with the optical access trocar for safe and rapid entry in the performance of laparoscopic gastric bypass. *Surg Endosc.* July 24 2006.

54. Cogliandolo A, Manganaro T, Saitta FP, Micali B. Blind versus open approach to laparoscopic cholecystectomy – a randomized study. *Surgical Laparoscopy & Endoscopy.* 1998;8(5):353–355.

55. Leron E, Piura B, Ohana E, Mazor M. Delayed recognition of major vascular injury during laparoscopy. *Eur J Obstet Gynecol Reprod Biol.* 1998;79(1):91–93.

56. Palmer R. Safety in laparoscopy. *J Reprod Med.* 1974;13(1):1–5.

57. McMahon AJ, Baxter JN, O'Dwyer PJ. Preventing complications of laparoscopy. *Br J Surg.* 1993;80(12):1593–1594.

58. Roviaro GC, Maciocco M, Rebuffat C, et al. Complications following cholecystectomy. *J R Coll Surg Edinb.* 1997;42(5):324–328.

59. Pring DW. Inferior epigastric haemorrhage, an avoidable complication of laparoscopic clip sterilization. *Br J Obstet Gynaecol.* 1983;90(5):480–482.

60. Nezhat F, Brill A, Nezhat C. Traumatic hypogastric artery bleeding controlled with bipolar desiccation during operative laparoscopy. *J Am Assoc Gynecol Laparosc.* 1994;1(2):171–173.

61. Honda T, Tokushige M, Uda S, Egawa H, Suginami H. A case of laparoscopic complication: injury of the left common iliac vessels and subsequent acute compartment syndrome of the left leg. *J Obstet Gynaecol.* 1995;21(3):273–275.

62. Tsai FP, Cheng PJ, Lee CL, Soong YK, Chang MY. Major complications during laparoscopy-assisted vaginal hysterectomy—report of four cases and review of the literature. *Changgeng Yi Xue Za Zhi.* 1995;18(1):52–57.

63. Bateman BG, Kolp LA, Hoeger K. Complications of laparoscopy–operative and diagnostic. *Fertil Steril.* 1996;66(1):30–35.

64. Jansen FW, Kapiteyn K, Trimbos-Kemper T, Hermans J, Trimbos JB. Complications of laparoscopy: a prospective multicentre observational study. *Br J Obstet Gynaecol.* 1997;104(5):595–600.

65. Lin P, Grow DR. Complications of laparoscopy. Strategies for prevention and cure. *Obstet Gynecol Clin North Am.* 1999;26(1):23–38, v.

66. Reid GD, Cooper MJ, Parker J. Implications for port placement of deep circumflex iliac artery damage at laparoscopy. *J Am Assoc Gynecol Laparosc.* 1999;6(2):221–223.

67. Ruiz A, Ramirez JC, Arbelaez F. Management of injuries to great vessels during laparoscopy. *J Am Assoc Gynecol Laparosc.* 1999;6(1):101–104.

68. Vilos GA. Litigation of laparoscopic major vessel injuries in Canada. *J Am Assoc Gynecol Laparosc.* 2000;7(4):503–509.

69. Chandler JG, Corson SL, Way LW. Three spectra of laparoscopic entry access injuries. *J Am Coll Surg.* 2001;192(4):478–490; discussion 490–471.

70. Corson SL, Chandler JG, Way LW. Survey of laparoscopic entry injuries provoking litigation. *J Am Assoc Gynecol Laparosc.* 2001;8(3):341–347.

71. Munro MG. Laparoscopic access: complications, technologies, and techniques. *Curr Opin Obstet Gynecol.* 2002;14(4):365–374.

72. Sharp HT, Dodson MK, Draper ML, Watts DA, Doucette RC, Hurd WW. Complications associated with optical-access laparoscopic trocars. *Obstet Gynecol.* 2002;99(4):553–555.

73. Liauw L, Chung YN, Tsoi CW, Pang CP, Cheung KB. Laparoscopy for the treatment of women with endometrial cancer. *Hong Kong Med J.* 2003;9(2):108–112.

74. Milad MP, Sokol E. Laparoscopic morcellator-related injuries. *J Am Assoc Gynecol Laparosc.* 2003;10(3):383–385.

75. Kohler C, Klemm P, Schau A, et al. Introduction of transperitoneal lymphadenectomy in a gynecologic oncology center: analysis of 650 laparoscopic pelvic and/or paraaortic transperitoneal lymphadenectomies. *Gynecol Oncol.* 2004;95(1):52–61.

76. Tarik A, Fehmi C. Complications of gynaecological laparoscopy–a retrospective analysis of 3572 cases from a single institute. *J Obstet Gynaecol.* 2004;24(7):813–816.

77. Madrigal V, Edelman DA, Goldsmith A. Laparoscopic sterilization as an outpatient procedure. *J Reprod Med.* 1977;18(5):261–264.

78. Riedel HH, Lehmann-Willenbrock E, Conrad P, Semm K. German pelviscopic statistics for the years 1978–1982. *Endoscopy.* 1986;18(6):219–222.

79. Wright TB, Bertino RB, Bishop AF, et al. Complications of laparoscopic cholecystectomy and their interventional radiologic management. *Radiographics.* 1993;13(1):119–128.

80. Genyk YS, Keller FS, Halpern NB. Hepatic artery pseudoaneurysm and hemobilia following laser laparoscopic cholecystectomy. A case report. *Surg Endosc.* 1994;8(3):201–204.

81. Stewart BT, Abraham RJ, Thomson KR, Collier NA. Postcholecystectomy haemobilia: enjoying a renaissance in the laparoscopic era? *Aust N Z J Surg.* 1995;65(3):185–188.

82. Bergey E, Einstein DM, Herts BR. Cystic artery pseudoaneurysm as a complication of laparoscopic cholecystectomy. *Abdom Imaging.* 1995;20(1):75–77.

83. Meshikhes AW, al-Dhurais S, Bhatia D, al-Khatir N. Laparoscopic cholecystectomy: the Dammam Central Hospital experience. *Int Surg.* 1995;80(2):102–104.

84. Thompson JE, Jr., Bock R, Lowe DK, Moody WE, 3rd. Vena cava injuries during laparoscopic cholecystectomy. *Surg Laparosc Endosc.* 1996;6(3):221–223.

85. Yelle JD, Fairfull-Smith R, Rasuli P, Lorimer JW. Hemobilia complicating elective laparoscopic cholecystectomy: a case report. *Can J Surg.* 1996;39(3):240–242.

86. Modini C, Mingoli A, Castaldo P, Sgarzini G, Marzano M, Nardacchione F. Aortic laceration during laparoscopic cholecystectomy that required delayed emergency laparotomy. *Eur J Surg.* 1996;162(9):739–741.

87. Kapoor R, Agarwal S, Calton R, Pawar G. Hepatic artery pseudoaneurysm and hemobilia following laparoscopic cholecystectomy. *Indian J Gastroenterol.* 1997;16(1):32–33.

88. Balsara KP, Dubash C, Shah CR. Pseudoaneurysm of the hepatic artery along with common bile duct injury following laparoscopic cholecystectomy. A report of two cases. *Surg Endosc.* 1998;12(3):276–277.

89. Nishio H, Kamiya J, Nagino M, et al. Right hepatic lobectomy for bile duct injury associated with major vascular occlusion after laparoscopic cholecystectomy. *J Hepatobiliary Pancreat Surg.* 1999;6(4):427–430.

90. Misawa T, Koike M, Suzuki K, et al. Ultrasonographic assessment of the risk of injury to branches of the middle hepatic vein during laparoscopic cholecystectomy. *Am J Surg*. 1999;178(5): 418–421.

91. Uenishi T, Hirohashi K, Tanaka H, Fujio N, Kubo S, Kinoshita H. Right hepatic lobectomy for recurrent cholangitis after bile duct and hepatic artery injury during laparoscopic cholecystectomy: report of a case. *Hepatogastroenterology*. 1999;46(28):2296–2298.

92. Koffron A, Ferrario M, Parsons W, Nemcek A, Saker M, Abecassis M. Failed primary management of iatrogenic biliary injury: incidence and significance of concomitant hepatic arterial disruption. *Surgery*. 2001;130(4):722–728; discussion 728–731.

93. Bachellier P, Nakano H, Weber JC, et al. Surgical repair after bile duct and vascular injuries during laparoscopic cholecystectomy: when and how? *World J Surg*. 2001;25(10):1335–1345.

94. Wong MD, Lucas CE. Liver infarction after laparoscopic cholecystectomy injury to the right hepatic artery and portal vein. *Am Surg*. 2001;67(5):410–411.

95. Schmidt SC, Langrehr JM, Raakow R, Klupp J, Steinmuller T, Neuhaus P. Right hepatic lobectomy for recurrent cholangitis after combined bile duct and right hepatic artery injury during laparoscopic cholecystectomy: a report of two cases. *Langenbecks Arch Surg*. 2002;387(3–4):183–187.

96. Mathisen O, Soreide O, Bergan A. Laparoscopic cholecystectomy: bile duct and vascular injuries: management and outcome. *Scand J Gastroenterol*. 2002;37(4):476–481.

97. Shen BY, Li HW, Chen M, et al. Color Doppler ultrasonographic assessment of the risk of injury to major branch of the middle hepatic vein during laparoscopic cholecystectomy. *Hepatobiliary Pancreat Dis Int*. 2003;2(1):126–130.

98. Alves A, Farges O, Nicolet J, Watrin T, Sauvanet A, Belghiti J. Incidence and consequence of an hepatic artery injury in patients with postcholecystectomy bile duct strictures. *Ann Surg*. 2003;238(1):93–96.

99. Bilge O, Bozkiran S, Ozden I, et al. The effect of concomitant vascular disruption in patients with iatrogenic biliary injuries. *Langenbecks Arch Surg*. 2003;388(4):265–269.

100. Chigot V, Lallier M, Alvarez F, Dubois J. Hepatic artery pseudoaneurysm following laparoscopic cholecystectomy. *Pediatr Radiol*. 2003;33(1):24–26.

101. Battaglia L, Bartolucci R, Berni A, Leo E, De Antoni E. Major vessel injuries during laparoscopic cholecystectomy: a case report. *Chir Ital*. 2003;55(2):291–294.

102. Shamiyeh A, Wayand W. Laparoscopic cholecystectomy: early and late complications and their treatment. *Langenbecks Arch Surg*. 2004;389(3):164–171.

103. Stewart L, Robinson TN, Lee CM, Liu K, Whang K, Way LW. Right hepatic artery injury associated with laparoscopic bile duct injury: incidence, mechanism, and consequences. *J Gastrointest Surg*. 2004;8(5):523–530; discussion 530–531.

104. Schmidt SC, Settmacher U, Langrehr JM, Neuhaus P. Management and outcome of patients with combined bile duct and hepatic arterial injuries after laparoscopic cholecystectomy. *Surgery*. 2004;135(6):613–618.

105. Singh R, Kaushik R, Sharma R, Attri AK. Non-biliary mishaps during laparoscopic cholecystectomy. *Indian J Gastroenterol*. 2004;23(2):47–49.

106. Guloglu R, Dilege S, Aksoy M, et al. Major retroperitoneal vascular injuries during laparoscopic cholecystectomy and appendectomy. *J Laparoendosc Adv Surg Tech A*. 2004;14(2):73–76.

107. Miguel PR, Reusch M, daRosa AL, Carlos JR. Laparoscopic hernia repair—complications. *Jsls*. 1998;2(1):35–40.

108. Kemppainen E, Kiviluoto T. Fatal cardiac tamponade after emergency tension-free repair of a large paraesophageal hernia. *Surg Endosc*. 2000;14(6):593.

109. Hsu TH, Su LM, Ratner LE, Kavoussi LR. Renovascular complications of laparoscopic donor nephrectomy. *Urology*. 2002;60(5):811–815; discussion 815.

110. Parsons JK, Varkarakis I, Rha KH, Jarrett TW, Pinto PA, Kavoussi LR. Complications of abdominal urologic laparoscopy: longitudinal five-year analysis. *Urology*. 2004;63(1):27–32.

111. McAllister M, Bhayani SB, Ong A, et al. Vena caval transection during retroperitoneoscopic nephrectomy: report of the complication and review of the literature. *J Urol*. 2004;172(1):183–185.

112. Corcione F, Esposito C, Cuccurullo D, et al. Vena cava injury. A serious complication during laparoscopic right adrenalectomy. *Surg Endosc*. 2001;15(2):218.

113. Gregori A, Simonato A, Lissiani A, Bozzola A, Galli S, Gaboardi F. Laparoscopic radical prostatectomy: perioperative complications in an initial and consecutive series of 80 cases. *Eur Urol*. 2003;44(2):190–194; discussion 194.

114. Montero M, Tellado MG, Rios J, et al. Aortic injury during diagnostic pediatric laparoscopy. *Surg Endosc*. 2001;15(5):519.

Section 20.2. Ureteral Injury

Tatum Tarin and Thomas H. S. Hsu

URETERAL INJURIES

Ureteral injury during laparoscopic surgery has become more common as a result of the increased number of laparoscopic hysterectomies and retroperitoneal procedures that are being performed.[1] In a review published by Ostrzenski and colleagues [1], the incidence of ureteral injuries was found to fall between 0.3% and 2.0%. Consequently, prevention of ureteral injuries should be a priority during laparoscopic gynecologic surgery.

ANATOMY

Detailed anatomic knowledge of the retroperitoneum is necessary to prevent ureteral injuries. The ureters are retroperitoneal tubular structures that extend from the renal pelvis, coursing medially and inferiorly to the bladder. Each ureter travels inferiorly along the psoas muscle and crosses the iliac vessels at approximately the level of the bifurcation of the common iliac arteries.[2] In females, the ureter is crossed anteriorly by the ovarian vessels as they enter the pelvis. Inferiorly, they are crossed anteriorly by the uterine artery. At this point, they enter the cardinal ligament, approximately 1.5 to 2.0 cm lateral to the cervix before their insertion into the trigone of the bladder.[3]

The ureters derive their blood supply from the renal artery, aorta, gonadal artery, and common iliac artery while they traverse intra-abdominally. These vessels approach the ureter from its medial side and course longitudinally within the periureteral adventitia. In the pelvis, the ureter derives its blood supply from the internal iliac artery or its branches. These vessels approach the ureter from its lateral side and also course longitudinally within the periureteral adventitia.[2]

LOCATION AND CAUSE OF INJURIES

Intraoperative ureteral injury may result from transection, ligation, angulation, crush, ischemia, or resection. Chan et al. identified three specific anatomic locations for potential ureteral injury during gynecologic laparoscopy: at the infundibulopelvic ligament, the ovarian fossa, and the ureteral canal.[3] In Ostrzenski's review of 70 cases of ureteral injury, 14.3% occurred at or above the level of the pelvic brim, 11.4% occurred at or above the uterine artery, and 8.6% occurred at the level of the bladder.[1] The initial procedure in 20% of these cases was laparoscopic-assisted vaginal hysterectomy. Alterations to normal anatomy may also hinder identification of the ureters as in severe endometriosis, which may involve the ureter and also cause intraperitoneal adhesions.[2,4]

PREVENTION

Injury to the ureters can be prevented by meticulous surgical technique and adequate visualization. Techniques to enhance visualization include hydrodissection and resection of the affected peritoneum.[5] By making a small opening in the peritoneum and injecting 50 to 100 mL of lactated Ringer's solution along the course of the ureter, one can displace the ureter laterally and create a safe plane within which to operate.[5] Preoperative intravenous pyelogram (IVP) has been used to locate the ureters in high-risk patients with potentially distorted anatomy; however, this did not decrease the risk of ureteral injury.[3] Ureteral catheterization has also been used to help identify the ureters. However, in a large review of major gynecologic surgeries, Kuno et al. [6] found that ureteral catheterization did not substantially reduce the risk of ureteral injury. The surgeon must practice meticulous surgical technique and have intimate knowledge of the ureter's course to prevent ureteral injury.

RECOGNITION

According to Ostrzenski et al. [1], intraoperative diagnosis of ureteral injury was made in only 8.6% of the reported cases. Once a ureteral injury is suspected, the ureter must be identified to assess the severity of the injury. Ureteral injury should be suspected with the presence of hematuria or urinary extravasation. Intravenous indigo carmine may be given to aid in the diagnosis and localization of the site of injury. Unfortunately, the majority of ureteral injuries are diagnosed in the postoperative period. Patients who present with postoperative fever, flank pain, and leukocytosis should undergo evaluation for ureteral injury.

MANAGEMENT

Once the diagnosis of ureteral injury is made, a urologic consultation should be obtained. Management of ureteral injuries depends on the severity of the injury, location of the injury, and comfort level of the surgeon. Minor injuries have been managed with cystoscopic stent placement; however, more severe injuries may require surgical intervention. Whether the injury can be repaired laparoscopically versus by open laparotomy depends on the comfort level of the surgeon. Modi et al. [7] reported a case series of six patients with distal ureteral injury secondary to gynecologic procedures that were managed with laparoscopic psoas hitch with ureteroneocystostomy without any complications. Ou et al. [8] reported a case series of four patients with upper ureteral strictures treated with laparoscopic ureteroureteral anastomosis without any complications. Although laparoscopic repair of ureteral injuries is possible, the majority of injuries are treated with open laparotomy.[1] Reconstruction of the urinary system is dependent on the severity and location of the injury and may be accomplished by ureteral reimplantation, psoas hitch, Boari flap, or primary end-to-end anastomosis.

REFERENCES

1. Ostrezenski A, Radolinski B, Ostrzenska K. A review of laparoscopic ureteral injury in pelvic surgery. *Obstet Gynecol Surv*. 2003;58:794–799.

2. Kabalin J. Surgical anatomy of the retroperitoneum, kidneys and ureters. In: Walsh P, Retik A, Wein A, eds. *Campbell's Urology*. 8th ed. Philadelphia: WB Saunders; 2002:36–40.

3. Chan J, Morrow J, Manetta A. Prevention of ureteral injuries in gynecologic surgery. *Am J Obstet Gynecol*. 2003;188:1273–1277.

4. Grainger DA, Soderstrom RM, Schiff SF, Glickman MG, DeCherney AH, Diamond MP. Ureteral injuries at laparoscopy: insights into diagnosis, management, and prevention. *Obstet Gynecol*. 1990;75:839–843.

5. Nezhat C. Complications. In: Nezhat CR, Luciano AA, Seidman DS, eds. *Operative Gynecologic Laparoscopy: Principles and Techniques*. 2nd ed. New York: McGraw-Hill Professional Publishing; 2000.

6. Kuno K, Menzin A, Kauder H, Sison C, Gal D. Prophylactic ureteral catheterization in gynecologic surgery. *Urology*. 1998;52:1004–1008.

7. Modi P, Goel R, Dodiya S. Laparoscopic ureteroneocystostomy for distal ureteral injuries. *Urology*. 2005;66:751–753.

8. Ou CS, Huang IA, Rowbotham, R. Laparoscopic ureteroureteral anastomosis for repair of ureteral injury involving stricture. *Int Urogynecol J Pelvic Floor Dysfunct*. 2005;16:155–157; discussion 157.

Section 20.3. Laparoscopic Management of Intestinal Endometriosis

Andrew A. Shelton

The reported incidence of intestinal endometriosis varies from 3% to 34% of women affected with the disease.[1–5] Endometriomas on the bowel typically involve the serosa and muscularis propria, rarely involving the submucosa or mucosa. The bowel reacts with significant fibrosis and overgrowth of the muscularis propria, often leading to narrowing or structuring of the lumen of the bowel. Symptoms of intestinal endometriosis may be nonspecific and include abdominal and pelvic pain, dyschezia, cyclic hematochezia, dyspareunia, obstructive symptoms, or a change in bowel habits, including both diarrhea and constipation. Pelvic pain, rectal pain, and dyspareunia are the most commonly reported symptoms of endometriosis involving the gastrointestinal tract.[6,7] These symptoms may often be difficult to differentiate from the discomfort felt from endometriosis not involving the gastrointestinal tract or from conditions unrelated to endometriosis. The differential diagnosis of intestinal endometriosis is wide and includes primary carcinoma of the gastrointestinal tract (colorectal cancer), metastatic cancer with a Blumer's shelf, diverticulitis, inflammatory bowel disease, pelvic inflammatory disease, radiation colitis, and ischemic stricture of the colon, among others.[6,8]

SITE OF INVOLVEMENT

Endometriosis may involve any portion of the gastrointestinal tract but most frequently involves the structures of the gastrointestinal tract that normally reside in the pelvis. The rectum, rectosigmoid colon, and rectovaginal septum are most commonly involved, accounting for 70% to 88% of cases of gastrointestinal endometriosis.[6] Deep retroperitoneal endometriosis preferentially involves the rectovaginal space. These implants can reach the upper limit of the rectovaginal septum, although magnetic resonance imaging (MRI) studies show that the septum itself is typically uninvolved.[9] Involvement of the small intestine by endometriosis typically occurs in the terminal ileum, usually within 10 cm of the ileocecal valve. A 20-year review from the Mayo Clinic found small intestinal endometriosis in 38 of 7200 cases of endometriosis (0.53%).[10] Autopsy studies have shown the prevalence of endometriosis involving the vermiform appendix to be 0.054%.[11] Not infrequently, more than one site is involved, so a careful laparoscopic examination of the colon and small bowel is important.[12]

DIAGNOSIS OF INTESTINAL ENDOMETRIOSIS

Endometriosis has been called the "great masquerader" because the symptoms of gastrointestinal involvement can be so nonspecific and similar to so many different gastrointestinal conditions.[13] The diagnosis may be suggested by symptoms and physical examination, but not infrequently a diagnostic laparoscopy is required. Studies such as MRI, barium enema, colonoscopy, or endorectal ultrasound rarely contribute to the diagnosis or alter the operative plan in cases of superficial endometriosis involving the gastrointestinal tract. They can, however, be useful in cases of deeply infiltrating endometriosis or to rule out alternative causes of a patient's symptoms.

Physical Examination

The most common finding on physical examination of a patient with colorectal endometriosis is modularity and tenderness in the cul-de-sac and along the uterosacral ligaments and adherence of the rectal wall to the cul-de-sac. This is often best appreciated on bi-digital examination.[6]

Endoscopy

Endometriotic implants occur on the serosal surface of the bowl and can involve the muscularis propria, but rarely is the mucosa involved.[14] Biopsies obtained endoscopically will rarely be able to confirm the diagnosis of colorectal endometriosis, although patients with cyclic hematochezia are more likely to have mucosal abnormalities and biopsies revealing endometriosis.[15] The frequent symptom of cyclic rectal bleeding has been attributed to transient breaks in the mucosa that occur with swelling of the endometriotic implant during menses.[16] Because of this, direct endoscopic visualization of colorectal endometriosis is uncommon, and the main utility of colonoscopy is in ruling out alternative sources for the patient's symptoms, such as primary colorectal cancer or inflammatory bowel disease.[17,18] There are, however, indirect findings at endoscopy that suggest involvement of the colon by endometriosis. Extrinsic compression may be found as well as a fixed area of narrowing. Secondary changes may be seen in the mucosa, such as edema, flattening or puckering of the mucosa, or loss of mobility of the mucosa from the underlying muscularis. These findings are frequently subtle and may be easily overlooked if the endoscopist is not anticipating or looking for them.

Imaging Studies

A number of imaging studies are available in the diagnosis of gastrointestinal endometriosis, including barium enema, ultrasonography, and MRI.

Barium Enema

The simple, old-fashioned double-contrast barium enema may be a useful tool in evaluating women with symptoms suggestive of colonic endometriosis. The finding most suggestive of colonic endometriosis on barium enema is extrinsic mass effect with fine mucosal crenulations or a serrated, wavy outline of the colonic mucosa. Although this finding is not specific for colonic endometriosis, it is a characteristic finding. Annular strictures or polypoid masses may be seen in more advanced cases.[19] Landi et al. [20] reported on the routine use of preoperative double-contrast barium enema in 108 women with symptoms and physical findings suggestive of colonic endometriosis. Radiographic abnormalities suggestive of colonic endometriosis were found in 53 women, and these findings were confirmed at laparoscopy in all but one woman. Use of barium enema to confirm suspected colonic endometriosis may be a useful tool in preoperative planning.

Ultrasound

Transabdominal ultrasound for colorectal endometriosis has limited clinical utility, but both transvaginal and endorectal ultrasound are useful tools in the evaluation of suspected endometriosis of the gastrointestinal tract. Diagnostic criteria at sonography for bowel endometriosis include a hypoechoic irregular-shaped area corresponding to a layer of hypertrophic muscularis propria, surrounded by a hyperechoic rim corresponding to the mucosa and submucosa. Nodular masses located within the outer rectal wall are readily identified by both transrectal and transvaginal sonography.[21] Recent studies have demonstrated a sensitivity of 97% and a specificity of 89% in the diagnosis of rectal wall involvement in patients with histologically proven rectal endometriosis.[22] Transvaginal and endorectal ultrasound are valuable tools in the evaluation of patients suspected of having rectal endometriosis; however, they provide limited information regarding the gastrointestinal tract proximal to the rectosigmoid colon.

MRI

Magnetic resonance imaging is increasingly being used for the evaluation of pelvic endometriosis. It is more specific than transabdominal ultrasonography in the evaluation of the bladder, ovaries, uterus, uterosacral ligaments, vagina, rectovaginal septum, and pararectal region. However, it is less effective than endorectal ultrasound in the evaluation of depth of infiltration of endometriosis into the rectal wall.[22,23] Diagnostic criteria for rectal wall involvement by MRI include colorectal wall thickening with anterior triangular attraction of the rectum toward the torus uteri or asymmetric thickening of the lower sigmoid wall. MRI has been reported to have a sensitivity of 77% to 93% and specificity of 99% for the detection of colorectal endometriosis.[22,24,25] Use of an endorectal coil has been reported to increase the sensitivity of MRI, but this technique may be painful and is not widely used.

ANATOMY OF THE GASTROINTESTINAL TRACT

Endometriotic implants may potentially involve any portion of the gastrointestinal tract. The small bowel, colon, and rectum are the most frequent sites involved and are discussed below.

Small Bowel

The small intestine in adults from the ligament of Treitz to the ileocecal valve is 5 to 6 m long. The proximal two fifths of small intestine is jejunum, and the distal three fifths is ileum, although there is no sharp line of demarcation between the two. As the small intestine proceeds distally, the lumen of the bowel narrows and the mesenteric vascular arcades become more complex. In general, the jejunum resides in the left side of the abdomen and the ileum in the right side and pelvis. The most terminal portion of the ileum can be easily identified from the remainder of the small intestine by its veil of antimesenteric fat.

The small intestine is attached to the posterior abdominal wall by its mesentery, which runs obliquely from just to the left of the midline in the left upper quadrant, to the right lower quadrant. The blood supply of the small intestine is from the superior mesenteric artery and its jejunal and ileal arcades. Venous drainage of the small intestine is into the superior mesenteric vein.

Colon

The colon extends from the terminal ileum to the rectum. The length of the colon varies depending on the size of the patient but on average is approximately 5 ft long. It is divided into the cecum, ascending colon, hepatic flexure, transverse colon, splenic flexure, descending colon, and sigmoid colon. The ascending and descending portions of the colon are fixed in the retroperitoneal space, whereas the transverse and sigmoid portions are suspended in the peritoneal cavity by their mesenteries. The colon is easily distinguished from the small bowel or rectum by the presence of the three taeniae coli, haustra, and epiploic fat. The taeniae coli are bandlike condensations of the outer longitudinal layer of the muscularis propria. Haustra are not fixed anatomic structures but rather are the result of contractions of the taeniae coli and the inner circular layer of the colon wall. The caliber of the lumen of the colon is greatest at the cecum and diminishes distally, making the left colon more susceptible to obstruction.

Embryologically, the colon is derived from both the midgut (cecum to mid-transverse colon) and the hindgut (mid-transverse colon to rectum) and therefore receives arterial blood supply from both the superior and inferior mesenteric arteries. Colonic branches from the superior mesenteric artery are the ileocolic, right, and middle colic arteries. The inferior mesenteric artery arises from the aorta and gives off the left colic artery and the sigmoidal branches before becoming the superior rectal artery. The colic arteries bifurcate and form an anastomotic arcade approximately 2.5 cm from the mesocolic called the marginal artery of Drummond. The vasa recta are the terminal arterial branches to the colon. Venous drainage from the right and proximal transverse colon is to the superior mesenteric vein (SMV). The distal transverse colon, descending colon, and sigmoid colon drain into the inferior mesenteric vein (IMV). The IMV drains into the splenic vein. The splenic vein and SMV then converge to form the portal vein.

The vermiform appendix arises from the base of the cecum at the convergence of the taeniae coli. The appendix is fixed retrocecally in 16% of adults and is freely mobile in the remainder.

Rectum

The rectum is the terminal 12 to 15 cm of the gastrointestinal tract lying between the sigmoid colon and anal canal. The rectum typically starts at approximately the level of the sacral promontory but anatomically is distinguishable from the sigmoid colon by the absence of taeniae coli. The taeniae coli diverge at the rectosigmoid junction to form a circumferential outer longitudinal layer of smooth muscle. The rectum contains both intraperitoneal and extraperitoneal portions. The upper rectum is invested by peritoneum anteriorly and laterally, but posteriorly it is extraperitoneal up to the rectosigmoid junction. The distal rectum is completely extraperitoneal. The peritoneal reflection between the anterior rectal wall and posterior vaginal wall (pouch of Douglas) occurs approximately 7 cm from the anal verge, although this distance may be shorter in women with pelvic floor relaxation.

The rectum receives a rich triple-arterial blood supply from the terminal branch of the inferior mesenteric artery (the superior rectal artery), bilateral branches of the internal iliac arteries (the middle rectal arteries), and bilateral branches of the internal pudendal artery (the inferior rectal arteries). The venous drainage of the rectum is into the IMV.

A layer of fat known as the mesorectum surrounds the rectum posteriorly and laterally. Surrounding this is a condensation of endopelvic fascia known as the fascia propria of the rectum. The mesorectum contains the perirectal lymph nodes and descending and ascending branches of the superior and middle rectal arteries. The middle rectal artery runs along the pelvic floor after branching from the internal iliac artery, entering and ascending in the mesorectum. The rectum and mesorectum sit in the hollow of the sacrum, turning anteriorly in the distal third of the rectum. These anatomic relationships are important to keep in mind during surgical mobilization of the rectum. After entering the presacral space below the level of the superior rectal artery, it is possible to mobilize the rectum circumferentially down to the level of the pelvic floor in a completely loose areolar, avascular plane as long as the surgeon dissects just outside the fascia propria of the rectum. Bleeding occurring during rectal mobilization implies dissection either too close to the rectum (within the mesorectum) or too far from the rectum. As the rectal mobilization continues distally, posterior dissection must change in an anterior direction, or bleeding from anterior sacral veins may occur.

A note on the normal function of the rectum is important in the context of surgical procedures that may involve removing a portion of the rectum. Rectal reservoir capacity and compliance are integral to the maintenance of continence. Rectal distention with gas or stool leads to relaxation of the rectal wall. With increasing volumes in the rectum, the rectum relaxes to maintain a low rectal pressure until an appropriate time to defecate. Disease conditions that alter rectal compliance or decreased reservoir capacity, such as partial surgical excision of the rectum, may lead to alterations in bowel habits with fecal urgency and impaired continence.

LAPAROSCOPIC COLORECTAL SURGERY

General surgeons were relative latecomers to the field of minimally invasive surgery. Muhe performed the first human laparoscopic cholecystectomy in 1985, but it was not until the late 1980s and early 1990s that the technique was widely accepted. This was soon followed by the adoption of minimally invasive techniques for splenectomy, adrenalectomy, inguinal hernia repair, and the treatment of gastroesophageal reflux disease (Nissen fundoplication). Reports of laparoscopically assisted colon resection were in the surgical literature as early as 1989 [26,27], but laparoscopic colon resection has not had the same rapid rise in popularity as have many of the other surgical techniques because of the complexity of the procedure. When compared with other surgical procedures for which laparoscopy rapidly became the technique of choice, a number of differences are apparent. Laparoscopic colectomy requires operating in several different quadrants, the ligation of major vascular pedicles, removal and extraction of a segment of intestine, and creation of an anastomosis. In addition, retraction and exposure may become difficult after mobilization of the segment of intestine. Despite these difficulties, with increased experience and the advances in technology and development of new minimally invasive instruments, laparoscopic procedures are increasingly being performed for a variety of benign and malignant conditions, including colorectal cancer, diverticulitis, inflammatory bowel disease, and endometriosis involving the gastrointestinal tract.[28–35]

SURGICAL TREATMENT OF INTESTINAL ENDOMETRIOSIS

The surgical management of intestinal endometriosis is somewhat controversial, especially regarding the question of when to intervene. Most authors recommend resection in the setting of symptomatic partial obstruction of the bowel. This is based on the finding that most obstructing endometrial implants are fibrotic and unresponsive to hormonal therapy.[2,6,36,37] Historically, surgical treatment of intestinal endometriosis has been performed at the time of laparotomy. One of the first series to report the successful use of laparoscopic techniques to treat colonic endometriosis was reported by Nezhat et al. in 1992.[38] Since that time, minimally invasive techniques to treat intestinal endometriosis have been increasingly used and reported in the literature.[7,12,39–53] Although the ability to treat intestinal endometriosis laparoscopically is feasible, this fact should not change the indications for the mode of surgical treatment. Not uncommonly, additional gynecologic surgical treatment is required at the time of surgical treatment of intestinal endometriosis, so a multidisciplinary team approach between the general or colorectal surgeon and gynecologist is essential.[6,7]

Appendectomy

Endometriosis of the appendix can mimic acute appendicitis, and therefore appendectomy is recommended.[54] Laparoscopic appendectomy is readily performed using a 5-mm umbilical port for a 5-mm camera, a 10-mm suprapubic port, and a 5-mm port in the patient's left lower quadrant. The surgeon operates from the patient's left side. The appendix is mobilized as necessary. The plane between the mesoappendix and appendix at the base of the appendix is developed. The mesoappendix can then be divided with the LigaSure (Valleylab) or an Endo GIA stapler (United States Surgical) with a vascular cartridge. The appendix is then divided at its base with the Endo GIA. If necessary, a portion of the base of the cecum may also be resected, as long as care is taken not to impinge and narrow the ileocecal valve. The appendix may then be placed in a bag and retracted through the 10-mm left lower quadrant port site.

Ileocolic Resection and Small Bowel Resection

Endometriotic implants involving the distal ileum frequently require mobilization of the distal ileum and right colon to facilitate a laparoscopically assisted ileocolic resection with an ileo-ascending colostomy or a laparoscopically assisted ileal resection with an ileo-ileostomy. The patient is placed in a modified lithotomy position in Allen stirrups after having received a mechanical bowel preparation. Antibiotics covering gram-negative rods and anaerobes are given within 60 minutes of the incision. Ten-millimeter trocars are placed in the right and left lower quadrants and suprapubically in the midline with an umbilical camera port. The patient is placed in steep Trendelenburg with the left side down to facilitate mobilization of the small bowel out of the pelvis and operative field. The first assistant, standing on the patient's left side, retracts the small bowel out of the pelvis, exposing the posterior attachment of the distal ileal mesentery in the patient's right lower quadrant. The surgeon, standing between the legs or on the patient's right side, then grasps the cecum or appendix, retracting it toward the patient's head and exposing the retroperitoneal attachments and placing them on tension. The peritoneum of the ileal mesentery is then scored with electrocautery from the third portion of the duodenum to the cecum. The ileal and right colon mesentery can then be mobilized free from the retroperitoneum using blunt and sharp dissection, exposing the right gonadal vessels, the right ureter, the second and third portions of the duodenum, and the right kidney. The colon is mobilized up to the level of the hepatic flexure. Leaving the lateral attachments of the ascending colon intact to this point facilitates placing traction on the right colon. After completing the posterior mobilization of the colon, the lateral peritoneal attachment of the right colon is easily divided with electrocautery with medial retraction of the colon. If necessary, the attachment of the hepatic flexure and the right side of the gastrocolic ligament can be divided with the LigaSure, completely mobilizing the right colon.

After fully mobilizing the colon and ileal mesentery, the bowel is ready to be resected. This may be accomplished entirely intracorporeally using the LigaSure for mesenteric division and the Endo GIA for division of the bowel and creation of a stapled side-to-side functional end-to-end anastomosis. However, because an incision must be made for retraction of the specimen, we favor enlarging the midline or right lower quadrant incision, extracting the segment of bowel to be resected, and creating an extracorporeal anastomosis. After fully mobilizing the colon and distal small bowel mesenteries, the right colon and terminal ileum are generally easily prolapsed out through a small 4- to 5-cm incision in the right lower quadrant or midline. The bowel proximal and distal to the endometriotic implant is then divided with an Endo GIA stapler, the mesentery is divided with the LigaSure, and the specimen is removed. The antimesenteric corners of the staple lines are then cut off, and a side-to-side anastomosis is created with a third firing of the Endo GIA stapler. The remaining enterotomy can then be sutured or stapled closed with another firing of

the Endo GIA or a TA (Tyco Healthcare Group) stapler and the bowel placed back intraperitoneally.

Segmental Colon Resection

The most common segment of colon requiring resection is the sigmoid colon, so the technique of laparoscopic sigmoid colectomy will be described. The patient is placed in a modified lithotomy position in Allen stirrups after a mechanical bowel preparation using polyethylene glycol (GoLYTELY, Braintree Laboratories) or sodium phosphate (Phospho-soda, C. B. Fleet Company). Intravenous antibiotics covering gram-negative rods and anaerobes should be given within 60 minutes before incision. Port placement depends somewhat on what additional procedures need to be performed, but in general, 10-mm ports are placed in the right and left lower quadrants and right and left upper quadrants. The patient is then placed in steep Trendelenburg with the right side down, facilitating mobilization of the small bowel out of the pelvis and operative field. The first assistant, standing on the patient's left side, grasps the sigmoid colon or its mesentery using traumatic graspers, such as the Endo Babcock instrument (United States Surgical), and retracts the sigmoid colon in a ventral fashion toward the patient's abdominal wall, placing traction on the medial portion of the sigmoid mesentery. The peritoneum of the sigmoid mesentery is then scored using electrocautery from the sacral promontory to the take-off of the left colic artery. Using blunt and sharp dissection, the sigmoid mesentery is then mobilized off the retroperitoneum, exposing the gonadal vessels and the left ureter. The superior rectal artery can then be isolated and divided with a device such as the LigaSure or an Endo GIA stapler with a vascular cartridge without injury to the ureter. The descending colon can then be bluntly mobilized free from the retroperitoneum. Leaving the lateral attachments of the sigmoid and descending colon intact to this point preserves the ability to provide traction to the otherwise mobile colon and facilitates this dissection. The colon can then be retracted medially and the lateral peritoneal attachments divided as far proximally as necessary. If necessary, the splenic flexure can be mobilized laparoscopically. The mesentery at the level of the rectosigmoid junction can then be divided with the LigaSure and the rectosigmoid junction divided with an Endo GIA–type stapler passed through the right lower quadrant port site. If the patient is undergoing a simultaneous laparoscopic hysterectomy, the vaginal cuff may be left open (with a sterile surgical glove in the vagina to maintain pneumoperitoneum) and the proximal end delivered out the vagina. The mesentery of the colon proximal to the endometrioma and the colon are divided, and the specimen can be passed from the field. The anvil of a circular stapler is then placed in the open end of the descending colon and secured in place with a purse-string suture, and the colon is retracted back intraperitoneally. If a hysterectomy is not being performed, the left lower quadrant port is removed, the incision is enlarged 4 to 5 cm, and the colon is removed and similarly resected. The head of the stapler is then passed transanally by the assistant and opened through the apex of the stapled-off rectum. Laparoscopic anvil graspers are useful in facilitating connection of the anvil and the stapler, which is then closed and fired, creating a double-stapled colorectal anastomosis. Both proximal and distal rings should be inspected to ensure they are intact. A "leak test" test is performed by inflating the rectum through a rigid proctoscope under water with the proximal bowel occluded. Any air leak can then be reinforced with laparoscopically placed sutures. Care should be taken to adhere to sound surgical principles, including creation of a well-vascularized, tension-free anastomosis to minimize the risk of anastomotic leak.

Procedures for Rectal Endometriosis

The rectum is the part of the gastrointestinal tract most commonly involved with endometriosis. A variety of surgical techniques are available for the treatment of rectal endometriosis. The choice of which technique to use depends on the size of the implant as well the degree and depth of involvement of the endometriosis. As a general rule, less is better when it comes to the removal of rectal endometriosis as long as the implant can be completely removed with the technique in question. There is no need to perform a difficult low anterior resection when a shave excision or disc excision of the anterior rectal wall is all that is necessary. This is done in order to minimize potential complications and preserve normal rectal function.

Shave Excision

Rectovaginal endometriosis superficially involving the rectal wall can be shaved off the rectal wall without entering the mucosa of the rectum. The lateral peritoneal attachments of the rectum are incised, as is the peritoneal reflection at the pouch of Douglas. The rectum and vagina can then be separated and the endometrial implant dissected free from the anterior rectal wall and posterior vaginal wall. This portion of the rectum is extraperitoneal, so there is no serosal surface. The dissection of the endometrioma may involve resection of a portion of the muscularis propria of the rectum. If the dissection is very superficial, nothing further need be done. For deeper lesions, the anterior rectal wall can be imbricated with laparoscopically placed sutures. A proctoscopy should be performed upon completion of the excision to ensure that an inadvertent proctotomy was not created. If one is noted, it can be repaired.

Anterior Disc Excision

Deeper lesions on the anterior rectal wall require more extensive resection, but a formal low anterior resection is not necessarily required. A full-thickness excision of the anterior rectal wall can be performed using electrocautery or CO_2 laser after laparoscopic mobilization of the rectum. The resulting proctotomy is then closed transversely with an Endo GIA stapler or sutures placed laparoscopically.

Woods et al. [45] described the technique of partial anterior wall disc excision of the rectal wall using a circular stapler. This technique is useful for anterior rectal endometriomas that occupy less than one third of the circumference of the rectal wall and are less than 2 cm in size. The rectum is laparoscopically mobilized anteriorly and laterally, encompassing the endometriosis lesion on the anterior rectal wall. Sufficient mobilization of the vagina off the rectal wall is done down to normal, healthy, soft, supple rectum. The circular stapler is inserted transanally with the anvil in place. The stapler is then opened, with the area to be excised placed in the hollow between the anvil and the shoulder of the stapler. A suture or tie held by graspers on either side of the rectum is then used to place downward pressure on the portion of the rectum to be excised while upward pressure is then placed on the stapler. This places the area to be excised within the stapler. The stapler is then closed and fired, excising a portion of the anterior rectal wall without narrowing the lumen of the rectum. The specimen should be examined to confirm excision of the nodule with a margin or normal rectum. A leak test can then be performed by instilling air or Betadine into the rectum through a proctoscope. Larger lesions can be treated in a similar fashion if the lesion is partially transected, leaving a portion on the posterior vaginal or uterine wall and only 2 cm on the anterior rectal wall. Woods et al. [45] reported results using this technique on 30 patients. Although they reported morbidity in 13%, only one documented anastomotic leak occurred, presenting as a rectovaginal fistula. The other complications included difficulty with stapler extraction; minor bleeding from the staple line, requiring no further treatment; and a patient who presented with pelvic pain and fevers but no radiographic evidence of an anastomotic leak. At no time is the gastrointestinal tract "open," avoiding potential contamination, and there is no need for potentially difficult suture closure of the anterior rectal wall deep in the pelvis.[45] Similar success using this technique has been reported by others, with no anastomotic leaks.[7]

Anterior Resection and Low Anterior Resection

An anterior resection is defined as an anastomosis between the colon and the intraperitoneal rectum, whereas a low anterior resection implies an anastomosis between the colon and the extraperitoneal rectum. The operation proceeds similar to that described for segmental resection of the sigmoid colon. However, rather than stapling the rectosigmoid junction, the rectum is mobilized below the level of the endometriosis. As described in the section on rectal anatomy, the blood supply of the rectum travels within the mesorectum, entering the mesorectum proximally as the superior rectal artery or inferiorly from the pelvic floor as the inferior rectal artery. The mesorectum is contained within a layer of fascia known as the fascia propria. Therefore, after incising the lateral and anterior peritoneal attachment of the rectum, if one is in the correct plane, it is possible to mobilize the rectum posteriorly, laterally, and anteriorly to the level of the levator ani muscles in an avascular plane with appropriate traction and countertraction on the rectum. Once the rectum is sufficiently mobilized below the involved segment, the mesorectum must be divided with a device such as the LigaSure and the rectum transected with a stapling device. The bowel is resected and the anastomosis is created and checked as described in the section on sigmoid resection.

SURGICAL RESULTS

An evaluation of any surgical treatment, especially one for benign disease, must take into consideration both its effectiveness in relief of symptoms and the rate of significant postoperative complications.

Symptoms

Laparoscopic treatment of intestinal endometriosis is a relatively new technique, and only recently have quality-of-life and outcome studies appeared in the literature.[55] Most studies report an improvement in symptoms after resection of

Table 20.3.1: Complication Rates after Laparoscopic Treatment of Colorectal Endometriosis

Author	Year	Patients, no.	Morbidity, %	Leak, %	Fistula, %
Dubernard [40]	2006	58	15.5	10.3	10.3
Jatan [7]	2005	98	8	0	0
Darai [42]	2005	40	10	7.5	7.5
Campagnacci [43]	2005	7	0	0	0
Abrao [44]	2005	8	0	0	0
Marpeau [59]	2004	32		6.3	6.3
Ford[56]	2004	48		2	0
Duepree [46]	2002	51	10.3	2	0
Redwine [47]	2001	84	0	0	0
Varol [49]	2000	2	0	0	0
Jerby [12]	1999	30	13	3	3
Nezhat [60]	1994	8	12	0	0
Sharpe [52]	1992	8	0	0	0
Nezhat [38]	1992	16	0	0	0

intestinal endometriosis of at least 80% to 90% and a complete "cure" in 50%.[24,42,43,56] Ford et al. [56] reported on quality of life after resection of rectovaginal endometriosis (12 treated by laparotomy and 48 by laparoscopy) and found improvement in quality of life in 86% of women, with 61% having pain completely gone or significantly improved. Fedele et al. [57] reported on 83 women who underwent surgery for rectovaginal endometriosis (only 25% treated laparoscopically). They found that segmental resection of the bowel improved outcome in terms of pain, disease recurrence, and need for further treatment of symptomatic endometriosis when compared with those who did not undergo bowel resection. Dubernard [40] reported on the results of 58 women undergoing surgical resection of colorectal endometriosis (88% completed laparoscopically) evaluated postoperatively with the short form SF-36 quality-of-life indicator. A significant improvement in dysmenorrhea, dyspareunia, dyschezia, diarrhea, and asthenia was found. There was no improvement in rectal pain, tenesmus, or constipation. There is a paucity of data on improvement in fertility with treatment of colorectal endometriosis, although some studies have demonstrated an improvement in pregnancy rates after surgical resection.[58]

Complications of Laparoscopic Surgery for Intestinal Endometriosis

The benefit of any surgical procedure, especially a relatively new technique, must be weighed against the morbidity of the procedure and its potential complications. (See Table 20.3.1.) Potential complications of laparoscopic colorectal resection include bleeding; wound infection; injury to adjacent normal organs such as the ureter, bladder, or small bowel; and anastomotic stricture.

However, probably the complication most feared by the patient is the potential for an anastomotic leak. Consequences of anastomotic leak include pelvic and intra-abdominal abscess, peritonitis, fistulas, and the potential need for fecal diversion with a colostomy or ileostomy. In 1994, Bailey et al. [6] reported the results of 130 women undergoing open surgical resection of colorectal endometriosis. In their series, 90% of the anastomoses were to the extraperitoneal rectum. They observed no clinical or radiographic anastomotic leaks and no rectovaginal fistulas, although there was a 1% rate of pelvic abscess, suggesting the possibility of an occult microscopic leak. These are enviable results because the anastomotic leak rate for colorectal resection with low pelvic anastomoses to the extraperitoneal rectum for other conditions, such as cancer, inflammatory bowel disease, and diverticulitis, may be as high as 5% to 15%. It is this bar to which laparoscopic resection for colorectal endometriosis must be compared. Significant complication rates have been reported in some series. Darai et al. [42] reported a 10% major complication rate in 40 women undergoing laparoscopic resection. Three women developed rectovaginal fistulas and one a pelvic abscess. Marpeau et al. [59] reported their results with 32 women; 6.3% developed a rectovaginal fistula requiring treatment with colostomy. However, Jatan [7] recently reported the largest series in the literature of the laparoscopic treatment of colorectal endometriosis, with 98 patients treated. Their overall morbidity was 8.3%, but there were no anastomotic leaks or fistulas.

These results show that although there is potential for significant morbidity with the laparoscopic treatment of colorectal endometriosis, it is possible to perform the procedure with acceptably low overall and anastomotic complication rates. It is important that these potential complications be discussed with the patient preoperatively so that appropriate informed consent can be obtained.

CONCLUSIONS

Involvement of the gastrointestinal tract by endometriosis occurs in a minority of affected women but may be a significant source of the patient's symptoms. The rectum, rectovaginal septum, and sigmoid colon are the sites most frequently involved. A number of surgical techniques are available for the treatment of endometriosis in this region, including shave excision, disc excision, and segmental resection. These procedures may be performed laparoscopically with an acceptable morbidity and anastomotic complication rate and with the expectation of significant symptom relief for the patient.

REFERENCES

1. Sakamoto K, Maeda T, Yamamoto T, et al. Simultaneous laparoscopic treatment for rectosigmoid and ileal endometriosis. *J Laparoendosc Adv Surg Tech A.* 2006;16:251–255.
2. Kratzer GL, Salvati EP. Collective review of endometriosis of the colon. *Am J Surg.* 1955;90:866–869.
3. Macafee CH, Greer HL. Intestinal endometriosis. A report of 29 cases and a survey of the literature. *J Obstet Gynaecol Br Emp.* 1960;67:539–555.

4. Williams TJ, Pratt JH. Endometriosis in 1000 consecutive celiotomies: incidence and management. *Am J Obstet Gynecol.* 1977;129:245–250.

5. Gustofson RL, Kim N, Liu S, Stratton P. Endometriosis and the appendix: a case series and comprehensive review of the literature. *Fertil Steril.* 2006;86:298–303.

6. Bailey HR, Ott MT, Hartendorp P. Aggressive surgical management for advanced colorectal endometriosis. *Dis Colon Rectum.* 1994;37:747–753.

7. Jatan AK, Solomon MJ, Young J, Cooper M, Pathma-Nathan N. Laparoscopic management of rectal endometriosis. *Dis Colon Rectum.* 2006;49:169–174.

8. Shah M, Tager D, Feller E. Intestinal endometriosis masquerading as common digestive disorders. *Arch Intern Med.* 1995;155:977–980.

9. Chapron C, Liaras E, Fayet P, et al. Magnetic resonance imaging and endometriosis: deeply infiltrating endometriosis does not originate from the rectovaginal septum. *Gynecol Obstet Invest.* 2002;53:204–208.

10. Martimbeau PW, Pratt JH, Gaffey TA. Small-bowel obstruction secondary to endometriosis. *Mayo Clin Proc.* 1975;50:239–243.

11. Collins DC. A study of 50,000 specimens of the human vermiform appendix. *Surg Gynecol Obstet.* 1955;101:437–445.

12. Jerby BL, Kessler H, Falcone T, Milsom JW. Laparoscopic management of colorectal endometriosis. *Surg Endosc.* 1999;13:1125–1128.

13. Skoog SM, Foxx-Orenstein AE, Levy MJ, Rajan E, Session DR. Intestinal endometriosis: the great masquerader. *Curr Gastroenterol Rep.* 2004, 6:405–409.

14. Rowland R, Langman JM. Endometriosis of the large bowel: a report of 11 cases. *Pathology.* 1989;21:259–265.

15. Bozdech JM. Endoscopic diagnosis of colonic endometriosis. *Gastrointest Endosc.* 1992;38:568–570.

16. Levitt MD, Hodby KJ, van Merwyk AJ, Glancy RJ. Cyclical rectal bleeding in colorectal endometriosis. *Aust N Z J Surg.* 1989;59:941–943.

17. Farinon AM, Vadora E. Endometriosis of the colon and rectum: an indication for peroperative coloscopy. *Endoscopy.* 1980;12:136–139.

18. Caccese WJ, McKinley MJ, Bronzo RL, Bronson R. Endoscopic confirmation of colonic endometriosis. *Gastrointest Endosc.* 1984;30:191–193.

19. Gordon RL, Evers K, Kressel HY, Laufer I, Herlinger H, Thompson JJ. Double-contrast enema in pelvic endometriosis. *AJR Am J Roentgenol.* 1982;138:549–552.

20. Landi S, Barbieri F, Fiaccavento A, et al. Preoperative double-contrast barium enema in patients with suspected intestinal endometriosis. *J Am Assoc Gynecol Laparosc.* 2004;11:223–228.

21. Koga K, Osuga Y, Yano T, et al. Characteristic images of deeply infiltrating rectosigmoid endometriosis on transvaginal and transrectal ultrasonography. *Hum Reprod.* 2003;18:1328–1333.

22. Chapron C, Vieira M, Chopin N, et al. Accuracy of rectal endoscopic ultrasonography and magnetic resonance imaging in the diagnosis of rectal involvement for patients presenting with deeply infiltrating endometriosis. *Ultrasound Obstet Gynecol.* 2004;24:175–179.

23. Bahr A, de Parades V, Gadonneix P, et al. Endorectal ultrasonography in predicting rectal wall infiltration in patients with deep pelvic endometriosis: a modern tool for an ancient disease. *Dis Colon Rectum.* 2006;49:869–875.

24. Thomassin I, Bazot M, Detchev R, Barranger E, Cortez A, Darai E. Symptoms before and after surgical removal of colorectal endometriosis that are assessed by magnetic resonance imaging and rectal endoscopic sonography. *Am J Obstet Gynecol.* 2004;190:1264–1271.

25. Bazot M, Darai E, Hourani R, et al. Deep pelvic endometriosis: MR imaging for diagnosis and prediction of extension of disease. *Radiology.* 2004;232:379–389.

26. Jacobs M, Verdeja JC, Goldstein HS. Minimally invasive colon resection (laparoscopic colectomy). *Surg Laparosc Endosc.* 1991;1:144–150.

27. Nezhat C, Nezhat FR. Safe laser endoscopic excision or vaporization of peritoneal endometriosis. *Fertil Steril.* 1989;52(1):149–151.

28. Clinical Outcomes of Surgical Therapy Study Group. A comparison of laparoscopically assisted and open colectomy for colon cancer. *N Engl J Med.* 2004;350:2050–2059.

29. Lacy AM, Garcia-Valdecasas JC, Delgado S, et al. Laparoscopy-assisted colectomy versus open colectomy for treatment of non-metastatic colon cancer: a randomised trial. *Lancet.* 2002;359:2224–2229.

30. Milsom JW, Hammerhofer KA, Bohm B, Marcello P, Elson P, Fazio VW. Prospective, randomized trial comparing laparoscopic vs. conventional surgery for refractory ileocolic Crohn's disease. *Dis Colon Rectum.* 2001;44:1–8; discussion 8–9.

31. Marcello PW, Milsom JW, Wong SK, et al. Laparoscopic restorative proctocolectomy: case-matched comparative study with open restorative proctocolectomy. *Dis Colon Rectum.* 2000;43:604–608.

32. Milsom JW, Bohm B, Hammerhofer KA, Fazio V, Steiger E, Elson P. A prospective, randomized trial comparing laparoscopic versus conventional techniques in colorectal cancer surgery: a preliminary report. *J Am Coll Surg.* 1998;187:46–54; discussion 54–55.

33. Schmitt SL, Cohen SM, Wexner SD, Nogueras JJ, Jagelman DG. Does laparoscopic-assisted ileal pouch anal anastomosis reduce the length of hospitalization? *Int J Colorectal Dis.* 1994;9:134–137.

34. Dwivedi A, Chahin F, Agrawal S, et al. Laparoscopic colectomy vs. open colectomy for sigmoid diverticular disease. *Dis Colon Rectum.* 2002;45:1309–1314; discussion 1314–1315.

35. Alves A, Panis Y, Slim K, Heyd B, Kwiatkowski F, Mantion G. French multicentre prospective observational study of laparoscopic versus open colectomy for sigmoid diverticular disease. *Br J Surg.* 2005;92:1520–1525.

36. Weed JC, Ray JE. Endometriosis of the bowel. *Obstet Gynecol.* 1987;69:727–730.

37. Prystowsky JB, Stryker SJ, Ujiki GT, Poticha SM. Gastrointestinal endometriosis. Incidence and indications for resection. *Arch Surg.* 1988;123:855–858.

38. Nezhat F, Nezhat C, Pennington E, Ambroze W, Jr. Laparoscopic segmental resection for infiltrating endometriosis of the rectosigmoid colon: a preliminary report. *Surg Laparosc Endosc.* 1992;2:212–216.

39. Langebrekke A, Istre O, Busund B, Johannessen HO, Qvigstad E. Endoscopic treatment of deep infiltrating endometriosis (DIE) involving the bladder and rectosigmoid colon. *Acta Obstet Gynecol Scand.* 2006;85:712–715.

40. Dubernard G, Piketty M, Rouzier R, Houry S, Bazot M, Darai E. Quality of life after laparoscopic colorectal resection for endometriosis. *Hum Reprod.* 2006;21:1243–1247.

41. Ford J, English J, Miles WF, Giannopoulos T. A new technique for laparoscopic anterior resection for rectal endometriosis. *JSLS.* 2005;9:73–77.

42. Darai E, Thomassin I, Barranger E, et al. Feasibility and clinical outcome of laparoscopic colorectal resection for endometriosis. *Am J Obstet Gynecol.* 2005;192:394–400.

43. Campagnacci R, Perretta S, Guerrieri M, et al. Laparoscopic colorectal resection for endometriosis. *Surg Endosc.* 2005;19:662–664.

44. Abrao MS, Sagae UE, Gonzales M, Podgaec S, Dias JA Jr. Treatment of rectosigmoid endometriosis by laparoscopically assisted

vaginal rectosigmoidectomy. *Int J Gynaecol Obstet*. 2005;91:27–31.

45. Woods RJ, Heriot AG, Chen FC. Anterior rectal wall excision for endometriosis using the circular stapler. *ANZ J Surg*. 2003;73:647–648.

46. Duepree HJ, Senagore AJ, Delaney CP, Marcello PW, Brady KM, Falcone T. Laparoscopic resection of deep pelvic endometriosis with rectosigmoid involvement. *J Am Coll Surg*. 2002;195:754–758.

47. Nezhat C, Nezhat F, Pennington E. Laparoscopic treatment of infiltrative rectosigmoid colon and rectovaginal septum endometriosis by the technique of videolaparoscopy and CO_2 laser. *Br J Obstet Gynecol*. 1992;99(8):664–667.

48. Nezhat F. Laparoscopic segmental resection for infiltrating endometriosis of rectosigmoid colon: a preliminary report. *Surg Laparosc Endosc Percutan Tech*. 2001;11:67–68.

49. Varol N, Maher P, Woods R. Laparoscopic management of intestinal endometriosis. *J Am Assoc Gynecol Laparosc*. 2000;7:405–409.

50. Mohr C, Nezhat FR, Nezhat CH, Seidman DS, Nezhat CR. Fertility considerations in laparoscopic treatment of infiltrative bowel endometriosis. *JSLS*. 2005;9(1):16–24.

51. Redwine DB, Sharpe DR. Laparoscopic surgery for intestinal and urinary endometriosis. *Baillieres Clin Obstet Gynaecol*. 1995;9:775–794.

52. Sharpe DR, Redwine DB. Laparoscopic segmental resection of the sigmoid and rectosigmoid colon for endometriosis. *Surg Laparosc Endosc*. 1992;2:120–124.

53. Redwine DB, Sharpe DR. Laparoscopic segmental resection of the sigmoid colon for endometriosis. *J Laparoendosc Surg*. 1991;1:217–220.

54. Pittaway DE. Appendectomy in the surgical treatment of endometriosis. *Obstet Gynecol*. 1983;61:421–424.

55. Emmanuel KR, Davis C. Outcomes and treatment options in rectovaginal endometriosis. *Curr Opin Obstet Gynecol*. 2005;17:399–402.

56. Ford J, English J, Miles WA, Giannopoulos T. Pain, quality of life and complications following the radical resection of rectovaginal endometriosis. *BJOG*. 2004;111:353–356.

57. Fedele L, Bianchi S, Zanconato G, Bettoni G, Gotsch F. Long-term follow-up after conservative surgery for rectovaginal endometriosis. *Am J Obstet Gynecol*. 2004;190:1020–1024.

58. Darai E, Marpeau O, Thomassin I, Dubernard G, Barranger E, Bazot M. Fertility after laparoscopic colorectal resection for endometriosis: preliminary results. *Fertil Steril*. 2005;84:945–950.

59. Marpeau O, Thomassin I, Barranger E, Detchev R, Bazot M, Darai E. Laparoscopic colorectal resection for endometriosis: preliminary results [in French]. *J Gynecol Obstet Biol Reprod (Paris)*. 2004;33:600–606.

60. Nezhat C, Nezhat F, Pennington E, Nezhat CH, Ambroze W. Laparoscopic disk excision and primary repair of the anterior rectal wall for the treatment of full-thickness bowel endometriosis. *Surg Endosc*. 1994;8:682–685.

21 | ADDITIONAL PROCEDURES FOR PELVIC SURGEONS

Section 21.1. Cystoscopy

Ceana Nezhat and Deidre T. Fisher

Cystoscopy, the gold standard for diagnosis of disorders and injuries of the lower urinary tract, provides another tool for prevention and active management of urologic pathology and surgical complications by allowing the surgeon to assess the integrity and function of the urethra, bladder, and ureters. At our center, we have incidentally detected bladder endometriosis, polyps, malignant lesions, diverticula, duplicated ureter, and interstitial cystitis. One case of complete ureteral obstruction and renal necrosis due to invasive endometriosis was detected during an incidental cystoscopy. Contralateral periureteral disease was treated, resulting in successful conservation of the other kidney.

Cystoscopic technique, unfortunately, is not routinely taught during obstetrics/gynecology residency training; therefore, many gynecologists do not feel comfortable performing the procedure. This is unfortunate as gynecologists deal with urogynecologic issues daily with conditions such as urinary incontinence, pelvic organ prolapse, and severe endometriosis involving the lower urinary tract. Two large multicenter studies demonstrated that 66% to 80% of patients with chronic pelvic pain had evidence of bladder-origin pain due to bladder epithelial damage or interstitial cystitis.[1] In the gynecologic literature, chronic pelvic pain is associated with endometriosis in 30% to 87% of cases as well.[2] The surgical treatment of pelvic pain is the most frequent indication for operative laparoscopy, although in as many as 40% of patients, no pathology is found.[3] By the time a diagnosis is made, these patients have undergone various diagnostic procedures and surgeries and have often been given various unsuccessful empiric treatments. Because there is a high prevalence of coexisting interstitial cystitis and endometriosis, it is absolutely imperative that evaluation for both be undertaken in a timely manner to ensure a proper and timely diagnosis. In addition, because the vast majority of ureteral injuries occur during the half million hysterectomies performed annually, it is imperative that gynecologists master the prevention, recognition, and management of lower urinary tract injuries. The focus of this section is to introduce instruments and techniques used during basic cystoscopy as a tool to help achieve these goals.

INDICATIONS

The list of indications for cystoscopy is extensive and may include hematuria, calculus, polyps (Figure 21.1.1), suspected bladder cancer, large leiomyomatous uterus (Figure 21.1.2), urogenital fistula, cervical cancer staging, and persistent or atypical urinary tract infections. However, more commonly, the gynecologic surgeon will conduct this procedure to evaluate the anatomy and function of the lower urinary tract either before or after a urogynecologic procedure for incontinence and/or prolapse.

In addition, cystoscopy may be part of the evaluation for a disease or disorder such as severe endometriosis with suspected bladder involvement (Figure 21.1.3), interstitial cystitis, chronic pelvic pain, or persistent urinary symptoms.

On cystoscopy, interstitial cystitis can be diagnosed by the presence of characteristic petechial hemorrhages called glomerulations or Hunner's ulcers, which are pathognomonic, although infrequently seen in this disorder.[4] Because during urogynecologic procedures the lower urinary tract is at risk for injury, intraoperative cystoscopy is especially helpful if there is any suspicion about the integrity of the ureters, bladder, or urethra. It is unfortunate that many of these injuries are never detected, leading to complications such as fistulae, infection, and loss of kidney function. With intraoperative cystoscopy, Harris and coworkers [5] noted a complication rate of 4% among 224 patients undergoing a Burch colposuspension or culdoplasty. Most injuries were related to sutures and could be corrected by removal of the offending suture without further sequelae. Pettit and Petrou [6] evaluated patients after vaginal surgery including urogynecologic procedures, anterior repair, and culdoplasty. Among 236 patients, seven injuries were detected by cystoscopy with indigo carmine injection. In conclusion, one could recommend cystoscopic evaluation after all urogynecologic procedures. In cases of suspected injuries, or when persistent symptoms cannot be explained, referral to a specialist should be made.

INSTRUMENTS

The first attempt to visualize the human bladder was in 1806, when Bozzini presented his device, the Lichtleiter, which consisted of a urethral speculum and candle, to the Academy of Medicine in Vienna.[7] Since then, we have seen the advent of fiberoptic technology, the rod–lens system, accessory instrumentation, and flexible endoscopy.

There are four major advantages to the use of the rigid cystoscope: (1) traditionally better visualization; (2) larger lumen for medium flow, which translates into a clearer view; (3) a larger operative channel for the introduction of instruments; and (4) easier manipulation and maintenance of orientation, especially in the short female urethra. However, in certain cases, flexible cystoscopy may allow for ease of passage in an extremely exaggerated urethral angle (e.g., secondary to an aggressive sling procedure or postradiation urethral scarring).

The size of cystoscopes is usually given using the French (F) scale and refers to the outside diameter of the instrument in millimeters multiplied by 3. When instrumentation is necessary, sheaths with accessory ports are available as well. For adult patients, the typical caliber of the telescope can range from 16F to

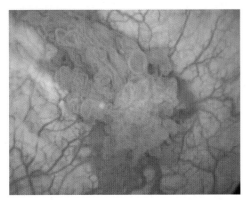

Figure 21.1.1. Bladder polyp.

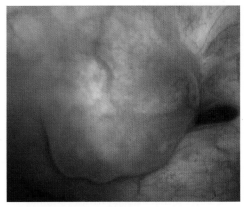

Figure 21.1.3. Bladder endometriosis.

25F, and the sheaths range from calibers of 17F to 28F. However, for our gynecologic population, a 15F telescope is usually more than adequate with a 19F sheath and will allow for adequate diagnostic cystoscopy without placing undue tension on the urethra. In cases in which instrumentation is necessary, a sheath of at least 21F to 24F is usually adequate.

Most systems consist of a telescope, bridge, and outer sheath (Figure 21.1.4). The telescope transmits light into the bladder cavity and provides a view of this cavity to the operator. The telescope slides through the sheath, which allows for introduction of both the telescope and distention media into the bladder. The bridge serves as a connector between the telescope and sheath and forms a watertight seal, and allows passage of ureteral catheters, tiny biopsy forceps, and other instruments. The distal end of the bridge has two ports to allow both influx and egress of distention media and bladder fluid, respectively. The distal end of the cystoscope is usually beveled to allow for more comfort with insertion into the urethra. An obturator may be placed into the sheath to provide a blunt, smooth tip for insertion into the urethra when a large sheath is necessary for certain instrumentation.

Distention of the bladder can be accomplished with three media types: conductive fluids (e.g., lactated Ringer's, normal saline), nonconductive fluids (e.g., sterile water, glycine), and gas. Although cystoscopy is feasible with CO_2 gas, most surgeons prefer fluids (either sterile water or normal saline) for diagnostic procedures because of better visualization and ease of monitoring distention volumes. In cases in which electrosurgery is anticipated, a nonconductive media such as glycine is preferred.

The choice of distention media should largely be based on the indication for, as well as length of, the proposed procedure. All distention fluids should ideally be warmed before infusion. It is also prudent to limit the height from which the medium is infusing to 60 cm above the bladder.[7,8] This will limit the distention pressure to minimize inadvertent overdistention while still providing adequate flow. The benefit of normal saline and lactated Ringer's solution during diagnostic cystoscopy is that they can be used in larger volumes without the risk of electrolyte imbalance.

Telescope cables, which are either fiberoptic or fluid filled, serve as the illuminating system. Fluid-filled cables tend to be more durable; fiberoptic cables are more common because they are far less expensive. The lens at the tip of the telescope collects the light of the image and transmits this image to the eyepiece through the rod–lens system. The telescopes are available in various angles to allow for optimal view of certain structures. For instance, a 0° and 12° lens focuses largely straight ahead and is usually inadequate for visualization of the entire bladder but optimal for view of the urethra. A 30° lens allows the optimal visualization of both the posterior wall and base of the bladder. According to some, this is the most versatile instrument. Used frequently, the 70° lens allows for visualization of the bladder dome, anterolateral walls, and into an elevated urethrovesical junction, such as after colposuspension procedures. Finally, 120°

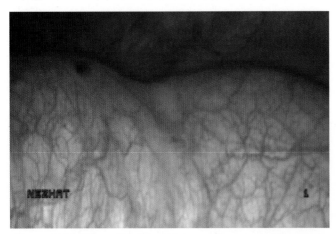

Figure 21.1.2. Normal bladder with external myoma impingement.

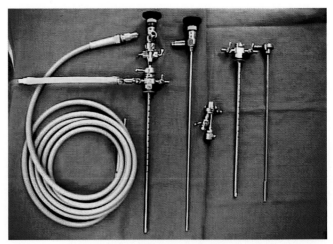

Figure 21.1.4. Cystoscopic equipment (assembled and unassembled), including light cord, tubing, telescope, bridge, sheath, and obturator.

retro-lenses, which are usually unnecessary in visualization of the female bladder and urethra, allow for ease in visualization of the bladder neck.

In conclusion, to perform a diagnostic cystoscopy, whether in the office or operative suite, one needs the following items:

1. Fiberoptic cables and a light source; the xenon light source is usually the most efficient lamp in use
2. An intravenous pole, connection tubing, and distention media
3. Cystoscope (usually 30° or 70°) with sheath, bridge, and obturator
4. Camera system with TV monitor, if desired
5. Container bin for instrument sterilization

ANATOMY

The female external urethra is a 5-mm vertical orifice between the clitoris and vagina. The internal urethra extends 3 to 4 cm at an upward angle and lies over the anterior vaginal wall; it is made of skeletal muscle and is firmly supported by the pubourethral ligament. The urethral blood supply is derived from the vaginal arteries; however, the venous drainage is via the pelvic veins. The hypogastric nerves of the pelvic plexus provide innervation to the smooth muscles of the urethra, whereas the pudendal nerve supplies the striated muscle fibers of the external urethral sphincter.

Although the bladder is a pelvic structure, it can rise impressively to the level of the umbilicus when extremely overdistended. The bladder is bordered anteriorly by the space of Retzius, rectus abdominis muscles, and pubic symphysis; inferiorly by the levator ani muscles and obturator internus muscles; posteriorly by the lower uterine segment, cervix, and vagina; and superiorly by the anteverted uterus. The bladder neck is directly above the urogenital diaphragm. The arterial blood supply is mainly distributed by the hypogastric artery through the superior, middle, and inferior vesicle arteries. In addition, the vaginal arteries supply the bladder neck. The primary venous drainage is via the hypogastric vein. The nerve supply includes the hypogastric sympathetic plexus and the pelvic splanchnic nerves, which accompany the vessels. Although the bladder is triangular in shape when empty, it becomes a sphere when filled. The bladder wall is composed of three muscle layers: inner longitudinal, middle circular, and external longitudinal. Where these muscle layers converge comprises the trigone. Between the ureteral orifices lies the interureteric fold, which also comprises the roof of the trigone. The mucosa is made of transitional epithelium.[8–10]

TECHNIQUE

Whether performed in the office or in the operating room, the overall principles of cystoscopy are essentially the same. Depending on the indication for the cystoscopy, a comprehensive examination may include careful inspection for costovertebral angle tenderness, bladder tenderness, or distention; a gynecologic examination; and urine microscopic and culture studies. After the procedure has been discussed and proper consent obtained, care should be taken to make the patient as comfortable as possible. The buttocks should be positioned at the edge of the table. The legs should be supported optimally in well-padded knee crutches or stirrups, with the help of an attentive assistant. It is extremely important that the hips are not excessively abducted, especially if the patient is sedated.

Before beginning the procedure, it is imperative to make sure all necessary instruments are available and in working order and that sterile technique is observed. Inspection of the external urethra and vagina should be performed at this point. If a sterile urine specimen is to be collected, this should be done at the beginning of the procedure. After allowing an anesthetic lubricant to take effect, the cystoscope should be flushed to ensure that no air is introduced into the bladder. With the media running briskly, the cystoscope should then be placed under direct visualization gently into the urethral meatus, aiming cephalad toward the umbilicus. Any urethral or bladder mucosal abnormalities, as well as the urethral length and width, should be noted. At times, urethral dilatation is necessary. Gradual dilatations with Hegar dilators may be done. Care should be taken not to overdilate the urethra in the rare cases when dilation is necessary. The bladder can generally accommodate 300 to 350 mL of fluid.[7–9] Once the cystoscope is inside the bladder and one has optimal visualization, systemic evaluation should take place. One such technique would be to evaluate the entire length of the urethral wall mucosa, noting stenosis, diverticula, or lesions such as microabscess or calculus. To maintain orientation, it should be remembered that the light cord is 180° opposite the direction the lens is illuminating. For instance, the light cord will be at 11 o'clock if one is visualizing the bladder at 5 o'clock. The surgeon should note the relationship of the urethra to the bladder neck, as a sharp drop or decline at the junction of the posterior urethra with the bladder neck confirms the presence of a cystocele. One should inspect the bladder using an imaginary clock, noting in a systematic fashion the color, lesions, and any aberrant vessels. The trigone and ureteral orifices should be examined, demonstrating brisk jets of urine bilaterally. Intravenous infusion of indigo carmine dye approximately 5 minutes before initiating cystoscopy may facilitate the visualization of the ureteral jets (Figure 21.1.5).

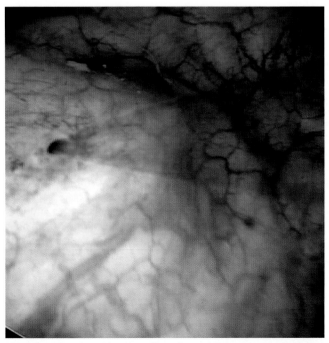

Figure 21.1.5. Ureteral urine efflux from right ureter using indigo carmine dye.

Table 21.1.1: Bacterial Endocarditis Prophylaxis for Genitourinary Procedures

Situation	Agent	Regimen
High-risk patient	Ampicillin + gentamicin	Ampicillin 2 g IM/IV with gentamicin 1.5 mg/kg (not to exceed 120 mg)*; repeat in 6 hours 1 g IV/IM or amoxicillin 1 g orally
High-risk patients allergic to penicillin	Vancomycin + gentamicin	Vancomycin 1 g IV over 1–2 hours + gentamicin 1.5 mg/kg IV/IM (not to exceed 120 mg)*
Moderate-risk patients	Amoxicillin or ampicillin	Amoxicillin 2 g orally 1 hour before procedure or ampicillin 2 g IM/IV*
Moderate-risk patients allergic to penicillin	Vancomycin	Vancomycin 1 g IV over 1–2 hours*

*Complete injection/infusion within 30 minutes of starting procedure. IM, intramuscularly; IV, intravenously.

Visualization of the bladder base may be difficult in a patient with a large cystocele. In this case, placing a finger into the vagina to elevate the wall and reduce the cystocele may be helpful.[8] A gas bubble is a sure sign that one is visualizing the bladder dome. Lastly, the anterior bladder is easier to see before the bladder is fully distended, and application of suprapubic pressure may help facilitate visualization. At the conclusion of the procedure, the fluid should be discontinued and the cystoscope should gently be removed while leaving the sheath in place by disconnecting it at the bridge to allow the bladder to drain. It is prudent to have the patient void before discharge.

ANTIBIOTIC PROPHYLAXIS

Antibiotics are not routinely necessary for cystoscopic procedures. However, bacteriuria has been described after cystoscopy in 3% to 16% of patients and may be transient or lead to symptomatic infection.[11] The recommendations concerning prophylactic treatment are varied. Some believe that if one adheres to sterile technique and there is an adequate antiseptic prep, antibiotics are unnecessary. Others advocate a single dose of trimethoprim-sulfamethoxazole, double-strength (160/800 mg), or ampicillin 500 mg.[12] Antibiotic use is advisable, however, if the procedure is performed while the patient has a diagnosed urinary tract infection. In these cases, a complete course of a third-generation cephalosporin or penicillin is usually prescribed. In a patient at risk for bacterial endocarditis, the American Heart Association recommendations should be followed (Table 21.1.1).[13]

CONCLUSION

In the evaluation of many disorders presented to the gynecologic surgeon, such as chronic pelvic pain, severe endometriosis, interstitial cystitis, and incontinence, cystoscopy has been proven to be a helpful assessment tool. In fact, injuries of the bladder and ureters will continue to be of utmost importance to the obstetric and gynecologic surgeon. The importance of urinary tract evaluation for the prevention, timely detection, and treatment of surgical complications cannot be overstated.[14–17] As previously stated, many advocate that cystoscopy should be an integral part of urogynecologic and pelvic reconstructive procedures.

REFERENCES

1. Stanford EJ, Koziol J, Feng A. The prevalence of interstitial cystitis, endometriosis, adhesions, and vulvar pain in women with chronic pelvic pain. *J Minim Invasive Gynecol.* 2005;12:43–49.
2. Chung MK, Chung RP, Gordon D, Jennings C. The evil twins of chronic pelvic pain syndrome: endometriosis and interstitial cystitis. *JSLS.* 2002;6:311–314.
3. Howard FM. The role of laparoscopy in chronic pelvic pain: promise and pitfalls. *Obstet Gynecol Surv.* 1993;48:357–387.
4. Portera G. Equipment for cystoscopy. In: Miller BE, ed. *An Atlas of Sigmoidoscopy and Cystoscopy.* New York: Parthenon Publishing; 2002:57–59.
5. Harris RL, Cundiff GW, Theofrastous JP, Yoon H, Bump RC, Addison WA. The value of intraoperative cystoscopy in urogynecologic and reconstructive pelvic surgery. *Am J Obstet Gynecol.* 1997;177:1367–1369.
6. Pettit PD, Petrou SP. The value of cystoscopy in major vaginal surgery. *Obstet Gynecol.* 1994;84:318–320.
7. Cundiff GW, Bent AE. Endoscopic evaluation of the lower urinary tract. In: Walters MD, Karram MM, eds. *Urogynecology and Reconstructive Pelvic Surgery.* 2nd ed. Philadelphia: Mosby; 1999:111–121.
8. Miller BE, Katsanis WA. The cystoscopy examination in the female. In: Miller BE, ed. *An Atlas of Sigmoidoscopy and Cystoscopy.* New York: Parthenon Publishing; 2002:65–72.
9. Weinberger MW. Cystourethroscopy for the practicing gynecologist. *Clin Obstet Gynecol.* 1998;41:764–776.
10. Bent AE, Cundiff GW. Cystourethroscopy. In: Baggish MS, Karram MM, eds. *Atlas of Pelvic Anatomy and Gynecologic Surgery.* Philadelphia: WB Saunders; 2001:721–746.
11. Miller BE. Patient preparation for cystoscopy. In: Miller BE, ed. *An Atlas of Sigmoidoscopy and Cystoscopy.* New York: Parthenon Publishing; 2002:61–63.
12. Carter HB. Evaluation of the urologic patient. In: Walsh PC, Retik AB, Stamy TA, Vaughan ED, eds. *Campbell's Urology.* 6th ed. Philadelphia: WB Saunders; 1992:335–337.
13. American Heart Association. Prevention of infective endocarditis. Guidelines from the American Heart Association. *Circulation,* Apr 2007; doi: 10.1161/CIRCULATIONAHA.106.183095.
14. Hibbert ML, Salminen ER, Dainty LA, Davis GD, Perez, RP. Credentialing residents for intraoperative cystoscopy. *Obstet Gynecol.* 2000;96:1014–1017.
15. Gearhart JP. Surgical complications. In: Marshall FF, ed. *Urologic Complications, Medical and Surgical, Adult and Pediatric.* 2nd ed. Philadelphia: Mosby Yearbook; 1990:380–381.
16. Lawson RK, Taylor AJ. Anatomy, physiology, and examination. In: Buchsbaum HJ, Schmidt JD, eds. *Gynecologic and Obstetric Urology.* 3rd ed. Philadelphia: WB Saunders; 1993:80–81.
17. Gowri V, Krolikowski A. Chronic pelvic pain: laparoscopic and cystoscopic findings. *Saudi Med J.* 2001;22:769–770.

Section 21.2. Intraoperative Sigmoidoscopy in Gynecologic Surgery

Ceana Nezhat and Andrew DeFazio

Bowel injury is one of the most serious complications of laparoscopy.[1] The estimated risk of gastrointestinal injuries during gynecologic laparoscopy is between 0.6 and 1.6 per thousand [2–6]; however, most of these injuries (69%) [7] are not recognized at the time of surgery. Intraoperative detection and treatment of such injuries are greatly enhanced by the use of sigmoidoscopy.

Sigmoidoscopy is a very effective tool in gynecologic surgery. It can be used intraoperatively to evaluate bowel integrity following procedures involving the rectosigmoid colon or rectovaginal septum. Sigmoidoscopy may also be used as an adjunct to laparoscopy and intraoperative rectovaginal examination to determine the extent of invasion of endometriosis in this area. When used concomitantly during operative laparoscopy, it can be used as a probe to delineate the boundaries of diseased areas and assist in identifying the proper plane of dissection. Intraoperative sigmoidoscopy is a safe procedure and adds little to preoperative preparation and operative procedure length.

INSTRUMENTATION

The rigid sigmoidoscope used intraoperatively is available in either reusable or disposable forms. Sigmoidoscopy kits include a sigmoidoscope, obturator, light handle, insufflation bulb, and transformer (Figure 21.2.1). The sigmoidoscopes are made of stainless steel and have a fiberoptic light source providing excellent visualization. The sigmoidoscope has discrete markings every centimeter to allow measurements from either the dentate line or anal verge. The light source is usually either at the handle or at the connection of the scope. The insufflation bulb should be maintained as close to the scope as possible to allow for better control and ease of insufflation. The obturator is placed through the scope to allow insertion of the instrument into the rectum with minimal trauma.[8–10]

PROCEDURE

In a study published in 1980, Wheeless [11] provided a complete description of the technique needed to demonstrate rectosigmoid integrity following repair by laparotomy. To demonstrate rectosigmoid integrity, one must first observe the pieces of transected colon. Wheeless stated, "Two complete circles of colon must be identified before one can be certain that the colon anastomosis is intact and complete."[11] Then direct visualization of the anastomosis must be achieved with a sigmoidoscope using a 360° transanal view. Lastly, the pelvis should be filled with saline,

at which point air is injected through the sigmoidoscope into the rectum and sigmoid colon while compressing the colon proximal to the site of repair. If a defect is present, bubbles will emerge, and the exact site is then identified and repaired.[12]

To perform a sigmoidoscopy, the device is first attached to its light source and insufflation bulb, and the obturator, with its tip lubricated, is placed through the scope. The surgeon then performs a rectal exam to lubricate the anus and distal rectum and relax the sphincter muscles.

The sigmoidoscope is then typically held in the left hand, and the insufflating bulb is squeezed with the right hand. The obturator and scope are inserted together in a direction pointing toward the umbilicus. Once the scope is felt to be within the rectum, the obturator is removed. Air insufflation is then performed by squeezing the bulb to allow visualization of the colonic and rectal lumen. Care should be taken to avoid excessive dilation of the colon. Once the lumen is seen, the scope can be advanced under direct visualization. Typically, the low and mid-rectum is midline, requiring the surgeon to direct the scope in a posterior direction. As the scope is advanced through a visualized lumen to the upper rectum, it should be directed toward the left to follow the normal course of the rectum (Figure 21.2.2). At the region of the rectosigmoid junction, the colon turns to the right. A complete exam usually requires examination up to a level of 20 to 25 cm. Intraoperatively, however, an adequate exam requires that the involved portion of bowel be visualized and examined completely. At the completion of the examination, the air is removed and the sigmoidoscope retracted.[8–10]

INDICATIONS

Intraoperative proctosigmoidoscopy is indicated in cases of severe disease involving the bowel, such as endometriosis, adhesions, fibrosis, or certain malignant implants (Figures 21.2.3–21.2.5). The proctosigmoidoscope is used as a probe to delineate the boundaries of the lesions, identify planes of dissection, and facilitate their removal. This is done by gently moving the sigmoidoscope within the bowel, with or without the use of air, in the vertical and horizontal planes under direct laparoscopic visualization.

Proctosigmoidoscopy should also be used at the completion of procedures such as extensive dissections involving the bowel, shaving and resection of bowel wall lesions (Figure 21.2.6), and bowel resections or repair to assure bowel integrity. This is accomplished by simultaneous examination and direct visualization of the area in question with the sigmoidoscope and laparoscope. The pelvis is then filled with an isotonic solution, such as normal

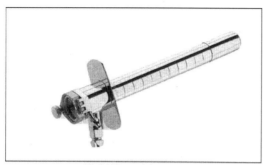

Rigid Sigmoidoscope

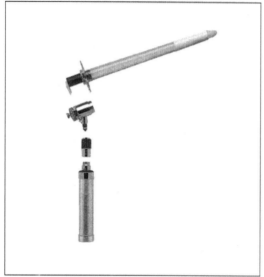

53130 KleenSpec® Disposable Sigmoidoscope, Shown with 3.5v Halogen Illumination System

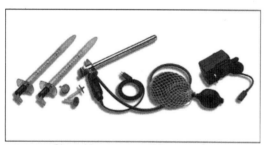

Sigmoidoscopes and Accessories

Figure 21.2.1. Sigmoidoscopes and accessories. Reproduced with permission from Welch Allyn, Inc.

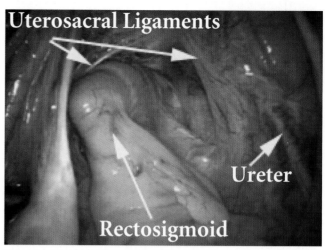

Figure 21.2.2. Normal rectosigmoid deviated to left by sigmoidoscope.

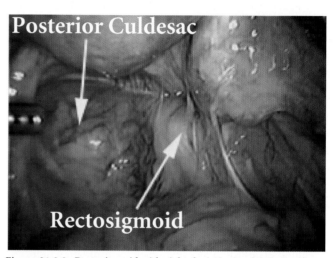

Figure 21.2.3. Rectosigmoid with right deviation and stricture due to endometriosis and fibrosis.

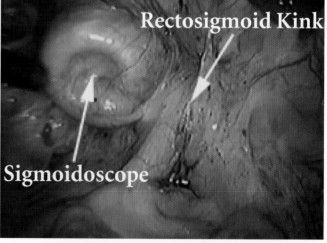

Figure 21.2.4. Rectosigmoid with right deviation and stricture due to endometriosis and fibrosis with distal sigmoidoscope placement.

saline, and air is insufflated into the bowel via the sigmoidoscope. The site of bowel dissection or repair is then submersed in the fluid while the proximal bowel is gently compressed with a blunt instrument (Figure 21.2.7). The production of air bubbles in the fluid denotes a lack of bowel integrity as air can escape even through very small defects. When this occurs, the defect is repaired and the procedure is repeated.[10,11]

A recent study showed the utility and safety of intraoperative proctosigmoidoscopy.[13] Two hundred sixty-two consecutive patients who underwent operative laparoscopy for rectosigmoid endometriosis and severe adhesions had a sigmoidoscopy

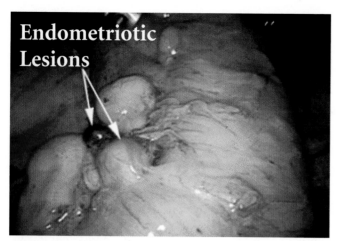

Figure 21.2.5. Rectosigmoid with sigmoidoscope tip at the level of endometriotic lesions.

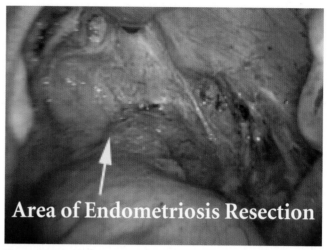

Figure 21.2.7. Underwater exam after shaving of endometriosis from rectosigmoid with no air bubble production.

performed at the end of the procedure. Intraoperative findings during laparoscopy included pelvic endometriosis in 30.3%, pelvic adhesions in 20.2%, and both in 43.5% of the patients. Sigmoidoscopy was used because of treatment of lesions involving the rectum or sigmoid in 60.7%, the large bowel in 11.1%, and the posterior cul-de-sac in 28.3% of the cases. Forty-four (16.8%) of the patients had an enterotomy. All cases of bowel injury were diagnosed intraoperatively. In four patients (1.5%), the bowel injury was identified only during sigmoidoscopy. The enterotomies were all repaired by intracorporeal laparoscopic suturing. One incomplete repair was detected by intraoperative sigmoidoscopy, and one incidental benign rectal polyp was also detected. There were no postoperative bowel perforations.

Intraoperative sigmoidoscopy is an invaluable tool during laparoscopic surgery involving the rectosigmoid colon, rectovaginal septum, or posterior cul-de-sac. The depth of penetration of endometriosis can be ascertained, proper planes of dissection identified, and rectosigmoid integrity evaluated, following manipulation or repair. A very safe procedure, it can detect intraoperative gastrointestinal complications, thereby preventing serious adverse postoperative outcomes. It is a simple

procedure that can be easily learned and has minimal, if any, risk of injury or complication. It is not associated with a significant increase in intraoperative time or additional cost. By decreasing the risk of severe postoperative complications, the benefit of its use significantly outweighs the risks.

REFERENCES

1. Schrenk P, Woisetschlager R, Rieger R, Wayand W. Mechanism, management, and prevention of laparoscopic bowel injuries. *Gastrointest Endosc.* 1996;43:572–574.
2. Harkki-Siren P, Kurki T. A nationwide analysis of laparoscopic complication. *Obstet Gynecol.* 1997;89:108–112.
3. Peterson HB, Hulka JF, Phillips JM. American Association of Gynecologic Laparoscopists' 1988 membership survey on operative laparoscopy. *J Reprod Med.* 1990;35:587–589.
4. Lehmann Willenbrock E, Riedel HH, Mecke H, Semm K. Pelviscopy/laparoscopy and its complications in Germany, 1949–1988. *J Reprod Med.* 1992;37:671–677.
5. Jansen FW, Kapiteyen K, Trimbos-Kemper T, et al. Complications of laparoscopy: a prospective multicentre observational study. *Br J Obstet Gynaecol.* 1997;104:595–600.
6. Chapron C, Pierre F, Harchaoui Y, et al. Gastrointestinal injuries during gynaecologic laparoscopy. *Hum Reprod.* 1999;14:333–337.
7. Bishoff JT, Allaf ME, Kirkels W, Moore RG, Kavoussi LR, Schroder F. Laparoscopic bowel injury: incidence and clinical presentation. *J Urol.* 1999;161:887–890.
8. Corman ML. *Colon and Rectal Surgery.* Philadelphia: Lippincott Williams & Wilkins; 1998:52.
9. Beck D. *Complications of Colon and Rectal Surgery.* Baltimore: Williams & Wilkins; 1996:79.
10. Beard JD, Nicholson ML, Sayers RD, et al. Intraoperative air testing of colorectal anastomosis: a prospective, randomized trial. *Br J Surg.* 1990;77:1095.
11. Wheeless CR, Dorsey JH. Use of the automatic surgical stapler for intestinal anastomosis associated with gynecologic malignancy: review of 283 procedures. *Gynecol Oncol.* 1981;11:1–7.
12. Rock JA, Thompson JD, eds. *Te Linde's Operative Gynecology.* 8th ed. Philadelphia: Lippincott-Raven Publishers; 1997:1297–1298.
13. Nezhat CH, Seidman D, Nezhat F, Nezhat CR. The role of intraoperative proctosigmoidoscopy in laparoscopic pelvic surgery. *J Am Assoc Gynecol Laparosc.* 2004;11:47–49.

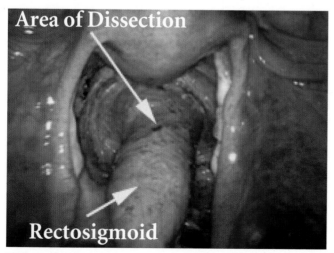

Figure 21.2.6. Rectosigmoid with sigmoidoscope after vaporization and shaving of endometriosis.

Section 21.3. Appendectomy

Bulent Berker, Farr Nezhat, Ceana Nezhat, and Camran Nezhat

Although diagnostic laparoscopy to examine abdominal pathology has been available for a substantial length of time, it has only been in the last two decades that gynecologists and general surgeons have been performing the procedure in large numbers. This is mainly because of advances in technology and surgical ingenuity, and general acceptance of the safety of laparoscopy.[1] As gynecologic and general surgeons do more endoscopic procedures, the advantages of laparoscopic appendectomy should be considered. Kurt Semm performed the first laparoscopic appendectomy in 1980.[2] Before the laparoscopic revolution of the 1980s and 1990s, appendicitis had been well treated by open appendectomy for at least 100 years. The completion of more than two dozen prospective randomized trials shows that the laparoscopic technique produces better outcomes for patients with suspected acute appendicitis than does conventional open appendectomy.[3,4]

This section describes the value of laparoscopy in the diagnosis of appendicitis, discusses the indications for laparoscopic appendectomy, and illustrates the techniques.

WHY LAPAROSCOPY?

The indications for surgical intervention, whether open or laparoscopic, in acute appendicitis depend on the degree of suspicion for the disease as well as its pathologic presentation. If the degree of suspicion is low, observation with serial abdominal examinations is justified. A moderate to high degree of suspicion warrants surgical exploration. Furthermore, acute appendicitis may be difficult to diagnose, especially in women, because many gynecologic disorders cause symptoms and signs indistinguishable from those of appendicitis.[5] The type and location of pain or discomfort associated with ovulation, ovarian cysts, endometriosis, salpingitis, and urinary tract disorders cannot be differentiated easily from those of acute appendicitis. In the general population, 15% to 20% of appendixes removed by laparotomy for suspected appendicitis show no abnormality compared with 30% to 45% in young women.[6] Accurate diagnosis and prompt management help prevent complications from perforation, including significant postoperative morbidity and an increased risk of tubal infertility.[7–9]

When the cause of right iliac fossa pain cannot be determined clinically and radiologically, laparoscopy has high specificity for the diagnosis and reduces the negative appendectomy rate. The diagnosis of acute appendicitis is difficult in women of childbearing age, and diagnostic laparoscopy is particularly useful in this group of women. It affords excellent exposure of the appendix regardless of its position and allows a thorough examination of the rest of the peritoneal cavity. In young women who complain of right lower abdominal pain, laparoscopy can give a precise diagnosis and reduce the rate of unnecessary appendectomies. Laine and associates [10] did a randomized study to compare laparoscopic and open appendectomy in 50 young female patients with suspected acute appendicitis. They reported that the diagnosis was established accurately in 96% of the patients in the laparoscopic group and 72% in the open group. There were 11 (44%) unnecessary appendectomies in the open group but only one (4%) in the laparoscopic group. The impact of laparoscopic appendectomy on the incidence of histologically normal appendixes recently was evaluated by Barrat and associates [11], who found that in 930 patients operated on using the classic McBurney approach, the incidence of histologically normal appendixes was 25.1%. The incidence was only 8.2% in 290 patients who underwent laparoscopic exploration, with an appendectomy carried out if there were macroscopic abnormalities. The risk of false positives and false negatives was approximately 10%. The diagnostic difficulties usually occurred in the initial phase of the disease, with acute mucosal involvement in a morphologically normal appendix. Those authors concluded that laparoscopy reduced the number of histologically normal appendixes compared with a laparotomy. This was achieved by not removing macroscopically normal appendixes. A small proportion (5% to 10%) could be patients with early appendicitis with only mucosal involvement. Moberg and coauthors [12] summarized the results of diagnostic laparoscopy in 1043 patients with symptoms and signs of acute appendicitis. They showed that diagnostic laparoscopy is safe and can be recommended in patients with suspected acute appendicitis, particularly in women. Their data also suggested that a macroscopically normal-looking appendix need not be removed.

Laparoscopy provides superior visualization of the entire abdominal cavity, a distinct advantage when a diagnosis is uncertain. In cases in which high clinical suspicion for appendicitis lacks corroborating radiologic evidence, exploratory laparoscopy can confirm appendicitis or identify other reasons for abdominal pain. Clearly, laparoscopy has a vital role in providing diagnostic information in unclear or atypical cases. Reiertsen and coworkers [13] did a randomized controlled trial with sequential design of laparoscopic and conventional appendectomy in 272 patients with suspected appendicitis. They found that the risk of unnecessary appendectomy was significantly lower after laparoscopy and concluded that an initial laparoscopy may reduce the rate of errors.

The sequelae from appendectomies by laparotomy that reveal a normal appendix usually are not serious, although a 1% to 17% morbidity rate from such operations has been reported.[2,13]

These observations and concern about postoperative adhesions have increased the use of laparoscopy for the diagnosis of the cause of pelvic and abdominal pain before definitive therapy. [14–17] In a patient with suspected appendicitis, laparoscopy can reduce the need for laparotomy because the surgeon can inspect the peritoneal cavity and pelvis thoroughly with the laparoscope and avoid even a McBurney or small laparotomy incision.[18,19] However, observation of the entire appendix by laparoscopy is possible in only 90% to 95% of patients.[20] In addition, some visually normal appendixes have been removed in which histologic examination revealed acute or chronic inflammation.[17,21] In a series of 100 incidental appendectomies, 52 appendixes were normal, 28 had adhesions, 14 showed foci of endometriosis, four showed focal chronic inflammation, one contained a benign mucocele, and one had a carcinoid.[3] These findings demonstrate the potential yield of appendiceal disease associated with a grossly normal appendix. A similar abnormality rate was reported by Krone [22] in his series of 1718 incidental appendectomies: 21.4% were normal, but 65.1% showed evidence of chronic disease and 5.6% had a carcinoid, a mucocele, or endometriosis. Women with chronic right lower quadrant (RLQ) pain also have a high rate of gross or microscopic appendiceal abnormalities. In a series of 62 laparoscopic appendectomies done for acute and chronic pain [23], 38 were associated with entrapping adhesions, 12 showed evidence of chronic inflammation, and five were involved with endometriosis. Only seven were normal. Of the 55 patients with predominantly RLQ or flank pain, 53 had complete or significant pain relief on long-term follow-up (1 to 6 years). In addition, in a patient who has chronic RLQ pain and no obvious appendiceal abnormality, prophylactic laparoscopic appendectomy should be considered. The procedure eliminates the chance of missing early appendicitis or other appendiceal abnormalities. Prolonging laparoscopy for 4 to 21 minutes to carry out an appendectomy imposes minimal stress to the patient.[3]

Cervini and colleagues [24] demonstrated that the decision to perform laparoscopic appendectomy is strongly influenced by a surgeon's training and experience with laparoscopy. Most investigators agree that the populations that benefit most from a laparoscopic approach are obese patients and women in the childbearing years.[25] Contraindications to laparoscopic appendectomy are few and coincide with those of laparoscopy in general: severe cardiopulmonary disease, uncorrected coagulopathy, and patient refusal.

INCIDENTAL APPENDECTOMY BY LAPAROSCOPY

Prophylactic laparoscopic appendectomy is relatively easy and safe. It is similar in principle to appendectomy by laparotomy. With the expansion of laparoscopic procedures, the transition from laparoscopic diagnosis to laparoscopic appendectomy is logical. Removal of a normal-appearing appendix while operating for suspected acute appendicitis has been the standard of care. It has been suggested that the introduction of operative laparoscopy should not alter this practice. Others contend that a normal-looking appendix may be left in place.[12,13] Laparoscopy can prevent unnecessary appendectomies.[10,13] Laparoscopic removal of the normal appendix caused no increase

in morbidity or length of hospitalization compared with diagnostic laparoscopy.[26] This observation shows the cost-effectiveness of laparoscopic appendectomy in terms of preventing missed and future appendicitis. Incidental laparoscopic appendectomy may be the preferred treatment option. The decision to remove a normal appendix is likely best made upon each surgeon's consideration of the risk–benefit ratio for an individual patient, taking into account such factors as age, immunocompetence, comorbidities, and perceived degree of technical difficulty. The surgeon should discuss with the patient before surgery the likelihood that a normal-appearing appendix will be removed if discovered.

Laparoscopy plays a critical role in the diagnostic work-up of patients with chronic pelvic pain, especially in patients with nonspecific clinical or radiologic findings. Diagnostic laparoscopy may be helpful in ruling out endometriosis. In addition to the excellent exposure of the pelvic cavity, it allows a thorough examination of the abdominal cavity.[1] Endometriosis traditionally has been included in the differential diagnosis of chronic pelvic pain, particularly in women of reproductive age.[27] In one study, endometriosis was documented in up to 80% of patients undergoing laparoscopic surgery for chronic pelvic pain.[28] However, in patients with endometriosis, the assumption that chronic pelvic pain is solely the result of pelvic endometriosis may be flawed. Among other disorders, appendiceal pathology also should be considered.[29] Reports evaluating gastrointestinal endometriosis suggest that the appendix is the second most common site of involvement, with only the rectosigmoid colon being more commonly affected.[30,31] In one study, we evaluated appendiceal pathology in women with endometriosis and chronic pelvic pain without solely RLQ pain.[32] Of the 231 patients with pelvic endometriosis, concomitant appendiceal pathology was found in 115. Notably, of the 231 patients with pelvic endometriosis, 51 (22.1%) had histologic evidence of appendiceal endometriosis. Pathology other than endometriosis was found in 64 (27.7%) of all patients.

The appendix itself may be a cause of chronic pelvic pain. The laparoscopic appearance of chronic or recurrent appendicitis was studied prospectively in 42 women with long-term or recurrent lower abdominal pain.[33] Appendectomy was done when at least two of the following pathologic changes were present at diagnostic laparoscopy: vascular injection of appendiceal peritoneum, periappendiceal adhesions, and induration of the appendix. During a mean observation of 13 months, 74% of women had no abdominal pain, 12% had partial relief in a mean of 15 months of observation, and 12% experienced no change in abdominal pain. New laparoscopic techniques with associated local anesthesia and conscious sedation allow operative laparoscopic procedures to be achieved while the patient is awake. Such evaluation of the appendix with intraoperative patient feedback concerning the presence and absence of pain allows more accurate diagnosis of chronic appendicitis during conscious pain mapping.[34]

Prophylactic antibiotics are administered preoperatively to patients who complain of RLQ pain. The operation is carried out under general anesthesia. Appendectomy is advisable after other laparoscopic procedures have been completed. Copious irrigation is advisable to minimize bacterial contamination.

After the pelvis is inspected, the appendix is identified, mobilized, and examined. Periappendiceal or pericecal adhesions are

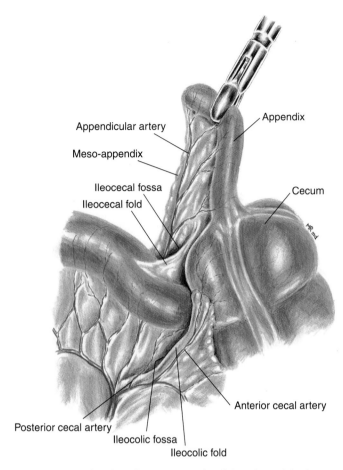

Figure 21.3.1. After the pelvis is inspected and the other pelvic abnormalities have been treated, the appendix is identified, mobilized, and examined.

lysed, using the laser or scissors, because adequate mobilization and good exposure are essential, particularly if the appendix is adherent to the pelvic side wall or is retrocecal. The mesoappendix is coagulated with bipolar forceps or clipped and cut with laparoscopic scissors or a laser to skeletonize the appendix (Figures 21.3.1–21.3.3). Fecal contents are milked toward the tip of the appendix by using a grasper over an area 2 cm from the cecum. Two Endoloop sutures (Ethicon) are passed sequentially through one of the 5-mm suprapubic trocar sleeves and looped around the base of the appendix next to each other (Figure 21.3.4). A third Endoloop suture is applied 5 mm distal to the first two sutures. Hulka tubal clips (used for tubal sterilization) also may be used to secure the proximal and distal portions of the appendix.[15,35] The appendix is cut between the two sets of sutures, using the laser or laparoscopic scissors (Figure 21.3.5). The luminal portion of the appendiceal stump is seared with the CO_2 laser, povidone–iodine (Betadine) solution may be applied, and the tissues are irrigated copiously with lactated Ringer's solution (Figure 21.3.6). A pursestring or Z-suture may be placed in the cecum to bury the appendiceal stump [36], although there appears to be no advantage to its invagination.[37] Countersinking the stump does not guarantee that adhesions or complications will be avoided. If the stump is to be buried, a polydioxanone Endosuture (Ethicon) is used with two needle holders or graspers inserted through

the suprapubic trocar sleeves. The stump is invaginated with a grasper, and the pursestring suture is tied using an instrument-tying method or extracorporeal suturing. A significant difference was found in the incidence of postoperative small bowel obstruction when invagination was compared with stump ligation. In the invagination group, there were six instances of bowel obstruction (1.6%), whereas the stump ligation group included only one patient who became obstructed postoperatively (0.3%). This difference in complications may be related to the high incidence of adhesions found in more than 70% of patients with pursestring or Z-suture placement.[21] Simple ligation simplifies the technical procedure and shortens the operating time. It produces no deformation of the cecal wall that might arouse suspicion of a neoplasm in subsequent contrast radiography.

An Endoloop suture may be placed around the distal tip of the appendix as a substitute for a grasping instrument during initial mobilization and excision of the appendix. Once the appendix is free, the suture is used to pull the appendix into a 5- or 10-mm accessory trocar sleeve. The trocar sleeve is removed from the suprapubic incision with the appendix contained within it. Endobags (Ethicon) that minimize contact between contaminated tissue and the pelvis are available. Traction on the pursestring of the bag allows it to be drawn through a small skin incision without contaminating it. The appendix also can be removed from the abdomen with long grasping forceps placed through the operating channel of the laparoscope. However, this method contaminates both the graspers and the operating channel.

Stapling devices make laparoscopic appendectomy easier and faster. The multi-fire stapler is introduced through a 12-mm suprapubic midline incision and applied directly across the entire mesoappendix and appendix. In a single motion, the entire appendix and its mesoappendix are clipped and cut (Figure 21.3.7). The stapler's operation should not be hindered by contact with surrounding tissue, and the cecum must be free from attachments. Appendiceal contents do not leak intraperitoneally, and the larger trocar sleeve allows easier removal of the separated appendix. Two disadvantages to the stapling device are its cost and the need to use a 12-mm trocar.

Patients are discharged on the same day or after an overnight stay. They should avoid solid food for 24 hours. In a series of 100 patients at the Center for Special Pelvic Surgery, all were discharged within 24 hours, although seven remained overnight because of their own preference or a delayed surgery.[3] Although the procedure has a favorable cost/benefit ratio, complications include stump blowout, wound infection, hemorrhage, and postoperative ileus.[38,39] Laparoscopic appendectomy can be achieved safely by using instruments smaller than 3 mm that leave practically no scars.[40] This technique may appeal to pediatric surgeons [41] and possibly be of value in the office setting with local anesthesia and conscious sedation.[34]

APPENDICITIS IN PREGNANCY AND LAPAROSCOPIC MANAGEMENT

Advanced operative laparoscopy is being performed increasingly for various indications and in diverse patient populations, including gravid women. In the United States, approximately 1.6% to 2.2% of pregnant women require nonobstetric

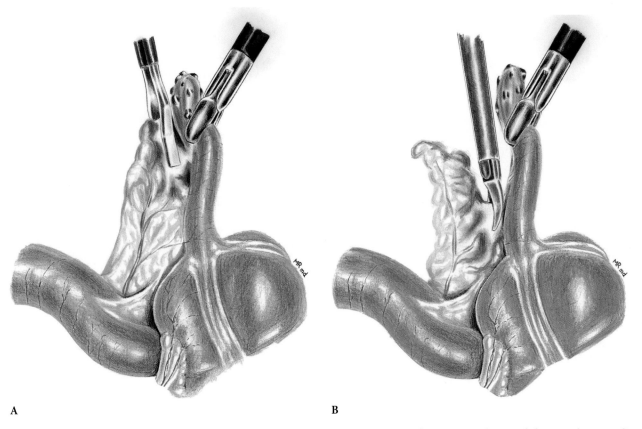

A   **B**

Figure 21.3.2. (**A**) The mesoappendix is coagulated with bipolar forceps. (**B**) It is cut with scissors or a laser to skeletonize the appendix.

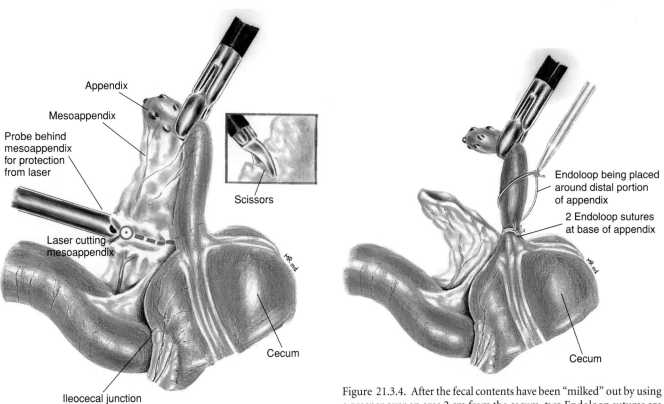

Appendix

Mesoappendix

Probe behind
mesoappendix
for protection
from laser

Scissors

Laser cutting
mesoappendix

Ileocecal junction

Cecum

Figure 21.3.3. Alternatively, the base of the mesoappendix may be cut with the CO_2 laser or a scissors (*inset*). The tip of the appendix contains endometrial implants.

Endoloop being placed
around distal portion
of appendix

2 Endoloop sutures
at base of appendix

Cecum

Figure 21.3.4. After the fecal contents have been "milked" out by using a grasper over an area 2 cm from the cecum, two Endoloop sutures are passed sequentially through one of the 5-mm trocar sleeves around the base of the appendix close to each other. A third Endoloop suture is applied 5 mm distal to the first two sutures.

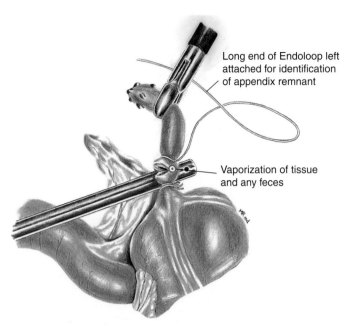

Long end of Endoloop left attached for identification of appendix remnant

Vaporization of tissue and any feces

Figure 21.3.5. The appendix is cut between two sets of sutures, using either the laser or laparoscopic scissors.

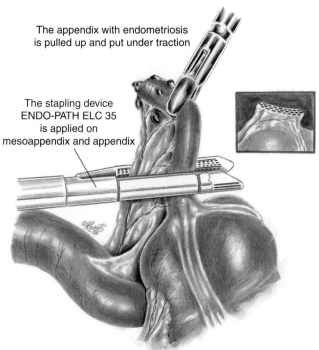

The appendix with endometriosis is pulled up and put under traction

The stapling device ENDO-PATH ELC 35 is applied on mesoappendix and appendix

Figure 21.3.7. The multi-fire stapler is inserted through a 12-mm trocar sleeve and applied directly across the mesoappendix and appendix. In a single motion, the entire appendix and the mesoappendix are clipped and cut. The appendix can be removed from the abdomen with long grasping forceps placed through the trocar sleeve. The trocar sleeve is removed with the appendix contained within it. Alternatively, an Endobag may be used as the receptacle for the detached appendix. *Inset* shows the line of staples.

surgery for abdominal and pelvic pathology. Increasing numbers of case reports suggest the feasibility and safety of operative laparoscopy during pregnancy.[42] Acute appendicitis is the most common extrauterine condition requiring an abdominal operation during pregnancy, occurring in approximately one in 1500 deliveries.[43] The diagnosis of acute appendicitis is difficult in pregnant women, and much of the morbidity and mortality of appendicitis in pregnancy stems from a delay in diagnosis. Therefore, pregnant patients with suspected appendicitis should receive expedient surgical exploration, and diagnostic laparoscopy may allow a timely diagnosis. Pregnancy was a relative contraindication to laparoscopy until recently because of the belief that the

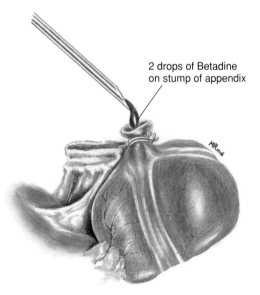

2 drops of Betadine on stump of appendix

Figure 21.3.6. The luminal part of the stump is seared with either the laser or electrosurgery, Betadine is applied, and the tissue is irrigated copiously with lactated Ringer's solution.

procedure would decrease uterine and fetal blood flow and result in abortion or possibly influence fetal development.[44] Other operative risks are premature labor, premature rupture of membranes, and thromboembolism. In many recent studies, however, laparoscopy was safe in pregnancy, with minimal fetal and maternal morbidity. Lachman and colleagues [45] reviewed the English literature regarding laparoscopic surgery during pregnancy and reported 518 procedures, 15% of which were appendectomies. Thirty-three percent were performed in the first trimester, 56% in the second trimester, and 11% in the third trimester. This review demonstrates that laparoscopy in pregnancy appears to be safe when performed by experienced practitioners. In a study, 19 pregnant women underwent laparoscopic surgery, 26.3% of them for appendectomies. No adverse perinatal outcome occurred, although one woman had irregular uterine contractions that promptly resolved with tocolytics. One patient delivered at 35 weeks' gestation, and the rest carried their pregnancy to term, all delivering normal infants.[46]

Thus, appendicitis in pregnancy can be successfully managed by laparoscopic appendectomy.[47,48] Potential advantages of laparoscopic appendectomy in pregnancy include less abdominal wall trauma to an expanding abdomen, reducing the risk of ventral hernias; less pain, resulting in less narcotic analgesia and decreased fetal depression; faster return to normal activity; and earlier mobilization, decreasing the risk of thromboembolism.[49,50] Care must be exercised in establishing abdominal access in the second and especially third trimesters.

LAPAROSCOPIC APPENDECTOMY FOR APPENDICITIS

Acute RLQ abdominal pain frequently represents a diagnostic dilemma for surgeons and gynecologists. In clinical practice, the diagnostic accuracy in identifying the cause of a lower quadrant abdominal pain still remains low, despite the improved technology of computed tomography and ultrasound. Hence, it is not infrequent that a gynecologist operating on a woman of childbearing age for suspected adnexal pathology finds an appendicular disease instead. The laparoscopic approach has been proven to be useful in the evaluation of acute RLQ pain either for a benign gynecologic disease or for acute appendicitis.[51] The following features of right iliac fossa pain favor appendicitis rather than a gynecologic cause: (1) initial diffuse abdominal pain in the epigastrium or around the umbilicus and shifting to and localizing in the right iliac fossa; (2) association with anorexia, nausea, or vomiting; and (3) percussion tenderness with involuntary guarding over McBurney's point (signs of peritoneal irritation). The clinical diagnosis of appendicitis is fairly unreliable. The rate of normal appendixes in women with the clinical diagnosis of acute appendicitis is 22% to 47%, whereas in men it is only 7% to 15%.[1,52]

The procedure is similar to an incidental appendectomy except that the appendix is edematous and possibly more fragile. The presence of gross inflammation, ease of excision, and absence of abscess formation influence the decision to do an appendectomy. Two or three accessory trocars are required, with the laparoscope in the umbilical position. Adhesions are lysed with the laser or scissors so that the appendix is mobile. In removing the appendix at its base, a sufficient stump is left to prevent spillage of luminal contents from the pedicle. An alternative procedure [35] is to place Hulka clips at the base of the inflamed appendix and then control the blood supply in the mesoappendix with electrocoagulation, hemoclips, or a multi-fire stapling device. If an inflamed appendix is removed laparoscopically, a larger trocar may be needed to ease its removal [53] and the operative site is irrigated copiously.

A retrocecal appendicitis makes laparoscopic appendectomy more difficult. Gotz and coworkers [54] noted that complications requiring laparotomy (including bleeding, adhesions, and an abnormal position of the appendix) occurred early in their series of 388 patients with appendicitis who had a laparoscopic appendectomy. These findings prompted them to emphasize the significant learning curve and the long period needed to become proficient in laparoscopic appendectomy for a ruptured appendix in the presence of extensive adhesions, or if the appendix is relatively inaccessible. Laparoscopically assisted appendectomy has been described for cases in which the proper endoscopic instruments and sutures are unavailable.[53] The laparoscope facilitates the definitive diagnosis of appendicitis, and a grasper is passed through an accessory trocar located over McBurney's point. The tip of the appendix is grasped and then pulled from the trocar insertion along with the trocar sleeve and grasper. Routine appendectomy can be done through a small abdominal incision. The procedure usually requires 5 to 20 minutes but takes longer if the appendix is ruptured or an abscess is present.

Complicated appendicitis is defined as acute appendicitis in which perforation or an intra-abdominal abscess is present. Although a few retrospective studies of varying methodologic quality have discussed the feasibility and anecdotal success of the laparoscopic approach, it was not until Wullstein et al. [55] reported a large case series that any objective advantage of a minimally invasive technique for complicated appendicitis was established. Few authors also concluded from their experience that the procedure is equally suitable for perforated and gangrenous appendixes.[56,57] Laparoscopy may increase the risk of spreading infected material in the peritoneal cavity, although it allows adequate suction and irrigation of the entire peritoneal cavity. Bacterial translocation from the peritoneal cavity to the systemic circulation is a concern.[58] The safety and efficacy of laparoscopic appendectomy in perforated and gangrenous appendicitis remain to be established in randomized, controlled trials.[59] Successful conservative management of appendicular mass with broad-spectrum antibiotics with or without percutaneous catheter drainage followed by laparoscopic appendectomy was reported.[60] Ball and coworkers [61] studied the use of laparoscopic appendectomy for complicated appendicitis. In their study, of the 233 laparoscopic procedures performed, 161 (69%) were for uncomplicated and 72 (31%) for complicated appendicitis. The operating times, lengths of hospital stay, return to activity times, complication rates, and analgesia requirements, both in the hospital and after discharge, were equivalent. Furthermore, tenuous comparison of the laparoscopic appendectomy cohort with an open appendectomy group in cases of complicated disease also has shown the minimally invasive approach to be superior in terms of complication rates and length of hospital stay. The investigators concluded that in addition to its diagnostic advantage, the laparoscopic technique is safe and efficient on a therapeutic level. It should be the initial procedure of choice for nearly all cases of complicated appendicitis.

Laparoscopic appendectomy appears to be as safe as open appendectomy and seems to have the advantage of allowing a quicker recovery.[62] A meta-analysis that included multiple randomized controlled trials found that laparoscopic appendectomy reduced the time to full recovery by 5.5 days, reduced postoperative pain at 24 hours, and decreased the absolute risk for wound infection by 3.2%.[4] There was no difference between the two techniques in regard to length of hospitalization, readmission rate, and intra-abdominal abscess formation. The longer operative time for the laparoscopic approach had been attributed to the learning curve associated with the procedure and was not found to increase morbidity.[63] The operating time was increased on average by 17 minutes.[34] Moberg and Montgomery [64] suggested that at the price of a longer operation, the laparoscopic technique offered significant benefits over the conventional approach. Decreased trauma, better diagnostic accuracy, and superior cosmetic results were achieved.

Laparoscopic appendectomy has been associated with higher hospital costs. In 1997, the average total charge for an open appendectomy was $9670 whereas that for a laparoscopic appendectomy was $11,290.[65] However, laparoscopic appendectomy offers significant cost savings for working patients.[66,67]

CONCLUSION

Studies over the past 20 years have shown laparoscopic appendectomy to be safe and effective for both simple and complicated appendicitis. Clinical trials have demonstrated that laparoscopic appendectomy provides certain advantages over open appendectomy, including a shorter length of stay, lower rate of wound infections, decreased postoperative pain, and faster return to normal activities. In addition, laparoscopy affords superior visualization of surrounding structures, which is particularly valuable in cases of diagnostic uncertainty. For these reasons, laparoscopic appendectomy should be the approach of choice to appendiceal diseases.

REFERENCES

1. Kumar R, Erian M, Sinnot S, Knoesen R, Kimble R. Laparoscopic appendectomy in modern gynecology. *J Am Assoc Gynecol Laparosc*. 2002;9:252–263.
2. Litynski GS. Kurt Semm and the fight against skepticism: endoscopic hemostasis, laparoscopic appendectomy, and Semm's impact on the "laparoscopic revolution." *J Soc Laparoendosc Surg*. 1998;2:309.
3. Nezhat C, Nezhat F. Incidental appendectomy during videolaseroscopy. *Am J Obstet Gynecol*. 1991;165:559.
4. Garbutt JM, Soper NJ, Shannon WD, et al. Meta-analysis of randomized controlled trials comparing laparoscopic and open appendectomy. *Surg Laparosc Endosc*. 1999;9:17.
5. Bongard F, Landers DV, Lewis F. Differential diagnosis of appendicitis and pelvic inflammatory disease: a prospective analysis. *Am J Surg*. 1985;150:90.
6. Condon RE. Appendicitis. In: Sabiston DG, ed. *Textbook of Surgery*. 13th ed. Philadelphia: WB Saunders; 1986.
7. Mueller BA, Daling JR, Moore DE, et al. Appendectomy and the risk of tubal infertility. *N Engl J Med*. 1986;315:1506.
8. Geerdsen J, Hansen JB. Incidence of sterility in women operated on in childhood for perforated appendicitis. *Acta Obstet Gynecol Scand*. 1977;56:523.
9. Powley PH. Infertility due to pelvic abscess and pelvic peritonitis in appendicitis. *Lancet*. 1965;1:27.
10. Laine S, Rantala A, Gullichsen R, Ovaska J. Laparoscopic appendectomy – is it worthwhile? A prospective, randomized study in young women. *Surg Endosc*. 1997;11:95.
11. Barrat C, Catheline JM, Rizk N, Champault GG. Does laparoscopy reduce the incidence of unnecessary appendicectomies? *Surg Laparosc Endosc*. 1999;9:27.
12. Moberg AC, Ahlberg G, Leijonmarck CE, et al. Diagnostic laparoscopy in 1043 patients with suspected acute appendicitis. *Eur J Surg*. 1998;164:833.
13. Reiertsen O, Larsen S, Trondsen E, et al. Randomized controlled trial with sequential design of laparoscopic verus conventional appendicectomy. *Br J Surg*. 1997;84:842.
14. Chang FC, Hogle HH, Welling DR. The fate of the negative appendix. *Am J Surg*. 1973;126:752.
15. Leahy PF. Technique of laparoscopic appendectomy. *Br J Surg*. 1989;76:616.
16. Paterson-Brown S, Thompson JN, Eckersley JRT, et al. Which patients with suspected appendicitis should undergo laparoscopy? *Br Med J*. 1988;296:1363.
17. Whitworth CM, Whitworth PW, Sanfilippo J, et al. Value of diagnostic laparoscopy in young women with possible appendicitis. *Surg Gynecol Obstet*. 1988;167:187.
18. Deutsch AA, Zelikovsky A, Reiss R. Laparoscopy in the prevention of unnecessary appendectomies: a prospective study. *Br J Surg*. 1982;69:336.
19. Leape LL, Ramenofsky MD. Laparoscopy for questionable appendicitis – can it reduce the negative appendectomy rate? *Ann Surg*. 1980;191:410.
20. Nowzaradan Y. Laparoscopic appendectomy for acute appendicitis: indications and current use. *J Laparoendosc Surg*. 1991;7:247.
21. Schrieber JH. Early experience with laparoscopic appendectomy in women. *Surg Endosc*. 1987;1:211.
22. Krone HA. Preventive appendectomy in gynecologic surgery: report of 1718 cases. *Geburtshilfe Frauenheilkd*. 1989;49:1035.
23. Bryson K. Laparoscopic appendectomy. *J Gynecol Surg*. 1991;7:93.
24. Cervini P, Smith LC, Urbach DR. The surgeon on call is a strong factor determining the use of a laparoscopic approach for appendectomy. *Surg Endosc*. 2002;16:1774–1777.
25. Wilcox RT, Traverso LW. Have the evaluation and treatment of acute appendicitis changed with new technology? *Surg Clin North Am*. 1997;77:1355–1370.
26. Greason KL, Rappold JF, Liberman MA. Incidental laparoscopic appendectomy for acute right lower quadrant abdominal pain: its time has come. *Surg Endosc*. 1998;12:223.
27. Milingos S, Protopapas A, Drakakis P, et al. Laparoscopic management of patients with endometriosis and chronic pelvic pain. *Ann N Y Acad Sci*. 2003;997:269–273.
28. Carter JE. Combined hysteroscopic and laparoscopic findings in patients with chronic pelvic pain. *J Am Assoc Gynecol Laparosc*. 1994;2:43–47.
29. Harris RS, Foster WG, Surrey MW, et al. Appendiceal disease in women with endometriosis and right lower quadrant pain. *J Am Assoc Gynecol Laparosc*. 2001;8:536–541.
30. Cameron IC, Rogers S, Collins MC, et al. Intestinal endometriosis: presentation, investigation, and surgical management. *Int J Colorectal Dis*. 1995;10:83–86.
31. Redwine DB. Ovarian endometriosis: a marker for more extensive pelvic and intestinal disease. *Fertil Steril*. 1999;72:310–315.
32. Berker B, Lashay N, Davarpanah R, Marziali M, Nezhat CH, Nezhat C. Laparoscopic appendectomy in patients with endometriosis. *J Minim Invasive Gynecol*. 2005;12:206–209.
33. Popp LW. Gynecologically indicated single-endoloop laparoscopic appendectomy. *J Am Assoc Gynecol Laparosc*. 1998;5:275.
34. Almeida OD Jr, Val-Gallas JM, Rizk B. Appendectomy under local anaesthesia following conscious pain mapping with microlaparoscopy. *Hum Reprod*. 1998;13:588.
35. Schultz LS, Pietrafitta JJ, Graber JN, et al. Retrograde laparoscopic appendectomy: report of a case. *J Laparoendosc Surg*. 1991;1:111.
36. Semm K. Endoscopic appendectomy. *Endoscopy*. 1983;15:59.
37. Engstrom L, Fenyo G. Appendectomy: assessment of stump invagination versus simple ligation: a prospective, randomized trial. *Br J Surg*. 1985;72:971.
38. Fisher KS, Ross DS. Guidelines for therapeutic decision in incidental appendectomy. *Surg Gynecol Obstet*. 1990;171:95.
39. Nezhat C, Baggish M, Nezhat F. Operative gynecology (minimally invasive surgery): state of the art. *J Gynecol Surg*. 1992;8:111.
40. Gagner M, Garcia-Ruiz A. Technical aspects of minimally invasive abdominal surgery performed with needlescopic instruments. *Surg Laparosc Endosc*. 1998;8:171.
41. Schier F. Laparoscopic appendectomy with 1.7-mm instruments. *Pediatr Surg Int*. 1998;14:142.
42. Tazuke SI, Nezhat FR, Nezhat CH, Seidman DS, Phillips DR, Nezhat CR. Laparoscopic management of pelvic pathology during pregnancy. *J Am Assoc Gynecol Laparosc*. 1997;4:605–608.
43. Babaknia A, Parsa H, Wooddruff JD. Appendicitis during pregnancy. *Obstet Gynecol*. 1977;50:40–44.

44. Hunter JG, Swanstrom L, Thornbury K. Carbon dioxide pneumoperitoneum induces fetal acidosis in pregnant ewe model. *Surg Endosc.* 1995;9:272–274.

45. Lachman E, Schienfeld A, Voss E, et al. Pregnancy and laparoscopic surgery. *J Am Assoc Gynecol Laparosc.* 1999;6:347–351.

46. Andreoli M, Servakov M, Meyers P, Mann WJ Jr. Laparoscopic surgery during pregnancy. *J Am Assoc Gynecol Laparosc.* 1999; 6:229–233.

47. Nezhat FR, Tazuke S, Nezhat CH, et al. Laparoscopy during pregnancy: a literature review. *J Soc Laparoendosc Surg.* 1997;1: 17.

48. Thomas SJ, Brisson P. Laparoscopic appendectomy and cholecystectomy during pregnancy: six case reports. *J Soc Laparoendosc Surg.* 1998;2:41.

49. McKinlay R, Mastrangelo MJ Jr. Current status of laparoscopic appendectomy. *Curr Surg.* 2003;60:506–512.

50. Fatum M, Rojansky N. Laparoscopic surgery during pregnancy. *Obstet Gynecol Surv.* 2001;56:50–59.

51. Ghezzi F, Raio L, Mueller MD, Franchi M. Laparoscopic appendectomy: a gynecological approach. *Surg Laparosc Endosc Percutan Tech.* 2003;13:257–260.

52. Cox MR, McCall JL, Toouli J, et al. Prospective randomized comparison of open versus laparoscopic appendectomy in men. *World J Surg.* 1996;20:263–266.

53. Fleming JS. Laparoscopically directed appendicectomy. *Aust N Z Obstet Gynecol.* 1985;25:238.

54. Gotz F, Pier A, Bacher C. Modified laparoscopic appendectomy in surgery: a report on 388 operations. *Surg Endosc.* 1990;4:6.

55. Wullstein C, Barkhausen S, Gross E. Results of laparoscopic vs conventional appendectomy in complicated appendicitis. *Dis Colon Rectum.* 2001;44:1700–1705.

56. Johnson AB, Peetz ME. Laparoscopic appendectomy is an acceptable alternative for the treatment of perforated appendicitis. *Surg Endosc.* 1998;12:940–943.

57. Stringel G, Zitsman JL, Shehadi I, et al. Laparoscopic appendectomy in children. *J Soc Laparoendosc Surg.* 1997;1:37–39.

58. Cuschieri A. Appendectomy – laparoscopy or open? *Surg Endosc.* 1997;11:319–320.

59. Yao CC, Lin CS, Yang CC. Laparoscopic appendicectomy for ruptured appendicitis. *Surg Laparosc Endosc Percutan Tech.* 1999;9:271–273.

60. Nguyen DB, Silen W, Hodin RA. Interval appendectomy in the laparoscopic era. *J Gastointest Surg.* 1999;3:189–193.

61. Ball CG, Kortbeek JB, Kirkpatrick AW, Mitchell P. Laparoscopic appendectomy for complicated appendicitis: an evaluation of postoperative factors. *Surg Endosc.* 2004;18:969–973.

62. Hellberg A, Rudberg C, Kullman E, et al. Prospective randomized multicentre study of laparoscopic versus open appendicectomy. *Br J Surg.* 1999;86:48.

63. Tarnoff M, Atabek U, Goodman M, et al. A comparison of laparoscopic and open appendectomy. *J Soc Laparoendosc Surg.* 1998;2:153.

64. Moberg AC, Montgomery A. Appendicitis: laparoscopic versus conventional operation: a study and review of the literature. *Surg Laparosc Endosc.* 1997;7:459.

65. Mushinski M. Laparoscopic and open appendectomies – average charges. *Stat Bull Metrop Insur Co.* 1999;80:23.

66. Wagaman R, Williams RS. Conservative therapy for adnexal torsion. A case report. *J Reprod Med.* 1990;35:833.

67. Heikkinen TJ, Haukipuro K, Hulkko A. Cost-effective appendectomy: open or laparoscopic? A prospective randomized study. *Surg Endosc.* 1998;12:1204.

22 | LAPAROSCOPY SIMULATORS FOR TRAINING BASIC SURGICAL SKILLS, TASKS, AND PROCEDURES

Wm. LeRoy Heinrichs

Videoendoscopic surgery has changed everything! Surgeons don't operate on patients any more; they operate on (their) images.

Heinrichs, 2005

A variety of surgical simulators are available to assist surgeons in learning and practicing the technical skills needed for conducting laparoscopic surgery. Some are low-fidelity and others are high-fidelity systems that have been validated as effective surgical training systems for novice users. Proficiency and safety are unequivocally improved in the subsequent surgical performances of users.

Teaching and learning the basic technical skills required for performing laparoscopic procedures by surgical trainees has been greatly facilitated with today's surgical simulators. Published evaluation data on learning outcomes from the use of surgical simulators clearly indicate their value in surgical education. Simulators can be characterized by their fidelity to authentic surgical environments:

- Box trainers using physical objects (such as cotton string, pegs, latex tubes, and rings, some with haptics)
- Computer-based with either physical objects or virtual images of tubes, bands, balls, and so on, and instruments projected onto monitors/displays
- Virtual three-dimensional (3D) models of simulated and real tissues and organs

Some devices provide authentic surgical instruments for manipulating real objects, and others have interfaces that provide touch sensations (haptics) for virtual objects; both afford practice of the basic skills, gestures, and instrument–tissue manipulations. Two important features for learning differentiate them: haptics and metrics, both of which earn the designation as high-fidelity systems. A few incorporate virtual 3D models of human anatomy for conducting parts of surgical procedures, and three systems are for learning endovascular procedures. Benchmark data have been established by experienced surgeons for describing proficiency scores on 26 learning modules in five commercially available basic skills trainers.

INTRODUCTION

The Accreditation Council for Graduate Medical Education (ACGME) Outlook Project seeks to broadly improve medical training of all physicians. The six competencies of physicians recently identified by ACGME [1,2] are patient care, medical knowledge, practice-based learning and improvement, interpersonal and communication skills, professionalism, and systems-based practice; the acquisition and maintenance of surgical technical skills are included in patient care and practice-based learning and improvement requirements. The integration of technical skills into the performance of procedures extends to systems-based practice.

Several in vitro methods to prepare trainees for the operating room (OR) have been implemented in recent years, mainly because of the advantages for patients from changing from open surgical procedures to minimal access surgery (MAS; or minimally invasive surgery [MIS]). Teaching, developing, and practicing basic surgical skills of laparoscopic surgery via the apprenticeship model of training is considered inappropriate in ORs of today.[3] New modes of preparatory training for OR practice (e.g., the use of synthetic objects, animal models, and video training) have supplanted the apprentice-style learning in the OR. Accordingly, "clinical skills labs," "part-task trainers" (defined later), and "animal surgery" have been introduced into surgical training programs with increasing frequency for providing hands-on instruction of technical skills. Because today's surgical practice requires acquisition of new technical skills and greater emphasis on the issues of patient safety [3,4], MAS training requires alternative methods of instruction.

Simulator development follows from a new assessment method of surgical skills with objective, structured assessments of technical skills (OSATS).[5,6] First evaluated among general surgical trainees, this formative assessment method has also been used to guide learning and for assessing performance of trainees in obstetrics and gynecology.[7]

Many anecdotes indicate that surgeons have constructed simple trainers for personal use using variations of cardboard boxes, camcorders connected to TV sets, and disposable ports and instruments. Nails, screws, marbles, string, and foam objects have been used as targets to be placed into dishes or cups or onto pegs to support the self-perceived need for practice of surgical skills. Professor Kurt Semm's legendary Pelvi-Trainer marketed by WISAP Corp. pre-dated Ethicon Endo-Surgery's development of a collapsible box for use by its representatives demonstrating new surgical equipment. Hundreds of these low-fidelity "box" trainers were provided for residency programs to be used by surgical trainees. The trainers could be used with many animate objects, including animal parts, to support a large variety of surgical skills. Recent development and marketing of simple box trainers include those of 3DMed and Simulab and the Society of American Gastrointestinal Endoscopic Surgeons (SAGES) FLS (Fundamentals of Laparoscopic Surgery) Trainer.[8,9,10] These systems measure neither performance data nor incorporate anatomically relevant objects (except optional animal parts), but afford the "natural" haptics of physical instruments and objects. Their use involves tutors and observers trained in the methods of subjective assessment. These practical, low-cost method trainers have been superseded by several high-fidelity systems,[11,12] thus the need for description and categorization.

A NEW DEFINITION OF TRAINERS AND SIMULATORS

Agreement has not been reached on the distinguishing features of trainers and simulators, but the issues are becoming clearer. Most agree with the term *part-task trainer*, adopted from its original use in the psychology field, where psychomotor procedures were deconstructed into their component parts and identified as tasks.[13] Tasks are equivalent to the eight fundamental manipulations of tissues by surgical instruments that have been taught since 500 BC, first described by Sushruta, the Father of Surgery.[14,15] These are exploration (both visual and haptic [touch]), aspiration/injection, incision, excision, extraction, evacuation, scarification (purposeful injury), and closure (e.g., suturing, clips). Implantation/transplantation, a new manipulation developed during the 20th century, has been added as the ninth. Vascular cannulation, another modern procedure, is considered an extension of the aspiration/injection manipulation. Each of these manipulations comprises several eye–hand and foot coordination skills that must be acquired for performing the more complex manipulations.

Part-task trainers include two types of simulators: (1) those that afford practicing basic skills, the psychomotor actions of surgery, and (2) those that focus on more complex tasks of surgical procedures, such as suturing, that rely on several basic skills. An example of a "basic-skills" trainer is one that teaches the eye–hand coordination required for using surgical instruments. Navigating cameras, grasping tissue, and picking, placing, and handling of objects between instruments can be learned and must be practiced for proficient surgical performance. These skills are also called the "surgical gestures" [13] of surgery that must be replicated during surgical procedures, much as a mime goes through prescribed motions to mimic real-life actions. In practice, basic skills represent the *enabling* skills that must be learned before conducting the more complex tasks that require learning *target* skills. At the level of target skills, one calls upon higher levels of cognition necessary for implementation. Not all basic-skills trainers afford the fidelity needed for the more complex tasks, such as dissection or suturing, that involve more than one basic skill. Several basic-skills trainers have added modules that support practicing manipulations of increasing complexity. For them, the exercise of deconstructing tasks into their individual components is beneficial because practicing these technically demanding components is critical in the performance of instrument–tissue manipulations. As part-task trainers continue to evolve, this separation is likely to diminish and be less important than at present. Indeed, a few "part-procedure" modules are present in today's simulators.

Table 22.1 provides an example of the basic skills that comprise the tasks afforded by the LTS3e (RealSim Systems). Deconstructing the "tasks" into the basic skills used for performing them illustrates the relationship of these terms.

Based upon the designation of fidelity to authentic surgical environments, five categories of trainers have been identified:

Table 22.1: Relationships of Skills and Tasks Using the LTS3e

LTS3e "Tasks"	Basic Skills
Peg manipulation	Navigate, grasp, transfer, place, release
Ring manipulation	Navigate, grasp, rotate, traverse, guide, stretch, place, release
Ductal cannulation	Navigate, grasp, push to cannulate, grasp, extract
Lasso loop formation & cinching	Navigate, place, grasp for counter traction, pull to cinch
Intracorporeal suturing	Navigate, grasp, penetrate target, rotate, grasp, tie knot, test
Tissue "disc" dissection	Navigate, grasp, incise, rotate, elevate, release

four for laparoscopy and one for endoluminal vascular interventions. Physical trainers are subdivided to represent their evolving development.

Laparoscopy Trainers

1. Physical trainers: low fidelity (no electronic user data, nonhaptic)
   a. First-generation box trainers
   b. Second-generation box trainers
2. Physical trainers: low fidelity (electronic user data, nonhaptic)
3. Virtual reality trainers: high fidelity (electronic user data with or without haptics)
4. Virtual reality trainers: high fidelity (electronic user data and haptics)

Endoluminal Vascular Trainers

5. Virtual reality trainers: high fidelity (electronic user data and haptics)

Tables 22.2 to 22.7 indicate the basic skills that each of the listed types of trainers may provide, based upon the creativity of users who choose the objects that serve as targets. Low-fidelity systems that offer simple surgical "environments" provide no electronic assessment but have the advantage of using real instruments. Most of the first-generation systems are available for less than $500, including a "box," most with model objects, but offer no camera or monitor to display the performance. Second-generation systems cost up to $2000 and afford a camera and monitor. Both types of trainers require replenishment of objects that become frayed or torn. Some instructors have used animal parts such as animal bowel and pigs' feet as objects, but these also must be replenished and are messy to use.

The first box was the Semm Pelvi-Trainer, patented in 1986. The trainer shown in Figure 22.1, as the present model, is a distant comparison to the original Lucite box with eight rubber dams on the top through which ports and instruments could be inserted. Examples of these second-generation box trainers follow (Figure 22.2).

Table 22.2: Physical Trainers: Low Fidelity (No Electronic User Data, Nonhaptic)

A. First-generation box trainers	Construction materials: e.g., cardboard, wood, Lucite, plastic View: directly or by camcorder, endoscope, periscope (mirrors) Surgical instruments: authentic reusable, or disposable Objects/targets: physical objects, e.g., string, pegs; animal parts

Simulator: Basic Skills in 1) Physical Trainers: Low Fidelity

	Navigate – go to target	Grasp – take a hold of	Transfer – between instruments	Traverse – location to location	Guide – move/direct object	Pull/Stretch – retract by pulling	Place – put into position	Rotate – about instrument axis	Release – let go	Cannulate – push object thru	Extract – remove	Penetrate – with sharp object	Elevate – lift upward	Incise/Cut into – open sharply	Excise – incise entirely	Tissue manipulation	Dissection	Suturing – endo, extracorporeal	Educational objectives	Electronic data collection	Haptics
Semm (WISAP)	√	√	√	√	√	√	√	√	√	√	√	√	√	√	√	√	√	√	0	0	0

The skills with a √ can be incorporated into all of the following systems: Ethicon Endo-Surgery, Pietro (LTT), Blacker, Tower–Simulab Corp., 3DMed

Table 22.3:

B. Second-generation box trainers	Construction materials: e.g., Lucite, plastic View: directly or by camcorder, endoscope Surgical instruments: authentic reusable, or disposable (nonhaptic) Objects/targets: physical objects, foam, plastic, wood, animal parts

	Navigate – go to target	Grasp – take a hold of	Transfer – between instruments	Traverse – location to location	Guide – move/direct object	Pull/Stretch – retract by pulling	Place – put into position	Rotate – about instrument axis	Release – let go	Cannulate – push object thru	Extract – remove	Penetrate – with sharp object	Elevate – lift upward	Incise/Cut into – open sharply	Excise – incise entirely	Tissue manipulation	Dissection	Suturing – endo, extracorporeal	Educational objectives	Electronic data collection	Haptics
3-DMed trainer	√	√	√	√	√	√	√	√	√	√	√	√	√	√	√	√	√	√	0	0	0
Lap Trainer	√	√	√	√	√	√	√	√	√	√	√	√	√	√	√	√	√	√	0	0	0
FLS	√	√	√	√	√	√	√	√	√	√	√	√	√	√	√	√	√	√	0	0	0
Endo Tower	√	0	0	√	0	0	0	0	0	0	0	0	0	0	0	0	0	0	0	0	0
RapidFire	√	√	√	√	√	√	√	√	√	√	√	√	√	√	√	√	√	√	0	0	0
LTS2000	√	√	√	√	√	√	√	√	√	√	√	√	√	√	√	√	√	√	0	0	0
Top-Gun	√	√	√	√	√	√	√	√	√	0	0	√	0	0	0	0	0	√	0	0	0
ICSAD*	√	√	√	√	√	√	√	√	√	√	√	√	√	√	√	√	√	√	0	0	0

*Hand-tracking sensors.

Table 22.4: Physical Trainers: Low Fidelity (Electronic User Data, Nonhaptic)

Physical trainers	Construction materials: e.g., Lucite, plastic, etc. View: directly or by camcorder, endoscope Surgical instruments: authentic reusable, or disposable (nonhaptic) Objects/targets: physical objects, foam, plastic, wood, fabric, etc.

Simulator: Basic Skills in Physical Trainers – Low Fidelity with Electronic User Data

	Navigate – go to target	Grasp – take a hold of	Transfer – between instruments	Traverse – location to location	Guide – move /direct object	Pull/Stretch – retract by pulling	Place – put into position	Rotate – about instrument axis	Release – let go	Cannulate – push object thru	Extract – remove	Penetrate – with sharp object	Elevate – lift upward	Incise/Cut into – open sharply	Excise – incise entirely	Tissue manipulation	Dissection	Suturing – endo, extracorporeal	Educational objectives	Electronic data collection	Haptics
LTS3e	√	√	√	√	√	√	√	√	√	√	√	√	√	√	√	√	√	√	√	√	0
ProMIS	√	√	√	√	√	√	√	√	√	√	√	√	√	√	√	√	√	√	√	√	0

Table 22.5: Virtual Reality Trainers: High Fidelity (Electronic User Data with or without Haptics)

Virtual reality trainers	Construction: computers (desk- or laptop), software, with or without haptics interface View: directly on monitor Surgical instruments: virtual tips, real handles, haptically enabled or not Objects/targets: virtual objects, e.g., tubes, balls, bands, arrows

Simulator: Basic Skills in VR Trainers – High Fidelity with Electronic User Data

	Navigate – go to target	Grasp – take a hold of	Transfer – between instruments	Traverse – location to location	Guide – move /direct object	Pull/Stretch – retract by pulling	Place – put into position	Rotate – about instrument axis	Release – let go	Cannulate – push object thru	Extract – remove	Penetrate – with sharp object	Elevate – lift upward	Incise/Cut into – open sharply	Excise – incise entirely	Tissue manipulation	Dissection	Suturing – endo, extracorporeal	Educational objectives	Electronic data collection	Haptics
MIST–VR ± H	√	√	√	√	√	√	√	√	√	√	√	√	√	√	√	√	√	√	√	√	0
SKA	√	√	√	√	√	√	√	√	√	√	√	√	√	√	√	√	√	√	√	√	0
Lap Mentor ± H	√	√	√	√	√	√	√	√	√	√	√	√	√	√	√	√	√	√	√	√	0
LapSim ± H	√	√	√	√	√	√	√	√	√	√	√	√	√	√	√	√	√	√	√	√	0
SurgicalSim ± H	√	√	√	√	√	√	√	√	√	√	√	√	√	√	√	√	√	√	√	√	0
PERCMentor ± H	√	√	√	√	√	√	√	√	√	√	√	√	√	√	√	√	√	√	√	√	0

Table 22.6: Virtual Reality Trainers: High Fidelity (Electronic User Data and Haptics)
Simulator: Procedures in Virtual Reality Trainers – High Fidelity with Electronic User Data

Virtual reality trainers: procedures	Construction: computers (desk or laptop), software, with or without haptics interface
	View: on monitor, either integrated into OR table design or desktop
	Surgical instruments: virtual-tips, real handles, haptically enabled or not
	Objects/targets: virtual objects, e.g., tissues, membranes, organs, vessels

Name	*Procedure*	*Tissue/Organ*
Uro Mentor	Biopsy, desiccation	Kidney, ureter, bladder
GI Mentor	Biopsy, desiccation	
LapSim A. General surgery	Dissection, clipping, desiccation, cutting	Gallbladder, angle of Calot
B. Gynecologic surgery	Desiccation Dissection, desiccation, excision Suturing wound	a. Tubal sterilization b. Ectopic (tubal) pregnancy c. Uterine myoma excision site
SurgicalSIM	Dissection, desiccation	Gallbladder from liver "bed"
Hysteroscopy Trainer	Electrosurgical extraction of lesions	
		a. Polyp b. Myoma
ProMIS	Dissection, dessication, and extraction	Colon

As the value of simulation has begun to be understood, instructors' desire for documenting performances has come into focus for the benefit of trainees and for assessment alike. Two physical box simulators, the ProMIS and the LTS3e (Figures 22.3, 22.4), incorporate metrics supported by laptop computers. As with all box trainers, these use real surgical instruments, providing opportunity for practicing with them. The FLS trainer is a portable unit that can be used in the user's environment of choice. This trainer includes a set of accessories used to simulate specific surgical techniques that have been validated by Dr. Gerald Fried through the MISTELS Program at McGill University. Evaluation of user performance is conducted by trained proctors who rate various features of performance.

One of the earliest virtual reality trainers, the MIST-VR (minimally invasive surgery trainer – virtual reality), developed by Sullivan in the United Kingdom and now available from Mentice Corp., has been validated by numerous studies. This system can be used as a nonhaptic system or a haptic system, depending upon the type of interface purchased. Immersion Medical Corp. sells both types, the nonhaptic for about $12,500, and the 5-dof Surgical Workstation for about $40,000. Other trainers in this group incorporate virtual objects of many types. One, the PERC Mentor, is a transcutaneous simulator for invasive procedures, such as renal calyx inspection. These systems, too, are available with or without haptics interfaces. The cost of these systems, including computers, monitors, and software, ranges from $20,000 to $90,000. The haptics interface is not included in the lower-priced systems but is integrated into those most expensive.

As interest and technical capabilities have increased, more complex manipulations have been developed. An example of a high-fidelity, part-task trainer supporting complex instrument–tissue manipulations is one that focuses on a component of a laparoscopic cholecystectomy, such as dissection of the triangle of Calot. This anatomic region, where the cystic duct and cystic artery emerge adjacent to each other, may present in unpredictable configurations and elevates risk for inadvertent injury during dissection.

The skills necessary for doing the manipulations necessary for exposure of these structures are grasping and retracting, incising sharply with a scissors or with a selected energy modality (electrosurgery, ultrasound, or laser), pushing and/or pulling (retracting) to extend an initial incision and to separate the fibrous tissues that encase them, elevation of the identified tubular structures to assure their separation/isolation, clipping or suturing to interrupt the lumina, and cutting to divide the structures. Inspection for hemostasis and irrigation and/or aspiration of blood and possibly bile from the dissection site are additional necessary manipulations. The actions required to accomplish them exceed those offered by basic-skills trainers. Trainers that enable users to perform more than part-tasks can be considered part-procedure trainers. They support multiple part-tasks but do not afford, at this time, the conduct of entire procedures. Thus, simulators are increasing in their complexity as they incorporate additional features, just as surgeons learn and practice basic skills that they choreograph into procedures during surgical procedures in the operating room.

Three systems, the LapSim trainer of Surgical-Science AB, SurgicalSIM from METI, and Lap Mentor from Simbionix, Ltd, (see Figures 22.5–22.8), have labeled this above exercise as *Dissection*, a part of a procedure of cholecystectomy. The requisite set of surgical manipulations requires using target skills (see below), but this dissection component of the surgical procedure is but one part of a laparoscopic cholecystectomy; therefore, we label the more advanced devices as part-procedure simulators.

Table 22.7: Virtual Reality Trainers: High Fidelity (Electronic User Data and Haptics)
Simulator: Cannulation and Stent placement in Virtual Reality Trainers – High Fidelity with Electronic User Data

Virtual reality trainers: endovascular	Construction: desktop computers, software, haptics interface
	View: on fluoroscopy monitor, integrated into radiologic procedure table
	Virtual catheters, instruments, haptically enabled or not
	Objects/targets: virtual objects, e.g., vascular lumina

Name	Procedure	Vascular System	Therapy
Angio Mentor	Cannulation	Carotid, coronary, renal, iliac, hypogastric, intracranial	Stent, balloon introduction, cardiac rhythm management, embolization
Endovascular Accutouch System	Lead placement, vascular cannulation	Carotid, coronary, renal, iliac, intracranial	Stent introduction, cardiac rhythm management
Vascular Interventional System Trainer (VIST)	Lead placement, vascular cannulation	Carotid, coronary, renal, iliac, intracranial	Stent introduction, cardiac rhythm management

Exploration by endoscopy or radiography of the common bile duct may be needed as another component. Dissection of the gallbladder from the liver and removal of the excised structure is the manipulation simulated by the SurgicalSIM dissection module. Many simulators designed to support dissection of Calot's triangle have been offered as LapChole simulators, but most are part-procedure trainers and are not comprehensive for all of the necessary actions/manipulations of a LapChole. Simulation of the introduction of trocars into surgical spaces, the

chest and abdomen, has recently been introduced in the SurgicalSIM device as an additional part of the cholecystectomy procedure.

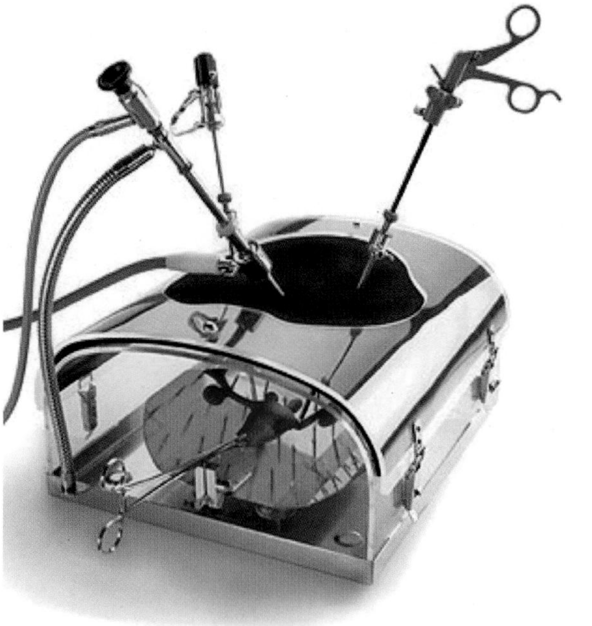

The category of trainers for endoluminal vascular procedures represents a parallel development that is important for two reasons that prompt its inclusion: (1) these systems are similar to laparoscopy in that these procedures require manipulations inside cavities, in this case vessels, and (2) the training systems have been developed in response to a pressing clinical training need. Vascular simulators also offer to a large number of clinicians, interventional radiologists, cardiologists, and cardiovascular surgeons a method for reducing patient complications from endoluminal manipulations, including stent placement. Three systems have been developed and are available for $35,000 to $90,000. (See Figures 22.8–22.11.)

Figure 22.1. WISAP Pel/Lap Trainer. With the increasing interest in laparoscopic surgery and recognition of the need for preparation for intra-operative dexterity, a second generation of systems emerged to provide increased fidelity. Most have evolved from the laboratories of academic surgeons and are available commercially either by companies or professional organizations. http://www.wisap.de/lap-pel/pel-lap-trainer.html

VALIDATION STUDIES

Nowadays, basic MAS/MIS maneuvers can be learned and practiced by students, residents, and instructors using computer-based physical or virtual environments, and performances can be monitored objectively before proceeding to patients in the OR. Recently reported studies [6,8–12] with simulation-based instruction using first- and second-generation part-task trainers have demonstrated enhanced performance of trainees in either animal or human OR settings. In one study [12] in which safety was considered, the number of surgical errors was also reduced. Several "V-R to OR" studies have validated the merit of training with surgical simulators to enhance surgical performance in the OR.[11,12,15,16] One outstanding example of the development of a training curriculum and validation among a number of surgeons has been the 7-year effort of the SAGES organization to implement the FLS box trainer, using the MISTELS program developed by Gerald Fried, MD, of McGill University.[8]

Heretofore, neither program directors nor trainees had training benchmarks by which to guide and direct their practice effort with the various systems available. Most of those that recorded performance data electronically devised simulator-specific

SAGES' FLS Trainer

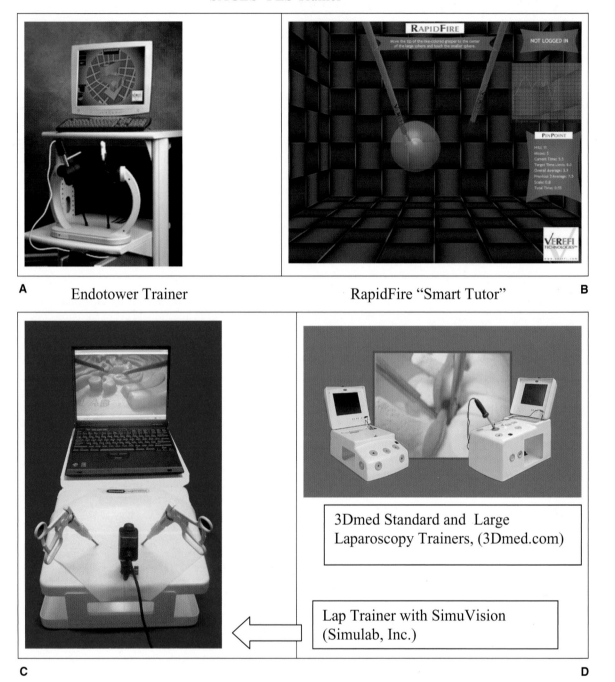

Figure 22.2. SAGES FLS Trainer (**A**) Endotower Trainer (**B**) RapidFire "Smart Tutor," (**C**) Lap Trainer with SimuVision (Simulab, Inc.) and (**D**) 3Dmed standard and large laparoscopy Trainers (3Dmed.com).

measures in their training modules, and many calculated a performance metric. With the revelation that surgical simulation improved surgical performance in the OR and that patient safety could be enhanced, surgical leaders began to cautiously acquire simulation systems and began requiring surgical resident physicians to use them. In addition, in 2005 the American College of Surgery introduced a set of criteria for characterizing two levels of regional training centers. The types of simulators to be used were left to the discretion of individual centers. A significant void

remained in setting the benchmarks that address the move toward criterion-based training, compared with the traditional time-in-residency–based training.

The vision of creating such a database derived from the performances of experienced laparoscopic surgeons on the available surgical simulators was from Dr. Richard Satava and the Simulation Committee of the Society of Laparoendoscopic Surgeons (SLS). Beginning in 2004, this vision was implemented, with the financial support of DARPA and TATRC. The author and colleagues

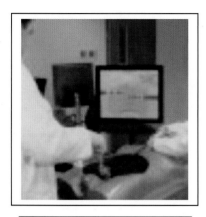

ProMIS Trainer, Haptica, Inc.

Figure 22.3. ProMIS Trainer, Haptica, Inc.

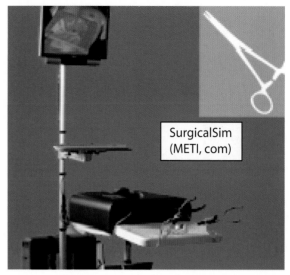

SurgicalSim (METI, com)

Figure 22.6. SurgicalSim (METI.com).

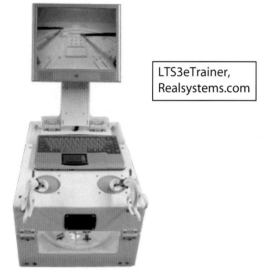

LTS3eTrainer, Realsystems.com

Figure 22.4. LTS3eTrainer, Realsystems.com

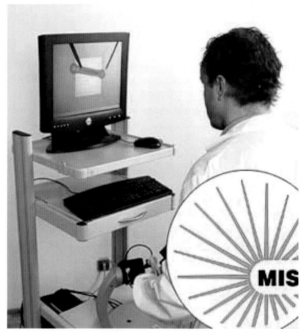

Figure 22.7. MIST.

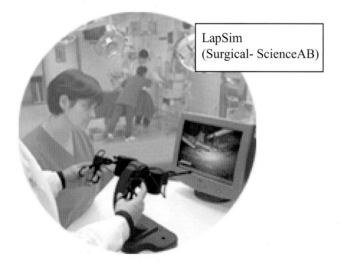

LapSim (Surgical- ScienceAB)

Figure 22.5. LapSim (Surgical-Science AB).

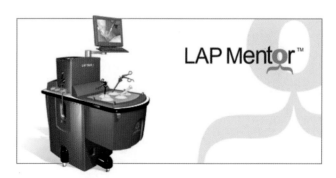

LAP Mentor™

Figure 22.8. LAP Mentor.

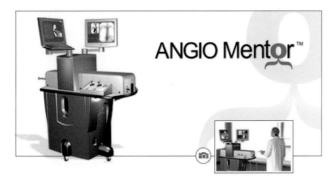

Figure 22.9. ANGIO Mentor.

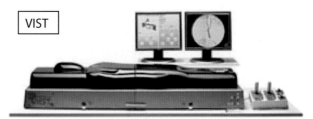

Figure 22.11. VIST.

at SUMMIT (Stanford University Medical Media and Information Technologies), a research group known for developing and assessing learning technologies in medicine, were commissioned to conduct a research study on available surgical simulators. In formative research at annual meetings of the SLS and at those of the American Association of Gynecological Laparoscopists (AAGL), interested surgeons (a convenience sample) were invited to perform a basic-skills module on each of four different systems. This experience with about 150 laparoscopic surgeons led to the design of a rigorous controlled study in which 17 experienced laparoscopic surgeons were recruited by committee members to demonstrate their skills on 26 modules selected from five systems that produced electronic data for statistical analysis. Representatives were included from general surgery, gynecology, and urology. Random assignments to modules, each system with a trained simulator assistant, and time allocations enabled the acquisition of performance data on 204 measures contained in the selected modules. Summative research was initiated in September 2005 and a preliminary report submitted to the committee in March 2006. A challenge in this project was finding a statistical method with which to generate proficiency scores across multiple systems that employed different measures, and diverse units of measure such as meters, millimeters, angles, instances; only time was consistently measured in seconds.

The SLS Simulation Committee agreed with consultants in statistics and educational evaluation about the form in which to present the data at the SLA Annual Meeting in September 2006. Such data was recently published.[17]

SOURCES OF SUPPORT

This work was supported in part by contract NLM/NIH 185N034 and grants from DARPA and TATRC.

REFERENCES

1. Kavic MS. Competency and the six core competencies [editorial]. *JSLS*. 2002;6:95–97.
2. ACGME Outcome Project. Available at: http://www.acgme.org/outcome/comp/compFull.asp. Accessed September 2006.
3. Bridges M, Diamond DL. The financial impact of teaching surgical residents in the operating room. *Am J Surg*. 1999;177:28–32.
4. Sachdeva AK. Acquisition and maintenance of surgical competence. *Semin Vasc Surg*. 2002;15:182–190.
5. Martin JA, Regehr G, Reznick RK, et al. Objective structured assessment of technical skill (OSATS) for surgical residents. *Br J Surg*. 1997;84:273–278.
6. Wanzel KR, Ward M, Reznick RK. Teaching the surgical craft: from selection to certification. *Curr Probl Surg*. 2002;39:573–659.
7. Goff BA, Lentz GM, Lee D, Fenner D, Morris J, Mandel LS. Development of bench stations for objective, structured assessment of technical skills. *Obstet Gynecol*. 2001;98;412–416.
8. Fried GM, DeRossis AM, Bothwell J, Sigman HH. Comparison of laparoscopic performance in vivo with performance in a laparoscopic simulator. *Surg Endosc*. 1999;13:1077–1081.
9. Scott DJ, Bergen PC, Rege RV, et al. Laparoscopic training on bench models: better and more cost effective than operating room experience? *J Am Coll Surg*. 2000;191:272–283.
10. Hamilton EC, Scott DJ, Fleming JB, et al. Comparison of video trainer and virtual reality training systems on acquisition of laparoscopic skills. *Surg Endosc*. 2002;16:406–411.
11. Hyltander A, Liljegren E, Rhodin PH, Lonroth H. The transfer of basic skills learned in a laparoscopic simulator to the operating room. *Surg Endosc*. 2002;16:1324–1329.
12. Seymour NE, Gallagher AG, Roman SA, et al. Virtual reality performance improves operating room performance: results of a randomized, double-blinded trial. *Ann Surg*. 2002;236:458–464.
13. Heinrichs WL, Srivastava S, Montgomery K, Dev P. The fundamental manipulations of surgery: a structured vocabulary for designing surgical curricula and simulators [special article]. *J Am Assoc Gynecol Laparosc*. 2004;11:450–456.
14. Garrison FE. An introduction to the history of medicine, 4th ed. WB Saunders, Co., Philadelphia, PA 1929, p. 70–73.
15. Youngblood P, Wren S, Srivastava S, et al. Training in laparoscopic surgery: a comparison of virtual reality (VR) and traditional simulation methods. *J Am Coll Surg*. 2005:200:546–551.
16. Gallagher AG, Ritter EM, Champion H, et al. Virtual reality simulation for the operating room: proficiency-based training as a paradigm shift in surgical skills training. *Ann Surg*. 2005;241:364–372.

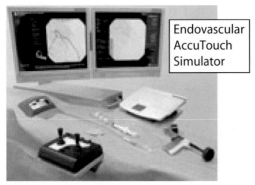

Figure 22.10. Endovasular AccuTouch Simulator.

17. Heinrichs WL, Lukoff B, Youngblood P, Shavelson R, Dev P, et al. Criterion-based technical training for surgeons. *JSLS* 2007;11: 273–302.

ACKNOWLEDGMENTS

My colleagues at SUMMIT – Kevin Montgomery, PhD; Sakti Srivastava, MBBS, MS; Kenneth Waldron, PhD; Camillan Huang, PhD; and Parvati Dev, PhD – have taught me about computer-based systems. Patricia Youngblood, PhD, has taught me about validation and assessment. Fortunate collaborations with Camran Nezhat, MD, and Mary T. Jacobson, MD, provide curious fellows and residents for simulator-based studies.

23 | ROBOT-ASSISTED LAPAROSCOPY

Section 23.1. Computer-Assisted Surgery and Surgical Robotics

Sanjeev Dutta and Thomas M. Krummel

The development of surgical robotics is a dynamic process, a constant interplay between clinical need and technologic capability. As both of these factors are constantly changing, it is unlikely that the form the surgical robot takes today will be the form it takes in 20 years. In many aspects, the technology has progressed beyond perceived clinical need. This has created a novel challenge for the surgeon – to determine whether a technologic innovation with apparent benefit has meaningful clinical application. This process has defined the incorporation of robotic technologies into many surgical disciplines, including gynecologic, cardiothoracic, urologic, abdominal, and pediatric surgeries. In whatever way this interplay of technology and clinical need progresses, surgeons are left with the task of guiding its impact on patient care.

The term *robot* is a misnomer when describing this surgical device. Derived from the Czech *robota* meaning "drudgery," this term implies autonomous function [1], which most surgical robots do not have. Instead, they are better described as *computer-assisted telemanipulators*, implying that they are subject to human control. The complexity of surgical procedures does not currently allow for devices that work entirely autonomously. Nevertheless, the term *robot* has added a flare of futurism to the endeavor and has been the one most commonly used in the literature.

Surgical robots follow on the heels of conventional minimal-access surgery (MAS), bringing solutions to two-dimensional vision, fulcrum effect, reduced degrees of freedom, and other limitations of MAS. Satava [2] has suggested that laparoscopic instruments are a transitional technology to robotics. At the least, robotic systems have reduced the technical difficulty of complex minimal-access procedures currently performed with conventional laparoscopic equipment.

CLASSIFICATION OF SURGICAL ROBOTIC PLATFORMS

Surgical robotic systems can be classified according to the role they play in a procedure [3] and their application.[4] The Bio-Robotics Group at Stanford University has developed a procedural role–based taxonomy [5] of robotic involvement in surgery that ranges in levels of autonomy:

1. Passive role: These robots are typically composed of a "master" console and "slave" console. The master console provides telemanipulators that can be used to guide the robotic arms of the slave console. The slave has no autonomous function. This type of robot carries minimal risk.

2. Restricted role: In this semi-active role, the robot is responsible for some invasive tasks but is controlled by the surgeon for higher-risk procedures or for guidance.

3. Active role: Through use of artificial intelligence, the robot performs the procedure under the supervision of the surgeon. This type of robot carries high responsibility and risk.

In terms of clinical application, three types of robotic systems have been developed: (1) robotic assistants, (2) stereotactic localizers, and (3) neuronavigators.[4]

Master–slave systems are *passive-role robotic assistants* that are generally used for thoracic and abdominopelvic operations, including those for gynecology, general surgery, urology, cardiothoracics, and pediatric surgery. The slave unit is composed of the robotic arms performing the surgery, and the separate master console is outfitted with telemanipulation devices that allow the surgeon to control the slave. There are currently two platforms in clinical use: the Zeus (Computer Motion Inc., Goleta, CA; Figure 23.1.1) and the da Vinci (Intuitive Surgical, Inc., Sunnyvale, CA). Since the acquisition of Computer Motion by Intuitive Surgical in 2003, the Zeus system is no longer in production, though its parts and service support is ongoing.

The Zeus slave console is composed of two robotic arms and a telescopic camera. Using an ergonomic command module, the surgeon electronically controls robotically activated instruments while surveying the operative field by three-dimensional video feed. The camera is operated by a voice-command system that controls a separate robotic arm designed for camera manipulation (Automated Endoscopy System for Optimal Placement [AESOP], Computer Motion Inc.). The separate slave components are attached to the operating table, allowing multiple configurations for arm placement. The operating table and arms can be moved as a single unit. Zeus visualization systems are either two-dimensional or three-dimensional (stereoscopic). When introduced in 1998, the Zeus system had standard laparoscopic instruments with four degrees of freedom.[6] Subsequently in 2002, Computer Motion introduced Microwrist instruments with unidirectional articulation and six degrees of freedom.

The primary difference with the da Vinci system is that the robotic arms are not individual units but instead hang off a single tower structure. This tower is positioned over the patient. The da Vinci is equipped with a camera arm and two robotic arms, with an optional fourth operative arm. A stereoscopic camera provides up to a $10\times$ magnified three-dimensional view, and

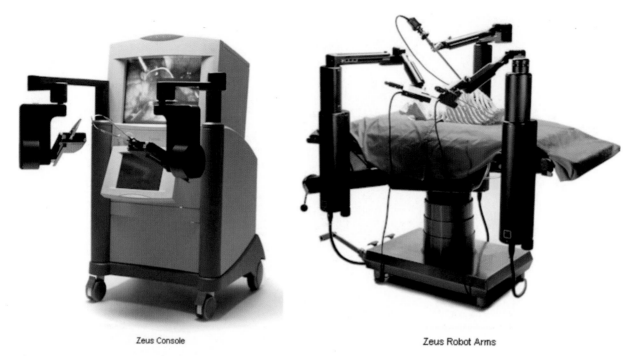

Zeus Console   Zeus Robot Arms

Figure 23.1.1. Zeus Surgical Robot – console and robotic arms. Photo courtesy of Intuitive Surgical/Computer Motion, Goleta, CA.

Intuitive Surgical's Endowrist technology (Figure 23.1.2) with bidirectional articulation allows for seven degrees of freedom (including grip). The design goal of the master console is to mimic the movements of a surgeon's hand and give the sense of directly operating on the patient.

In orthopedic surgery, the RoboDoc system (Integrated Surgical Systems Inc., Sacramento, CA) is a *stereotactic localizer* that uses anatomic landmarks calibrated from computed tomography (CT) scan data to map and drill a femoral cavity that accepts a hip prosthesis.[7] RoboDoc plays a *restricted role* in that it has some autonomous function, despite requiring data input from the surgeon. The Acrobot (Acrobot Company Ltd., London, England; Figure 23.1.3) is a similar device used to drill holes for knee arthroplasty that defines its drill path based on limitations set by preoperative imaging.[8] Another stereotactic localizer is the PAKY-RCM system developed by the urorobotics group at Johns Hopkins University for percutaneous renal needle placement.[4] PAKY (percutaneous access of the kidney) consists of an automated needle advancement system mounted in a remote center-of-motion (RCM) robotic arm that can work within the confines of a fluoroscopic C-arm.

The first reports of robot use in neurosurgery were by Kwoh et al. [9] in 1988 and Drake et al. [10] in 1991. Both groups used the Programmable Universal Machine for Assembly (PUMA; Advanced Research Robotics, Oxford, CT). Kwoh used the PUMA to hold and direct a biopsy cannula, whereas Drake used it as a retraction device during resection of a thalamic astrocytoma. Widespread application of robotics came with the introduction of NeuroMate (Integrated Surgical Systems, Sacramento, CA), which is a *passive-role neuronavigator* that uses preoperative imaging to constrain surgeon movement within a safe zone.[11,12] In order to allow real-time imaging that accounts for tissue shift, neurosurgical robots have evolved to be compatible with computed tomography and magnetic resonance imaging.

THE PROS AND CONS OF CURRENT SURGICAL ROBOTIC TECHNOLOGY

There are a number of features that offer potential benefit to the surgeon.[13] The high resolution, three-dimensional image provides an excellent image of the operative field, with the added benefits of depth perception and high magnification. The robot can correct for hand tremor and can scale movements such that a large hand movement can be translated to a small one on the robot. Unlike standard laparoscopic instruments, robotic instruments have added degrees of freedom with an articulated wrist joint. The robot can be operated remotely at a distance (telesurgery), allowing for use in remote locations or in hostile environments (battlefield or contaminated areas) where surgeon safety may otherwise be compromised. Finally, the robot offers ergonomic benefits as the surgeon sits comfortably at a console to perform the operation.

Despite these benefits, current surgical robots suffer from certain limitations. The operating surgeon receives no force feedback at the console and must rely on visual cues to determine the tensile strength of tissue and sutures (lack of *haptics*). It is necessary to have a specially trained dedicated operating room staff familiar with device setup, and the complexity of this setup can add considerably to total operative time. Current robotic platforms can be large and cumbersome, and instrument selection is limited. Perhaps the greatest limitation is the high cost of the robot; the initial purchase price of a da Vinci is $1.2 million, with

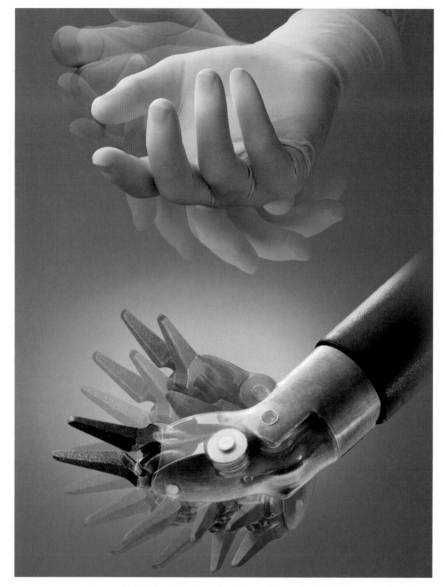

Figure 23.1.2. Endowrist technology with seven degrees of freedom. Photo courtesy of Intuitive Surgical, Sunnyvale, CA.

individual tools designed for finite usage costing approximately $200/tool/case.

SURGICAL ROBOTICS IN GYNECOLOGY

Whereas laparoscopy is now a widely accepted modality for gynecologic operations [14], the role of robotics in gynecology is still in evolution. Gynecologic surgeons at the Cleveland Clinic were the first to report a robotic gynecologic procedure, using the Zeus system to perform microsurgical tubal reanastomosis in an animal model.[15] They subsequently reported a series of 10 human patients.[16] The procedures were completed robotically in all cases, with a mean operative time of 159 minutes for both tubes. Hysterosalpingograms performed 6 weeks after surgery demonstrated an 89% patency, and pregnancy rate was 50%. When com-

pared with their laparoscopic experience, operative times were up to 2 hours longer with the robot, with no difference in tubal patency or pregnancy rates.

The same group assessed the feasibility of robotic solid organ gynecologic surgery by performing adnexal surgery and hysterectomy in a porcine model.[17] Completing all operations with the robotic arms, they reported mean operative times of 170 $\pm$ 44 minutes for adnexectomy and 200 $\pm$ 57 minutes for hysterectomy. There were no complications.

Diaz-Arrastia and colleagues [18] subsequently performed robotic hysterectomy and bilateral salpingo-oophorectomy on 11 human patients using a four-port technique (one for the scope, one for the assistant, and two for the robotic arms) with the da Vinci system. Ovarian and uterine vessels were tied with sutures, an anterior colpotomy was created, and the hysterectomy was completed transvaginally. Operative times ranged from 4.5 to

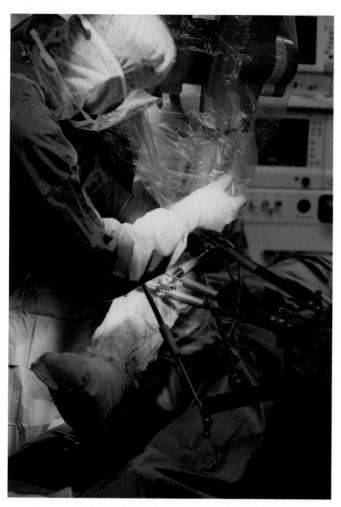

Figure 23.1.3. Acrobot Active Constraint Knee Arthroplasty System. Photo courtesy of The Acrobot Company Limited.

10 hours and blood loss from 50 to 1500 mL, with one conversion due to bleeding from an ovarian vessel. All patients were reported to have tolerated the procedure well.

Elliot and colleagues [19] performed robotic-assisted laparoscopic sacrocolpopexy for vaginal vault prolapse in a series of 20 patients. They used the da Vinci system to attach a Prolene mesh to the sacral promontory and to the apex of the vaginal vault. The initial vaginal and sacral dissection was carried out using standard laparoscopy, after which the robot was used to suture the graft to the vagina and sacrum. The mean total operative time was 3.2 hours, and 95% of patients were discharged on the first postoperative day. One patient was converted to an open procedure because of unfavorable anatomy. Two patients had minor complications (port-site infection), and there were no major complications. One patient had a recurrent rectocele. The authors noted that the difficulty of this laparoscopic procedure was reduced with the use of robotic instruments. Further details of robotic applications in gynecology are described in Section 23.2.

THE FUTURE OF ROBOTICS IN SURGERY

The future of robotic surgery lies in its ability to transcend human capability. The ability to control multiple robotic arms and see around corners with a flexible endoscope will allow a single surgeon to perform maneuvers that are currently not possible in open and laparoscopic surgery. High-fidelity force sensors will allow surgeons to manipulate delicate tissue with tactile sensation beyond human capability.[5] Overlaying of imaging data onto the operative visualization system, known as augmented reality, will guide the surgeon through preoperatively planned dissection paths programmed with spatial constraints to prevent inadvertent injury. Furthermore, the surgeon can use the imaging data on the robotic platform to rehearse a complex operation before actually performing it.

Device miniaturization will allow surgeons to access remote anatomy without extensive dissection. When taken to a nanoscale level, these devices could be transported through the body's circulatory systems and act at a cellular scale.[5] Microelectrical mechanical systems (MEMs) are a first step toward achieving this.[20] Smaller than the diameter of a single hair, MEMs are inexpensive and mass-producible silicon-based mechanical devices that perform at the micron level.

Some surgeons have leveraged the separation of surgeon and patient inherent in surgical robotics to develop distance telesurgery and telementoring systems. With the use of high-quality telecommunications lines such as asynchronous transfer mode, robotic surgery offers the ability to perform an operation at great distance (telerobotics) without significant latency, thus allowing remote regions access to this sort of expertise without the need for the physical presence of the surgeon. Marescaux and colleagues [21] demonstrated this potential with the first transatlantic telesurgical cholecystectomy, dubbed "operation Lindbergh." Using a commercial fiberoptic network, Anvari and colleagues [22] have established a telesurgery program, having successfully performed 21 telerobotic laparoscopic surgeries between Hamilton and North Bay, Canada (a distance of 400 km), including 13 fundoplications, three sigmoid resections, two right hemicolectomies, one anterior resection, and two inguinal hernia repairs. Other groups have tested the robotic platform for the purpose of mentoring less experienced surgeons at a distance and providing expert care to remote locations.[23,24] Current limitations to telesurgery and telementoring include latency inherent to the network (Anvari's group successfully managed latencies of up to 140 milliseconds), communication failure, and robotic failure. Furthermore, measures must be taken to ensure secure transmission to maintain patient confidentiality.

CONCLUSION

Although still in the experimental stages, particularly with respect to gynecology, robotic surgery has the potential to be a valuable adjunct in the clinical care of our surgical patients. This utility will result in part from judicious application to surgical problems, and in part from technologic evolution driven by clinical need. It is vital that, as surgeons, we take an active role in the development of this and other novel technologies so that we may ensure their effective and safe application in our patients.

REFERENCES

1. Woo R, Le D, Krummel TM, Albanese C. Robot-assisted pediatric surgery. *Am J Surg*. 2004;188(4A suppl):27S–37S.

2. Satava RM. Emerging technologies for surgery in the 21st century. *Arch Surg.* 1999;134:1197–1202.

3. Schneider O, Troccaz J. A six-degree-of-freedom passive arm with dynamic constraints (PADyC) for cardiac surgery application: preliminary experiments. *Comput Aided Surg.* 2001;6:340–351.

4. Stoianovici D. Robotic surgery. *World J Urol.* 2000;18:289–295.

5. Camarillo DB, Krummel TM, Salisbury JK Jr. Robotic technology in surgery: past, present, and future. *Am J Surg.* 2004;188(4Asuppl):2S–15S.

6. Eichel L, Ahlering TE, Clayman RV. Role of robotics in laparoscopic urologic surgery. *Urol Clin North Am.* 2004;31:781–792.

7. Bargar WL, Bauer A, Borner M. Primary and revision total hip replacement using the Robodoc system. *Clin Orthop Relat Res.* 1998(354):82–91.

8. Jakopec M, Harris SJ, Rodriguez y Baena F, et al. The first clinical application of a "hands-on" robotic knee surgery system. *Comput Aided Surg.* 2001;6:329–339.

9. Kwoh YS, Hou J, Jonckheere EA, Hayati S. A robot with improved absolute positioning accuracy for CT guided stereotactic brain surgery. *IEEE Trans Biomed Eng.* 1988;35:153–160.

10. Drake JM, Joy M, Goldenberg A, Kreindler D. Computer- and robot-assisted resection of thalamic astrocytomas in children. *Neurosurgery.* 1991;29:27–33.

11. Benabid AL, Cinquin P, Lavalle S, et al. Computer-driven robot for stereotactic surgery connected to CT scan and magnetic resonance imaging. Technological design and preliminary results. *Appl Neurophysiol.* 1987;50:153–154.

12. Varma TR, Eldridge PR, Forster A, et al. Use of the NeuroMate stereotactic robot in a frameless mode for movement disorder surgery. *Stereotact Funct Neurosurg.* 2003;80:132–135.

13. Lorincz A, Langenburg S, Klein MD. Robotics and the pediatric surgeon. *Curr Opin Pediatr.* 2003;15:262–266.

14. Falcone T, Goldberg JM. Robotics in gynecology. *Surg Clin North Am.* 2003;83:1483–1489, xii.

15. Margossian H, Garcia-Ruiz A, Falcone T, et al. Robotically assisted laparoscopic tubal anastomosis in a porcine model: a pilot study. *J Laparoendosc Adv Surg Tech A.* 1998;8:69–73.

16. Goldberg JM, Falcone T. Laparoscopic microsurgical tubal anastomosis with and without robotic assistance. *Hum Reprod.* 2003;18:145–147.

17. Margossian H, Falcone T. Robotically assisted laparoscopic hysterectomy and adnexal surgery. *J Laparoendosc Adv Surg Tech A.* 2001;11:161–165.

18. Diaz-Arrastia C, Jurnalov C, Gomez G, Townsend C Jr. Laparoscopic hysterectomy using a computer-enhanced surgical robot. *Surg Endosc.* 2002;16:1271–1273.

19. Elliott DS, Frank I, Dimarco DS, Chow GK. Gynecologic use of robotically assisted laparoscopy: sacrocolpopexy for the treatment of high-grade vaginal vault prolapse. *Am J Surg.* 2004;188(4A suppl):52S–56S.

20. Salzberg AD, Bloom MB, Mourlas NJ, Krummel TM. Microelectrical mechanical systems in surgery and medicine. *J Am Coll Surg.* 2002;194:463–476.

21. Marescaux J, Leroy J, Gagner M, et al. Transatlantic robot-assisted telesurgery. *Nature.* 2001;413:379–380.

22. Anvari M, McKinley C, Stein H. Establishment of the world's first telerobotic remote surgical service: for provision of advanced laparoscopic surgery in a rural community. *Ann Surg.* 2005;241:460–464.

23. Latifi R, Peck K, Satava R, Anvari M. Telepresence and telementoring in surgery. *Stud Health Technol Inform.* 2004;104:200–206.

24. Mendez I, Hill R, Clarke D, Kolyvas G. Robotic long-distance telementoring in neurosurgery. *Neurosurgery.* 2005;56:434–440.

Section 23.2. Minimally Invasive Gynecologic Surgery: The Evolving Role of Robotics

Arnold P. Advincula and Tommaso Falcone

A physician by the name of Bozzini was credited with the first documented endoscopic procedure. This report from 1807 described the use of a candle and simple tube-like device to view the urethra. In 1936, Boesch described the first gynecologic use of laparoscopy with tubal sterilization. Eventually, these rudimentary beginnings evolved into a surgical approach that revolutionized gynecology in the early 1970s. Since then, minimally invasive surgery has become increasingly popular among both surgeons and patients.

Technical advancements have clearly changed the face of modern-day laparoscopy, particularly in the area of minimally invasive gynecologic surgery. These include multi-chip cameras, high-intensity xenon and halogen light sources, and improved endomechanical instrumentation. Laparoscopy has moved from being just a diagnostic procedure to one in which operative interventions can be performed. Studies have clearly shown that laparoscopic surgery allows faster recovery with improved cosmesis, decreased blood loss, and less postoperative pain. Despite these technologic advancements and benefits, more complex procedures, such as the management of advanced endometriosis and pelvic cancer, and procedures that require extensive suturing, such as myomectomy, pelvic reconstructive surgery, and tubal reanastomosis, are typically still managed by laparotomy.

One major obstacle to the more widespread acceptance and application of minimally invasive surgical techniques to gynecologic surgery has been the limitations encountered with conventional laparoscopy. These include counterintuitive hand movement, two-dimensional visualization, limited degrees of instrument motion within the body, and poor surgeon ergonomics. Another major obstacle has been the steep learning curve associated with assimilating advanced laparoscopic techniques. In an attempt to overcome these obstacles, robotics has evolved into the armamentarium of minimally invasive gynecologic surgeons.

ROBOTICS IN GYNECOLOGY

The concept of robotic technology was born through the collaborative efforts of the Stanford Research Institute (SRI), the Massachusetts Institute of Technology (MIT), and International Business Machines (IBM) in conjunction with agencies such as the Department of Defense and the National Aeronautics and Space Administration (NASA).[1] The impetus for this concept was the need to be able to provide immediate operative care to wounded soldiers by way of remote battlefield surgery. Soon thereafter, this technology became commercialized and robots were making their presence known in civilian operating rooms. Although early applications of robotic technology were in the area of cardiac surgery [2], it was not long before these developments were applied to the field of gynecology.

One of the early predecessors and first applications of robotic technology to the field of gynecology was with a voice-activated robotic arm known as AESOP (Computer Motion Inc., Goleta, CA). The primary role of AESOP was to operate the camera during laparoscopic surgery. A study by Mettler et al. [3] compared the system to a surgical assistant holding the laparoscope during gynecologic surgery. The authors found that the time required to perform surgery was faster with the robotic camera holder because it allowed the two surgeons to use both hands for operating, thereby improving efficiency. The system did have the disadvantage of requiring frequent voice commands.

Another predecessor to the current platform of surgical robots was Zeus (Computer Motion Inc., Goleta, CA). Although no longer in production, this system comprised three remotely controlled robotic arms that were attached to the surgical table and a workstation called a robotic console. The console consisted of a video monitor, a touch screen display, and two handles that controlled the robotic arms holding the surgical instruments. Three-dimensional vision was obtained with the aid of special glasses that contained a polarizing filter. Two of the robotic arms possessed interchangeable "microwrist" instruments, such as needle holders and graspers, that could be manipulated by the surgeon seated at the console whereas the third was a voice-activated robotic arm that operated the laparoscope.

A separate touch screen display at the console allowed the surgeon to adjust how the robotic instruments functioned. One such parameter was motion scaling. For example, a scaling ratio of 10:1 meant that for every 1 cm the surgeon moved the handles at the console, the robotic surgical instruments would move 1 mm at the surgical site. Tremors and small, unintended hand motions could be filtered out, thereby providing improved dexterity and precision throughout the procedure. There was no observable delay between the movement of the handles and the movement of the instruments. Although these microwrist instruments more closely mimicked the movements of the human wrist through articulation at their tips, when compared with conventional laparoscopic instruments, their movements were not totally instinctive.

Significant advantages to this surgical platform were its small profile and ability to easily attach to the surgical table. Surgical assistants could move around the patient and have ready access to the abdomen and vagina.

Early studies reported on the successful application of Zeus to tubal reanastomosis. In one prospective study, pregnancy rates were evaluated in 10 patients with previous tubal ligations who underwent laparoscopic tubal reanastomosis using the identical technique incorporated at laparotomy.[4] A postoperative tubal patency rate of 89% was demonstrated in 17 of the 19 tubes anastomosed. A pregnancy rate of 50% was noted at 1 year. There were no complications or ectopic pregnancies.

The use of robotics in gynecology has continued to increase over the past 5 years, particularly with the introduction of the latest Food and Drug Administration (FDA)-approved platform in surgical robotics, the da Vinci surgical system (Intuitive Surgical, Sunnyvale, CA). The da Vinci surgical system is currently the only actively produced robotic surgical system incorporating an immersive telepresence environment. As of April 2005, the da Vinci surgical system gained FDA clearance for its use in gynecologic laparoscopic procedures.

The da Vinci surgical system comprises three components (Figure 23.2.1). The first component is the surgeon console where the surgeon controls the robotic system remotely through a computer interface that translates the movements of the surgeon and transmits them to the mechanical arms that hold the surgical instruments. A stereoscopic viewer and hand and foot controls are housed in this unit. The second component of the da Vinci surgical system is the InSite vision system, which provides the three-dimensional imaging through a 12-mm endoscope containing stereoscopic cameras and dual optical lenses. The third component of the da Vinci surgical system is the patient-side cart with telerobotic arms and Endowrist instruments. Currently this sys-

tem is available with either three or four robotic arms. One of the arms holds the laparoscope while the other two to three arms hold the various Endowrist instruments. These laparoscopic surgical instruments are unique in that they possess seven degrees of freedom, replicating the full range of motion of the surgeon's hand, while also eliminating the fulcrum effect seen with conventional laparoscopy (Figure 23.2.2). These seven degrees of freedom are (1) in and out movement, (2) axial rotation, (3) opening and closing of instrument, (4) lateral movement at the articulation, (5) vertical movement at the articulation, (6) right movement at each articulation, and (7) left movement at each articulation. A variety of laparoscopic instruments are available, such as needle drivers, DeBakey forceps, and round tip scissors (Figure 23.2.3). In contrast, conventional laparoscopic instruments are only able to offer four degrees of freedom.[5] The significant improvement over earlier prototypes is that the added degrees of freedom obtained at the surgeon console allow instrument manipulation to be instinctive.

In numerous studies across various disciplines, the da Vinci surgical system has been shown to be a safe and effective alternative to conventional laparoscopic surgery, particularly when dealing with complex pathology. In the area of gynecology, there are reports of robot-assisted laparoscopy for both complex and suture-based procedures, in which improved dexterity and precision coupled with advanced imaging are a huge benefit to the surgeon.

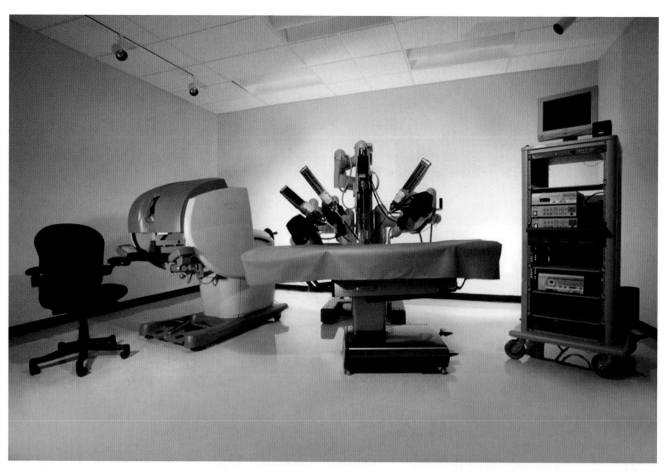

Figure 23.2.1. Photograph of the da Vinci Robotic System. From left to right: surgeon's console, patient-side surgical cart, and InSite vision tower. Photo courtesy of Intuitive Surgical, Inc.

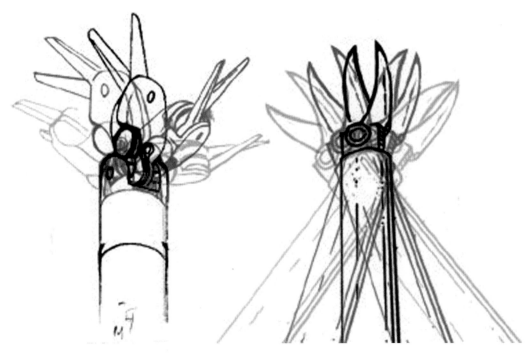

Figure 23.2.2. Schematic comparison of Endowrist instrument on left with conventional laparoscopic instrument demonstrating fulcrum effect on right.

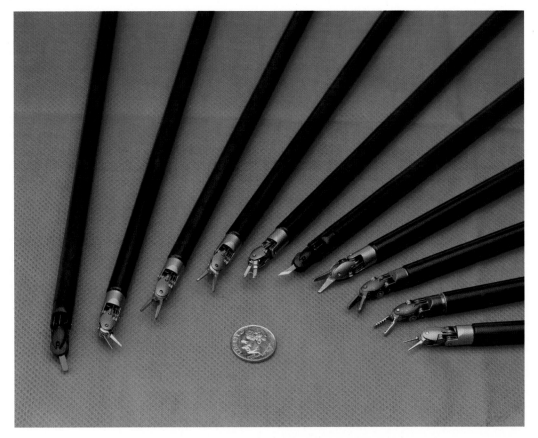

Figure 23.2.3. Selection of available Endowrist instruments.

GENERAL APPROACH TO ROBOTICS IN GYNECOLOGY

Before discussing the various applications of robotics in gynecology with the da Vinci surgical system, it is worthwhile to describe an overall approach to cases that has proven successful to Advincula and colleagues at the University of Michigan. First of all, surgeons must complete a 2-day training course to understand the setup, maintenance, and various applications of the da Vinci surgical system as required by the FDA. After completion of this certification process, additional training and preparation are obtained through case observations and proctored cases. Each hospital will have its own credentialing requirements that must be completed before any case is performed. Team training and education are important. It is a group effort that involves integration of field service engineers, nurses, biomedical technicians, operating room coordinators, anesthesiologists and surgeons, because all members are critical to the success of a robotic case.

Once a robotics program is ready to be implemented, the operating room layout must be determined. Floor dimensions need to be large enough to accommodate the footprint of the da Vinci surgical system without compromising patient care or the flow of operating room personnel throughout the room. To properly determine the layout of a room, the system cable connections and their lengths must be taken into consideration along with the physical dimensions of the da Vinci surgical system itself.[6]

Before the start of any robotic case, all patients are placed in low dorsal lithotomy position with arms padded and tucked at their sides after general endotracheal anesthesia is administered. The bladder is drained with a Foley catheter, and either a ZUMI or RUMI uterine manipulator (Cooper Surgical, Trumbull, CT) is placed (Figure 23.2.4). Four trocars are typically used after pneumoperitoneum is obtained. A long 12-mm trocar is placed either at or above the umbilicus depending on the size of the pelvic pathology (Figure 23.2.5). This trocar accommodates the endoscope with stereoscopic cameras and dual optical lenses. Occasionally a left upper quadrant entry with a 3-mm microlaparoscope is performed to help guide operative trocar placement in patients with markedly enlarged pelvic pathology or who are at risk for abdominal and/or pelvic adhesions. Two 8-mm trocars that mount directly to the surgical cart's two operating arms are placed in the left and right lower quadrants, respectively. A

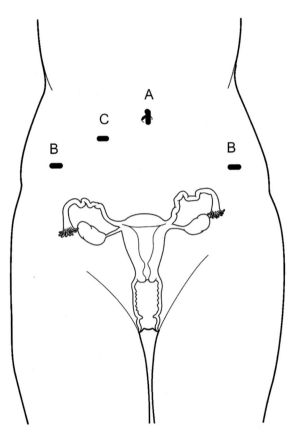

Figure 23.2.5. Port placement. (**A**) The camera port (12-mm) either at the umbilicus or above, depending on the size of the uterus. (**B**) The lateral ports: 8-mm da Vinci ports in the right and left lower quadrants of the abdomen. (**C**) The assist port (12–15 mm) placed between the camera port and the right lower quadrant port.

fourth trocar that serves as an accessory port is placed between the camera port and the right lower quadrant port. This trocar is typically 12 to 15 mm to facilitate introduction of suture, a tissue morcellator, or suction–irrigation instruments in addition to traction/countertraction.

Once all four trocars are in place, the patient is placed in steep Trendelenburg and the surgical cart with three robotic arms is brought between the patient's legs and docked, meaning that each trocar is attached to the assigned robotic arm with the exception of the accessory port that is manipulated by the bedside surgical assistant. The right and left operating arms are attached directly to the right and left lower quadrant trocars, respectively, whereas the camera arm is attached to the umbilical or supraumbilical trocar. From this point forward, cases are modified depending on the procedure performed while adhering to the basic principles of open surgical technique.

MYOMECTOMY

The primary surgical management of symptomatic leiomyomas for women desiring uterine conservation or future fertility is myomectomy. Many cases of intramural and subserous leiomyomas are managed with laparoscopic myomectomy. Despite several comparative trials showing postoperative morbidity to be

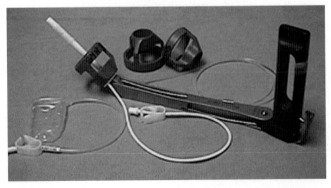

Figure 23.2.4. RUMI uterine manipulator in conjunction with Koh colpotomy rings and a vaginal pneumo-occluder balloon (all Cooper Surgical, Trumbull, CT).

less and recovery faster in the laparoscopic cases compared with laparotomy cases, the vast majority of myomectomies are still performed through laparotomy.[7–9]

The management of leiomyomas endoscopically is one of the more challenging procedures in minimally invasive surgery and requires a skilled surgeon. In the past, surgeons have suggested the need to limit laparoscopic myomectomy based on size, number, and/or location of leiomyomas, particularly as a result of inherent technical problems such as hemostasis, uterine closure, and tissue extraction. Critical to the success of a laparoscopic myomectomy is the ability to enucleate leiomyomas and repair the uterus with a multilayer sutured closure. For many surgeons, this technically challenging aspect of a laparoscopic myomectomy has been thought to affect conversion rates to laparotomy and possibly play a role in cases of uterine rupture. This ability to adequately repair a uterine defect laparoscopically continues to be a subject of debate. In fact, laparoscopically assisted myomectomy has been suggested in the past. Nezhat et al. [10] described a technique in which enucleation of myomas is performed laparoscopically and uterine closure is done through a minilaparotomy incision.

In an attempt to overcome many of the concerns and obstacles inherent in a laparoscopic myomectomy, Advincula et al. [11] described a technique that successfully applied robotics to 32 of 35 attempted myomectomies. Based on their experience, uteri with solitary symptomatic leiomyomas were best served with a robot-assisted approach. Factors such as size greater than or equal to 5 cm, intramural myomas, and anterior location, which have traditionally affected conversion rates and precluded a laparoscopic approach, did not significantly impact their ability to perform a robot-assisted laparoscopic myomectomy. Additionally, an adequate surgical field with room to manipulate instruments and uterine mobility were important factors to consider when determining candidacy for the robotic approach. In other words, a 7-cm leiomyoma was not universally a robotic candidate based on the conglomeration of these variables. Each patient was evaluated individually.

Once the robot-assist device is docked, a dilute concentration of vasopressin is infiltrated via a 7-inch 22-gauge spinal needle transabdominally into the myometrium as an adjunct for hemostasis. A variety of Endowrist instruments are attached to the right and left operating arms and used to enucleate the leiomyoma(s) (Figure 23.2.6). Countertraction is provided by the bedside surgical assistant through the accessory port. Once the leiomyoma(s) are enucleated, attention is directed toward a multilayered closure of the myomectomy resection bed(s). If the endometrial cavity is entered, confirmation is apparent based on visualization of the uterine manipulator balloon. The repair is readily completed with robotic assistance. Endowrist instruments are used to perform a closure that is modeled after traditional open surgical technique. Interrupted sutures of 3-0 Vicryl on an SH needle (cut to 6 inches) are used to repair the endometrial cavity if entered. Interrupted figure-of-eight sutures of 0 Vicryl on CT-2 needles (cut to 6 inches) are used to close the first two myometrial layers followed by a running baseball stitch of 3-0 Vicryl on an SH needle (cut to 11 inches) for the serosa. The sutures are tied with the Endowrist DeBakey forceps and large needle driver via instrument tying techniques (Figure 23.2.7). Once the uterine defect(s) are repaired, a power tissue morcellator is used to extract the specimen through the accessory port.

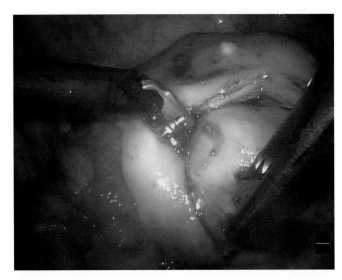

Figure 23.2.6. Photo of a fibroid being enucleated robotically. Countertraction is provided by a bedside surgical assistant with a myoma grasper.

Adhesion prevention measures can be undertaken before the end of the procedure. Throughout the myomectomy, adequate hemostasis is obtained with the combination of pneumoperitoneum, vasopressin, and electrocautery.

Interestingly in their series, there were no conversions to laparotomy as a result of suturing difficulty during repair of the uterine defect. The mean number of myomas removed per patient was 1.6 (range, 1 to 5). The average diameter of myomas removed was 7.9 ± 3.5 cm (95% CI, 6.63–9.13) with the majority greater than 5 cm. The mean myoma weight was 223.2 ± 244.1 g (95% CI, 135.8–310.6). Mean operating time was 230.8 ± 83 minutes (95% CI, 201.6–260) with a trend toward decreased operative times with experience. The average estimated blood loss was 169 ± 198.7 mL (95% CI, 99.1–238.4).

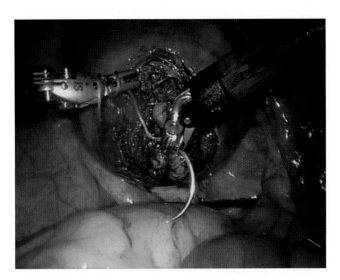

Figure 23.2.7. Instrument tying with Endowrist instruments (DeBakey forceps and needle driver) during multilayer sutured closure of a uterine defect.

Although there are no published comparative clinical trials of robotic versus conventional laparoscopic myomectomy, the preliminary results confirm feasibility to this approach and demonstrate outcomes similar to those seen with traditional laparoscopy. As experience with this approach grows, robotics will either prove to be advantageous or a bridge to laparoscopy for individuals performing myomectomies by laparotomy.

HYSTERECTOMY

Hysterectomy is the most common non–pregnancy-related procedure performed in the United States. Approximately 600,000 cases are performed annually, with the majority done because of benign conditions.[12,13] Since the introduction of laparoscopically assisted vaginal hysterectomy in the late 1980s by pioneers such as Reich, the surgical approach to hysterectomy is no longer strictly vaginal or abdominal.[14] Over the years, this endoscopic approach has evolved to include both subtotal and total laparoscopic hysterectomy. In the 1990s, a definite trend was seen toward laparoscopic hysterectomy: An increase from 0.3% to 9.9% was observed over a 7-year period in the United States.[15] Despite the introduction of advanced laparoscopic techniques, the vast majority of hysterectomies are still approached by either a vaginal or abdominal route. In fact in 2002, Farquhar and Steiner [15] reported that only approximately 10% of hysterectomies are performed with the assistance of laparoscopy.

One explanation for the slow acceptance of laparoscopic approaches to hysterectomy is the learning curve with conventional laparoscopy and its associated complications.[16] In an attempt to provide solutions to the inherent limitations of conventional laparoscopy, several investigators have applied robot-assisted technology in their approach to hysterectomy.[17–20] One of the earliest reports by Diaz-Arrastia et al. [17] did not convey encouraging results, with operative times as long as 10 hours and blood loss as high as 1500 mL. Interestingly, in this series, all hysterectomies were completed in a fashion consistent with a laparoscopically assisted vaginal hysterectomy or American Association of Gynecologic Laparoscopists (AAGL) type IIB.[21] The remaining investigators were able to demonstrate shorter operative times and a trend toward completion of the hysterectomy in a totally endoscopic fashion (AAGL type IVE). In a study by Advincula [19], all hysterectomies were approached with suture ligation of all vascular pedicles and sutured closure of the vaginal cuff robotically (Figure 23.2.8). The indications spanned the gamut of both benign and malignant disease for all investigators (Table 23.2.1).

GYNECOLOGIC ONCOLOGY

The acceptance of minimally invasive surgical techniques in the treatment of gynecologic cancers has been slow. Several reasons are the steep learning curves for specific procedures, the concern for port-site metastases, and the overall long-term outcome. As an extension of the hysterectomy experiences already described, robotics has also been applied to cancer staging (Table 23.2.2). Reynolds et al. [22] successfully completed seven attempted robotic staging procedures for endometrial, ovarian, and fallopian tube cancers. Overall results were promising, with a median

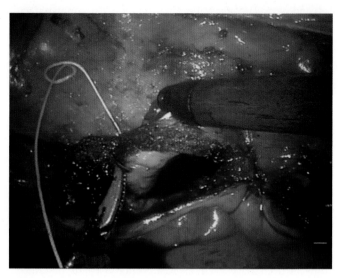

Figure 23.2.8. Closure of the vaginal cuff with interrupted sutures of 0 Vicryl on CT-2 needles.

lymph node count of 15, minimal blood loss, and a shortened hospital stay. Similar results were seen in 12 robotic cancer cases by the group out of Belgium and France.[20]

Along the lines of cancer-related applications, Molpus et al. [23] reported a case of robotic ovarian transposition. Ovarian function was successfully preserved in a young woman treated with radiotherapy for stage 1-B1 squamous cell carcinoma of the cervix.

UROGYNECOLOGY

The preliminary experience with robotics in pelvic reconstructive surgery has centered on sacrocolpopexy. In a study by DiMarco et al. [24], robotic technology was viewed as a way to overcome the difficulties described in the initial reports of conventional laparoscopic sacrocolpopexy.[25,26] The initial dissection was completed with conventional laparoscopic means followed by the use of the robot for suturing the graft in place. Although no recurrent vaginal vault prolapse was noted at the limited follow-up of only 4 months, the feasibility of this approach was demonstrated.

TUBAL REANASTOMOSIS

The first gynecologic procedure attempted with a robotic system was reported by Falcone and colleagues in 1999.[27] Because these robotic systems were designed with coronary bypass surgery in mind, it was thought that the fine suturing required for the vascular anastomosis could be applied to a tubal reversal procedure. Tubal reversal procedures are performed with sutures that are between 6-0 and 8-0 in size.

The main advantage of the robot for tubal surgery is the extreme precision allowed by the combination of the three-dimensional view and the Endowrist capability. The surgeon can precisely place a suture no matter how awkward the angle. The main disadvantage of the robotic system is the lack of haptic

Table 23.2.1: Comparison of Robot-Assisted Hysterectomy

	Diaz-Arrastia [17]	Beste [18]	Advincula [19]	Marchal [20]
Type of hysterectomy (no.)	IIB (10) Staging (1)	IVE	IVE (5) III (1)	IIB (23) IVE (6)
Study subjects, no.	11	11	6	30
Age, years	55	38	40	53
BMI		26	26 kg/m^2	
Indications for surgery	Recurrent CIN 3, pelvic mass, endometrial CA, postmenopausal bleeding, ovarian CA	Menorrhagia, dysmenorrhea, pelvic pain, symptomatic fibroids	Endometriosis, abnormal uterine bleeding, symptomatic fibroids	Endometrial CA, cervical CA, benign pathologies
EBL, mL	300 (50–1500)	25–350	87.5 (50–150)	83 (0–900)
Blood transfusions, no.	1	0	0	
Uterine weight, g		49–227	121.7	
Operating time, min.	270–600	148–277	254 (170–368)	185 (43–315)
Hospital stay, days	2	1	1.3	8
Complications (no.)	Conversion to minilaparotomy (1)	Conversion to open case (1) Cystotomy (1)	Vaginal cuff hematoma (1)	Venous phlebitis (1) Lymph collection (1) Pelvic hematoma (1) UTI (1) Vaginal hemorrhage (1)

BMI, body mass index; CA, cancer; CIN 3, cervical intraepithelial neoplasia; EBL, estimated blood loss; American Association of Gynecologic Laparoscopists (AAGL) classifications IIB, IVE; UTI, urinary tract infection.

Table 23.2.2: Comparison of Robot-Assisted Cancer Staging

	Diaz-Arrastia [17]	Marchal [20]	Reynolds [22]
Study subjects, no.	11	30	7
Age, years	55	53	48
BMI			27 kg/m^2
Indication for surgery (no.)	Recurrent CIN 3 or pelvic mass (6) Endometrial CA or postmenopausal bleeding (4) Ovarian CA (1)	Endometrial CA (5) Cervix CA (7) Benign pathologies of the uterus (18)	Endometrial CA (4) Ovarian CA (2) Fallopian tube CA (1)
EBL, mL	300 (50–1500)	83 (0–900)	50
Operating time, min.	270–600	185 (43–315)	257 (174–345)
Lymph node count		11 (4–21)	15 (4–29)
Blood transfusions, no.	1		0
Hospital stay, days	2	8	2 (1–6)
Complications (no.)	Conversion to minilaparotomy (1)	Venous phlebitis (1) Lymph collection (1) Pelvic hematoma (1) UTI (1) Vaginal hemorrhage (1)	Sinusitis (1)

feedback that necessitates the use of visual cues to manipulate tissue without damaging it. The lumen of the proximal isthmus is 1 to 2 mm, and the mucosa is easily sheared. Tissue damage can easily result. The use of small needles without haptic feedback may result in needles bending or in avulsion from the suture.

The case starts with the patient in lithotomy position. A uterine manipulator that allows injection of dilute indigo carmine dye is inserted. A conventional laparoscopy is performed to confirm that there is adequate length of uterine tube and no other pathology, such as chronic pelvic inflammatory disease, that would not allow an optimal result. Dilute vasopressin is then injected into the mesosalpinx below the anastomosis site.

Three accessory ports are used. Two are placed lateral to the rectus muscle a few centimeters below the level of the umbilicus for the robotic arms. One suprapubic port is placed for introduction or removal of needles. The advantage of this port for the needles is that the laparoscope has to be moved minimally to directly observe the insertion and removal of small needles that are very hard to find.

The proximal and distal anastomosis sites are then prepared and confirmed patent with injection of indigo carmine dye through the cervix and through the fimbriae. Monopolar current set at 18 W and microscissors are used. The robot is placed between the patient's legs and the robot arms are engaged. All the sutures placed are interrupted single stitches. 6-0 Vicryl is used to reapproximate the mesosalpinx. Then a two-layered closure is performed using 8-0 Vicryl. The mucosal muscularis layer usually requires three or four separate stitches. The first is placed at a 6 o'clock position and tied (Figure 23.2.9). A stitch is placed at 3 and 9 o'clock but not tied so as not to obscure visibility of the lumen for subsequent stitches (Figure 23.2.10). The final 12 o'clock stitch is placed and tied. The muscularis serosal layer requires two to three stitches. Patency is confirmed at the end with injection of indigo carmine dye through the cervix.

The robotic procedure is performed in the same manner as an open microsurgical procedure. However, it is possible that

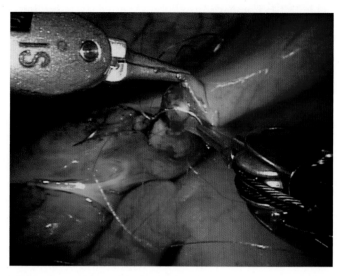

Figure 23.2.10. The 6 o'clock stitch has been tied. The 9 o'clock stitch has been placed but not tied. The needle is seen in the foreground. The 3 o'clock stitch is being placed.

the precision that is offered by the robot may not be essential. In a retrospective case control study, outcomes were similar whether the procedure was carried out by conventional or robotic laparoscopy.[28] However, the robot was an early prototype of the Zeus that did not have an articulation at the distal end of the instrument.

OTHER ROBOTIC APPLICATIONS

Although many of the limitations encountered with conventional laparoscopic instrumentation are overcome with robotics, other challenges remain that center on the training and acquisition of advanced skills. Specifically, access to surgical training, the surgeon's skill level, and the lengthy training interval to attain laparoscopic competence have been known to affect the application of minimally invasive surgical techniques to procedures such as hysterectomy.[16] In an interesting report by Chapron et al. [29] from Europe, training was found to be a major factor in the choice of technique when a review of the rate of laparoscopic hysterectomy in 23 French medical centers revealed that only nine centers carried out total laparoscopic hysterectomies.

Even when access to surgical training is available, the learning curve for conventional laparoscopy and prevention of associated complications are still significant limitations to the widespread application of minimally invasive surgical techniques. Although there are no absolute contraindications to many of the laparoscopic procedures in gynecology, a surgeon's experience and the pathology encountered remain the limiting factors for performing successfully. The technical advantages gained with robotics may provide a way to improve surgical training and the acquisition of advanced skills. Several investigators have identified the increased precision and accuracy of robotics as an advantage when compared with conventional laparoscopy.[30–33] A recent study by Sarle et al. [34] confirmed this belief. The authors assessed the impact of robotics on surgical skills by comparing conventional laparoscopy with the da Vinci surgical system in the performance

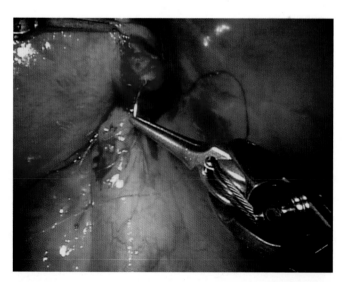

Figure 23.2.9. The first interrupted stitch has been placed through the distal site through the serosa and exits through the mucosa into the lumen. The suture will then be placed through the mucosa and exit through the serosa of the proximal site.

of four training drills. Surgeons completed drills faster with the robotic system. Most importantly, the study found that the playing field between novice and expert laparoscopic surgeons was leveled with use of the robotic system.

In an interesting study of surgical training by Ferguson and colleagues [35], a bilateral tubal ligation was used as a transition procedure when adopting robotics in gynecology. In order to obtain credentialing and gain experience with the da Vinci surgical system, the surgeons applied robotic assistance to the completion of tubal ligations using the Parkland method in four women. Although feasibility was proven, operative times were lengthy at 85 to 151 minutes. Costs were not addressed.

COMPLICATIONS OF ROBOTIC SURGERY

No specific complications unique to robotic surgeries have been reported so far. All the complications associated with conventional laparoscopic surgery are possible with robotic assistance. This is evident in the complications noted in Tables 23.2.1 and 23.2.2.

CONCLUSION

The role of robotics in gynecology holds much promise. Today's platforms of robotic surgical systems are able to provide improved instrument dexterity and precision along with three-dimensional imaging. Preliminary experience thus far seems to indicate that many of the technical difficulties encountered with conventional laparoscopy are overcome. However, proper clinical trials comparing robotics with conventional laparoscopic approaches must be performed to truly evaluate advantages and disadvantages.

The use of robot-assisted laparoscopy may also rapidly bridge the gap between the assimilation of new techniques and the actual application of the procedure. Although learning curves may be shortened with improvements in training efficiency and precision, this has yet to be translated to the operating room.

Despite all the advantages seen thus far, the economics surrounding this technology remain prohibitive. The cost of the da Vinci surgical system is on the order of $1 million, with an additional cost for disposables per case. Although current cost is high, as with any new technology, cost is likely to decrease over time. Additionally, the absence of tactile feedback remains a limitation. Overall, evolving robotic technology may further improve patient outcomes and facilitate the transition between traditional open surgical and laparoscopic techniques in gynecology.

REFERENCES

1. Satava RM. Robotic surgery: from past to future – a personal journey. *Surg Clin North Am.* 2003;83:1–6.
2. Diodato MD, Damiano RJ. Robotic cardiac surgery: overview. *Surg Clin North Am.* 2003;83:1351–1367.
3. Mettler L, Ibrahim M, Jonat W. One year of experience working with the aid of a robotic assistant (the voice-controlled optic holder AESOP) in gynecologic endoscopic surgery. *Hum Reprod.* 1998;13:2748–2750.

4. Falcone T, Goldberg JM, Margossian H, Stevens L. Robotically assisted laparoscopic microsurgical anastomosis: a human pilot study. *Fertil Steril.* 2000;73:1040–1042.
5. Sturges RH, Wright PK. A quantification of manual dexterity. *Robot Comput Integr Manuf.* 1989;6:237–252.
6. Sprague RA, Hayes CS, Advincula AP. Integration of robot-assisted laparoscopy in the minimally invasive management of symptomatic uterine fibroids. *Biomed Instrum Technol.* 2005;suppl:55–60.
7. Falcone T, Bedaiwy MA. Minimally invasive management of uterine fibroids. *Curr Opin Obstet Gynecol.* 2002;14:401–407.
8. Mais V, Ajossa S, Guerriero S, et al. Laparoscopic versus abdominal myomectomy: a prospective randomized trial to evaluate benefits in early outcome. *Am J Obstet Gynecol.* 1996;174:654–658.
9. Seracchioli R, Rossi S, Govoni F, et al. Fertility and obstetric outcome after laparoscopic myomectomy of large myomata: a randomized comparison with abdominal myomectomy. *Hum Reprod.* 2000;15:2663–2668.
10. Nezhat C, Nezhat F, Bess O, et al. Laparoscopically assisted myomectomy: a report of a new technique in 57 cases. *Int J Fertil Menopausal Stud.* 1994;39:39–44.
11. Advincula AP, Song A, Burke W, Reynolds RK. Preliminary experience with robot-assisted laparoscopic myomectomy. *J Am Assoc Gynecol Laparosc.* 2004;11:511–518.
12. Wilcox LS, Koonin LM, Pokras R, Strauss LT, Xia Z, Peterson HB. Hysterectomy in the United States, 1988–1990. *Obstet Gynecol.* 1994;83:549–555.
13. Lepine LA, Hillis SD, Marchbanks PA, et al. Hysterectomy surveillance – United States, 1980–1993. *MMWR CDC Surveill Summ.* 1997;46:1–15.
14. Reich H, Decaprio J, McGlynn F. Laparoscopic hysterectomy. *L Gynecol Surg* 1989;5:213–216.
15. Farquhar CM, Steiner CA. Hysterectomy rates in the United States 1990–1997. *Obstet Gynecol.* 2002;99:229–234.
16. Wattiez A, Cohen SB, Selvaggi L. Laparoscopic hysterectomy. *Curr Opin Obstet Gynecol.* 2002;14:417–422.
17. Diaz-Arrastia C, Jurnalov C, Gomez G, Townsend C. Laparoscopic hysterectomy using a computer-enhanced surgical robot. *Surg Endosc.* 2002;16:1271–1273.
18. Beste TM, Nelson KH, Daucher JA. Total laparoscopic hysterectomy using a robotic surgical system. *JSLS.* 2005;9:13–15.
19. Advincula AP, Reynolds RK. The use of robot-assisted laparoscopic hysterectomy in the patient with a scarred or obliterated anterior cul de sac. *JSLS.* 2005;9:287–291.
20. Marchal F, Rauch P, Vandromme J, et al. Telerobotic-assisted laparoscopic hysterectomy for benign and oncologic pathologies; initial clinical experience with 30 patients. *Surg Endosc.* 2005;19:826–831.
21. Olive DL, Parker WH, Cooper JM, Levine RL. The AAGL classification system for laparoscopic hysterectomy. *J Am Assoc Gynecol Laparosc.* 2000;7:9–15.
22. Reynolds RK, Burke WM, Advincula AP. Preliminary experience with robot-assisted laparoscopic staging of gynecologic malignancies. *JSLS.* 2005;9:149–158.
23. Molpus KL, Wedergren JS, Carlson MA. Robotically-assisted endoscopic ovarian transposition. *JSLS.* 2003;7:59–62.
24. Dimarco DS, Chow GK, Gettman MT, Elliott DS. Robotic-assisted laparoscopic sacrocolpopexy for treatment of vaginal vault prolapse. *Urology.* 2004;63:373–376.
25. Ostrzenski A. Laparoscopic colposuspension for total vaginal prolapse. *Int J Gynecol Obstet.* 1996;55:147–152.
26. Cosson M, Rajabally R, Bogaert E, et al. Laparoscopic sacrocolpopexy, hysterectomy, and Burch colposuspension: feasibility and short-term complications of 77 procedures. *JSLS.* 2002;6:115–119.

27. Falcone T, Goldberg J, Garcia-Ruiz A, Margossian H, Stevens L. Full robotic assistance for laparoscopic tubal anastomosis. First case report. *J Laparoendosc Adv Surg Tech*. 1999;9:107–113.

28. Goldberg JM, Falcone T. Laparoscopic microsurgical tubal anastomosis with and without robotic assistance. *Hum Reprod*. 2003;18:145–147.

29. Chapron C, Laforest L, Ansquer Y, Fauconnier A, et al. Hysterectomy techniques used for benign pathologies: results of a French multicenter study. *Hum Reprod*. 1999;14:2464–2470.

30. Nio D, Bemelman WA, den Boer KT, et al. Efficiency of manual vs. robotical (Zeus) assisted laparoscopic surgery in the performance of standardized tasks. *Surg Endosc*. 2002;16:412–415.

31. Prasad SM, Maniar HS, Soper NJ, et al. The effect of robotic assistance on learning curves for basic laparoscopic skills. *Am J Surg*. 2002;183:702–707.

32. De Ugarte DA, Etzioni DA, Gracia C, et al. Robotic surgery and resident training. *Surg Endosc*. 2003;17:960–963.

33. Yohannes P, Rotariu P, Pinto P, et al. Comparison of robotic versus laparoscopic skills: is there a difference in the learning curve? *Urology*. 2002;60:39–45.

34. Sarle R, Tewari A, Shrivastava A, et al. Surgical robotics and laparoscopic training drills. *J Endourol*. 2004;18:63–67.

35. Ferguson JL, Beste TM, Nelson KH, Daucher JA. Making the transition from standard gynecologic laparoscopy to robotic laparoscopy. *JSLS*. 2004;8:326–328.

24 | HYSTEROSCOPY AND ENDOMETRIAL CANCER

William H. Bradley and Farr Nezhat

The use of hysteroscopy in the setting of endometrial carcinoma raises two major concerns: that distention of the uterus will propel cancerous cells into the abdomen via the fallopian tubes and that those cells will seed the abdomen and either increase the risk of recurrence of the cancer or cause implants to be viable and grossly present at the time of staging. Hysteroscopy improves the likelihood of diagnosing endometrial pathology by affording the surgeon a direct visualization of the cavity and therefore any lesions that may be present. Quantifying this benefit must be weighed against the potential risks and costs of the procedure. Some have described protocols for managing endometrial cancer in the setting of fertility preservation or a poor surgical candidate using hysteroscopy as a tool for either following a lesion treated with progesterones or resecting the lesion altogether with a hysteroscopic resectoscope. In this chapter we review the use of hysteroscopy in endometrial cancer, focusing on diagnosis, treatment, and possible impact on the disease.

HYSTEROSCOPY AND DIAGNOSIS OF ENDOMETRIAL CANCER

Since its introduction in 1869 by Pantaleoni to treat abnormal bleeding from an endometrial polyp [1], hysteroscopy has been utilized in the diagnosis and treatment of abnormal vaginal bleeding. Endometrial cancer presents as abnormal bleeding in approximately 93% of cases [2], and a reported 5% to 15% of postmenopausal women with abnormal bleeding will have endometrial carcinoma. [3,4] The most common gynecologic cancer in the United States, endometrial cancer is typically diagnosed while confined to the uterus. In these early stages, it is frequently treated with a simple hysterectomy and the occasional use of adjunctive radiation. As abnormal vaginal bleeding is the most common presentation, a sampling of the endometrial tissue is warranted in all cases of postmenopausal bleeding.

Hysteroscopy entered its modern era in the 1970s, and its increasing popularity and usefulness has led to its status as a preferred technique for the evaluation of abnormal vaginal bleeding. For years, dilatation and curettage (D&C) had been considered the gold standard for detection of intrauterine pathology, although the sampling of the endometrial lining represents only approximately 60% of the total surface.[3]

Hysteroscopy and Dilatation and Curettage

Hysteroscopy is often used in conjunction with D&C, but a number of authors have evaluated how each modality adds to the other. A hysteroscopic diagnosis can be made with visualization and directed biopsy or by performing a D&C before or after hysteroscopy. When hysteroscopy with directed biopsy has been compared to D&C, pathologic diagnosis was increased.[4] In 16% of cases, a hysteroscopic biopsy was more useful than tissue gathered by D&C. However, in this study no cases of endometrial cancer were missed by D&C. These findings were recapitulated by Loffer [5] when he reported on 151 patients evaluated for abnormal bleeding. A negative hysteroscopic view was associated with disease in only 1 of 102 cases. A positive view had a 100% positive predictive value. Blind D&C missed 17 of 49 cases of endometrial pathology. Ben-Yehuda et al. found that a hysteroscopic impression did not improve the sensitivity of D&C, but the D&C was performed after a visualization of the cavity with hysteroscopy, possibly improving its sensitivity. Negative hysteroscopic impression did not assure absence of carcinoma in this study.[6]

The most concerning cases of endometrial pathology reported involve focal abnormalities. Epstein et al. reported on 105 women with postmenopausal bleeding and an endometrial stripe ≥ 5 mm who underwent hysteroscopy with D&C and then hysteroscopic resection of any residual focal lesion. The D&C missed 2 of 19 endometrial cancers and 3 of 5 atypical hyperplastic endometrial lesions that were diagnosed by directed biopsy. Again, a high correlation between hysteroscopy and final pathology was noted (94%).[6,7]

Hysteroscopy and Endometrial Biopsy

Endometrial biopsy can be accomplished in the office, making it a less costly and invasive technique than D&C. The combination of transvaginal sonography with biopsy may rule out most intrauterine pathology. An endometrial stripe of <4 mm can rule out most, but not all, cases of endometrial carcinoma.[8] In cases of known endometrial carcinoma, biopsy can be extremely accurate. Stovall et al. [9] were able to detect 39 of 40 known endometrial carcinomas via office Pipelle biopsy.

In undiagnosed cases of abnormal bleeding, an important distinction exists between pre- and postmenopausal women. Not only is the rate of carcinoma higher in postmenopausal women with abnormal bleeding, but also the rate of detection is improved. In a meta-analysis, Dijkuizen et al. reported a sensitivity of 99.6% for Pipelle detection of endometrial cancer, whereas the Vabra device showed a sensitivity of 97.1%. When premenopausal women were included in studies reviewed, the sensitivity dropped to 91% for Pipelle and 80% for Vabra. The authors observed that sensitivity dropped in studies that used

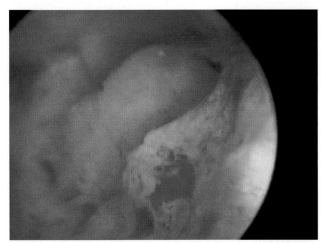

Figure 24.1. Endometrium with well-differentiated endometrioid carcinoma.

hysterectomy specimen as the gold standard rather than D&C. The hysteroscope detected more pathology than a curetting.

Hysteroscopic Observation

A number of authors have reviewed their experience diagnosing endometrial cancer by hysteroscopic impression [10–15], with a sensitivity ranging from 68% to 100% for detection of carcinoma. In the studies with lower sensitivity, only one case of carcinoma was felt to be normal endometrium. Other false impressions were simple polyps, hyperplasia, or atrophy, all diagnoses that resulted in a tissue biopsy (Figures 24.1 and 24.2). Generally a high degree of accuracy is seen with hysteroscopic diagnosis, with false negatives often coming from studies that had to be discontinued or were challenged by technical factors. In a meta-analysis, Clark et al. confirmed the finding that hysteroscopy is effective for diagnosing endometrial cancer but cannot exclude the diagnosis in a negative view. The higher prevalence of endometrial cancer in

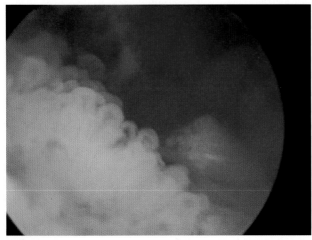

Figure 24.2. Endometrium with well-differentiated endometrioid carcinoma.

postmenopausal women with abnormal bleeding again made for a more accurate test in this population.[16]

HYSTEROSCOPY AND IMPLICATIONS FOR PERITONEAL CYTOLOGY

The most concerning criticism raised against hysteroscopy in the setting of endometrial cancer is the risk of dissemination of cancerous cells into the abdomen. A number of authors have described the retrograde flow of endometrial tissue under the pressure of hysteroscopic distending media (either liquid or CO_2).[17, 18] That benign endometrial tissue can exfoliate and spread beyond the endometrial cavity is less concerning, but the transmission and dissemination of malignant endometrial tissue into the abdomen, bloodstream, or lymphatics could have a number of consequences. Endometrial cancer with cytology that is positive for malignant cells that are otherwise confined to the uterus is by convention staged as IIIA. In a Gynecologic Oncology Group (GOG) study of pathologic spread in endometrial cancer, positive cytology was noted in 9% of cases. However, this finding is associated with other evidence of extrauterine spread, such as with pelvic or periaortic lymph node involvement.[19, 20]

Hysteroscopy Increases the Risk of Positive Peritoneal Cytology

In the 1990s a number of case reports were published that raised the concern that identified extra-uterine disease could be associated with hysteroscopy.[21–23] Retrospective reviews have offered evidence confirming the association between use of preoperative hysteroscopy and positive peritoneal cytology [24–28], but these findings have not been born out by other reviews.[29–32] The possibility of a diagnostic study potentially worsening the prognosis of patients raises a number of concerns. Leveque et al. [25] and Obermair et al. [27] reported on patients who otherwise had disease confined to the uterus. In Obermair's review the increased risk of positive cytology was not associated with other pathologic factors, such as invasion, grade, or histological subtype. Leveque did not analyze these variables but reported on a homogenous group of patients with IA and IB cancers, each of whom had grade 1 histology. The follow-up of patients with positive cytology was extended for a median of 25 months, and, interestingly, none of these patients recurred.

Both Bradley et al. [28] and Zerbe et al. [26] reported on larger groups (256 and 222 patients, respectively). Both of these articles reported an increased odds ratio for malignant cytology if hysteroscopy was used, although in Zerbe's group, the risk was confined to patients with other risk factors such as grade, lymphvascular invasion, and ovarian involvement. A higher risk of malignant cytology was confirmed after adjusting for these confounding factors. Bradley et al. noted an increased odds ratio after controlling for grade and stage. Both of these studies included higher stage patients with other evidence of extra-uterine carcinoma, and neither evaluated the recurrence risk.

Although it is sufficient in itself to upstage a patient with endometrial cancer otherwise confined to the uterus, the management of malignant cytology is controversial in itself. A number of reports argue that cytology is a prognostic factor only if it is associated with other evidence of extrauterine disease.[33]

However, a recent survey of gynecologic oncologists in the Society of Gynecologic Oncologists (SGO) indicated that over half would recommend some form of adjuvant therapy if malignant cytology were the only evidence of extrauterine disease.[34] That hysteroscopy may have been associated with the positive cytology would not change the need for adjuvant therapy for the majority of respondents.

Hysteroscopy Does Not Increase the Risk of Positive Peritoneal Cytology

Not all reports of peritoneal cytology after hysteroscopic diagnosis of endometrial cancer have shown an increased in the risk of malignant cells. Gu et al. [31] reviewed the experience at Memorial Sloan-Kettering and found that the risk of malignant cytology after endometrial biopsy or D&C was 9.5%, whereas hysteroscopy was associated with a 13% rate of malignant cytology ($P = 0.79$). This study included 284 patients, but did not control for stage and grade. A smaller, but more comprehensive, study was published by Selvaggi et al. [30] They compared 147 patients diagnosed with D&C, hysteroscopy with D&C, or hysteroscopy alone and found no difference in the rate of malignant cytology. The overall rate of positive cytology was only 6%, which is lower than most rates published in pathologic reviews.

A prospective, nonrandomized study was carried out by Kudela et al. [35] in which patients who underwent hysteroscopy had a culdocentesis performed immediately after hysteroscopy with cytology sent. This cytology was compared with washings at definitive staging. The rate of malignant cytology was comparable in both the D&C control group and the hysteroscopy group. This study included patients in all pathologic stages. Although regression was not carried out to adjust for the variables of stage and grade, it was reported by the authors that there was no statistical differences between the two groups.

The effect of dispersing endometrial cells at hysteroscopy has begun to be elucidated. Arikan et al. [36] cultured and analyzed the adherence of carcinomatous endometrial cells flushed via hysteroscopy from fresh pathological specimens. Functional viability after culturing cells on a matrix was appreciated from 42% (10/24) of specimens. Interestingly, fluid was not recovered from every flushing, and of those that did malignant cells were found in 17 of 20.

The follow-up of patients who underwent hysteroscopy generally shows encouraging signs. Early-stage endometrial carcinoma patients have not shown a worsened outcome after undergoing preoperative hysteroscopy. Obermair et al. [37] followed 135 patients who underwent hysteroscopy prior to staging surgery and compared them with a control group of 127 patients diagnosed with D&C. Cytology was analyzed in 111 patients, but the primary outcome studied was disease-free survival, and patients were followed for a median of 23 months. There was no difference noted in disease-free survival in that time. However, patients who underwent hysteroscopy received systemic adjuvant therapy more often than those who did not. A small study by Gucer et al. [38] followed 33 patients after diagnosis with hysteroscopy and found no recurrence difference from 27 matched controls. Follow-up was for a median of 30 months.

The question of whether hysteroscopy causes dissemination of tumor cells in the abdomen does not have a definitive answer. A randomized trial that could potentially worsen the outcome of one arm would not be undertaken. More retrospective data will continue to be published to complement the work available. Outcome data are still immature and need to be augmented, but thus far it appears that hysteroscopy does not carry high risks of either early or distant metastasis, even if an increased risk of malignant cytology is accepted. It must be noted, however, that there may be an increase in treatment-related morbidity due to systemic therapy being given to those patients with positive cytology as the only evidence of extrauterine disease.

MINIMALLY INVASIVE MANAGEMENT OF EARLY-STAGE ENDOMETRIAL CANCER: THE ROLE OF HYSTEROSCOPY

The management of endometrial cancer utilizing minimally invasive techniques has typically been reserved for two types of patients: those who desire maintenance of fertility and those not felt to be appropriate surgical candidates. Thus far, published reports on this topic are restricted to case reports and small series. Although it may be useful to have some of these techniques available for patients who are unwilling to undergo hysterectomy or for whom the risks of surgery outweigh the risks of less definitive treatment, the information to guide patient counseling is limited. Treatment regimens have included early-stage and grade cancers that are hormonally driven and can reasonably be expected to respond to progesterone therapy.

Montz et al. [39] treated 16 patients with grade 1 endometrial cancer without evidence of invasion with intrauterine progesterone. Each of these patients was considered to be a high surgical risk (American Society of Anesthesia III or IV). Prior to placement of the progesterone-containing IUD, each patient underwent maximal tissue reduction via D&C after having their endometrial cavities assessed by hysteroscopy. After 1 year these patients had their endometrial cavities reevaluated with hysteroscopy. Although two of eight patients had persistence of endometrial cancer at 1 year, none developed systemic disease, and there was no evidence of malignant cytology in those patients who ultimately underwent definitive therapy.

Both Kung et al. [40] and Mazzon et al. [41] described cases of endometrial cancer arising in women at 22 and 31 years of age, respectively. Both patients were treated with tamoxifen and megace after an evaluation of the endometrial cavity by hysteroscopy and, in the case described by Mazzon, a hysteroscopic resection of the visible lesion. Both of the cases described were of grade 1 adenocarcinomas without evidence of invasion, and both patients had a cancer that was related to unopposed endogenous estrogen exposure.

CONCLUSION

The ability to directly visualize the endometrial cavity to diagnose or treat abnormalities has been an important addition to the gynecologist's tools to increase the health of women. Many of the causes of abnormal bleeding have benign etiologies that respond well to local, minimally invasive treatment. The risks of hysteroscopy in the setting of endometrial carcinoma are ill defined. Our best estimate is that hysteroscopy increases the risk of tumor spillage. This has not been shown to increase the risk of distant metastasis or disease recurrence, but data are still maturing. Regardless of risk, the majority of gynecologic oncologists in the United States would offer some form of systemic treatment in the face of positive cytology. Risks associated with adjuvant therapy alone should cause physicians to hesitate to use hysteroscopy as a frontline diagnostic agent when there are a number of other modalities usually adequate for assessing the uterine cavity. If a diagnostic question persists, the use of hysteroscopy after endometrial biopsy, sonogram, or D&C is more reasonable. Situations in which a tissue diagnosis has been made and is negative for carcinoma are clearly appropriate for hysteroscopic treatment. Currently, any treatment of known carcinoma without hysterectomy and utilizing hysteroscopy should be considered experimental and be made available to the literature to increase the data available.

REFERENCES

1. Pantaleoni DC. On endoscopic examination of the cavity of the womb. *Med Press Circ.* 1869;8:26.

2. Giusa-Chiferi MG, Goncalves WJ, Baracat EC, et al. Transvaginal ultrasound, uterine biopsy and hysteroscopy for postmenopausal bleeding. *Int J Gynecol Obstet.* 1996;55:39–44.

3. Danero S, Ricci MG, La Rosa R, et al. Critical review of dilation and curettage in the diagnosis of malignant pathology of the endometrium. *Curr J Gynecol Oncol.* 1986;7:162–164.

4. O'Connell LP, Fries MH, Zeringue E, et al. Triage of abnormal postmenopausal bleeding: a comparison of endometrial biopsy and transvaginal sonohysterography versus fractional curettage with hysteroscopy. *Am J Obstet Gynecol.* 1998;178:956–961.

5. Loffer FD. Hysteroscopy with selective endometrial sampling compared with D&C for abnormal uterine bleeding: the value of a negative hysteroscopic view. *Obstet Gynecol.* 1989;73:16–20.

6. Ben-Yehuda OM, Kim YB, Leuchter RS. Does hysteroscopy improve upon the sensitivity of dilatation and curettage in the diagnosis of endometrial hyperplasia or carcinoma? *Gynecol Oncol.* 1998;68:4–7.

7. Epstein E, Ramirez A, Skoog L, et al. Dilatation and curettage fails to detect most focal lesions in the uterine cavity in women with postmenopausal bleeding. *Acta Obstet Gynecol Scand.* 2001;80:1131–1136.

8. Goldstein SR, Nachtigall M, Snyder JR, et al. Endometrial assessment of vaginal ultrasonography before endometrial sampling in patients with postmenopausal bleeding. *Am J Obstet Gynecol.* 1990;163:119–123.

9. Stovall TG, Photopulos GJ, Poston WM, et al. Pipelle endometrial sampling in patients with known endometrial carcinoma. *Obstet Gynecol.* 1991;77:954–956.

10. Triolo O, Antico F, Palmara V, et al. Hysteroscopic findings of endometrial carcinoma: evaluation of 104 cases. *Eur J Gynaecol Oncol.* 2005;26:434–436.

11. Litta P, Merlin F, Saccardi C, et al. Role of hysteroscopy with endometrial biopsy to rule out endometrial cancer in postmenopausal women with abnormal uterine bleeding. *Maturitas.* 2005;50:117–123.

12. Marchetti M, Litta P, Lanze P, et al. The role of hysteroscopy in early diagnosis of endometrial cancer. *Eur J Gynaecol Oncol.* 2002;23:151–153.

13. Iossa A, Cianferoni L, Ciatto S, et al. Hysterosocpy and endometrial cancer diagnosis: a review of 2007 consecutive examinations in self-referred patients. *Tumori.* 1991;77:479–483.

14. Birinyi L, Darago P, Torok P, et al. Predictive value of hysteroscopic examination in intrauterine abnormalities. *Eur J Obstet Gynecol.* 2004;115:75–79.

15. Garuti G, Sambruni I, Colonnelli M, et al. Accuracy of hysteroscopy in predicting histopathology of endometrium in 1500 women. *J Am Assoc Gynecol Laparosc.* 2001;8:207–213.

16. Clark TJ, Voit D, Gupta JK, et al. Accuracy of hysteroscopy in the diagnosis of endometrial cancer and hyperplasia. *JAMA.* 2002;288:1610–1621.

17. Nagele F, Wieser F, Deery A, et al. Endometrial cell dissemination at diagnostic hysteroscopy: a prospective randomized cross-over comparison of normal saline and carbon dioxide uterine distension. *Hum Reprod.* 1999;14:2739–2742.

18. Lo KWK, Cheung TH, Yim, SF, et al. Hysteroscopic dissemination of endometrial carcinoma using carbon dioxide and normal saline: a retrospective study. *Gynecol Oncol.* 2002;84:394–398.

19. Creasman WT, Morrow CP, Bundy BN, et al. Surgical pathologic spread patterns of endometrial cancer. *Cancer.* 1987;60:2035–2041.

20. Gy M, Shi W, Barakat RR, et al. Peritoneal washings in endometrial carcinoma. *Acta Cytol.* 2000;44:783–789.

21. Romano S, Shimoni Y, Muralee D, et al. Retrograde seeding of endometrial carcinoma during hysteroscopy. *Gynecol Oncol.* 1992;44:116–118.

22. Egarter C, Krestan C, Kurz C. Abdominal dissemination of malignant cells with hysteroscopy. *Gynecol Oncol.* 1996;63:143–144.

23. Rose PG, Mendelsohn G, Kornbluth I. Hysteroscopic dissemination of endometrial carcinoma. *Gynecol Oncol.* 1998;71:145–146.

24. Alcazar JL, Errasti T, Zornoza A. Saline infusion sonohysterography in endometrial cancer: assessment of malignant cells dissemination risk. *Acta Obstet Gynecol Scand.* 200;79:321–322.

25. Leveque J, Goyat F, Dugast J, et al. Value of peritoneal cytology after hysteroscopy in surgical stage I adenocarcinoma of the endometrium. *Oncol Rep.* 1998;5:712–715.

26. Zerbe MJ, Zhang J, Bristow RE, et al. Retrograde seeding of malignant cells during hysteroscopy in presumed early endometrial cancer. *Gynecol Oncol.* 2000;79:55–58.

27. Obermair A, Geramou M, Gucer F, et al. Does hysteroscopy facilitate tumor cell dissemination? *Cancer.* 2000;88:139–143.

28. Bradley WH, Boente MP, Brooker D, et al. Hysteroscopy and cytology in endometrial cancer. *Obstet Gynecol.* 2004;104:1030–1033.

29. Gutman G, Almog B, Lessing JB, et al. Diagnosis of endometrial cancer by hysteroscopy does not increase the risk for microscopic extrauterine spread in early-stage disease. *Gynecol Surg.* 2005;2:21–23.

30. Selvaggi L, Cormio G, Ceci O, et al. Hysteroscopy does not increase the risk of microscopic extrauterine spread in endometrial carcinoma. *Int J Gynecol Cancer.* 2003;13:223–227.

31. Gu M, Shi W, Huang J, et al. Association between initial diagnostic procedure and hysteroscopy and abnormal peritoneal washings in patients with endometrial carcinoma. *Cancer Cytol.* 2000;90:143–147.

32. Biewenga P, de Blok S, Birnie E. Does diagnostic hysteroscopy in patients with stage I endometrial carcinoma cause positive peritoneal washings? *Gynecol Oncol.* 2004;93:194–198.

33. Kadar N, Homesley H, Malfetano J. Positive peritoneal cytology is an adverse risk factor in endometrial carcinoma only if there is other evidence of extrauterine disease. *Gynecol Oncol.* 1992;46:145–149.

34. Lee CM, Slomovitz BM, Greer M, et al. Practice patterns of SGO members for IIIA endometrial cancer. *Gynecol Oncol.* 2005;98:77–83.

35. Kudela M, Pilka R. Is there a real risk in patients with endometrial carcinoma undergoing diagnostic hysteroscopy? *Eur J Gynaecol Oncol.* 2001;22:342–344.

36. Arikan G, Reich O, Weiss U, et al. Are endometrial carcinoma cells disseminated at hysteroscopy functionally viable? *Gynecol Oncol.* 2001;83:221–226.

37. Obermair A, Geramou M, Gucer F, et al. Impact of hysteroscopy on disease-free survival in clinically stage I endometrial cancer patients. *Int J Gynecol Cancer.* 2000;10:275–279.

38. Gücer F, Tamussino K, Reich O, et al. Two-year follow up of patients with endometrial carcinoma after preoperative fluid hysteroscopy. *Int J Gynecol Cancer.* 1998;8:476–480.

39. Montz FJ, Bristow RE, Bovicelli A, et al. Intrauterine proges-terone treatment of early endometrial cancer. *Am J Obstet Gynecol.* 2002;186:651–657.

40. Kung FT, Chen WJ, Chou HH, Ko SF, et al. Conservative man-agement of early endometrial adenocarcinoma with repeat curet-tage and hormone therapy under assistance of hysteroscopy and laparoscopy. *Hum Reprod.* 1997;12:1649–1653.

41. Mazzon I, Corrado G, Morricone D, et al. Reproductive preser-vation for treatment of stage IA endometrial cancer in a young woman: hysteroscopic resection. *Int J Gynecol Cancer.* 2005;15:974–978.

25 | OVERVIEW OF COMPLICATIONS

Camran Nezhat, Farr Nezhat, and Ceana Nezhat

Despite the degree of caution used, complications occur during operative laparoscopy. Because sequelae can result from even relatively easy procedures, a surgeon must be able to recognize them promptly and carry out proper management. The risks increase with the complexity of the procedure, the relative inexperience of the surgeon, and the amount of deviation from standard technique. As laparoscopic operations become more complex, the ability to handle them endoscopically becomes important.

Diagnostic laparoscopy and laparoscopic tubal sterilization involve few risks. The rate of intraoperative and postoperative complications is less than 1% (Table 25.1). Most reports are from large practices with experienced gynecologists [1], surveys of American Association of Gynecologic Laparoscopists (AAGL) members [2–6], and tertiary referral clinics.[7]

The intraoperative and postoperative complication rates in 361 women who underwent laparoscopic hysterectomy for benign pathologic conditions were evaluated.[8] The overall complication rate for hysterectomy carried out by laparoscopy was 11.1%. Most of the complications were minor, including cystitis (1.66%), transient high fever (1.39%), abdominal wall ecchymosis (1.12%), and pneumonia and bronchitis (1.12%). There was no correlation between the type of laparoscopic hysterectomy and the complication rate. Complication rates associated with laparoscopic hysterectomy compare favorably with published complication rates for vaginal and abdominal hysterectomy.[9]

Although most gynecologists are taught traditional operations under supervision during residency, advanced laparoscopic procedures often are learned in clinical practice. The learning curve for laparoscopic operations is lengthy. The risk of complications is greatest early in a surgeon's experience and increases when new techniques or equipment is utilized. In 17,521 diagnostic and operative procedures done at seven centers, a complication rate of 3.2 per 1000 was found (Table 25.2).[10] The rate for diagnostic and minor procedures was 1.1 per 1000, and it was 5.2 per 1000 for major and advanced operations. Laparotomies were done for hemorrhage in 17 instances and for visceral injuries in 40 patients. One fatality was reported. Three national surveys conducted in The Netherlands [11], France [12], and Finland [13] included, respectively, 25,764, 29,966, and 70,607 laparoscopic procedures. The total complication rates were 5.7 [11], 4.6 [12], and 3.613 per 1000 procedures. Laparotomy was needed in 3.3 per 1000 operations.

PREVENTION

Avoiding complications is the best form of prevention. Thorough preoperative evaluation, consultation, and proper patient selection help lessen the possibility of injury and subsequent legal action. A successful operation depends on the gynecologist's familiarity with normal and abnormal anatomy, a thorough evaluation of abnormal findings, meticulous dissection and vaporization, familiarity with instruments and energy sources, training under the supervision of a qualified surgeon, and a properly trained operation room (OR) staff and assistant.

Soderstrom and Butler [14] reported that the complication rate for laparoscopic sterilization was highest among physicians who had done fewer than 100 procedures. It requires 4 to 7 years to gain adequate laparoscopic skills by doing several procedures each week with gradually increasing levels of complexity.[15]

CONTRAINDICATIONS

In some patients, laparoscopy may not be appropriate (Table 25.3). However, improvement in laparoscopic skills and experience, combined with the availability of the proper instruments, has reduced the number of conditions that were previously considered absolute contraindications for laparoscopy to relative contraindications. These conditions include obesity [16,17], severe adhesions [18], previous abdominal operations [19], cancer [20–22], abdominal hernia [23], pregnancy [24,25], hypovolemic shock [26], and bowel perforation with generalized peritonitis.[27–29]

In patients who have generalized peritonitis, the bowel frequently is matted and adherent to the abdominal wall. However, laparoscopic treatment of generalized peritonitis secondary to perforated sigmoid diverticulitis has been a safe alternative to conventional operations.[27] Laparoscopy was found to be safe and effective in the diagnosis and treatment of patients with peritonitis.[28] Laparoscopic treatment was practical in a patient who had an appendicular and gastroduodenal perforation.[29] Hemoperitoneum in an unstable patient has been considered a contraindication because the bleeding source may be difficult to find and treat laparoscopically. However, laparoscopy offers many theoretical advantages for the immediate diagnosis and management of a patient presenting with hemodynamic instability and suspected active intra-abdominal bleeding caused by an ectopic pregnancy.[26] These features include superior observation of the entire abdominal cavity, decreased intra-abdominal bleeding because of compression by the creation of a pneumoperitoneum, and ability to control the source of bleeding effectively with minimal tissue damage. Thus, it seems appropriate, when an optimal setup is available, to diagnose and treat suspected intra-abdominal bleeding caused by ectopic pregnancies or a bleeding hemorrhagic corpus luteum.

Table 25.1: Major Complications per 1000 Operative Laparoscopy Procedures

Intestinal	1.1–2.6
Bladder	0.2–1.7
Ureteral	0.1–1.4
Vascular	0.4–2.5
Laparotomy	3.3

Sources: Jansen et al.,[11] Chapron et al.,[12] Harkkl-Stren and Kurki.[13]

Intestinal obstruction and bowel distention are associated with an increased risk of perforation. Although laparoscopy is less invasive than laparotomy and often is the better of the two approaches, bowel obstruction not relieved by conservative decompression techniques may require laparotomy.

Patients with class IV cardiac disease have a high risk of cardiac arrhythmias and failure as a result of Trendelenburg positioning, even for relatively short procedures. Anesthesia for laparoscopic cholecystectomy may be achieved safely in elderly American Society of Anesthesiology (ASA) class III patients with increased cardiac risk.[30] Laparoscopic cholecystectomy appears to be safer than open cholecystectomy in all eligible patients, especially elderly individuals and patients in higher ASA classes.[31,32]

PROCEDURAL FAILURES

It is better to complete a procedure by laparotomy than to risk injury to the patient or be forced to proceed with an emergency laparotomy because of a complication. This deviation from the surgical plan raises concerns about the adequacy of the presurgical evaluation, the patient's consent, and the surgeon's skill.

The possibility of complications is increased during the insertion of the Veress needle and primary and secondary trocars in patients with multiple previous laparotomies, those with a body mass index >30, and very thin patients. Bowel preparation is recommended if there is a risk of bowel injury. Veress needle and trocar insertion is modified in the presence of a large pelvic mass.

The most critical point of laparoscopy is abdominal cavity entry of the Veress needle and the primary and secondary trocars. In a series of 2324 laparoscopies, there were more complications

Table 25.2: Complications of Gynecologic Laparoscopy

Laparoscopic Procedures	No. of Procedures	Laparotomies for Complications	Rate/100
Diagnostic	4130	7	1.7
Minor	4213	2	0.5
Major extensive adhesiolysis	1910	16	8.4
Other	6370	24	3.8
Advanced	898	8	8.9

Table 25.3: Relative Contraindications to Laparoscopy

Generalized peritonitis

Hypovolemic shock

Intestinal obstruction

Class IV cardiac disease

Large pelvic or abdominal mass

Pelvic abscess

Multiple prior abdominal surgical procedures

Diaphragmatio hernia

Chronic pulmonary disease

Extremes of body weight

from Veress needle and trocar insertion than from the actual operative procedures.[33] Another study suggested that about half the complications occur during the insertion of the Veress needle and laparoscopic trocars.[34]

The frequency of adhesions between the abdominal wall and the underlying omentum and bowel was assessed in 360 women undergoing operative laparoscopy after a previous laparotomy.[35] Patients with prior midline incisions had more adhesions than did those with prior Pfannenstiel incisions. Patients with midline incisions carried out for gynecologic indications had more adhesions than did those with all types of incisions done for obstetric indications. Adhesions to the bowel were more common after midline incisions above the umbilicus. Twenty-one women had direct injury to adherent omentum and bowel during the laparoscopic procedure. Intra-abdominal adhesions between the abdominal scar and the underlying viscera are a common consequence of laparotomy. When patients undergo laparoscopy after a previous laparotomy, the presence of adhesions between the old scar and the bowel and omentum must be considered.

Veress Needle

Intra-abdominal placement of the Veress needle is required to establish a pneumoperitoneum. Because the Veress needle is inserted "blindly," it can enter inappropriate spaces or puncture organs. Further instillation of CO_2 under pressure through the Veress needle can create serious complications.

Prevention

Factors increasing the risk of perforation or laceration include bowel adhesions; lateral displacement of the needle during its insertion; too steep an insertion angle; and uncontrolled, sudden entry. The patient must be in a horizontal position so the sacral promontory and sacral curve are identified easily. A premature Trendelenburg position should be avoided.

When an upper abdominal site is used to establish a pneumoperitoneum, the needle can puncture the pleural cavity, stomach, liver, or spleen. The stomach becomes distended after prolonged manual ventilation with a mask or when endotracheal intubation is difficult. The stomach can be punctured even with

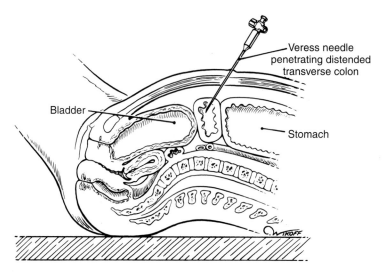

Figure 25.1. A distended stomach can displace the transverse colon toward the lower abdomen, increasing the possibility of puncture of the colon.

umbilical placement of the Veress needle. A distended stomach displaces the transverse colon toward the lower abdomen and increases the probability of an intestinal puncture (Figure 25.1). A nasogastric tube lessens the risk of gastric distention. An overdistended bladder also is at risk for injury. Routine placement of a Foley catheter before the procedure should eliminate the risk of inadvertent vesical injury.

Recognition

Veress needle injuries generally are not apparent until CO_2 insufflation or after the insertion of the laparoscope. Abnormally high insufflation pressures are encountered if the needle is misplaced. During the initial examination of the pelvis, one should survey the middle and upper abdomen for signs of needle-induced trauma, such as hematomas, needle trauma, and collections of gas.

Management

Puncture of a hollow viscus with the Veress needle generally requires examination of the puncture site to look for a bleeding vessel or leakage from the viscus. If the needle punctures the viscus, repair is indicated. The route of repair depends on the organ involved (small or large bowel, bladder, stomach, or major blood vessels), the nature of the leaking fluid, and the operator's skill. Many injuries require immediate laparotomy for repair and copious irrigation of the abdomen, whereas some surgeons can repair injuries laparoscopically. Postoperatively, the patient is instructed to call the physician if there is increasing abdominal pain or fever.

Establishing a Pneumoperitoneum

Complications developing as a result of insufflating a space other than the abdominal cavity vary, depending on the perforated structure and the amount of CO_2 instilled.

Prevention

Placement of a Foley catheter preoperatively virtually eliminates the risk of a vesical injury. Aspiration facilitates early recog-

nition of stomach or bowel penetration, but this method is fallible. Stomach or bowel insufflation is suspected if there is asymmetric abdominal distention, belching, or passing of flatus. If these signs develop, the gas is allowed to escape. Once a proper pneumoperi-toneum is established, the laparoscope is inserted and the suspected perforation site is examined.

If a large vessel entry is not noticed on insertion of the Veress needle, intravascular insufflation with CO_2 may lead to a gas embolism and even death.[36] This event usually occurs in patients with a previous abdominal or pelvic surgical history.[37] Transuterine insufflation is associated with a risk of gas embolism.[38] Gas embolism initially presents as cardiorespiratory distress with cardiac bradycardia or arrhythmia and an associated classic "mill wheel" murmur. Sudden bilateral mydriasis is the earliest neurologic sign.[37] Once it is recognized, the patient needs to be placed in the left lateral decubitus position for a possible immediate cardiac puncture to release the gas.[38]

Recognition

Signs of potential complications include elevated CO_2 filling pressures; continued liver dullness after the instillation of 1 L of CO_2; subcutaneous crepitation; belching or passing of flatus; asymmetric abdominal distention; hematuria or air bubbles in the Foley catheter line; a sudden drop in blood pressure, tachycardia, or cardiac arrest; and difficulty in ventilating the patient.

However, the absence of these signs does not confirm proper placement. Preperitoneal placement of the Veress needle with sufficient insufflation of CO_2 leads to the disappearance of liver dullness. If the Veress needle enters the bowel, the condition may not be recognized immediately because the bowel's large capacity allows low filling pressures. Even though the needle is placed correctly, the increased abdominal pressure and peritoneal irritation associated with the instillation of CO_2 can cause bradycardia and hypotension. These signs respond readily to supportive measures.

Treatment

When the initial flow rate or intra-abdominal pressure is high, elevating the abdominal wall can correct the placement of the needle, particularly if initially it was placed within the omentum. If the pressure does not fall immediately to normal levels, the needle is withdrawn and examined to confirm that the spring action of the device works properly and no tissue is occluding the tip. If a second placement attempt fails, consideration is given to insertion of the needle at another site, open laparoscopy, or direct trocar entry.

The most common extraperitoneal site insufflated is the preperitoneal space. If this is recognized early, the CO_2 line is disconnected and the gas is allowed to escape. The needle is removed and reinserted with attention to the "pop" that occurs as the needle pierces the peritoneum. If this is not recognized early and enough gas is instilled, the preperitoneal gas collection will be discovered after trocar placement and insertion of the laparoscope. The spiderweb appearance of the tissue becomes apparent, and gas is allowed to escape before the surgeon attempts to reinsert the needle. Preperitoneal insufflation can extend to the mediastinum and endanger cardiac function. If this occurs, the laparoscopy is stopped and the gas is allowed to escape.

Pneumo-omentum is a common, benign occurrence unless a vessel is lacerated. Omental trauma from the needle is associated with higher than normal filling pressures. Slight withdrawal of the needle or traction on the abdominal wall releases the omentum. Because this occurs frequently, the omentum and other structures in the path of the needle and trocars are examined at initial exploration of the pelvis to search for laceration of omental vessels. If a large vascular injury is missed on insertion of the Veress needle, intravascular insufflation with CO_2 can cause a gas embolism and mortality.

Primary Trocar Injuries

Punctures or lacerations of pelvic structures during trocar insertion are potentially serious because of the large diameters of trocars.

Prevention

An adequate pneumoperitoneum provides a safe distance between the anterior abdominal wall and the pelvic viscera, but trocar injuries can result from poor technique or adherent bowel (Figure 25.2).[39] Excessive force while inserting the trocar can be caused by an inadequate umbilical incision, scar tissue, or a dull trocar. Uncontrolled sudden entry of the trocar, its lateral displacement during insertion, and too steep an angle for placement increase the risk of injury. Even with meticulous technique, abdominal wall bleeding, hollow viscus perforation, blood vessel laceration, and liver and spleen injury can occur. The use of a minilaparoscope allows the gynecologist to observe and carry out adhesiolysis at the entry site before the insertion of an umbilical cannula. Minilaparoscopy reduced serious vascular or visceral injury from the insertion of the primary cannula in patients who had had previous pelvic and abdominal operations.[40]

The trocar should be sharp to penetrate muscle and fascia. Establishing a large pneumoperitoneum and elevating the abdominal wall to increase the distance between the abdominal

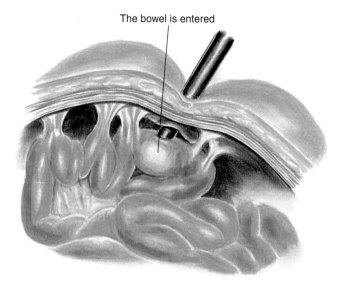

The bowel is entered

Figure 25.2. The trocar has penetrated the adherent bowel.

wall and the viscera decreases the chance of intestinal and vascular injury. The syringe test can indicate the presence of adhesions. Nezhat and co-workers [41] showed that direct insertion of the umbilical trocar without prior pneumoperitoneum is safe. The benefits of direct trocar insertion have been demonstrated by several authors.[41–43] The operating time was reduced; in tubal ligations, there was less gas inflated and the duration of exposure of the patient to the gas and anesthesia was lessened.

Woolcott [44] reviewed the records of 6173 laparoscopies that used the technique of direct insertion of the umbilical trocar and insufflation of CO_2 under vision. He found that there were 4 perforating bowel injuries (0.06%) that required laparotomy (2 small intestine, 2 large intestine). Three of the 4 patients who had bowel injury had undergone prior abdominal operations and had midline vertical subumbilical incisions. There were no instances of major vascular injury or gas embolus necessitating operative or resuscitative measures. Woolcott concluded that bowel or vessel perforation rates (requiring laparotomy or resuscitation) were 1 in 1000 regardless of whether the method of gaining peritoneal access was the open (Hasson) technique, Veress needle insufflation, or direct trocar insertion. The latter method may reduce the risk of gas embolism by insufflating only after intraperitoneal replacement has been confirmed; it allows immediate recognition and rapid treatment of major blood vessel lacerations, which is crucial in reducing laparoscopy-associated mortality. A large retrospective French study [45] evaluated the incidence of serious trocar accidents in 103,852 laparoscopic operations involving almost 390,000 trocars. The results identified 7 perioperative deaths (mortality, 0.07 per 1000) arising almost exclusively from vascular injuries. The open insertion of the first trocar appeared to be the best means of preventing these accidents. Each method has advantages, disadvantages, and similar morbidity when done by experienced operators with appropriate indications.

The disposable trocar with its sharp tip and spring-loaded safety shield should allow a controlled entry but does not prevent injury to intra-abdominal structures.[46] No large-scale clinical trial has established its advantages, and the unexpected ease of insertion could result in accidental damage. One study compared patients treated in a nonrandomized design with either sharp cutting single-use trocars or cone-shaped noncutting reusable trocars.[47] The data suggested that patients treated with a sharp trocar tip had more trocar-related bleeding events at the insertion site in the abdominal wall than did those treated with the conic tip design. The relative risk of vessel injury was increased by the use of pyramidal-tipped trocars compared with conical-tipped trocars, especially when larger diameter trocars were used.[48]

The first trocar is inserted with the patient in a horizontal position because a premature Trendelenburg position can alter the relation of the sacral promontory and sacral hollow. The abdominal wall is elevated on both sides of the umbilicus with towel clips. As the trocar is inserted, it is advanced toward the sacral hollow to provide the greatest distance between the trocar tip and solid tissue. With this technique, the bowel slides away from the advancing trocar.

In an obese patient, the trocar is angled almost perpendicular to the skin so the distance among the sacral promontory, blood vessels, and trocar is large. In thin patients, the distance between the anterior abdominal wall and sacral promontory is small (Figure 25.3). The force required to introduce the trocar often is less than anticipated, so a controlled angle entry is essential.

In a prospective study [49] the cephalocaudal relationship among the umbilicus, aortic bifurcation, and iliac vessels was measured during laparoscopy in 97 patients. The distance from the aortic bifurcation relative to the umbilicus was assessed in both the supine and Trendelenburg positions with a marked suction–irrigator probe. Patients were stratified into three groups on the basis of body mass index (kg/m^2). The position of the aortic bifurcation ranged from 5 cm cephalad to 3 cm caudal to the umbilicus in the supine position and from 3 cm cephalad to 3 cm caudal in the Trendelenburg position. In the supine position, the aortic bifurcation was located caudal to the umbilicus in only 11% of patients compared with 33% in the Trendelenburg position. This difference was significant for the total study population and for the nonoverweight group. In both positions, no correlation was found between the distance from the aortic bifurcation to the umbilicus and body mass index. Mean $\pm$ SI distance of the aortic bifurcation from the umbilicus in the supine position was 0.1 $\pm$ 1.2 cm for the nonoverweight group, 0.7 $\pm$ 1.5 cm for the overweight group, and 1.2 $\pm$ 1.5 cm for the very overweight group. Respective values in the Trendelenburg position were 1.0 $\pm$ 1.1, –0.4 $\pm$ 1.2, and –0.2 $\pm$ 1.3 cm. The common iliac artery was caudal to the umbilicus in four women. The space between common iliac arteries always was occupied, at least partly, by the left common iliac vein and was filled completely in 19 women (28%). The cephalocaudal relationship between the aortic bifurcation and the umbilicus varies widely and is not related to body mass index in anesthetized patients. Regardless of body mass index, the aortic bifurcation more likely is located caudal to the umbilicus in the Trendelenburg position compared with the supine position. The presumed location of the aortic bifurcation can be misleading during Veress needle or primary cannula insertion, and a more reliable guide is necessary for this procedure to avoid major retroperitoneal vascular injury.

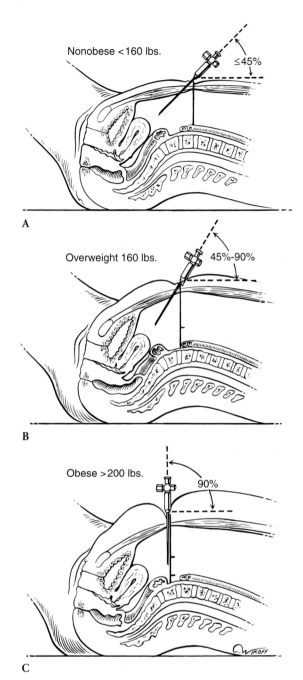

Figure 25.3. Angles of the Veress needle and umbilical insertion of the trocar. (**A**) Nonobese patient. (**B**) Overweight patient. (**C**) Obese patient.

A distended bowel increases the risk of trocar injury. This condition can be iatrogenic, resulting from intraluminal placement of the Veress needle. The surgeon may be unaware of this complication because the filling pressure of the small bowel is the same as that of the abdominal cavity.

Recognition

When the trocar is removed, signs of complications requiring immediate evaluation are bleeding from the trocar sleeve or a fecal odor. Insertion of the laparoscope allows assessment of the injury.

If the laparoscope enters the bowel lumen, the instrument is left in place to prevent the escape of bowel contents and to help locate the injury (Figure 25.2). In the presence of excessive bleeding, immediate laparotomy is indicated.

Treatment

See "Bleeding" and "Bowel Injuries," below.

Accessory Trocar Injuries

Prevention

Intra-abdominal injury is less likely to occur during insertion of accessory trocars because they are inserted under direct observation. The structures most frequently injured are the inferior epigastric vessels that run lateral to the rectus muscles.[11] The most common complication of multipuncture operative laparoscopy is inferior epigastric vessel injury. Two methods are utilized to avoid injuring these vessels. First, the position of the superficial vessels often can be ascertained with transillumination of the abdominal wall, particularly in thin women. Second, the courses of the inferior epigastric vessels are seen through the parietal peritoneum laparoscopically. As the trocar is advanced through the abdominal wall, the direction of the trocar is altered to avoid laceration of those vessels.

Quint and colleagues [50] did a prospective study to ascertain the efficacy of transillumination for locating abdominal wall vessels before trocar placement during laparoscopy. They showed that in women of normal weight, a single vessel could be seen approximately 5 cm from the midline in >90% of the patients and a second vessel could be seen approximately 8 cm from the midline in 51%. The more medial vessels did not correlate with the course of the inferior epigastric vessels seen laparoscopically. The ability to see vessels was decreased significantly by the patients' weight but not by skin color. Superficial abdominal wall vessels were located by transillumination in most women of normal weight regardless of skin color, but this technique is less useful in overweight and obese women. However, the deep (inferior) epigastric vessels cannot be located effectively by transillumination, and other techniques should be used to minimize the risk of injury to those vessels.

Despite these safeguards, the inferior epigastric vessels can be injured intraoperatively. Inferior epigastric injury was the most common complication of laparoscopically assisted vaginal hysterectomy in an AAGL survey.[4] Retroperitoneal bleeding may spread and accumulate before it is recognized. Significant damage to large retroperitoneal blood vessels may not be apparent during laparoscopy.[51] This injury occurs mostly in thin patients and those who have had abdominal surgery or have lax abdominal walls.

Long procedures are associated with moving, dislocating, and enlarging the trocar sleeve. Inserting clamps and other instruments through accessory trocar incisions or enlargement of the incision to remove large tissue pieces can damage these vessels. The risk of complications increases if the trocar is not aimed toward the sacral hollow; it may go down the pelvic side wall or puncture the posterior peritoneum. In inserting the accessory trocars, sudden, uncontrolled entry or the use of excessive force can result in laceration of the bladder, uterus, or bowel.

Recognition

If a vessel is damaged, the surgeon may notice blood running down the cannula or the formation of an abdominal wall hematoma.[1] Trocar sleeves can tamponade bleeding from a small laceration that does not become apparent until the trocar sleeve is removed. Profuse bleeding from the incisional site or significant local swelling can be observed postoperatively.

Injuries to iliac vessels are associated with profuse hemorrhage or a rapidly enlarging retroperitoneal hematoma, both of which require immediate laparotomy. Retroperitoneal bleeding can spread and accumulate before it is recognized. This injury mostly occurs in thin patients, those who have had abdominal operations, and those with lax abdominal walls.

Uterine lacerations are not life-threatening, and the bleeding usually is controlled easily. Bladder injury can occur if that organ is displaced because of a previous laparotomy or if an accessory trocar is placed less than 4 cm above the pubic symphysis.

Management

Bleeding from an inferior epigastric artery can be controlled by sutures, electrocoagulation, or pressure. With the trocar in place, using 0 absorbable suture on a CT-1 needle, a figure-of-eight is placed on either side of the trocar. Alternatively, a straight needle can be passed transabdominally on the distal side of the trocar and pulled through the abdominal wall again, using laparoscopic forceps. The suture is tied within the trocar incision and buried beneath the skin (Figure 25.4A). The suture is removed within 24 hours postoperatively. Control of inferior epigastric artery hemorrhage caused by cannula injury from percutaneous transabdominal placement of polypropylene sutures allows the procedure to be completed with the cannula in place.[52] However, cutaneous necrosis requiring debridement and delayed primary closure may occur if the sutures are not removed less than 24 hours postoperatively. If these two methods fail to control bleeding, the trocar incision is extended and a grasping forceps is used to apply pressure to the inferior epigastric artery to help find the bleeding point. Sutures are applied. A blunt instrument placed through a contralateral accessory trocar can be used to apply pressure to the bleeding point. Bipolar forceps are applied at the source of the bleeding (Figure 25.4B). Finally, an expandable trocar can be placed and used to apply pressure at the site from the skin and parietal surfaces or the bleeding sites can be tied with Carter-Thomason, Valley, or J needles.

ANESTHESIA

Increased intra-abdominal pressures caused by the pneumoperitoneum, absorption of CO_2 gas or fluid, and the Trendelenburg position concern anesthesiologists. A vasovagal reaction and cardiac arrhythmias developing from CO_2 absorption are avoided by administering atropine preoperatively. Difficulties in ventilation result from a steep Trendelenburg position, high intra-abdominal pressures, and obesity. The risk of carbon monoxide (CO) poisoning caused by smoke generated by laser and bipolar electrosurgery

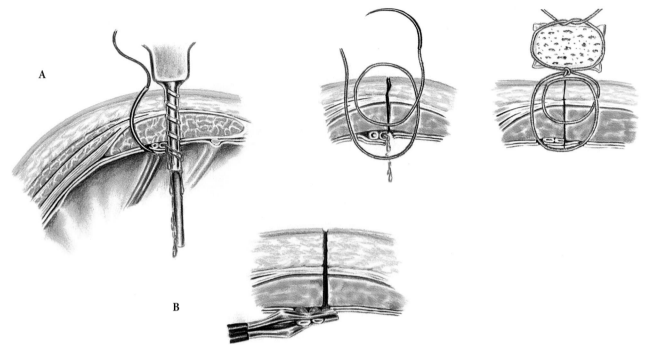

Figure 25.4. Methods to control bleeding from the inferior epigastric vessel. (**A**) A figure-of-eight suture is placed on either side of the trocar and tied above the incision. (**B**) Bipolar forceps is introduced through the opposite trocar sleeve, and the vessel is coagulated.

during prolonged laparoscopic operations was studied.[53] A decrease in carboxyhemoglobin concentrations was found intra-operatively. The carboxyhemoglobin level was increased at the end of the operation in one woman. In one patient, the levels exceeded 1% (1.33%), well below the human threshold tolerance level of 2%. CO poisoning is not associated with even prolonged laparoscopy. This observation was attributed to high-flow CO_2 insufflation and intensive evacuation of intra-abdominal smoke that minimize exposure to CO and active elimination of CO by controlled ventilation with high oxygen concentrations.

Fluid overload and high molecular weight dextran used as a distention medium for hysteroscopy are circumvented by accurately measuring input and output. Pulmonary edema is a rare complication of absorbing crystalloid irrigating fluid during laparoscopy.[54] Lavage with large volumes of room temperature irrigation fluid can be associated with hypothermia, so the fluid should be warmed or a heating blanket should be used. The use of warmed irrigation fluid decreased the drop in core temperature associated with laparoscopy.[55]

Reconditioning laparoscopic gas by filtering, heating, and hydrating the gas may reduce or eliminate laparoscopically induced hypothermia, shortening recovery room length of stay and reducing postoperative pain.[56] Warming the insufflation gas reduced the postoperative intraperitoneal cytokine response.[57] However, the heat-preserving effect of humidified gas insufflation during prolonged laparoscopic procedures has been questioned.[58]

Arrhythmias, including junctional rhythm, bradycardia, bigeminy, and asystole, have been associated with CO_2 insufflation of the abdomen. Bradycardia results from pressure on the peritoneum with an increased vagal response.

ELECTROSURGICAL INJURIES

Improper use of electrosurgery during a procedure, unfamiliarity with the equipment, and use of incompatible components contribute to many injuries. The first response to electrosurgical equipment failure should never be to increase the current. Because equipment malfunction is rarely the sole reason for injury, each component is checked systematically to localize the problem. Even properly functioning equipment can result in injury. Attempts to control a bleeding vessel with the bipolar forceps can damage nearby structures if the surgeon fails to identify them. Although some injuries are evident intraoperatively, others become clinically apparent postoperatively.

When unipolar current is used, the grounding pad must be applied. One should not use mixed trocars (half plastic and half metal) that will result in undesired capacitation and contribute to burns. Energy sources used without proper understanding and caution can cause significant vascular injury.[59]

BLEEDING

Uncontrolled bleeding and hemorrhage are the cause of most emergency laparotomies.[60,61] Bleeding occurs during sharp dissection of adhesions, transection of vessels during laser excision or dissection (the laser effectively coagulates very small vessels), uterosacral ablation, and rough handling of tissues. Lacerations of the oviduct, mesosalpinx, and infundibulopelvic ligament can bleed profusely. Distorted anatomy is an important compounding factor in many cases of major retroperitoneal vascular injury.[58]

When pressure gradients return to normal, bleeding into the retroperitoneal space may begin, eventually leading to hematoma and hypovolemic shock.[52] All exposed vessels should be evaluated at the end of the procedure with the patient supine and intra-abdominal pressure reduced. Blood clots in the pelvic side wall should be evacuated before complete hemostasis is confirmed.

An injury to the hypogastric artery was managed laparoscopically with bipolar electrodesiccation.[62] Those authors did 3 laparotomies to control bleeding after the treatment of dense adhesions in their first 2000 operations but only 1 in the last 5000. The adequacy and safety of laparoscopic control of major vessel bleeding should be investigated further, and consultation with a vascular surgeon should be considered in all cases.[59]

Unipolar and bipolar electrocoagulators, vasopressin, clips, sutures, and loop ligatures should be available to control bleeding. The choice of methods depends on the surgeon's preference. Pressure allows evacuation of blood and reduces blood loss until the necessary equipment is placed in the abdomen. Most bleeding is controlled with bipolar forceps. Fine bipolar forceps are employed near the fallopian tube to lessen thermal damage and subsequent adhesions.

UTERINE INJURIES

Complications involving the uterus include cervical lacerations or uterine perforation from sounding the uterus, and the use of a uterine dilator or uterine manipulator. Cervical lacerations are treated with pressure from a sponge stick or are sutured. Bleeding from uterine perforations is controlled with bipolar electrocoagulation or observed. Because a CO_2 laser beam can lacerate the uterine serosa, the uterus cannot be used as a backstop.

BLADDER INJURIES

Vesical injury is rare and occurs in patients who have had laparotomies [63] or whose bladders are not empty. Under these conditions, trocars, uterine anteverters, and blunt instruments can perforate or lacerate the bladder, and electrosurgery and lasers can cause thermal injury. Certain laparoscopic procedures increase the risk of vesical injury.

Prevention

The Veress needle can perforate a distended bladder. A misplaced Rubin's cannula can perforate the vagina and bladder with upward pressure.[64] Insertion of accessory trocars can injure a full bladder or one with distorted anatomy from a previous pelvic operation, endometriosis, or adhesions. Coagulation or laser ablation of endometriosis implants or adhesiolysis in the anterior cul-de-sac can predispose a patient to bladder injury unless hydrodissection or a backstop is used with the CO_2 laser. During laparoscopic hysterectomy (LH) or laparoscopically assisted vaginal hysterectomy (LAVH), the bladder can be lacerated or torn if blunt dissection is used to free it from the pubocervical fascia, particularly in women with prior cesarean delivery, severe endometriosis, or lower segment myomas. Also, a vesical injury can occur while entering and dissecting the space of Retzius before laparoscopic bladder neck suspension.

To prevent injuries, a Foley catheter is placed to drain the bladder. The position of the bladder should be assessed during the initial examination with the laparoscope. If the boundaries of the bladder are not clear, particularly when the pelvic anatomy is distorted, the bladder should be filled with 350 mL of normal saline to delineate its position. When one is doing an LH or LAVH, the assistant should push the uterus up during bladder dissection.

Recognition

Signs of intraoperative bladder injury include the following:

1. Air is seen in the urinary catheter and bag during insufflation.
2. The bladder appears to be pushed by the accessory trocar as the trocar is advanced through the abdominal wall.
3. Hematuria develops during the procedure.
4. Urine drainage is noted from the accessory trocar incision.
5. The amount of urine obtained during catheterization is less than anticipated.
6. Leakage of indigo carmine is seen from the injured site.
7. Suprapubic bruising.
8. Mass in the abdominal wall or pelvis.
9. Abdominal swelling.
10. Azotemia or peritonitis.

Because trocar injury often involves entry and exit punctures, locating both is important. Some bladder complications become apparent postoperatively, particularly those caused by electrocoagulation. If a vesical injury is suspected, a retrograde cystogram may reveal the defect.

Management

Small holes in the bladder generally heal without sequelae. Trocar injuries to the bladder dome require closure followed by urinary drainage for 5 to 7 days. Drainage promotes healing, encourages spontaneous closure, and reduces further complications. Lacerations may require a laparotomy, although some laparoscopists repair the laceration laparoscopically. Care should be used when doing an LH or LAVH, and the assistant should push the uterus up during bladder dissection.[8]

One report described the laparoscopic closure of intentional or unintentional bladder lacerations during operative laparoscopy in 19 women.[65] The defect was repaired laparoscopically in one layer using interrupted absorbable polyglycolic suture (17 patients) or polydioxanone suture (2 patients) and was followed by 7 to 14 days of transurethral drainage. Complications were limited to one vesicovaginal fistula that required reoperation. After 6 to 48 months of follow-up, all the patients were well with a good outcome. Because urinary bladder injury is one of the most common complications associated with LAVH, laparoscopists are becoming more familiar with laparoscopic management of urinary bladder injury.[66] An experienced laparoscopic surgeon may elect in selected cases of bladder injury to repair the laceration laparoscopically.

URETERAL INJURIES

Prevention

Knowledge of the ureter's path through the pelvis and the vulnerable points is the key to preventing injuries. The intrapelvic

Table 25.4: Laparoscopic Procedures Associated with Increased Risk of Ureteral Injury

Oophorectomy

Pelvic side wall adhesions

Presacral neurectomy

Endometriosis ablation

Severe bowel adhesions

Uterosacral nerve transection

Uterosacral plication

Hysterectomy

Vaginal cuff closure

Bladder neck suspension

segment of the ureter is near the broad ligament, ovaries, and uterosacral ligaments, and injuries occur in those areas (Table 25.4).[67] The ureter is at risk during laparoscopic surgery when the cardinal ligament is dissected and divided below the uterine vessels.[68] Endometriosis and severe pelvic adhesions can thicken the peritoneum, obscuring the location of the ureter, especially near the uterosacral ligaments.[69]

Laparoscopic placement of transmural sutures at the bladder neck also has been reported to lead to entrapment of the intramural portion of the ureter.[70] Ureteral injury can occur in the course of sharp dissection of an ovary adherent to the pelvic side wall; uterosacral transection; ligation, transection, and coagulation of the uterine arteries; removal of endometriotic implants or fibrosis from the ureter [71–73]; and attempts to control bleeding vessels.

To prevent such injuries, the ureter must be identified before irreversible action is taken. Precise and continuous attention to the location of the ureter will reduce the incidence of complications. Methods to protect the ureter include using hydrodissection and resecting affected peritoneum.[74] A small opening is made in the peritoneum, and 50 to 100 mL of lactated Ringer's solution is injected along the course of the ureter. This displaces it laterally, providing a plane for safe ablation of endometriotic implants, lysis of adhesions, or resection of involved peritoneum (Figure 25.5). Fluid absorbs laser energy and decreases the risk of thermal damage to underlying tissue.[75] This procedure is applicable if the peritoneum is not adherent to the underlying ureter. During uterosacral transection, a backstop is placed between the lateral aspect of the uterosacral ligament and the ureter. Before the bipolar forceps is used during an adnexectomy, the infundibulopelvic ligament is put under traction to identify the ureter and avoid thermal damage. No prospective study has substantiated the routine use of preoperative intravenous pyelography to prevent ureteral injury. In selected patients, it can help diagnose ureteral obstruction and allow appropriate surgical planning. In patients who have severe endometriosis and adhesions the ureters are difficult to see; ureteral catheters may be useful. Lighted ureteral catheters are available and are supposed to provide a visual road map of the ureter during laparoscopy.[76] The prophylactic use of ureteral catheters, including the use during laparoscopy of lighted catheters, is safe and technically simple. Ureteral catheters enhance identification of ureters and facilitate ureteral dissection.[77] However, prophylactic ureteral catheters did not reduce the rate of ureteral injury.[78] The routine use of ureteric catheters in laparoscopic hysterectomy may result in unnecessary complications.[79] As long as surgical techniques meticulously avoid ureteral injury, routine catheterization during laparoscopic hysterectomy is not warranted. Ureteral catheters are useful in some instances of severe endometriosis and adhesions.[69]

The gynecologist should note the ureter's course through the peritoneum. Endometriosis and severe pelvic adhesions can thicken the peritoneum, obscuring the location of the ureter, especially near the uterosacral ligaments. If the ureter is not identified clearly through the peritoneum, it must be located by retroperitoneal dissection. Using hydrodissection, a horizontal incision is made in the peritoneum midway between the ovary and the uterosacral ligament. The lower edge of the peritoneum is grasped and pulled medially. Blunt dissection with the suction–irrigator probe helps locate the ureter lateral to the peritoneum. If the peritoneum is involved with endometriosis and there is retroperitoneal fibrosis, the ureter can be attached to the peritoneum. The horizontal incision in the peritoneum is extended as necessary.

Until recently, most reported instances of ureteral injury during laparoscopic procedures involved electrocoagulation because that is the most reliable technique to arrest bleeding. As the use of stapling devices increases, additional injuries to the ureters are being reported.[80–82]

Nezhat and co-workers [69] reported six ureteral injuries. Four of the six injuries were intentional, occurring in the course of treating partial or complete obstruction. Unrecognized anomalies in ureteral location can predispose a patient to injury.[83]

Recognition

Early recognition intraoperatively is critical to successful treatment. Intraoperative ureteral damage is suspected if urine leakage or blood-tinged urine is noted or indigo carmine dye is seen intraperitoneally after its intravenous administration. When surgical procedures involve the ureter, postoperative ureteral patency is detected by cystoscopy, ureteral catheterization, or an intravenous retrograde pyelogram. Intraoperative recognition of these complications will minimize additional operations.[84] A technique using transvaginal color Doppler ultrasound has been described for postoperative detection of ureteral jets into the bladder when ureteral integrity is in question.[85] Stenting of the ureter or repair by laparotomy is indicated, but laparoscopic repair of partial- and full-thickness injuries is an option for some laparoscopists.[72,83] Unfortunately, a diagnosis of ureteral injury usually is made postoperatively by intravenous pyelography.[67] Fever, flank pain, peritonitis, and abdominal distention within 48 to 72 hours postoperatively should alert the clinician to possible ureteral injury. Leukocytosis and hematuria can be present. Some of the symptoms are present in patients who

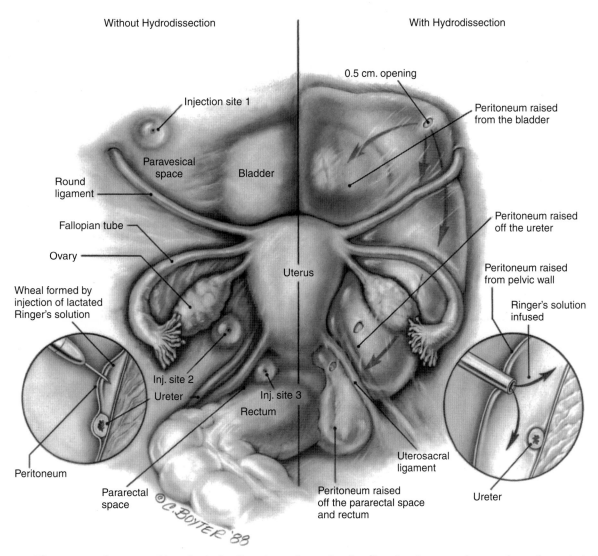

Without Hydrodissection

With Hydrodissection

0.5 cm. opening

Injection site 1

Peritoneum raised
from the bladder

Paravesical
space

Bladder

Round
ligament

Peritoneum raised
off the ureter

Fallopian tube

Peritoneum raised
from pelvic wall

Ovary

Uterus

Ringer's solution
infused

Wheal formed by
injection of lactated
Ringer's solution

Inj. site 2

Ureter

Inj. site 3

Rectum

Uterosacral
ligament

Peritoneum

Ureter

Pararectal
space

Peritoneum raised
off the pararectal space
and rectum

Figure 25.5. The ureter can be protected by using hydrodissection and resecting the affected peritoneum when treating endometriosis. The inset shows the forced injection of lactated Ringer's solution.

develop ileus or bowel injury so that an intravenous pyelogram (IVP) is important for diagnosis.

Management

Whether the discovery of ureteral complications is immediate or delayed, a urologist should be consulted. If the IVP indicates ureteral injury, initial therapy should involve attempts at retrograde or antegrade stenting. Therapeutic options by laparotomy include ureteroureterostomy and ureteroneocystostomy. Both require stenting and drainage with a ureteral catheter. There have been several reports of conservative and laparoscopic treatment of ureteral injuries.

Gomel and James [86] reported ureteral injury during needle electrosurgical ablation of the left uterosacral ligament. While they were examining the pelvic structures at the end of the procedure, a transverse laceration was found over the anterior aspect of the ureter, extending over more than one half of its circumference. Notably, the ureter was medial to the uterosacral ligament, a

significant variation from its normal lateral position. The edges of the laceration appeared healthy, with no blanching or irregularity. No leakage of blue-stained urine was observed after intravenous injection of methylene blue. A whistle-tip ureteral catheter was introduced through a cystoscope. The edges of the laceration were approximated with a single 4-0 plain catgut suture. Pelvic drainage was not employed, and the patient was given prophylactic antibiotics. Two weeks after the procedure, the stent was removed, and an IVP done 10 weeks postoperatively did not indicate ureteral dilation or stenosis.

A patient who had long-term ureteral obstruction caused by endometriosis needed an incidental partial resection of the ureter laparoscopically.[87]

The ureter's course was distorted by a 2-cm fibrotic nodule approximately 4 cm above the bladder, corresponding to the level of obstruction. Hydrodissection aided in entering the retroperitoneal space at the pelvic brim. The ureter was dissected with the CO_2 laser. Under cystoscopic guidance, a 7F ureteral catheter was passed through the ureterovesical junction. The catheter was advanced through the proximal portion of the ureter to the left renal pelvis. The edges of the ureter were approximated using four interrupted 4-0 polydioxanone sutures. The postoperative course was uncomplicated, and a postoperative IVP confirmed ureteral patency.

In one woman, during the treatment of severe pelvic wall endometriosis, a 1.5-cm segment of the ureter was unintentionally completely resected midway between the pelvic brim and the ureterosacral ligament.[72] After the location of the injury was identified by injecting indigo carmine intravenously, the 2 to 3 cm of the proximal and distal ureteral ends was freed from the periureteral attachments. The ends were approximated with a 4-0 polydioxanone suture (Ethicon), and a stay ureteral stent was introduced cystoscopically and passed through the proximal end of the injury into the renal pelvis.[23] The stent was secured outside and placed on continuous drainage. Repair was carried out by placing four 4-0 polydioxanone sutures at 12, 6, 9, and 3 o'clock. The lacerated edges were approximated. A Jackson-Pratt drain was inserted, and an indwelling Foley catheter was introduced into the bladder. The duration of the entire procedure was 3 hours, whereas the repair required 35 minutes. One gram of cefoxitin was given preoperatively and continued postoperatively until the patient was discharged from the hospital.

On the first postoperative day, there was no drainage from the Jackson-Pratt drain, and it was removed. No postoperative complications were noted. The patient remained afebrile with normal renal function tests and sterile urine. Although the ureteral stent stayed in place, the Foley catheter was removed. The patient was discharged on the second postoperative day and was prescribed prophylactic antibiotics (Septran DS; Burroughs Wellcome, Research Triangle Park, NC). Six weeks postoperatively, the ureteral catheter was removed, and no evidence of ureteral dilation or stenosis was seen. An IVP was normal.

Of the four patients who had partial resections of injured ureters, one occurred during separation of an adherent endometrioma from the pelvic side wall. The ureter was distorted, and despite retroperitoneal dissection, a 1-cm perforation was noted in the midpelvic area between the pelvic brim and the uterosacral ligament. After the ovary was removed, the ureter was freed and a stay ureteral stent was placed. The perforation was repaired with one 4-0 polydioxanone suture. No drainage was used. The patient was discharged the following day. The ureteral stent was removed 2 weeks later, after an IVP had confirmed that no leakage or stenosis was present. The other three patients had severe right pelvic side wall endometriosis with ureteral involvement, resulting in some degree of stenosis and hydroureter. The endometriosis and fibrosis were excised and removed, but ureteral resection was required. In two women, the ureter was repaired with two sutures. In one of them, the perforation was small. It was treated by inserting the stay ureteral stent for 2 weeks. No long-term complications were described by any of the six patients.

Therapeutic options with laparotomy include ureteroureterostomy and ureteroneocystostomy.[69] A patient who had a long-term ureteral obstruction caused by endometriosis needed an incidental partial resection of the ureter laparoscopically.[87] A laparoscopist familiar with delicate laparoscopic suturing can repair ureteral injuries laparoscopically with good results.[69,88]

SMALL BOWEL INJURIES

Small bowel injuries occur if the bowel is immobilized by adhesions.[15] The bowel can be injured during insertion of the Veress needle or trocar, bowel manipulation, or enterolysis. Electrosurgery and stray laser beams can result in unrecognized thermal injuries to the bowel. Injury to the gastrointestinal tract is a serious complication. Whether discovered intraoperatively or postoperatively, small bowel injuries may necessitate a laparotomy to avoid serious morbidity and even mortality.[3]

Prevention

Direct mechanical and electrical trauma can injure the gastrointestinal tract, but a consistent difference in injury pattern has been noted. The characteristics of each pattern distinguish between the two causes.[89] Thermal burns, sharp dissection, and needle punctures create most of these injuries.[90,91]

Intestinal lacerations occur with trocars, scissors, the laser, or electricity. The risk of injury is higher if adhesions are dense and tissue planes are poorly defined. Traction on the bowel with serrated graspers can cause abrasions and lacerations. An inadvertent small bowel biopsy specimen was taken during a hysteroscopic procedure, and the diagnosis of the tissue was made by the pathologist.[92]

Intestinal inspection after sharp dissection that shows bleeding or a hematoma should alert the operator to potential intestinal injury. Manipulation of the bowel from the pelvis with a blunt metal probe is done cautiously, and blunt dissection should be avoided. Intestines trapped in incisions as trocars are withdrawn increase the risk for small bowel obstruction.[93] Some laparoscopists recommend opening the valve of the umbilical trocar as it is withdrawn to prevent the creation of a vacuum that can draw the bowel into the incision. Using a Z-track insertion may eliminate this complication.[94]

Adhesions between the small bowel and the anterior abdominal wall are associated with a risk of trocar injury, especially in patients who have had a bowel resection or exploratory laparotomy for trauma. Women who undergo a second-look laparoscopy after treatment for ovarian carcinoma by laparotomy have adhesions from previous omentectomy and debulking.[95]

Despite the use of open laparoscopy, bowel lacerations can occur when the peritoneum is entered.[96] It is difficult to decide which patients should have an open laparoscopy. In one series, all 16 patients who had small bowel injuries also had had previous laparotomies and small bowel adhesions. Six were trocar injuries, 8 occurred during adhesiolysis, and 2 occurred during open laparoscopy. When a patient is at risk for bowel adhesions, it is prudent to prepare her with a mechanical and possibly antibiotic bowel preparation preoperatively.

Recognition

Electrical injuries to the intestine are not always apparent intraoperatively, or their appearance leads the surgeon to choose conservative management.[49] Most intestinal burns less than 5 mm in diameter can be treated expectantly. If the area of blanching on the intestinal serosa exceeds 5 mm, the extent of thermal damage will exceed the apparent damage, and therapy is instituted immediately. The actual area of injury can extend up to 5 cm from the apparent injury.[97] If the small bowel is lacerated by a trocar, the laparoscopist views the mucosal surface to search for leaking intestinal contents or a hematoma on the serosa.

If the small bowel injury is not recognized intraoperatively, the patient generally presents on the third or fourth postoperative day with lower abdominal pain, fever, nausea, and anorexia. By the fifth or sixth postoperative day, increases occur in abdominal pain, nausea, vomiting, fever, and white blood cell count.[97] Radiograms reveal multiple air and fluid levels or air under the diaphragm. An unusual postoperative presentation of laparoscopic bowel injuries that were not recognized intraoperatively was reported in four patients.[98] Those patients had severe pain in a single trocar site, abdominal distention, diarrhea, and leukopenia followed by acute cardiopulmonary collapse secondary to sepsis within 96 hours. Persistent focal pain in a trocar site with abdominal distention, diarrhea, and leukopenia can present with the symptoms and signs of an unrecognized perforation.

Management

Complications from small bowel injury are related to the extent of damage and the time that elapses before the damage is discovered. Sharp trocar wounds can be limited to the serosa or involve the entire wall. Small punctures or superficial lacerations seal readily and require no further treatment, assuming that careful inspection of the affected bowel reveals no leakage or bleeding. Small (<5 mm) superficial lacerations are inspected to assure that only the serosa is involved. These patients are treated conservatively and discharged the day of the operation with instructions to report any untoward reaction.

Patients who have obvious leakage require intervention and perhaps laparotomy. The intestine should be inspected on both sides to search for through-and-through injuries, especially injuries created by a trocar. If only one entry is found and repaired, peritonitis can develop postoperatively. If the laparoscope is inserted through the laceration and a laparotomy is done, the defect is identified and closed by a purse-string suture as the laparoscope is withdrawn to decrease peritoneal contamination.[99,100]

The small intestine is repaired in one or two layers by placing an initial row of interrupted sutures to approximate the mucosa and muscularis. A reinforcing layer of 3-0 silk Lembert sutures may be used to approximate the muscularis and serosal edges.[101] All lacerations are closed transversely to lessen the occurrence of stenosis of the bowel lumen. This closure is appropriate only if the laceration is less than one half the diameter of the bowel. When the laceration exceeds one half the diameter of the lumen, segmental resection and anastomosis are done. If the mesenteric blood supply is interrupted by the puncture, a resection is done regardless of the size or length of the laceration to maintain blood supply to that segment of bowel.[99]

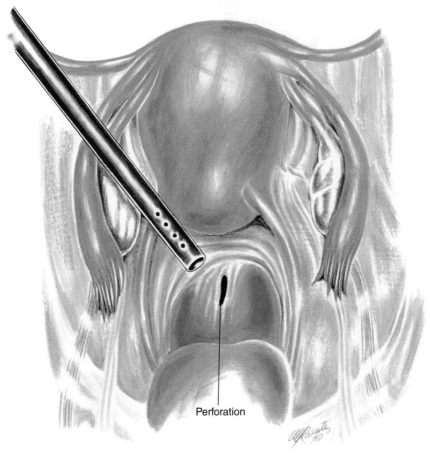

Perforation

A

Figure 25.6. (**A**) A small laceration is noted in the rectosigmoid. (*Continued*)

Intraoperative consultation with a general surgeon is appropriate whenever significant bowel trauma occurs. Small bowel injuries caused by trocars or the CO_2 laser can be repaired in one layer by using 3-0 silk or 4-0 polydioxanone without complication or laparotomy.[102] Injuries less than 2 cm (small or large bowel) may be repaired transversely or longitudinally; however, injuries more than 2 cm should be repaired transversely. Repair of bowel perforation should be done with intra-abdominal laparoscopic suturing (Figure 25.6A,B).

After repair of a bowel laceration, the entire abdomen is irrigated. A nasogastric tube may be placed and then removed when drainage has decreased, indicating that bowel function has resumed. The patient is not given anything by mouth until she passes flatus.

When possible bowel laceration becomes apparent after the patient has been discharged, conservative management is successful in patients who have not developed peritonitis. In-hospital management consists of hydration, nothing by mouth, and close observation with white blood cell count and physical examination every 6 hours. Wheeless [97] reported that over one half the patients treated conservatively required no surgical intervention. Patients whose condition deteriorated during observation underwent laparotomy and had no complications attributable to delayed surgery.

Immediate surgical intervention and possible laparotomy are indicated in patients who present with fever, severe abdominal pain, nausea, vomiting, obstipation, or peritonitis and those whose clinical condition worsens. Surgical considerations for managing bowel injuries that are discovered postoperatively differ somewhat from those for injuries discovered and managed intraoperatively. The damaged bowel must be repaired or resected. In addition, resection of all necrotic tissue in the pelvis is mandatory even if this requires a hysterectomy and bilateral salpingo-oophorectomy. If burned or necrotic tissue that has been bathed in intestinal contents, blood, or serum is not excised, a pelvic abscess will develop.[97]

Wheeless [97] presented a seven-point plan to manage patients with peritonitis secondary to bowel perforation:

1. Preoperative stabilization with fluids, electrolytes, and nasogastric suction
2. Exploratory laparotomy with repair or resection of the injured bowel
3. Resection of all necrotic tissue

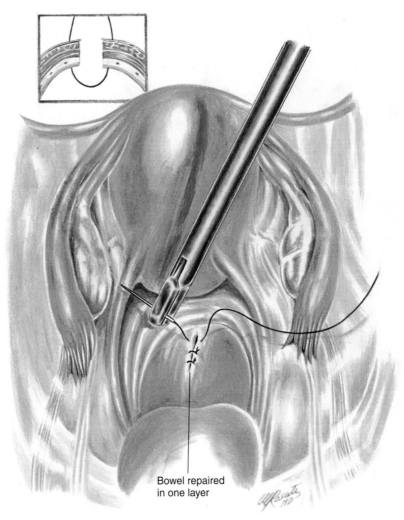

B

Figure 25.6. (*Continued*) (**B**) The bowel is repaired in one layer. The inset shows a through-and-through suture.

4. Copious and repeated saline lavage of the abdomen
5. Pelvic drainage through the vagina using a closed drainage system
6. Aggressive antibiotic therapy
7. Embolus prophylaxis with minidose heparin (5000 U three times daily).

In an AAGL membership poll, the two deaths reported from 36,928 procedures were attributed to bowel injuries. In one instance, the patient had extensive adhesions from the abdominal wall to the bowel. Although the bowel injury was recognized and repaired, the patient developed a persistent postoperative ileus and died of peritonitis. The second death was attributable to sepsis after an unrecognized small bowel perforation.[3]

LARGE BOWEL INJURIES

Colon entry is a major complication, particularly if the bowel is unprepared or the injury is not recognized. Even small perforations, such as those from the Veress needle, require attention because the high bacterial concentration of minor leaks can cause infection and abscess formation.

Prevention

Factors that contribute to an increased risk of large bowel injuries include (1) failure to establish an adequate pneumoperitoneum; (2) the use of dull trocars that require excessive force; (3) uncontrolled, sudden entry of sharp instruments; and (4) gastric distention. Poorly controlled or sudden trocar entry can result in rectosigmoid laceration. Gastric distention can displace the transverse colon toward the pelvis, where it can be punctured by the Veress needle or lacerated with the trocar. This complication can be eliminated by using a nasogastric tube intraoperatively.

The rectosigmoid can be injured if the depth of penetration by endometriosis domestriosis is underestimated or the cul-de-sac is obliterated. When the rectum is adherent to the posterior aspect of the cervix or uterosacral ligaments, blunt dissection may lacerate the rectum. Sharp dissection with scissors or the CO_2 laser is recommended. The combination of high-power superpulse or ultrapulse CO_2 laser and hydrodissection is relatively safe for working around the bowel.

When the cul-de-sac is dissected, identification of the vagina and rectum is facilitated by placing a probe or an assistant's finger in both the vagina and the rectum. Dissection should begin lateral to the uterosacral ligaments, where the anatomy is less distorted, and proceed toward the obliterated cul-de-sac.[103,104] Similarly, when a posterior culdotomy is done for tissue removal or during laparoscopic hysterectomy, correct identification of the vagina and rectum is important.[80,105]

When a difficult pelvic operation is contemplated, such as cul-de-sac nodularity in a patient with endometriosis or a history suggesting significant pelvic adhesions, preoperative bowel preparation is indicated.

Recognition

Perforation of the large bowel with the Veress needle sometimes can be recognized with the saline aspiration test; recovery of brownish fluid is pathognomonic. Fecal odor may be detected. If large bowel entry is suspected on the basis of these two tests, the needle should be withdrawn promptly and another sterile Veress needle should be reinserted. Once the laparoscope is inserted, the entry site should be sought and examined. Because of the high bacterial concentration, minor leaks of fecal material into the peritoneal cavity can be the source of serious infection. Intraoperative sigmoidoscopy is useful in identifying large bowel injury.[106] The "underwater" examination with sigmoidoscopy is recommended after the treatment of severe endometriosis and adhesions of the rectum and rectosigmoid colon.

Large bowel injuries can be serious because they may not be recognized at operation. Under these circumstances, the patient generally presents on the third or fourth postoperative day with lower abdominal pain, mild fever, slight nausea, and anorexia. By the fifth or sixth postoperative day, these symptoms progress to include fever, severe abdominal pain, nausea, vomiting, obstipation, increased white blood cell count, and peritonitis.[107]

Management

For small colonic wounds associated with minimal contamination, laparotomy with primary suture closure has been the accepted therapy. In addition, copious lavage of the peritoneal cavity, broad-spectrum antibiotics, and drainage minimize the risk of infection. Under the proper circumstances, a small wound to the colon may be closed through the laparoscope. This procedure was carried out in 25 of 26 large bowel injuries without complication.[108] Copious irrigation and antibiotic coverage are essential.

Electrical injury to the right colon is managed by resecting the injured segment and doing a primary anastomosis. Diverting ileostomy facilitates healing and reduces morbidity and mortality. Injury to the descending colon, sigmoid, or rectum in unprepared bowel is not amenable to primary closure or resection with primary anastomosis. Diverting colostomy with resection of the injured portion is recommended.

Colonic lacerations in prepared bowel can be repaired laparoscopically after excising endometriosis nodules and identifying the extent of the laceration. A single-layer repair using 4-0 silk, 4-0 polydioxanone, or 0 polyglactin sutures is done.

The knowledge that the bowel can be repaired successfully by laparoscopic techniques in a properly prepared patient should increase the confidence of a surgeon operating in the deep pelvis.

POSTOPERATIVE COMPLICATIONS

Bleeding

Hemostasis that appears adequate before closure because of the Trendelenburg position, high intra-abdominal pressures, and relative hypotension may change once the patient resumes an upright position. If the patient does not respond to intravenous hydration, a repeat hematocrit may suggest hemorrhage and a physical exam may reveal abdominal distention.

Of four instances of intra-abdominal bleeding,[1] one was caused by persistent ectopic pregnancy, two resulted from a blood disorder, and no source of bleeding was found for the fourth. Only two of these patients had a laparotomy. The patient with persistent ectopic pregnancy presented at another center with signs of intra-abdominal bleeding and underwent a laparotomy. She had a leaking, persistent ectopic pregnancy, which was removed. A patient who had storage pool disease presented with intra-abdominal bleeding 24 hours postoperatively. At laparoscopy, the source of bleeding was not located, and so a laparotomy was done. However, laparotomy failed to reveal the site. It was generalized oozing from the pelvic cavity. Postoperatively, she was treated with blood products and coagulation factors.

Nerve Injuries

Postoperative ilioinguinal neuralgia has been reported after laparoscopic ilioinguinal nerve damage caused by direct trauma from a secondary trocar placed in the right iliac fossa.[109] Neuropathy of the genitofemoral nerve may be differentiated from ilioinguinal neuralgia by diagnostic blocks and managed by laparoscopy.[110] Common postoperative neurologic syndromes include sciatic nerve injury, brachial palsy (shoulder-hand syndrome), and perineal nerve palsy. Allowing the buttocks to protrude too far off the end of the operating table may cause back injury.

Pain

Many patients still complain of moderate abdominal and shoulder pain during the first 48 to 72 hours postoperatively. Based on the theory of "dorsal horn hypersensitivity," several clinical trials have shown diminished pain with preincisional infiltration of a local anesthetic. Injection with 0.5% bupivacaine at the surgical site before incision and insertion of the trocars resulted in decreased postoperative pain.[111] Infiltrating bupivacaine at time of incision closure did not offer similar benefits in the control of pain postoperatively. Another study showed that pain is no better controlled with preincisional infiltration than with postincisional infiltration of bupivacaine.[112]

The beneficial effect of flushing 0.5% bupivacaine down the laparoscopy trocar over the peritoneal folds and into the abdominal wall after laparoscopy was small.[113] In women undergoing laparoscopic tubal sterilization with silastic bands, topical bupivacaine decreased postoperative pain compared with placebo.[114] The addition of periportal injection of bupivacaine at the level of the parietal peritoneum under direct vision was effective in reducing pain.[112] The CO_2 commonly used for insufflation is a peritoneal irritant. Intraoperatively, this irritation can manifest as a vasovagal reaction. Postoperatively, residual gas accumulates under the diaphragm when an upright position is maintained, thus irritating the diaphragm. The pain is referred to the shoulder by the phrenic nerve.

Warming the insufflation CO_2 gas reduces postoperative pain.[55,56] Complete removal of intra-abdominal CO_2 is difficult but may be facilitated by leaving the patient in the Trendelenburg position. Pressure exerted on the abdomen toward the symphysis allows the gas trapped in the lower abdomen to be expressed through the umbilical or suprapubic trocars. If pain develops, the patient can assume a supine position and use a pillow to elevate the lower abdomen, allowing gas to accumulate in the pelvis. The efficacy of intraperitoneal irrigation with a long-acting anesthetic into the subdiaphragmatic space after laparo-

scopic procedures reduced both the frequency and the intensity of postoperative shoulder-tip pain.[115,116] However, the effect tends to be transient and has little impact on the patient's convalescence.[117]

Infection

Urinary tract infections can be caused by instrumentation or asymptomatic bacteria. The use of advanced techniques such as laparoscopic Burch colposuspension using permanent surgical mesh can cause abscess formation.[118]

Postoperative infection is unusual after laparoscopic procedures, although the risk appears to be higher after prolonged, intricate procedures. Most infections are limited to skin or stitch abscesses and require incision and drainage. Occasionally, a pelvic infection occurs after a tubal operation, but it is not clear whether this is caused by a preexisting condition or contamination or is secondary to tissue destruction and necrosis. Urinary tract infections can be caused by instrumentation or asymptomatic bacteria.

Incisional Hernia

Herniation of the omentum or small bowel at the umbilical incision site has been reported with 5-mm or larger trocars. Patients at increased risk are those who are very thin (especially the elderly), those with chronic coughs, and those with a history of hernias. A survey of AAGL members revealed 933 hernias from an estimated 4,385,000 laparoscopic procedures, an incidence of 21 per 100,000.[119] Over two thirds of these patients underwent subsequent surgical repair. The average time to reoperation was 8.5 days in one report.[120]

Possible preventive measures, although not proven, include Z-track insertion, avoiding trocar insertion directly through the umbilicus, and careful withdrawal of the umbilical trocar. Incisional hernia was more common in patients treated with a sharp-tip cutting single-use trocar compared with a cone-shaped noncutting reusable trocar, an incidence of 1.83% compared with 0.17%, respectively.[44]

The use of instruments for the closure of subcutaneous tissue in laparoscopic sites is gaining popularity because of the risk of incisional hernia at trocar sites.[121] However, in the AAGL survey [119] almost one fifth of the reported hernias occurred despite fascial closure. In such situations, incisional hernia may be attributed to infection, premature suture disruption, or failure to approximate fascial wound edges adequately.[122]

Incisional hernias occur mostly in sites where trocars 10 mm in diameter or larger were used.[119,120] Among 5300 patients who underwent laparoscopy [123] 11 hernias occurred, an incidence of 0.2%. The 10-fold higher incidence of this complication compared with the AAGL survey was attributed to the more advanced and prolonged nature of the laparoscopic procedures in this study. Omentum herniated in 7, and bowel herniated in 4 others. In one patient, the sigmoid epiploica irreducibly herniated through the peritoneum, not the fascia. Six women required a laparoscopic operation to retract the entrapped omentum or bowel, and in 1 a laparoscopically assisted bowel resection was necessary. The hernias occurred through a 5-mm trocar incision site in half the women, so whenever extensive manipulation is done through a 5-mm trocar port that causes extension of the incision, these ports should be closed as is done with the 10-mm ports.

A subclinical hernia with adhesions between the peritoneal incision site and the bowel may place a patient at significant risk of bowel perforation if she requires another laparoscopy. Some gynecologists advocate removing the umbilical trocar under laparoscopic observation to avoid entrapment of the bowel or removing the trocar with the valve open to avoid negative pressure that could draw omentum or small bowel into the defect.

Vaginal Cuff Dehiscence

Vaginal vault rupture with intestinal herniation is a postoperative complication of total hysterectomy. It can occur spontaneously or postcoitally. Three women, ages 40 to 43 years, presented to the emergency room with bleeding and pain 2 to 5 months after total laparoscopic hysterectomy.[124] The small bowel was visible through the introitus or protruding into the vagina. One rupture occurred after vaginal intercourse, and the other two were spontaneous. Inspection of the bowel revealed no evidence of trauma. Two vaginal cuff repairs were completed transvaginally and one laparoscopically, all with interrupted sutures of 0 polydioxanone or polyglactin.

Mortality

The 1991 AAGL membership reported 1 death from 56,536 laparoscopic procedures, a low death rate of 1.8 per 100,000 procedures.[5] The 1993 AAGL membership reported 1 death from 22,966 sterilizations and none from 36,482 diagnostic procedures.[6] The death rates remained essentially unchanged in subsequent AAGL surveys.[4]

In a retrospective review of the literature and the authors' experience, data revealed 15 deaths in 501,779 laparoscopic procedures, a death rate of 3 per 100,000.[125] Surveys from France [12] and The Netherlands [11] revealed 3 deaths among 55,730 laparoscopic operations, a mortality rate of 5.4 per 100,000 procedures. However, in a Finnish national study of laparoscopic complications, no deaths were reported in connection with 70,607 gynecologic laparoscopies.[13]

Peterson and associates [126] identified 29 deaths (3.6 per 100,000) associated with tubal sterilization: 11 resulted from anesthesia, 7 from sepsis after unrecognized bowel injury, 4 from hemorrhage after major vessel laceration, and 3 from myocardial infarction; 4 were related to other causes. Some deaths might have been prevented by the use of endotracheal intubation for general anesthesia, safer use of unipolar coagulation or alternative techniques, and careful insertion of the Veress needle and trocar.

REFERENCES

1. Nezhat F, Nezhat C, Levy JS. A report of laparoscopic injuries and complications over a 10-year period. Paper presented at: 41st annual clinical meeting of the American College of Obstetricians and Gynecologists; January 3, 1993; Washington, DC.
2. Hulka JF, Levy BS, Luciano AA, et al. 1997 AAGL membership survey: practice profiles. *Am Assoc Gynecol Laparosc*. 1998;5:344.
3. Peterson HB, Hulka JF, Phillips JM. American Association of Gynecologic Laparoscopists' 1988 membership survey on operative laparoscopy. *J Reprod Med*. 1990;35:587.
4. Hulka JF, Levy BS, Parker WH, Phillips JM. Laparoscopic-assisted vaginal hysterectomy: American Association of Gynecologic Laparoscopists' 1995 membership survey. *J Am Assoc Gynecol Laparosc*. 1997;4:167.
5. Hulka JF, Peterson HB, Phillips JM, Surrey MW. Operative laparoscopy: American Association of Gynecologic Laparoscopists' 1991 membership survey. *J Reprod Med*. 1993;38:569.
6. Hulka JF, Phillips JM, Peterson HB, Surrey MW. Laparoscopic sterilization: American Association of Gynecologic Laparoscopists' 1993 membership survey. *J Am Assoc Gynecol Laparosc*. 1995;2:137.
7. Lehmann-Willenbrock E, Riedel HH, Mecke H, Semm K. Pelviscopy/laparoscopy and its complications in Germany 1949–1988. *J Reprod Med*. 1992;37:671.
8. Nezhat F, Nezhat CH, Admon D, et al. Complications and results of 361 hysterectomies performed at laparoscopy. *J Am Coll Surg*. 1995;180:307.
9. Reich H. Total laparoscopic hysterectomy: indications, techniques, and outcomes. *Curr Opin Obstet Gynecol*. 2007;19:337.
10. Querleu D, Chapron C, Chevallier L, Bruhat MA. Complications of gynecologic laparoscopic surgery—a French multicenter collaborative study (letter). *N Engl J Med*. 1993;328:1355.
11. Jansen FW, Kapiteyn K, Trimbos-Kemper T, et al. Complications of laparoscopy: a prospective multicentre observational study. *Br J Obstet Gynaecol*. 1997;104:595.
12. Chapron C, Querleu D, Bruhat MA, et al. Surgical complications of diagnostic and operative gynaecological laparoscopy: a series of 29,966 cases. *Hum Reprod*. 1998;13:867.
13. Harkki-Siren P, Kurki T. A nationwide analysis of laparoscopic complications. *Obstet Gynecol*. 1997;89:108.
14. Soderstrom RM, Butler JC. A critical evaluation of complications in laparoscopy. *J Reprod Med*. 1973;10:245.
15. Nezhat C, Nezhat F, Nezhat CH. Operative laparoscopy (minimally invasive surgery): state of the art. *J Gynecol Surg*. 1992;8:111.
16. Fried M, Peskova M, Kasalicky M. The role of laparoscopy in the treatment of morbid obesity. *Obes Surg*. 1998;8:520.
17. O' Hanlon KA, Dibble SL, Fisher DT. Total laparoscopic hysterectomy for uterine pathology: impact of bodymass index on outcomes. *Gynecol Oncol*. 2006;103:938.
18. Clough KB, Ladonne JM, Nos C, et al. Second look for ovarian cancer: laparoscopy or laparotomy?: a prospective comparative study. *Gynecol Oncol*. 1999;72:411.
19. Brill Al, Nezhat F, Nezhat CH, Nezhat C. The incidence of adhesions after prior laparotomy: a laparoscopic appraisal. *Obstet Gynecol*. 1995;85:269.
20. Amara DP, Nezhat C, Teng NN, et al. Operative laparoscopy in the management of ovarian cancer. *Surg Laparosc Endosc*. 1996;6:38.
21. Nezhat C, Seidman DS, Nezhat F, Nezhat CH. Laparoscopic surgery for gynecologic cancer. In: Szabo Z, Lewis JE, Fanini GA, eds. *Surgery Technology International IV*. San Francisco, CA: Universal Medical Press; 1995.
22. Chi DS, Curtin JP. Gynecologic cancer and laparoscopy. *Obstet Gynecol Clin North Am*. 1999;26:201.
23. Crawford DL, Phillips EH. Laparoscopic repair and groin hernia surgery. *Surg Clin North Am*. 1998;78:1047.
24. Nezhat FR, Tazuke S, Nezhat CH, et al. Laparoscopy during pregnancy: A literature review. *J Soc Laparoendosc Surg*. 1997;1:17.
25. Cohen-Kerem R, Railton C, Oren D. et al. Pregnancy outcome following non-obstetric surgical intervention. *Am J Surg*. 2005;190:467.

26. Soriano D, Yefet Y, Oelsner G, et al. Operative laparoscopy for management of ectopic pregnancy in patients with hypovolemic shock. *J Am Assoc Gynecol Laparosc.* 1997;4:363.

27. Rizk N, Barrat C, Faranda C, et al. Laparoscopic treatment of generalized peritonitis with diverticular perforation of the sigmoid colon: report of 10 cases. *Chirurgie.* 1998;123:358.

28. Pokala N, Sadhasivam S, Kiran RP, et al. Complicated appendicitis – is the laparoscopic approach appropriate? A comparative study with the open approach: outcome in a community hospital setting. *Am Surg.* 2007;73:737.

29. Cueto J, Diaz O, Garteiz D, et al. The efficacy of laparoscopic surgery in the diagnosis and treatment of peritonitis: experience with 107 cases in Mexico City. *Surg Endosc.* 1997;11:366.

30. Zollinger A, Krayer S, Singer T, et al. Haemodynamic effects of pneumoperitoneum in elderly patients with an increased cardiac risk. *Eur J Anaesthesiol.* 1997;14:266.

31. Carroll BJ, Chandra M, Phillips EH, Margulies DR. Laparoscopic cholecystectomy in critically ill cardiac patients. *Am Surg.* 1993;59:783.

32. Massie MT, Massic LB. Marrangoni AG, et al. Advantages of laparoscopic cholecystectomy in the elderly and in patients with high ASA classifications. *J Laparoendosc Surg.* 1993;3:467.

33. Bateman BG, Kolp LA, Hoeger K. Complications of laparoscopy—operative and diagnostic. *Fertil Steril.* 1996;66:30.

34. Mac Cordick C, Lecuru F, Rizk E, et al. Morbidity in laparoscopic gynecological surgery: results of a prospective single-center study. *Surg Endosc.* 1999;13:57.

35. Brill AI, Nezhat F, Nezhat CH, Nezhat C. The incidence of adhesions after prior laparotomy: a laparoscopic appraisal. *Obstet Gynecol.* 1995;85:269.

36. Servais D, Althoff H. Fatal carbon dioxide embolism as a complication of endoscopic interventions. *Chirurgie.* 1998;69:773.

37. Cottin V, Delafosse B, Viale JP. Gas embolism during laparoscopy: a report of seven cases in patients with previous abdominal surgical history. *Surg Endosc.* 1996;10:166.

38. Lantz PE, Smith JD. Fatal carbon dioxide embolism complicating attempted laparoscopic cholecystectomy—case report and literature review. *J Forensic Sci.* 1994;39:1468.

39. Vilos GA, Ternamian A, Dempster J et al. The Society of Obstetricians and Gynecologist of Canada. Laparoscopic entry: a review of techniques, technologies, and complications. *J Obstet Gynaecol Can.* 2007;29:433.

40. Lee PI, Chi YS, Chang YK, Joo KY. Minilaparoscopy to reduce complications from cannula insertion in patients with previous pelvic or abdominal surgery. *J Am Assoc Gynecol Laparosc.* 1999;6:91.

41. Nezhat FR, Silfen SL, Evans D, Nezhat C. Comparison of direct insertion of disposable and standard reusable laparoscopic trocars and previous pneumoperitoneum with Veress needle. *Obstet Gynecol.* 1991;78:148.

42. Agresta F, De Simone P, Ciardo LF, et al. Direct trocar insertion vs veress needle in nonobese patients undergoing laparoscopic procedures: a randomized prospective single-center study. *Surg Endosc.* 2004;18:1778.

43. Byron JW, Markenson G, Miyazawa K. A randomized comparison of Veress needle and direct trocar insertion for laparoscopy. *Surg Gynecol Obstet.* 1993;177:259.

44. Woolcott R. The safety of laparoscopy performed by direct trocar insertion and carbon dioxide insufflation under vision. *Aust N Z J Obstet Gynaecol.* 1997;37:216.

45. Champault G, Cazacu F, Taffinder N. Serious trocar accidents in laparoscopic surgery: a French survey of 103,852 operations. *Surg Laparosc Endosc.* 1996;6:367.

46. Bhroyrul S, Vierra MA, Nezhat CR et al. Trocar injuries in laparoscopic surgery. *J Am Coll Surg.* 2001;192:677.

47. Leibl BJ, Schmedt CG, Schwarz J, et al. Laparoscopic surgery complications associated with trocar tip design: review of literature and own results. *J Laparoendosc Adv Surg Tech.* 1999;9:135.

48. Hurd WW, Wang L, Schemmel MT. A comparison of the relative risk of vessel injury with conical versus pyramidal laparoscopic trocars in a rabbit model. *Am J Obstet Gynecol.* 1995;173:1731.

49. Nezhat F, Brill AI, Nezhat CH, et al. Laparoscopic appraisal of the anatomic relationship of the umbilicus to the aortic bifurcation. *J Am Assoc Gynecol Laparosc.* 1998;5:135.

50. Quint EH, Wang FL, Hurd WW. Laparoscopic transillumination for the location of anterior abdominal wall blood vessels. *J Laparoendosc Surg.* 1996;6:167.

51. Seidman DS, Nasserbakht F, Nezhat F, Nezhat C. Delayed recognition of iliac artery injury during laparoscopic surgery. *Surg Endosc.* 1996;10:1099.

52. Spitzer M, Golden P, Rehwaldt L, Benjamin F. Repair of laparoscopic injury to abdominal wall arteries complicated by cutaneous necrosis. *J Am Assoc Gynecol Laparosc.* 1996;3:449.

53. Nezhat C, Seidman DS, Vreman HJ, et al. The risk of carbon monoxide poisoning after prolonged laparoscopic surgery. *Obstet Gynecol.* 1996;88:771.

54. Healzer JM, Nezhat C, Brodsky JB, et al. Pulmonary edema after absorbing crystalloid irrigating fluid during laparoscopy. *Anesth Analg.* 1994;78:1207.

55. Moore SS, Green CR, Wang FL, et al. The role of irrigation in the development of hypothermia during laparoscopic surgery. *Am J Obstet Gynecol.* 1997;176:598.

56. Ott DE, Reich H, Love B, et al. Reduction of laparoscopic-induced hypothermia, postoperative pain and recovery room length of stay by pre-conditioning gas with the Insuflow device: a prospective randomized controlled multi-center study. *J Soc Laparoendosc Surg.* 1998;2:321.

57. Puttick MI, Scott-Coombes DM, Dye J, et al. Comparison of immunologic and physiologic effects of CO_2 pneumoperitoneum at room and body temperatures. *Surg Endosc.* 1999;13:572.

58. Mouton WG, Bessell JR, Millard SH, et al. A randomized controlled trial assessing the benefit of humidified insufflation gas during laparoscopic surgery. *Surg Endosc.* 1999;13:106.

59. Nezhat C, Childers J, Nezhat F, et al. Major retroperitoneal vascular injury during laparoscopic surgery. *Hum Reprod.* 1997;12:480.

60. Chapron CM, Pierre F, Lacroix S, et al. Major vascular injuries during gynecologic laparoscopy. *J Am Coll Surg.* 1997;185:461.

61. Guloglu R, Dilepe S, Aksoy M, et al. Major retroperitoneal vascular injuries during laparoscopic cholecystectomy and appendectomy. *J Laparoendo Adv Surg Tech A.* 2004;14:73.

62. Nezhat F, Brill A, Nezhat C. Traumatic hypogastric artery bleeding controlled with bipolar desiccation during operative laparoscopy. *J Am Assoc Gynecol Laparosc.* 1994;1:171.

63. Georgy FM, Fetterman HH, Chefetz MD. Complications of laparoscopy: two cases of perforated urinary bladder. *Am J Obstet Gynecol.* 1974;120:1121.

64. Sherer DM. Inadvertent transvaginal cystotomy during laparoscopy. *Int J Gynaecol Obstet.* 1990;32:77.

65. Nezhat CH, Seidman DS, Nezhat F, et al. Laparoscopic management of intentional and unintentional cystotomy. *J Urol.* 1996;156:1400.

66. Lee CL, Lai YM, Soong YK. Management of urinary bladder injuries in laparoscopic assisted vaginal hysterectomy. *Acta Obstet Gynecol Scand.* 1996;75:174.

67. Ostrzenski A, Radolmski B, Ostrzenski KM. A review of laparoscopic uretal injury in pelvic surgery. *Obstet Gynecol Surv.* 2003;58:794.

68. Tamussino KF, Lang PF, Breinl E. Ureteral complications with operative gynecologic laparoscopy. *Am J Obstet Gynecol.* 1998;178:967.

69. Nezhat C, Nezhat F, Nezhat CH, et al. Urinary tract endometriosis treated by laparoscopy. *Fertil Steril.* 1996;66:920.

70. Ferland RD, Rosenblatt P. Ureteral compromise after laparoscopic burch colpopexy. *J Am Assoc Gynecol Laparosc.* 1999;6:217.

71. Cheng YS. Ureteral injury resulting from laparoscopic fulguration of endometriotic implants. *Am J Obstet Gynecol.* 1976;126:1045.

72. Nezhat C, Nezhat F. Laparoscopic repair of resected ureter during operative laparoscopy to treat endometriosis: a case report. *Obstet Gynecol.* 1992;80:543.

73. Chaffkin L, Luciano LA. Ureteral injuries. In: Corfman RS, Diamond WP, DeCherney AH, eds. *Complications of Laparoscopy and Hysteroscopy.* Cambridge, UK: Blackwell; 1993.

74. Nezhat C, Nezhat F. Safe laser excision or vaporization of peritoneal endometriosis. *Fertil Steril.* 1989;52:149.

75. Cook AS, Rock JA. The role of laparoscopy in the treatment of endometriosis. *Fertil Steril.* 1991;55:663.

76. Teichman JM, Lackner JE, Harrison JM. Comparison of lighted ureteral catheter luminance for laparoscopy. *Tech Urol.* 1997;3:213.

77. Quinlan DJ, Townsend DE, Johnson GH. Are ureteral catheters in gynecologic surgery beneficial or hazardous? *Am Assoc Gynecol Laparosc.* 1995;3:61.

78. Kuno K, Menzin A, Kauder HH, et al. Prophylactic ureteral catheterization in gynecologic surgery. *Urology.* 1998;52:1004.

79. Wood EC, Maher P, Pelosi MA. Routine use of ureteric catheters at laparoscopic hysterectomy may cause unnecessary complications. *J Am Assoc Gynecol Laparosc.* 1996;3:393.

80. Nezhat C, Nezhat F, Gordon S, Wilkins E. Laparoscopic versus abdominal hysterectomy. *J Reprod Med.* 1992;37:247.

81. Woodland MB. Ureter injury during laparoscopy-assisted vaginal hysterectomy with the endoscopic linear stapler. *Am J Obstet Gynecol.* 1992;176:756.

82. Nezhat C, Nezhat F, Bess O, Nezhat CH. Injuries associated with the use of a linear stapler during operative laparoscopy: review of diagnosis, management and prevention. *J Gynecol Surg.* 1993;9:145.

83. Tulinkangas PK, Gill IS, Falcone T. Laparoscopic repair of uretal injuries. *J Am Assoc Gynecol Laparosc.* 2001;8:259.

84. Saidi MH, Sadler RK, Vancaillie TG, et al. Diagnosis and management of serious urinary complications after major operative laparoscopy. *Obstet Gynecol.* 1996;87:272.

85. Timor-Tritsch IE, Haratz-Rubinstein N, Monteagudo A, et al. Transvaginal color Doppler sonography of the ureteral jets: a method to detect ureteral patency. *Obstet Gynecol.* 1997;89:113.

86. Gomel V, James C. Intraoperative management of ureteral injury during operative laparoscopy. *Fertil Steril.* 1991;55:416.

87. Nezhat C, Nezhat F, Green B. Laparoscopic treatment of obstructed ureter due to endometriosis by resection and ureteroureterostomy: a case report. *J Urol.* 1992;148:865.

88. Nezhat CH, Malik S, Nezhat F, et al. Laparoscopic ureteoneosystotomy and vesicopsoas hitch for infiltrative endometriosis. *JSLS.* 2004;8:3.

89. Levy BS, Soderstrom RM, Dail DH. Bowel injuries during laparoscopy: gross anatomy and histology. *J Reprod Med.* 1985;30:168.

90. Chapron C, Pierre F, Harchaoui Y, et al. Gastrointestinal injuries during gynaecological laparoscopy. *Hum Reprod.* 1999;14:333.

91. Schrenk P, Woisetschlager R, Rieger R, Wayand W. Mechanism, management, and prevention of laparoscopic bowel injuries. *Gastrointest Endosc.* 1996;43:572.

92. Gentile GP, Siegler AM. Inadvertent intentional biopsy during laparoscopy and hysteroscopy: a report of two cases. *Fertil Steril.* 1981;36:402.

93. Sauer M, Jarrett JC. Small bowel obstruction following diagnostic laparoscopy. *Fertil Steril.* 1984;42:653.

94. Corson SL, Bolognese RJ. Laparoscopy overview and results of a large series. *J Reprod Med.* 1972;9:148.

95. Loffer FD, Pent D. Indications, contraindications and complications of laparoscopy. *Obstet Gynecol Surv.* 1975;30:407.

96. Penfield AJ. How to prevent complications of open laparoscopy. *J Reprod Med.* 1985;30:660.

97. Wheeless CR. Gastrointestinal injuries associated with laparoscopy. In: Phillips JM, ed. *Endoscopy in Gynecology.* Santa Fe Springs, CA: AAGL; 1978.

98. Bishoff JT, Allaf ME, Kirkels W, et al. Laparoscopic bowel injury: incidence and clinical presentation. *J Urol.* 1999;161:887.

99. DeCherney AH. Laparoscopy with unexpected viscus penetration. In: Nichols DH, ed. *Clinical Problems, Injuries and Complications of Gynecologic Surgery.* Baltimore, MD: Williams & Wilkins; 1988.

100. Corson SL, Batzer FR, Gocial B, Maislin G. Measurement of the force necessary for laparoscopic trocar entry. *J Reprod Med.* 1989;34:282.

101. Borton M. *Laparoscopic Complication: Prevention and Management.* Philadelphia, PA: Decker, 1986.

102. Nezhat C, Nezhat F, Ambroze W, Pennington E. Laparoscopic repair of small bowel, colon, and rectal endometriosis: a report of twenty-six cases. *Surg Endosc.* 1993;7:88.

103. Nezhat C, Nezhat F, Pennington E. Laparoscopic treatment of lower colorectal and infiltrative rectovaginal septum endometriosis by the technique of videolaseroscopy. *Br J Obstet Gynaecol.* 1992;99:664.

104. Redwine D. Laparoscopic en bloc resection for treatment of the obliterated cul-de-sac in endometriosis. *J Reprod Med.* 1992;37:696.

105. Nezhat F, Brill Al, Nezhat CH, Nezhat C. Adhesion formation after endoscopic posterior colpotomy. *J Reprod Med.* 1993;38:534.

106. Mohr C, Nezhat FR, Nezhat CH, et al. Fertility considerations in laparoscopic treatment of infiltrative bowel endometriosis. *JSLS.* 2005;9:16.

107. El-Bama M, Abdel-Atty M, El-Meteini M, et al. Management of laparoscopic-related bowel injuries. *Surg Endosc.* 2000;14:779.

108. Kirkpatrick JR, Rajpal SG. The injured colon: therapeutic considerations. *Am J Surg.* 1975;129:187.

109. Parker J, Hayes C, Wong F, Carter J. Laparoscopic ilioinguinal nerve injury. *Gynecol Endosc.* 1998;7:327.

110. Perry CP. Laparoscopic treatment of genitofemoral neuralgia. *J Am Assoc Gynecol Laparosc.* 1997;4:231.

111. Ke RW, Portera SG, Bagous W, Lincoln SR. A randomized, double-blinded trial of preemptive analgesia in laparoscopy. *Obstet Gynecol.* 1998;92:972.

112. Alexander DJ, Ngoi SS, Lee L, et al. Randomized trial of periportal peritoneal bupivacaine for pain relief after laparoscopic cholecystectomy. *Br J Surg.* 1996;83:1223.

113. Johnson N, Onwude JL, Player J, et al. Pain after laparoscopy: an observational study and a randomized trial of local anesthetic. *J Gynecol Surg.* 1994;10:129.

114. Tool AL, Kammerer-Doak DN, Nguyen CM, et al. Postoperative pain relief following laparoscopic tubal sterilization with silastic bands. *Obstet Gynecol.* 1997;90:731.

115. Weber A, Munoz J, Garteiz D, Cueto J. Use of subdiaphragmatic bupivacaine instillation to control postoperative pain after laparoscopic surgery. *Surg Laparosc Endosc.* 1997;7:6.

116. Cunniffe MG, McAnena OJ, Dar MA, et al. A prospective randomized trial of intraoperative bupivacaine irrigation for management of shoulder-tip pain following laparoscopy. *Am J Surg.* 1998;176:258.

117. Szem JW, Hydo L, Barie PS. A double-blinded evaluation of intraperitoneal bupivacaine vs saline for the reduction of

postoperative pain and nausea after laparoscopiccholecystectomy. *Surg Endosc.* 1996;10:44.

118. Balaloski SP, Richards SR, Singh E. Conservative management of delayed suprapubic abscess after laparoscopic burch colposuspension using nonabsorbable polypropylene mesh. *J Am Assoc Gynecol Laparosc.* 1999;6:225.

119. Montz FJ, Holschneider CH, Munro MG. Incisional hernia following laparoscopy: a survey of the American Association of Gynecologic Laparoscopists. *Obstet Gynecol.* 1994;84:881.

120. Coda A, Bossotti M, Ferri F, et al. Incisional hernia and fascial defect following laparoscopic surgery. *Surg Laparosc Endosc Percutan Tech.* 2000;10:34.

121. Carter JE. A new technique of fascial closure for laparoscopic incisions. *J Laparosc Surg.* 1994;4:143.

122. Jones DB, Callery MP, Soper NJ. Strangulated incisional hernia at trocar site. *Surg Laparosc Endosc.* 1996;6:152.

123. Nezhat C, Nezhat F, Seidman DS, Nezhat C. Incisional hernias after operative laparoscopy. *J Laparoendosc Adv Surg Tech.* 1997;7:111.

124. Nezhat CH, Nezhat F, Seidman DS, Nezhat C. Vaginal vault evisceration after total laparoscopic hysterectomy. *Obstet Gynecol.* 1996;87:868.

125. Bonjer HJ, Hazebroek EJ, Kazemier G, et al. Open versus closed establishment of pneumoperitoneum in laparoscopic surgery. *Br J Surg.* 1997;84:599.

126. Peterson HB, DeStefano F, Rubin GL, et al. Deaths attributable to tubal sterilization in the United States, 1977 to 1981. *Am J Obstet Gynecol.* 1983;146:135.

Appendix A   The Informed Consent and Malpractice

A surgeon is required by law and bound by moral and ethical standards to explain a planned operation, its risks, and the expected outcome to the patient preoperatively. The purpose of this Appendix is to (1) provide a guide for discussing a proposed laparoscopic operation with the patient and (2) describe the informed consent as it relates to laparoscopy.

Diagnostic laparoscopy has gained widespread acceptance among gynecologic and general surgeons, but patients' expectations and the actual results from advanced operative laparoscopic procedures frequently do not coincide. For example, some patients believe that lasers are essential for a thorough operation, although most surgeons acknowledge that scissors and electrosurgical instruments are equally effective. Patients tend to consider laparoscopic procedures minor operations. This idea is reinforced by terms such as *same-day surgery, Band-Aid surgery, minimal invasive surgery,* and *laser surgery.* Patients and physicians underestimate the risks of complex operative endoscopy, which are potentially as serious as those associated with laparotomy.

The Informed Consent

Since 1914, surgeons have been required to obtain a patient's written consent before an operative procedure. This process allows the patient to participate in decisions with an understanding of the factors relevant to the proposed operation. The proper consent requires that the patient be informed of the diagnosis, the proposed treatment, the probability of success, alternative forms of therapy, and the risks of the planned operation. The information should be precise and presented understandably. Audiovisual material can be used to supplement the physician's explanation. This exchange forms an intrinsic part of the doctor–patient relationship. Through these discussions, the physician can make intraoperative decisions that are consistent with the patient's desires and goals. The circumstances under which the consent is obtained are also important. The patient should not be under the influence of a medication that might interfere with his or her rational judgment.

Although the principle of obtaining an informed consent is the same in any operation, the following discussion concerns issues in laparoscopic procedures. Operative laparoscopy often is done immediately after a diagnostic laparoscopy. Sometimes a precise diagnosis cannot be made preoperatively, particularly in infertile women and those complaining of pelvic pain. The preoperative discussion should include possible diagnoses because some infertile patients have no clinical evidence of adhesions, endometriosis, or pelvic abnormalities, and significant disease that is found laparoscopically requires an extensive operation. Anticipated procedures should be explained so that the patient

has realistic expectations about the type and duration of the anesthesia, the planned operation, and the length of hospitalization. The surgeon provides information about the procedure's chance of success and the possible need for follow-up therapy. If a patient declines the proposed operation, alternatives are described. Patients undergoing operations for the relief of pelvic pain require extensive preoperative evaluation and counseling because these women may be disappointed if they experience postoperative pain.

Postoperative complaints after laparoscopic operations vary with the type of procedure[1] and are influenced by the geographic setting.[2] For example, expectations regarding pain and discomfort postoperatively may differ between women in Europe and America and can be influenced culturally. Most women are informed that they can return to normal activity within a week after advanced operative procedures and a few days after a diagnostic laparoscopy.

If the findings provide a range of options, the patient can elect to have only diagnostic laparoscopy. A woman suspected of having an ectopic pregnancy needs to understand the relative risks and benefits of expectant or medical management and salpingectomy or salpingostomy. Her obstetric history, clinical findings, and desire for fertility and acceptance as well as the financial availability of assisted reproductive technology influence the type of operation. Myomectomies done by laparoscopy can be associated with bleeding or injury to adjacent organs, and a laparotomy may be required. The patient should be made aware of the possible risk of uterine rupture in future pregnancies.[3] When initial laparoscopy reveals severe pelvic adhesions or when there is a known history of severe endometriosis, particularly in women with cul-de-sac obliteration, the risk of complications, especially bowel injury, is increased. The importance of the laparoscopie surgeon's experience in such cases is stressed.

Ideally, most questions are answered in the physician's office during the preoperative consultation, but the patient should be given ample time preoperatively to discuss additional concerns, such as fertility, in case intraoperative decisions affect future childbearing. If the abnormalities cannot be corrected laparoscopically, some patients will request a laparotomy under the same anesthesia, while others will want to schedule a laparotomy later.

Adequacy of the Informed Consent

Legal standards define the adequacy of an informed consent.[4] With the majority rule, disclosure is decided by a professional medical standard on the basis of the customary disclosure practices of physicians in the same specialty. The minority rule requires physicians to divulge the risks that a prudent patient

CONSENT TO LAPAROSCOPIC SURGERY

Patient's Name_____ Date_____

I authorize and direct_____M.D., and/or associates or assistants of his or her choice to treat the condition/s believed to exist in my case.

The laparoscope, a surgical instrument similar to a telescope is inserted through a small incision in the belly button. The abdomen is distended with a gas called carbon dioxide. The scope allows the doctor to visualize the pelvic organs and allows other instruments to be used under direct vision. Small second, third and fourth incisions are occasionally made at the pubic hairline for scissors, coagulator, or laser to perform major closed surgery at laparoscopy.

Hysteroscopy (the use of a small optical tube that is inserted through the vagina into the uterus without incision to visualize the uterine cavity) is usually performed with laparoscopy in order to determine: (1) the size and depth of the uterine cavity; (2) the presence of congenital abnormalities within the uterus, such as a septum that divides the inside of the uterus, or a double uterus; (3) the presence of polyps or fibroid tumors in the uterine cavity; (4) whether specific abnormalities of the endometrium (lining of the uterus) are present, e.g. hyperplasia (build up lining of the uterus), tuberculosis, or cell changes that indicate early cancer. D&C (dilatation and curettage) may also be performed if indicated.

Video and/or pictures may be taken during surgery and used to show you what was seen and done. They are also used for teaching other patients and other surgeons these techniques.

Your doctor performs advanced laparoscopic surgery that includes procedures considered investigational and may include modified instrumentation. These are relatively new techniques not commonly undertaken elsewhere and can include laparoscopic oophorectomy, hysterectomy, and tubal reversal. Laparoscopic treatment of ovarian neoplasms, benign or malignant is considered investigational.

Antibiotics, anticoagulants, and other medications may be used with surgery to aid in healing. These medications are not labeled (neither approved nor disapproved) by the FDA for adhesion prevention.

Although laparoscopy is generally an outpatient procedure, you may be asleep from 1-4 hours, occasionally longer.

1. Plan to avoid any activities that will require concentration for at least 2 days.
2. You can usually return to work and moderate activities by the third day.
3. You may need 1-3 weeks to return to heavy activities and for full recovery.

Shoulder pain from the carbon dioxide gas and abdominal distention are common. Your throat may be sore from the endotracheal tube. About 1 in 40 patients are admitted for overnight stay due to nausea, drowsiness, or pain.

Complications from laparoscopic surgery are very uncommon, but they do sometimes occur. It is also possible that because of complications, or because of the discovery of life-threatening abnormalities, immediate major abdominal surgery might be necessary. The chance of severe complications such as hysterectomy, colostomy, paralysis, or death is rare. With respect to your life, this operation is six times safer than driving a car and two to three times safer than being pregnant.

Some of the possible complications are the same as those of regular surgery. Complications include bleeding; infection, particularly of the navel; generalized disease; inflammation of the lining of the abdomen; injury to the stomach or intestines; gas embolism to the lining from the carbon dioxide; abnormal gas collections underneath the skin and in the chest; ruptures or hernias in the surgical wound and through the breathing muscles (diaphragm); burns on the skin of the abdomen and inside the abdomen; damage to the kidney and urinary system; blood clots in the pelvis and lungs; damage to the kidney and urinary systems; blood clots in the pelvis and lungs; and allergic and other bad reactions to one or more substances used in the procedure.

Some of the complications of this procedure may require major surgery; some of the complications can cause poor healing wounds, scarring and permanent disability, and very rarely, some of the complications can even cause death.

The alternative procedure to the laparoscopic surgery is major surgery. However, this alternative method also carries the same risks, and requires a much longer period to recover and more pain and discomfort. Therefore, in those patients in whom laparoscopic surgery is possible, the procedures provide the patient with diagnosis and treatment at low risk and less discomfort. Your doctor cannot and does not guarantee the success of this procedure, but believes that the procedure is in your best interest.

I further understand that during the course of the operations or treatment, unforeseen conditions may be revealed requiring an extension of the original procedure/s or different procedures than those specifically discussed. I hereby authorize the above named surgeon, his or her associates, and assistants to perform such other laparoscopic surgical procedures and if necessary laparotomy (abdominal surgery) and to remove any tissue or organs that may be necessary or medically desirable as determined by the surgeons professional judgement. This authority shall extend to treatment of conditions; not previously known by my physicians.

My signature below constitutes my acknowledgment: 1. that I have read or had read to me the contents of this form, 2. that I understand and I agree to the foregoing, 3. that the proposed operation/s or procedure/s have been satisfactorily explained to me including possible risks and alternatives, 4. that I have all the information that I desire and have had ample opportunity to ask questions on specific points, 5. and that I hereby give my authorization and consent.

DO NOT SIGN THIS FORM UNLESS YOU HAVE READ IT, UNDERSTAND IT, AND AGREE WITH WHAT IT SAYS.

Date: Signature:

Time: Witness:

Figure A.1. This consent form is used for laparoscopic operations.

PHOTOGRAPH CONSENT AND RELEASE FORM

I,_____, hereby irrevocably authorize
_____, their successors, assigns, and those acting with their permission upon their authority to copyright, use and publish for art, advertising, medical, trade, commercial and other lawful purpose, any depiction or likeness for me or which I may be included in whole or part, including, but not limited to, motion pictures, video tapes and still photographs, and further including any composite photograph or photograph distorted in character or in form, and any motion picture or video tape edited by addition thereto or deletion of any part thereof, whether in conjunction with my name, a fictitious name or no name, or any reproduction or variation thereof by whatever medium made, taken at _____ Hospital during the period of_____.

I hereby waive any right which I may have to inspect or approve any such photograph, motion picture, video tape or other likeness or the use to which it is put, and acknowledge that except for the consideration recited I shall receive no payment or remuneration for the use of any such photograph, motion picture, or video tape or likeness.

I hereby release _____ their successors and assigns, and those acting with their permission and upon their authority, of and from every liability, responsibility and claim which may arise by reason of any exercise of the authority granted above or any blurring, distortion, alteration, optical illusion, or use in composite form, whether intentional or otherwise, which may occur or result in the taking or publication of such photograph, motion picture, video tape or other likeness unless it can be shown that publication _____ thereof was for the purpose of subjecting me to conspicuous ridicule, scandal or indignity.

I understand that my tape(s) may be used for medical studies and instructional purposes for the advancement and increased expertise of videolaseroscopy.

The condition of the pelvis will be videotaped before, in some parts during, and after the procedure. This tape could be misplaced or erased. If I personally receive a tape, it will be an edited version, approximately 5-10 minutes in length, and the _____ and staff cannot be held responsible for any mechanical failure that might occur during the original filming or reproduction of the video.

_____   _____
SIGNATURE   DATE

_____   _____
WITNESS   DATE

Figure A.2. Photographic consent and release form.

CONSENT AND APPLICATION FOR OBSERVATION OF MEDICAL
PROCEDURE RELEASE AND INDEMNITY

PATIENTS CONSENT TO OBSERVER

I hereby authorize_____Hospital to permit the presence of such observers as they may deem fit while I am undergoing surgery, childbirth, examination, or other treatment or diagnostic procedure at the Hospital. I hereby consent to being observed by any such persons.

This consent and authorization is expressly limited to the following conditions:

_____
_____
_____

_____   _____
Patient's Signature   Date/Time   Witness   Date/Time

_____
Patient's Representative   Date/Time   Patient unable to consent
                                                     because_____

I. OBSERVER'S REQUEST AND RELEASE

I_____, hereby request_____Hospital to permit me to observe certain medical and/or surgical procedures to be performed at the Hospital. I understand that I will be under the physician's direct supervision and agree to follow the physician's instructions to abide by all Hospital rules and regulations governing such observations. I recognize that I will be under the supervision of the physician, and not the hospital.

In consideration for the physician and hospital allowing me to observe, I hereby expressly release the physician, the hospital, their agents and employees of and from any and all claims, damages, responsibilities and liabilities which may arise, directly or indirectly, from or in connection with my activities at the Hospital. I further agree to indemnify and hold harmless the physician, the hospital, their agents and employees from and against any and all claims, liabilities and damages arising directly or indirectly out of or in connection with my observation of medical and/or surgical procedures at the Hospital.

If I am under eighteen years of age, my parent or legal guardian has consented to my observation of the medical and/or surgical procedures and agrees to release, indemnify and hold harmless the physicians, the hospital, their agents and employees from and against any and all claims, liabilities and damages arising directly or indirectly out of or in connection with my observation of medical and/or surgical procedures at the Hospital.

_____   _____
Observer   Date   Witness   Date
_____   _____
Parent or Guardian   Date   Witness   Date

II. PHYSICIAN'S INDEMNITY FOR OBSERVER

I have agreed to let_____(the "observer") accompany me during certain medical and/or surgical procedures at the Hospital and to observe such procedures. I agree that I will be completely responsible for the Observer and that he or she will be within my control at all times and will abide by all Hospital rules and regulations relating to his or her observing such procedures at the hospital.

In consideration of the Hospital's permitting the observer to accompany me, I agree to indemnify and hold harmless the hospital, its agents and employees from and against any and all claims, liabilities and damages arising, directly or indirectly, out of or in connection with the observation by such observer of medical and/or surgical procedures at the Hospital.

_____   _____
Physician   Date   Witness   Date

Figure A.3. A sample consent and application form for observation of medical procedures release and indemnity.

needs to understand to make a decision. The minority rule has been modified to either a subjective test or the informational requirements of a specific patient: the plaintiff.

The consumers' movement in health care and the proliferation of consumer-directed information, including the Internet information "superhighway," have contributed to the growing participation of patients in medical decision making.[5] This new attitude is consistent with both the ethical principle of patient autonomy and the legal requirement of informed consent. Patients are not expected to be passive and compliant and are encouraged to participate in surgical decision making. The traditional unilateral process of informed consent is evolving into one of informed collaborative choice.[5,6] More patient participation and opportunity for choice of treatment options will improve patient satisfaction and may decrease the risk of malpractice claims.[7,8]

Patient communication must be free from inappropriate outside influences to obtain adequate informed consent.[9] Studies have shown that physicians often fail during the informed consent process to communicate pertinent information, including the rationale of the procedure, its benefits and risks, and alternative procedures.[10] Failure to share information with the patient is a major barrier to informed consent. The process of decision making and the importance of patient participation are recognized in many fields of medicine.[9,11] Appropriately, the American College of Obstetricians and Gynecologists' computer-based interactions series has developed a program that provides insight on clinical decision making.[12] When asked to provide informed consent, many patients lack the self-confidence needed to make complex decisions about the operation. The rushed setting, the fear of limited access to costly care in the managed care era, and the difficulty of putting into perspective the risks of nontreatment often prevent the patient from reaching a thoughtful decision in considering an operation. It is essential to provide the patient with simple and accurate information in a comfortable and safe environment.

Sensitivity to the patient and a commonsense approach to the informed consent are practical. Good communication is essential and is encouraged. The patient expects her physician to assess the problem, propose treatment, and address her concerns with compassion. Patients are anxious preoperatively; the physician can ease that apprehension by carefully explaining the procedure's anticipated consequences. When describing the frequency of complications, one should use terms such as *rare, uncommon,* and *unusual.* One should not attempt to provide precise complication rates. It is important to explain the precautions that will be taken to lessen the risks. Additional consent is required for photographic documentation.

Exceptions to the Informed Consent
Clinical conditions such as life-threatening situations can create exceptions to a full disclosure. Other possible exceptions are an unconscious patient and a situation in which the risks of failure to treat are greater than the risks of treatment. Whenever possible, the patient's family should be informed. Obtaining an informed consent implies that the patient is competent to give it. No clear standard exists for competency, but patients with severe mental retardation or psychiatric disorders, and those intoxicated by drugs or alcohol are unable to give an informed consent. Crite-

ria for discovering incompetency include inability to make decisions, making decisions for irrational reasons, irrational decision, and inability to know, appreciate, or understand the information provided. If the physician believes a patient is partially or totally incompetent, it is important to involve the family, a guardian, or even the courts to get a proper informed consent. A patient can waive her right for full disclosure of the risks, but the reasons must be documented and discussed with the family. However, the physician should not decide that disclosing some or all of the risks would upset the patient and prevent her from making a rational decision. Such a claim can be difficult to prove. The courts may view the physician's self-interest as an overriding factor.[13]

Malpractice (Civil Liability)

Regardless of the type or route of the surgical procedure, the basis for malpractice is the same. Most cases begin after the patient experiences an unanticipated unfavorable result.[14] Operations more likely to result in a lawsuit are those in which the doctor did not discuss with the patient the possibility of an adverse outcome.[14] Knowing when to stop a complicated procedure represents common sense and good judgment. Despite proper training and skill, sequelae can occur. To prevent untoward results, gynecologists must improve their competence in operative laparoscopy with postgraduate courses and by gradually undertaking increasingly complex procedures. The cause of the complication should be explained to the patient. When the surgeon does not communicate adequately, the patient may seek another physician to explain the untoward result. Physicians should be restrained in criticizing colleagues unless all the facts are known. In a review of adverse outcomes, less than 2 percent resulted in a malpractice claim.[15]

Proof of Malpractice
The elements needed to legally prove malpractice are as follows:

1. *Duty.* The physician's duty in a legal sense is decided by the community standard of practice for a particular procedure.
2. *Dereliction of duty (negligence).* Negligence is a deviation from the accepted standard of care, custom, or common practice. It can result from several acts or failures to act, including failure to conduct adequate examinations and tests, careless execution of medical and surgical procedures, inappropriate prescription or administration of drugs, inadequate monitoring of the patient, failure to refer patients to other specialists as needed, and unethical conduct that harms a patient.
3. *Damage and direct causality.* If injury results, the patient needs to prove that the negligence was the proximate cause of the damage.

As operative laparoscopy becomes more complex, the levels of experience and expertise vary widely. Often, the standard of care is not defined clearly. Surgeons must be aware of their level of skill, as some laparoscopic operations may be done safely by laparotomy. In other instances, a colleague with more endoscopic experience can help or the patient can be referred to a more accomplished endoscopist.

The relation between the number of malpractice claims and personal, educational, and practice characteristics was studied in a sample of 427 surgeons, including 115 gynecologists.[16] Surgeons who were terminated because of a high number of claims were found to be less likely to have completed a fellowship, belong to a clinical faculty, be members of professional societies, have specialty board certification, or be in a group practice. These findings were interpreted to suggest that manifest exemplary modes of professional peer relationships and responsible clinical behavior are likely to be related to a lower rate of malpractice claims.

Audiotape analysis has identified significant differences in the communication actions of no-claims and claims physicians in primary care. Compared with claims primary care physicians, no-claims primary care physicians used more statements of orientation, laughed and used humor more, tended to use more facilitation, and spent more time in routine visits. Interestingly, a similar association between communication behaviors and malpractice claims was not found for surgeons.[17]

Malpractice cases usually are caused by delayed diagnosis, failure to recognize a complication, or inadequate treatment. Many injuries can be identified intraoperatively and repaired. For instance, delayed recognition of bowel injury can result in a catastrophic outcome of a complication that could have been repaired during the primary operation. Once the injury is identified, the physician can either repair it or seek proper consultation.[18] Failure to call for consultation and inappropriate repair of a laparoscopic injury have been recognized as a major cause of litigation.[19] Patients who complain postoperatively of increasing abdominal pain should be examined promptly, and their clinical condition should be evaluated. Postoperative infection is rare, and a careful examination is needed to discover the cause of fever. Significant abdominal discomfort and vomiting postoperatively can be associated with an incisional hernia even in small 5-mm ports that are left unsutured.[20] Hypotension caused by intraoperative hemorrhage is managed by promptly diagnosing and locating the vascular injury, obtaining hemostasis, and replacing blood as needed.[21,22]

Doing an appendectomy incidental to other authorized abdominal and pelvic operations is acceptable, as the long-term benefits of appendectomy have been shown in women with chronic pelvic pain even when the appendix is histologically normal.[23] However, the physician can be liable for assault and battery if proper consent is not obtained. If a complication arises, the lack of consent can become the source of a malpractice claim.

Medical errors that harm patients should be brought to their attention. Such full disclosure is clearly in the best interest of patients because it allows them to understand what has occurred and gain appropriate compensation for the harm they have suffered.[24] However, not infrequently surgeons find it difficult to admit errors, especially to those who have been harmed by them. Yet physicians' ethical responsibilities sometimes differ from their legal and risk-management responsibilities. It is therefore argued that the physician must continue to respect the patient and communicate honestly with him or her throughout the relationship even if the patient has been injured. Moreover, offering an apology for harming a patient should be considered one of a surgeon's ethical responsibilities. Monetary compensation alone should not be offered as a charitable gesture; instead, it should be accompanied by an apology to demonstrate the responsibility of the physician to the trusting patient. Full and honest disclosure

of errors is most consistent with the mutual respect and trust patients expect from their physicians.

Avoiding Malpractice

While it is impossible to guarantee that a surgeon can avoid malpractice claims, Roberts and colleagues[8] suggest several steps to reduce the risk:

1. Engage in good-quality careful medical practice.
2. Be sure that you are trained adequately before attempting a diagnostic procedure or treatment.
3. Refer a patient to other physicians for care or consultation if the care required is not within your area of expertise.
4. Make sure that your knowledge is current, especially in the rapidly advancing areas of diagnostic and operative laparoscopy.
5. Do the procedure only if the facility in which care is given is equipped to provide good emergency care if a complication occurs during treatment.
6. When using nonstandard treatments (those not generally condoned and employed by the medical community), exercise caution.
7. Obtain adequate informed consent. Sample consent forms are illustrated below (Figures A.1, A.2, and A.3).

REFERENCES

1. Azizz R, Steinkampf MP, Murphy A. Postoperative recuperation: Relation to the extent of endoscopic surgery. *Fertil Steril* 1989;51:1061.
2. Semm K: *Operative Manual for Endoscopic Abdominal Surgery.* Chicago: Year Book, 1987.
3. Stenchever MA. Too much informed consent? *Obstet Gynecol* 1991;77:631.
4. Meisel A. The "exceptions" to the informed consent doctrine: Striking a balance between competing values in medical decision making. *Conn Med* 1981;45:107 (pt 1) and 45:27 (pt 2).
5. Barr JR. Following a few simple rules may help prevent malpractice claims. *Can Med Assoc J* 1991;114:355.
6. Localio AR, Lawhters AG, Brennan TA, et al. Relation between malpractice claims and adverse events due to negligence: Results of the Harvard Medical Practice Study III. *N Engl J Med* 1991; 325:245.
7. Mills HM. Medical lessons from malpractice cases. *JAMA* 1963;183:1073.
8. Roberts DK, Shane JA, Roberts ML. *Confronting the Malpractice Crisis: Guidelines for the Obstetrician-Gynecologist.* Kansas, City: Eagle Press, 1985.
9. Pelosi MA III, Pelosi MA. Spontaneous uterine rupture at thirty-three weeks subsequent to previous superficial laparoscopic myomectomy. *Am J Obstet Gynecol* 1997;177:1547.
10. Gambone JC, Reiter RC. Hysterectomy: Improving the patient's decision making process. *Clin Obstet Gynecol* 1997;40:868.
11. DiMatteo MR. The physician-patient relationship: Effects on the quality of health care. *Clin Obstet Gynecol* 1994;37:149.
12. Ballard-Reisch DS. A model of participative decision making for physician-patient interaction. *Health Comm* 1990;2:91.
13. Greenfield S, Kaplan R, Ware JE. Expanding patient involvement in care: Effects on patient outcomes. *Ann Intern Med* 1985; 102:520.

14. Wagener J, Taylor SE. What else could I have done? Patients' responses to failed treatment decisions. *Health Psychol* 1986; 5:481.

15. Honde CJ, Reiter RC. Decision making in women's health care. *Obstet Gynecol* 1994;37:162.

16. Wu WC, Pearlman RA. Consent in medical decision making: The role of communication. *J Gen Intern Med* 1988;3:9.

17. Gambone JC, Reiter RC, Pitts J. *Interactions: Programs in Clinical Decision Making.* American College of Obstetricians and Gynecologists. Hamilton, Ontario: Decker Electronic Publishing, 1996.

18. Adamson TE, Baldwin DC Jr, Sheehan TJ, Oppenberg AA. Characteristics of surgeons with high and low malpractice claims rates. *West J Med* 1997;166:37.

19. Levinson W, Roter DL, Mullooly JP, et al. Physician-patient communication: The relationship with malpractice claims among primary care physicians and surgeons. *JAMA* 1997;277:553.

20. Sutton CJG. Medico-legal implications of keyhole surgery. *Medico-Legal J* 1996;64:101.

21. Nezhat C, Nezhat F, Seidman DS, Nezhat C. Incisional hernias after operative laparoscopy. *J Laparoendosc Adv Surg Tech* 1997;7:111.

22. Seidman DS, Nasserbakht F, Nezhat F, et al. Delayed recognition of iliac artery injury during laparoscopic surgery. *Surg Endosc* 1996;10:1099.

23. Nezhat C, Childers J, Nezhat F, et al. Major retroperitoneal vascular injury during laparoscopic surgery. *Hum Reprod* 1997;12: 480.

24. Protopapas A, Shushan A, Hart R, et al. Is laparoscopic appendectomy a gynaecological procedure? *Lancet* 1998;351:500.

Atlas

The Atlas consists of illustrations that were selected either because they are characteristic of a specific condition or they amplify material found in the text. Serous cystadenomas, polycystic ovaries, and ovarian malignancy seen at laparoscopy are illustrated. Endometriomas, implants of endometriosis involving the bowel, ureter, bladder, uterosacral ligaments, appendix, ovaries, and cul-de-sac are revealed. The laparoscopic technique for ovarian cystectomy, ovarian "drilling' myomectomy, and uterosacral ablation are shown.

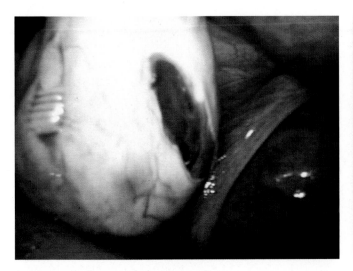

1. A hemorrhagic corpus luteum is noted.

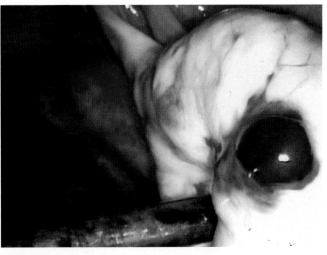

2. Endometriotic implant is present on the ovary.

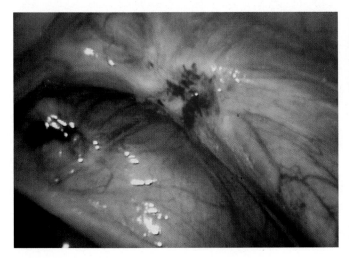

3. Endometriotic implants are seen over the ureter.

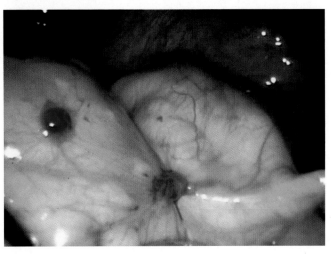

4. The rectosigmoid is involved with endometriosis.

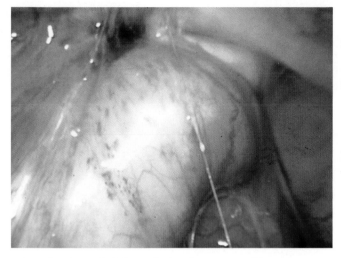

5. Rectal endometriosis is attached to the uterosacral ligaments.

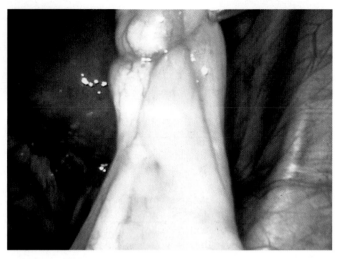

6. The appendix is involved with endometriosis.

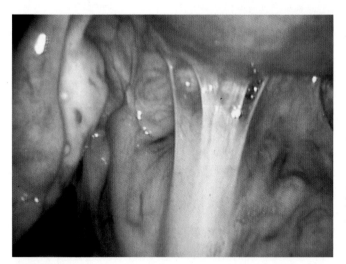

7. The cul-de-sac has been obliterated with endometriotic implants and adhesions.

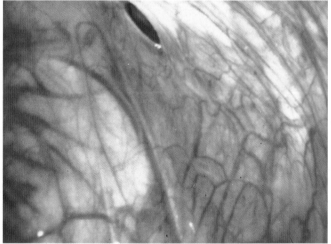

8. The peritoneal defect contained endometriosis.

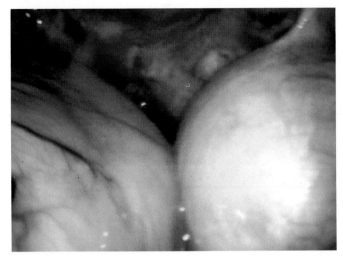

9. Endometriomas are seen in both ovaries.

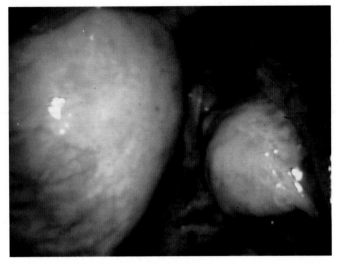

10. Cystic teratomas are present in both ovaries.

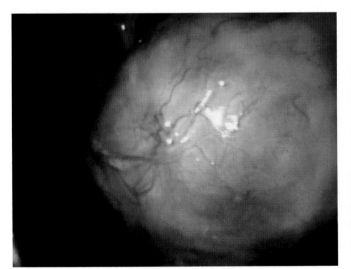

11. A benign cystadenoma was found on histologic examination.

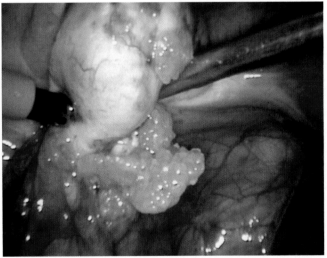

12. An ovarian malignancy is seen with excrescences.

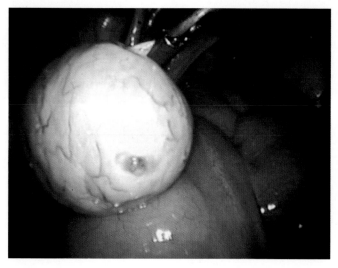

13. A polycystic ovary is noted with characteristic superficial blood vessels.

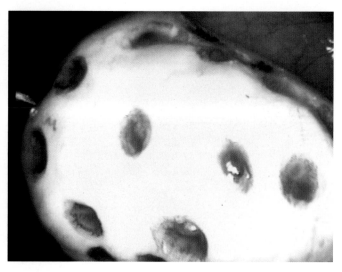

14. The appearance of the ovarian surface is seen after "drilling" with the CO_2 laser.

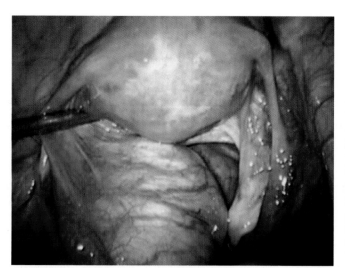

15. A large ovarian cyst was found in the left ovary.

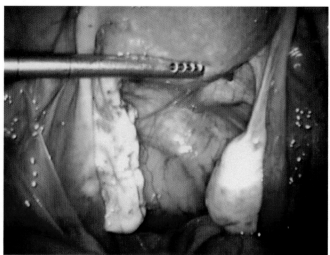

16. The cyst has been removed.

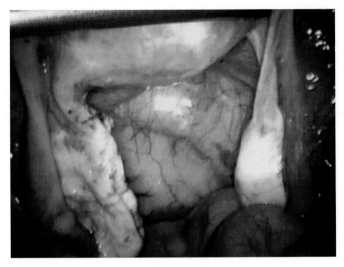

17. The ovarian edges were approximated.

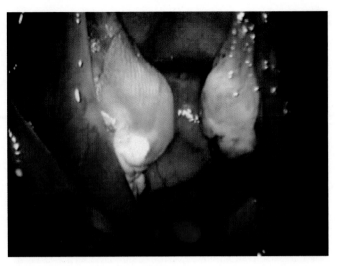

18. Interceed was placed over the ovary.

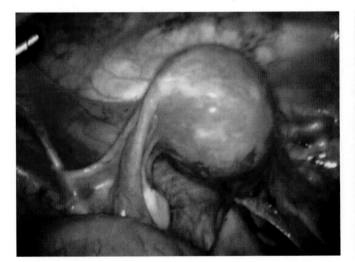

19. A unicornuate uterus is noted.

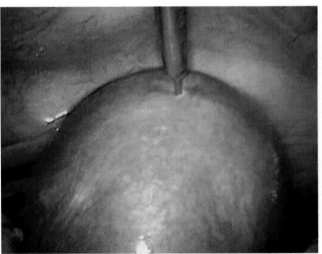

20. A "corkscrew" device is inserted into the fundal myoma.

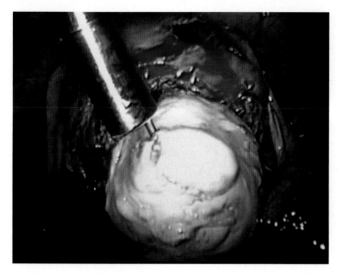

21. The myoma is being enucleated.

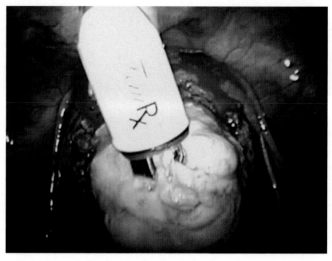

22. Myoma morcellation is beginning.

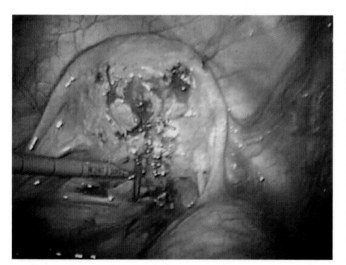

23. The uterine edges have been approximated.

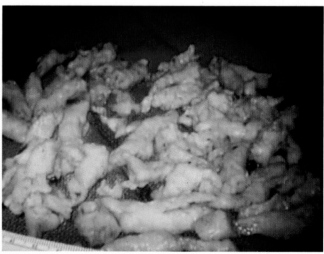

24. Myomatous fragments are seen.

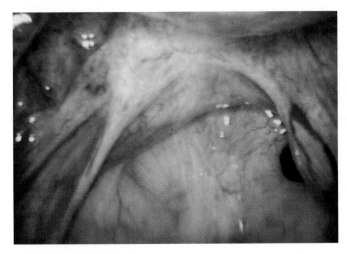

25. The uterosacral ligaments are observed.

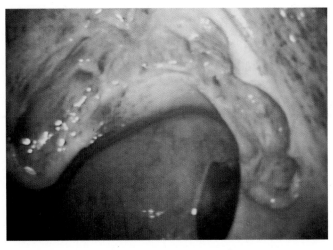

26. Note the extent of ablation of the uterosacral ligaments.

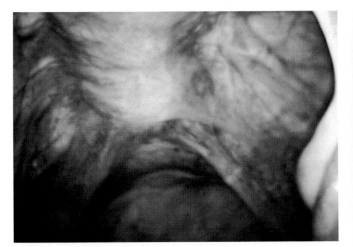

27. Two years later the area was healed without the formation of adhesions.

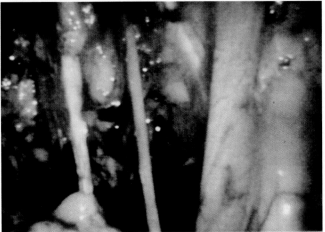

28. External iliac artery and vein are seen on the right; the obturator nerve is in the middle; the obliterated hypogastric artery is on the left.

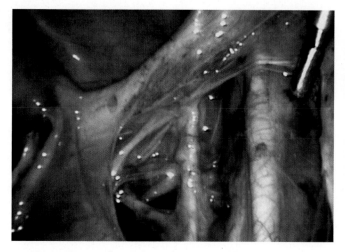

29. The uterine artery has been dissected from the hypogastric artery. The external iliac artery is on the right; the right round ligament appears in the foreground; the infundibuopelvic ligament is medial.

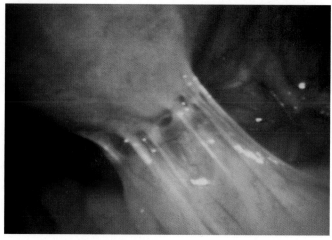

30. Avascular adhesions between the uterus and omentum are stretched before dissection with scissors.

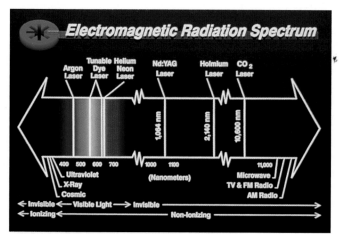

31. Laser light is unique and uniform unlike regular light which is divided into colors of the spectrum.

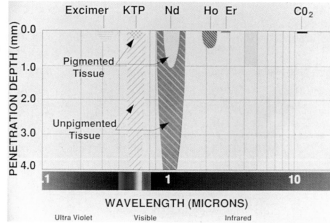

32. Argon, KTP, and Nd-YAG lasers are absorbed by pigmented tissues containing hemoglobin but pass through water and clear tissues.

Index

Page numbers followed by "*t*" indicates tables and "*f*" indicates figures.